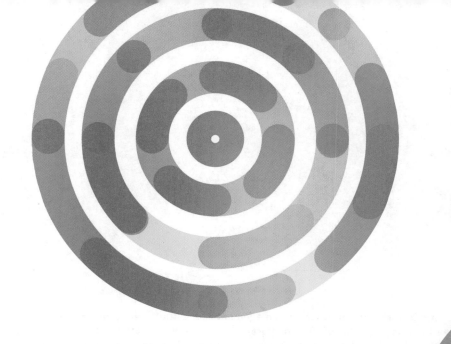

Health Information Management Technology

An Applied Approach

Sixth Edition

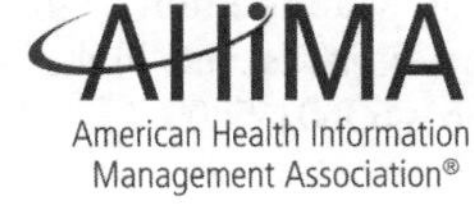

ISBN: **978-1-58426-720-1**
AHIMA Product No.: AB103118

AHIMA Staff:
Megan Grennan, Managing Editor
Kimberly Wilson, Production Development Editor
James Pinnick, Vice President, Content and Product Development
Rachel Schratz, MA, Assistant Editor

Cover image: sollia ©Shutterstock

For more information, including updates, about AHIMA Press publications, visit http://www.ahima.org/education/press.

American Health Information Management Association
233 North Michigan Avenue, 21st Floor
Chicago, Illinois 60601-5809
ahima.org

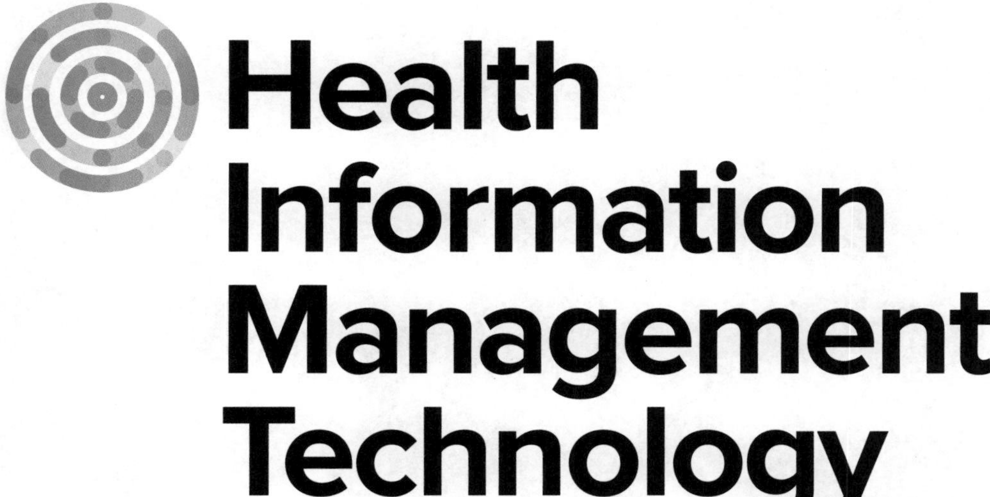

Health Information Management Technology

An Applied Approach

Sixth Edition

Volume Editors

Nanette B. Sayles, EdD, RHIA, CCS, CDIP, CHDA, CHPS, CPHI, CPHIMS, FAHIMA

Leslie L. Gordon, MS, RHIA, FAHIMA

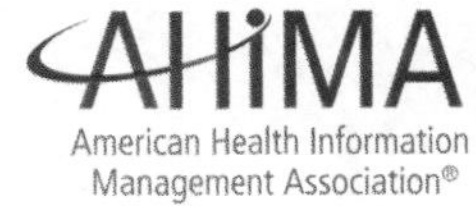

Brief Table of Contents

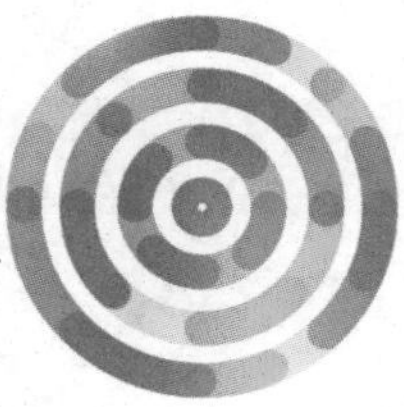

Table of Contents

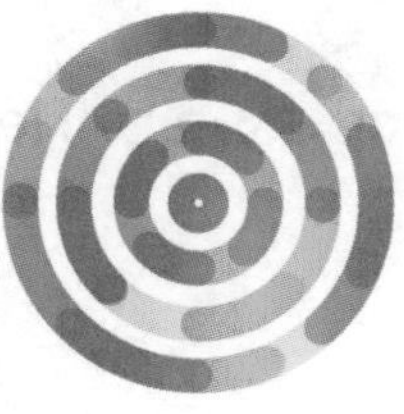

About the Volume Editors and Chapter Authors

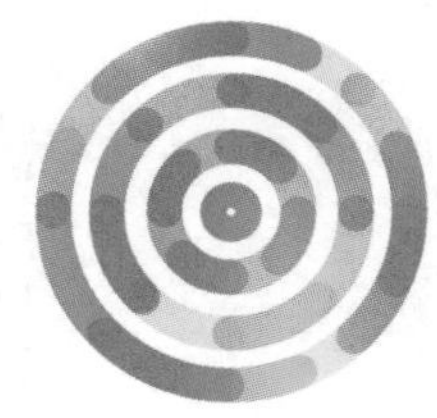

Volume Editors

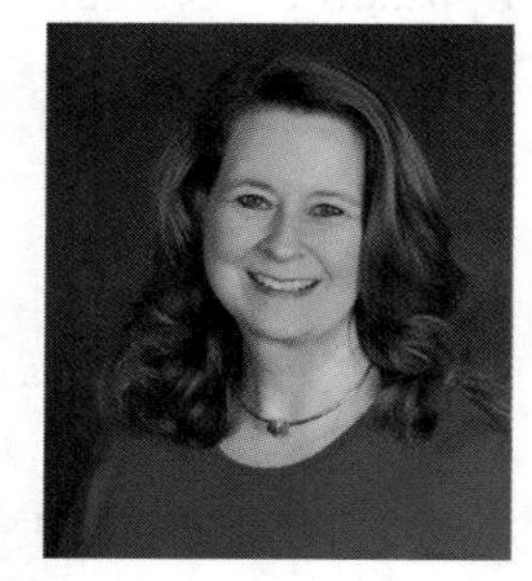

Nanette B. Sayles, EdD, RHIA, CCS, CDIP, CHDA, CHPS, CPHI, CPHIMS, FAHIMA, is a professor in the health information management program at East Central College in Union, MC. She has a BS in medical record administration, an MS in health information management, a master's degree in public administration, and a doctorate of education in adult education. Dr. Sayles has more than 10 years of experience as a health information management practitioner with experience in hospitals, a consulting firm, and a computer vendor. She was the 2005 American Health Information Management Association Triumph Educator award recipient. She has held numerous volunteer roles for the American Health Information Management Association (AHIMA), the Georgia Health Information Management Association (GHIMA), the Alabama Association of Health Information Management (AAHIM), Middle Georgia Health Information Management Association (MGHIMA), and Birmingham Regional Health Information Management Association (BRHIMA). These positions include: AHIMA Educational Strategies Committee, AHIMA co-chair RHIA Workgroup, GHIMA director, and president of MGHIMA. Dr. Sayles is the author of *Professional Review Guide for the CHP, CHS, and CHPS Examinations* and *Case Studies for Health Information Management*. She is an editor for two chapters in the *PRG Professional Review Guide* for the RHIA and RHIT examinations.

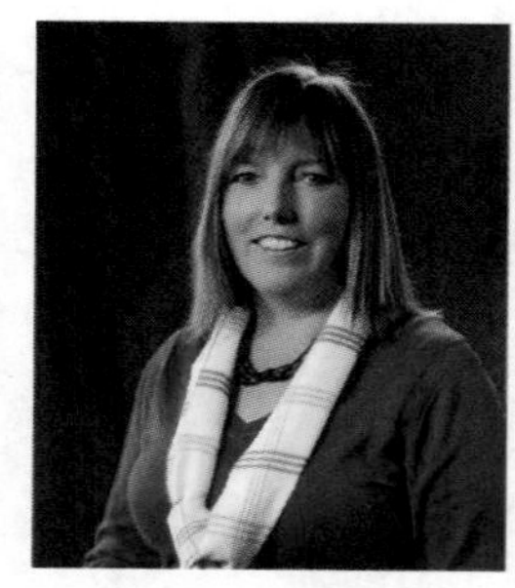

Leslie L. Gordon, MS, RHIA, FAHIMA, is the director of performance improvement for the Southeast Alaska Regional Health Consortium. She earned a BA and an MS from the College of St. Scholastica. She taught at the University of Alaska Southeast for many years. Before teaching she worked as a coder, reimbursement manager, and data analyst at a hospital in Sitka, Alaska. Ms. Gordon is an active member of the Alaska CSA (AKHIMA) and has served in several positions on the AKHIMA Board. She is a Fellow of AHIMA and currently serves on the Council of Accreditation of Health Informatics and Information Management Education (CAHIIM) Health Information Management Accreditation Council (HIMAC).

Chapter Authors

Margret K. Amatayakul, MBA, RHIA, CHPS, CPEHR, FHIMSS, is president of Margret\A Consulting, LLC, in West Linn, Oregon, a consulting firm specializing in electronic health records (EHRs) and health information, including implementing standards and regulations. She has been a leading authority on health IT strategies for over 40 years. She has extensive national and international experience in EHR optimization and workflow redesign, HIPAA privacy, security, and transactions/code sets, and adoption of value-based care. She helped form and served as executive director of the Computer-based Patient Record Institute (CPRI), was associate executive director of AHIMA, associate professor at the University of Illinois at Chicago, and director of medical record services at the Illinois Eye and Ear Infirmary. She holds a clinical associate professorship at the University of Illinois at Chicago, and she is serves as adjunct faculty at the College of St. Scholastica. She is a highly sought-after speaker, has published extensively, serves on several boards, and has earned numerous professional service awards.

Hertencia Bowe, EdD, MSA, RHIA, FAHIMA, is an assistant professor at Fisher College in the undergraduate health information management. Dr. Bowe is also the principal consultant at Bowe Academic Consulting, LCC. In this role, she coaches academic programs challenged by applying professional competencies and navigating accreditation standards. Dr. Bowe has extensive experience in teaching and developing health information management (HIM) curricula and has a depth of knowledge in academic programmatic accreditation solutions. She has held numerous appointed and volunteer positions with the American Health Information Management Association (AHIMA), the Commission on Accreditation of Health Information and Informatics Management (CAHIIM), and the Florida HIM Association (FHIMA). She served on the 2017-2018 CAHIM Board while chairing its HIM Accreditation Council. Dr. Bowe has served as a health information technology advisory board member for Paradigm Education Solutions in 2015-2019. Other volunteer experiences include being a member of the AHIMA Council for Excellence in Education (CEE) HIMR Strategic Oversight Committee, the AHIMA Commission on Certification for Health Informatics and Information Management (CCHIIM), the Registered Health Information Technician Construction Committee and several AHIMA CEE workgroups. Dr. Bowe has also served as a CAHIIM accreditation peer reviewer.

Megan R. Brickner, MSA, RHIA, serves as the director of compliance programs and privacy officer for the Kettering Health Network in Dayton, Ohio. She is responsible for daily and strategic operations of the Kettering Health Network's information security and privacy program, titled PROTECT. Her PROTECT Program was highlighted at the 2012 Annual Ohio Hospital Association Meeting as a program of best practice and at the 2016 Ohio Health Information Management Association's 36th Annual Meeting and Trade Show. Most recently, her privacy program was highlighted as an industry best practice in the customer success story published by the FairWarning company in 2019. Ms. Brickner has over 20 years of experience in the area of healthcare compliance. She holds a bachelor's in healthcare administration and health information management as well as a master's in healthcare administration. Ms. Brickner is a registered health information administrator (RHIA) and has served as an adjunct faculty member for the health information management department at Sinclair Community College in Dayton for over 15 years.

Danika E. Brinda, PhD, RHIA, CHPS, HCISPP, is an associate professor in the health informatics and information management department at the College of St. Scholastica. She teaches a variety of courses in the health information management and health informatics programs related to legal issues in healthcare, HIPAA privacy and security, compliance, EHRs in healthcare, and research. Dr. Brinda is the CEO of TriPoint Healthcare Solutions and Planet HIPAA, which focus on helping organizations understand, operationalize, and implement the complex healthcare privacy and security regulations. She enjoys making privacy and security regulations fun and understandable to all organizations and specialties in healthcare. Dr. Brinda is a well-known speaker in healthcare privacy and security. She is a 2010 recipient of the AHIMA Rising Star Triumph Award.

Darcy Carter, DHSc, MHA, RHIA, earned her doctorate degree in health science with an emphasis in leadership and organizational behavior and her master's degree in healthcare administration. She is currently assistant professor and MHA program director at Weber State University where she teaches courses in coding, reimbursement, and database management. Dr. Carter is coauthor of *Quality and Performance Improvement in Healthcare: Theory, Practice, and Management* published by AHIMA.

Darline Foltz, RHIA, CHPS, CPC, is assistant professor-educator in the online health information systems technology program at the University of Cincinnati Clermont College. She is currently pursuing her master's degree in educational studies from the University of Cincinnati. Ms. Foltz has a bachelor's degree in health information management (HIM) from The Ohio State University and a bachelor's degree in information systems from the University of Cincinnati. Prior to joining UC Clermont, Ms. Foltz spent her career in many facets of HIM including owning her own consulting business; director of HIM at Deaconess Hospital, Cincinnati; director of HIM at the Drake Center; and director of IS and telecommunications at Deaconess Hospital, Cincinnati. Ms. Foltz has been a consultant for long-term and acute-care hospitals, nursing homes, dialysis clinics, physician offices, mental health agencies, drug and alcohol rehab centers, and rehab hospitals and she is the coauthor of the textbook, *Exploring the Electronic Health Records*.

Kathy Giannangelo, MA, RHIA, CCS, CPHIMS, FAHIMA, is a medical informaticist with Language and Computing, Inc (L&C). In this position, she supports the ontology, modeling, sales, and product development activities related to the creation and implementation of natural language-processing applications where clinical terminology and classification systems are utilized. Ms. Giannangelo has a comprehensive background in the field of clinical terminologies and classification, with over 30 years of experience in the health information management (HIM) field. Prior to joining L&C, she was director of practice leadership with AHIMA. She has served as senior nosologist for a health information services company and worked in various HIM roles, including vice president of product development, education specialist, director of medical records, quality assurance coordinator, and manager of a Centers for Disease Control and Prevention research team. Ms. Giannangelo has developed classification, grouping, and reimbursement systems products for healthcare providers; conducted seminars; and provided consulting assessments throughout the United States as well as in Canada, Australia, Ireland, Bulgaria, and the United Kingdom. She has authored numerous articles and created online continuing education courses on clinical terminologies. As an adjunct faculty at the College of St. Scholastica, she teaches a graduate course in clinical vocabularies and classification systems. She is an active volunteer in the HIM profession at the international, national, state, and local levels. Ms. Giannangelo holds a master's degree in HIM from the College of St. Scholastica.

Morley L. Gordon, RHIT, is a clinical informatics specialist for Home Health and Hospice at Evergreen Health Hospital in Kirkland, Washington. Prior to that role, she was the director of health information management (HIM) at a long-term care facility in Central Washington. She graduated from the Western Governors University with her bachelor's degree in health informatics. She also studied health information technology at the University of Alaska. She credits her mom, Leslie Gordon, with introducing her to the field of health information management and for recommending that she pursue a career in HIM. Ms. Gordon is grateful for the opportunities that she is afforded because of it.

Misty Hamilton, MBA, RHIT, is a professor and director of health information management technology at Zane State College for the past 13 years. She teaches courses in introduction to health information management, legal aspects in health care, clinical classification I, II, and III, health care quality improvement, and management of health information services. Ms. Hamilton is also a member of the Ohio Educator's Day Committee as well as the curricula workgroup through AHIMA.

Karen M. Lankisch, PhD, MHI, RHIA, CHDA, CPC, CPPM, holds a bachelor's degree in business, a master's degree in health informatics, a master's degree in education, and a doctorate degree in education. Dr. Lankisch has has over 10 years of experience in the health information management. Dr. Lankisch is a registered health information administrator (RHIA), a certified data analyst (CHDA), and an active member of the American Health Information Management Association (AHIMA). She holds certified professional coder (CPC) and a certified physician practice management (CPPM) credentials through the American Association of Professional Coders (CPC). Dr. Lankisch has worked in higher education for over 20 years. Dr. Lankisch is a Quality Matters Master Peer Review and has completed reviews both nationally and internationally. Dr. Lankisch has served on the panel of reviewers for the Commission on Accreditation for Health Informatics and Information Management Education (CAHIIM) since 2016. Dr. Lankisch is a co-author of two textbooks and a contributing co-author of a health-related textbook for health information technology. In 2013, she received the University of Cincinnati Faculty Award for Innovative Use of Technology in the Classroom. In 2016, Dr. Lankisch was selected as a member of the Academy of Fellows of Teaching and Learning at the University of Cincinnati. In 2018, she received the UC Clermont Faculty Mentoring Award.

Marjorie H. McNeill, PhD, RHIA, CCS, FAHIMA, serves as the interim associate dean of the School of allied health sciences at Florida A&M University. Dr. McNeill earned her bachelor's degree in medical record administration from the Medical College of Georgia, a master's degree in health education from Florida State University, and PhD in educational leadership from Florida A&M University. Dr. McNeill has over 30 years of experience as a health information management educator, rising to the academic rank of professor. She is the former director of the division of health informatics and information management. Dr. McNeill has several educational publications to her credit, including research articles in *Perspectives in Health Information Management, Journal of Allied Health,* and the *Journal of the American Health Information Management Association*. She is an active member and has served in leadership roles of the Northwest Florida Health Information Management Association, Florida Health Information Management Association, and American Health Information Management Association (AHIMA). Dr. McNeill is the recipient of the Florida Health Information Management Association 2008 Distinguished Service Award, the 2010 Literary Award, and the 2015 Educator Award. Dr. McNeill is the recipient of the 2015 American Health Information Management Association Educator Triumph Award. She is also a Fellow of AHIMA.

Kelly Miller, MA, RHIA, is an assistant professor and program coordinator for the health information management (HIM) program at Regis University. She is currently pursuing her doctorate in health administration with a focus in health care quality analytics. She has worked in various HIM roles including assistant director at an acute care hospital, director of records management for a large hospital network and HIM director at a Specialty Hospital. In these roles, she oversaw all HIM operations including a system-wide records retention/destruction project, scanning and archiving of medical records and an EHR implementation. Ms. Miller served as a member of AHIMA's Council for Excellence in Education from 2015-2018. In this role she chaired the curriculum workgroup. She has served in numerous roles within the Colorado HIM Association; including director, education committee chair and delegate. She is a recipient of CHIMA's Distinguished Member and Outstanding Volunteer award.

Miland N. Palmer, MPH, RHIA, earned his master's degree in public health from the University of Utah and is currently pursuing his PhD in public health. Mr. Palmer is a full-time faculty member at Weber State University in the health administrative services department where he teaches courses in health administration, health information management, healthcare data governance, epidemiology, and biostatistics. Mr. Palmer has over 10 years experience in public health, health administration, and health information management, spending time at the Utah Department of Health and the Department of Veterans Affairs Salt Lake City Healthcare System.

Valerie S. Prater, MBA, RHIT, FAHIMA, is a retired clinical assistant professor in the HIM program, department of biomedical and health information sciences, College of Applied Health Sciences, University of Illinois at Chicago (UIC), where she continues to teach as an adjunct instructor. Ms. Prater has been recognized by students and peers at UIC for her commitment as an educator, including being the recipient of the University's Silver Circle Award and the Educator of the Year for the College of Applied Health Sciences. She serves on the Health Information Management Council of the Commission on Accreditation for Health Informatics and Information Management Education (CAHIIM) and is a member of Society for Human Resource Management (SHRM). Ms. Prater has extensive experience developing curricula for health information programs at UIC and in her previous positions as program director, DeVry University, Corporate Academics, and as adjunct faculty for the University of Connecticut. Prior to entering education, Ms. Prater held healthcare management positions with responsibilities encompassing operations, strategic planning, quality management, business development, and HIM. She has delivered numerous presentations to national professional groups, including AHIMA's Assembly on Education.

Laurie A. Rinehart-Thompson, JD, RHIA, CHP, FAHIMA, is professor and director of the health information management (HIM) and systems program at The Ohio State University. She earned a bachelor's degree in medical record administration and a Juris Doctor degree, both from The Ohio State University. In addition to education, her professional experiences include behavioral health, home health, and acute care. She has served as an expert witness in civil litigation regarding the privacy and confidentiality of health information/HIPAA compliance. She has served on numerous AHIMA committees and is a member of AHIMA's Council for Excellence in Education. She is a member of the board of directors of the Ohio Health Information Management Association (OHIMA). She is a recipient of the AHIMA Triumph Award and the OHIMA Distinguished Member Award. A speaker on the HIPAA Privacy Rule, she is a coeditor and coauthor of AHIMA's *Fundamentals of Law for Health Informatics and Information Management*, the author of AHIMA's *Introduction to Health Information Privacy and Security*, and a contributing author in *Health Information Technology: An Applied Approach* (AHIMA), *Documentation for Health Records* (AHIMA), *Documentation for Medical Practices* (AHIMA), and *Ethical Health Informatics: Challenges and Opportunities* (Jones & Bartlett Learning). She has been published in the *Journal of AHIMA* and in AHIMA's *Perspectives in Health Information Management*.

Marcia Y. Sharp, EdD, MBA, RHIA, is associate professor and program director at the University of Tennessee Health Science Center in the department of health informatics and information management. She teaches leadership, information technology, and healthcare information systems. Prior to teaching, Dr. Sharp served in leadership roles in health information management for over 15 years. She is a former human resources director and a retired member of the US Navy Reserve. Previously, Dr. Sharp served as member of AHIMA's Council for Excellence in Education. Additionally, she served on the CEE's faculty development workgroup and as a delegate for the Tennessee Health Information Management

Association. Currently, Dr. Sharp is a reviewer for AHIMA's *Perspectives in Health Information Management*. She holds a PhD in higher and adult education from the University of Memphis, an MBA from Webster University, and a bachelor's degree in health information management from the University of Tennessee.

Lynette M. Williamson, EdD, RHIA, CCS, CPC, FAHIMA, is a full-time assistant professor-educator in the health information management (HIM) department at the University of Hawai'i-West O'ahu. She teaches a variety of courses related to HIM, medical coding, and healthcare administration. Previously, she served as program director for the medical coding specialist certificate program at Santa Barbara City College. Dr. Williamson has served in various volunteer capacities including the Registered Health Information Technician Exam Construction Committee, peer reviewer for CAHIIM, CAHIIM board member, and most recently a member of CAHIIM's Health Information Management Accreditation Council. In 2011, Dr. Williamson was awarded fellowship from AHIMA. In 2017, she received the merit scholarship for leadership from AHIMA. Currently, she serves on the Commission on Certification for Health Informatics and Information Management (CCHIM).

Preface

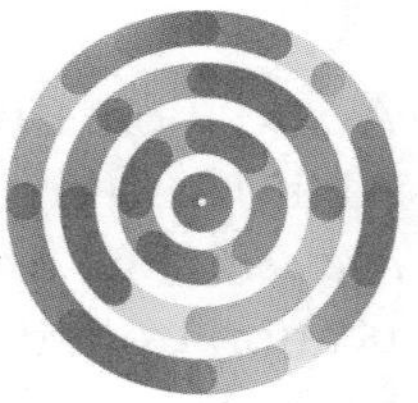

Health information management (HIM) professionals play an integral role on the healthcare team. They serve the healthcare industry and the public by using best practices in managing healthcare information to support quality healthcare delivery. Whether stored on paper or in electronic file format, reliable health information is crucial to quality healthcare. One of the primary goals of the HIM professional and profession is to enhance the individual patient care through timely and relevant information.

The American Health Information Management Association (AHIMA) represents more than 103,000 health information professionals who work throughout the healthcare industry. AHIMA has a long history of commitment to HIM education. Among other contributions, AHIMA has developed and maintained a rigorous accreditation process for academic programs, continuously developed up-to-date curriculum models, supported faculty development, and continued to research and study the needs and future directions of HIM education.

This textbook is specifically developed for associate degree programs in health information technology (HIT) and serves as an outgrowth of AHIMA's ongoing commitment to provide valuable resources for the education and training of new HIM professionals. Its subject matter is based on AHIMA's HIM associate degree program entry-level competencies and AHIMA's registered health information technician (RHIT) certification examination content domains. AHIMA made a significant change to the entry-level competencies in 2018 and this curriculum change created the need for modifications to this edition. This edition follows the prescribed curricular content found in the HIM associate degree entry-level competencies and covers the information and topics considered essential for every entry-level HIT practitioner. Although the primary audience for this book is students enrolled in two-year HIT programs, students in other HIM disciplines and allied health programs will find its content highly valuable and useful.

The fundamental organization of the book is built on the curricular content of the HIM associate degree entry-level competencies. Each of the content areas is represented in this textbook except those relating to the biomedical sciences and to technical aspects of classification systems such as the International Classification of Diseases. To provide maximum flexibility for instructional delivery, the content of each chapter is designed to stand on its own, providing maximum coverage of specific domains and competencies. Because of the interdependency of content areas that support knowledge and skills for performing many of the competencies, this approach has necessitated some duplication of material throughout the text. In these cases, the predominant content is covered in depth and is supplemented by a high-level overview of other supporting knowledge. Where appropriate, students are referred to other chapters for additional information or detail to round out necessary knowledge.

The organizing framework for content of the text is arranged in order by the six domains contained in the HIM Associate Degree Entry-Level Competencies. These domains are: Data Content Structure and Standards; Information Protection: Access, Disclosure, Archival, Privacy, and Security; Informatics, Analytics, and Data Use; Revenue Management; Compliance; and Leadership. This organization does not presuppose a pedagogical progression of presenting basic foundations and then progressing to advanced concepts. Therefore, given its student population, mission and goals, and other variables, each academic program must assess the appropriate sequence of presentation of the chapters within its curriculum. Additional information and models of chapter sequencing can be found in the instructor's manual.

The book's underlying structure is to translate basic theory into practice. A review of the cognitive and competency levels of the entry-level competencies reveals that HIT programs are applied in nature. Outcome expectations are that students understand theory at a basic level with a major emphasis on skill building to perform day-to-day operational tasks in health information management.

Therefore, the pedagogical tools used throughout the book focus on translating basic theory into practice. To accomplish this, each chapter contains the following features to reinforce comprehension:

Check Your Understanding This active learning review feature includes multiple-choice, matching, and true-and-false questions. These review quizzes appear throughout each chapter to reinforce concepts covered in the sections the students have just read. Students are asked to pause and review these concepts to ensure they understand the key concepts before moving ahead.

Real-World Cases Two real-world cases appear at the end of each chapter. These cases present two actual situations faced by HIM professionals. The cases are designed to help students develop the critical skills they need to be successful.

This text is divided into six parts that correspond with the domains from the 2018 AHIMA Associate Degree Entry-Level Competencies. Where appropriate, chapter content has been expanded in this new edition to prepare students for transitional and changing roles in an electronic health information environment. All chapters have been updated to reflect current trends, practices, standards, and legal issues.

Part I, Foundational Concepts These chapters provide a vital foundational base to the understanding of HIM in general. This part concentrates on the roles of the health information manager; the content, function, structure, and uses of health information; the healthcare delivery system; and how health information is managed. Chapter 1, *Health Information Management Profession*, introduces the concept of HIM. The discussion focuses on the history of the HIM profession and the evolution of the roles and functions of HIM professionals over the years. Particular emphasis is placed on HIM future roles and their relationship to the movement toward an electronic health record (EHR). Chapter 2, *Healthcare Delivery Systems*, introduces the history, organization, financing, and delivery of health services in the United States. Chapter 3, *Health Information Functions, Purpose, and Users*, introduces the function and purpose of the health record function as well as who uses the record.

Part II, Data Content Structure and Standards Part II reflects Domain I of the 2018 AHIMA competencies and explores the content related to diagnostic and procedural classification and terminologies, health record documentation requirements, data accuracy and integrity, data integration and interoperability, and the needs for data, information standards, and data management policies and procedures. Chapter 4, *Health Record Content and Documentation*, introduces students to standards for the content of the health record and requirements for documentation. Chapter 5, *Clinical Terminologies, Classifications, and Code Systems*, provides an introduction to clinical vocabularies and classification systems. Its purpose is to introduce the characteristics of prominent systems and help students understand how they are used throughout the healthcare system. Chapter 6, *Data Management*, is an essential part of the day-to-day operations of a healthcare organization. It includes understanding data sources and where they exist, how they are transmitted, and where they are stored. Chapter 7, *Secondary Data Sources*, explains the uses of the health record beyond patient care, such as registries and administrative functions.

Part III, Information Protection: Access, Disclosure and Archival, Privacy and Security This part contains healthcare law including theory of all healthcare law excluding what is covered by compliance, privacy, security, and confidentiality policies and procedures, in addition to the infrastructure and education of staff on information protection methods, risk assessment, access, and disclosure management and falls under Domain II of the 2018 AHIMA competencies. Chapter 8, *Health Law*, discusses legal issues associated with health information and includes an overview of sources of law and legal system. Chapter 9, *Data Privacy and Confidentiality*, are defined in terms of the legal rights of patients and the responsibility of healthcare organizations to protect those rights. Chapter 10, *Data Security*, examines the concept of data security, which encompasses measures and tools to safeguard data and the information systems on which they reside from unauthorized access, use, disclosure, disruption, modification, or destruction.

Part IV, Informatics, Analytics and Data Use Part IV addresses the creation and use of business health intelligence, including the review of selection implementation, use and management of technology solutions, system and data architecture, interface consideration, information management planning, data modeling systems, testing technology, benefit realization analytics and decision support, data visualization techniques, trend analysis administrative reports, statistics, data quality and covers Domain III of the 2018 AHIMA competencies. Chapter 11, *Health Information Systems*, defines the scope of health information technology and how it has evolved into its current state in healthcare settings. The systems development life cycle is explored in terms of management of health IT. Chapter 12, *Healthcare Information*, discusses the importance of healthcare information to the healthcare industry and the strategic uses of that information. Chapter 13, *Research and Data Analysis*, provides methods to analyze and present healthcare data and information in an understandable and useful fashion. Chapter 14, *Healthcare Statistics*, discusses common statistical measures and types of data used by organization in different healthcare settings.

Part V, Revenue Cycle and Compliance This part reflects Domains IV and V of the 2018 AHIMA competencies and includes healthcare reimbursement, as well as revenue cycle regulations and activities related to revenue management and compliance. Chapter 15, *Revenue Cycle and Reimbursement*, explores the billing and payment methodologies. Chapter 16, *Fraud and Abuse Compliance*, addresses federal laws that mandates all healthcare organizations comply with standards of quality care and proper billing practices.

Part VI, Leadership This part covers leadership models, theories and skills, change management, workflow analysis, design tools and techniques, human resources management training and development strategic planning, financial management, ethics and project management and reflects Domain VI of the 2018 AHIMA competencies. In Chapter 17, *Management*, explores the process of planning, controlling, leading, and organizing the activities of a healthcare organization Chapter 18, *Performance Improvement*, is the continuous study and adaptation of a healthcare organization's functions and processes to increase the likelihood of achieving desired outcomes. Chapter 19, *Leadership*, leadership theories and styles are explored and the impact of change management on processes, people, and systems. Chapter 20, *Human Resources Management and Professional Development*, help students understand the laws and regulations related to human resource management and the need for employee training and development. Chapter 21, *Ethical Issues in Health Information Management*, discusses the ethical issues associated with health information management and presents the concepts of stewardship and the HIM professional's core ethical obligations.

A complete glossary of HIM terms is provided at the end of the book. **Boldface** type is used in the text chapters to indicate the first substantial reference to each glossary term. The bolded terms in a chapter are listed at the beginning of the chapter and are identified as key terms.

An answer key, glossary, and a detailed content index complete the book.

AHIMA provides supplemental materials for educators who use this book in their classes. Instructor materials for this book include lesson plans, lesson slides, RHIT competency map, test bank, and other useful resources.

Student and Instructor Online Resources

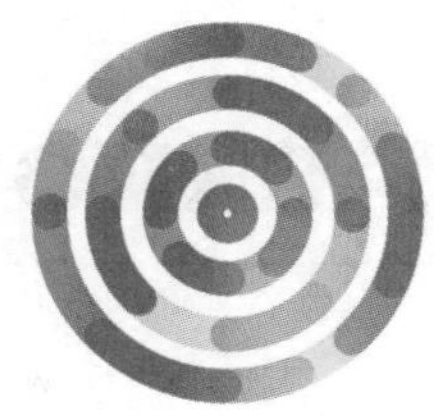

For Students

Visit http://www.ahimapress.org/sayles7201/ and register your unique student access code that is provided on the inside front cover of this text to downlaod the following valuable study and practice resources: Information about a *new* optional digital adaptive learning tool to strengthen comprehension of key concepts; student workbook with real-world cases and case discussion questions, application exercises, and review quizzes; and AHIMA's Code of Ethics, and AHIMA's Standards of Ethical Coding.

For Instructors

Instructor materials for this textbook are provided only to approved educators. In addition to the student resources, instructors can access the following educator resources: instructor's manual, presentation slides, *new* adaptive learning tool, course curriculum map, and a test bank instructor's manual and PowerPoint slides. Please visit http://www.ahima.org/publications/educators.aspx for further instruction. If you have any questions regarding the instructor materials, please contact AHIMA Customer Relations at (800) 335-5535 or submit a customer support request at https://my.ahima.org/messages.

AHIMA's *new* responsive **adaptive learning tool** for health information management programs

What is Adaptive Learning?

AHIMA Press has partnered with adaptive learning systems leader, Area9 Lyceum, to bring this powerful technology to health information management academic programs. This adaptive learning tool automatically customizes instructional content based on need. Students receive incremental assistance in areas where they struggle, facilitating both mastery and confidence.

Technology will never replace a student's hard work nor an experienced educator's training and intuition. But innovation can improve how we approach and deliver education. Learn more at ahima.org/adapt.

Acknowledgments

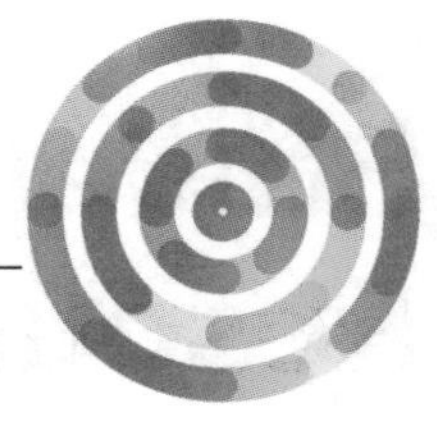

Many health information management professionals contributed to the development of the sixth edition of this landmark textbook. The volume editors and AHIMA press extend their sincere thank you to **Merida L. Johns, PhD, RHIA,** for pioneering this textbook through the first three editions. We thank all the chapter authors for sharing their expertise and time revising this text with the most up-to-date content and the best examples and resources.

No publication is ever complete without the diligent efforts of the subject expert reviewers. Their careful reviews and insightful suggestions have helped us ensure the quality and integrity of this edition. We also want to thank the following reviewers for their time and critical technical review to this endeavor:

Nora Blankenbecler, MBA, RHIA
Dana D. Carcamo, RHIA, CCS
Valerie D. Brock, RHIA, RHIT, CPC, CDIP, CPAR
Angela Campbell, RHIA, CHEP

We also want to acknowledge the following chapter authors who contributed to past editions of this text:

Sandra Bailey, RHIA
Cathleen A. Barnes, RHIA, CCS
Mary Jo Bowie, MS, RHIA
Elizabeth D. Bowman, MPA, RHIA
Sheila Carlon, PhD, RHIA, CHPS, FAHIMA
Bonnie S. Cassidy, MPA, RHIA, FHIMSS, FAHIMA
Lisa A. Cerrato, MS, RHIA
Michelle L. Dougherty, RHIA, CHP
Chris Elliott, MS, RHIA
Sandra R. Fuller, MA, RHIA
Michelle A. Green, MPS, RHIA, CMA, CHP
Laurinda B. Harman, PhD, RHIA, FAHIMA
Anita C. Hazelwood, MLS, RHIA, FAHIMA
Terrill Herzig, MSHI
Beth M. Hjort, RHIA
Joan Hicks, MSHI, RHIA
Cheryl V. Homan, MBA, RHIA
Merida L. Johns, PhD, RHIA
Kathleen M. LaTour, MA, RHIA, FAHIMA
Joan Ludwig, RHIA
Carol E. Osborn, PhD, RHIA
Bonnie Petterson, PhD, RHIA
Harry B. Rhodes, MBA, RHIA
Jane Roberts, MS, RHIA
Karen S. Scott, MEd, RHIA, CCS-P, CPC
Martin Smith, MEd, RHIT, CCA
Carol A. Venable, MPH, RHIA, FAHIMA
Karen A. Wager, DBA, RHIA
Frances Wickham Lee, DBA, RHIA
Susan B. Willner, RHIA
Andrea Weatherby White, PhD, RHIA

Foreword

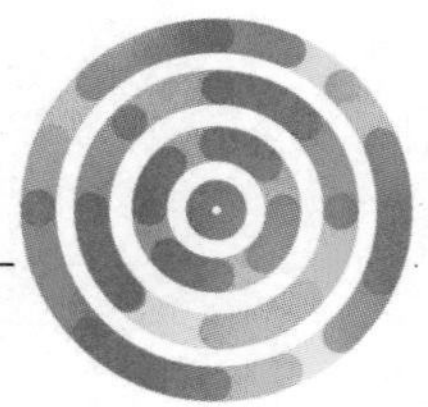

Health Information Management Technology: An Applied Approach continues as the foundational text for the education and training of health information management (HIM) students. For the sixth edition, the volume editors, Nanette B. Sayles and Leslie L. Gordon, have updated the competency coverage for the data management, data security, and fraud and abuse compliance topics. They have also expanded on ethical issues in the health information management profession.

The healthcare ecosystem continues to evolve. Healthcare delivery, practice, regulation, laws, and employment have and continue to change. These changes have required innovation from all corners of healthcare, but information remains the most important component of quality healthcare. This text will help prepare the next generation of HIM professionals handling vitally important healthcare information, ensuring that quality information is passed on to students seeking to learn new knowledge or update their skills.

There are several trends happening now in the professional development arena that will have an impact on the health information sector: professionalized learning paths, micro-learning/stackable learning, collaborative leaning, peer-to-peer learning, and augmented reality. Every decade brings with it changes in learning and changes in the demands placed on it by the workforce. As technology continues to evolve, so do the skills required to manage healthcare information. Nonetheless, healthcare information will always need people to handle it and employers will need people in place to analyze the information and manage the systems. It is the Health Information professional that is needed to ensure that the information is rich in accuracy and reliable.

It is expected that the next decade will bring both predictable and unpredictable changes in all areas of healthcare management. However, we remain securely grounded knowing that this book is anchored in solid facts, principles, and directives to help ensure your success as you progress through your career.

In closing, I wish you the best that life has to offer, and I hope this book helps you in your HIM goals, whether you are just starting your career or you are a seasoned veteran using this book as reference.

Amy Mosser
Chief Operating Officer

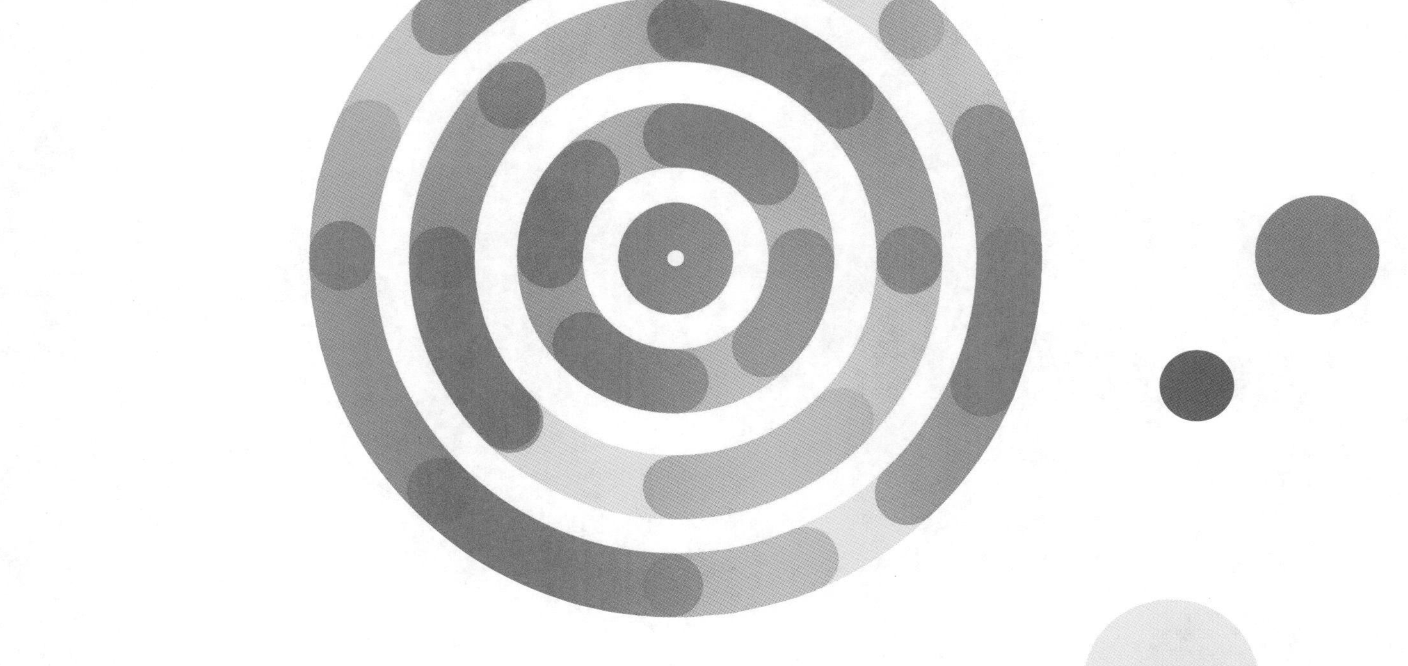

PART I

Foundational Concepts

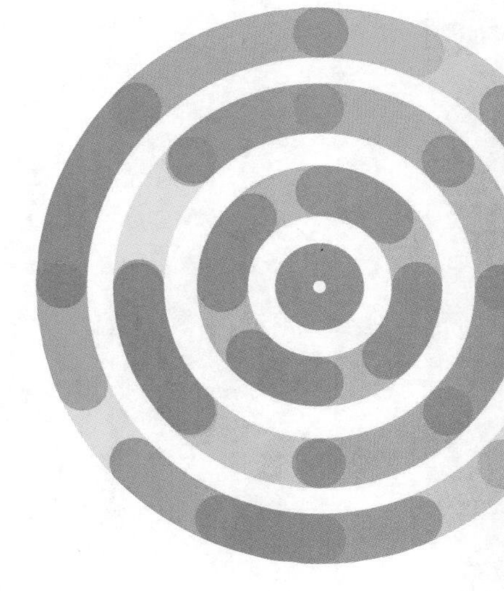

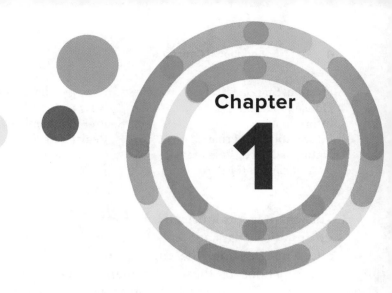

Health Information Management Profession

Nanette B. Sayles, EdD, RHIA, CCS, CDIP, CHDA, CHPS, CPHI, CPHIMS, FAHIMA

Learning Objectives

- Summarize the development of the health information management (HIM) profession from its beginnings to the present
- Discuss how professional practice must evolve to accommodate changes in the healthcare environment
- Identify the roles of HIM professionals
- Describe the purpose and structure of the American Health Information Management Association (AHIMA)
- Explain AHIMA's certification processes
- Discuss the accreditation process of the Commission on Accreditation for Health Informatics and Information Management Education
- Identify the appropriate professional organizations for the various specializations of HIM

Key Terms

Accreditation
Active membership
AHIMA Foundation
American Academy of Professional Coders (AAPC)
American Association of Medical Record Librarians (AAMRL)
American College of Surgeons (ACS)
American Health Information Management Association (AHIMA)
American Medical Record Association (AMRA)
Association for Healthcare Documentation Integrity (AHDI)
Association of Record Librarians of North America (ARLNA)
Board of directors
Certification
Chief executive officer
Code of ethics
Commission on Accreditation for Health Informatics and Information Management Education (CAHIIM)
Commission on Certification for Health Informatics and Information Management (CCHIIM)
Component state associations (CSAs)
Continuing education units (CEUs)
Council for Excellence in Education (CEE)
Credential
Data analytics
Data use
Emeritus membership
Engage
Fellowship program
Global membership
Group membership
Health information management (HIM)
Healthcare Information and Management Systems Society (HIMSS)

Hospital Standardization Program
House of Delegates
Informatics
Information governance
National Cancer Registrars Association (NCRA)
New graduate membership
New to AHIMA membership
Premier membership
Registered Health Information Administrator (RHIA)
Registered Health Information Technician (RHIT)
Registration
Student membership

This chapter introduces the history of the health information management (HIM) profession and offers insights into the current and future roles and functions of those who manage health information. The role of HIM professionals is even more important now than it was when the Association of Record Librarians of North America (ARLNA) was created in 1928 due to the complexity of today's information- and technology-driven healthcare environment.

Early History of Health Information Management

The commitment, wisdom, and efforts of HIM pioneers are reflected in what we see today as the HIM profession. Four distinct steps influenced development of the HIM profession. These steps include the hospital standardization movement, the organization of record librarians, the approval of formal educational processes, and an educational curriculum for medical record (now known as health information) librarians.

Hospital Standardization

Before 1918, the creation and management of hospital health records were the sole responsibilities of the attending physician. Physicians of that time often disliked doing paperwork. Unless the physician was interested in medical research, the medical records in the early 20th century were "practically worthless and consisted principally of nurse's notes" (Huffman 1941, 101).

Health records of that time did not contain graphical records or laboratory reports. Because there was no general management of health record processes, hospitals made no effort to ensure missing or incomplete portions of the health records were completed. Furthermore, no standardized vocabulary was used to document why the patient was admitted to the hospital or the final diagnosis upon discharge.

In 1918, the hospital standardization movement was inaugurated by the American College of Surgeons (ACS). The purpose of the resulting Hospital Standardization Program was to raise the standards of surgery by establishing minimum quality standards for hospitals. The ASC realized one of the most important items in the care of every patient was a complete and accurate report of the care and treatment provided during hospitalization. The health record should contain test results, identification information, diagnoses, treatment, and more (Huffman 1941).

It was not long before hospitals realized that to comply with the hospital standards, new health record processes had to be implemented. In addition, staff had to be hired to ensure the new processes were appropriately carried out. Furthermore, hospitals recognized health records must be maintained and filed in an orderly manner. Cross-indexes of diseases, operations, and physicians must be compiled. Thus, the job position of health record clerk was established.

Organization of the Association of Record Librarians

In 1928, 35 members of the Club of Record Clerks met at the Hospital Standardization Conference in Boston. Near the close of the meeting, the Association of Record Librarians of North America (ARLNA) was formed. During its first year the association had a charter membership of 58 individuals. Members were admitted from 25 of the

48 states, the District of Columbia, and Canada (Huffman 1985). ARLNA was the original name of the American Health Information Management Association (AHIMA), which is discussed later in this chapter.

Approval of Formal Education and Certification Programs

Early HIM professionals understood that for an occupation to be recognized as a profession there must be preliminary training. They also understood such training needed to be distinguished from mere skill. This training needed to be intellectual in character, involving knowledge and learning. Therefore, work began on the formulation of a prescribed course of study as early as 1929. In 1932, the association adopted the first formal curriculum for HIM education.

The first schools for medical record librarians were surveyed and approved by ARLNA in 1934. By 1941, 10 schools had been approved to provide training for medical record librarians. This formal approval process of academic programs was the precursor to the current accreditation program managed by the Commission on Accreditation for Health Informatics and Information Management Education (CAHIIM). Accreditation is a determination by an accrediting body that an eligible organization, network, program, group, or individual complies with applicable standards. In the case of CAHIIM, it is academic educational programs.

The Board of Registration, a certification board, was instituted in 1933 and developed the baseline by which to measure qualified health record librarians. "Certification is a credential earned by demonstrating specific skills or knowledge usually tied to an occupation, technology, or industry. Certifications are usually offered by a professional organization or a company that specializes in a particular field or technology" (CareerOneStop 2018). The Board of Registration developed the eligibility criteria for registration and developed and administered a national qualifying examination. Registration is the act of enrolling; in this case, enrolling in AHIMA's certifications (this process is discussed later in this chapter). Today, AHIMA's Commission on Certification for Health Informatics and Information Management (CCHIIM) functions as the Board of Registration. CCHIIM's role and function are discussed later in this chapter.

The professional membership of the association of HIM professionals grew over the subsequent decades. Although the name of the association changed several times, the fundamental elements of the profession—formal training requirements and certification by examination—have remained the same.

Evolution of Practice

The various names given to the health record association and its associated credentials reveal a lot about the evolution of the profession and its practice. A credential is a formal agreement granting an individual permission to practice in a profession, usually conferred by a national professional organization dedicated to a specific area of healthcare practice; or the accordance of permission by a healthcare organization to a licensed, independent practitioner (physician, nurse practitioner, or other professional) to practice in a specific area of specialty within that organization. It usually requires an applicant to pass an examination to obtain the credential initially and then to participate in continuing education activities to maintain the credential thereafter. The health record association was known as ARLNA until Canadian members formed their own organization in 1944. At that time, the name of the professional organization was changed to the American Association of Medical Record Librarians (AAMRL). In 1970, the professional organization changed its name again to eliminate the term *librarian*. The professional organization's name became the American Medical Record Association (AMRA). The professional organization underwent another name change in 1991 to become American Health Information Management Association (AHIMA).

The changes in the professional organization's name in 1970 and 1991 reflected the changing nature of the roles and functions of the association's professional membership. In 1970, the term *administrator* mirrored the work performed by members more accurately than the term *librarian*. Similarly, in 1991, association leaders believed that the management of *information*, rather than the management of *records*, would be the primary function of the profession in the future.

In 1999, AHIMA's House of Delegates (HOD) approved a credential name change. Registered Record Administrator (RRA) became **Registered Health Information Administrator (RHIA)**, and Accredited Record Technician (ART) became **Registered Health Information Technician (RHIT)**. These certifications are discussed later in this chapter. This section will address the traditional practice of HIM, the current information-oriented management practice, as well as the future of HIM.

Traditional Practice

The original practice of HIM emphasized the need to ensure that complete and accurate health records were compiled and maintained for every patient. Accurate records were needed to support the care and treatment provided to the patient as well as to conduct various types of clinical research.

Traditional practices of HIM involved planning, developing, and implementing systems designed to control, monitor, and track the quantity of record content and the flow, storage, and retrieval of health records. In other words, activities centered primarily on the health record or reports within the record as a physical unit rather than on the data elements that make up the information within the health record.

In 1928, very few standards "addressed issues relating to determination of the completion, significance, organization, timeliness, or accuracy of information contained in the medical record or its usefulness to decision support" (Johns 1991, 57).

Traditionally, HIM professionals worked in a hospital HIM department. Today, HIM professionals are found in many settings and in many roles. Some of the more common settings and some HIM roles are listed in table 1.1.

Table 1.1 HIM profession's job setting

Setting	Roles
Acute-care hospital	HIM director Cancer registrar Discharge analyst Systems analyst Privacy officer Compliance
Integrated healthcare delivery sytem	HIM director Privacy officer Coder Compliance officer
Other provider setting (such as long-term care and psychiatric)	HIM director Privacy officer Coder Compliance officer
Vendor	Sales Systems analyst Consultant Systems implementation Trainer
Insurance companies	Claims coordinator Auditor Privacy officer
Consulting	Consultant
Educational institution	Professor
Law firm	HIM director
Government agency	Reimbursement specialist Data manager Data mapper
Pharmaceutical companies	Research assistant

Source: ©AHIMA.

Information-Oriented Management Practice

The traditional model of practice roles is not appropriate for today's information-intensive and automated healthcare environment. The traditional model of practice is department focused with an emphasis on tasks. These tasks include the processing and tracking of records rather than processing and tracking information.

In today's information age, information crosses departmental boundaries and is broadly disseminated throughout the organization and beyond. Because of the focus on information, information governance is crucial. **Information governance** is "an organization-wide framework for managing information throughout its lifecycle and for supporting the organization's strategy, operations, regulatory, legal, risk, and environmental requirements" (IG Advisors 2018). In other words, the information must be managed to ensure the needs of the organization are met. See chapter 6, *Data Management*, for more on information governance.

Information grows out of data manipulation using data from a variety of shared data sources, both internal and external to the healthcare organization. For the HIM professional to manage this information, informatics skills, data analytics skills, and data use skills are required (Dooling et al. 2016). **Informatics** is a field of study that focuses on the use of technology to improve access to, and utilization of, information. Informatics uses software applications, databases, managing processes, and more (Dooling et al. 2016). To learn more about informatics, refer to chapter 13, *Research and Data Analysis*. **Data analytics** is the science of examining raw data with the purpose of drawing conclusions about that information. For example, the data may be analyzed to determine what services increase revenue for the healthcare organization and which ones incur a loss. Data analytics includes healthcare statistics, research methods, and interpretation. **Data use** is the ability to use technology to collect, store, analyze, and manage information, including the ability to use data visualization methods (Dooling et al. 2016). For example, a graph or chart may be created to show the trends of inpatient admissions over time. Information on graphs and charts is found in chapter 13, *Research and Data Analysis*.

The Future of HIM

Research shows the HIM profession is continuing to evolve from the traditional HIM roles to roles focused on information. Many of these changes result from the conversion to the electronic health record (EHR), but other factors including regulations, new technologies, and engaged consumers also influence the changes (The Caviart Group 2015). The EHR is an electronic record of health-related information about an individual that conforms to nationally recognized interoperability standards and can be created, managed, and consulted by authorized clinicians and staff across more than one healthcare organization. The EHR has dramatically increased the amount of information available and the ability to manipulate and interpret information. With a paper health record, collecting and analyzing data is very resource intensive so there are many limitations. Data analytics and informatics, discussed earlier in the chapter, will be important in the future for managing the increased data and information created by the EHR and other changes, such as changes in regulations and in technology. The 2015 Work Force Study, a research study on the roles and opportunities for HIM professions, identified the top 10 skills required by HIM professionals both today and into the future (The Caviart Group 2015). Table 1.2 shows these skills in order of importance.

Table 1.2 Comparison of the most important present and future HIM skills

Today's most important skills	Future's most important skills
1. Medical record coding	**1.** Electronic health record (EHR) management
2. Managing information privacy and security	**2.** Managing information privacy and security
3. Analytical thinking	**3.** Analytical thinking
4. Ensuring data integrity	**4.** Critical thinking
5. Critical thinking	**5.** Ensuring data integrity
6. Clinical documentation integrity	**6.** Problem solving
7. Electronic health record (EHR) management	**7.** Communication (written, spoken, or presentation)
8. Communication (written, spoken, or presentation)	**8.** Clinical documentation integrity
9. Problem solving	**9.** Leadership
10. Developing and promoting HIM standards	**10.** Analyzing big data

Source: Adapted from The Caviart Group 2015.

Check Your Understanding 1.1

Answer the following questions.

1. The hospital standardization movement was initiated by the:
   a. American Health Information Management Association
   b. American College of Surgeons
   c. Record Librarians of North America
   d. American College of Physicians

2. The healthcare organization wants to examine raw data to make conclusions about the future of the healthcare organization. This is known as:
   a. Data use
   b. Data analytics
   c. Informatics
   d. Information governance

3. The HIM profession is changing due to:
   a. Changes in technology
   b. Demands of physicians
   c. Changes in medical staff bylaws
   d. Changes at AHIMA

4. The new model of HIM practice is:
   a. Information focused
   b. Record focused
   c. Department focused
   d. Traditional focused

5. A formal agreement granting an individual permission to practice in a profession is known as:
   a. Registration
   b. Certification
   c. Informatics
   d. Information governance

6. The organization that accredits HIM education programs is:
   a. Joint Commission
   b. CAHIIM
   c. AHIMA
   d. CCHIIM

Today's Professional Organization

AHIMA is a membership organization representing more than 103,000 health information professionals. These professionals serve the healthcare industry and the public by managing, analyzing, and utilizing information vital for patient care and making it accessible to healthcare providers when and where it is needed.

AHIMA strives to foster the professional development of its members through education, certification, and lifelong learning. AHIMA also advocates for the HIM profession by working with legislators, stakeholders, and others to address issues related to HIM. The intent of this advocacy is to promote the development of high-quality information that benefits the public, healthcare consumers, healthcare providers, and other users of clinical data. The organization has certification programs that set high standards to ensure the minimum qualifications of the individuals who practice as health information managers and technicians. In addition, AHIMA supports numerous continuing education (CE) programs to help its credentialed members and others maintain their knowledge base and skills.

As previously described, AHIMA's name has changed several times over the years to reflect changes in the organization and the profession. The sections that follow discuss the mission, membership, and organizational structure of AHIMA.

AHIMA Mission and Vision

Before studying AHIMA's structure, it is important to understand why the organization exists and what contributions it makes to its members and the healthcare system in general. The mission of an organization explains what the organization is and what it does. In other words, it describes the organization's distinctive purpose. A vision is a futuristic view of where the organization is going. Figure 1.1 shows AHIMA's current mission and vision.

All organizations have values but these values may or may not be written. The values provide guidance to the organization when making decisions and establishing a culture (Tutorialspoint nd).

To accomplish its mission, AHIMA expects its members to follow a code of professional ethics (a complete discussion of ethical principles and AHIMA's Code of Ethics is provided in chapter 21, *Ethical Issues in Health Information Management*.) A code of ethics is a statement of ethical principles regarding business practices and professional behavior. The AHIMA Code of Ethics requires members of AHIMA, CCHIIM, credentialed nonmembers (certificants), and students enrolled in a formal certificate- or degree-granting programs directly relevant to AHIMA's purpose to act in an ethical manner and comply with all laws, regulations, and standards governing the practice of HIM. Just as professionals, members, certificants, and students are expected to continually update their knowledge base and skills through CE and lifelong learning, HIM professionals and managers are expected to promote high standards of HIM practice, education, and research. Additionally, they are expected to promote and protect the confidentiality and security of health records and health information.

Figure 1.1 AHIMA's mission and vision

Mission	**Vision**
Empowering people to impact health	A world where trusted information transforms health and healthcare by connecting people, systems, and ideas

Source: AHIMA 2019a.

AHIMA Membership

To accommodate the diversity in AHIMA membership, the organization has established the following seven membership categories: active membership, premier membership, student membership, new graduate membership, emeritus membership, global membership, and group membership (AHIMA 2019b).

Active membership is open to all individuals who are interested in AHIMA's purpose and willing to abide by the code of ethics. Active members in good standing are entitled to all membership privileges including the right to vote and to serve in the House of Delegates (discussed later in this chapter). Active membership provides HIM professionals the opportunity to participate in the organization and to offer input to the current and future practices of the profession.

Premier membership provides all the benefits described in active membership plus additional benefits such as unlimited recertification and additional discounts.

Student membership includes any student who does not have an AHIMA credential, has not previously been an active member of AHIMA, and who is formally enrolled in a Professional Certificate Approval Program or an Approved Committee for Certificate Program, or in a CAHIIM-accredited HIM program. The student membership category gives entry-level professionals an opportunity to participate on a national level in promoting sound HIM practices. Student members can serve on committees and subcommittees in designated student positions with a voice, but they do not have a vote.

New graduate membership is for student members who are recent graduates of accredited associate, bachelor's, and master's degree programs as well as AHIMA-approved coding programs. This membership level allows the students to continue their membership at a reduced rate for one year. This membership level has all membership rights including voting.

Emeritus membership allows AHIMA members who are 65 years or older to be a member at a reduced rate. This membership level has all membership rights including the right to vote.

Global membership is for people who are interested in HIM but live outside of the United States.

Group membership allows multiple individuals from an organization to join at one time. Student and business groups are eligible for this membership type.

New to AHIMA membership offers those who have never been a member of AHIMA a discounted rate for two years. This membership receives the same benefits as the Active Member (AHIMA 2019b).

AHIMA Structure and Operation

Every organization needs a management structure to operate effectively and efficiently. AHIMA is made up of two components—volunteer and staff. The volunteer structure establishes the organization's mission and goals, develops policy, and provides oversight for the organization's operations. Figure 1.2 shows AHIMA's volunteer structure. The staff component of the organization carries out the operational tasks necessary to support the organization's mission and goals. The staff works within the policies established by the volunteer component.

Association Leadership

As a nonprofit membership association, AHIMA depends on the participation and direction of volunteer leaders from the HIM community. AHIMA's members elect those who serve in the governing bodies of the organization.

The AHIMA **board of directors** governs the association. They set the organizational strategy, maintain fiscal oversight, and act as trustees of the organization (AHIMA 2019c). The business and affairs of AHIMA are managed by or under the direction of the Board of Directors. Its members include the president/chair, the president/chair-elect, the past president/chair, speaker of the House of Delegates, nine elected directors, the chief executive officer of the organization, and the advisor to the board. Except for the chief executive officer and the advisor, who are selected by the board of directors, all members of the board of directors are elected by the membership and serve three-year terms of office; members must be active members of the association. The president/chair must be a certificant and the majority of the directors must also be certificants.

In addition to the board of directors, CCHIIM is elected by the membership. CCHIIM is an AHIMA commission that is dedicated to assuring the competency of professionals practicing HIIM. It is a standing commission of AHIMA that is empowered with the responsibility and authority related to certification and recertification of HIIM professionals (AHIMA 2019c).

Engage

Engage is a community website managed by AHIMA for members to communicate on HIM topics. Engage has communities open to all HIM professionals and some specific for AHIMA members only. Engage provides the following benefits:

- Opportunities for members to contact other members to gain knowledge, share information, and learn best practices
- Opportunities to identify members with similar interests and backgrounds
- Gives members the ability to share and retrieve resources (AHIMA 2019d)

National Committees

AHIMA's president/chair oversees the appointment of members of the association's national committees, practice councils, and workgroups. These groups support the mission of the organization and work on specific projects as designated by the president/chair and the board of directors. Examples of the national committees include the

Figure 1.2 AHIMA's volunteer structure

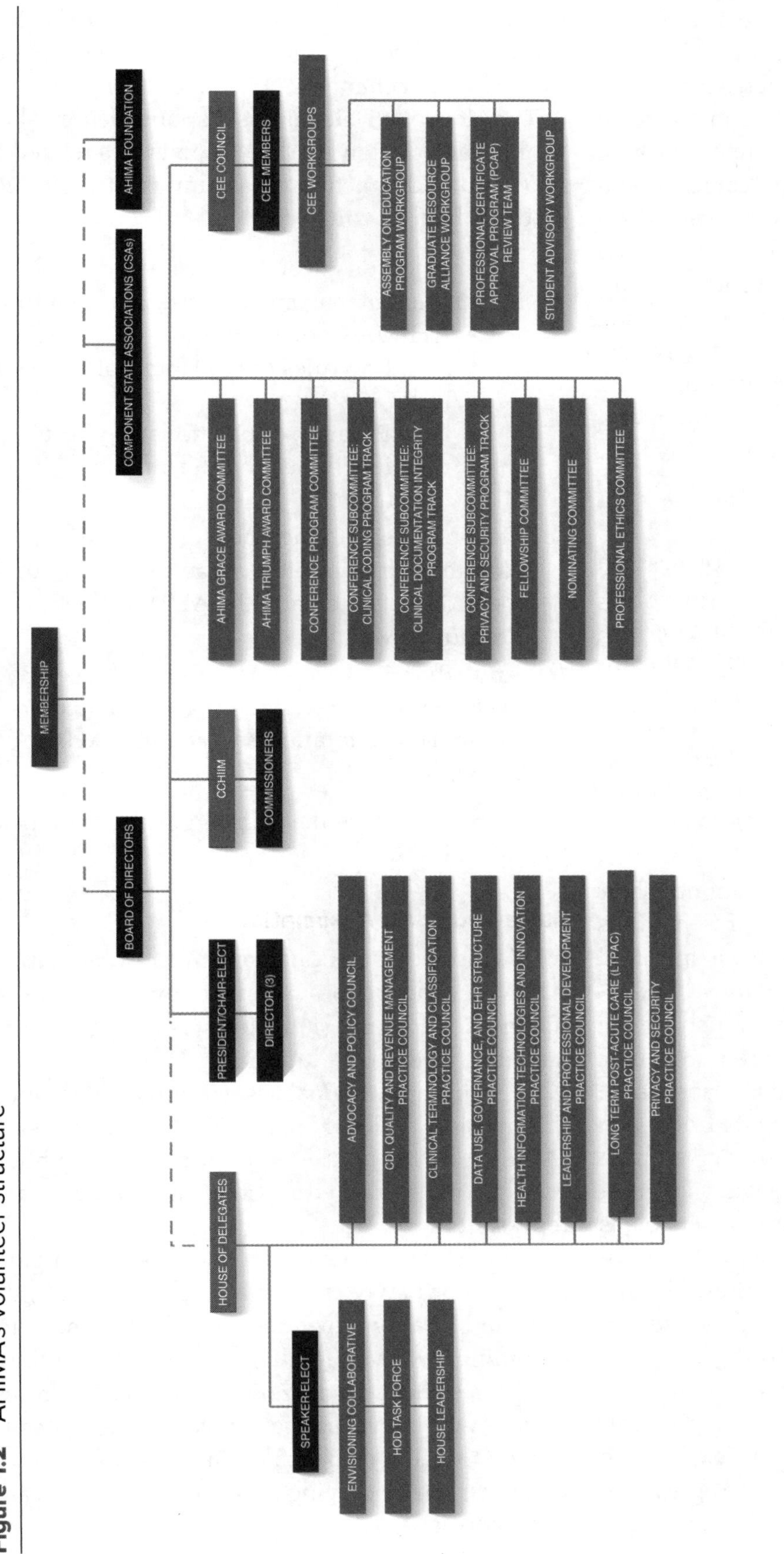

Source: AHIMA 2019b.

Conference Program Committee, the Fellowship Committee, and the Professional Ethics Committee. Practice councils are established as thought leadership groups to develop HIM content for a specific topic. Examples of practice councils include clinical classification and terminology, clinical documentation integrity, and privacy and security. Practice councils and committees are created to meet a specific need and may continue for years. In addition, AHIMA addresses challenges by establishing workgroups for short-term projects and then disbanding them. An example of a workgroup is the LGBTQ (lesbian, gay, bisexual, transgender and queer equality) Volunteer Workgroup.

House of Delegates

The House of Delegates governs the profession of health information management by providing a forum for membership and professional issues and to establish and maintain professional standards of the membership. For this reason, it is an important component of the volunteer structure (AHIMA 2019c). The House works virtually year-round with one annual face-to-face business meeting held in conjunction with AHIMA's conference.

Each component state association, defined later in this chapter, elects or appoints representatives to the House of Delegates to serve for a specified term of office. For this reason, the House of Delegates is similar to the legislative branch of the US government. Under the House are two teams: House Leadership and Envisioning Collaborative. The teams are made up of one delegate from each state. The Envisioning Collaborative serves as a "think tank." It is composed of delegates, subject matter experts, and industry leaders. Their role is to bring forward an exchange of viewpoints, innovation, and ideas. The outcomes of these discussions are the development of strategies used to advance the profession (AHIMA 2019d).

The House Leadership team ensures effective House operations through alignment with strategy and fosters the overall delegate experience and provides oversight of task force progression. Ad hoc task forces are created under the House to address topics that are important to the profession. These task forces change over time as the needs of the profession change.

The House of Delegates is responsible for establishing the position of AHIMA on issues related to HIM and taking action on a number of topics, including the following:

(a) "The standards governing the health information management profession, including:
- AHIMA Code of Ethics
- Standing rules of the House of Delegates
- Development of positions and best practices in health information management

(b) Election of six (6) members of the AHIMA Nominating Committee in accordance with the process set forth in the AHIMA Policy and Procedure Manual.

(c) Any other matters put before the House of Delegates by the AHIMA Board of Directors for final consideration and action" (AHIMA 2019d, 14).

Figure 1.3 shows the formal governance structure of AHIMA.

State and Local Associations

In addition to its national volunteer organization, AHIMA supports a system of component organizations in every state, plus Washington, DC, and Puerto Rico. Component state associations (CSAs) are professional associations that support the mission and views of AHIMA in their state (AHIMA 2019d). CSAs provide their members with professional education, networking, and representation.

Many states also have local or regional organizations. For newly credentialed professionals, the state and local organizations are ideal avenues for becoming involved with volunteer work within the professional organization. Most HIM professionals who serve in the House of Delegates or serve on AHIMA's Board of Directors began their volunteerism by serving at the local, regional, and state associations.

Figure 1.3 Governance structure of AHIMA

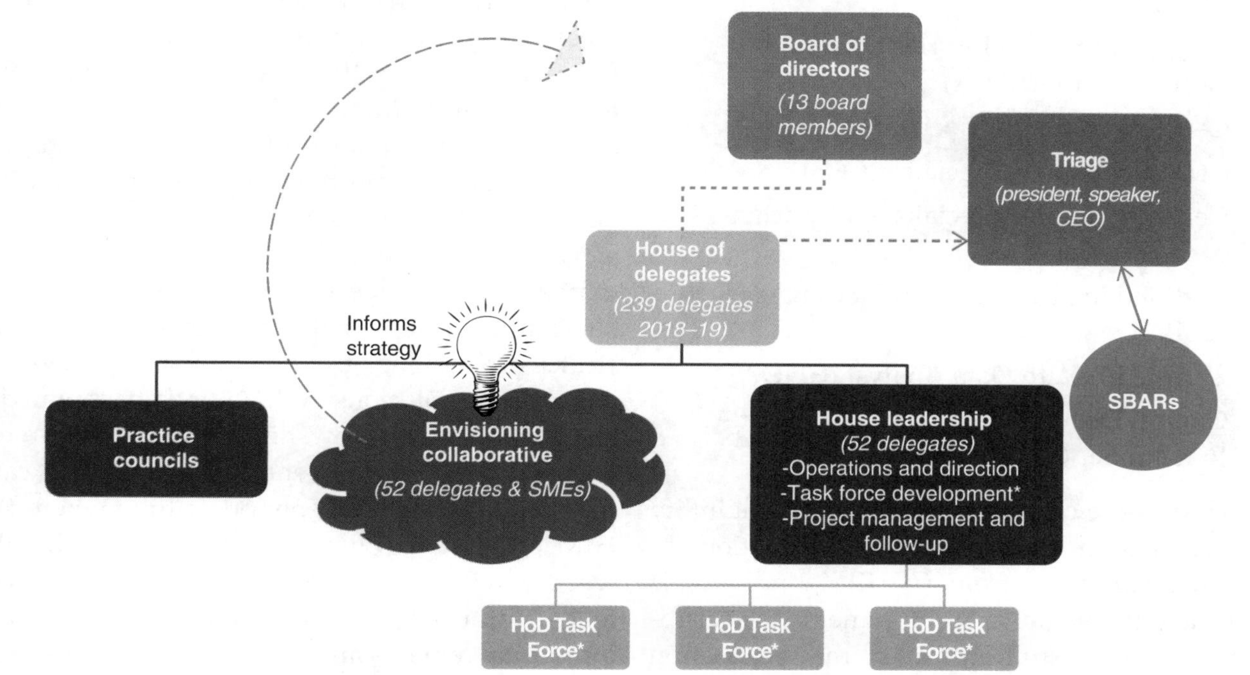

Source: AHIMA 2019.

Staff Structure

The AHIMA headquarters is located in Chicago, Illinois. The chief executive officer (CEO) is given the authority and responsibility to operate AHIMA in all its activities, subject to the policies and directions of the Board of Directors. The CEO undertakes his or her duties in accordance with a job description approved by the Board (AHIMA 2019d). The CEO is responsible for overseeing day-to-day operations. A team of executives, managers, and staff support the CEO. These executives include a chief knowledge officer and chief operating officer. Examples of the staff departments include, among others, member services, professional practice services, AHIMA Press, marketing, and policy and government relations.

Accreditation of Educational Programs

AHIMA has a long tradition of commitment to HIM education. As discussed previously, the first prescribed educational curriculum for the training of health record professionals was proposed in 1929. The first educational programs were accredited in 1934. Since then, the association has developed and maintained a rigorous accreditation process for academic programs, continuously developed up-to-date curriculum models, and supported educational programs in a variety of ways. Accreditation is discussed in more detail later in this chapter.

Certification and Registration Program

As the field of HIM became more complex, the association recognized the need to regulate its credentialing program. In 2008, CCHIIM was established. CCHIIM is dedicated to ensuring the competency of HIM professionals. CCHIIM serves the public by establishing, implementing, and enforcing standards and procedures for certification and recertification of HIM professionals. CCHIIM provides strategic oversight of all AHIMA certification programs. This standing commission of AHIMA is empowered with the sole and independent authority in all matters pertaining to both the initial certification and ongoing recertification (certification maintenance) of HIM professionals.

Today, AHIMA's certification program encompasses several credentials, including the following:

- Registered Health Information Technician (RHIT)
- Registered Health Information Administrator (RHIA)
- Certified Coding Associate (CCA)
- Certified Coding Specialist (CCS)
- Certified Coding Specialist—Physician-based (CCS-P)
- Certified in Healthcare Privacy and Security (CHPS)
- Certified Health Data Analyst (CHDA)
- Clinical Documentation Improvement Practitioner (CDIP)

Each of these credentials has specific eligibility requirements and a certification examination. To achieve certification from CCHIIM, individuals must meet the eligibility requirements for certification and successfully complete the certification examination.

Because the HIM profession is constantly changing, certified individuals must demonstrate they are continuing to maintain their knowledge and skill base. Therefore, to maintain their certification, individuals who hold any of AHIMA's credentials must complete a designated set of continuing education units (CEUs). Activities that qualify for CEUs include participation in workshops and seminars, taking college courses, participating in independent study activities, and engaging in self-assessment activities. The CCHIIM website provides information on the most recent requirements for maintenance of certification.

Fellowship Program

AHIMA's fellowship program is a program of earned recognition for AHIMA members who have made significant and sustained contributions to the HIM profession through meritorious service, excellence in professional practice, education, and advancement of the profession through innovation and knowledge sharing (AHIMA 2019e). Individuals who earn fellowship use the designation Fellow of the American Health Information Management Association (FAHIMA).

Fellowship is open to any individual who is an active or Emeritus member of AHIMA and who meets the eligibility requirements. Fellows must have a minimum of 10 years full-time professional experience in HIM or a related field, a minimum of 10 years continuous AHIMA membership at the time they submit their application (excluding years as a student member), hold a minimum of a master's degree, hold an active CCHIIM credential and provide evidence of sustained and substantial professional achievement that demonstrates professional growth and use of innovative and creative solutions. AHIMA members who desire to apply for fellowship but do not yet meet the eligibility requirements may apply for candidacy. Candidacy is a period of time where the HIM professional, who is not currently eligible, works toward the recognition. Once conferred, fellowship is a lifetime recognition as long as the individual remains an AHIMA member and complies with AHIMA's Code of Ethics. At the time of this writing, 200 members have been awarded fellowship status.

AHIMA Support of Training and Education

AHIMA supports training and education in a number of ways including educational webinars and face-to-face meetings for HIM professionals. AHIMA has also created self-assessments for HIM professionals to evaluate their skills in comparison to the skills required for current HIM practices.

AHIMA provides HIM educational programs with a number of resources. For example, the Virtual Lab provides HIM educational programs access to a number of information systems, such as the EHR and data visioning, that students will see in practice. AHIMA publishes HIM textbooks and creates entry-level competencies used in HIM educational programs. AHIMA also provides courses in a number of topics related to HIM.

AHIMA created the Council for Excellence in Education (CEE) to bring together representatives of the HIM education stakeholders, including industry representatives, to address issues related to the future of the profession and HIM education.

Figure 1.4 Career Map

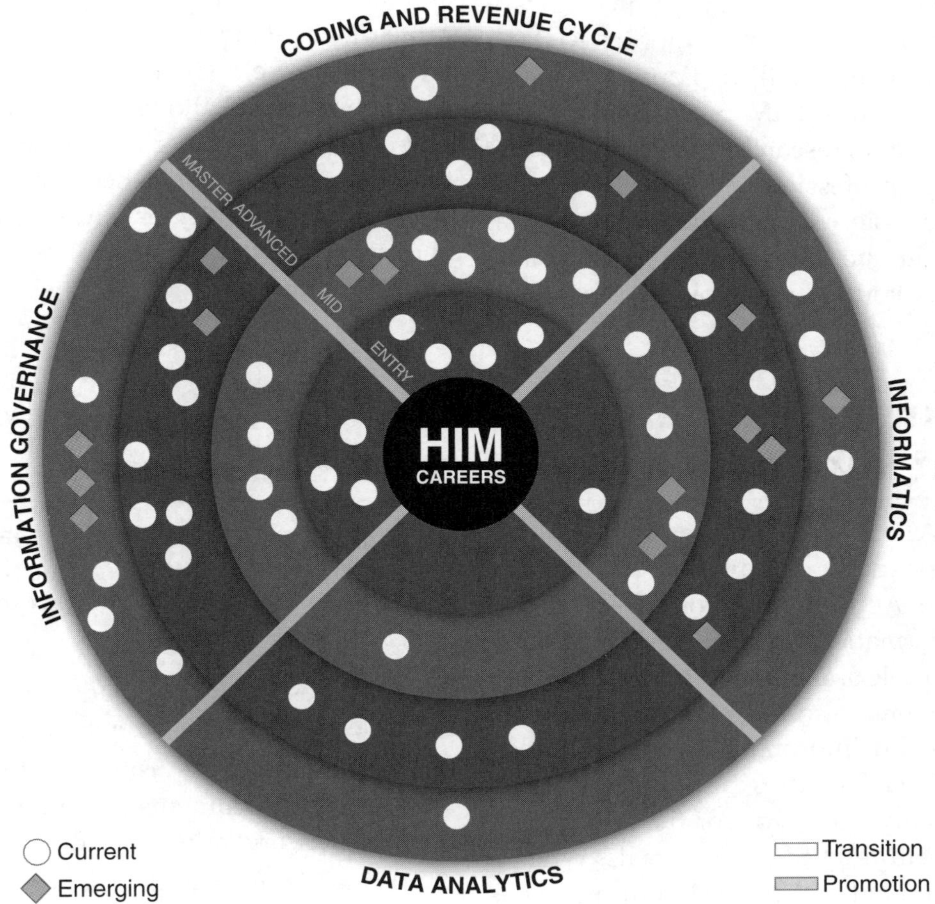

Source: AHIMA 2019g.

The CEE works to "ensure that education is positioned as the cornerstone of health information professions through communication, collaboration, innovation, and research" (AHIMA 2019f). The CEE board is elected by the AHIMA membership for a three-year term.

The CEE has a number of workgroups to conduct the work of the council. These workgroups include curricula, educational programming, graduate resources, student advisory, and workforce (AHIMA 2019f). These workgroups help strengthen members by identifying the future needs of the profession and then setting the college curriculum required to ensure future HIM professionals have those skills. They also assist educators by helping educators keep skills current and by assisting with establishing standards for professional practice experiences.

AHIMA Career Map

AHIMA created the interactive Career Map. This Career Map provides a synopsis of current and emerging HIM careers (roles) in four categories: Coding and Revenue Cycle, Data Analytics, Informatics, and Information Governance. These roles are categorized into four tiers: entry, mid, advanced, and master level. The Career Map shows common paths a HIM professional might take as he or she moves from entry-level roles to master-level roles. This path may jump from category to category. For example, the Informatics mid-level of implementation support analyst can jump to the Information Governance advanced role of HIM manager (AHIMA nd). The Career Map is shown in figure 1.4. To access the Career Map, visit http://www.ahima.org/careermap.

AHIMA Foundation

Founded in 1962, AHIMA Foundation is a separate entity from AHIMA but supports AHIMA in a multitude of ways. AHIMA Foundation supports people (including HIM professionals, HIM students, and others), research, and resources that enhance the HIM profession.

The HIM profession is based on the belief that high-quality healthcare requires high-quality information. AHIMA Foundation provides leadership in research, workforce development, scholarships, and competency-based education for the HIM professional. One of the ways that it supports workforce development is through an apprenticeship program that allows recent HIM graduates to obtain real-world experience. Its role is to envision the future direction and needs of the field and to respond with strategies, information, planning, and programs that will keep the HIM profession on the cutting edge.

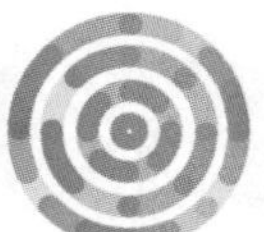

Commission on Accreditation for Health Informatics and Information Management Education

In 2004, AHIMA's House of Delegates voted to establish an independent accreditation commission, Commission on Accreditation for Health Informatics and Information Management Education (CAHIIM), with sole and independent authority in all matters pertaining to accreditation of educational programs in health informatics and information management. CAHIIM serves the public interest by establishing quality standards for the educational preparation of future HIM professionals. When a program is accredited by CAHIIM, it means it has voluntarily undergone a rigorous review process and has been determined to meet or exceed the accreditation standards established by CAHIIM. CAHIIM accreditation recognizes and publicizes best practices for HIM education programs.

CAHIIM reviews formal applications from college programs that apply for candidacy status, which is a preliminary approval process. After a successful review of the application documentation, a program may be deemed a candidate for accreditation for up to two years. Students enrolled in programs placed in candidacy status are eligible to join AHIMA as student members. The steps of the accreditation process are the following:

1. The college program prepares a self-assessment document that helps the college identify its strengths and weaknesses.
2. Accreditation site visitors visit the campus to review documents and interview faculty, students, and administration.
3. A final determination is made as to the ability of the college program to meet the accreditation standards for curriculum, facility, resources, and other requirements.

The accreditation of educational programs is important because only those individuals who graduate from an approved program may sit for the national credentialing examinations for the RHIT and RHIA. At the time this chapter was written, an exception has been made that allows RHITs who have a bachelor's degree in any subject to qualify to sit for the RHIA exam.

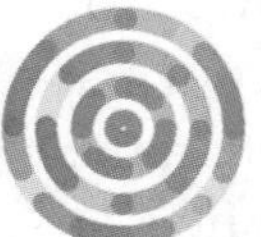

Health Information Management Specialty Professional Organizations

Health information management professionals frequently specialize in an area of the HIM profession. Examples of these specialties include clinical documentation integrity, coding, tumor registry, medical transcription, information governance, privacy and security, standards, and information systems. A number of specialty organizations support these areas.

Healthcare Information and Management Systems Society

Healthcare Information and Management Systems Society (HIMSS) is a not-for-profit organization that supports "the information of health through the application of information and technology" (HIMSS 2018a). The HIMSS sponsors exams for health information and information systems professionals—the certified professional in Healthcare Information and Management Systems (CPHIMS) certification and Certified Associate Professional in Healthcare Information and Management Systems (CAHIMS). The CPHIMS exam covers topics such as healthcare environment, technology environment, system analysis, system design, system selection and implementation, privacy and security, and administration (HIMSS 2018b). The CAHIMS certification covers administration, healthcare information and systems management, organization environment, and the technology/organizational environment (HIMSS 2018c).

Association for Healthcare Documentation Integrity

The Association for Healthcare Documentation Integrity (AHDI) is a professional organization dedicated to the capture of health data and documentation (AHDI 2018a). AHDI sponsors the Registered Healthcare Documentation Specialist (RHDS) and Certified Healthcare Documentation Specialist (CHDS) credentials. The RHDS is the entry-level certification sponsored by AHDI. The CHDS determines if the candidate is qualified to be a transcriptionist in a multidisciplinary environment. Both certification exams address basic transcription concepts including transcription standards and style, clinical medicine, and health information technology (AHDI 2018b).

American Academy of Professional Coders

The American Academy of Professional Coders (AAPC) educates and certifies medical coders, billers, medical auditors, revenue cycle managers, and other administrative specialties. The AAPC sponsors certifications in these specialty areas. Some of the certifications include the following:

- Certified Professional Coder (CPC)
- Certified Professional Medical Auditor (CPMA)
- Certified Professional Compliance Officer (CPCO)
- Certified Inpatient Coder (CIC)
- Certified Outpatient Coder (COC)
- Certified Risk Adjustment Coder (CRC)
- Certified Documentation Expert Outpatient (CDEO)
- Certified Physician Practice Manager (CPPM)

(AAPC 2018)

National Cancer Registrars Association

The National Cancer Registrars Association (NCRA) represents cancer registrar professionals. Their mission is to "serve as the premier education, credentialing, and advocacy resource for cancer data professionals" (NCRA 2018). The NCRA sponsors the Certified Tumor Registrar (CTR) certification. This exam includes information on registry organization and operations, abstracting, coding, follow-up, data analysis, and interpretation as well as coding and staging.

Check Your Understanding 1.2

Answer the following questions.

1. Our college has applied to become accredited by CAHIIM and we have completed the initial steps. Identify the name of the initial stage of accreditation that we are in.
   a. Certification
   b. Candidacy
   c. Fellowship
   d. Credentialing

2. I would like to consult with other HIM professionals on what to do in a situation. I should utilize:
   a. Engage
   b. Fellowship
   c. House of Delegates
   d. CEE
3. I would like to propose a change to the HIM profession. I should go to:
   a. Board of Directors
   b. House of Delegates
   c. CCHIIM
   d. CAHIIM
4. I would like to apply for AHIMA Fellowship. I have been a member of AHIMA for eight continuous years of HIM experience. I have a master's degree and I have worked in a number of volunteer roles for AHIMA. Determine if I am eligible for the designation. If not, determine why.
   a. I am currently eligible for AHIMA Fellowship.
   b. I am not eligible for AHIMA Fellowship because I need a minimum of 10 years of HIM experience.
   c. I am not eligible for AHIMA Fellowship because I need to publish in journals as well as volunteer for AHIMA.
   d. I am not eligible for AHIMA Fellowship because I must have a doctorate degree.
5. I need to decide which CCHIIM credential to apply for. I am graduating with an associate degree in health information management from a CAHIIM-accredited program. The best credential for me to take is:
   a. Registered Healthcare Documentation Specialist
   b. Registered Health Information Technician
   c. Certified Professional in Healthcare Information and Management Systems
   d. Certified Professional Coder

Real-World Case 1.1

The electronic health record (EHR) is causing many changes in both the health information management (HIM) profession and the structure of the HIM department. Because of the EHR, many functions of the HIM department can be performed remotely. Some HIM staff such as coders and transcriptionists are now working from home. The file areas where the paper records are housed are disappearing as more and more of the health records are electronic. These changes enable the healthcare organization to use the space previously occupied by the HIM staff and the file areas to be used for other purposes. Some healthcare organizations with multiple locations have centralized their HIM functions, enabling them to standardize the HIM functions and to share staff among the healthcare organizations. The HIM staff at the central location can perform most of the functions of the HIM department. There may be some staff at the healthcare organization to attend committee meetings, take authorization for release of information from patients, and perform other functions that require staff on site. Whether employees work from home or at a centralized location, the privacy and security of patient information must always be ensured at all the locations and employee productivity must meet the standards established by the organization.

Real-World Case 1.2

One of the strengths of the HIM profession is the opportunity for the HIM professional's career path to evolve over time. Kathryn has a registered health information technician (RHIT) credential. She began her HIM career immediately after college working in utilization review. After a year or two, she transitioned to HIM department management and worked at hospitals ranging in size from 60 beds to 900+ beds. After 15 years of working in hospitals she was ready for a change, so she left the hospital and worked first in a HIM consulting firm and then for an information system vendor. In both roles, she traveled around the country working with clients. Kathryn quickly tired of the travel and decided to change the focus of her career path once again. Now, she is a HIM educator and writes HIM textbooks on the side. While Kathryn has earned both a master's degree and a doctorate degree, it was her HIM degree and skills that allowed her to move from one career path to another.

References

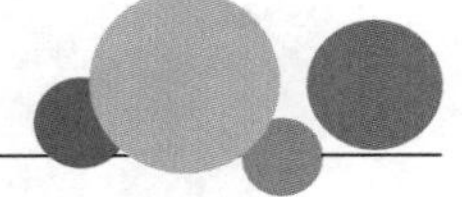

American Academy of Professional Coders. 2018. Medical Billing and Coding Certification. http://www.aapc.com/certification.

American Health Information Management Association. 2017. *Pocket Glossary of Health Information Management and Technology*, 5th ed. Chicago: AHIMA.

American Health Information Management Association. 2019a. Who We Are. https://www.ahima.org/about/aboutahima.

American Health Information Management Association. 2019b. About the Commission. http://www.ahima.org/certification/cchiim.

American Health Information Management Association. 2019b. AHIMA Membership. http://www.ahima.org/membership.

American Health Information Management Association. 2019c. AHIMA House of Delegates Policy and Procedure Management. http://bok.ahima.org/PdfView?oid=302856

American Health Information Management Association. 2019d. Bylaws of American Health Information Management Association. http://bok.ahima.org/PdfView?oid=302856.

American Health Information Management Association. 2019d. How to Guide. https://engage.ahima.org/helpfaqs1/tutorials.

American Health Information Management Association. 2019e. Fellowship Program. http://www.ahima.org/about/recognition?tabid=fellowship.

American Health Information Management Association. 2019e. House of Delegates. http://www.ahima.org/about/governance?tabid=hod.

American Health Information Management Association. 2019e. Volunteer organization. http://www.ahima.org/volunteers.

American Health Information Management Association. 2019f. CEE Workgroups. http://ahima.org/education/academic-affairs/council-for-excellence.

American Health Information Management Association. 2019g. Career Map. https://my.ahima.org/careermap.

American Health Information Management Association. 2019g. What is the CEE. http://www.ahima.org/education/academic-affairs/council-for-excellence.

Association for Healthcare Documentation Integrity. 2018a. About AHDI. https://www.ahdionline.org/page/about.

Association for Healthcare Documentation Integrity. 2018b. https://cdn.ymaws.com/ahdionline.site-ym.com/resource/resmgr/Credentialing-Downloads/CredentialingCandidateGuide.pdf.

CareerOneStop. 2018. Earning a certification can help you enter or advance in many careers. https://www.careeronestop.org/FindTraining/Types/certifications.aspx.

The Caviart Group. 2015. A Workforce Study of the Future Direction and Skill Set for HIM Professionals. http://bok.ahima.org/PdfView?oid=300801.

Dooling, J.A., S.H. Houser, R. Mikaelian, C.P. Smith. 2016. Transitioning to a Data-Driven Informatics-Oriented Department. *Journal of AHIMA* 87(10): 58-62.

Healthcare Information Management Systems Society. 2018a. About HIMSS. http://www.himss.org/aboutHIMSS/.

Healthcare Information Management Systems Society. 2018b. CPHIMS Candidate Handbook. https://www.himss.org/health-it-certification/cphims/handbook.

Healthcare Information Management Systems Society. 2018c. CAHIMS Candidate Handbook. https://www.himss.org/health-it-certification/cahims/handbook.

Huffman, E.K. 1985. *Medical Record Management*, 8th ed. Berwyn, IL: Physicians' Record Company.

Huffman, E.K. 1941. Requirements and advantages of registration for health record librarians. *Bulletin of the American Association of Medical Record Librarians.*

IG Advisors. 2018. Information Governance Glossary. http://www.ahima.org/topics/infogovernance/ig-glossary.

Johns, M.L. 1991. Information management: A shifting paradigm for medical record professionals? *Journal of the American Medical Record Association* 62(8):55–63.

National Cancer Registrars Association. 2018. Membership. http://www.ncra-usa.org/Membership.

Tutorialspoint. nd. Mission, Vision and Values. https://www.tutorialspoint.com/management_principles/management_principles_mission_vision_values.htm.

Healthcare Delivery Systems

Kelly Miller, MA, RHIA

Learning Objectives

- Differentiate the roles of various healthcare providers throughout the healthcare delivery system
- Determine the basic organization and operation of various types of hospitals and other healthcare organizations and services
- Examine the use and functions of telehealth services in healthcare
- Examine the influence of artificial intelligence in the delivery of healthcare
- Identify the various policy making influences in the delivery of healthcare
- Examine healthcare delivery in the United States

Key Terms

Accountable care organizations (ACOs)
Allied health professional
Ambulatory care
American Recovery and Reinvestment Act (ARRA)
Artificial intelligence (AI)
Average length of stay (ALOS)
Big data
Case management
Centers for Disease Control and Prevention (CDC)
Chief executive officer (CEO)
Chief financial officer (CFO)
Chief information officer (CIO)
Chief nursing officer (CNO)
Chief operating officer (COO)
Clinical privileges
Continuum of care
Critical access hospital (CAH)
Extended care facility
Health Information Technology for Economic and Clinical Health (HITECH) Act
Home healthcare
Hospice
Hospital
Hospitalist
Integrated delivery network (IDN)
Integrated delivery system (IDS)
Managed care organization (MCO)
Medicaid
Medical home
Medical staff bylaws
Medical staff classification
Medicare
Patient Protection and Affordable Care Act (ACA)
Peer review organization (PRO)
Quality improvement organization (QIO)
Safety net hospital (SNH)
Skilled nursing facility (SNF)
Social determinants of health (SDOH)
Subacute care
Telehealth
Utilization review (UR)
Utilization Review Act

A broad array of healthcare services is available in the United States today, from simple preventive measures such as vaccinations to complex life-saving procedures such as heart transplants. An individual's contact with the healthcare delivery system often begins before he or she is born, with family planning and prenatal care, and continues through the end of life, when long-term care or hospice care may be needed.

Health information is a vital component of the healthcare system. Therefore, it is crucial for health information management professionals to have a comprehensive understanding of healthcare delivery. This chapter discusses healthcare delivery in the United States and how political, societal, and other factors have influenced its development. Well-known legislation affecting healthcare and healthcare information systems in the United States is examined. Different healthcare providers and types of delivery facilities and the services they provide are explained.

Healthcare Providers

The US healthcare system employs an estimated 16 million workers in the roles of health practitioners, practitioner support, technologists, technicians, and support roles (BLS 2017a). Physicians, nurses, and other clinical providers deliver healthcare services in a variety of healthcare settings. Those care settings include ambulatory, acute care, rehabilitative, psychiatric, long-term care, hospice, home care, assisted living centers, industrial medical clinics, and public health clinics. In other words, wherever people need access to the healthcare system, there are healthcare professionals providing that care.

Medical Practice

There are many providers included under the term *medical practice*, all of which are referred to as "doctor." It should be noted that *doctor* is an educational degree, not a profession. Some of the most common healthcare practitioners are the following:

- Chiropractor (DC—Doctor of Chiropractic) focuses on the diagnosis, treatment, and prevention of disorders of the neuromusculoskeletal system.
- Dentist (DDS or DMD—Doctor of Dental Surgery or Doctor of Medicine in Dentistry) focuses on the diagnosis, prevention, and treatment of diseases and conditions of the oral cavity.
- Medical (MD—Doctor of Medicine) focuses on the diagnosis, treatment, and education of any human disease or condition.
- Optometrist (OD—Doctor of Optometry) focuses on vision and visual systems and is trained to prescribe and fit lenses to improve vision.
- Osteopath (DO—Doctor of Osteopathic Medicine) not only focuses on manipulation of muscles and bones but also incorporates the diagnosis and treatment of diseases.
- Podiatrist (DPM—Doctor of Podiatric Medicine) focuses on the treatment of disorders of the foot, ankle, and lower extremities.

All states require physicians be licensed to practice. Licensure requires graduating from a medical school with a Doctor of Medicine (MD) or a Doctor of Osteopathy (DO), successful completion of a licensing examination, and completion of a supervised residency program. Residencies are paid, on-the-job training that may last two to six years. Both MDs and DOs utilize acceptable treatment practices, including prescribing medications or performing surgeries.

The main difference between a DO and MD is in the philosophy and approach to medical treatment. The DO practices osteopathic medicine, which places an emphasis on the muscular system, stresses preventive medicine, and takes a holistic approach to patient care (Shi and Singh 2019). MDs practice allopathic medicine, which utilizes medical treatment as an active intervention to counteract and neutralize the effects of disease (Shi and Singh 2019). MDs may utilize preventive medicine combined with allopathic medicine. A 2016 census of active licensed physicians in the US identified 953,695 allopathic and osteopathic physicians serving a population of 323 million people. More than 90 percent of actively licensed physicians are MDs, compared to DOs (Young et al. 2016)

Physicians can be categorized as generalists or specialists. A generalist is trained in family medicine, general practice, general internal medicine, and general pediatrics. Generalists are considered primary care physicians. Non–primary care physicians are specialists. Specialists must obtain additional certification in their specialty. Medical specialties are divided into six major categories: 1) subspecialties of internal medicine 2) broad medical specialties 3) obstetrics and gynecology 4) surgery, 5) hospital-based radiology anesthesiology, and (6) psychiatry (Shi and Singh 2019). Some of the medical specialties and subspecialties are defined in figure 2.1. Some subspecialties can be included in more than one specialty category. For example, there is a subspecialty of pediatrics for most specialties.

Figure 2.1 Medical specialties and subspecialties

Medical Specialties and Subspecialties	
Allergy and Immunology	Diagnoses and manages disorders involving immune conditions such as asthma, anaphylaxis, rhinitis, and eczema as well as adverse reactions to drugs, food, and insects. In addition, they diagnose and manage immune deficiency diseases and problems related autoimmune diseases, organ transplantation, or malignancies of the immune system.
Anesthesiology	Provides anesthesia for patients undergoing surgical, obstetric, diagnostic, or therapeutic procedures while monitoring the patient's condition and supporting vital organ functions. Anesthesiologists also provide resuscitation and medical management for patients with critical illnesses and severe injuries.
Pediatric	Provides anesthesia for neonates, infants, children, and adolescents undergoing surgical, diagnostic, or therapeutic procedures as well as appropriate pre- and post-operative care, advanced life support, and acute pain management.
Colon and Rectal Surgery	Diagnoses and treats various diseases of the small intestine, colon, rectum, anal canal, and perianal area including the organs and tissues related to primary intestinal diseases.
Dermatology	Provides diagnosis and medical/surgical management of diseases of the skin, hair and nails, and mucous membranes.
Dermatopathology	Diagnoses and monitors diseases of the skin, including infectious, immunologic, degenerative, and neoplastic diseases
Emergency Medicine	Focuses on the immediate decision-making and action necessary to prevent death or any further disability both in the pre-hospital setting by directing emergency medical technicians and in the emergency department.
Family Medicine	Delivers a range of acute, chronic, and preventive medical care services to individuals of all ages, families, and communities. In addition to diagnosing and treating illness, these personal physicians manage chronic illness and provide preventive care, including routine checkups, health risk assessments, immunization and screening tests, and personalized counseling on maintaining a healthy lifestyle.
Geriatric Medicine	Includes special knowledge of the aging process and special skills in the diagnostic, therapeutic, preventive, and rehabilitative aspects of illness in the elderly.
Hospice and Palliative Medicine	Provides care to prevent and relieve the suffering experienced by patients with life-limiting illnesses.

continued

Figure 2.1 Medical specialties and subspecialties *(continued)*

Specialty	Description
Internal Medicine	Provides long-term, comprehensive care in the office and in the hospital, managing both common and complex illnesses of adolescents, adults, and the elderly. Internists are trained in the diagnosis and treatment of cancer, infections, and diseases affecting the heart, blood, kidneys, joints, and the digestive, respiratory, and vascular systems. They are also trained in the essentials of primary care internal medicine.
Cardiovascular Disease	Specializes in diseases of the heart and blood vessels and manages complex cardiac conditions, such as heart attacks and life-threatening, abnormal heartbeat rhythms.
Critical Care Medicine	Specializes in the diagnosis, treatment, and support of critically ill and injured patients, particularly trauma victims and patients with multiple organ dysfunction.
Neurocritical Care	Provides comprehensive multisystem care of the critically ill patient with neurological diseases and conditions.
Endocrinology, Diabetes, and Metabolism	Specializes in the diagnosis and management of disorders of hormones and their actions, metabolic disorders, and neoplasia of the endocrine glands.
Gastroenterology	Specializes in diagnosis and treatment of diseases of the digestive organs including the stomach, bowels, liver, and gallbladder.
Hematology	Specializes in diseases of the blood, spleen, and lymph.
Infectious Disease	Provides care for infectious diseases of all types and in all organ systems. Infectious disease specialists may also have expertise in preventive medicine and travel medicine.
Interventional Cardiology	Uses specialized imaging and other diagnostic techniques to evaluate blood flow and pressure in the coronary arteries and chambers of the heart, and uses technical procedures and medications to treat abnormalities that impair the function of the cardiovascular system.
Medical Oncology	Diagnoses and treats all types of cancer and other benign and malignant tumors.
Nephrology	Treats disorders of the kidney, high blood pressure, fluid and mineral balance, and dialysis of body wastes when the kidneys do not function.
Pulmonary Disease	Treats diseases of the lungs and airways. Diagnoses and treats cancer, pneumonia, pleurisy, asthma, occupational and environmental diseases, bronchitis, sleep disorders, emphysema, and other complex disorders of the lungs.
Rheumatology	Treats diseases of joints, muscle, bones, and tendons. Diagnoses and treats arthritis, back pain, muscle strains, common athletic injuries, and collagen diseases.
Medical Genetics and Genomics	Specializes in medicine that involves the interaction between genes and health. Medical geneticists are trained to evaluate, diagnose, manage, treat, and counsel individuals of all ages with hereditary disorders. These specialists use modern cytogenetic, molecular, genomic, and biochemical genetic testing to assist in specialized diagnostic evaluations, implement needed therapeutic interventions, and provide genetic counseling and prevention through prenatal and preimplantation diagnosis.
Neurological Surgery	Treats adult and pediatric patients for pain or pathological processes that may modify the function or activity of the central nervous system, the peripheral nervous system, the autonomic nervous system, the supporting structures of these systems, and their vascular supply.
Neurology	Evaluates and treats all types of diseases or impaired functions of the brain, spinal cord, peripheral nerves, muscles, and autonomic nervous system, as well as the blood vessels that relate to these structures.
Brain Injury Medicine	Focuses on the prevention, evaluation, treatment, and rehabilitation of individuals with acquired brain injury.
Clinical Neurophysiology	Evaluates and treats central, peripheral, and autonomic nervous system disorders using a combination of clinical evaluation and electrophysiologic testing such as electroencephalography (EEG), electromyography (EMG), and nerve conduction studies (NCS). Practitioners may be neurologists, pediatric neurologists, or psychiatrists.
Epilepsy	Evaluates and treats adults and children with recurrent seizure activity and seizure disorders. Neurologists and pediatric neurologists provide epilepsy care.
Obstetrics and Gynecology	Focuses on the health of women before, during, and after childbearing years, diagnosing and treating conditions of the reproductive system and associated disorders.

continued

Figure 2.1 Medical specialties and subspecialties *(continued)*

Specialty	Description
Complex Family Planning	Diagnoses and treats women with medically and surgically complex conditions.
Maternal–Fetal Medicine	Focuses on patients with complications of pregnancy and the effects on both the mother and the fetus.
Reproductive Endocrinology and Infertility	Concentrates on hormonal functioning as it pertains to reproduction as well as the issue of infertility. These specialists also are trained to evaluate and treat hormonal dysfunctions in females outside of infertility.
Ophthalmology	Prescribes eyeglasses and contact lenses, dispenses medications, diagnoses and treats eye conditions and diseases, and performs surgeries. Ophthalmologists are the only physicians medically trained to manage the complete range of eye and vision care.
Orthopaedic Surgery	Focuses on the preservation, investigation, and restoration of the form and function of the extremities, spine, and associated structures by medical, surgical, and physical means.
Otolaryngology – Head and Neck Surgery	Provides medical and surgical therapy for the prevention of diseases, allergies, neoplasms, deformities, disorders, and injuries of the ears, nose, sinuses, throat, respiratory, and upper alimentary systems, face, jaws, and the other head and neck systems.
Pain Medicine	Provides care for patients with acute, chronic, or cancer pain in both inpatient and outpatient settings while coordinating patient care needs with other specialists.
Pathology	Deals with the causes and nature of disease and contributes to diagnosis, prognosis, and treatment through knowledge gained by the laboratory application of the biological, chemical, and physical sciences.
Pediatrics	Focuses on the physical, emotional, and social health of children from birth to young adulthood. Pediatric care encompasses a broad spectrum of health services ranging from preventive healthcare to the diagnosis and treatment of acute and chronic diseases.
Adolescent Medicine	Focuses on the unique physical, psychological, and social characteristics of adolescents, and their healthcare problems and needs.
Physical Medicine and Rehabilitation	Evaluates and treats patients with physical or cognitive impairments and disabilities that result from musculoskeletal conditions (such as neck or back pain, or sports or work injuries), neurological conditions (such as stroke, brain injury, or spinal cord injury), or other medical conditions. Also called a physiatrist.
Plastic Surgery	Deals with the repair, reconstruction, or replacement of physical defects of form or function involving the skin, musculoskeletal system, craniomaxillofacial structures, hand, extremities, breast and trunk, and external genitalia or cosmetic enhancement of these areas of the body. Cosmetic surgery is an essential component of plastic surgery
Preventive Medicine	Focuses on the health of individuals and defined populations to protect, promote, and maintain health and well-being and to prevent disease, disability, and premature death.
Addiction Medicine	Concerned with the prevention, evaluation, diagnosis, and treatment of persons with the disease of addiction, of those with substance-related health conditions, and of people who show unhealthy use of substances including nicotine, alcohol, prescription medications, and other licit and illicit drugs.
Clinical Informatics	Collaborates with other healthcare and information technology professionals to analyze, design, implement, and evaluate information and communication systems that enhance individual and population health outcomes, improve patient care, and strengthen the clinician–patient relationship.
Medical Toxicology	Specializes in the prevention, evaluation, treatment, and monitoring of injury and illness from exposures to drugs and chemicals, as well as biological and radiological agents.
Psychiatry	Evaluates and treats mental, addictive, and emotional disorders such as schizophrenia and other psychotic disorders, mood disorders, anxiety disorders, substance-related disorders, sexual and gender-identity disorders, and adjustment disorders.
Radiology	Utilizes imaging methodologies to diagnose and manage patients and provide therapeutic options.
Diagnostic	Utilizes x-rays, radionuclides, ultrasound, and electromagnetic radiation to diagnose and treat disease.
Interventional Radiology and Diagnostic Radiology	Combines competence in imaging, image-guided minimally invasive procedures, and peri-procedural patient care to diagnose and treat benign and malignant conditions of the thorax, abdomen, pelvis, and extremities.

continued

Figure 2.1 Medical specialties and subspecialties *(concluded)*

Radiation Oncology	Uses ionizing radiation and other modalities to treat malignant and some benign diseases.
Neuroradiology	Diagnoses and treats disorders of the brain, sinuses, spine, spinal cord, neck, and the central nervous system, such as aging and degenerative diseases, seizure disorders, cancer, stroke, cerebrovascular diseases, and trauma.
Nuclear Radiology	Uses the administration of trace amounts of radioactive substances (radionuclides) to provide images and information for making a diagnosis.
Sleep Medicine	Diagnoses and manages clinical conditions that occur during sleep, that disturb sleep, or that are affected by disturbances in the wake-sleep cycle. Includes the analysis and interpretation of comprehensive polysomnography, and practitioners are well versed in emerging research and management of a sleep laboratory.
Sports Medicine	Focuses on the prevention, diagnosis, and treatment of injuries related to participating in sports or exercise.
Surgery (General)	Provides diagnosis and care of patients with diseases and disorders affecting the abdomen, digestive tract, endocrine system, breast, skin, and blood vessels. General surgeons are skilled in the use of minimally invasive techniques and endoscopies. Common conditions treated by general surgeons include hernias, gallstones, appendicitis, breast tumors, thyroid disorders, pancreatitis, bowel obstructions, colon inflammation, and colon cancer.
Thoracic Surgery	Encompasses the operative, perioperative, and surgical critical care of patients with acquired and congenital pathological conditions within the chest.
Congenital Cardiac Surgery	Refers to the procedures that are performed to repair the many types of heart defects that may be present at birth and can occasionally go undiagnosed into adulthood.
Urology	Focuses on diagnosing and treating disorders of the urinary tracts of males and females, and on the reproductive system of males. Manages nonsurgical problems such as urinary tract infections, as well as surgical problems such as the correction of congenital abnormalities.
Female Pelvic Medicine and Reconstructive Surgery	Provides consultation and comprehensive management of women with complex benign pelvic conditions, lower urinary tract disorders, and pelvic floor dysfunction.

Source: Adapted from American Board of Medical Specialties (ABMS).2019. ABMS Guide to Medical Specialties. https://www.abms.org/media/194925/abms-guide-to-medical-specialties-2019.pdf

Another specific role for physicians is that of a hospitalist. A **hospitalist** is a physician who specializes in the care of inpatient hospital patients (Shi and Singh 2019). Typically, hospitalists do not have a relationship with the patient prior to providing care during the hospitalization. In the traditional inpatient model, the patient's primary care physician would oversee their care. In the hospitalist model, the hospitalist oversees the patient's care until discharge; then the patient returns to the care of their primary care physician.

Hospitalists were first utilized to provide care for unassigned patients on general medicine floors and to cover for community-based primary care physicians. As hospitals began to focus on managed care, hospitalists were viewed as a means for hospitals to gain greater efficiency (Furci and Furci 2017). With the use of hospitalists, primary care physicians can devote more time to their office practices. There are approximately 50,000 hospitalists practicing in 75 percent of US Hospitals (Wachter and Goldman 2016).

Physician Assistants

Some physicians and healthcare facilities employ physician assistants (PAs) to help carry out clinical responsibilities. PAs practice medicine with teams of physicians, surgeons, and other healthcare workers to examine, diagnose, and treat patients. They work in a variety of clinical settings. A PA is licensed to provide care and perform medical procedures only under the supervision of a physician. In most states PAs have the authority to prescribe medications. Employment of PAs is projected to grow 37 percent from 2016 to 2026 (BLS 2018).

Nursing Practice

Nurses represent the largest number of healthcare professionals with four million registered nurses (RNs) (ANA 2019). Nurses are the primary caregivers for sick and injured patients. They use their judgment to integrate objective data with subjective observation of the patient's biological, physical, and behavioral needs. Nurses work in a variety of health settings, from providing critical care to vaccinations in a physician practice. The American Nurses Association (2019) provides the following four key responsibilities of registered nurses (ABMS 2019):

1. Perform physical exams and health histories before making critical decisions
2. Provide health promotion, counseling, and education
3. Administer medications and other personalized interventions
4. Coordinate care in collaboration with a wide array of healthcare professionals

Most RNs have either a two-year associate degree or a four-year bachelor of science degree from a state-approved nursing school, though some schools offer a master's degree that allows the graduate to sit for the licensure examination. Nurse practitioners, researchers, educators, and administrators generally have a four-year degree in nursing and additional postgraduate education in nursing. The postgraduate degree may be a master of science or a doctorate in nursing. Nurses who graduate from nonacademic training programs are called licensed practical nurses (LPNs) or licensed vocational nurses (LVNs). Non-degreed nursing personnel work under the direct supervision of RNs. Nurses must be licensed in the state in which they are working. They may be licensed in more than one state through examination or endorsement of a license issued by another state.

Today's RNs are highly trained clinical professionals. Many nurses specialize in specific areas of practice such as surgery, psychiatry, or intensive care. Nurse-midwives complete advanced training and are certified by the American College of Nurse-Midwives. Similarly, nurse-anesthetists are certified by the Council on Certification/Council on Recertification of Nurse Anesthetists. Nurse practitioners also receive advanced training at the master's level that qualifies them to provide primary care services to patients. They are certified by several organizations (for example, the National Board of Pediatric Nurse Practitioners) to practice in the area of their specialty.

The need for RNs is expected to rise over the next decade. Hospitals in the US report continued vacancies for RNs. The Bureau of Labor Statistics estimates that between the years 2016 and 2026 approximately 438,100 more RNs will be needed over the projected supply (BLS 2017b).

Allied Health Professions

After World War I, many roles previously assumed by nurses and nonclinical personnel began to change. With the advent of modern diagnostic and therapeutic technology in the mid-20th century, the complex skills needed by ancillary medical personnel fostered the growth of specialized training programs and professional accreditation and licensure.

According to the Association of Schools of Allied Health Professions (ASAHP), allied health encompasses a broad group of health professionals who use scientific principles and evidence-based practice for the diagnosis, evaluation, and treatment of acute and chronic diseases; promote disease prevention and wellness for optimum health; and apply administration and management skills to support healthcare systems in a variety of settings. The Health Professions Education Extension Amendment of 1992, which amended the Public Health Service Act, describes **allied health professionals** as health professionals (other than registered nurses, physicians, and physician assistants) who have received a certificate, an associate degree, a bachelor degree, a master degree, a doctorate, or postdoctoral training in a healthcare-related science. Such individuals share responsibility for the delivery of healthcare services with clinicians (physicians, nurses, and physician assistants).

Allied health plays an essential role in the delivery of healthcare. It is estimated that as much as 60 percent of the US healthcare workforce can be classified as allied health (ASAHP 2018). Professions that fall in the category of allied health are the non-nurse, non-physician healthcare providers. The formal education requirements for these professions range from certifications through postsecondary education to postgraduate degrees. Technicians and assistants such as a physical therapist assistant, dental assistant, or laboratory technician typically receive less than two years postsecondary education and must work under the supervision of a therapist or technologist. Therapists such as a physical or speech therapist receive more advanced training.

The following list briefly describes some of the major occupations usually considered to be allied health professions:

- *Audiology*. Audiology is the branch of science that studies hearing, balance, and related disorders. Audiologists treat those with hearing loss and proactively prevent related damage. According to the American Speech-Language-Hearing Association, audiologists provide comprehensive diagnostic and treatment or rehabilitative services for auditory and related impairments. These services are provided to all individuals regardless of age, socioeconomic status, ethnicity, or cultural backgrounds (ASHA 2016).
- *Clinical laboratory science*. Originally referred to as medical laboratory technology, this field is now known as clinical laboratory science. Clinical laboratory technicians perform a wide array of tests on body fluids, tissues, and cells to assist in the detection, diagnosis, and treatment of diseases and illnesses. The clinical laboratory is divided into two sections—anatomic pathology and clinical pathology. Anatomic pathology deals with human tissues and provides surgical pathology, autopsy, and cytology services. Clinical pathology deals mainly with the analysis of body fluids—principally blood, but also urine, gastric contents, and cerebrospinal fluid. Physicians who specialize in performing and interpreting the results of pathology tests are called pathologists. Laboratory technicians are allied health professionals trained to operate laboratory equipment and perform laboratory tests under the supervision of a pathologist.
- *Diagnostic medical sonography or imaging technology*. Originally referred to as x-ray technology and then radiologic technology, this field is now referred to as diagnostic imaging. The field continues to expand to include nuclear medicine, radiation therapy, and echocardiography. Physician specialists (radiologists) and technologists including radiation therapists, cardiosonographers (ultrasound technologists), and magnetic resonance imaging technologists provide these services. Nuclear medicine involves the use of ionizing radiation and small amounts of short-lived radioactive tracers to treat disease, specifically neoplastic disease (that is, nonmalignant tumors and malignant cancers). Radiation therapy uses high-energy x-rays, cobalt, electrons, and other sources of radiation to treat human disease. In current practice, radiation therapy is used alone or in combination with surgery or chemotherapy (drugs) to treat many types of cancer. In addition to external beam therapy, radioactive implants (as well as therapy performed with heat—hyperthermia) are available.
- *Dietetics and nutrition*. Dietitians (also clinical nutritionists) are trained in nutrition. They are responsible for providing nutritional care to individuals and for overseeing nutrition and food services in a variety of settings, ranging from hospitals to schools.
- *Emergency medical technology*. Emergency medical technicians (EMTs) and paramedics provide a wide range of services on an emergency basis for cases of traumatic injury and other emergency situations and in the transport of emergency patients to a healthcare organization.
- *Health information management*. Health information management (HIM) professionals. Registered Health Information

Administrators (RHIAs) and Registered Health Information Technicians (RHITs) are the credentials for HIM professions. They are responsible for ensuring the availability, accuracy, and protection of the clinical information that is needed to deliver healthcare services and to make appropriate healthcare-related decisions.

- *Occupational therapy*. Occupational therapists (OTs) use work and play activities to improve patients' independent functioning, enhance their development, and prevent or decrease their level of disability. Occupational therapy activities may involve the adaptation of tasks or the environment to achieve maximum independence and to enhance the patient's quality of life and improve his or her activities of daily living (ADL). An occupational therapist may treat developmental deficits, birth defects, learning disabilities, traumatic injuries, burns, neurological conditions, orthopedic conditions, mental deficiencies, and psychiatric disorders. Working under the direction of physicians, occupational therapy is made available in acute-care hospitals, clinics, and rehabilitation centers.
- *Optometry*. Optometry is a health profession that is focused on the eyes and related structures, as well as vision, visual systems, and vision information processing in humans. Optometrists provide treatments such as contact lenses and corrective and low-vision devices and are authorized to use diagnostic and therapeutic pharmaceutical agents to treat anterior segment disease, glaucoma, and ocular hypertension. As primary eye care practitioners, optometrists often are the first ones to detect such potentially serious conditions as diabetes, hypertension, and arteriosclerosis.
- *Pharmacy*. Traditionally the role of a pharmacist was to dispense medications and to provide consultation on the proper selection and use of medications. Prior to 2005, the bachelor's degree was the standard for pharmacists. The current standard is a PharmD, which requires six years of postsecondary education. The scope of practice for a pharmacist is expanding into specialty areas such as pharmacotherapy. Pharmacotherapists work closely with physicians and specialize in drug therapy. Pharmacists take an active role in pharmaceutical care of patients by assisting prescribers in appropriate drug choices, by effecting distribution of medications to patients, and by assuming direct responsibility to collaborate with other healthcare providers and the patient to achieve a desired therapeutic outcome (Shi and Sing 2019).
- *Physical therapy*. Physical therapists (PTs), who work under the direction of a physician, evaluate and treat patients to improve functional mobility, reduce pain, maintain cardiopulmonary function, and limit disability. PTs treat movement dysfunction resulting from accidents, trauma, stroke, fractures, multiple sclerosis, cerebral palsy, arthritis, and heart and respiratory illness. Treatment modalities include therapeutic exercise, therapeutic massage, biofeedback, and applications of heat, low-energy lasers, cold, water, electricity, and ultrasound.
- *Respiratory therapy*. Respiratory therapists (RTs) evaluate, treat, and care for patients with acute or chronic lung disorders. They work under the direction of qualified physicians and provide services such as emergency care for stroke, heart failure, and shock. In addition, they treat patients with emphysema and asthma. Respiratory treatments include the administration of oxygen and inhalants such as bronchodilators and setting up and monitoring ventilator equipment.
- *Speech-language pathology*. Speech-language pathologists and audiologists identify, assess, and provide treatment for individuals with speech, language, or hearing problems.
- *Surgical technologist*. Surgical technologists provide surgical care to patients in a variety

Figure 2.2 Largest occupations in healthcare and the social assistance industry

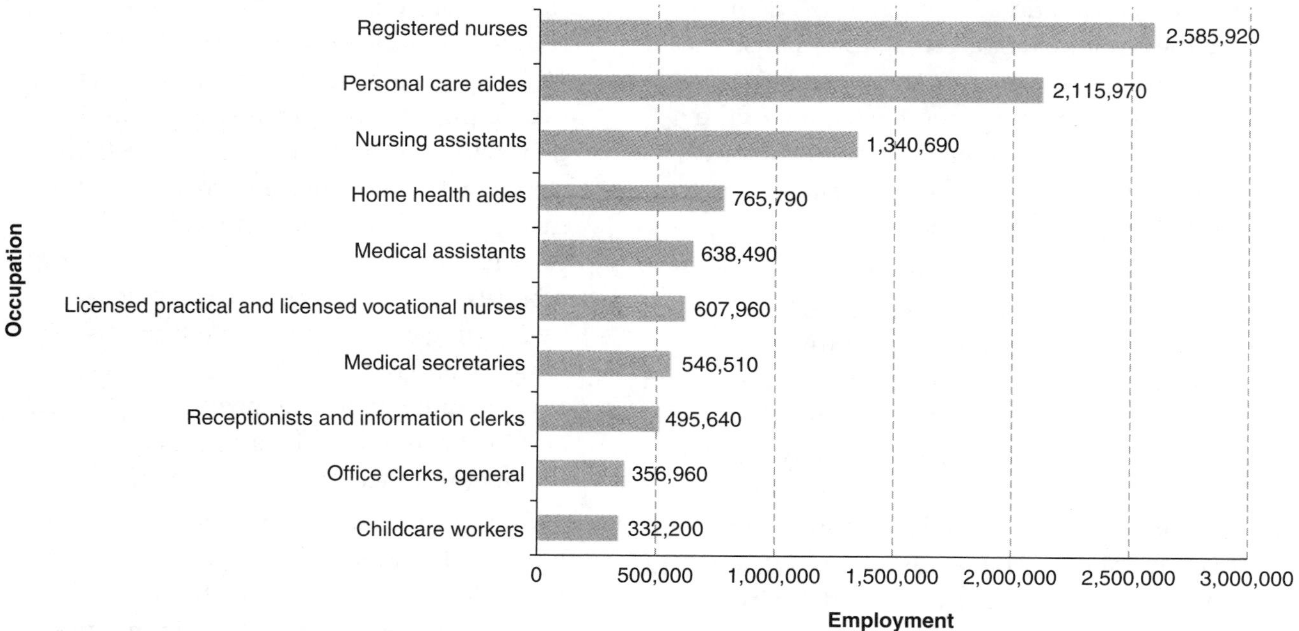

Source: BLS 2017c.

of settings; the majority are hospital operating rooms. Surgical technologists work under medical supervision to facilitate the safe and effective conduct of invasive surgical procedures (Kickman and Kovner 2015).

The occupations in the healthcare industry with the largest number of employees include RNs and personal care aides. Figure 2.2 shows the number of employees by field in healthcare and the social assistance industry.

Check Your Understanding 2.1

Answer the following questions.

1. Which of the following is a physician specializing in the care of inpatient hospital patients?
   a. Hospitalist
   b. Internist
   c. Critical care specialist
   d. Hospice physician
2. Which healthcare professional is licensed to practice medicine with physician supervision?
   a. Diagnostic medical sonographer
   b. Health information manager
   c. Clinical laboratory technician
   d. Physician assistant
3. Which service diagnoses and treats patients who have acute or chronic lung disorders?
   a. Occupational therapy
   b. Physical therapy
   c. Respiratory therapy
   d. Clinical laboratory services

4. Which healthcare provider utilizes ultrasound, computed tomography, or magnetic resonance imaging?
   a. Nuclear medicine technologist
   b. Orthodontist
   c. Podiatrist
   d. Radiologic technologist
5. Which of the following is a surgical specialty?
   a. Internal medicine
   b. Oncology
   c. Neurology
   d. Orthopedics
6. Which of the following statements is true about registered nurses (RNs)?
   a. RNs only provide clinical services within a healthcare entity.
   b. RNs are required to have a license in the state in which they practice.
   c. RNs are graduates of nonacademic training programs.
   d. RNs must have a bachelor's degree from an approved nursing school.
7. Which of the following perform a wide array of tests on body fluids, tissues, and cells to assist in the detection, diagnosis, and treatment of diseases and illnesses?
   a. Clinical laboratory scientists
   b. Sonographers
   c. Licensed practical nurses
   d. Surgical technologists
8. True or false: HIM professionals are responsible for ensuring the availability, accuracy, and protection of clinical information.
9. True or false: Audiologists provide comprehensive diagnostic and treatment and rehabilitative services for auditory, vestibular, and related impairments.
10. True or false: Physical therapists and occupational therapists are the only members of the rehabilitation service team

Organization and Operation of Modern Hospitals

During the 1990s, hospitals in the United States faced growing pressure to contain costs, improve quality, and demonstrate how they contributed to the health of the communities they served. Hospitals responded to these pressures in various ways. Some hospitals merged with other hospitals and healthcare facilities, or they were bought out. Other hospitals created **integrated delivery systems (IDSs)**. These are healthcare systems that combine the financial and clinical aspects of healthcare and use a group of healthcare providers, selected on the basis of quality and cost management criteria, to furnish comprehensive health services across the continuum of care. The IDSs were created to provide a full range of healthcare services along the continuum of care, from ambulatory care to inpatient care to long-term care. The **continuum of care** places an emphasis on treating individual patients at the level of care required by their course of treatment and extends from their primary care providers to specialists and ancillary providers. In 2014, the American Hospital Association released "Your Hospital's Path to the Second Curve: Integration and Transformation." This paper discusses the shift in the healthcare field from the "first curve," where hospitals operate in a volume-based environment to the "second curve" where they build value-based care systems (AHA 2014). Hospitals and care systems need to redesign how care is delivered to eliminate inefficiencies within the system that will lead to better, integrated care, and lower total cost of care. The establishment of IDSs, the greater use of teams, and leveraging the skills and capabilities of all providers in different settings within the IDS is a step towards achieving patient-centered care and the second curve environment.

Others have concentrated on improving the care they provide by focusing on patients as customers. Many hospitals responded to local competition by quickly entering into affiliations and other risk-sharing agreements with acute- and nonacute-care providers, physicians' groups, and **managed care organizations (MCOs)**—a type of healthcare organization that delivers medical care and manages all aspects of patient care or the payment for care by limiting providers of care, discounting payments to providers of care, or limiting access to care.

While most hospitals are integrated into their communities through ties with area physicians and other healthcare providers, clinics and outpatient facilities, and other practitioners, almost half the nation's hospitals also are tied to larger organizational entities such as multihospital and integrated healthcare systems (IHCSs), **integrated delivery networks (IDNs)**, and alliances. An IDN comprises a group of hospitals, physicians, other providers, insurers, or community agencies that work together to deliver health services. In 2015, 55 percent of all hospitals in the US belonged to an IDN (AHA 2015).

By the end of 2010, healthcare organizations faced the challenges of a stressed economy. Hospital reimbursement payments continued to shrink as a result of higher unemployment and more uninsured individuals throughout the nation. At that time, hospitals reached out for opportunities to control costs, streamline operations, implement efficient information technologies, engage in quality initiatives, and pursue joint ventures and consolidation. Today, hospitals are a dominant player in the healthcare system and have a significant impact on the US economy. According to the American Hospital Association (AHA), in 2016 hospitals treated 143 million people in their emergency departments, provided 605 million outpatient visits, performed over 27 million surgeries, and delivered nearly 4 million infants. In addition to providing vital healthcare services, hospitals employ nearly 6 million people and are one of the top sources of private-sector jobs (AHA 2018b). In 2017, healthcare expenditures in the United States were approximately \$3.5 trillion, which represented 17.9 percent of the total American economy (CMS 2018a). According to Centers for Medicare and Medicaid Services (CMS) projections, national health spending is projected to grow an average rate of 5.5 percent each year and reach \$5.7 trillion by 2026 (CMS 2018b). Figure 2.3 shows the national health expenditures in 2017 were \$3.5 trillion dollars, with 45 percent going toward hospital care.

The term **hospital** can be applied to any healthcare facility that does the following:

- Has an organized medical staff
- Provides permanent inpatient beds
- Offers around-the-clock nursing services
- Provides diagnostic and therapeutic services

Most hospitals provide acute-care services to inpatients. Acute care is the short-term care provided to diagnose or treat an illness or injury. The individuals who receive acute-care services in hospitals are considered inpatients. Inpatients receive room-and-board services in addition to continuous nursing services. Generally, patients who spend more than 24 hours in a hospital are considered inpatients.

Hospitals that have an **average length of stay (ALOS)** of 25 days or less are considered acute-care

Figure 2.3 National health expenditures in 2017

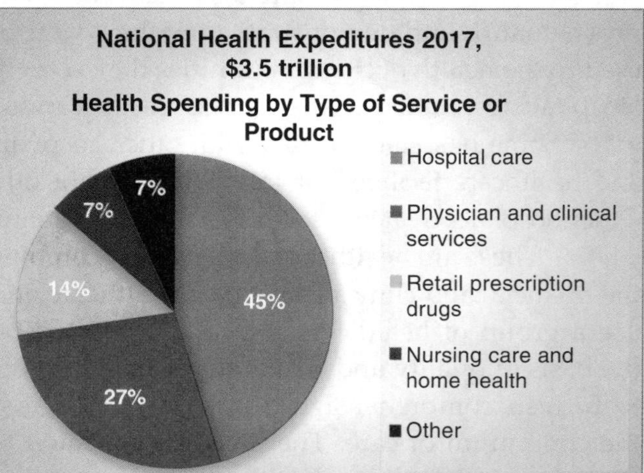

Source: Adapted from CMS 2018a.

hospitals. Hospitals that have ALOSs longer than 25 days are considered long-term acute-care facilities. Long-term care is discussed in detail later in this chapter. The ALOS is the mean length of stay for hospital inpatients discharged during a given period of time. With recent advances in surgical technology, anesthesia, and pharmacology, the ALOS in an acute-care hospital is much shorter today than it was only a few years ago. In addition, many diagnostic and therapeutic procedures that once required inpatient care now can be performed on an outpatient basis.

For example, before the development of laparoscopic surgical techniques, a patient might be hospitalized for 10 days after a routine appendectomy (surgical removal of the appendix). Today, a patient undergoing a laparoscopic appendectomy might spend only a few hours in the hospital's outpatient surgery department and go home the same day. The influence of managed care and the emphasis on cost control in the Medicare or Medicaid programs also have resulted in shorter hospital stays. More information on healthcare statistics can be found in chapter 14, *Healthcare Statistics*.

In large acute-care hospitals, hundreds of clinicians, administrators, managers, and support staff must work closely to provide effective and efficient diagnostic and therapeutic services. Most hospitals provide services to both inpatients and outpatients. A hospital outpatient is a patient who receives hospital services without being admitted for inpatient (overnight) hospital care. Outpatient care is considered ambulatory care. (Ambulatory care is discussed later in this chapter.)

Types of Hospitals

There are many types of hospitals providing care within the US healthcare system. The five major criteria used to classify hospital types are the following:

1. Functionality
2. Location
3. Number of beds
4. Specialization
5. Types of ownership

Functionality

This refers to how the hospitals function within the communities they serve. They could be general, teaching, acute care, long term, community, and research or trauma centers.

Location

Hospitals can be classified by their location. Rural hospitals may have limited access to advanced equipment or specialized procedures. Urban hospitals serve larger metropolitan areas and often offer a wide degree of versatility when it comes to treatment options.

Number of Beds

A hospital's number of beds refers to the beds that are equipped and staffed for patient care. The term *bed capacity* sometimes is used to reflect the maximum number of inpatients for which the hospital can care. *Licensed beds* are the number of beds that the state has authorized the hospital to have available for patients and *staffed beds* refers to the number of beds for which the hospital has nursing staff to cover patient treatment. A hospital is usually considered small if it has fewer than 100 beds. Most US hospitals fall into this category. Some large, urban hospitals may have more than 500 beds. The number of beds is usually broken down by adult and pediatric beds. The number of maternity beds and other special categories may be listed separately. Hospitals also can be categorized according to the number of outpatient visits per year.

Specialization

A hospital may specialize in certain types of services and treatment of specific illnesses. The following are examples:

- *Rehabilitation hospitals* generally provide long-term care services to patients recuperating from debilitating or chronic illnesses and injuries such as strokes, head and spine injuries, and gunshot wounds. Patients often stay in rehabilitation hospitals for several months.
- *Psychiatric hospitals* provide inpatient care for patients with mental and developmental

disorders. In the past, the ALOS for psychiatric inpatients was longer than it is today. Rather than months or years, most patients now spend only a few days or weeks per stay. However, many patients require repeated hospitalization for chronic psychiatric illnesses.

- *General hospitals* provide a wide range of medical and surgical services to diagnose and treat most illnesses and injuries.
- *Specialty hospitals* provide diagnostic and therapeutic services for a limited range of conditions such as burns, cancer, tuberculosis, obstetrics, or gynecology.
- *Long-term acute-care hospitals (LTACHs)* specialize in the treatment of patients with serious medical conditions that require care on an ongoing basis. These patients do not require intensive care or extensive diagnostic procedures but require more care than they can receive in a rehabilitation center, skilled nursing facility, or home.

Types of Ownership

The most common ownership types for hospitals and other kinds of healthcare organizations in the United States include the following:

- *Government-owned hospitals* which are operated by a specific branch of federal, state, or local government as not-for-profit organizations. (Government-owned hospitals sometimes are called public hospitals.) They are supported, at least in part, by tax dollars. Examples of federally owned and operated hospitals include those operated by the Department of Veterans Affairs (VA) to serve retired military personnel. The Department of Defense operates facilities for active military personnel and their dependents. Many states own and operate psychiatric hospitals. County and city governments often operate public (municipal) hospitals to serve the healthcare needs of their communities, especially those residents who are unable to pay for their care.
- *Proprietary hospitals* may be owned by private foundations, partnerships, or investor-owned corporations. Large corporations may own a number of for-profit hospitals, and the stocks of several large US hospital chains are traded publicly.
- *Voluntary hospitals* are not-for-profit hospitals owned by universities, churches, charities, religious orders, unions, and other not-for-profit entities. They often provide free care to patients who otherwise would not have access to healthcare services.

Hospitals also can be classified based on their ownership and profitability status. Not-for-profit healthcare facilities use excess funds to improve their services and to finance educational programs and community services. For-profit healthcare organizations are privately owned. Excess funds are paid back to the managers, owners, and investors in the form of bonuses and dividends.

Safety Net Hospitals

A safety net hospital (SNH) is defined as a hospital with the highest number of inpatient stays paid by Medicaid. Uninsured safety net organizations play a major role in providing services to medically and socially vulnerable populations. When compared with non-SNHs, SNHs are more likely to be teaching hospitals, have a large number of inpatient beds, and just over 27 percent are located in large central metropolitan areas (Sutton et al. 2016).

Critical Access Hospitals

As part of the Balanced Budget Act of 1997 (discussed later in this chapter), CMS was authorized to allow certain healthcare organizations the designation of critical access hospital (CAH). By meeting certain requirements these hospitals are allowed a separate payment system that allows reimbursement for Medicare patients at 101 percent of reasonable costs and are not subject to the inpatient prospective payment system (IPPS) or the hospital outpatient prospective payment system (OPPS). The criteria to qualify as a CAH are as follows (see chapter 15, *Revenue Management and Reimbursement* for more details on IPPS and OPPS):

- Be located in a state that accepted a grant under the Medicare Rural Hospital Flexibility Program, which helps states to strengthen their rural healthcare infrastructure
- Be located in a rural area
- Furnish 24-hour emergency care services 7 days a week
- Maintain no more than 25 inpatient beds that may also be used as swing beds (hospital beds that can be either acute-care or skilled nursing facility beds)
- Have an annual length of stay of 96 hours or less per patient for acute-care services
- Be located more than a 35-mile distance from any other hospital
- Be certified as a CAH prior to January 1, 2006 (CMS 2014)

Organization of Hospital Services

The organizational structure of every hospital is designed to meet its specific needs. For example, most acute-care hospitals are comprised of a professional medical staff and hospital administrative services, which include an executive administrative staff, medical and surgical services, patient care (nursing) services, diagnostic and laboratory services, and support services (for example, nutritional services, environmental safety, and HIM services). Hospitals are overseen by a board of directors.

Board of Directors

The board of directors (also known as the governing board or board of trustees) has primary responsibility for setting the overall direction of the hospital. The board works with the chief executive officer (CEO) and the leaders of the organization's medical staff to develop the hospital's strategic direction as well as its mission (statement of the hospital's purpose and the customers it serves), vision (description of the hospital's ideal future), and values (descriptive list of the organization's fundamental principles or beliefs). Chapter 17, *Management*, covers mission, vision, and values in more detail.

The board of directors' other responsibilities include the following:

- Establishing bylaws in accordance with the organization's legal and licensing requirements
- Selecting qualified administrators
- Approving the organization and makeup of the clinical staff
- Monitoring the quality of care

Board members are elected or appointed to serve a specific term (for example, five years). Boards may elect officers, commonly a chairman, vice-chairman, president, secretary, and treasurer. The size of the board varies. Individual board members are called directors, board members, or trustees. Individuals serve on one or more standing committees such as the executive committee, joint conference committee, finance committee, strategic planning committee, and building committee.

The makeup of the board depends on the type of hospital and the form of ownership. For example, the board of a community hospital is likely to include local business leaders, representatives of community organizations, and other people interested in the welfare of the community. The board of a teaching hospital, on the other hand, is likely to include medical school alumni and university administrators, among others.

Increased competition among healthcare providers and limits on managed care and Medicare or Medicaid reimbursement have made the governing of hospitals especially difficult in the past two decades. In the future, boards of directors will continue to face strict accountability in terms of cost containment, performance management, and integration of services to maintain fiscal stability and to ensure the delivery of high-quality patient care.

Medical Staff

The medical staff consists of physicians who have received extensive training in various medical disciplines (internal medicine, pediatrics, cardiology, gynecology and obstetrics, orthopedics, surgery, and so on). The medical staff's primary objective is to provide high-quality patient care to the patients who come to the hospital. The physicians on the hospital's medical staff diagnose illnesses and develop patient-centered treatment regimens. Moreover, they may serve on the hospital's governing board, where they provide critical insight relevant to strategic and operational planning and policy making.

The medical staff is the aggregate of physicians who have been granted permission to provide clinical services in the hospital. This permission is called clinical privileges. An individual physician's privileges are limited to a specific scope of practice. For example, an internal medicine physician would be permitted to diagnose and treat a patient with pneumonia, but not to perform a surgical procedure. Traditionally, most members of the medical staff have not been employees of the hospital, although this is changing as many hospitals are purchasing physician practices.

Medical staff classification refers to the organization of physicians according to clinical assignment. Depending on the size of the hospital and on the credentials and clinical privileges of its physicians, the medical staff may be separated into departments such as medicine, surgery, obstetrics, pediatrics, and other specialty services. Typical medical staff classifications include active, provisional, honorary, consulting, courtesy, and medical resident assignments.

Officers of the medical staff usually include a president or chief of staff, a vice president or chief of staff elect, and a secretary. These officers are authorized by a vote of the entire active medical staff. The president presides over all regular meetings of the medical staff and is an ex officio member of all medical staff committees. The secretary keeps the minutes from the meetings and ensures they are accurate and complete. The secretary also handles correspondence appropriately.

The medical staff operates according to a predetermined set of policies called the medical staff bylaws. The bylaws state the specific qualifications a physician must demonstrate before he or she can practice medicine in the hospital. The bylaws are considered legally binding. The medical staff and the hospital's governing body must vote to approve any changes to the bylaws.

Administrative Staff

The CEO or chief administrator is the leader of the administrative staff. The CEO implements the policies and strategic direction set by the hospital's board of directors. The CEO is also responsible for building an effective executive management team and coordinating the hospital's services. Today, healthcare organizations commonly designate the following roles as the executive management team: chief financial officer (CFO), the senior manager responsible for the fiscal management of an organization; a chief operating officer (COO), the executive responsible for high-level, day-to-day operations; and a chief information officer (CIO), the senior manager responsible for the management of the information resources.

The executive management team is responsible for managing the hospital's finances and ensuring the hospital complies with the federal, state, and local rules, standards, and laws that govern the delivery of healthcare services. Depending on the size of the hospital, the CEO's staff may include healthcare administrators with job titles such as vice president, associate administrator, department director or manager, or administrative assistant. Department-level administrators manage and coordinate the activities of the highly specialized and multidisciplinary units that perform clinical, administrative, and support services in the hospital.

Healthcare administrators may hold advanced degrees in healthcare administration, nursing, public health, or business management. A growing number of hospitals are hiring physician executives to lead their executive management teams.

Patient Care Services

Most direct patient care delivered in hospitals is provided by professional nurses. Modern nursing requires a diverse skill set, advanced clinical competencies, and postgraduate education. In almost every hospital, patient care services constitute the largest clinical department in terms of staffing, budget, specialized services offered, and clinical expertise required.

Nurses are responsible for providing continuous, around-the-clock treatment and support for hospital inpatients. The quantity and quality of nursing care available to patients is influenced by a number of factors, including the nursing staff's educational preparation and specialization, experience, and skill level. The level of patient care staffing also is a critical component of quality.

Traditionally, physicians alone determined the type of treatment each patient would receive. However, today's nurses are playing a wider role in treatment planning and **case management**. They perform an ongoing, concurrent review to ensure the necessity and effectiveness of the clinical services being provided to patients. Their responsibilities include performing patient assessments, creating care plans, evaluating the appropriateness of treatment, and evaluating the effectiveness of care. At the same time, they provide technical care and offer personal care that recognizes the concerns and emotional needs of patients and their families.

An RN who is qualified by advanced education and clinical and management experience usually administers patient care services. Although the title may vary, this role is usually referred to as the **chief nursing officer (CNO)** or vice president of nursing or patient care. The CNO is a member of the hospital's executive management team and usually reports directly to the CEO.

Diagnostic Services

The services provided to patients in hospitals go beyond the clinical services provided directly by the medical and nursing staff. Many diagnostic and therapeutic services involve the work of allied health professionals. Allied health professionals receive specialized education and training, and their qualifications are registered or certified by a number of specialty organizations.

Diagnostic and therapeutic services are critical to the success of every patient care delivery system. Diagnostic services include clinical laboratory, radiology, and nuclear medicine. Therapeutic services include clinical laboratory services, radiology, and radiation therapy.

Rehabilitation Services

Rehabilitation services are dedicated to eliminating the patient's disability or alleviating it as fully as possible. The goal is to improve the cognitive, social, and physical abilities of patients impaired by chronic disease or injury. Rehabilitation services can be provided within the acute-care setting or in specialty hospitals dedicated to providing many forms of rehabilitation to patients to facilitate their return to work or home. The rehabilitation team may include physicians, nurses, occupational therapists, physical therapists, respiratory therapists, speech therapists, social workers, and other healthcare personnel.

Ancillary Support Services

The ancillary units of the hospital provide vital clinical and administrative support services to patients, medical staff, visitors, and employees.

The clinical support units provide the following services:

- Pharmaceutical services (provided by registered pharmacists and pharmacy technologists)
- Food and nutrition services (managed by registered dietitians who develop general and special-diet menus and nutritional plans for individual patients)
- Health information services (managed by RHIAs and RHITs)
- Social work and social services (provided by licensed social workers and licensed clinical social workers)
- Patient advocacy services (provided by several types of healthcare professionals, most commonly registered nurses and licensed social workers)
- Environmental (housekeeping) services
- Purchasing, central supply, and materials management services
- Engineering and plant operations (maintenance)

In addition to clinical support services, hospitals need administrative support services to operate effectively. Administrative support services

Figure 2.4 Hospital structure – example organizational chart

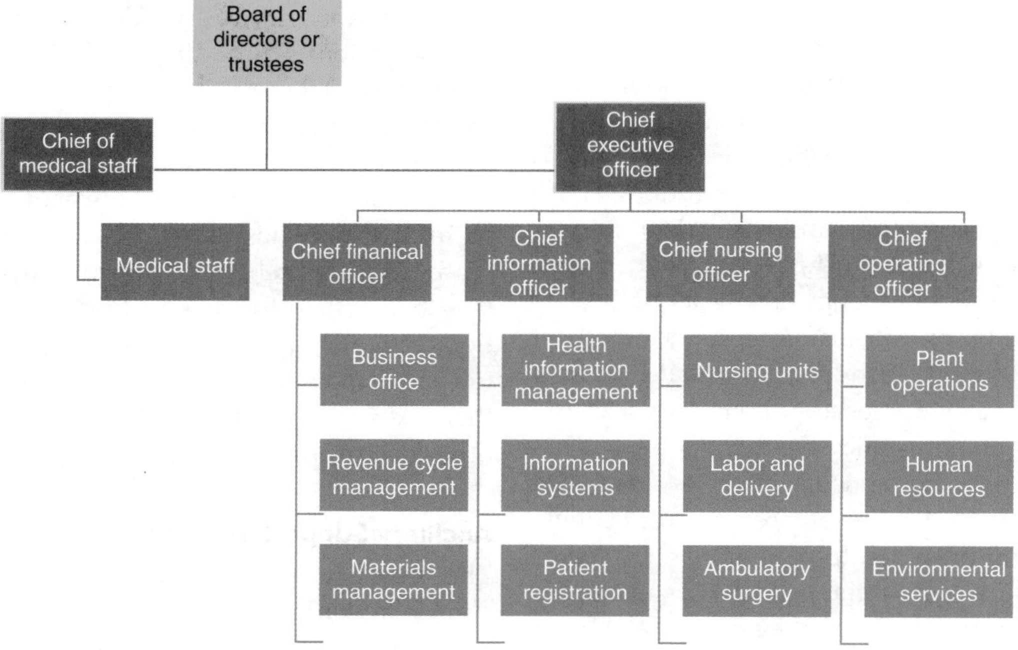

Source: ©AHIMA.

provide business management and clerical services in several key areas, including the following:

- Admissions and central registration
- Claims and billing (business office)
- Accounting
- Information services
- Human resources
- Public relations
- Fund development
- Marketing

Figure 2.4 is an example of a healthcare organizational chart showing the reporting structure for departments within the organization. The board of directors has the ultimate responsibility for the organization.

Check Your Understanding 2.2

Answer the following questions.

1. The emphasis on treating individual patients at the level of care required by their treatment across all healthcare services refers to:
   a. Managed care
   b. Continuum of care
   c. Primary care
   d. Palliative care
2. Who has the primary responsibility to guide the direction of the hospital?
   a. Board of directors
   b. Chief executive officer
   c. Medical staff
   d. Chief operating officer

3. Which of the following is an example of a federally run hospital?
   a. Veterans Administration
   b. Psychiatric
   c. Not-for-profit
   d. Community
4. This type of hospital has the majority of its inpatient visits paid for through Medicaid.
   a. Safety net hospital
   b. Critical access hospital
   c. Proprietary hospital
   d. General hospital
5. Dr. Smith has been granted permission by community hospital to perform cardiac catheterizations. This permission is called:
   a. Clinical privileges
   b. Clinical assignment
   c. Clinical classification
   d. Case management
6. True or false: Acute-care hospitals provide short-term care to diagnose or treat an illness.
7. True or false: Case management is the ongoing, concurrent review to ensure the necessity and effectiveness of clinical services provided to patients.
8. True or false: Pharmaceutical services are considered part of the clinical support services.
9. True or false: Critical access hospitals specialize in the treatment of patients with serious medical conditions that require care on an ongoing basis.

Other Types of Healthcare Services

Healthcare delivery is more than hospital-related care. It can be viewed as a continuum of services that cuts across care settings, including ambulatory, acute, subacute, long-term, and residential care, among others.

Managed Care Organizations

Managed care is a generic term for a healthcare reimbursement system that manages cost, quality, and access to services. Most managed care plans do not provide healthcare directly. Instead, they enter into service contracts with the physicians, hospitals, and other healthcare providers who provide medical services to enrollees in the plans.

Managed care systems control costs primarily by presetting payment amounts and restricting patient access to healthcare services through precertification and utilization review processes. (Managed care is discussed in more detail in chapter 15, *Revenue Management and Reimbursement*.)

Managed care delivery systems also attempt to manage cost and quality by doing the following:

- Implementing various forms of financial incentives for providers
- Promoting healthy lifestyles
- Identifying risk factors and illnesses early in the disease process
- Providing patient education

There are three basic types of managed care plans. The following are the three types of managed care plans:

1. Health maintenance organizations (HMOs), which provide healthcare within a closed network
2. Preferred provider organizations (PPOs), which provide reduced costs if the plan member stays within the network but will contribute at a reduced cost if the member goes outside the network

3. Point of service (POS), which allows patients to choose between an HMO or PPO each time they have a medical encounter (NIH 2015).

Accountable Care Organizations

The Patient Protection and Affordable Care Act of 2010 has had a significant impact on physicians and hospitals, namely in the establishment of accountable care organizations (ACOs). An ACO generally describes groups of providers who are willing and able to take responsibility for improving the overall health status, care efficiency, and healthcare experience for a defined population (DeVore and Champion 2011). The law allows CMS to create ACOs by developing voluntary partnerships between hospitals and physicians to coordinate and deliver quality care to patients and allow the participating organizations to share the savings that would result from improvement of care for those Medicare populations. CMS has established three primary ACO programs whereby participating ACOs would assume the accountability for improving quality care while reducing costs for a defined Medicare patient population. The beneficiaries will be assigned to the ACO based on utilization of primary care services provided by primary care physicians. The following are the three ACO models:

1. Medicare Shared Savings program that gives Medicare fee-for-service providers an opportunity to become an ACO
2. Advance Payment ACO model designed as a supplementary incentive program for selected participants
3. Pioneer ACO model created for early adopters of coordinate care, though CMS is no longer accepting applications for this model

CMS has outlined a series of 33 quality measures in four categories (patient or caregiver experience; care coordination or patient safety; preventative health; and at-risk population) to assess the quality of care furnished by the ACO (RTI International 2015). As of 2018, there are 561 ACOs with 10.5 million beneficiaries (CMS 2018c).

Ambulatory Care

Ambulatory care is defined as the preventive or corrective healthcare provided in a practitioner's office, a clinic, or a hospital on a nonresident (outpatient) basis. The term usually implies that patients go to locations outside their homes to obtain healthcare services and return the same day.

Ambulatory care encompasses all the health services provided to individual patients who are not residents in a healthcare facility. Such services include the educational services provided by community health clinics and public health departments. Primary care, emergency care, and ambulatory specialty care (which includes ambulatory surgery) all may be considered ambulatory care. Ambulatory care services are provided in a variety of settings, including urgent care centers, school-based clinics, public health clinics, and neighborhood and community health centers.

Current medical practice emphasizes performing healthcare services in the least costly setting possible. This change in thinking has led to decreased utilization of emergency services, increased utilization of nonemergency ambulatory facilities, decreased hospital admissions, and shorter hospital stays. The need to reduce the cost of healthcare also has led primary care physicians to treat conditions they once would have referred to specialists.

Physicians who provide ambulatory care services fall into two categories—physicians working in private practice and physicians working for ambulatory care organizations. Physicians in private practice are self-employed. They may work solo, in partnership, and in group practices set up as for-profit organizations.

Alternatively, physicians who work for ambulatory care organizations are employees of those organizations. Ambulatory care organizations include HMOs, hospital-based ambulatory clinics, walk-in and emergency clinics, hospital-owned group practices and health promotion centers, freestanding surgery centers, freestanding urgent care centers, freestanding emergency care centers, health department clinics, neighborhood clinics, home care agencies, community mental health centers, school and workplace health services, and prison health services.

Ambulatory care organizations also employ other healthcare providers, including nurses, laboratory technicians, podiatrists, chiropractors, physical therapists, radiology technicians, psychologists, and social workers.

Private Medical Practice

Private medical practices are physician-owned entities that provide primary care or medical or surgical specialty care services in a freestanding office setting. The physicians have medical privileges at local hospitals and surgical centers but are not employees of the other healthcare entities.

Medical Home

The medical home is a model of primary care physician practices that is patient-centered, comprehensive, team-based, coordinated, accessible, and focused on quality and safety. This has become a model for how primary care should be delivered. It is sometimes referred to as a patient-centered medical home (PCPCC 2019). Many hospitals have established medical home programs to provide the patient with a direct relationship with the provider responsible for providing their care. Between 2012 and 2016, the percentage of hospitals with a medical home grew from 18 percent to 28 percent (AHA 2018).

Hospital-Based Ambulatory Care Services

In addition to providing inpatient services, many acute-care hospitals provide various ambulatory care services such as the following.

Emergency Services and Trauma Care More than 90 percent of community hospitals in the US provide emergency services. Hospital-based emergency departments provide specialized care for victims of traumatic accidents and life-threatening illnesses. In urban areas, many also provide walk-in services for patients with minor illnesses and injuries who do not have access to regular primary care physicians.

Many physicians on the hospital staff also use the emergency care department as a setting to assess patients with problems that may either lead to an inpatient admission or require equipment or diagnostic imaging facilities not available in a private office or nursing home. Emergency services function as a major source of unscheduled admissions to the hospital.

Outpatient Surgical Services Generally, the term *ambulatory surgery* refers to any surgical procedure that does not require an overnight stay in a hospital. It can be performed in the outpatient surgery department of a hospital and in a freestanding ambulatory surgery center.

Outpatient Diagnostic and Therapeutic Services Outpatient diagnostic and therapeutic services are provided in a hospital or one of its satellite facilities. Diagnostic services are those services performed by a physician to identify the disease or condition from which the patient is suffering. Therapeutic services are those services performed by a physician to treat the disease or condition that has been identified.

Hospital outpatients fall into different classifications according to the types of services they receive and the location of the service. For example, emergency outpatients are treated in the hospital's emergency or trauma care department for conditions that require immediate care. Clinic outpatients are treated in one of the hospital's clinical departments on an ambulatory basis. Referral outpatients receive special diagnostic or therapeutic services in the hospital on an ambulatory basis, but responsibility for their care remains with the referring physician.

Observation Services An observation patient visit is a type of outpatient visit. While they may be in the same units as inpatients, they are considered an outpatient visit. Observation services are used when physicians need to determine if the patient is sick enough to need inpatient treatment.

Community-Based Ambulatory Care Services

Community-based ambulatory care services are those services provided in freestanding facilities that are not owned by or affiliated with a hospital.

Such facilities can range in size from a small medical practice with a single physician to a large clinic with an organized medical staff.

Among the organizations that provide ambulatory care services are specialized treatment facilities. Examples of these community-based ambulatory care services facilities include birthing centers, cancer treatment centers, renal dialysis centers, and rehabilitation centers.

Freestanding Ambulatory Care Centers Freestanding ambulatory care centers provide emergency services and urgent care for walk-in patients. Urgent care centers provide diagnostic and therapeutic care for patients with minor illnesses and injuries. They do not serve seriously ill patients, and most do not accept patients arriving by ambulance.

Two groups of patients find these centers attractive. The first group consists of patients seeking the convenience and access of emergency services without the delays and high costs associated with using hospital services for nonurgent problems. The second group consists of patients whose insurance treats urgent care centers preferentially compared with physicians' offices.

As they have increased in number and become familiar to more patients, many freestanding ambulatory care centers now offer a combination of walk-in and appointment services.

Freestanding Ambulatory Surgery Centers Freestanding ambulatory surgery centers generally provide surgical procedures that take anywhere from 5 to 90 minutes to perform and require less than a four-hour recovery period. Patients must schedule their surgeries in advance and be prepared to return home on the same day. Patients who experience surgical complications are sent to an inpatient facility for care.

Most ambulatory surgery centers are for-profit entities. Individual physicians, MCOs, or entrepreneurs may own them. Generally, ambulatory care centers can provide surgical services at lower cost than hospitals can because their overhead expenses are lower.

Public Health Services

The states have constitutional authority to implement public health measures, and many of them are assisted by a wide variety of federal programs and laws. The Department of Health and Human Services (HHS) is the principal federal agency that ensures health and provides essential human services. HHS has eleven operating divisions, including eight agencies in the US Public Health Services and three human services agencies. These operating divisions are responsible for a wide variety of health and human services, including prevention and conducting research for the nation. HHS coordinates closely with state and local government agencies and many HHS-funded services are provided by these agencies as well as by private-sector and nonprofit organizations.

Two units in the Office of the Secretary of HHS are important to public health—the Office of the Surgeon General of the United States and the Office of Disease Prevention and Health Promotion (ODPHP). The surgeon general is appointed by the president of the United States and provides leadership and authoritative, science-based recommendations about the public's health. He or she has responsibility for the public health service (PHS) workforce and the ODPHP provides an analysis and leadership role for health promotion and disease prevention. Figure 2.5 shows the agencies that exist within HHS.

Home Healthcare Services

Home healthcare is the fastest-growing sector to offer services for recipients. Home healthcare is limited part-time or intermittent skilled nursing care and home health aide services, physical therapy, occupational therapy, speech-language therapy, medical social services, durable medical equipment, supplies and other services (CMS 2017a). The primary reason for this is increased economic pressure from third-party payers who want patients released from the hospital more quickly than they were in the past. Moreover, patients generally prefer to be cared for in their own homes. In fact, most patients prefer home care, no matter how complex their medical problems.

In 1989, Medicare rules for home care services were clarified to make it easier for Medicare beneficiaries to receive them. Patients are eligible to receive home health services from a qualified Medicare provider when they are homebound, under the care of a specified physician who will

Figure 2.5 Department of Health and Human Services agencies

Administration for Children and Families (ACF)	ACF promotes the economic and social well-being of families, children, individuals, and communities.
Administration for Community Living (ACL)	ACL increases access to community support and resources for the unique needs of older Americans and people with disabilities.
Agency for Healthcare Research and Quality (AHRQ)	AHRQ's mission is to produce evidence to make healthcare safer, higher quality, more accessible, equitable, and affordable, and to work within HHS and with other partners to make sure that the evidence is understood and used.
Agency for Toxic Substances and Disease Registry (ATSDR)	ATSDR prevents exposure to toxic substances and the adverse health effects and diminished quality of life associated with exposure to hazardous substances from waste sites, unplanned releases, and other sources of environmental pollution.
Centers for Disease Control and Prevention (CDC)	CDC, part of the US Public Health Service (PHS) protects the public health of the nation by providing leadership and direction in the prevention and control of diseases and other preventable conditions, and responding to public health emergencies.
Centers for Medicare & Medicaid Services (CMS)	CMS combines the oversight of the Medicare program, the federal portion of the Medicaid program and State Children's Health Insurance Program, the Health Insurance Marketplace, and related quality assurance activities.
Food and Drug Administration (FDA)	FDA, part of the PHS ensures food is safe, pure, and wholesome; human and animal drugs, biological products, and medical devices are safe and effective; and electronic products that emit radiation are safe.
Health Resources and Services Administration (HRSA)	HRSA, part of the PHS provides healthcare to people who are geographically isolated or economically or medically vulnerable.
Indian Health Service (IHS)	IHS, part of the PHS provides American Indians and Alaskan Natives with comprehensive health services by developing and managing programs to meet their health needs.
National Institutes of Health (NIH)	NIH, part of the PHS, supports biomedical and behavioral research within the US and abroad, conducts research in its own laboratories and clinics, trains promising young researchers, and promotes collecting and sharing medical knowledge.
Substance Abuse and Mental Health Services Administration (SAMHSA)	SAMHSA, part of the PHS, improves access and reduces barriers to high-quality, effective programs and services for individuals who suffer from or are at risk for addictive and mental disorders, as well as for their families and communities.

Source: Adapted from HHS 2019.

establish a home health plan, and when they need physical or occupational therapy, speech therapy, or intermittent skilled nursing care.

Skilled nursing care is defined as technical procedures, such as tube feedings and catheter care, and skilled nursing observations. *Intermittent* is defined as up to 28 hours per week for nursing care and 35 hours per week for home health aide care. Many hospitals have formed their own home healthcare agencies to increase revenues and at the same time to enable them to discharge patients from the hospital earlier.

Voluntary Agencies

Voluntary agencies provide healthcare and healthcare planning services, usually at the local level and to low-income patients. Their services range from giving free immunizations to offering family planning counseling. Funds to operate such agencies come from a variety of sources, including local or state health departments, private grants, and funds from different federal bureaus.

One common example of a voluntary agency is the community health center. Sometimes called neighborhood health centers, community health centers offer comprehensive, primary healthcare services to patients who otherwise would not have access to them. Often patients pay for these services on a sliding scale based on income or according to a flat rate, discounted fee schedule supplemented by public funding.

Some voluntary agencies offer specialized services such as counseling for battered and abused women. Typically, these are set up within local communities. An example of a voluntary agency that offers services on a much larger scale is the Red Cross.

Subacute Care

Patients needing ongoing rehabilitative care or treatment using advanced technology sometimes are eligible to receive subacute care. Subacute care offers patients access to constant nursing care while recovering at home. In the past, patients could receive comprehensive rehabilitative care only while in the hospital. Today, however, the availability of subacute-care services allows patients to optimize their functional gain in a familiar and more comfortable environment. In essence, subacute care in most IDNs emphasizes patient independence. The patient is given an individualized care plan developed by a highly trained team of healthcare professionals. Patients considered appropriate for subacute care are those recovering from stroke, cardiac surgery, serious injury, amputation, joint replacement, or chronic wounds.

Long-Term Care

In general, long-term care is the healthcare rendered in a non-acute-care facility to patients who require inpatient nursing and related services for more than 30 consecutive days. Skilled nursing facilities, nursing homes, and rehabilitation hospitals are the principal facilities that provide long-term care. Rehabilitation hospitals provide recuperative services for patients who have suffered strokes and traumatic injuries as well as other serious illnesses. Specialized long-term care facilities serve patients with chronic respiratory disease, permanent cognitive impairment, and other incapacitating conditions.

Long-term care encompasses a range of health, personal care, social, and housing services provided to people of all ages with health conditions that limit their ability to carry out normal daily activities without assistance. People who need long-term care have many different types of physical and mental disabilities. Moreover, their need for the mix and intensity of long-term care services can change over time.

Long-term care is mainly rehabilitative and supportive rather than curative. Moreover, healthcare workers other than physicians can provide long-term care in the home or in residential or institutional settings.

Long-Term Care in the Continuum of Care

The availability of long-term care is one of the most important health issues in the United States today. There are two principal reasons for this. First, people are living longer today than they did in the past as a result of advances in medicine and healthcare practices. The number of people who survive previously fatal conditions is growing, and more and more people with chronic medical problems can live reasonably normal lives. Second, there was an explosion in the birthrate after World War II. Children born during that period (1946 to 1964), the "baby-boomer" generation, are today in their late 1950s to 1970s. These factors combined mean that the need for long-term care will only increase in the years to come.

As discussed earlier, healthcare is now viewed as a continuum of care. In the case of long-term care, the patient's continuum of care may have begun with a primary provider in a hospital and then continued with home care and eventually care in a skilled nursing facility. The patient's care is coordinated from one care setting to the next.

Moreover, the roles of the different care providers along the patient's continuum of care are continuing to evolve. Health information managers play a key part in providing consultation services to long-term care facilities with regard to developing systems to manage information from a diverse number of healthcare providers.

Delivery of Long-Term Care Services

Long-term care services are delivered in a variety of settings, including skilled nursing facilities or nursing homes, residential care facilities, hospice programs, and adult day-care programs.

Skilled Nursing Facilities or Nursing Homes The most important providers of formal, long-term care services are nursing homes, or skilled nursing facilities (SNFs), which provide medical, nursing, or rehabilitative care, in some cases, around the clock. Most SNFs have residents over the age 65 and provide care for those who can no longer live independently.

Many SNFs are owned by for-profit organizations. However, SNFs also may be owned by not-for-profit groups as well as local, state, and federal governments. In recent years, there has been a decline in the total number of nursing homes in the US, but an increase in the number of nursing home beds.

Nursing homes are no longer the only option for patients needing long-term care. Various factors play a role in determining which type of long-term care facility is best for a particular patient, including cost, access to services, and individual needs.

Residential Care Facilities New living environments that are more homelike and less institutional are the focus of much attention in the current long-term care market. Residential care facilities now play a growing role in the continuum of long-term care services. Having affordable and appropriate housing available for elderly and disabled people can reduce the level of need for institutional long-term care services in the community. Institutionalization can be postponed or prevented when the elderly and disabled live in safe, accessible settings where assistance with daily activities is available.

Hospice Programs Hospice care is provided mainly in the home to patients who are diagnosed with a terminal illness with a limited life expectancy of six months or less. **Hospice** is based on a philosophy of palliative care imported from England and Canada that holds that during the course of terminal illness, the patient should be able to live life as fully and as comfortably as possible, but without artificial or mechanical efforts to prolong life. Hospice care is not focused on cure. It is palliative; focusing on pain relief, comfort, and enhanced quality of life for the terminally ill.

In the hospice approach, the family is the unit of treatment. An interdisciplinary team provides medical, nursing, psychological, therapeutic, pharmacological, and spiritual support during the final stages of illness, at the time of death, and during bereavement. The main goals are to control pain, maintain independence, and minimize the stress and trauma of death.

Hospice services have gained acceptance as an alternative to hospital care for the terminally ill. The number of hospices is likely to continue to grow because this philosophy of care for people at the end of life has become a model for the nation.

Adult Day-Care Programs Adult day-care programs offer a wide range of health and social services to elderly persons during the daytime hours. Adult day-care services are usually targeted to elderly members of families in which the regular caregivers work during the day. Many elderly people who live alone also benefit from leaving their homes every day to participate in programs designed to keep them active. The goals of adult day-care programs are to delay the need for institutionalization and to provide respite for caregivers.

Data on adult day-care programs are still limited, but there were about 5,000 programs in 2015 providing services to 260,000 participants in a variety of programs (NADSA 2019).

Biomedical and Technological Advances in Medicine

Advances in technology in the healthcare industry have made it possible for care to be delivered to patients closer to their home or even in their home. The sections that follow will explore and describe the benefits of telehealth technologies and electronic health records and health data and the effects they have made on the delivery of healthcare.

Telehealth

The Health Resources and Services Administration (HRSA) of HHS defines **telehealth** as the use of electronic information and telecommunications technologies to support and promote long-distance clinical healthcare, patient and professional health-related education, public health, and health administration. Technologies include videoconferencing, the internet, store-and-forward imaging, streaming media, and terrestrial and wireless communications (ONCHIT 2019). Figure 2.6 shows the types of telehealth applications.

Figure 2.6 Types of telehealth applications

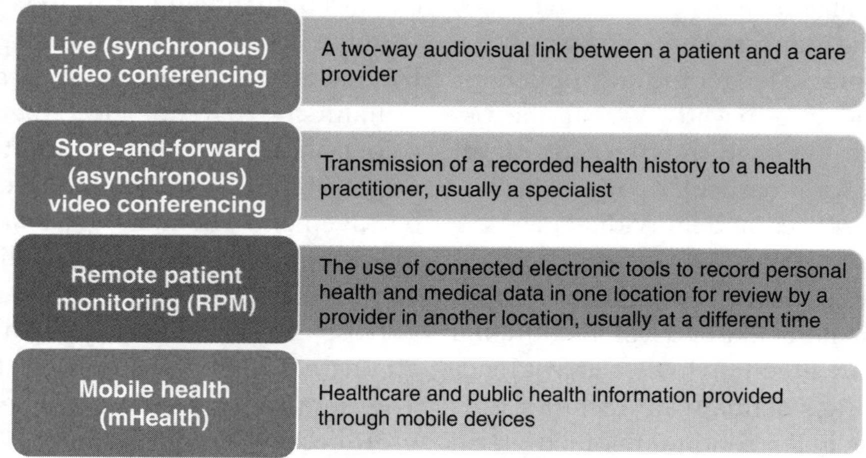

Source: Adapted from ONCHIT 2019.

Electronic Health Records and Health Data

Electronic health records (EHRs) and the ability to record, capture, and manipulate health data have had a tremendous impact on the delivery of healthcare. **Big data** refers to large amounts of data that are collected from sources and then processed and used for analytics. Collected and analyzed health data have multiple benefits including the following:

- Reducing healthcare costs
- Predicting epidemics
- Avoiding preventable deaths
- Improving quality of life
- Reducing healthcare waste
- Improving efficiency and quality of care
- Developing new drugs and treatments (Banova, 2018)

The American Recovery and Reinvestment Act of 2009, the Patient Protection and Affordable Care Act, and other quality-of-care programs represent the movement from a volume-based delivery model to a data-driven, value-based approach. Data collected from EHRs is utilized to measure outcomes performance that is directly tied to reimbursement. In addition, data collected from EHRs is utilized by clinical researchers to develop new treatments for common health problems. The collection and evaluation of data in a centralized system can identify a viral or bacterial infection to give insights into how widespread an outbreak is.

Ninety-six percent of hospitals in the United States have a federally tested and certified EHR program (Reisman 2017). The next challenge for the use of EHRs is ensuring interoperability. Interoperability refers to more than the exchange of information; it requires that the data exchanged are usable. This means that the receiving system must be able to interpret the data. With the variety of government certified EHR products in use, each one has its own clinical terminologies, technical specifications, and functional capabilities. This makes it very difficult to create one standard interoperability format to share data.

Artificial Intelligence

The increasing availability of healthcare data and rapid development of big data analytic methods have made possible the recent successful applications of **artificial intelligence (AI)** in healthcare. AI is the ability of a computer program or machine to think and learn. AI uses sophisticated algorithms to learn trends or features from large volumes of health data to make judgments. It can be equipped with learning and self-correcting abilities to improve accuracy based on feedback. AI is not meant to replace the physician, but to assist the physician in making better clinical decisions or replace human judgment in functional areas of healthcare such as radiology (Jiang et al. 2017).

Before AI systems can be successfully utilized, they have to be trained through data that are generated from clinical activities so they can learn the group of subjects and associations. There are two major categories of AI: machine learning (ML) and natural language processing (NLP). Machine learning analyzes structured data such as imaging and genetic results, then attempts to cluster the patient's traits or infer the probability of the disease outcomes (Jiang et al. 2017). NLP methods extract information from unstructured data such as clinical notes to supplement the structured data. NLP focuses on turning the text into machine-readable structured data that can be analyzed by ML techniques.

One of the most common uses of AI in healthcare has been the use of speech recognition. It is also being used in radiology to assist in the diagnostic process by analyzing images such as MRIs, x-rays, and CT scans and providing feedback on what it detects. AI is being utilized in medical monitoring devices to transform them into smart medical devices. Traditional medical devices monitor and record data to be reviewed by a clinician at a later time. Smart medical devices can analyze and respond to the recorded data. For example, an insulin pump utilizing AI can predict how much insulin the patient will need and when they will need it rather than just responding to spikes in blood sugar.

Check Your Understanding 2.3

Answer the following questions.

1. The healthcare organization provides healthcare services to low-income patients in the local community at a:
   a. Freestanding ambulatory care center
   b. Private medical practice
   c. Subacute care
   d. Voluntary agency
2. My daughter fell and cut herself tonight. Though it is not an emergency, I believe she needs stitches and she should see healthcare practitioner tonight for treatment. Which type of setting would I most likely access?
   a. Hospital emergency department
   b. Community-based ambulatory care services
   c. Private medical practice
   d. Freestanding ambulatory care center
3. Most patients in long-term care facilities require inpatient nursing and related services for more than how many consecutive days?
   a. 14
   b. 30
   c. 60
   d. 100
4. Which healthcare organization offers palliative care for end-of-life care so that the patient may live life as fully and as comfortably as possible?
   a. Hospice
   b. Adult day-care
   c. Skilled nursing facility
   d. Nursing home

5. The ability of a computer to think and learn is:
   a. Artificial intelligence
   b. Big data
   c. Interoperability
   d. Telehealth

Match the descriptions with the terms.

6. ______ Managed care
7. ______ Freestanding ambulatory care centers
8. ______ Human Genome Project
9. ______ Subacute care
10. ______ Continuum of care

   a. A 13-year-long international effort with three principal goals: (1) to determine the sequence of the three billion DNA subunits, (2) to identify all human genes, and (3) to enable genes to be used in further biological study
   b. Provides emergency services and urgent care for walk-in patients
   c. Care that offers patients access to constant nursing care while recovering at home
   d. Care provided by different caregivers at several different levels of the healthcare system
   e. Manages cost, quality, and access to services

Policy Making and Healthcare Delivery

The American healthcare system is a patchwork of independent and governmental entities that provide healthcare services to those in need. Institutions ranging from not-for-profits, for-profits, and governmental agencies provide not only services but also policy on how Americans are to receive and pay for their healthcare.

The government's role in healthcare services is extensive from the federal level down to the county and local levels. By setting policies on how healthcare is provided, delivered, and reimbursed, government agencies have a significant impact on our healthcare delivery system.

The following sections list five ways that healthcare policies affect the American people. All the policies are dedicated to providing the best services in a system that is constrained by increasing costs generally at the expense of access and quality.

Healthy People 2020

Launched in December 2010 by the Office of Disease Prevention and Heath Promotion of HHS, Healthy People 2020 sets out a plan to improve the nation's health with a vision of "a society in which all people live long, healthy lives" (Healthy People 2015). Healthy People provides users with access to data on changes in the health status of the US population and informs of each new decade's goals and objectives. Communities may adopt the Healthy People goals and objectives and may alter them to set the priorities for their region and population groups. Since it was launched, Healthy People has noted significant achievements in reducing causes of death such as heart disease and cancer; reducing infant and maternal mortality; reducing risk factors like tobacco smoking, hypertension, and elevated cholesterol; and increasing childhood vaccinations (Healthy People 2019a).

Healthy People 2020 is the third initiative (starting with Healthy People 2000) since its inception 30 years ago. The overall goals of Healthy People 2020 are to do the following:

- Attain high-quality, longer lives free of preventable disease, disability, injury, and premature death

- Achieve health equity, eliminate disparities, and improve the health of all groups
- Create social and physical environments that promote good health for all
- Promote quality of life, healthy development, and healthy behaviors across all life stages (Healthy People 2015)

One topic area of Healthy People 2020 is social determinants of health. **Social determinants of health (SDOH)** are conditions such as environment and age that impact a wide range of health, functioning, and quality-of-life outcomes and risks. Examples of social determinants include:

- Availability of resources to meet daily needs
- Access to educational, economic, and job opportunities
- Availability of community-based resources
- Exposure to crime, violence, and social disorder
- Socioeconomic conditions
- Language and literacy
- Access to mass media and emerging technologies
- Culture (Healthy People 2019b)

Healthy People 2020 established a place-based organizing framework reflecting five determinants areas of SDOH. This framework reflects the importance of the relationship between how population groups experience "place" and the impact of "place" on health. This includes both social and physical determinants. The five key determinants are economic stability, education, social and community context, health and healthcare, and neighborhood and built environment (Healthy People 2019b). Figure 2.7 shows the five key social determinants of health, including economic stability, education, social and community context, health and healthcare and neighborhood and built environment.

Healthy People 2020 also recognizes that health information technology and health communication are integral parts of the implementation process of the initiative.

The next phase of Healthy People is Healthy People 2030. The framework for the Healthy People 2030 initiative has been developed. HHS solicited comments on the proposed framework and these comments were used to finalize the framework. The Healthy People 2030 framework was approved by the HHS Secretary in June 2018. The overarching goals of the framework include the following:

Figure 2.7 Healthy People 2020 five key social determinants of health

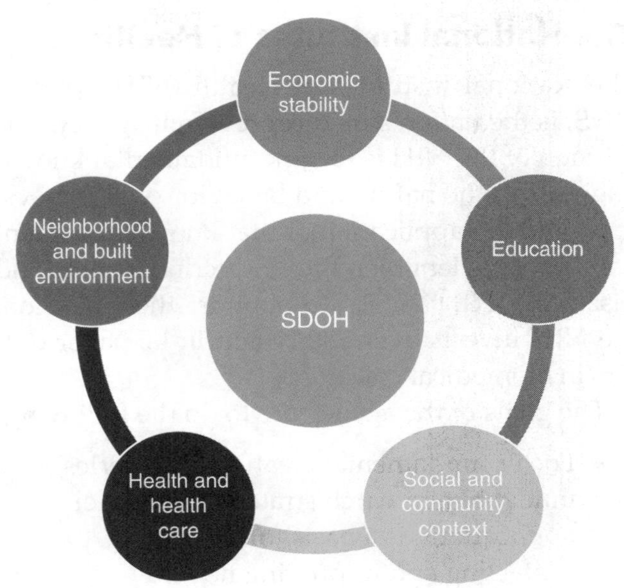

Source: Adapted from Healthy People 2019b.

- Attain healthy, thriving lives and well-being, free of preventable disease, disability, injury, and premature death
- Eliminate health disparities, achieve health equity, and attain health literacy to improve the health and well-being of all
- Create social, physical, and economic environments that promote attaining full potential for health and well-being for all
- Promote healthy development, healthy behaviors and well-being across all life stages
- Engage leadership, key constituents, and the public across multiple sectors to take action and design policies that improve the health and well-being of all (Healthy People 2019a)

The ultimate goal of Healthy People 2020 is to develop a feasible, public health information technology infrastructure in conjunction with the national health information network.

The National Institutes of Health

The National Institutes of Health (NIH), part of HHS, is the nation's medical research agency. The mission of the NIH is to seek fundamental knowledge about the nature and behavior of living systems and the application of that knowledge to enhance health, lengthen life, and reduce illness and disability (NIH 2017). To support their mission, the NIH invests over $30 billion in taxpayer dollars in biomedical research.

The goals of the agency are to do the following:

- Foster fundamental creative discoveries, innovative research strategies, and their applications as a basis for ultimately protecting and improving health
- Develop, maintain, and renew scientific human and physical resources that will ensure the nation's capability to prevent disease
- Expand the knowledge base in medical and associated sciences to enhance the nation's economic well-being and ensure a continued high return on the public investment in research
- Exemplify and promote the highest level of scientific integrity, public accountability, and social responsibility in the conduct of science

Surgical procedures were performed before the development of anesthesia, requiring surgeons to work quickly on conscious patients to minimize the risk and pain. The availability of anesthesia made it possible for surgeons to develop more advanced surgical techniques. Ether, nitrous oxide, and chloroform were used as anesthetics by the middle of the 19th century. By the 1860s, the physicians who treated the casualties of the American Civil War on both sides had access to anesthetic and painkilling drugs.

During the late 1800s, significant improvements in healthcare were being made. In 1885, Louis Pasteur developed a vaccine that prevented rabies. Joseph Lister was the first to apply Pasteur's research to the treatment of infected wounds. His discovery was called the antiseptic principle, which helped reduce the mortality rate in Lister's own hospital. At the end of the 19th century, German physicist Wilhelm Rontgen was studying the effects of passing an electrical current through gases at low pressure. While doing this, he accidentally discovered x-rays (The Scientist 2011).

Diagnostic radiology and radiation therapy have undergone huge advances in the past 50 years. In 1971 an imaging modality called computed tomography (CT) was first invented. The first CT scanners were used to create images of the skull. Whole-body scanners were introduced in 1974. In the 1980s, another powerful diagnostic tool was added—magnetic resonance imaging (MRI). An MRI is a noninvasive technique that uses magnetic and radio-frequency fields to record images of soft tissues.

Surgical advances have been remarkable as well. Cardiac bypass surgery and joint replacement surgery were developed in the 1970s. Organs are now successfully transplanted, and artificial organs are being tested. New surgical techniques have included the use of lasers in ophthalmology, gynecology, and urology. Microsurgery is now a common tool in the reconstruction of damaged nerves and blood vessels.

The future of surgery could include physicians using advanced robots, virtual reality, augmented reality, and 3D printing and simulations in preoperative planning and education (The Medical Futurist 2017).

Today, it is human genetics and progress toward sequencing the human genome that promise to change the healthcare paradigm. New research on cellular and molecular changes underlying disease processes will necessitate new approaches to diagnosis and treatment.

The current paradigm for treating disease is to meet with the patient, diagnose the patient's symptoms, and prescribe therapy to treat them. The hope is that genetic medicine will enable the provider to identify gene patterns that underlie the process of cellular dysfunction that leads to injury before even meeting with the patient. Thus, diseases will be diagnosed much earlier, enabling physicians to provide treatment to stop or slow the disease process.

The study of cell-based technologies is controversial. Cell-based technologies include the following:

- Tissue engineering, which involves the use of biomaterials to develop new tissue and even whole organs with or without transplanting cells
- Human embryonic stem cells or adult stem cells used for transplantation and in regenerative medicine
- Gene therapy or cell transplantation

The National Human Genome Research Institute (NHGRI) was established in 1989 to carry out the role of the NIH in the International Human Genome Project (HGP). The HGP began in 1990 to map the human genome. Since the completion of the human genome sequence in 2003, the NHGRI expanded its role to apply genome technologies to the study of specific diseases (NHGRI 2018). In fall 2020, NHGRI will launch its newest strategic plan aimed at accelerating scientific and medical breakthroughs. Through its strategic plan, the NHGRI will prioritize discussions in emerging areas of genomics that are not well defined and that are not specific to particular diseases or physiological systems. These include broadly applicable areas such as genomic technology development; using genomic information in patient care; and the ethical, legal, and social implications of genomics.

National Academy of Medicine Reports

The National Academy of Medicine (NAM), formerly known as the Institute of Medicine, was established in 1970 as a nongovernmental agency to provide unbiased advice to decision makers and the public. NAM has written over 1,000 reports since 1970. A selection of quintessential publications dealing with the public's health include the following publications:

- *To Error is Human* (1999) reported that as many as 98,000 people die each year from preventable medical errors (IOM 1999).
- *Crossing the Quality Chasm* (2001) identified gaps in the delivery of patient care services resulting from a complex medical system as well as the rapid advancement in medical knowledge (IOM 2001).
- *Envisioning a National Health Care Quality Report* (2001) addressed the collection, measurement, and analysis of quality data (Hurtado et al. 2001).
- *Leadership by Example* (2002) addressed the duplication and contrasting approaches to performance measures by the six major governmental healthcare programs that serve nearly 100 million Americans (IOM 2002).
- *Priority Areas for National Action* (2003) recognized priorities from earlier reports and suggested a framework for action (IOM 2003).
- *Health IT and Patient Safety* (2012) stated that the improvement in safety of health IT is essential and can help improve healthcare providers' performance, improve communication between patients and providers, and enhance patient safety (IOM 2012).
- *Human Genome Editing: Science, Ethics and Governance* (2017) considered important questions about the human application of genome editing.
- *Optimizing Strategies for Clinical Decision Support* (2017) identified the need for a continuously learning health system driven by the seamless and rapid generation, processing, and practical application of the best available evidence for clinical decision-making.
- *Procuring Interoperability: Achieving High-Quality, Connected, and Person-Centered Care* (2018) identified data exchanges determined to be critical to achieving interoperability and identified the key characteristics of information exchange involved in health and healthcare.

Centers for Disease Control and Prevention

Founded in 1946, the **Centers for Disease Control and Prevention (CDC)** is the leading federal agency charged with protecting the public health and safety through the control and prevention of disease, injury, and disability. The CDC leads the nation in the following services:

- Detecting and responding to diseases and conditions (attention deficit hyperactivity disorder, sexually transmitted diseases, cancer, heart disease, diabetes, flu)
- Promoting healthy living (adolescents and school health, food safety, tobacco and alcohol use, overweight and obesity, vaccines and immunizations)
- Providing information for travelers' health (destinations, travel notices, find a clinic)
- Educating for emergency preparedness (natural disasters and severe weather, recent outbreaks and incidents, bioterrorism, chemical emergencies, radiation emergencies, mass casualties)

The CDC headquarters is in Atlanta, GA and there are 10 additional locations in the United States. With over 14,000 employees, the CDC collects, analyzes, and creates national statistical databases and publishes papers on important health issues (CDC 2019).

Local, State, and Federal Policies

All levels of government create policies affecting the nation's healthcare. At the local and community level, leaders decide where public funds will finance community health centers and municipal hospitals, which provide care regardless of the patient's ability to pay.

At the state level, decisions on access, eligibility, and level of treatments for Medicaid recipients, where state and federal dollars will be spent on items like tobacco cessation and gambling addiction centers (for those states with casinos), and how to provide services to people with special needs, as well as funding for mental health facilities are a large component of most state budgets.

At the federal level, six agencies provide healthcare to over 100 million Americans (Medicare, Medicaid, State Children's Health Insurance Program [SCHIP], Veterans Health Administration [VHA], TRICARE, and Indian Health Service [IHS]). All three branches of government have input on the cost, access, and quality of care provided to Americans through these federal agencies as well as the various policy-making institutions that provide carefully considered input to the decision makers.

Unfortunately, the American healthcare system was not developed from a master plan but is instead a patchwork quilt of measures passed not from thought as to how they would affect the whole, but rather based on ideology. Much attention today is focused on the cost of healthcare often at the expense of patient access and the quality of care provided.

Patient-Centered Outcomes Research Institute

The Patient-Centered Outcomes Research Institute (PCORI) was created in 2010 from the passage of the Patient Protection and Affordable Care Act (ACA) as a nonprofit, nongovernmental organization mandated to improve the quality and applicability of evidence available to help all stakeholders (patients, caregivers, clinicians, employers, insurers, and policy makers) to make knowledgeable healthcare choices. While PCORI is not the first organization focusing on patient-centered care, it is the largest single research funder that has comparative effectiveness research (CER) as its main focus and incorporates patients and other stakeholders throughout the process more consistently and intensively than others have before. In its strategic plan, PCORI has outlined the following three overarching goals:

1. Substantially increase the quantity, quality, and timeliness of useful, trustworthy information available to support health decisions
2. Speed the implementation and use of patient-centered outcomes research (PCOR) evidence.
3. Influence clinical and healthcare research funded by others to be more patient centered (PCORI 2017)

Check Your Understanding 2.4

Answer the following questions.

1. According to the publication *To Error Is Human,* how many patients die each year from preventable medical mistakes?
   a. 10,000
   b. 46,000
   c. 72,000
   d. 98,000
2. To "create social and physical environments that promote good health for all" is a goal of:
   a. CDC
   b. Healthy People 2020
   c. PCORI
   d. VHA
3. Identify a nonprofit, nongovernmental organization from the following.
   a. SCHIP
   b. CDC
   c. National Academy of Medicine
   d. Healthy People 2020
4. The federal agency that monitors healthy precautions for international travelers is the:
   a. CDC
   b. VHA
   c. IHS
   d. PCORI
5. A report from the National Academy of Medicine addressing the duplication and contrasting approaches to performance measures by the six major governmental healthcare programs that serve nearly 100 million Americans is:
   a. *To Error is Human*
   b. *Leadership by Example*
   c. *Envisioning a National Health Care Quality Report*
   d. *Priority Areas for National Action*
6. True or false: The National Academy of Medicine is the largest single research funder hospitals and care systems use to redesign how care is delivered, to eliminate inefficiencies within the system that will lead to better, integrated care, and lower total cost of care.
7. True or false: Healthcare policy is only formulated at the federal level.
8. True or false: Hospitals and care systems need to redesign how patient care is delivered so inefficiencies can be eliminated within the system.
9. True or false: The organization that collects, analyzes, and creates national statistical databases and publishes papers on important health issues is the CDC.
10. True or false: Social determinants of health are environmental issues that impact a wide range of health, functioning, and quality-of-life outcomes and risks.

Modern Healthcare Delivery in the United States

Until World War II, most healthcare was provided in the home. Quality in healthcare services was considered a product of appropriate medical practice and oversight by physicians and surgeons. Even the minimum standards used to evaluate the performance of hospitals were based on factors directly related to the composition and skills of the hospital medical staff.

The 20th century was a period of tremendous change in American society. Advances in medical science promised better outcomes and increased the demand for healthcare services. But medical care has never been free. Even in the best economic times, many Americans have been unable to take full advantage of what medicine has to offer because they cannot afford it.

Concern over access to healthcare was especially evident during the Great Depression of the 1930s. During the Depression, America's leaders were forced to consider how the poor and disadvantaged could receive the care they needed. Before the Depression, medical care for the poor and elderly had been handled as a function of social welfare agencies. However, during the 1930s, few people were able to pay for medical care. The problem of how to pay for the healthcare needs of millions of Americans became a public and governmental concern. Working Americans turned to prepaid health plans to help them pay for healthcare, but the unemployed and the unemployable needed help from a different source.

During the 20th century, Congress passed many pieces of legislation that had a significant impact on the delivery of healthcare services in the United States.

Social Security Act of 1935

The Great Depression revived the dormant social reform movement in the United States as well as more radical currents in American politics. The Depression also brought to power the Democratic administration of Franklin D. Roosevelt, which was more willing than any previous administration to involve the federal government in the management of economic and social welfare.

Although old-age pension and unemployment insurance bills were introduced into Congress soon after his election, Roosevelt refused to give them his strong support. Instead, he created a program of his own and appointed a Committee on Economic Security to study the issue comprehensively and report to Congress in January 1935.

Sentiment in favor of health insurance was strong among members of the Committee on Economic Security. However, many members of the committee were convinced that adding a health insurance amendment would spell defeat for the entire Social Security legislation. Ultimately, the Social Security bill included only one reference to health insurance as a subject that the new Social Security Board might study. The Social Security Act was passed in 1935.

Public Law 89–97 of 1965

In 1965, passage of a number of amendments to the Social Security Act brought Medicare and Medicaid into existence. The two programs have greatly changed how healthcare organizations are reimbursed. Recent attempts to curtail Medicare and Medicaid spending continue to affect healthcare organizations.

Medicare (Title XVIII of the Social Security Act) is a federal program that provides healthcare benefits for people age 65 and older who are covered by Social Security. The program was inaugurated on July 1, 1966. Over the years, amendments have extended coverage to individuals who are not covered by Social Security but are willing to pay a premium for coverage, to the disabled, and to those suffering from end-stage renal disease (ESRD).

The companion program, **Medicaid** (Title XIX of the Social Security Act), was established at the same time to support medical and hospital care for persons classified as medically indigent. Originally targeting recipients of public assistance (primarily single-parent families and the aged, blind, and disabled), Medicaid has expanded to additional groups so that it now targets poor children, the disabled, pregnant women, and very poor adults, including those age 65 and older.

Today, Medicaid is a federally mandated program that provides healthcare benefits to low-income people and their children. Medicaid programs are administered and partially paid for by individual states. Medicaid is an umbrella for 50 different state programs designed specifically to serve the poor. Beginning in January 1967, Medicaid provided federal funds to states on a cost-sharing basis to ensure welfare recipients would be guaranteed medical services. Coverage of four types of care was required: inpatient and outpatient services, other laboratory and x-ray services, physician services, and nursing facility care for persons over 21 years of age.

Many enhancements have been made in the years since Medicaid was enacted. Services now include family planning and 31 other optional services such as prescription drugs and dental services. With few exceptions, recipients of cash assistance are automatically eligible for Medicaid. Medicaid also pays the Medicare premium, deductible, and coinsurance costs for some low-income Medicare beneficiaries. More information on Medicaid can be found in chapter 15, *Revenue Management and Reimbursement*.

Medicaid spending has also increased 13.9 percent over that time period. The increase in spending is attributed to the growth in enrollment, increased provider rates, increased prescription costs, and other costs spread out over the healthcare system (Kaiser Family Foundation 2015). This represented a peak in enrollment. Since 2015, enrollment growth has slowed, in part, to the tapering of ACA enrollment growth (Kaiser Family Foundation 2019).

Public Law 92–603 of 1972

To curtail Medicare and Medicaid spending, additional amendments to the Social Security Act were instituted in 1972. Public Law 92–603 required concurrent review for Medicare and Medicaid patients. It also established the professional standards review organization (PSRO) program to implement concurrent review. PSROs performed professional review and evaluated patient care services for necessity, quality, and cost-effectiveness.

Utilization review (UR) is the process of determining whether the medical care provided to a specific patient is necessary according to pre-established objective screening criteria at time frames specified in the organization's utilization management plan. UR was a mandatory component of the original Medicare legislation. Medicare required hospitals and **extended care facilities**, which are facilities licensed by applicable state or local law to offer room and board, skilled nursing by a full-time RN, intermediate care, or a combination of levels on a 24-hour basis over a long period of time. Extended care facilities are required to establish a plan for UR as well as a permanent utilization review committee. The goal of the UR process is to ensure the services provided to Medicare beneficiaries are medically necessary.

Utilization Review Act of 1977

In 1977, the **Utilization Review Act** made it a requirement for hospitals to conduct continued-stay reviews for Medicare and Medicaid patients. Continued-stay reviews determine whether it is medically necessary for a patient to remain hospitalized. This legislation also included fraud and abuse regulations. More information on fraud and abuse can be found in chapter 16, *Fraud and Abuse Compliance*.

Peer Review Improvement Act of 1982

In 1982, the Peer Review Improvement Act redesigned the PSRO program and renamed the agencies **peer review organizations (PROs)**. At that time, hospitals began to review the medical necessity and appropriateness of certain admissions even before patients were admitted. PROs were given a new name in 2002 and now are called **quality improvement organizations (QIOs)**. They currently emphasize quality improvement processes. Each state and territory, as well as the District of Columbia, now has its own QIO. The mission of the QIOs is to ensure the quality, efficiency, and cost-effectiveness of the healthcare services provided to Medicare beneficiaries in its locale.

Tax Equity and Fiscal Responsibility Act of 1982

In 1982, Congress passed the Tax Equity and Fiscal Responsibility Act (TEFRA). TEFRA required extensive changes in the Medicare program. Its purpose was to control the rising cost of providing healthcare services to Medicare beneficiaries. Before this legislation was passed, healthcare services provided to Medicare beneficiaries were reimbursed on a retrospective, or fee-based, payment system. TEFRA required the gradual implementation of a prospective payment system (PPS) for Medicare reimbursement.

In a retrospective payment system, a service is provided, a claim for payment for the service is made, and the healthcare provider is reimbursed for the cost of delivering the service. In a PPS, a predetermined level of reimbursement is established before the service is provided. More information on PPSs can be found in chapter 15, *Revenue Management and Reimbursement*.

Public Law 98–21 of 1983

The PPS for acute hospital care (inpatient) services was implemented on October 1, 1983, according to Public Law 98–21. Under the inpatient PPS, reimbursement for hospital care provided to Medicare patients is based on diagnosis-related groups (DRGs). Each case is assigned to a DRG based on the patient's diagnosis at the time of discharge. For example, under the inpatient PPS, all cases of viral pneumonia would be reimbursed at the same predetermined level of reimbursement no matter how long the patients stayed in the hospital or how many services they received. PPSs for other healthcare services provided to Medicare beneficiaries have been gradually implemented since 1983.

Health Insurance Portability and Accountability Act of 1996

The Health Insurance Portability and Accountability Act of 1996 (HIPAA) addresses issues related to the portability of health insurance after leaving employment, establishment of national standards for electronic healthcare transactions, and national identifiers for providers, health plans, and employers. A portion of HIPAA addressed the security and privacy of health information by establishing privacy standards to protect health information and security standards for electronic healthcare information. HIPAA privacy and security standards are covered in chapter 9, *Data Privacy and Confidentiality*, and chapter 10, *Data Security*. Another provision of HIPAA was the creation of the Healthcare Integrity and Protection Data Bank (HIPDB) to combat fraud and abuse in health insurance and healthcare delivery. A purpose of the HIPDB is to inform federal and state agencies about potential quality problems with clinicians, suppliers, and providers of healthcare services. The American Recovery and Reinvestment Act (ARRA) includes important changes in HIPAA privacy and security standards that are also discussed in chapters 9 and 10.

American Recovery and Reinvestment Act of 2009

The American Recovery and Reinvestment Act of 2009 (ARRA) is considered one of the major health information technology laws that provided stimulus funds to the US economy in the midst of a major economic downturn. A substantial portion of the bill, Title XIII of the Act entitled the Health Information Technology for Economic and Clinical Health (HITECH) Act, allocated funds for implementation of a nationwide health information exchange and implementation of electronic health records. The bill provides for investment of billions of dollars in health information technology and incentives to encourage physicians and hospitals to use information technology; $19.2 billion was dedicated to implementing and supporting health information technology. ARRA requires the government to take a leadership role in developing standards for exchange of health information nationwide, strengthens federal privacy and security standards, and established the Office of the National Coordinator for Health Information Technology (ONC) as a permanent office (Rode 2009). Four major components of the bill include: meaningful use (that providers are using certified EHRs to improve patient outcomes); EHR standards and certifications; regional extension centers (used to assist providers with selection and implementation of EHRs); and breach notification guidance. Though challenged in court, the US Supreme Court upheld the law in a 6–3 decision. Meaningful use was changed in 2018 to the Promoting Interoperability incentive program. EHR incentive programs are discussed in chapter 16, *Fraud and Abuse Compliance*.

Patient Protection and Affordable Care Act of 2010

The Patient Protection and Affordable Care Act (ACA) was signed into law on March 23, 2010, and is the most significant healthcare reform legislation of the first decade of the 21st century. The Kaiser Family Foundation summarizes the following major provisions of the ACA:

- The Medicaid expansion to 138 percent of the federal poverty level ($15,415 for an individual and $31,809 for a family of four in 2012) for individuals under age 65
- The creation of health insurance exchanges through which individuals who do not have access to public coverage or affordable employer coverage will be able to purchase insurance with premium and cost-sharing credits available to some people to make coverage more affordable
- New regulations on all health plans that will prevent health insurers from denying coverage to people for any reason, including health status, and from charging higher premiums based on health status and gender
- The requirement that most individuals have health insurance beginning in 2014 with tax penalties for those without insurance
- The penalties to employers that do not offer affordable coverage to their employees, with exceptions for small employers (Kaiser Family Foundation 2012)

Since the ACA became law, the number of uninsured individuals in the United States has declined from 49 million in 2010 to 29 million in 2015 (JAMA 2016). The law's major coverage provisions combined with financial assistance for low- and moderate-income individuals to purchase their coverage and generous federal support for states that expand their Medicaid programs to cover more low-income adults have all contributed to the gains in health coverage. The law's provision allowing young adults to stay on a parent's plan until age 26 years has also played a contributing role, covering an estimated 2.3 million people after it took effect in late 2010 (JAMA 2016).

Since 2017, a number of proposals have been presented to repeal and replace the ACA. One includes the repeal of a 2.3 percent excise tax on the sale of certain medical devices by manufacturers. This tax was passed on to purchasers of devices, mainly hospitals and physicians, which filtered down to consumers. An executive order signed by President Trump on January 20, 2017, authorized the Secretary of the Department of Health and Human Services to repeal this tax at his discretion (Shi and Singh 2019).

Check Your Understanding 2.5 

Answer the following questions.

1. Identify the law that created the HITECH Act.
   a. Health Insurance Portability and Accountability Act
   b. American Recovery and Reinvestment Act
   c. Consolidated Omnibus Budget Reconciliation Act
   d. Healthcare Quality Improvement Act

2. Until World War II, most healthcare was provided:
   a. In a government clinic
   b. At a physician's office
   c. At home
   d. In a hospital

3. A HIM student has asked you why Medicare reimburses healthcare providers through prospective payment systems. Identify the piece of legislation that answers the student.
   a. Peer Review Improvement Act of 1982
   b. Consolidated Budget Reconciliation Act of 1986
   c. Tax Equity and Fiscal Responsibility Act of 1982
   d. Omnibus Budget Reconciliation Act of 1986

4. Identify the legislation that authorized the creation of the Office of National Coordinator for Health Information Technology.
   a. PPACA
   b. HIPAA
   c. ARRA
   d. TEFRA

5. Medicaid is a:
   a. Federal program targeted principally for those age 65 and older
   b. Federally mandated healthcare program for low-income people
   c. Healthcare program limited to those under age 65
   d. Healthcare program for low-income persons regardless of age that is totally financed and operated by the states

Match the description with the appropriate legislation.

6. ______ Tax Equity and Fiscal Responsibility Act of 1982
7. ______ Social Security Act of 1935
8. ______ Public Law 92–603 of 1972
9. ______ Patient Protection and Affordable Care Act of 2010
10. ______ Utilization Review Act of 1977
   a. Required that hospitals conduct continued-stay reviews for Medicare and Medicaid patients
   b. Required concurrent review of Medicare and Medicaid patients
   c. Provided an individual mandate to have minimum acceptable coverage or pay a tax penalty
   d. Gave the states funds on a matching basis for maternal and infant care, rehabilitation of crippled children, general public health work, and aid for dependent children under age 16
   e. Required the gradual implementation of a prospective payment system (PPS) for Medicare reimbursement

Real World Case 2.1

Steve is a 35-year-old, single male who lived in a one-bedroom apartment in a safe neighborhood. Steve worked as a maintenance technician for a local mill. Steve's job provided health insurance and he rarely needed to use it. Steve smoked half a pack of cigarettes each day and drank socially a few times a month.

One afternoon, Steve's company notified him that it was laying off more than one hundred employees, including him. Though he was devastated about losing his job, Steve was grateful that he had some savings that he could use for rent and other bills, in addition to the unemployment checks he would receive for a few months. For the next six months, Steve searched aggressively for a job but was unable to find one. With his savings depleted, he was not able to make ends meet, and he was evicted from his apartment. His self-esteem plummeted and he became depressed.

Steve stayed with various family members and friends and was able to pick up some odd jobs to make some money. However, his drinking and anger got worse and his hosts asked him to leave. When he ran out of people to call, he started sleeping at the park. One night when Steve was drunk, he fell and cut his shin. The injury became red and filled with pus. Steve was embarrassed about his situation and didn't want anyone to see him. But when he developed a fever and pain, he decided to walk to the nearest emergency department. He saw a provider who diagnosed him with cellulitis, a common but potentially serious bacterial skin infection, and gave him a copy of the patient instructions that read "discharge to home" and a prescription for antibiotics. Steve could not afford the entire prescription, but he was able to purchase half the tablets.

Steve began staying at a shelter. Each morning he had to leave the shelter by 6 am, and he walked the streets during the day and panhandled for money to buy alcohol. One day two men jumped Steve, kicked him repeatedly, and stole his backpack. A bystander called 911 and he was taken to the same emergency department where he had sought treatment for the shin injury. Again, the providers didn't screen him for homelessness, and he was discharged back to "home."

A few days later, an outreach team from a local nonprofit organization introduced themselves to Steve and asked if he was ok. He did not engage in conversation with them. They offered him a sandwich, a drink, and a blanket, which he took without making eye contact. The outreach team visited him over the next several days and noticed his shortness of breath and the cut on his leg.

After a couple of weeks, Steve began to trust the outreach team and agreed to go to the organization's medical clinic. The clinic provided primary care and behavioral health services through scheduled and walk-in appointments. Steve said the providers there treated him like a real person. He was able to have regular appointments with a therapist and began working on his depression and substance abuse. A year later, his health has improved. He is sober and working with a case manager to find housing.

Real-World Case 2.2

A municipal medical center in a city of 100,000 residents decided that they needed to diversify if they were going to survive the ups and downs of the economy. The board of directors met with the chief of the medical staff to determine the best course of action. They mutually decided to emphasize a cradle-to-grave approach by acquiring a few select physician practices and a local nursing home, starting a home health agency, and creating a hospice unit within the medical center. The board then decided to link all new acquisitions to the medical center's existing electronic health record (EHR) but ran into a problem with patient identification for health record purposes. The issue was that the same patient may have been or was going to be in multiple facilities within the new enterprise. However, at each of the present facilities (physician office, medical center, and nursing home), the same patient would have different health record numbers. A plan for an enterprise health record number was needed. The medical center administration decided to bring in the health information management director of the medical center to provide expertise and experience in resolving the problem.

References

American Board of Medical Specialties. 2019. ABMS Guide to Medical Specialties. https://www.abms.org/media/194925/abms-guide-to-medical-specialties-2019.pdf.

American Health Information Management Association. 2017. *Pocket Glossary of Health Information Management and Technology*, 5th ed. Chicago: AHIMA.

American Hospital Association. 2018b. Hospitals are Economic Drivers in Their Communities. https://www.aha.org/system/files/2018-06/econ-contribution-2018_0.pdf.

American Hospital Association. 2015. Fast Facts on US Hospitals. http://www.aha.org/aha/resource-center/Statistics-and-Studies/fast-facts.html.

American Hospital Association. 2014. Your Hospital's Path to the Second Curve: Integration and Transformation. https://www.aha.org/system/files/2018-01/your-hospitals-path-second-curve-integration-transformation-2014.pdf.

American Hospital Association. 2019. Promoting Healthy Communities. https://www.aha.org/ahia/promoting-healthy-communities.

American Nurses Association. 2019. What is Nursing? https://www.nursingworld.org/practice-policy/workforce/what-is-nursing/.

American Speech-Language-Hearing Association. 2016. http://www.asha.org/public/hearing.

Banova, B. 2018. The Impact of Technology on Healthcare. https://www.aimseducation.edu/blog/the-impact-of-technology-on-healthcare/.

Association of Schools of Allied Health Professions. 2019. What is Allied Health? http://www.asahp.org/what-is.

Bureau of Labor Statistics. 2018. Occupational Outlook Handbook, Physician Assistants. https://www.bls.gov/ooh/healthcare/physician-assistants.htm.

Bureau of Labor Statistics. 2017a. National Occupational Employment and Wage Estimates United States. https://www.bls.gov/oes/current/oes_nat.htm.

Bureau of Labor Statistics. 2017b. Occupational Outlook Handbook. http://www.bls.gov/ooh/healthcare/registered-nurses.htm.

Bureau of Labor Statistics. 2017c. Charts of the largest occupations in each industry, May 2018. https://www.bls.gov/oes/current/ind_emp_chart/ind_emp_chart.htm.

Caring for Communities: How Hospitals are Engaging in New Payment Models and Addressing Community Needs.

Centers for Disease Control and Prevention. 2019. Fast Facts about CDC. http://www.cdc.gov/24-7/CDCFastFacts/CDCFacts.html.

Centers for Medicare and Medicaid Services. 2018a. National Health Expenditures 2017 Highlights. https://www.cms.gov/Research-Statistics-Data-and-Systems/Statistics-Trends-and-Reports/NationalHealthExpendData/Downloads/highlights.pdf.

Centers for Medicare and Medicaid Services. 2018b. National Health Expenditure Projections 2017-2026 Forecast Summary. https://www.cms.gov/research-statistics-data-and-systems/statistics-trends-and-reports/nationalhealthexpenddata/downloads/forecastsummary.pdf.

Centers for Medicare and Medicaid Services. 2018c. Medicare Shared Savings Program Fast Facts. https://www.cms.gov/Medicare/Medicare-Fee-for-Service-Payment/sharedsavingsprogram/Downloads/SSP-2018-Fast-Facts.pdf http://www.ncsl.org/documents/health/privhlthins2.pdf.

Centers for Medicare and Medicaid Services. 2014. Critical Access Hospitals. http://www.cms.gov/Outreach-and-Education/Medicare-Learning-Network-MLN/MLNProducts/downloads/CritAccessHospfctsht.pdf.

Department of Health and Human Services. 2019. HHS Agencies & Offices. https://www.hhs.gov/about/agencies/hhs-agencies-and-offices/index.html.

DeVore, S. and R.W. Champion. 2011. Driving population health through accountable care organizations. *Health Affairs* 30(1): 41–50.

Furci, P.A. and S.J. Furci. 2017. Hospitalists continue to emerge. *Medical Staff Briefing* 27(11):6–9.

Healthy People. 2019a. Healthy People 2030 Framework. https://www.healthypeople.gov/2020/About-Healthy-People/Development-Healthy-People-2030/Framework.

Healthy People. 2019b. Social Determinants of Health. https://www.healthypeople.gov/2020/topics-objectives/topic/social-determinants-of-health.

Healthy People. 2015. http://www.healthypeople.gov/2020/About-Healthy-People.

Hurtado, M.P., E.K. Swift, and J.M. Corrigan. 2001. *Envisioning the National Health Care Quality Report*. Washington, DC: National Academies Press.

Institute of Medicine. 2012. Health IT and Patient Safety: Building Safer Systems for Better Care. http://iom.nationalacademies.org/Reports/2011/Health-IT-and-Patient-Safety-Building-Safer-Systems-for-Better-Care.aspx.

Institute of Medicine. 2003. Priority Areas for National Action: Transforming Health Care Quality. http://iom.

nationalacademies.org/reports/2003/priority-areas-for-national-action-transforming-health-care-quality.aspx.

Institute of Medicine. 2002. Leadership by Example: Coordinating Government Roles in Improving Health Care Quality. http://iom.nationalacademies.org/reports/2002/leadership-by-example-coordinating-government-roles-in-improving-health-care-quality.aspx.

Institute of Medicine. 1999. To Error is Human: Building a Safer Health System. http://iom.nationalacademies.org/~/media/Files/Report%20Files/1999/To-Err-is-Human/To%20Err%20is%20Human%201999%20%20report%20brief.pdf.

Institute of Medicine, Committee on Quality of Health Care in America. 2001. *Crossing the Quality Chasm: A New Health System for the 21st Century*. Washington, DC: National Academies Press.

JAMA. 2016. United States Health Care Reform: Progress to Date and Next Steps. 316(5):525-532. doi:10.1001/jama.2016.9797.

Jiang F., Y. Jiang, H. Zhi, Y. Dong, H. Li, S. Ma, Y. Wang, Q. Dong, H. Shen, and Y. Wang. 2017. *Stroke Vascular Neurology* 2(4):230–243. doi: 10.1136/svn-2017-000101. eCollection 2017 Dec. Review.

Kaiser Family Foundation. 2019. Medicaid Enrollment & Spending Growth: FY 2018 & 2019. https://www.kff.org/medicaid/issue-brief/medicaid-enrollment-spending-growth-fy-2018-2019/.

Kaiser Family Foundation. 2015. Medicaid Enrollment and Spending Growth: FY 2015 and 2016. http://kff.org/medicaid/issue-brief/medicaid-enrollment-spending-growth-fy-2015-2016.

Kaiser Family Foundation. 2012. Summary of Coverage Provisions in the Patient Protection and Affordable Care Act. https://www.kff.org/health-costs/issue-brief/summary-of-coverage-provisions-in-the-patient/.

Kickman, J.R. and A.R. Kovner. 2015. *Jonas and Kovner's Healthcare Delivery in the United States*, 11th ed. New York: Springer.

The Medical Futurist. 2017. The Technological Future of Surgery. https://medicalfuturist.com/the-technological-future-of-surgery.

National Academy on Medicine. 2018. Procuring Interoperability: Achieving High-Quality, Connected, and Person-Centered Care. https://nam.edu/wp-content/uploads/2018/10/Procuring-Interoperability_web.pdf.

National Adult Day Services Association. 2019. https://www.nadsa.org/research/.

The National Human Genome Research Institute. 2018. About NHGRI: A Brief History. https://www.genome.gov/10001763/about-nhgri-a-brief-history-and-timeline/.

National Institutes of Health. 2017. What We Do: Mission and Goals. https://www.nih.gov/about-nih/what-we-do/mission-goals.

National Institutes of Health. 2015. Managed Care. Medline Plus. https://www.nlm.nih.gov/medlineplus/managedcare.html#summary.

Office of the National Coordinator for Health Information Technology. 2019. https://www.healthit.gov/topic/health-it-initiatives/telemedicine-and-telehealth.

Patient-Centered Outcomes Research Institute. 2017. About Us. https://www.pcori.org/about-us/our-story.

Patient-Centered Primary Care Collaborative. 2019. https://www.pcpcc.org/about/medical-home.

Reisman, M. 2017. EHRs: The challenge of making electronic data usable and interoperable. *P&T: A Peer-Reviewed Journal for Managed Care & Formulary Management* 42(9): 572–575.

Rode, D. 2009. Recovery and privacy: Why a law about the economy is the biggest thing since HIPAA. *Journal of AHIMA* 80(5):42–44.

RTI International. 2015. Accountable Care Organization 2015: Program Analysis Quality Performance Standards Narrative Measure Specification. Prepared for CMS. https://www.cms.gov/medicare/medicare-fee-for-service-payment/sharedsavingsprogram/downloads/ry2015-narrative-specifications.pdf.

The Scientist. 2011. The First X-ray, 1895. https://www.the-scientist.com/foundations/the-first-x-ray-1895-42279.

Shi, L. and D. Sing. 2019. *Delivering Health Care in America: A Systems Approach*. 7th ed. Burlington, MA: Jones & Bartlett Learning.

Sutton, J.P., R.E.Washington, K.R. Fingar, and A. Elixhauser. 2016. Characteristics of Safety-Net Hospitals, 2014. https://www.hcup-us.ahrq.gov/reports/statbriefs/sb213-Safety-Net-Hospitals-2014.pdf.

Young, A., Chaudhry, H., Pei, X, Arnhart, K., Dugan, M., and Snyder, G. 2016. A Census of Activity Licensed Physicians in the United States, 2016. https://www.fsmb.org/siteassets/advocacy/publications/2016census.pdf.

Wachter, R. M. and L. Goldman. 2016. Zero to 50,000 - The 20th Anniversary of the Hospitalist. *The New England Journal of Medicine* 375(11):1009–11.

Health Information Functions, Purpose, and Users

Nanette B. Sayles, EdD, RHIA, CCS, CDIP, CHDA, CHPS, CPHI, CPHIMS, FAHIMA

Learning Objectives

- Identify the purposes of the health record
- Describe the different users of the health record and how they use it
- Utilize the master patient index
- Determine the appropriate format for the healthcare organization
- Justify the need to work with other departments in a healthcare organization
- Justify the use of the virtual health information management (HIM) department
- Educate others in the paper-based and electronic health records processes
- Justify the need for the use of information systems in the HIM department
- Explain the health information management information systems

Key Terms

Abstracting
Addendum
Aggregate data
Alphabetic filing system
Alphanumeric filing system
Amendment
Analysis
Assembly
Audit trail
Centralized unit filing system
Clinical coding
Clinical decision support (CDC)
Computer-assisted coding (CAC)
Concurrent review
Correction
Data
Data mining
Deficiency slip
Delinquent record
Demographics
Deterministic algorithm
Disclosure of health information
Document management system (DMS)
Duplicate health record
Electronic health record (EHR)
Encoder
Enterprise master patient index (EMPI)
Free-text data
Grouper
Guidelines
Health record
Hybrid health record
Index
Information

Input mask
Knowledge
Loose material
Master patient index (MPI)
Microfilm
Natural language processing (NLP)
Numeric filing system
Outguide
Overlap
Overlay
Paper health record
Patient account number
Primary purpose
Probabilistic algorithm
Qualitative analysis
Quantitative analysis
Record reconciliation
Registry
Requisition
Research
Retrospective review
Rules-based algorithm
Secondary purpose
Serial numbering system
Serial-unit numbering system
Standard
Statistics
Straight numeric filing system
Terminal-digit filing system
Turnaround time
Unit numbering system
Version control
Voice recognition technology

The health record contains information relating to the physical or mental health or condition of an individual, as made by or on behalf of a health professional in connection with the care ascribed that individual. In other words, the health record contains the who, what, where, when, why, and how of patient care and is used for many reasons and by many people. When discussing these usages and users, it is important to understand the difference between three terms—*data, information,* and *knowledge*. The terms *data* and *information* are often used interchangeably but they are distinctly different. Data are raw facts and figures such as Hospital A discharged 560 patients last month. Information is data that have been turned into something meaningful such as Hospital A discharged 560 patients last month, which was up 10 percent from the prior month and 20 percent from this time last year. Knowledge is the information, understanding, and experience that give individuals the power to make informed decisions. For example, investigation identified that the increase in patients was primarily due to an increase in obstetrics patients. This increase in obstetrics patients is why the healthcare organization decided to investigate ways to improve its obstetric services.

Purposes of the Health Record

The uses of a health record can be divided into primary and secondary purposes. The primary purposes are those for which the health record is developed and used—patient care. The secondary purposes are those where the health record is used for healthcare purposes not directly related to patient care.

Primary Purposes

The primary purposes of the health record are related to providing care to the patient. Patient care includes the direct care provided and the day-to-day business of the healthcare organization. These usages can be categorized in the following ways:

- *Patient care*. One of the most important uses of the health record for patient care is the documentation of the care provided by physicians, nurses, and allied health professionals such as physical therapists and dietitians. This documentation serves as a communication tool between these healthcare professionals, as discussed in chapter 2, *Healthcare Delivery Systems*, and may contain treatments and the patient's response to the treatment. For more information on health record documentation, see chapter 4, *Health Record Content and Documentation*.
- *Management of patient care*. The health record is an important part of managing patient care services performed at the healthcare organization. The health record is used to develop patient care standards; conduct research at the local, state, and national levels; and evaluate the quality of care

provided. For more on quality, see chapter 18, *Performance Improvement*.

- *Administrative purposes*. The health record is used for administrative purposes including billing for services provided, making decisions about the future of the healthcare organization, monitoring the fiscal health of the organization, and scheduling staffing. Many administrative purposes are discussed in detail in chapter 13, *Research and Data Analysis*, chapter 14, *Healthcare Statistics*, chapter 15, *Revenue Management and Reimbursement*, and chapter 18.

Secondary Purposes

Healthcare is a sophisticated industry and information from the health record is used for many purposes not related specifically to patient care. These secondary purposes include the following:

- *Education of healthcare professionals*. Health records are used by medical, nursing, and other allied health professionals including health information management (HIM) to teach present and future healthcare providers how to document care provided, and how to manage the healthcare information. See chapter 20, *Human Resources Management*, for more on training.
- *Legal, accreditation, and policy development*. The health record is used to protect the healthcare organization from medical malpractice and other lawsuits, to monitor compliance with laws and regulations, and to adhere to accreditation standards. Information from the health record is also used at the national level to determine where funding will be allocated, as well as the direction the healthcare industry should take. For additional information on how the record is used for legal purposes, see chapter 8, *Health Law*, chapter 9, *Data Privacy and Confidentiality*, and chapter 10, *Data Security*.
- *Public health and research*. Data in the health record are aggregated and turned into information that is used at the national level to establish best practices of patient care, conduct research on new medications and technologies, and study patient outcomes. New diseases are continuously identified while current ones evolve, sometimes making them resistant to traditional treatment. The information from the health record is used to determine what traditional and nontraditional treatments are effective for these new diseases and conditions. Registries are covered in chapter 7, *Secondary Data Sources*. Local health departments use health information to identify outbreaks in diseases early so the source of the disease can be managed, and epidemics can be managed or prevented. For additional information regarding public health and research usage, see chapter 14, *Healthcare Statistics*.

Formats of the Health Record

To understand how the health record is used, it is important to understand the three types of health records: paper, electronic, and hybrid. The paper health record is completely available in paper media. Some portions of it may have been created electronically, like lab results, but the lab results are printed and filed in the paper health record. The electronic health record (EHR) is a digital record of an individual's health-related information that conforms to nationally recognized interoperability standards and that can be created, managed, and consulted by authorized clinicians and staff across more than one healthcare organization. The hybrid health record, also known as hybrid record, is a combination of the paper health record and the EHR. In the hybrid health record, some documents are stored in the paper health record while others are stored in the EHR. The electronic documents may or may not be printed and stored in the paper health record. These three types of health records are discussed in more detail later in this chapter.

Users of the Health Record

Healthcare providers are the primary users of the health record; however, others use the health record to manage the healthcare organization and the healthcare industry. Some users of the health record access and use the health record directly while others use data or information that has been aggregated from multiple health records. Aggregate data are data that have been extracted from individual health records and combined to form deidentified information about groups of patients that can be compared and analyzed. For example, aggregate data can be used to determine survival rates for various kinds of cancer or to determine if a new drug is safe. Deidentification is the removal of all data elements that can identify the patient.

Individual Users

Individual users are those who depend on the health record to complete their jobs. The way the health record is used varies by individual user. For example, nurses use physician orders to know how to care for the patient. The following are descriptions of these individual users:

- *Patient care providers*. Patient care providers include physicians, nurses, and other allied health professionals who rely on information from the health record to make decisions about the care provided to the patient and for documentation of care. Allied health professionals include respiratory therapists, nutritionists, physical therapists, and many more. (Chapter 2, *Healthcare Delivery Systems*, covers allied health professionals in more detail.)
- *Patient care managers and support staff*. Patient care managers evaluate the services provided by their employees. As care is documented in the health record, it becomes a key resource in their evaluation of the quality of care provided. The managers look for patterns and trends to recommend changes to the process to improve outcomes and efficiency of the care provided. Support staff gathers information for the patient care managers to use.
- *Coding and billing staff*. Documentation in the health record is the basis for reimbursement, or payment, for the care provided. The coding staff at the healthcare organization must read the entire health record and assign the appropriate diagnoses and procedure codes for treatment received during the encounter. The billing staff obtains the codes from the coders and submits the bill to the insurance company. (Chapter 15, *Revenue Management and Reimbursement*, covers reimbursement in more detail.)
- *Patients*. Patients are informed consumers of their healthcare. As informed consumers, patients may obtain access to and be informed about their health record by obtaining a copy of their health record, accessing a patient portal, or maintaining a personal health record. Personal health records are discussed later in this chapter. (Chapter 9, *Data Privacy and Confidentiality*, covers patient rights and the health record in more detail.)
- *Employers*. Employers may use health records when processing health insurance claims and in managing wellness programs. Employers may also use the health record to determine when employees are well enough to return to work after an injury or illness, although this is generally limited to a note from the physician giving his or her approval. When an employee claims disability due to a work-related incident, it is the information found in the health record that supports or refutes the claim.
- *Lawyers*. Lawyers may need access to support a client (the patient) for life insurance claims and lawsuits such as those related to motor vehicle crashes, disability, and such. The lawyer must obtain consent from the patient to access the patient's health information. To protect themselves from medical malpractice and other lawsuits,

healthcare organizations may grant lawyers access to patient records.

- *Law enforcement officials.* Law enforcement officials need access to health record documentation to investigate gunshot wounds and other injuries resulting from a crime. They also may access documentation for information that will help protect the security of the country.
- *Healthcare researchers and clinical investigators.* Healthcare researchers use health records to study the safety and efficacy of drugs or the value of care provided. The researcher's aggregate data and information based on these findings are used to approve new treatments and to stop unsafe treatments. How the health record is used in research is covered in more detail in chapter 14, *Healthcare Statistics.*
- *Government policy makers.* The health record may be used to develop and evaluate current and future laws, regulations, and standards related to healthcare. The data collected can help determine best practices, gaps in current legislation, and other issues that need to be addressed to improve care and prevent fraud.

Institutional Users

Institutional users are organizations that need access to health records to accomplish their mission. Institutional users include healthcare organizations, third-party payers, medical review organizations, research organizations, educational organizations, accreditation organizations, government licensing agencies, and policy-making bodies.

- *Healthcare organizations.* Healthcare organizations—including hospitals, physician offices, home health agencies, and others—use the health record to provide care, submit claims for reimbursement, and evaluate the quality of care provided.
- *Third-party payers.* Third-party payers are organizations responsible for the reimbursement of healthcare services through an insurance program. These insurance programs include commercial insurance, managed care organizations, government insurance programs, accountable care organizations, as well as self-insured employers. The health record is used to justify the care provided and therefore the reimbursement. For additional information, refer to chapter 15, *Revenue Management and Reimbursement.*
- *Medical review organizations.* Medical review organizations evaluate the quality and appropriateness of the care provided to the patient. Medicare hires organizations known as quality improvement organizations to determine if the care provided to the patient was medically necessary. See chapter 18, *Performance Improvement,* for more information on quality improvement organizations.
- *Research organizations.* Research organizations conduct medical research and include state disease registries such as the cancer registry, research centers, and others who explore diseases and their treatment.
- *Educational organizations.* Colleges and universities train healthcare professionals. The students in these programs use the health records as case studies as a part of the educational program.
- *Accreditation organizations.* To be granted and maintain accreditation, a healthcare organization must show compliance with the accrediting body standards. This frequently requires review of the health record to determine compliance with documentation and patient care standards. For example, the accreditation organization may require the history and physical (refer to chapter 4, *Health Record Content and Documentation*) to be completed within 24 hours of admission. To learn more about accreditation, see chapter 8, *Health Law.*
- *Government licensing agencies.* Government agencies at the local, state, and federal level review the health record to ensure compliance with state licensing requirements and to verify

compliance with standards that enable the healthcare organization to receive federal funding. A more detailed discussion on licensing is also included in chapter 8, *Health Law*.

- *Policy-making bodies*. The data submitted for healthcare claims to governmental databases and other sources are analyzed and utilized for decision-making related to healthcare programs. For example, the Centers for Medicare and Medicaid Services (CMS) utilize a wide range of data to revise reimbursement systems each year.

Check Your Understanding 3.1

Answer the following questions.

1. Identify an example of a primary purpose of the health record.
   a. Education
   b. Policy making
   c. Research
   d. Patient care
2. Identify the institutional user that utilizes health record data to make decisions regarding healthcare programs.
   a. Educational organization
   b. Policy-making body
   c. Research organization
   d. Third-party payer
3. The entire health record at our healthcare organization is accessible online. We utilize a(n):
   a. Paper health record
   b. Personal health record
   c. EHR
   d. Hybrid health record
4. Identify a type of individual user.
   a. Policy-making body
   b. Government licensing agency
   c. Patient
   d. Accreditation organization
5. Deidentified data are used for:
   a. Education of healthcare professionals
   b. Public health and research
   c. Investigating gunshot wounds
   d. Patient care

Overview of HIM Functions

The HIM department performs many functions to support patient care and the healthcare organization. The functions focus on ensuring the quality, security, and availability of the health record. Some functions are performed in the HIM department, while others may be in their own department or outsourced. Outsourcing is the hiring of an individual or a company external to an organization to perform a function either on-site or off-site. Typical HIM functions include the following:

- Medical transcription and voice recognition
- Disclosure of health information
- Clinical coding and reimbursement
- Record storage and retrieval (paper and electronic)
- Statistics and research
- Master patient index
- Record storage and retrieval (paper and electronic)
- Record processing
- Registries (cancer, trauma, birth defects, and more)
- Birth and death certificate completion

The HIM department operates in conjunction with other departments to support and enhance their services including patient care, information governance, quality management, billing, and patient registration.

Medical Transcription and Voice Recognition

Medical transcription, the process of deciphering and typing medical dictation, may be a part of the HIM department or it may be a separate centralized department where all transcription services are performed. Transcription services may also be outsourced to another company. In that case, there should be a liaison between the HIM department and the transcription company. This liaison would work with physicians, monitor turnaround time, monitor the quality of the work, and more. Commonly transcribed reports include history and physical, discharge summary, pathology reports, procedure reports (such as colonoscopy and cardiac catheterization), and radiology reports. See chapter 4, *Health Record Content and Documentation*, for a description of these reports.

The transcription manager is responsible for monitoring the quality of the documents and services performed. The transcription supervisor should review a sample of the documents typed to ensure that proper formatting was used, there were no typographical or other errors, and it was transcribed in a timely manner. The date dictated and the date transcribed should be recorded on the document. The expected turnaround time is determined by the healthcare organization and may vary by document. For example, a radiology report may be transcribed within 24 hours and a discharge summary within three days of dictation.

Today, healthcare organizations may use speech recognition to go directly from dictation to a typed document. There are two strategies to be considered with speech recognition. Front-end speech recognition occurs when physicians review and edit the document directly upon dictation and then can sign it immediately. The document is available quickly with this strategy. The other strategy is back-end speech recognition. In this strategy, the transcriptionists become editors, making corrections to the document rather than typing it. Because they review and edit the document after dictation, the physician cannot sign the document until a later time. The advantage is that the physician can focus on patient care rather than correcting any issues in the document.

Disclosure of Health Information

One of the responsibilities of the HIM department is disclosure of health information. **Disclosure of health information** is the process of disclosing patient-identifiable information from the health record to another party. The HIM department receives a request for access to patient information, ensures that the request is appropriate for release, and then submits the information for use in patient care, insurance claims, legal claims, or other purpose. Disclosure of health information can be performed internally or can be outsourced to a disclosure of health information company. For more information on disclosure of health information and privacy requirements, see chapter 9, *Data Privacy and Confidentiality*.

The disclosure of health information supervisor is responsible for ensuring policies and procedures are followed, requests are processed in a timely manner, and the staff meets their productivity requirements. Quality control for the disclosure of health information function includes ensuring the health records are available first and foremost for patient care. It also includes ensuring the requested documents and only the requested documents are released or disclosed.

The supervisor is responsible for ensuring turnaround times are met. Turnaround time is the time between receipt of request and when the information is sent to the requester. The disclosure of health information system discussed later in this chapter can report this statistic.

The disclosure of health information staff is responsible for documenting to whom information is released, when it was released, and specifically what was released. This is known as an Accounting of Disclosure Log. This includes specific document(s) and the dates of service. A copy of the formal request for copies of patient information must be retained by the HIM department.

Clinical Coding and Reimbursement

Clinical coding, or assigning codes to represent diagnoses and procedures, is a key responsibility of the HIM department. Several coding systems can be used. During the coding process, data are abstracted into the information system. Abstracting can be either the process of extracting information from a document to create a brief summary of a patient's illness, treatment, and outcome, or the process of extracting elements of data from a source document or database and entering them into an automated system. The amount of data abstracted for coding purposes varies by healthcare organization but includes data such as date of surgery, surgeon, and disposition of patient upon discharge (went home, transferred to another hospital, and so forth). The codes are included on the bill and are used to determine reimbursement that the healthcare organization will receive. The coding supervisor must ensure the quality of code assignment and the timeliness of the coding process. If the coding process gets behind, the encounters cannot be billed, thus ensuring that reimbursement for patient care is delayed. For more information on coding, refer to chapter 15, *Revenue Management and Reimbursement*.

Record Storage and Retrieval Functions

A healthcare organization cannot move quickly from a paper-based record to an electronic record. The transition to the EHR can take years and often involves a hybrid record—part of the health record on paper and part of it electronic. During this time, some functions will be handled as described in the paper-based record environment while others may be handled electronically. As the percentage of the record digitized increases, more of the functions will be as described in the electronic record environment.

A common information system that is used during this transition period is the document management system (DMS). The DMS scans the paper record and stores it digitally. The user has the benefits of immediate access but unfortunately the user is not able to manipulate the data as the document is stored as a picture, not data. One of the advantages of a DMS is the ability to control the workflow electronically. The workflow is not limited to the HIM department but can be automatically routed to other users throughout the healthcare organization.

During the period of transition to an EHR, it is difficult to identify the legal health record as some of it is paper, some is electronic (and may be in a multitude of information systems), and some documents are created electronically but may be printed and stored in the paper health record. (Chapter 4, *Health Record Content and Documentation*, covers the legal health record in more detail.) This period is also challenging as the HIM department must manage both the paper and the electronic documents.

Master Patient Index

The master patient index (MPI) is the permanent record of all patients treated at a healthcare organization. It is used by the HIM department to look up patient demographics, dates of care, the patient's health record number, and other data. Demographics, also known as demographic data, are basic information about the patient such as their name, address, date of birth, and insurance information. The MPI is an important element of a numeric filing system (discussed later in this chapter) as it allows the user to look up the patient health record number so the record can be located. When a healthcare enterprise has more than one healthcare organization (such as hospital and ambulatory clinic) and the patient is seen at two or more places, the **enterprise master patient index (EMPI)** links the patient's information at the different healthcare facilities. The recommended core data elements for the EMPI are the following:

- Internal patient identification
- Person name
- Date of birth
- Gender
- Race
- Ethnicity
- Address
- Telephone number
- Alias, previous, or maiden names
- Social security number
- Facility identification
- Universal patient identifier
- Account or visit number
- Admission or visit number
- Admission, encounter, or visit data
- Discharge or departure date
- Encounter service type
- Encounter primary physician
- Patient disposition (AHIMA 2010)

Before computerization, the MPI was maintained on index cards; now the MPI is generally electronic, which allows for alphabetic and phonetic search capabilities, as well as the ability to search numerous data elements such as patient name, health record number, and billing number. A phonetic search retrieves names that sound the same; for example, Burgur, Burger, Berger, and Burgher. Figure 3.1 provides an example of an input screen for an electronic MPI system.

The health record number is created by the MPI and the numbers are issued in sequential numeric order. For example, Ms. Smith is admitted to the healthcare organization at 4:00 p.m. and is issued the health record number of 156876. When Ms. Jones, the next new patient, is admitted at 4:06 p.m., she is issued the health record number of 156877.

Figure 3.1 Input screen for an electronic MPI system

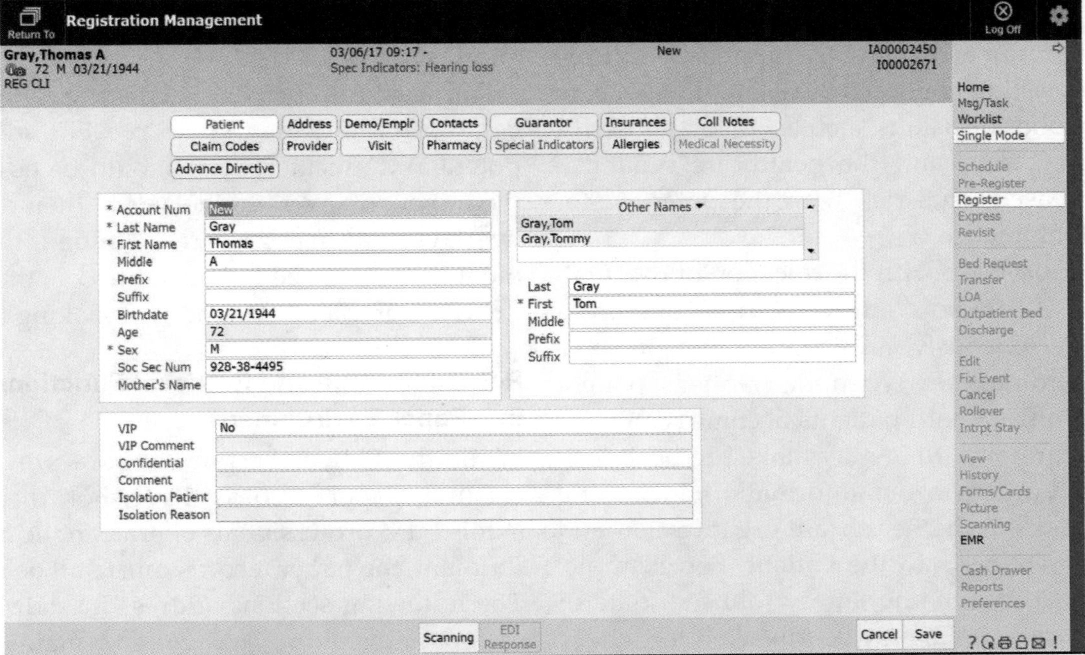

Source: MEDITECH Registration. Used with permission from MEDITECH Practice.

Unfortunately, there are data quality issues that result from improper issuance of health record numbers. Typographical errors, outdated demographic information, and other data quality issues are always present in the MPI. For example, patients change their name, identify themselves by their nickname, move, or change phone numbers. Some errors occur through data entry; for example, entering the birthday of January 1, instead of January 11. The erroneous information is then shared with other information systems, exacerbating the problem. It takes a lot of time to identify and correct the erroneous information. Some of the more common problems include duplicates, overlays, and overlaps.

When the patient is registered in the admissions department, previous MPI information may not be retrieved if the clerk does not conduct a thorough search for the patient or if the patient gives a different name. For example, the patient may give her new married name rather than her maiden name. The patient may also give a nickname, such as Bob, rather than his legal name, Robert. This results in a duplicate health record number being issued. A **duplicate health record** results when the patient has two or more health record numbers issued. The patient's health information becomes fragmented with some information under the first number and the remainder under the second number. When this happens, duplicate laboratory testing may occur, causing unnecessary expenses, poor decisions such as misdiagnoses or unnecessary tests, and the healthcare organization's increased legal risk with the potential for medical malpractice.

Another problem with the question of the quality of the MPI is an **overlay**. With an overlay, a patient is erroneously assigned another person's health record number. When this happens, patient information from both patients becomes commingled and care providers may make medical decisions based on erroneous information, increasing the legal risks to the healthcare organization and quality of care risks to the patient. For example, a patient with the name Jeffery Johnson, date of birth January 1, 1962, may be mistaken for Jeffery Johnson, date of birth January 1, 1957. One of the more common reasons for this is an error in selecting the correct patient by the hospital staff.

A third issue is an **overlap**, or when a patient has more than one health record number at different locations within an enterprise or healthcare organization. This frequently becomes an issue when healthcare organizations merge or create an EMPI.

A healthcare organization must work to protect the integrity of the data in the MPI. Most errors are human. The clerk may transpose numbers, make typographical errors or use poor search strategies that fail to find the patient in the information system, or the patient may give inaccurate information.

All healthcare organizations must have processes in place to maintain and correct the MPI against the quality issues of duplicates, overlays, and overlaps on a continuous basis. Algorithms are used to match patients so the patient information can be merged. There are three types of matching algorithms typically found in the MPI. The first, a **deterministic algorithm**, requires exact matches in data elements such as the patient name, date of birth, and social security number. The second, a **probabilistic algorithm**, uses mathematical probabilities to determine the possibility that two patients are the same. The third, a **rules-based algorithm**, assigns weights to specific data elements and uses those weights to compare one record to another (AHIMA 2010).

This clean-up process is ongoing. There should be a formal process to help prevent and identify potential duplicates. Staff should be educated on the impact of errors in the MPI. When duplicates, overlays, and overlaps are identified, the department managers need to be notified so they can address the problem with the staff making the errors.

Record Storage and Retrieval Functions in a Paper Environment

While the EHR is becoming more prevalent, the existing paper records have not disappeared. While HIM professionals operate in the EHR environment, the paper records must still be managed. The following sections address the HIM processes for the creation, storage, and maintenance of paper-based records.

The HIM department is responsible for the storage and retrieval of the paper-based record. Policies and procedures should be in place to ensure access to the health records for authorized users but to prevent access for unauthorized users. In a paper-based record, the documentation is typically stored alphabetically or numerically in a special file folder. Healthcare organizations may also file their paper-based records off-site, on microfilm, or digitally as scanned documents.

In a paper-based record filing system, the folders containing the health records are stored in shelving units or in filing cabinets based on the health record number or patient name. The filing systems used are the following alphabetic filing systems, numeric filing systems, and alphanumeric filing systems.

- ***Alphabetic Filing System*** In the alphabetic filing system, health records are filed in alphabetic order. This system works well with a small volume of health records such as in a physician practice. Employees are comfortable with it and the filing system is easy to create and use. A disadvantage is that there is no unique identifier as patients can have the same name. Another problem is the alphabetic filing system does not expand evenly. Statistically almost half of the files fall under the letters B, C, H, M, S, and W. Figure 3.2 contains rules for alphabetic filing.
- ***Numeric Filing Systems*** In a numeric filing system, the health records are filed by the health record number. The MPI is consulted to identify the health record number and then the number is used to locate the health record. This may seem like more work than the alphabetic system but there are many advantages to the numeric filing system. The most common types of numeric filing systems are the following:
  - The straight numeric filing system files the records in straight numeric order based on the health record number. This filing system is easy to teach to new employees; however, the most active area in the files is the higher numbers, which are the most current files, making it difficult to manage. Management problems include the higher number of department staff in one section of the file room and the space required by the health records may exceed the amount available.
  - The terminal-digit filing system may sound backward, but it is typically considered the most efficient of the numeric filing systems in part because it distributes health records evenly throughout the filing units. It is also effective for healthcare facilities with a heavy record volume. The health records are filed by the last two digits, called the terminal digits, then the middle two digits, known as the secondary unit. The health records are then filed by the first two or three numbers, known as the tertiary units. See figure 3.3 for an example.
- ***Alphanumeric Filing System*** As the name alphanumeric filing system indicates, both alphabetic and numeric characters are used to sort health records in this system. The first two letters of the patient's last name are followed by a unique numeric identifier such as SA2567. This filing system is appropriate for small healthcare facilities. Like numeric systems, alphanumeric filing systems require an MPI.

Paper health records are frequently filed in a centralized unit filing system. In a centralized unit filing system, any patient encounters are filed together in a single location. For example, a patient may be seen in radiology for a mammogram and in the laboratory for a urinalysis. These test results will be filed together. This type of filing system is usually associated with the unit numbering system; the unique identifiers can be alphabetic, alphanumeric, or numeric depending on the needs of the healthcare organization.

Storage Systems for Paper-Based Records Several options are available for storing paper records including filing cabinets, shelving units, microfilm, off-site storage, and image-based storage.

Figure 3.2 Rules for alphabetic filing

1. File each record alphabetically by the last name, followed by the first name and middle initial. For example:

   Brown, Michelle L.

   Brown, Michelle S.

   Brown, Robert A.

   When patients have identical last and first names and middle initials, order the records by date of birth, filing the record with the earliest birthdate first.
2. Last names beginning with a prefix or containing an apostrophe are filed in strict alphabetical order, ignoring any apostrophes or spaces. For example, the name D'Angelo would be filed as Dangelo.
3. Names beginning with the abbreviation St., such as St. Clair, are filed as S-a-i-n-t.
4. In hyphenated names such as Burchfield-Sayles, the hyphenation is ignored, and the record is filed as Burchfieldsayles.
5. If a name is given as an initial, the rule is "file nothing before something." For example, Smith, J would be filed before Smith, Jane.
6. Mac and Mc can be filed either way but there should be a policy stating whether Mac or Mc will be used.

Source: Huffman 1994.

Figure 3.3 Terminal-digit filing system example

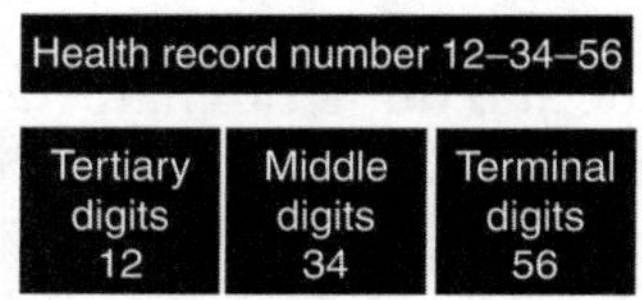

Source: ©AHIMA.

The storage choice for health records depends on the needs and storage capacity of the healthcare organization.

Vertical and lateral filing cabinets, open shelves, or compressible filing units can all be used for storage of records. Vertical and lateral filing cabinets are seen in most office settings and usually contain two or four drawers. These small filing cabinets are only appropriate for low-volume storage as it is challenging to quickly access health records from the drawers.

Typically, an HIM department uses open shelving units that resemble bookcases and can store large volumes of files that are easy to view and access. Multiple shelves separated by aisles large enough for a person to walk through to access the files can be used. A common variation is compressible filing units, where there is not an aisle between each shelving unit but instead one or two aisles while the rest of the units are collapsed together. These shelving units move and the aisles open and close as needed. The units are on tracks, which allow the units to be moved to open up the aisle.

Files of patients who have not been at the healthcare organization for a specified period, such as two years, may be purged or removed from the active filing area. The time period and frequency of purging depends on the space available, patient readmission rate, and the need for access to the health record. For more information on retention and destruction, see chapter 9, *Data Privacy and Confidentiality*.

An important role of the HIM professional is to determine the space requirements needed to store the paper health record by evaluating the volume indicators such as number of discharges, size of records, and the capacity of the storage units. For example, the space needed can be estimated with the following information:

Shelving unit shelf width = 36 inches

Number of shelves per unit = 8 shelves

Average record thickness = ½ inch

Average annual inpatient discharges = 10,200

The following demonstrates how these statistics are used to estimate the number of shelving units to store one year of health records.

1. Determine the linear inch capacity of each shelving unit.
   36 inches per shelf x 8 shelves per unit = 288 inches per shelving unit
2. Determine the linear filing inches needed for the volume of records.
   10,200 average annual inpatient discharges x ½ inch average record thickness = 5,100 inches required to store one year of inpatient discharge records
3. Determine the number of shelving units required by dividing the required filing space by the shelving unit linear inch capacity.
   5,100/288 = 17.7 = 18 shelving units

Since it is impossible to purchase a part of a shelving unit, the number of shelving units required should always be rounded up to a whole number. This example only included inpatient discharges for simplicity; however, outpatient health records would also have to be considered.

In vertical and lateral filing cabinets, open shelves, or compressible filing units, file folders are used to hold paper health records. File folders used for health records are usually purchased in one of two standard weights or thicknesses—11 points and 14 points—although the weight may be as much as 20 points. The higher the points, the more durable the file folder. The amount of filing and retrieval activity will impact the decision. Typically, side tabs are used for health records, but top tabs may be used in lateral shelving units. Two-pronged record fasteners should be placed at the top or sides of the file folder to hold the health record forms in place.

File folders should be color coded for easy filing and retrieval. For example, the tab on the file folder has a label that displays a single digit of the health record number in a specific color. This makes it easy to identify misfiled records. For example, a yellow label would stand out in a row of green and red. Typically, the file folders are purchased with the color-coding already applied, but labels can be applied manually.

Paper health records require a great deal of space. One way to reduce the amount of space required is to microfilm the health record, which is a photographic process that reduces an original paper document into a small static image on film. Microfilm has been used for decades by healthcare facilities and works well for inactive or infrequently used health records. A photo image is taken of each page of the health record and stored as a small negative. A microfilm viewer is required to read the image. The following are the different formats:

- *Roll microfilm*. The microfilm images are stored on a long roll of film. Each roll can store thousands of images for hundreds of patients. The major problem with this format is that patient encounters can be stored on multiple rolls, making retrieval difficult.
- *Jacket microfilm*. A roll of microfilm is cut and inserted into four-by-six-inch jackets with sleeves. Multiple jackets containing all episodes of care that have been microfilmed can be filed together to maintain the unit-record. The same type of filing systems that apply to paper records can be used.
- *Microfiche*. This format is a copy of the jacket microfilm. Microfiche is the same size as the microfilm jacket. Some facilities use microfiche rather than allow the original jacket microfilm outside of the HIM department (for example, microfiche would be sent to the nursing unit for patient care).

Inactive records can be stored off-site and copied on microfilm. The healthcare organization would define when a health record becomes inactive. The off-site location may be under the control of the healthcare organization or a commercial company that stores and retrieves the organization's health records for a fee. The healthcare organization must meet privacy and security regulations in terms of storage of health records. The vendor must be able to protect the health records from fire, pests, burglary, and other hazards. The commercial vendor must be able to return the records to the healthcare organization within a predetermined time. The health records can be faxed, scanned, and emailed, or hand-delivered to the healthcare organization.

Image-based storage is used when the document is scanned and storing it digitally on hard drives, CD, or another storage media. The file formats also vary but are typically picture file formats such as .tif or .jpg. The advantage of image-based storage over microfilm is that each document can be indexed or identified by patient or document type. The image itself cannot be searched but the indexed information is used to retrieve patient information. Retrieval of the images with a few keystrokes is a much quicker method than microfilm retrieval.

Retrieval and Tracking Systems for Paper-Based Records? Health records must be accessible to authorized users. A common way of tracking the location of a health record is the outguide. The outguide identifies where the health record is located and when it was removed. It is generally made of colored vinyl with two plastic pockets and it is placed in the shelving unit where the health record should be. The outguide is approximately the size of the health record. The larger plastic pocket can hold documentation that needs to be filed in the health record, known as loose material, which includes dictated reports, reports not filed on the nursing unit, and such. The small pocket can be used to hold a slip of paper that tells where the record has been moved to and when it was checked out.

Traditionally, when a patient care area or other department in the healthcare organization needs a health record, they submit a requisition, or request, for the health record. The requisition tells the HIM department the name, health record number, date of request, name of requester, and where the health record needs to be delivered. The requisition can be handwritten or be generated by an information system.

Today, automated systems frequently create the requisition and replace the outguide. In an automated chart tracking system, the computer keeps up with the location of the health record by "checking out" the health record to the nursing unit or other location. Because of this, an outguide is not needed to record the location of the health record but may still be used to hold the documents to be filed.

Record Processing of Paper-Based Records Record processing ensures health records are organized and meet standards. These functions help ensure the accessibility and completeness of the health record. When the quality of the health record is not maintained, patient care suffers due to missing, inaccurate, or incomplete information and it also impacts billing, research, and other purposes. Record processing includes the following processes:

- ***Admission and Discharge Record Reconciliation for Paper-Based Records*** When a patient is admitted to the healthcare organization, a search of the MPI is performed to identify if the patient has been at the healthcare organization before. If so, then the paper health record(s) from the previous encounters will be made available for patient care. Once the patient is discharged from the healthcare organization, the health record is taken to the HIM department for processing. The first task is to ensure all health records have been received. This process is known as record reconciliation.
- ***Record Assembly Function for Paper-Based Records*** Assembly is the process of ensuring each page in the health record is organized in a standardized format, which varies by healthcare organization. During the assembly process each page should be reviewed to ensure all the pages belong to the same patient and same encounter.
- ***Analysis for Paper-Based Records*** Analysis, or review, of the health record is performed by HIM department personnel to determine the completeness of the health record. Two types of analysis should be performed—qualitative and quantitative.

Qualitative analysis is monitoring the quality of the documentation. This is a collaborative effort among the HIM department, risk management, healthcare providers, and others. While the physicians must review the quality of physician documentation, nurses review nurse documentation, and so forth, HIM professionals can review legibility, timeliness of documentation, use of approved abbreviations, and other documentation standards.

Quantitative analysis is a review of the health record to determine if there are any missing reports, forms, or signatures. This analysis can be performed by concurrent review—in an ongoing manner while the patient is still in the healthcare organization. It can also be reviewed after discharge from the healthcare organization, known as retrospective review. The review involves the following:

- All forms and reports contain correct patient identification (name, health record number, encounter number, and date of service)
- All forms and reports are present
- Reports requiring signatures are signed

The healthcare organization would base their review on accreditation standards, state licensure, and other standards. When a document or signature is missing, a deficiency slip is created. The deficiency slip identifies the pertinent document and what needs to be done (dictated, completed, and signed), and is often created by a computer system. An example of a deficiency slip is shown in figure 3.4.

When a deficiency is identified in the health record, it must be corrected. This may require locating a missing document or asking the physician or other healthcare provider to either sign or complete a document. The specific analysis performed depends on the medical staff bylaws, rules, and regulations, as well as state licensing and accreditation requirements.

Monitoring Completion of Paper-Based Records

Physicians and other practitioners are notified when they have incomplete health records requiring their attention. They usually come to the HIM department to complete the necessary documentation in the health record. The health records are then reanalyzed to ensure everything has been completed. If no deficiencies are identified, the deficiency slip is removed, and the health record is filed away in the permanent file. If a health record remains incomplete for a specified number of days as defined in the medical staff rules and regulations, the record is considered a delinquent record. The specific number of days varies by healthcare organization but is generally 15 to 30 days.

Figure 3.4 Sample deficiency slip

Physician/Practitioner's Name: ______

Health Record Number: ______

Patient's Name: ______

Discharge Date: ______

Analyzed by: ______

Date: ______

Signatures required	**Dictation required**	**Missing reports**
____ History	____ History	____ History
____ Physical	____ Physical	____ Physical
____ Consultation	____ Consultation	____ Consultation
____ Operative report	____ Operative report	____ Operative report
____ Discharge summary	____ Discharge summary	____ Discharge summary
		____ Radiology report
Other	Other	____ Pathology report
____ ________	____ ________	____ Progress notes
____ ________	____ ________	
____ ________	____ ________	Other
		____ ________
		____ ________
		____ ________

Source: Cerrato and Roberts 2012.

Handling Corrections and Addendums in Paper-Based Records Occasionally, health records must be corrected, amended, or deleted. There are a number of reasons for this. Information may be written in the wrong patient's health record, information may have been omitted, or an error may have been made in documentation. Policies must be in place to ensure the integrity of the health record.

Corrections to the health record should be made by drawing a single line through the erroneous information and writing the word "error" above the mistake. The practitioner should sign, date, and time the correction. An **addendum** is additional information provided in the health record. The addendum should be dated the day it was written—not the date it is referencing. It should be signed, and the time of entry should be recorded. An **amendment** is a clarification made to healthcare documentation after the original document has been signed. It should be dated, timed, and signed.

Forms Design, Development, and Control for Paper-Based Records Forms should be designed using appropriate form design principles that will enhance the documentation on the form. The form must meet the needs of the end user, which means it should be easy to use and include all necessary data.

The purpose of the form should be identified before development of the form begins to ensure the appropriate data are included; and the form should not duplicate one that is already in use. Users should be involved in development of the form to ensure their needs are met. Effective form design principles include the following.

- All forms should contain a unique identifying number for positive identification and inventory control.
- Each form should include original and revised dates for the tracking and purging of obsolete forms.
- Each form should have a concise title that clearly identifies the form's purpose.
- The healthcare organization's name and logo should appear on each page of the form, preferably in the same location on each.
- For clinical forms, patient identification information (name, health record number, billing number, physician name and number, date of birth, admission date, and room number) should appear on every page.
- For clinical forms, a signature line should appear at the bottom and there should be no question about what has been authenticated. If initials are used, space also should be provided for the full name and title so that each set of initials is identified.
- Data-entry methodology should be considered when the information is to be keyed into a computer. The order of the form should mirror the data-entry order to ensure the information is entered consistently.
- Optical character reader codes and bar codes should be printed in the upper left-hand corner of the form when imaging the health record is a possibility.
- A standard of 8.5 by 11 inches is the best size for a document.
- Form colors should be black ink on white paper. If color coding is desired, a strip of color along one margin is the best option.
- Documents that contain punched holes should have a margin of at least 3/4 inch. All other margins should be at least 3/8-inch wide.
- Vertical and horizontal lines assist the user in completing and reviewing the form. Bold lines should be used to draw the reader's eye to an important field.
- Sufficient space should be provided to complete the entry (for example, 1/16 inch for typed letters and 1/3 inch for handwritten entries).
- Titles for boxes and fields should be located in the top left-hand corner of the box or field.
- Paper ranging from 20 to 24 pounds in weight is recommended for use in copiers, scanners, and fax machines.
- Type size should be no smaller than 9 points for lowercase letters and 10 points for uppercase letters (AHIMA 1997).

When a document management system is used, form design is critical as the color in both the paper and the ink can negatively impact the quality of the image and should be eliminated or reduced. Forms that will be scanned should have a bar code imprinted on them allowing the automatic indexing into the health record.

Every healthcare organization should have a clinical forms committee to establish standards for design and to approve new and revised forms. The committee should also have oversight of computer screens and other data capture tools. The committee should be comprised of users of health information and include representatives from the following areas:

- HIM
- Medical staff
- Nursing staff
- Purchasing
- Information services
- Performance improvement
- Support or ancillary departments
- Forms vendor representatives

Representatives from the area that will use the form should attend the committee meeting to explain the form and the need for it.

Without oversight the number of forms can become overwhelming to manage and there can be duplication. A forms control program includes the following:

- *Establishing standards.* Written standards and guidelines should ensure that effective forms design principles, as previously discussed, are used. These standards should be recorded in a forms manual. **Standards** are fixed rules that must be followed. A **guideline** provides general direction about the design of the form.
- *Establishing a number and tracking system.* As stated earlier, a unique number should be assigned to each form. There should be a master form index and a copy of all forms should be maintained. The master form index should include the title, number, origination date, revision dates, purpose, and legal requirements.
- *Establishing a testing and evaluation plan.* New and revised forms should be tested prior to their implementation to ensure data elements are not missing and that there is enough space to write.
- *Checking the quality of new forms.* A process should be in place to guarantee that the printed forms were printed correctly.
- *Systematizing storage, inventory, and distribution.* There must be a process to store and distribute the forms where and when they are needed.
- *Establishing a forms database.* An electronic database should be used to store and facilitate updating forms.

Quality Control Functions in Paper-Based Systems: There must be processes in place to safeguard the quality of analysis and forms design. Each function should have its own acceptable level of performance and monitoring should be performed to confirm the standards are met. If not, corrective actions should be taken. See chapter 18, *Performance Improvement,* for more on quality improvement.

Several components of storage and retrieval are monitored. Managers monitor misfiles, timeliness of storage and retrieval to calculate filing accuracy, and timeliness rates. Examples of standards include the following:

- An average of 50 health records will be filed in an hour
- Records for the emergency department will be retrieved within 10 minutes of the request
- Loose materials will be filed in either the health record or the outguide pocket within 24 hours of receipt in the HIM department

To complete health records in a paper media, the physician must come to the HIM department to dictate, sign, or otherwise complete the health record. If health records are unavailable to the physician when he or she tries to complete the health record, the completion of the health record is delayed. The manager monitors the number of health records not available to physicians, usually weekly.

Check Your Understanding 3.2

Answer the following questions.

1. Identify the microfilm format that is inefficient when retrieving multiple admissions for a patient.
   a. Roll
   b. Jacket
   c. Microfiche
   d. Both roll and jacket
2. The decision was made to choose a filing system that distributes health records evenly throughout the filing system. This is known as:
   a. Alphanumeric
   b. Alphabetic
   c. Straight numeric
   d. Terminal digit
3. _____ is used to assign weights to potential duplicate health records.
   a. Rules-based algorithm
   b. Deterministic algorithm
   c. Probabilistic algorithm
   d. Overlays
4. Form design standards should include:
   a. Using color to separate the various sections
   b. Using colored paper
   c. Using 8 1/2 by 13-inch paper
   d. Assigning a unique identifier
5. Differentiate between qualitative analysis and quantitative analysis.
   a. Qualitative analysis looks at the quality of documentation and quantitative analysis looks for the presence of documents or signatures.
   b. Quantitative analysis looks at the quality of documentation and qualitative analysis looks for the presence of documents or signatures.
   c. Qualitative analysis looks at the documentation standards and quantitative analysis looks for the presence of documents or signatures.
   d. Quantitative analysis looks for duplicates, overlays, and overlaps; qualitative analysis looks for the presence of documents or signatures.
6. The forms design committee:
   a. Provides oversight for the development, review, and control of forms and computer screens
   b. Is responsible for the EHR implementation and maintenance
   c. Is always a subcommittee of the quality improvement committee
   d. Is an optional function for the HIM department
7. In a paper-based system, individual health records are organized in a standardized order in which of the following processes?
   a. Retrieval
   b. Assembly
   c. Analysis
   d. Reordering

8. Extracting data from a health record and entering it into an information system is known as:
   a. Assembly
   b. Indexing
   c. Abstracting
   d. Coding
9. Two patients were given the same health record number. This is an example of a(n):
   a. Overlap
   b. Overlay
   c. Duplicate
   d. Purge
10. The physician did not complete the health record in the time frame required by the medical staff rules and regulations. These records are known as:
   a. Suspended
   b. Delinquent
   c. Loose
   d. Default

Record Storage and Retrieval in an Electronic Environment

The functions of the HIM department have changed dramatically with the introduction of the EHR. The EHR is an electronic record of health-related information on an individual that conforms to nationally recognized interoperability standards and that can be created, managed, and consulted by authorized clinicians and staff across more than one healthcare organization. Because of the changes, the paper health record is gradually being eliminated.

Record Filing and Tracking of EHRs Filing of health records is significantly reduced or even eliminated in the EHR environment. As more data are captured directly into the EHR, there is no need for paper or the storage of paper-based records. The EHR can track who has access to a record through the audit trail. An audit trail is a chronological set of computerized records that provides evidence of information system activity (log-ins and log-outs, file accesses) used to determine security violations. Audit logs are covered in more detail in chapter 10, *Data Security*.

Record Processing of EHRs In the EHR, the assembly process is eliminated; however, even if the healthcare organization does not use paper documents, they may receive papers from the patient or other sources. These loose reports are scanned and indexed for inclusion in the EHR. Indexing is the linking of patient name, health record number, document type, and other identifying information to the scanned document.

Record completion in the EHR is performed via computer so healthcare professionals can complete them from any accessible location. An electronic work queue, or workflow, allows the health record to be routed to all healthcare professionals who have deficiencies so that they can access, complete, and authenticate the health record. The work queue is also used to route the health record to HIM for processing. With a document management system, one function does not have to be completed before the next one, so the health record is available for all functions. For example, the health record does not have to be analyzed before it is coded. Also, if coding cannot be performed for some reason, workflow will reroute the health record to coding once the problem has been resolved.

Version Control of EHRs The health record may have multiple versions of the same document; for example, a signed and unsigned copy of a document. Additional versions are also created when addendums, corrections, or amendments are made to original documents. To address the issues that result from having multiple versions of the same document, policies and procedures addressing version control must be developed. Version control identifies which version(s) of the documents is available to the user. All versions must be maintained but access to all except the current version should be controlled so that there is no confusion about which version is correct.

Management of Free Text in EHRs Free-text data are the unstructured narrative data that are the result of a person typing data into an information system. Free-text data are undefined, unlimited, and unstructured, meaning that the typist can type anything into the field or document. The amount of free-text data in the EHR should be limited because the ability to manipulate data is diminished with its use. For example, terms used in structured data are consistent, whereas synonyms may be used in free-text data, making it more difficult to retrieve. The preferred data type is structured text where you point and click or otherwise select the data. For example, you would have two choices with the data element gender: male and female. The user simply points and clicks the appropriate choice rather than typing it in.

In the EHR, the user can copy and paste free text from one patient or patient encounter to another. This practice is dangerous as inaccurate information can easily be copied. Specific risks to documentation integrity of using copy functionality include the following:

- Inaccurate or outdated information
- Redundant information, which makes it difficult to identify the current information
- Inability to identify the author or intent of documentation
- Inability to identify when the documentation was first created
- Propagation of false information
- Internally inconsistent progress notes
- Unnecessarily lengthy progress notes (AHIMA 2014, 4)

Policies and procedures need to be in place to reduce some of the risks.

Management and Integration of Digital Dictation, Transcription, and Voice Recognition A common method to capture dictation in the EHR is digital dictation. The physician or other healthcare provider dictates a health report and the transcriptionist types what is said into an electronic, or digital, format. These reports are electronically transmitted into the EHR where the physician can sign the document.

With voice recognition technology, also called continuous speech recognition or continuous speech technology, a computer captures the dictation and converts what is said directly into text and no transcriptionist is needed. The transcriptionist becomes an editor and therefore focuses on data quality. More specifically, natural language processing (NLP) is a technology that converts human language (structured or unstructured) into data that can be translated then manipulated by computer systems. It is the software used for speech recognition.

Reconciliation Processes for EHRs As in the paper-record environment, the HIM professional must verify that there is a complete health record for every episode of care, including both inpatients and outpatients. HIM professionals also need to verify documents sent to the EHR from a transcription system and other information systems arrive in the EHR as expected. For example, all patients admitted to the hospital should have an EHR created for that admission.

Managing Other Electronic Documentation Many documentation sources not previously stored in the paper health record are included in the electronic health record. Examples of these documentation sources include email, voicemail, audio, monitoring strips, images (radiology, pathology), video (heart catheterization), and monitoring (fetal, electrocardiogram).

Email is being used in healthcare to share patient information. Policies and procedures need to be in place to address privacy and security as well as the creation, storage, and maintenance of the messages. The email management system should allow emails containing patient information to be stored in the EHR.

Voicemail containing patient information can also be included in the EHR. The message should include the provider and patient identification, date and time of message, and the date and time of message into the EHR.

Handling Materials from Other Healthcare Organizations When materials are received from other healthcare organizations such as paper health records or diagnostic images, they should be handled per organizational policy; these typically are added to the health records. Some states have laws that address these external health records. If state law does not address health records from other healthcare facilities, then the healthcare organization attorney should be consulted regarding whether to include them in the health record (AHIMA 2011).

Search, Retrieval, and Manipulation Functions of EHRs One of the advantages of the EHR is the ability to search, retrieve, and manipulate health data quickly and easily. This information can be used for patient care, research, and monitoring patient care. In the paper health record, each patient record had to be reviewed individually and data abstracted into a database or another data collection tool. In the EHR, data mining can be performed. Data mining is the process of extracting and analyzing large volumes of data from a database for the purpose of identifying hidden and sometimes subtle relationships or patterns and using those relationships to predict behaviors. Data mining could be used to determine why one physician's outcomes are better or which medication is the most effective.

Handling Amendments and Corrections in EHRs Policies and procedures need to be in place to address amendments and corrections in the EHR. Once a document is authenticated, the document should be locked to prevent changes. If an amendment, addendum, or deletion needs to be made, the document would then need to be unlocked for editing. Not everyone should have the ability to unlock the documents; the organizational policies should state who has the rights to unlock the document (Brown et al. 2012). The EHR should retain the previous version of the document and identify who made the change along with the date and time the change was made. If the change impacts data sent to other information systems, then the change must be made in the other information systems as well.

Quality Control Functions for EHRs Data are collected in several ways: scanning, data entry, bar codes, and transfer of data from other information systems. The information system should have measures in place to control the data entered into the EHR. For example, when entering fields such as the social security number (SSN), an input mask should be used. An input mask shows the format in which the data will be displayed. Entering the SSN, the user should be able to input the number 123456789 and it will appear in the system as 123-45-6789. This prevents one user from entering the SSN as 123456789 and the other as 123-45-6789. A drop-down box that is pre-populated with acceptable entries is another way of controlling what is entered. For example, a drop-down box can be used for states as there are a finite number of states as choices. A checkbox can be used for yes or no type entries. Radio buttons allow the user to select from a small number of choices such as male and female in the gender field.

Best practices for designing or evaluating the entry screens are as follows. All these features help ensure the quality of documentation and therefore the quality of patient care.

General guidelines

- Clear navigational buttons that direct the user to the next step in the documentation process and buttons to move from one screen to another
- Clear labeling of buttons and data fields
- Limited use of abbreviations on buttons and data fields
- Consistent location on the screen of navigation buttons
- Built-in alerts to notify the user of possible errors
- Availability of references at the appropriate data field
- Prompt for more information where appropriate
- Checks for warning signs or errors

Navigation design

- Ensure all controls are clear and placed in an intuitive location on the screen
- Use neutral colors and limit highlighting, flashing, and so forth to reduce eye fatigue
- Limit choices and label commands
- Provide undo buttons to make mistakes easy to override
- Use consistent grammar and terminology
- Provide a confirmation message for any critical function (such as deleting a file)
- Identify required fields

Input design

- Simplify data collection
- Sequence data input to follow workflow
- Provide a title for each screen
- Minimize keystrokes by using pop-up menus
- Use text-specific boxes to enter text
- Use number-specific boxes to enter numbers
- Use a selection box to allow the user to select a value from a predefined list:
    - Check boxes (used for multiple selections)
    - Radio buttons (used for single selections)
    - On-screen list boxes
        - Drop-down list boxes
        - Combo boxes

Data validation

- Perform a completeness check to ensure all the required data have been entered
- Perform a format check to ensure the data are the right type (numeric, alphabetic, and so on)
- Perform a range check to ensure the numeric data are in the correct range such as appropriate range for temperature
- Perform a consistency check to ensure the combinations of data are correct
- Perform a database check to compare data against a database or file to ensure data are correct as entered

Output design

- Minimize the number of clicks needed to reach data or a specific screen
- Combine data into a single, organized menu to eliminate layers of screens (Williams 2006)

Identification Systems

Identification systems link the patient to the health record. The health record number is a key data element in the MPI as it is a unique identifier for the patient. It is used to look up the patient's health record number. The health record number is typically assigned during the patient's initial registration encounter at the healthcare organization. The social security number should not be used for the health record due to confidentiality concerns.

There are several ways to identify records in a paper-based health record system. These include numeric, alphabetic, and alphanumeric systems. For numeric systems to work, the health record number must be accessed in the MPI before the health record can be retrieved. The identification systems are serial numbering systems, unit numbering systems, serial-unit numbering systems, and alphabetic filing systems. In the EHR, identifiers such as the health record number, patient name, and more are used.

Paper Health Record – Serial Numbering System

In the serial numbering system, a patient is issued a unique numeric identifier for every encounter at the healthcare organization. If a patient is admitted to the healthcare organization five times, he or she will have five different health record numbers. The documentation for each of the encounters is filed in the health record for that encounter so the information is filed separately, and all health records must be retrieved to view the complete health information. The serial numbering system is inefficient and more costly because of the extra costs to manage the folders as well as to purchase the folders.

Paper Health Record – Unit Numbering System

The unit numbering system is commonly used in large healthcare organizations because it does not have many of the inefficiencies of the serial numbering system. The patient is issued a health record number at the first encounter and that number is used for all subsequent encounters. This system consolidates all the information on the patient in one location and is therefore more efficient than the serial numbering system.

Paper Health Record – Serial-Unit Numbering System

The serial-unit numbering system is a combination of the serial and unit numbering systems. The patient is issued a new health record number with each encounter, but all the documentation is moved from the last number to the new number. It would have many of the same advantages and disadvantages as the serial and unit numbering systems.

Paper Health Record – Alphabetic Filing System

The alphabetic filing system is typically used by small clinics and physician offices. The folders are filed alphabetically by the patient's last name. If there is more than one person with the same last name, then the first and middle initial are used. The disadvantage of this system is that more than one person may have the same or similar name.

Electronic Health Record

The unit numbering system is the most common system used in the EHR. The advantage of the EHR is that identifiers other than the health record number—such as the patient name and patient account number—can be used to retrieve the information. The patient account number is a number assigned by a healthcare organization for billing purposes that is unique to a particular episode of care; a new account number is assigned each time the patient receives care or services at the healthcare organization. It is easy to select the wrong person in the EHR, so it is important to double-check to ensure the correct person is retrieved.

Statistics and Research

Statistics is a branch of mathematics concerned with collecting, organizing, summarizing, and analyzing data. Traditionally statistics utilized by HIM related to patient volume including the number of admissions, number of discharges, and length of stay as manual data collection was time consuming. With the implementation of the EHR, a healthcare organization can easily generate a wide range of statistics. These statistics can be used to manage the business of the healthcare organization as well as to evaluate and improve the quality of the care provided.

Research is an inquiry process aimed at discovering new information about a subject or revising old information. Research utilizes statistics and other methods to evaluate new medical treatments, new drugs, best practices, and so forth. HIM professionals can assist in research through data collection, generating statistics, and data analysis. For more on statistics and research, refer to chapter 13, *Research and Data Analysis*, and chapter 14, *Healthcare Statistics*.

Registries

A registry is a collection of care information related to a specific disease, condition, or procedure that makes health record information available for analysis and comparison. Common registries include cancer, trauma, birth defects, and organ transplant. These registries collect data, and generate reports, among other functions. For example, the cancer registry evaluates life expectancy, numbers of cases, and much more. Chapter 7, *Secondary Data Sources*, discusses registries in more detail.

Birth and Death Certificates

Today, information systems are used to collect and share the data in birth and death certificates. Some, but not all, HIM departments are involved in collecting and reporting that data. The birth certificate data collected include data about the birth, the pregnancy, the parents, and more. Death certificates collect data on the patient, the time of death, the cause of death, and more. Chapter 14, *Healthcare Statistics*, discusses birth and death certifications, in more detail.

HIM Interdepartmental Relationships

The HIM department cannot manage information in isolation. The HIM department must work with many departments to ensure they have the information that they need to perform their jobs. These departments include the following:

- *Patient registration*. The health record typically begins in patient registration with the capture of patient demographic information. This information is entered into the MPI as discussed earlier. The health record is assigned to new patients during the patient registration process. The HIM department works with patient registration to ensure the quality of the data collected and to correct duplicate and other issues with the MPI.
- *Billing department (also known as patient financial services)*. The billing department uses the codes assigned and data abstracted by the coders as part of the billing process. Because of this, the billing department cannot perform their responsibilities until the HIM department completes theirs. The two departments must work together to ensure that all the information required for billing is available.
- *Patient care departments*. The HIM department works closely with nursing units, the emergency department, and other patient care areas to ensure they have access to the patient's health records from previous encounters. In a paper-based environment, the records are delivered by the HIM staff or picked up by the patient care areas and then the records are returned once they are no longer needed. The departments may send loose reports to the HIM department for filing if the health record has already been returned.
- *Information systems*. The interaction between the HIM department and the information systems department will continue to increase as the EHR becomes more and more important to the organization. The HIM staff works with the information systems staff to plan, implement, and maintain information systems that impact the health record and other systems related to HIM. The information systems department also assists the HIM department with technical issues related to computers, printers, and other hardware. For more information, see chapter 11, *Health Information Systems*.
- *Quality management*. The quality management department depends on the health record to complete their functions. They need health records for committee meetings, audits, and outcome monitoring. HIM staff may collect some of the data needed, provide the records, generate statistics, write reports, mine data, or assist in other ways.

Virtual HIM

Much of the work of the HIM department can be performed remotely due to the implementation of the EHR. Some healthcare corporations have centralized their HIM services into a single location. Many healthcare facilities have employees who work at home. Common functions that can be performed from home include coding and transcription, but others can be performed remotely as well. The manager must ensure the employees are able to work independently so that productivity standards can still be met. Chapter 1, *Health Information Management Profession,* discusses the future of the HIM profession in more detail.

HIM Information Systems

The HIM department cannot perform the functions of the department efficiently without the use of information systems. These information systems assist in health record processing, provide access to patient information, and more. Some of these information systems are becoming more and more important with the implementation of the EHR while others will be phased out completely as the EHR makes them obsolete. The information systems include disclosure of health information, chart tracking, coding, registries, billing, quality improvement, and electronic health record.

Disclosure of Health Information

The systems that track the disclosure of health information track requests for information from patients, insurance companies, and other requesters. HIM staff enters basic information from the request such as the patient name, health record number, and who is requesting the health record. Once the patient information is released, the staff records what information is released and the date. The information system can bill requesters for the copies of records, when appropriate. It can monitor productivity, turnaround time, and more.

Chart Tracking

This information system currently tracks the location of the health record but will eventually become obsolete when paper health records are eliminated. The chart tracking information system records who checked it out, where it went, and how long it has been checked out. It also records when the health record returns to the HIM department.

Coding

Coders use two specialty information systems—encoders and groupers. An **encoder** assigns the diagnosis and procedure codes. The encoder assists in the coding process as it reminds coders to check for important diagnoses and procedures and provides easy access to coding resources. The **grouper** uses the codes assigned to determine the diagnostic-related group or another grouping. (See chapter 15, *Revenue Management and Reimbursement,* for specifics on diagnostic-related groups.) Some healthcare organizations are now using **computer-assisted coding (CAC)**, which uses EHR data to assign the codes. With computer-assisted coding, the HIM professional monitors the quality of the codes assigned by the information system rather than assigning the code.

Registries

As stated earlier in this chapter, registry is a database on specific diseases and procedures; for example, cancer and transplant registries are common ones. In the registry, data regarding the diagnosis, procedure, or other concept is captured and can be used for research, patient care, and quality monitoring. The data captured and functionality varies by the type of registry. Chapter 7, *Secondary Data Sources,* discusses registries in more detail.

Billing

The HIM department may or may not directly use the billing system. The encoder and grouper may submit the codes and other data directly to the billing system or it may be entered manually by the coder. The HIM department does not create the bill but rather provides information that is included on the bill.

Quality Improvement

Quality improvement systems go by many different names and perform a number of functions. Characteristically, they are repositories of data that are used to monitor trends, generate statistics, monitor outcomes, and improve the quality of the documentation in the EHR. The data may be collected from the EHR or be manually entered by HIM professionals.

Electronic Health Records

The EHR utilizes several information systems to capture patient information. These source systems supply the EHR with demographic information, test results, dictated reports, and more. The EHR also has clinical decision support (CDS), which assists physicians and other users when making decisions regarding medications, diagnoses, and such based on the information entered into the EHR. The EHR contains alerts and reminders to notify the user of medication allergies, tests that should be performed, immunizations due, and so forth. Benefits of the EHR include reduction in administrative costs and improvement in quality of care. The healthcare organization becomes more efficient with the improved accessibility to health information.

Personal Health Records

A personal health record (PHR) is an electronic or paper health record maintained and updated by an individual for himself or herself; a tool that individuals can use to collect, track, and share past and current information about their health or the health of someone in their care. The PHR provides a way for a patient to be involved in his or her healthcare. It is not the same as an EHR, but rather is a subset of the information that is available to and controlled by the patient. The patient can add information to the PHR, such as over-the-counter medications and self-administered blood glucose test results. The PHR is especially useful for patients with complex, chronic conditions. The healthcare provider or the insurance company may provide the PHR, or the patient may purchase or subscribe to it from a commercial vendor. Refer to chapter 12, *Healthcare Information*, for additional details.

Check Your Understanding 3.3

Answer the following questions.

1. Identify the type of health record that is controlled by patients.
   a. Electronic health record
   b. Health record in any format
   c. Personal health record
   d. Certified health record
2. Explain how amendments to the EHR are handled.
   a. Amendments are automatically appended to the original note. No additional signature is required.
   b. Amendments must be entered by the same person as the original note.
   c. Amendments cannot be entered after 24 hours of the event.
   d. The amendment must have a separate signature, date, and time.
3. Version control of documents in the EHR requires:
   a. The deletion of old versions and the retention of the most recent
   b. Policies and procedures to control which version(s) is displayed
   c. Signed and unsigned documents not to be considered two versions
   d. Previous versions to be accessible to administration only
4. The decision was made to not allow copying and pasting. Justification for this decision includes:
   a. Reduction in the time required to document
   b. Information system may not save data
   c. Copying outdated information
   d. The ease in identifying the author of the documentation
5. When I key in 10101963, the computer displays it as 10/10/1963. What enables this?
   a. Toolkit
   b. Input mask
   c. Checkbox
   d. Radio button

Real-World Case 3.1

General Hospital knew they had issues with duplicate health records and needed to clean up the master patient index (MPI) before the implementation date for the electronic health record (EHR) to get the best results. A consulting firm was hired, and a review of the data confirmed this problem when they identified over 3,000 potential duplicate health records issued over the past five years. The hospital started the MPI cleanup process by educating their patient registration staff on proper search strategies, questions to ask the patient, the importance of a unit health record, and other related topics. This education was an important first step so that additional duplicate health records would not be assigned while the cleanup process was going on. Once the training was complete, the consulting firm began cleaning up the MPI. The consultants reviewed the potential duplicate health records and merged the health records where appropriate. They ensured the health records were merged in other information systems used throughout the healthcare organization. They provided documentation to General Hospital showing which health records were and were not duplicates based on their review. They also provided statistics on which admission clerks created duplicate health records, and the departments (admissions, emergency department, outpatient services and others) that created the duplicates.

Real-World Case 3.2

Yale New Haven Health received the 2018 Grace Award from AHIMA. They received this prestigious award for their efforts to improve the documentation in the health record, reducing errors in the MPI, and analyzing data from the EHR. They were able to get patients involved in the management of their health information. Yale New Haven Health was able to make significant improvements such as reducing the errors in the MPI to less than two percent. They also centralized their staff. HIM professionals were leaders in these initiatives. Their efforts allowed them to make good business decisions due to their emphasis on the quality of data (AHIMA 2018).

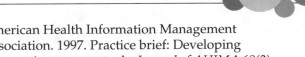

References

American Health Information Management Association. 2018. Grace W. Meyers Award. http://www.ahima.org/about/recognition.

American Health Information Management Association. 2014. Appropriate Use of the Copy and Paste Functionality in Electronic Health Records. http://bok.ahima.org/PdfView?oid=300306.

American Health Information Management Association. 2017. *Pocket Glossary of Health Information Management and Technology*, 5th ed. Chicago: AHIMA.

American Health Information Management Association. 2011. Fundamentals of the legal health record and designated record set. *Journal of AHIMA* 82(2):44–49.

American Health Information Management Association. 2010. Fundamentals for building a master patient index/enterprise master patient index (updated). *Journal of AHIMA*. http://bok.ahima.org/doc?oid=106227#.XSCh_Y8pCUk.

American Health Information Management Association. 1997. Practice brief: Developing information capture tools. *Journal of AHIMA* 68(3): supplement.

Brown, L., P. Komara, D. Warner, and L.A. Wiedemann. 2012. Amendments in the Electronic Health Record Toolkit. http://bok.ahima.org/PdfView?oid=105672.

Cerrato, L.A. and J. Roberts. 2012. Health Information Functions. Chapter 7 in *Health Information Management Technology: An Applied Approach*, 4th ed. Edited by N.B. Sayles. Chicago: AHIMA.

Huffman, E.K. 1994. *Health Information Management*. Berwyn, IL: Physician Record Co.

Williams, A. 2006. Design for better data: How software and users interact on screen matters to data quality. *Journal of AHIMA* 77(2):56–60.

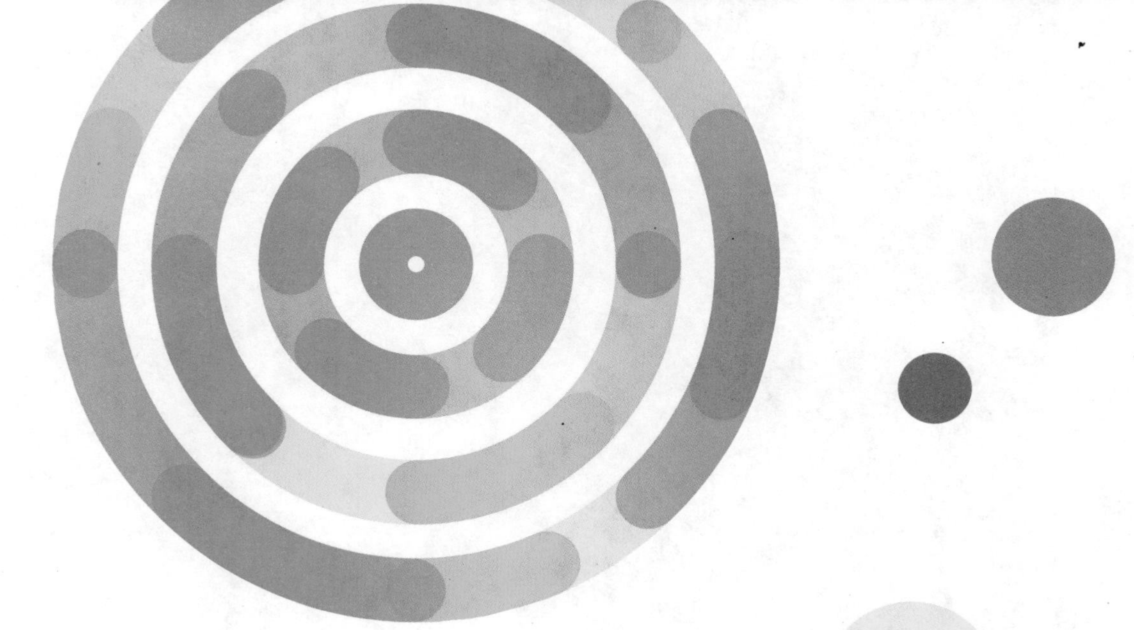

PART II

Data Content, Structures and Standards

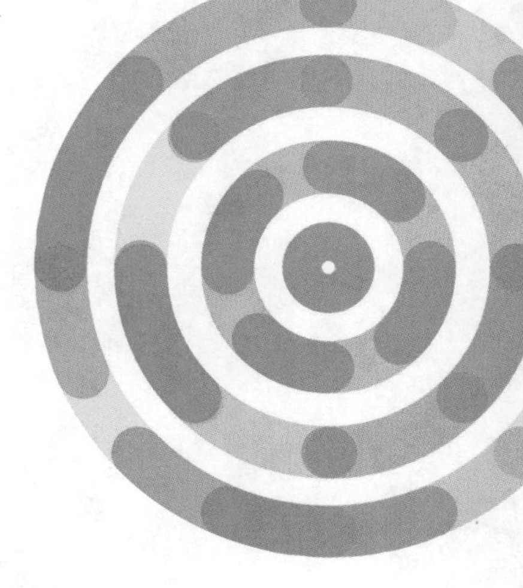

Health Record Content and Documentation

Megan R. Brickner, MSA, RHIA

Learning Objectives

- Define documentation standards.
- Describe how medical staff bylaws, accreditation entities, and state and federal regulations influence the documentation practice standards of healthcare provider organizations
- Articulate how documentation standards drive patient safety and quality within the healthcare industry
- Describe how the definition of a legal health record has changed as healthcare providers have more widely adopted electronic health record technologies
- Compare the documentation content of health records within different healthcare settings
- Evaluate the potential advantages and disadvantages of different health record media
- Describe the roles that various healthcare professionals play in health record documentation
- Evaluate documentation to determine if it meets the general documentation guidelines
- Justify the need for HIM professionals to be involved in health record documentation

Key Terms

Accreditation
Accreditation Association for Ambulatory Healthcare (AAAHC)
Accreditation organizations
Administrative data
Ambulatory surgery center/ambulatory surgical center (ASC)
Ancillary services
Anesthesia report
Authentication
Auto-authentication
Autopsy report
Care area assessments (CAAs)
Care plan
Centers for Medicare and Medicaid Services (CMS)
Certification
Clinical data
Clinical observations
Commission on Accreditation of Rehabilitation Facilities (CARF)
Conditions for Coverage (CfC)
Conditions of Participation (CoP)
Consultation report
Core measures
Data quality
Deemed status
Discharge summary
Documentation
Documentation standards

Document imaging
Healthcare Facilities Accreditation Program (HFAP)
History and physical (H&P)
Hybrid record
Integrated health record
Joint Commission
Legal health record
Licensure
Medical history
Medical staff
Medical staff bylaws
Medical staff privileges
Medicare Access and CHIP Reauthorization Act (MACRA)
Minimum Data Set
Operative report
Pathology report
Patient Driven Payment Model
Physical examination
Physician orders
Problem-oriented health record
Progress notes
Recovery room report
Resident assessment instrument (RAI)
Source-oriented health record
Subjective, objective, assessment, plan (SOAP)
Standard
Standing orders
Statute
Template
Transfer record
Universal chart order

The saying "If it wasn't documented, it wasn't done (or didn't happen)" succinctly conveys the level of importance all healthcare providers should place on health record documentation. **Documentation** is the recording of pertinent healthcare findings, interventions, and responses to treatment as a business record and form of communication among caregivers. Documentation takes various forms within the health record. Examples of health record documentation include progress notes, laboratory test results, radiology imaging reports, and operative reports, all of which provide a complete medical picture of the patient. The health record centralizes documentation regarding a patient's healthcare visit and treatment history in an official, permanent, and recorded format. For thousands of years, individuals have been documenting stories and events in written form to share and reshare with future generations. Healthcare documentation is no exception. The health record, specifically the documentation maintained within it, has historically allowed and presently enables the patient's healthcare providers to make well-informed concurrent treatment decisions for the patient and establishes a healthcare history for the patient for future reference.

It is important not only that there is documentation within the health record but that the documentation itself is appropriate, accurate, reliable, and readily accessible. **Data quality** is the reliability and effectiveness of data for its intended uses in operations, decision-making, and planning. Complete and accurate health record documentation drives high-quality patient care as well as appropriate coding and claims submission, resulting in appropriate reimbursement. Data quality applies not only to health record (clinical) information but also to billing and claims data, administrative and business data, and disease registry data. Documentation must be complete and accurate, support quality initiatives, and meet accreditation requirements. Chapter 6, *Data Management*, will address data quality in more depth.

When health record documentation is lacking in accuracy, reliability, and effectiveness, it may fail to appropriately describe the care and treatment of the patient. This lack of data quality can impact the quality of care the patient receives. Poor documentation impacts the assessment and evaluation of the patient and the communication among healthcare providers, results in medical errors, and contributes to poor patient outcomes. Poor documentation also impacts the accuracy of medical coding due to potential improper code assignment, resulting in inaccurate diagnosis and procedure codes. Inaccurate coding impacts billing, reimbursement, and claims submission for the care and treatment provided to the patient. If poor-quality documentation affects the accuracy of coding, billing, and claims submission, then state and federal regulatory compliance and accreditation standards of the healthcare organization can also be in jeopardy.

Role of Documentation

Health record documentation plays a variety of roles within the clinical healthcare setting. Documentation is a communication tool between and among healthcare providers. It allows for continuity in the care and treatment of the patient from one healthcare provider to the next and creates a permanent health record for all future care of the patient. The documentation that is generated during the care and treatment of the patient is the starting point for the revenue cycle, which facilitates the coding and billing of the care and treatment. When the documentation is of the appropriate quality, it serves as proof of care and services and demonstrates that documentation standards are met (or not met). The next section will discuss the principles, codes and beliefs, and guidelines related to documentation standards.

Documentation Standards

A **standard** is a set of principles, codes, beliefs, guidelines, and regulations that have been vetted and agreed upon by an individual or a group of individuals who are regarded as an authority on a particular subject matter. Standards must be based on generally accepted rules of the healthcare industry. Within the context of healthcare, **documentation standards** describe those principles, codes, beliefs, guidelines, and regulations that guide health record documentation. Documentation standards dictate how healthcare providers should document the treatment and services (rendered to the patient) within the health record. The basis for healthcare-related documentation standards is to promote healthcare quality and safety, as well as provide for optimized continuity of care for the patient. As the health record and health record documentation have become more computer based, documentation standards have become even more important, not only from a clinical documentation standpoint but also from an organizational standpoint. How health record documentation is used within the electronic health record (EHR) has become a focus of many health information management (HIM) professionals.

When the EHR first began replacing traditional paper-based health records, a common belief was that the standards addressing the documentation contained within the EHR (covered in chapter 11, *Health Information Technologies*) were somehow different from those standards addressing the documentation in a paper-based health record. This belief is incorrect. In general, the standards that traditionally applied to paper-based documentation hold true for documentation generated and maintained within the EHR. As healthcare providers have come to realize the great benefits of EHR technologies as they relate to documentation quality and overall patient safety, those same technologies have also presented some challenges. One example is the use of a template. A **template** is a pattern used in EHRs to capture data in a structured manner and specify the information to be collected. For example, a birth record template would require data such as date of birth, time of birth, APGAR scores, length, weight, and so forth. It helps the care provider ensure key information is not forgotten. It also certifies that the data are captured in a specific order and format. Whether the patient's health record is electronic or paper-based, accurate and appropriate documentation is key to meeting compliance standards—namely, those for medical necessity and the justification for treating the patient.

Standards

Over the years, documentation standards have become more detailed and focused on patient care quality, appropriate reimbursement, and the prevention of fraud and abuse from a regulatory perspective. The Centers for Medicare and Medicaid Services (CMS) defines *fraud* as the intentional deception or misrepresentation that an individual knows, or should know, to be false or does not believe to be true, knowing the deception could result in some unauthorized benefit to himself or some other person(s) and *abuse* describes practices that either directly or indirectly result in unnecessary costs to the Medicare Program (CMS 2017). Abuse includes any practice that is not consistent with the goals of providing patients with services that are medically necessary, meet professionally recognized standards, and are priced fairly. (See chapter 16, *Fraud and Abuse Compliance,* for more discussion on fraud and abuse.) The application of the standards varies depending upon the content of the health record; whether the record is an inpatient, ambulatory, behavioral health, or physician office record; and from where the standards originate. Sources for standards include insurance companies and payers, government regulatory agencies, licensing boards, accrediting bodies, healthcare organization policies and procedures, and healthcare provider organization medical staff bylaws.

With the healthcare industry focusing on patient care quality, appropriate reimbursement, and the prevention of fraud and abuse, the goal of documentation standards is to ensure what is documented in the health record is complete and accurately reflects the treatment provided to the patient. This provides an inherent level of acceptable quality so other healthcare providers have a clear and accurate understanding of the patient's condition and how the patient is responding to treatment. In addition, documentation standards drive appropriate healthcare reimbursement through accurate code capture during the revenue cycle process, reducing the chances that inaccurate or fraudulent claims are processed and sent to commercial or governmental payers for reimbursement.

Medical Staff Bylaws

A healthcare organization's medical staff bylaws are the standards that govern the practice of medical staff members. These medicals staff bylaws are typically voted upon by the organized medical staff and the medical staff executive committee and approved by the healthcare organization's board of directors. They play an important role in documentation standard mandates and development. Accreditation organizations measure the compliance of the healthcare organization with the standards developed by the accreditation organization. Licensure organizations are the legal authority or formal permission from the authorities to carry out certain activities that require such permission. For example, a hospital cannot treat patients without being licensed by the state. Federal and state regulatory agencies mandate the content, specifically the breadth and depth of these bylaws, as well as the application of the bylaws. Medical staff bylaws vary slightly from one healthcare organization to another as a result of differences in state laws and the needs of individual healthcare organizations. Before addressing medical staff bylaws, it is important to understand the function and responsibility of a healthcare organization's medical staff.

A healthcare organization's medical staff is a group of physicians and nonphysicians such as nurse practitioners and physician assistants who have medical staff privileges. Medical staff personnel go through a process that ensures the physician or other healthcare professional has the education and qualifications required to perform services and procedures in a healthcare organization. The result is a specific list of services and procedures (medical staff privileges) that the medical staff member may perform at a particular healthcare provider organization. The medical staff bylaws govern the business conduct, rights, and responsibilities of the medical staff; medical staff members must abide by the bylaws to practice in the healthcare organization. It is through the process of granting medical staff privileges and enforcing the medical staff bylaws that the overall quality of care and treatment provided to patients is governed (Adelman 2012). Credentialing is the process of reviewing and validating the qualifications (degrees, licenses, and other credentials) of physicians and other licensed independent practitioners for granting medical staff privileges to provide patient care services (AAFP 2019).

A number of accrediting, licensing, and regulatory entities drive the configuration of the medical staff and the content and application of the medical staff bylaws of a healthcare organization. The Centers for Medicare and Medicaid Services (CMS) is the federal agency within the Department of Health and Human Services (HHS) known for its operational oversight of the Medicare and Medicaid programs. The Joint Commission also plays an important regulatory role in a healthcare organization's medical staff makeup and the content of the medical staff bylaws by establishing standards for the medical staff bylaws. The Joint Commission is a common accreditation organization for hospitals and other healthcare organizations. (The Joint Commission is covered in more detail later in this chapter.)

Content required in medical staff bylaws includes the healthcare provider organization's processes for self-governance and general oversight obligations, due process rights as they relate to potential disciplinary action, peer review policies and procedures, and medical staff appointment, privileging, and credentialing (CMS 2018). CMS mandates the medical staff bylaws must do the following:

- Be approved by the governing body of the medical staff
- Address the duties and privileges of each type of medical staff member
- Describe the organization of the medical staff
- Describe the qualifications that must be met by any individual wishing to seek appointment to the medical staff (42 CFR 482.22(c))

CMS dictates that medical staff bylaws must address certain documentation requirements in the Medicare Conditions of Participation. The Medicare Conditions of Participation (CoP) are the standards that a healthcare organization must meet to receive Medicare funding. One of the requirements is that a medical history and physical (H&P) be documented for every patient no more than 30 days before or 24 hours after admission to the hospital. The H&P contains pertinent information about the patient, including chief complaint, past and present illnesses, family history, social history, and review of body systems, and must be documented in the health record prior to any surgery or procedure requiring the patient to receive anesthesia. If, however, the physical exam is completed within the 30 days of a surgery or procedure, an updated exam must be documented within 24 hours of admission and prior to the surgery or procedure. This updated exam must include any changes in the patient's condition since the time of the first exam (42 CFR 482.22(c)).

Accreditation

Accreditation is a voluntary process of institutional or organizational review in which a quasi-independent body created for this purpose periodically evaluates the quality of the entity's work against pre-established written criteria. CMS CoPs and Conditions for Coverage (CfCs) ensure patient care quality, safety, and improvement of clinical outcomes. CfCs are standards applied to healthcare organizations that choose to participate in federal government reimbursement programs such as Medicare and Medicaid (Ambulatory Surgery Center Association n.d.). For a healthcare provider to participate in federal government reimbursement programs, the healthcare provider must demonstrate they at least meet, or exceed, the CoPs and CfCs.

Auditing and monitoring are the main ways state and federal government measure a healthcare provider's compliance with the CoP and CfC standards and criteria. Healthcare providers that are accredited by an approved accreditation organization are exempt from direct government auditing and monitoring. The accreditation organization must go through its own CMS review to receive deemed status. Deemed status is an official designation indicating that a healthcare organization complies with the Medicare Conditions of Participation (ASHE n.d.). It is through this deemed status that the accreditation organization is permitted to evaluate other healthcare provider organizations for CoP and CfC compliance through its accreditation process. Currently nine national accreditation organizations have obtained deemed status and are responsible for surveying healthcare providers who are currently participating in the Medicare and Medicaid programs (see table 4.1).

Many healthcare providers seek accreditation because it gives the healthcare organization an opportunity to measure its own compliance as well as see what operational improvements it can make based upon the findings of the accreditation organization. Patients also want to know that the healthcare provider they entrust with their care complies with quality and clinical outcome measures. Accreditation enhances reputation among healthcare organizations that take part in the process. In most cases the accreditation process is voluntary, but the healthcare organization must be accredited by an accreditation organization to participate in specific programs and services. This is true for the Medicare and Medicaid programs. Because of the vast number of specialties within healthcare, there are a number of accreditation organizations that specialize in the surveying of particular types of healthcare facilities. These include:

- Healthcare Organizations Accreditation Program
- Commission on Accreditation of Rehabilitation Facilities
- Accreditation Association for Ambulatory Healthcare
- Joint Commission

The **Healthcare Facilities Accreditation Program (HFAP)** was initially created to evaluate osteopathic hospitals. A doctor of osteopathic medicine as well as a healthcare organization that identifies as an osteopathic entity, maintain a different philosophical and clinical approach to caring for the patient compared to the conventional (allopathic) approach to medicine. Due to these differences, these healthcare providers required a slightly different accreditation survey process. However, over time, HFAP began to evaluate all healthcare providers. Similar to other accreditation organizations, the requirements that healthcare providers must meet are based upon, for the most part, the CoPs. Most of the surveyors who perform the HFAP surveys are healthcare professionals themselves and survey and subsequently accredit acute-care facilities, critical access facilities, hospitals, ambulatory surgery centers, clinical labs, behavioral health facilities, and office-based surgery.

The **Commission on Accreditation of Rehabilitation Facilities (CARF)** was established in the 1960s as an independent, nonprofit accrediting organization to meet the survey needs of various rehabilitation-based healthcare providers. These rehabilitation-based healthcare providers include independent and nonprofit providers, aging services, behavioral health, and opioid treatment programs. CARF surveys the business operations, clinical processes, and rehabilitation program specialties, and subspecialties for compliance. As with all accreditation organizations, the

Table 4.1 CMS-approved accrediting organizations

Accreditation organization	Program
Accreditation Association for Ambulatory Health Care (AAAHC)	Ambulatory surgery centers
Accreditation Commission for Health Care (ACHC)	Home health, hospice
American Association for Accreditation of Ambulatory Surgery Facilities (AAAASF)	Ambulatory surgery centers, occupational therapy, rural health clinics
American Osteopathic Association/Healthcare Facilities Accreditation Program (HFAP)	Ambulatory surgery centers, critical access hospitals, hospital
Center for Improvement in Healthcare Quality (CIHQ)	Hospital
Community Health Accreditation Program (CHAP)	Home health, hospice
DNV GL Healthcare	Critical access hospitals, hospital
The Compliance Team	Rural health clinics
Joint Commission	Ambulatory surgery centers, critical access hospitals, hospital, home health, hospice, psychiatric hospital

Source: Adapted from Centers for Medicare and Medicaid Services, CMS 2018.

standards and evaluation methods are regularly reviewed and revised as necessary to meet the ever-changing regulatory standards environment in these areas of healthcare. CARF also assists healthcare providers with establishing best practices in these specialized areas of rehabilitation treatment.

The **Accreditation Association for Ambulatory Healthcare (AAAHC)** was established in the late 1970s. AAAHC surveys and subsequently accredits various ambulatory-based healthcare providers such as surgery centers, imaging centers, endoscopy centers, and women's health centers. Because of the variety of ambulatory specialties AAAHC accredits, the surveyor who is sent to survey for compliance typically has expertise in the specialty that is being surveyed. For example, a surveyor who reviews an ambulatory surgery center should have experience at an ambulatory surgery center. AAAHC's focus is on establishing, reviewing, and revising standards as well as measuring performance and providing education to those healthcare providers it surveys. The surveys evaluate the facility infrastructure and safety, as well as business operations, clinical operations, and patient documentation for compliance.

Joint Commission

The Joint Commission has already been introduced in this chapter. Although there are many high-quality accreditation organizations in existence today, all with the common goals of patient safety and the delivery of high-quality healthcare to patients, the Joint Commission has been an industry leader in the area of healthcare accreditation. The Joint Commission also provides organizations it accredits with education and compliance outreach services.

Over the years, the Joint Commission has expanded its accreditation program offerings and currently provides accreditation for ambulatory healthcare, behavioral health, critical access hospitals, home care, hospital, laboratory, nursing care centers, physician offices, and office-based surgery centers. In addition to the different types of healthcare provider organizations that can seek and obtain Joint Commission accreditation, specific programs addressing specific disease processes can also obtain accreditation through the Joint Commission certification process (Joint Commission 2016a).

Certification is the process by which a duly authorized body evaluates and recognizes an individual, institution, or educational program as meeting predetermined requirements. The more commonly known programs that often obtain certification address asthma, diabetes, and heart failure (Joint Commission 2016b–d).

Compliance, quality, and patient safety have become the focal points of the healthcare industry's clinical and operational practices. The Joint Commission responded to this shift in focus by moving from announced reviews that occurred once every three years to unannounced reviews, coupled with changes to the review process itself. The Joint Commission provides organizations that choose to obtain or maintain their accreditation with an accreditation manual. The manual is comprised of chapters addressing various areas of clinical and operational practice, including but not limited to:

- Environment of Care
- Leadership
- Provision of Care, Treatment, and Services
- Life Safety
- Information Management (Joint Commission 2016e)

The chapters in the Joint Commission accreditation manual contain specific standards and elements that describe in detail the continuous compliance expectations for the healthcare organization. Each standard and element has a corresponding explanation and scoring procedure associated with it. For example, within the Infection Control chapter, the Joint Commission describes when a healthcare provider should wear a gown when caring for a patient (contact precautions). When contact precautions are initiated, the Joint Commission expects that such activity will be documented appropriately in the patient's health record.

The Joint Commission emphasizes appropriate and standardized health record documentation. Those standards and elements address health record content, legibility and completeness, dating and timing of entries, order sets, abbreviations, history and physical component requirements, and informed consent, among many other standards and elements.

State Statutes

A statute is a piece of legislation written and approved by a state or federal legislature and then signed into law by the state's governor, or the President of the United States. State statutes, as they relate to health record documentation, vary by state in terms of what components of health record documentation are regulated and to what degree it is regulated by law. In many instances, state statutes address the documentation requirements according to the type of health record. For example, Ohio law addresses the specific documentation requirements for inpatient psychiatric service providers. For example, the Ohio Administrative Code describes how involved a patient should be in involved his or her care plan and how the care plan should be documented.

Legal Health Record

In the past, the terms *health record* and *legal health record* were used interchangeably, and the subtle nuances of these two terms provided little impact to the operations of a healthcare provider. The legal health record is the documents and data elements that a healthcare provider may include in response to legally permissible requests for patient information. Identifying the legal health record was simple when health records were primarily paper-based and included the contents of the paper health record in addition to diagnostic radiographic films or x-rays. During this time, the health record and the legal health record were one and the same. The legal health record became complicated when electronic health record technology was adopted and healthcare provider organizations moved from a strictly paper-based record to a more hybrid record model, and then to a fully electronic format since the health record became scattered and more information was available.

The current definition of the legal health record is complicated. Each healthcare organization must define what its legal health record contains. The legal health record is used to ensure compliance with laws and regulations, healthcare policies, accreditation standards, and any other requirements (HIMSS n.d.). Healthcare organizations with an EHR must determine what to do with health records that they receive from other healthcare providers. At one time, it was standard practice for a healthcare organization to incorporate another provider's health record into the legal health record and release that documentation as part of the healthcare organization's legal health record. Today, the healthcare organization should consult with legal counsel to assist with making a decision about whether or not to include another provider's records in the legal health record. Some state laws dictate what can and cannot be included in the healthcare organization's legal health record and, in many cases, the hospital's attorney is in the best position to decide whether to include or exclude the records from other providers. For the EHR to be a legal health record and meet the requirements, several concepts need to be considered. These concepts include how documentation is actually created and signed by healthcare providers; how the documentation is managed and preserved; how the documentation impacts and interacts with the revenue cycle functions of billing and claims submission; and how the documentation is displayed both electronically to the user as well as in hard copy form, should the data be printed (HIMSS 2011). Once a healthcare organization defines its legal health record, necessary policies and procedures should be developed to formalize the healthcare organization's approach to defining the health record. See chapter 8, *Health Law,* for more information about the legal health record.

Check Your Understanding 4.1

Answer the following questions.

1. Complete this statement: The patient's medical history can be completed within ___________ of admission to the hospital.
   a. 3 days
   b. 30 days
   c. 60 days
   d. 10 days
2. Justify the need for documentation standards.
   a. To ensure physicians have access to the health record information they need to care for the patient
   b. To ensure the healthcare provider organization is reimbursed appropriately by payers
   c. To ensure CMS does not find reason to fine the healthcare provider organization
   d. To ensure what is documented in the health record is complete and accurately reflects the treatment provided to the patient
3. A new hospital is town wants to accept Medicare patients. To receive Medicare funding, the hospital must meet:
   a. The medical bylaws of the healthcare provider organization
   b. The Medicare Conditions of Participation
   c. The accreditation organization
   d. The plan
4. The fact that ABC hospital is accredited by an accreditation organization that allows the hospital to also meet the Medicare Conditions of Participation is known as:
   a. Deemed status
   b. Certification
   c. Bylaws
   d. State statute
5. Dr. Smith admits patients to ABC hospital. There he is able to perform general surgery, order tests, and perform other services. This is known as:
   a. Certification
   b. Licensure
   c. Statutes
   d. Medical staff privileges

General Documentation Guidelines

General documentation guidelines apply to all categories of health records. These guidelines address the uniformity, accuracy, completeness, legibility, authenticity, timeliness, frequency, and format of health record entries. The American Health Information Management Association (AHIMA) developed the following general documentation guidelines:

- Every healthcare organization should have policies that ensure the uniformity of both the content and the format of the health record. The policies should be based on all applicable accreditation standards, federal and state regulations, payer requirements, and professional practice standards.
- The health record should be organized systematically to facilitate data retrieval and compilation.
- Only individuals (physicians, nurses, physical therapists, and more) authorized by

the healthcare organization's policies should be allowed to enter documentation in the health record.

- Organizational policy and medical staff rules and regulations should specify who may receive and transcribe verbal physician's orders.
- Health record entries should be documented at the time the services described are rendered.
- The authors of all entries should be clearly identified in the health record.
- Only abbreviations and symbols approved by the organization and medical staff rules and regulations should be used in the health record.
- All entries in the health record should be permanent (written in permanent ink).
- Errors in paper-based records should be corrected according to the following process: Draw a single line in ink through the incorrect entry. Then print the word "error" at the top of the entry along with a legal signature or initials, the date, time, and reason for change, and the title and discipline of the individual making the correction. The correct information is then added to the entry. Errors must never be obliterated. The original entry should remain legible, and the corrections should be entered in chronological order. Any late entries should be labeled as such.
- Any corrections or information added to the health record by the patient should be inserted as an addendum (a separate note). No changes should be made in the original entries in the record. Any information added to the health record by the patient should be clearly identified as a patient addendum (Smith 2001, 56).
- When errors in the EHR are corrected, the erroneous information should not be displayed; however, there should be a method to view the previous version of the document with the original data (Wiedemann 2010).

From a governmental regulatory perspective, CMS and federal regulations also address what would be considered general documentation guidelines and further explain what this guidance means.

- All health record entries must be legible. Orders, progress notes, nursing notes, or other entries in the health record that are not legible may be misread or misinterpreted and may lead to medical errors or other adverse patient events.
- All entries in the health record must be complete. A health record is considered complete if it contains enough information to identify the patient; support the diagnosis or condition; justify the care, treatment, and services; document the course and results of care, treatment, and services; and promote continuity of care among healthcare providers.
- The time and date of each entry (orders, reports, notes) must be accurately documented. Timing establishes when an order was given, when an activity happened, or when an activity is to occur. Entries must be timed and dated for patient safety and quality of care. Timed and dated entries establish a baseline for future actions or assessments and establishes a timeline of events.
- There must be a method to establish the identity of the author of each entry.
- There must be a method to require that each author takes a specific action to verify that the entry being authenticated is his or her entry or that he or she is responsible for the entry and the entry is accurate (42 CFR 482.24(c)(1)).

Authentication is the process of identifying the source of health record entries by attaching a handwritten signature, the author's initials, or an electronic signature. CMS defines what authentication methods are to be used for health record entries such as written signatures, initials, computer key, or other code; the requirements a healthcare provider needs to have in place; and controls to prevent any changes from being made to the health record after the entries have been authenticated (42 CFR 482.24(c)(1)).

Auto-authentication is a procedure that allows dictated reports to be considered automatically signed unless the HIM department is notified of needed revisions within a certain time limit or a process by which the failure of an author to review and affirmatively approve or disapprove an entry within a specified time period results in authentication. For example, a physician dictates an operation, the operative report is transcribed, but the physician never accesses the report to review it for accuracy and completeness. The EHR system is set up to show the physician signed the operative report even though he or she never reviewed the document. Auto-authentication does not meet standards for appropriate timing, dating, and signing-off of documentation by healthcare providers and therefore should not be used.

Check Your Understanding 4.2

Answer the following questions.

1. True or false: Only individuals authorized by the healthcare organization's policies should be allowed to enter documentation in the health record.
2. True or false: Auto-authentication is the preferred method of authentication.
3. Each entry in the health record should be:
   a. Signed only
   b. Signed and dated
   c. Reviewed by the patient
   d. Reviewed by another physician
4. True or false: When an error is made, the erroneous information can be obliterated.
5. True or false: Health record entries should be documented at the time the services they describe are rendered.

Documentation by Settings

Despite different settings in which healthcare can be provided—hospitals, ambulatory surgery centers, physician offices, long-term care facilities—health records contain two distinct types of information: *clinical* and *administrative* (defined later in the chapter). A healthcare organization must maintain a health record on every patient whom they treat. Hospitals frequently use a centralized health record. Having all patient care records stored together enables physicians and other healthcare providers to see the documentation of all the care provided to the patient by others. In a centralized health record, the inpatient and outpatient health record documentation is maintained in one health record rather than in separate health records. Whether the health record is paper-based, electronic, or hybrid, there are distinct differences in the documentation found in the health record. Inpatient, emergency department, ambulatory, ambulatory surgery, ancillary, physician office, long-term care, rehabilitation, and behavioral health settings are discussed in more detail in the section that follows.

Inpatient Health Record

The inpatient health record is generated when a patient is provided with room, board, and continuous general nursing care in an area of an acute-care healthcare organization, such as a hospital, where the patient generally stays overnight at that healthcare organization. The documents typically found in an inpatient health record include but are not limited to history and physical (H&P), consultation reports, physician's orders and progress notes, nursing assessments and progress notes, as well as a discharge summary. Over the years, there has been a dramatic shift in the delivery of healthcare treatment and services. Many services such as surgery, infusions, and other diagnostic procedures that once required a patient to stay overnight in the hospital can be performed on an outpatient basis. Only the most severely ill patients and the most invasive procedures require an overnight stay and therefore the inpatient health record is the most complex. A discussion of the three major health records categories within the inpatient care services continuum (medical and surgical, obstetric, and newborn) follows.

Medical and Surgical

The medical and surgical health record is found in a variety of settings including inpatient care units, long-term care facilities, home health, surgical centers, and ambulatory care units. Medical and surgical health record documentation pertains to adult patients with various acute and active disease processes or injuries. The medical and surgical health record contains documentation originating from physicians, nurses, diagnostic procedures, as well as from the dietary, pharmacy, social services, and other departments. The categories of information found in the medical and surgical record include clinical data, administrative data, and consents, authorizations, and acknowledgments. Consents and authorizations are discussed in chapter 8. An acknowledgment is a document that the patient' or the patient's authorized personal representative sign, confirming the receipt of important information.

Clinical Data Clinical data is the information that reflects the treatment and services provided to the patient as well as how the patient responded to such treatment and services; it is also the basis for the reimbursement of the treatment and service rendered to the patient. The clinical data portion of the acute-care record constitutes the largest portion of the health record and consists of nine separate and distinct parts. These parts are: medical history, physical exam, diagnostic and therapeutic procedure orders, clinical observations, diagnostic and procedure reports, surgical procedure documentation, consultation report, discharge summary, and patient instructions and transfer record.

Medical History The medical history portion of clinical data addresses the patient's current complaints and symptoms and describes his or her past medical, personal, and family history. In inpatient care, the medical history is the responsibility of the attending physician. The history generally focuses on the body systems involved in the patient's current illness. Table 4.2 shows the information that is usually included in a medical history.

Note that the *chief complaint* is a component of the medical history that is told to the healthcare provider by the patient and in the patient's own words. Examples of a chief complaint include vomiting, headache, and abdominal pain.

Physical Examination The physical examination represents the physician's assessment of the patient's current health status after evaluating the patient's physical condition. The physician performs the physical examination to ensure appropriate treatment and services are ordered for the patient. Table 4.3 lists the components of the physical examination documentation. Together the medical history and physical examination are commonly referred to as the history and physical (H&P).

CMS guidance and regulations, Joint Commission standards, and healthcare organization policies and procedures will dictate when the medical history and physical exam must be completed by the physician. There are also documentation standards that address when a previously completed H&P can be utilized when a patient is admitted to the hospital (discussed later in this chapter).

Diagnostic and Therapeutic Procedure Orders There are many diagnostic and therapeutic order types. Diagnostic orders include orders for x-rays, CT, MRI, lab tests, and more for the purpose of diagnosing a patient's symptoms of illness. Therapeutic orders are orders for treatment that either prevent or address illness by way of medication

Table 4.2 Information included in a complete medical history

Components of the history	Complaints and symptoms
Chief complaint	Nature and duration of the symptoms that caused the patient to seek medical attention as stated in his or her own words
Present illness	Detailed chronological description of the development of the patient's illness, from the appearance of the first symptom to the present situation
Past medical history	Summary of childhood and adult illnesses and conditions, such as infectious diseases, pregnancies, allergies and drug sensitivities, accidents, operations, hospitalizations, and current medications
Social and personal history	Marital status; dietary, sleep, and exercise patterns; use of coffee, tobacco, alcohol, and other drugs; occupation; home environment; daily routine
Family medical history	Diseases among relatives in which heredity or contact might play a role such as allergies, cancer, and infectious, psychiatric, metabolic, endocrine, cardiovascular, and renal diseases; health status or cause of and age at death for immediate relatives
Review of systems	Systemic inventory designed to uncover current or past subjective symptoms that includes the following types of data:
	• *General:* Usual weight, recent weight changes, fever, weakness, fatigue
	• *Skin:* Rashes, eruptions, dryness, cyanosis, jaundice; changes in skin, hair, or nails
	• *Head:* Headache (duration, severity, character, location)
	• *Eyes:* Glasses or contact lenses, last eye examination, glaucoma, cataracts, eyestrain, pain, diplopia, redness, lacrimation, inflammation, blurring
	• *Ears:* Hearing, discharge, tinnitus, dizziness, pain
	• *Nose:* Head colds, epistaxis, discharges, obstruction, postnasal drip, sinus pain
	• *Mouth and throat:* Condition of teeth and gums, last dental examination, soreness, redness, hoarseness, difficulty in swallowing
	• *Respiratory system:* Chest pain, wheezing, cough, dyspnea, sputum (color and quantity), hemoptysis, asthma, bronchitis, emphysema, pneumonia, tuberculosis, pleurisy, last chest x-ray
	• *Neurological system:* Fainting, blackouts, seizures, paralysis, tingling, tremors, memory loss
	• *Musculoskeletal system:* Joint pain or stiffness, arthritis, gout, backache, muscle pain, cramps, swelling, redness, limitation in motor activity
	• *Cardiovascular system:* Chest pain, rheumatic fever, tachycardia, palpitation, high blood pressure, edema, vertigo, faintness, varicose veins, thrombophlebitis
	• *Gastrointestinal system:* Appetite, thirst, nausea, vomiting, hematemesis, rectal bleeding, change in bowel habits, diarrhea, constipation, indigestion, food intolerance, flatus, hemorrhoids, jaundice
	• *Urinary system:* Frequent or painful urination, nocturia, pyuria, hematuria, incontinence, urinary infections
	• *Genitoreproductive system:* Male—venereal disease, sores, discharge from penis, hernias, testicular pain, or masses; female—age at menarche, frequency and duration of menstruation, dysmenorrhea, menorrhagia, symptoms of menopause, contraception, pregnancies, deliveries, abortions, last Pap smear
	• *Endocrine system:* Thyroid disease; heat or cold intolerance; excessive sweating, thirst, hunger, or urination
	• *Hematologic system:* Anemia, easy bruising or bleeding, past transfusions
	• *Psychiatric disorders:* Insomnia, headache, nightmares, personality disorders, anxiety disorders, mood disorders

Source: Petterson 2013, 79.

administration, surgery, or counseling. **Physician orders** are the instructions the physician gives to other healthcare professionals who perform diagnostic tests and treatments, administer medications, and provide specific services to a particular patient. For example, the physician might order a nurse to take the patient's temperature every two hours. Admission and discharge orders should be found for every patient unless the patient leaves the healthcare organizations against medical advice

Table 4.3 Information documented in the report of a physical examination

Report components	Content
General condition	Apparent state of health, signs of distress, posture, weight, height, skin color, dress and personal hygiene, facial expression, manner, mood, state of awareness, speech
Vital signs	Pulse, respiration, blood pressure, temperature
Skin	Color, vascularity, lesions, edema, moisture, temperature, texture, thickness, mobility and turgor, nails
Head	Hair, scalp, skull, face
Eyes	Visual acuity and fields; position and alignment of the eyes, eyebrows, eyelids; lacrimal apparatus; conjunctivae; sclerae; corneas; irises; size, shape, equality, reaction to light, and accommodation of pupils; extraocular movements; ophthalmoscopic exam
Ears	Auricles, canals, tympanic membranes, hearing, discharge
Nose and sinuses	Airways, mucosa, septum, sinus tenderness, discharge, bleeding, smell
Mouth	Breath, lips, teeth, gums, tongue, salivary ducts
Throat	Tonsils, pharynx, palate, uvula, postnasal drip
Neck	Stiffness, thyroid, trachea, vessels, lymph nodes, salivary glands
Thorax, anterior and posterior	Shape, symmetry, respiration
Breasts	Masses, tenderness, discharge from nipples
Lungs	Fremitus, breath sounds, adventitious sounds, friction, spoken voice, whispered voice
Heart	Location and quality of apical impulse, trill, pulsation, rhythm, sounds, murmurs, friction rub, jugular venous pressure and pulse, carotid artery pulse
Abdomen	Contour, peristalsis, scars, rigidity, tenderness, spasm, masses, fluid, hernia, bowel sounds and bruits, palpable organs
Male genitourinary organs	Scars, lesions, discharge, penis, scrotum, epididymis, varicocele, hydrocele
Female reproductive organs	External genitalia, Skene's glands and Bartholin's glands, vagina, cervix, uterus, adnexa
Rectum	Fissure, fistula, hemorrhoids, sphincter tone, masses, prostate, seminal vesicles, feces
Musculoskeletal system	Spine and extremities, deformities, swelling, redness, tenderness, range of motion
Lymphatics	Palpable cervical, axillary, inguinal nodes; location, size, consistency; mobility and tenderness
Blood vessels	Pulses, color, temperature, vessel walls, veins
Neurological system	Cranial nerves, coordination, reflexes, biceps, triceps, patellar, Achilles, abdominal, cremasteric, Babinski, Romberg, gait, sensory, vibratory
Diagnosis(es)	

Source: Petterson 2013, 80.

(AMA), but other orders will vary from patient to patient. All orders must be legible and include the date and the physician's signature. In electronic systems, signatures are attached via an authentication process discussed in chapter 10, *Data Security*.

Standing orders are orders the medical staff or an individual physician established as routine care for a specific diagnosis or procedure. Standing orders authorize other healthcare providers (such as nurses) to begin treating the patient before the physician examines the patient. Standing orders are commonly used for disease processes and injuries requiring prompt attention. For example, a standing order to all the physician's patients who are scheduled for an appendectomy would include all the orders commonly needed to get the patient ready for surgery. The physician can then add orders that are specific to a patient; for example, a patient who is scheduled for an appendectomy and who is also diabetic will have different standing orders than a patient with no underlying disease process. Like other physician orders, the standing orders must be signed, verified, and dated.

Physicians may communicate orders verbally or via telephone when the hospital's medical staff rules allow. State law and medical staff rules specify which practitioners can accept and execute verbal and telephone orders (for example, only registered nurses). How the orders are to be signed as well as the time period allowed for authentication also may be specified. Currently, there is technology that allows orders to be sent via mobile devices, such as smart phones and tablets, and healthcare organizations are beginning to explore the possibility of using this technology.

Clinical Observations In acute-care hospitals, the documentation of clinical observations is usually provided in a progress note. Clinical observations are the comments of physicians, nurses, and other caregivers that create a chronological report of the patient's condition and response to treatment during his or her hospital stay. Progress notes serve to justify further acute-care treatment in healthcare organizations. In addition, the progress notes document the appropriateness and coordination of the services provided. The patient's condition determines the frequency of the notes.

The rules and regulations of the hospital's medical staff specify which healthcare providers can enter progress notes in the health record. Typically, the patient's attending physician, consulting physicians who have medical staff privileges, house medical staff, nurses, nutritionists, social workers, and clinical therapists (such as physical therapists) are authorized to enter progress notes. Depending on the health record format used by the hospital, each discipline may maintain a separate section of the health record or the observations of all the providers may be combined in the same chronological or integrated health record. Guidelines for the frequency of notations may also be found in the medical staff rules and regulations.

Special types of notes are frequently found in a health record. For example, prior to the administration of any medication other than local anesthesia, the anesthesiologist visits the patient and documents important factors about the patient's condition that may have an impact on the anesthesia chosen or its route of administration. Allergies and drug reactions are noted. A post-anesthesia note that describes the patient's recovery from the anesthetic is required. Similarly, the surgeon responsible for a major procedure must document both pre- and post-surgical patient evaluations.

In the case of a death, the attending physician should add a summary statement to the patient's health record to document the circumstances surrounding the patient's death. The statement can take the form of a final progress note or a separate report. The statement should indicate the reason for the patient's admission, his or her diagnosis and course in the hospital, and a description of the events that led to his or her death.

Just as physician documentation begins with the H&P, nurses and allied health professionals may begin their care with assessments focused on understanding the patient's condition from the perspective of their specialized body of knowledge. Often a care plan— a summary of the patient's problems from the nurse or other professional's perspective with a detailed plan for interventions—may follow the assessment. In addition, nurses are responsible for specific patient admission and discharge notes and for documenting the patient's condition at regular intervals throughout the patient's stay. If a patient should die while hospitalized, nursing notes regarding the circumstances leading to and of death are important for quality and patient health outcomes improvement, risk management activities, and, in some cases, payer reimbursement considerations.

In certain situations, when the patient has died, an autopsy may be requested or required and a subsequent autopsy report, a description of the examination of a patient's body after he or she has died, is completed. Also called *necropsies*, autopsies are usually conducted when there is some question about the cause of death or when information is needed for educational or legal purposes. The purpose of the autopsy is to determine or confirm the cause of death or to provide more information about the course of the patient's disease.

The autopsy report is completed by a pathologist and becomes part of the patient's health record. The autopsy report content and the format of the content is standardized and governed by the National Association of Medical Examiners. Every autopsy report contains the diagnosis, toxicology, opinion, circumstances of death, identification of the decedent, general description of clothing and personal effects, evidence of medical intervention, external examination, external evidence of injury, internal examination, and samples obtained. Because reports from tissue examination or laboratory testing can take weeks or even months, a preliminary report including preliminary diagnoses is often documented until findings are received and the final report is completed. The authorization for the autopsy, signed by the patient's next of kin or by law enforcement authorities, must be obtained prior to the autopsy and should become part of the record.

Nursing professionals also maintain chronological records of the patient's vital signs (blood pressure, heart rate, respiration rate, and temperature) and documentation of medications ordered and administered. Other chronological monitors such as measures of a patient's fluid input and output may be ordered and recorded depending on the patient's diagnosis. Sometimes these records are referred to as flow records because they show trends over time, or the data may be represented in graphic form for ease of communication. Special interventions such as the use of restraints also require documentation. For example, restraint information must include the type of restraint used, time frame used, and regular vital sign monitors and descriptions of the patient's physical condition while restrained.

After an initial assessment, documentation by other allied health professionals varies by specialty. Each healthcare organization will define the appropriate content and frequency of documentation based on specific regulations and standards and the profession's practice guidelines. For example, respiratory therapy treatments may be documented via progress notes and social work interventions may appear as dictated reports.

Diagnostic and Therapeutic Procedure Reports The results of all diagnostic and therapeutic procedures become part of the patient's health record. Diagnostic procedures include the following:

- Laboratory tests performed on blood, urine, and other body fluids
- Pathological examinations of tissue samples and tissues or organs removed during surgical procedures
- Imaging procedures of the patient's body and specific organs (radiology, scans, ultrasounds, MRIs, PETs)
- Monitors and tracings of body functions

The results of most laboratory procedures are generated electronically by automated testing equipment. In contrast, the results of monitors, imaging, and pathology procedures require interpretation by specially trained physicians such as cardiologists, radiologists, and pathologists. These physicians document their findings in reports that then become part of the patient's permanent record, along with copies or samples of the tracing, images, and scans.

Surgical Procedure Documentation Any surgical procedure requires special documentation. Preoperative notes are made by the anesthesiologist and surgeon prior to the procedure, and nurses report preoperative patient preparations. The entire procedure itself is then recorded, along with an anesthesia record, an operative report, and a postanesthesia or **recovery room report**. When tissue is removed for evaluation, a pathology report also must be present.

The **anesthesia report** notes any preoperative medication and the response to it, the dosage of the anesthesia administered and the route of administration, the duration of administration, the patient's vital signs while under anesthesia, and any blood products administered to the patient during the procedure, and other preoperative information. The anesthesiologist or nurse anesthetist is responsible for this documentation.

The **operative report** describes in detail the surgical procedures performed on the patient. The content of the operative report is found in table 4.4.

The operative report should be written or dictated by the surgeon immediately after surgery and become part of the health record as soon as possible. When there is a delay in dictation or transcription, a progress note describing the surgery should be entered into the patient's health record. Reports of non-surgical other procedures or treatments

Table 4.4 Content of the operative report

• Patient's preoperative and postoperative diagnosis
• Descriptions of the procedure(s) performed
• Descriptions of all normal and abnormal findings
• Description of the patient's medical condition before, during, and after the surgical procedure
• Estimated blood loss
• Descriptions of any specimens removed
• Descriptions of any unique or unusual events during the surgical procedure
• Names of the surgeons and their assistants
• Date and duration of the surgical procedure

Source: ©AHIMA.

will require documentation as well. These may include administration of blood transfusions, chemotherapy documentation, and more.

Immediately after the procedure, the patient is evaluated for a period of time in a special unit called a recovery room. Monitoring is important to ensure the patient sufficiently recovers from the anesthesia and is stable enough to be moved to another location. The recovery room report includes the post-anesthesia note (if not found elsewhere), nurses' notes regarding the patient's condition and surgical site, vital signs, intravenous fluids, and other medical monitoring.

A pathology report is dictated by a pathologist after examination of tissue received for evaluation. This report usually includes descriptions of the tissue from a gross or macroscopic (with the eye) level and representative cells at the microscopic level along with interpretive findings. Sometimes an initial tissue evaluation occurs while the surgery is in progress to give the surgeon information important to the remainder of the operation. A full written pathology report would follow.

Consultation Reports The consultation report documents the clinical opinion of a physician other than the primary or attending physician. The consultation is usually requested by the primary or attending physician, but occasionally may be the request of the patient or the patient's family. The consultation report is based on the consulting physician's examination of the patient and a review of the patient's health record.

Some healthcare organizations allow consultation requests by telephone and provide the consultant with selected information from the patient's health record. The consultant then dictates his or her findings and returns them to the requesting physician.

Discharge Summary The discharge summary is a concise account of the patient's illness, course of treatment, response to treatment, and condition at the time of patient discharge (official release) from the hospital. The summary also includes instructions for follow-up care to be given to the patient or to his or her caregiver at the time of discharge. Because the summary provides an overview of the entire medical encounter, it is used for a variety of purposes, including the following:

- Ensures the continuity of future care by providing information to the patient's attending physician, referring physician, and any consulting physicians
- Provides information to support the activities of the medical staff review committee
- Provides concise information that can be used to answer information requests from authorized individuals or entities

The discharge summary is the responsibility of and must be signed by the attending physician. If the patient's stay is not complicated and lasts less than 48 hours or involves an uncomplicated delivery of a normal newborn, a discharge note in place of a full summary is often acceptable.

Patient Instructions and Transfer Records It is vital that the patient be given clear and concise instructions upon discharge, so the recovery progress begun in the hospital continues. Ideally, patient instructions are communicated verbally and in writing. The healthcare professional who delivers the instructions to the patient or caregiver should sign the health record to indicate that he or she has issued them. In addition, the person receiving the instructions should sign to verify that he or she has received and understands them.

A copy of these instructions should be filed in the health record.

When someone other than the patient assumes responsibility for the patient's aftercare, the record should indicate the instructions were given to the responsible party. Documentation of patient education may be accomplished by using formats that prompt the person providing instruction to cover important information.

When a patient is being transferred from the acute setting to another healthcare organization, a transfer record may be initiated. This documentation is also called a referral form. A brief review of the patient's acute stay along with current status, discharge and transfer orders, and any additional instructions will be noted. Social service and nursing personnel often complete portions of the transfer record.

Administrative Data Administrative data are coded information contained in secondary records (such as billing records) describing patient identification and insurance. Patient registration information would be considered administrative data as would patient account information.

Patient Registration Information Patient registration information includes those data elements obtained during the patient registration process. Most of the patient registration process usually takes place before the physician examines or begins treating the patient. During the registration, process, demographic data are collected. Demographic data are data that identify the patient and includes the following:

- Patient's full name (including any aliases the patient uses; for example, Bob instead of Robert)
- Patient's health record number if the patient was not seen at the healthcare organization before. as well as a patient's account number for this specific visit
- Patient's address
- Patient's contact phone number
- Patient's date of birth
- Patient's gender
- Patient's marital status
- Patient's religious affiliation (if patient has one and chooses to disclose it)
- Race (often this is optional)
- Next of kin information
- Healthcare power of attorney or advance directives (if the patient has these documents) (refer to chapter 8 for specifics)
- If the patient wants to be a private or confidential patient under HIPAA, where the patient opts-out of the healthcare organization's directory (discussed in chapter 9, *Data Privacy and Confidentiality*)

Figure 4.1 is an example of demographics in an EHR.

Ambulatory Surgery Record

Ambulatory facilities that perform surgery are called ambulatory surgery centers (ASC). Patients who have surgery in an ASC still must have a history and physical prior to surgery present within the health record. The patient must have signed the appropriate consent documentation prior to the procedure. Much like an inpatient health record containing a surgery component, an ambulatory surgery record must contain operative reports and notes, diagnostic and therapeutic documentation, consultations, and discharge notes at the conclusion of the treatment.

Ambulatory surgery centers will also perform discharge follow-up phone calls, where a nurse will call the patient within 24 to 48 hours postdischarge to check on the patient. The nurse will assess pain levels and address any immediate or future needs of the patient related to the treatment. This conversation must be documented in the health record. The Joint Commission and the American Association for Accreditation of Ambulatory Surgery Facilities (AAAASF) have requirements applicable to the ambulatory surgery center setting. CMS's Conditions for Coverage for ambulatory surgical centers govern those that seek Medicare reimbursement.

Ancillary Departments

Ancillary departments are the departments that provide treatment and services that support the

Figure 4.1 Demographics in an EHR

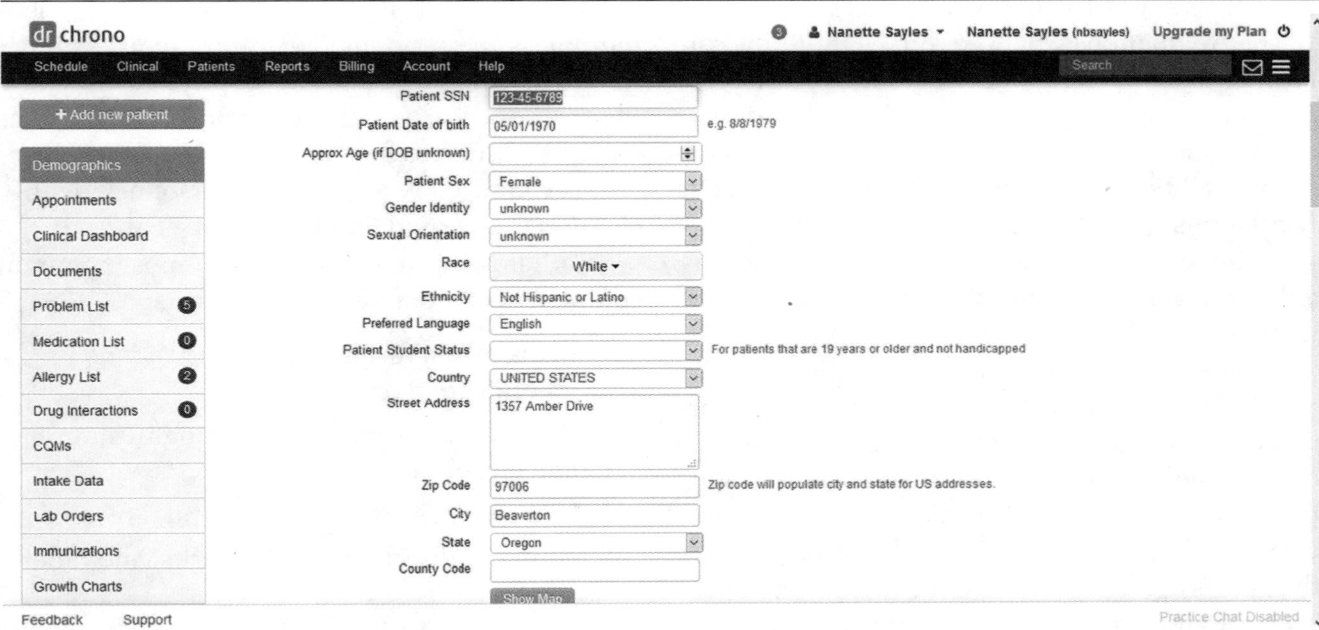

Source: ©drchrono. Used with permission.

patient's overall care plan. Ancillary departments perform ancillary services—tests and procedures sometimes ordered by a physician—and these services assist the physician with diagnosing and treating the patient. Ancillary departments also consist of departments that play an indirect patient care role but are necessary for the overall management of patient care. These departments include pharmacy, nutrition, HIM, social services, and patient advocacy and patient relations. Many ancillary departmental services must be documented within the patient health record according to the governing standards and regulations within a specific department.

Physician Office Record

Routine healthcare treatment commonly occurs within the physician office setting. Routine services include preventative services such as yearly physicals and blood tests, in addition to diagnosis and treatment of minor illnesses and injuries. In many instances, hospital-based health records can feed into the physician office record if the hospital and physician office records are electronic and information can be exchanged from one health record system to another. Much like a paper-based physician office record, the physician office record that is EHR-based, is often in an integrated health record format.

The physician office record content consists of the following:

- Medical history
- Family history
- Social history
- Vital signs
- Chief complaint
- Progress notes
- Allergies
- Medication list
- History of present illness
- Review of systems
- Assessment and diagnosis
- Plan of treatment

The next section will discuss the regulations that govern long-term care.

Long-Term Care

Long-term care is provided in a variety of healthcare organizations, including skilled nursing facilities (SNFs) or units; subacute-care facilities; nursing facilities (NFs) (nursing homes, long-term care facilities); and assisted-living facilities.

The regulations that govern long-term care facilities vary among these settings. Most SNFs and NFs are governed by both federal and state regulations, including the Medicare CoP. Assisted-living facilities are usually governed only by state regulations. Most long-term care providers do not participate in voluntary accreditation programs, although the Joint Commission does have long-term care facility standards.

Because the stay for a patient or resident in long-term settings can be lengthy, health records are based on ongoing assessments and reassessments of the patient's (or resident's) needs. An interdisciplinary team develops a plan of care for each patient upon admission to the healthcare organization, and the plan is updated regularly over the patient's stay. The team includes the patient's physician and representatives from nursing services, nutritional services, social services, and other specialty areas (such as physical therapy), as appropriate.

Assessments are a key component of the Patient Driven Payment Model (PDPM) used by Medicare for Skilled Nursing Facility reimbursement. The Minimum Data Set, Version 3 (MDS 3.0) Resident Assessment Instrument is used to group patients into a payment category. The MDS 3.0 includes diagnosis, therapeutic services such as physical therapy, data about the patient's level of functioning and more. This means that health record documentation is crucial to the PDPM documentation and, therefore, reimbursement. For more on the PDPM, refer to chapter 15. *Revenue Management and Reimbursement*.

Some of the data elements collected by the MDS 3.0 are used for the three assessments required by the PDPM. These assessments are the 5-Day Assessment (mandatory), Interim Payment Assessment (optional), and the Discharge Assessment (mandatory). The 5-Day Assessment and the Discharge Assessment will be performed on all Medicare SNF patients. The Interim Payment Assessment is performed when there is a significant change in the patient's situation.

The physician's role in a long-term care facility is not as visible as it is in other care settings. The physician develops a plan of treatment that includes the medications and treatments to be given to the resident. The physician visits the resident in the healthcare organizations on a 30- or 60-day schedule unless the resident's condition requires more frequent visits. At each visit, the physician reviews the plan of care and physician orders and makes changes as necessary. Between visits, the physician is contacted when nursing personnel identify changes in the resident's condition.

The following list identifies the most common components of long-term care records:

- Registration forms, including resident identification data
- Personal property list, including furniture and electronics
- History and physical and hospital records
- Advance directives, bill of rights, and other legal records
- Clinical assessments
- RAI and care plan
- Physician orders
- Physician's progress notes and consultations
- Nursing notes
- Rehabilitation therapy notes (physical, occupational, and speech therapy)
- Social services, nutritional services, and activities documentation
- Medication and records of monitors, including administration of restraints
- Laboratory, radiology, and special reports
- Discharge or transfer documentation

When paper-based records are found in a long-term setting, a process called record thinning may occur at intervals during the patient's stay. Records of patients whose stay extends to months or years become cumbersome to handle. Selected material may be removed and filed elsewhere according to the healthcare organization's guidelines. Any material removed must remain accessible when needed for patient care and service evaluation.

Rehabilitation

The focus of services in physical medicine and rehabilitation settings is increasing a patient's ability to function independently within the parameters of the individual's illness or disability. The documentation requirements for rehabilitation facilities vary based on the type of rehabilitation services provided.

Inpatient rehabilitation hospitals and units within hospitals are reimbursed by Medicare under a prospective payment system. A Patient Driven Payment Model is completed on Medicare patients shortly after admission and upon discharge. Based on the patient's condition, services, diagnosis, and medical condition, a payment level is determined for the inpatient rehabilitation stay. Comprehensive outpatient rehabilitation facilities have separate Medicare guidelines. For more information on the PAI, refer to chapter 15, *Revenue Management and Reimbursement*.

Many rehabilitation facilities are accredited through the Commission on Accreditation of Rehabilitation Facilities (CARF), although the Joint Commission or American Osteopathic Association (AOA) also can be chosen. CARF requires a facility to maintain a single case record for any patient it admits. The documentation standard for the health record includes the following requirements:

- Patient identification data
- Pertinent history, including functional history
- Diagnosis of disability and functional diagnosis
- Rehabilitation problems, goals, and prognosis
- Reports of assessments and program plans
- Reports from referring sources and service referrals
- Reports from outside consultations and laboratory, radiology, orthotic, and prosthetic services
- Designation of a manager for the patient's program
- Evidence of the patient's or family's participation in decision-making
- Evaluation reports from each service
- Reports of staff conferences
- Progress reports
- Correspondence related to the patient
- Release forms
- Discharge summary
- Follow-up reports (CARF 2016)

Behavioral Health

Behavioral health records contain much of the same content as a nonbehavioral health record such as discharge summary, H&P, or physician orders. Behavioral health records contain a treatment plan that often includes family and caregiver input and information as well as assessments geared toward the transition to outpatient, nonacute treatment. CMS requires that the social workers assigned to a patient assess and document the family or home environment and community services that are compatible with the patient's needs. The behavioral health record also contains a psychiatric evaluation that is performed by a healthcare provider appropriately trained to do such an evaluation and that evaluation consists of a patient history, current mental status, and cognitive function.

Home Health

Home health records contain documentation reflecting care and treatment provided to patients in the home setting. Home care itself takes many forms from very basic assistance that allows a patient to remain independent and live in his or her home, to short-term rehabilitation care, or comprehensive management of a chronic illness. The care provided in the home setting as well as the skill level of the healthcare professional providing the care is individualized based upon the needs of the patient.

The documentation that reflects the care and treatment in the home setting must be accurate and complete to ensure appropriate and quality care is provided to the patient, resulting in better patient outcomes. Quality home care documentation also drives appropriate coding, claims, and reimbursement for the treatment and care provided to the patient. Typically, the home health documentation itself includes an individualized treatment plan, general health assessment, problem list, treatment goals, interventions and outcomes, and communications with other healthcare providers.

Check Your Understanding 4.3

Answer the following questions.

1. True or false: The level and complexity of care a home care patient needs do not determine the skill level of the individual providing the care to the patient.
2. A summary of the patient's health record is found in the:
   a. Progress notes
   b. Discharge summary
   c. Care plan
   d. Physical examination
3. A patient's gender, phone number, address, next of kin, and insurance policyholder information would be considered what kind of data?
   a. Clinical data
   b. Authorization data
   c. Administrative data
   d. Consent data
4. The health record being reviewed documents the information from the family. The type of health record being reviewed is:
   a. Behavioral health records
   b. Ambulatory surgery health records
   c. Emergency department health records
   d. Obstetric health record
5. Recommend a method of facilitating documentation of orders for routine procedures and other common situations.
   a. Physician's office records
   b. Emergency care records
   c. Standing orders
   d. Order sets
6. True or false: Many services such as surgery, infusions, and other diagnostic procedures that once required an overnight hospital stay for the patient no longer require that level of care.
7. The assessment used by a rehabilitation center is known as:
   a. Care plan
   b. OASIS
   c. MDS
   d. PAI
8. Critique each statement to determine the true statement about behavioral health records.
   a. Behavioral health records are completely different from other health records.
   b. Behavioral health records are similar to other health records
   c. Behavioral health records do not record the input of family members
   d. Behavioral health records do not record the input of social workers.
9. The type of health record that records a nurse calling a patient 24 to 48 hours after they leave the healthcare setting.
   a. Behavioral health
   b. Ancillary services
   c. Ambulatory surgery center
   d. Long term care facility

10. When a patient goes into labor and subsequently delivers a newborn, what documentation will be found in the Labor and Delivery record?
   a. Apgar scores
   b. Fetal monitoring strips
   c. Obstetrical risks
   d. Medical history
11. A patient's registration forms, personal property list, RAI, care plan, and discharge or transfer documentation would be found most frequently in which type of health record?
   a. Rehabilitative care
   b. Ambulatory care
   c. Behavioral health
   d. Long-term care
12. The physician spoke to a patient about the risks and benefits of a treatment or procedure. This is known as:
   a. Consultation
   b. Clinical evaluation
   c. Implied consent
   d. Informed consent
13. An attending physician requests the advice of a second physician who then reviews the health record and examines the patient. The second physician records his or her evaluation documentation known as a(n):
   a. Consultation
   b. Progress note
   c. Operative report
   d. Discharge summary

Federal and State Initiatives on Documentation

As healthcare costs have steadily and, in many cases, dramatically increased over the years, the government, on state and federal levels, has focused its attention on alternative reimbursement and payment models. It has developed initiatives for the healthcare sector to follow with the goals of improving the quality of care provided and increasing efficiencies with an increased value of the care provided to patients. The alternative reimbursement and payment models, called pay-for-performance or value-based care, prioritize quality and efficiency rather than quantity. Healthcare providers such as hospitals and physicians are financially incentivized to put measures into place to continuously improve the quality and efficiency of the care they provide, resulting in better patient outcomes. Pay-for-performance programs have performance measures that healthcare providers must meet or exceed to receive financial payment. For example, Medicare may hold a percentage of reimbursement until the healthcare provider meets the quality standards. Clinical documentation plays a key role in demonstrating if a healthcare provider is meeting or exceeding these performance measures.

There are several federal and state initiatives related to quality and content of health record documentation. Two initiatives, however, are more commonly found across the entire healthcare continuum. These initiatives are the Medicare Access and CHIP Reauthorization Act (MACRA) and core measures. Both MACRA and core measures emphasize the quality and efficiency aspects of the treatment physicians and other healthcare providers provide to patients more than the quantity of the treatment provided.

MACRA was signed into law in 2015 by then President Barack Obama. Like other pay-for-performance initiatives, MACRA financially rewards healthcare providers for treatment. By meeting specific measures, the documentation generated by the treatment of Medicare beneficiaries demonstrates (or not) that the treatment provided was high-quality, efficient, and a good value for the patient. Moreover, greater emphasis is being placed on the patient outcomes over time. Healthcare providers are and will continue to be evaluated for patient outcomes and general management of specific conditions within the Medicare patient population.

Core measures are national treatment standards for specific healthcare conditions that were developed and continue to be developed and updated based on scientific clinical findings. Core measures have been proven to improve overall patient outcomes during treatment of these conditions. The goal of the core measures is to reduce patient adverse events and complications. The documentation of the treatment must reflect adherence to the core measures. Healthcare providers typically report core measures monthly or quarterly to the Joint Commission, CMS, or other agency. The documentation of the adherence to and subsequent reporting of the core measures demonstrates how frequently the healthcare provider follows the standards related to specific healthcare conditions. This reporting reflects, in part, the level of quality treatment and care the healthcare provider provides to his or her patient population.

Health Information Media

Over the years, healthcare documentation media has transformed from a paper-based health record that sat on a shelf to an EHR that can be shared. Many of the same rules, standards, and quality measures that held true for the paper-based health record hold true now for the EHR. Healthcare documentation integrity is paramount regardless of its form. In many respects, the rules, standards, and quality measures and indicators are available through EHR software enhancements that can leverage technology against what was once a manual process. Leveraging EHR features and technical capabilities in conjunction with strong and concise policies and procedures can ensure the integrity and accuracy of health record documentation (AHIMA 2013).

Paper Health Record Documentation

Some healthcare organizations still utilize the paper-based health records. The paper-based health record can take the **source-orientated health record** format in which the documentation is organized by source or originating department. For instance, all nursing notes are together, and all the physician progress notes are grouped together. With each source, the health record documentation is placed in reverse chronological order, where the most current or recent documentation is first. Reverse chronological order is kept while the patient is being treated. Many times post patient discharge, the health record is kept in its source orientation, but the documentation in each source section is rearranged and placed in chronological order. Other times, the health record post patient discharge is kept in reverse chronological order; this is called **universal chart order**.

In an **integrated health record**, the documentation is placed in chronological order regardless of source. This means that the lab results, nurses' notes, physician orders, and physician progress notes are placed in the order in which they occurred. The order of the health record is determined by when the documentation was entered into the health record, when the service or treatment was rendered, or when a test result was processed.

The **subjective, objective, assessment, plan (SOAP)** method is used to construct physician progress notes. Physicians use the acronym SOAP to remember what elements of documentation must be included in a progress note. The SOAP methodology came from the **problem-oriented health record** developed by Lawrence Reed in the 1970s, which defines and documents clinical problems individually (AAPC 2015). The problem-oriented health record consists of a problem list, the history and physical examination and initial lab findings (the database), the initial plan (tests, procedures), and progress notes. The HIM professional must be able to read and understand the documentation structure to locate information needed for coding, audits, and other usages.

As EHR technologies have advanced, the paper-based health record is considered antiquated by many. There are numerous shortcomings to the paper-based health record, notably the inability to share needed health information with multiple healthcare providers at one time (access and availability), as well as the lack of controls that can be placed in and around the paper-based health record in terms of data security. See chapter 10, *Data Security,* for more detail on data security.

Electronic Health Record Documentation

Computer-based health record documentation via EHRs has been in existence for 50 years. Over time, as EHR systems became more sophisticated, the way healthcare providers document the treatment and services they render to the patient also dramatically changed. Before EHR adoption, healthcare providers would carry paper-based health records into the patient's room to reference as they discussed and rendered treatment to the patient. The healthcare provider did not document what occurred until after seeing the patient. Today, EHRs allow point-of-care documentation to take place—the healthcare provider can log into the EHR in the exam or treatment room and document in the patient's health record during the exam or treatment. This change in the way healthcare documentation is captured has impacted treatment workflow in some of the most meaningful ways. See chapter 11, *Health Information Systems,* for additional information on the EHR.

Web-Based Document Imaging

Document imaging is the process by which paper-based documentation is captured, digitized, stored, and made available for retrieval by the end user (AIIM 2019). Although many healthcare provider organizations have an EHR, there remains a good deal of paper-based documentation that must be integrated and included in the patient's EHR. Current EHR systems contain documentation-imaging and document-management technologies that provide for the capture, digitization, integration, storage, and retrieval of paper-based health record documentation.

Check Your Understanding 4.4

Answer the following questions.

1. The originating department organizes the paper-based health record. This is an example of:
   a. Problem-oriented health record
   b. SOAP methodology
   c. Universal chart order
   d. Source-oriented health record
2. The S in SOAP is:
   a. Superior
   b. Subjective
   c. Simple
   d. Sample
3. As the government has shifted its focus towards quality, alternative reimbursement and payment models have developed. An example is:
   a. Bundled payments
   b. Managed care
   c. Pay-for-performance
   d. Fee-for-service

4. The healthcare organization needs to incorporate paper-based health records into the patient's EHR. It should use:
   a. Database management
   b. Document imaging
   c. Text processing
   d. Vocabulary standards
5. True or false: Pay-for-performance initiatives focus on treatment quality, efficiency, and value rather than the quantity of treatment provided.

Healthcare Providers in Documentation

Authenticated, accurate, legible, complete, and timely documentation is paramount to patient safety, quality of care provided to patients, and appropriate reimbursement. Healthcare providers have an obligation to document appropriately, reflecting a true picture of the treatment and services rendered to the patient. Not only does the health record documentation itself need to be of the highest quality, the health record also must be organized and available to the healthcare providers who need it to care for the patient. Physicians, nurses, allied health professionals, and HIM professionals all play vital roles in meeting the documentation standards from a healthcare organization's policy and procedural perspective and meeting regulatory requirements applicable to health record documentation.

Physicians

Patients place a significant level of trust in their physicians. Patients rely on their physicians to make sound medical decisions about them and document them accordingly. Payers and the government also trust physicians to document appropriately in the health record so quality care can be rendered and appropriate reimbursement issued by the payer. The information a physician documents in the health record impacts the patient first and foremost. All physicians caring for the patient and payers connected to the physicians need to coordinate their care and documentation. See chapter 16, *Fraud and Abuse Compliance,* for information on regulatory laws that directly and indirectly govern physician documentation. Those laws fall into the general category of fraud and abuse laws, but the False Claims Act and Anti-Kickback Statute have significant documentation compliance jurisdiction for physicians.

Nurses

Nurses play an important role in the day-to-day caregiving of a patient, and they are an important member of the patient care team. As with physicians, the way a nurse documents in the health record is based on the environment. Inpatient health record documentation looks slightly different from documentation in the operating room or in a long-term care facility. The elements or components that the nurse captures in the documentation also varies depending upon licensing and regulatory requirements, as well as the healthcare organization's internal policies and procedures. However, the same rules apply to nursing documentation as to physician documentation. Legible, complete, and timely entries are required. In addition, though the documentation of a physician is both subjective and objective, nursing documentation should only be objective in nature. In terms of the legal environment, nursing documentation standards tend to be more restrictive than physician documentation standards because physicians, not nurses, diagnose patients.

Allied Health Professionals

Some allied health professionals work more independently than others when providing treatment and services to the patient. Many follow a treatment plan developed by the patient's physician. In this case, the allied health professional documents the treatment and the patient's response to the treatment.

The allied health professional usually falls into one of two categories of practice—technician (assistant) and therapist or technologist. In both categories of practice, allied health professionals may have to meet certification and licensing requirements in addition to the standard documentation practices of an organization. Chapter 2, *Healthcare Delivery Systems,* discusses allied health professionals in more detail.

HIM and Documentation

While HIM professionals do not document in the health record, the documentation in the health record is important to them for coding, claim generation, data quality monitoring, disclosure of health information, and such. Complete, accurate, and available health record information is essential for quality care and patient safety. Other healthcare providers, the government, and payers expect the health record documentation to accurately reflect the treatment and services provided to the patient. This level of documentation is needed to ensure the patient receives the best quality healthcare available and that the appropriate reimbursement is received for the treatment and services provided. HIM professionals are often in charge of ensuring that physician documentation is complete and accurate and that the health record documentation is organized and readily accessible when needed for patient care. AHIMA defines information governance as "an organization-wide framework for managing information throughout its life cycle and supporting the organization's strategy, operations, regulatory, legal, risk, and environmental requirements" (AHIMA 2014, 70). The governance or management of health record information is a fundamental component of the overall information governance model. Information governance applies to many categories of data, including health record information. HIM professionals play vital and different roles in the overall governance of health record information. For information on data governance, see chapter 6, *Data Management*.

HIM professionals manage many aspects of the health record and its content. This includes the following activities:

- Scanning paper-based health record documentation into the EHR
- Organizing the content in the health record
- Analyzing the documentation for deficiencies like physician signatures
- Coding the health record documentation for appropriate reimbursement
- Controlling the access and disclosure of the health record and its content across a healthcare organization

Within an EHR environment, HIM professionals are viewed as the experts to develop workflows and infrastructure around the EHR. As EHR technology proliferates, traditional HIM job roles continue to be more information technology (IT) focused. Continuing to learn and expand knowledge within the computer technology field and continuing to learn the many ways IT can be leveraged to improve the EHR infrastructure to support information governance is paramount. HIM professionals and the roles they play will continue to evolve—as they will be involved in clinical documentation integrity (CDI), forms design, screen design, data quality, and so much more.

Check Your Understanding 4.5

Answer the following questions.

1. Documentation should be authenticated, accurate, legible, complete, and:
   a. Based solely on clinical care
   b. Based solely on reimbursement
   c. Electronic
   d. Timely
2. True or false: HIM professionals use the health record for coding.
3. True or false: HIM professionals are experts in the development of workflows related to the EHR.
4. Nursing documentation within the health record is:
   a. Subjective
   b. Objective
   c. Both subjective and objective
   d. Electronic
5. True or false: HIM professionals document in the health record.

HIM Roles

Health information management roles within healthcare have drastically changed over the past 10 to 15 years as the EHR has evolved. As more and more healthcare entities have transitioned from paper-based records to electronic-based records, traditional HIM roles have been impacted. HIM professionals have readily adapted to this impact and have taken more of a technical focus in response. An important role for HIM professionals is the clinical documentation integrity coordinator. The clinical documentation coordinator works with physicians to ensure the documentation is completed and contains enough information to assign diagnosis and procedure codes. For example, the documentation should identify whether the right or left radius was fractured.

Another role related to documentation is the analyst role. The analyst is responsible for ensuring the presence of key documents as defined by the healthcare organization and that the health record entries are authenticated and dated.

Real-World Case 4.1

The hospital clinical documentation improvement (CDI) specialist reports to you, the HIM manager of Anywhere hospital, that the hospital has been receiving reimbursement penalties. The physician documentation is not appropriately identifying specific conditions that CMS has identified as hospital-acquired conditions (HACs). In most cases, these conditions are present in patients before they are admitted. However, physicians are documenting these conditions later in the patients' stays, making it appear that the patients have acquired these conditions from the hospital. The hospital is being financially penalized because these conditions are considered to be preventable if the hospital follows national treatment standards and guidelines.

Anywhere hospital has a robust EHR. Many documentation improvement initiatives have been leveraged by the technological capabilities of the EHR. As the HIM manager, you wonder if something could be done from a technology standpoint that could assist physicians with identifying, upon admission, those conditions that are causing the reimbursement issue, and appropriately documenting the conditions. Physicians appropriately capturing and documenting these conditions would demonstrate that the hospital is following the national treatment standards and guidelines and the patients are not acquiring these conditions in the hospital.

You assemble a multidisciplinary team consisting of physicians, revenue cycle representatives, HIM, and information systems representation.

Real-World Case 4.2

You are a HIM professional working in Anywhere hospital's HIM department. You have been asked to review physician documentation within the hospital's new EHR system, implemented six months ago. The goal of the review is to catch any documentation issues early and work with the appropriate hospital leadership to fix those issues.

As you review the documentation in the EHR, you notice that physicians are utilizing the copy and paste functionality available in the EHR, which allows them to select health record documentation from one source or section of the EHR and replicate it in another source or section of the EHR. In one instance the health record identifies a patient as a 65-year-old male (as identified during the registration process), but in the progress notes the patient is described as a 25-year-old female who has given birth. Clearly, the physician utilized the copy and paste functionality inappropriately and accidentally copied health record information from the health record of a 25-year-old female and pasted that information into the health record of a 65-year-old male.

This type of error could have patient safety concerns, as well as billing and claims issues, and the use of this functionality could open up the facility to potential claims of fraud and abuse by the payer. You take this concern to your leadership and a multidisciplinary group of hospital employees including HIM professionals, nurses, physicians, and billing and revenue cycle employees to discuss and fix the problem. There are mixed opinions about the copy and paste functionality. Some individuals feel this feature is a time-saver and a productivity booster while others believe it only opens the hospital up to additional CMS scrutiny.

References

Adelman, T. 2012. Fundamentals of health law. *Fundamentals of Hospital Medical Staff Issues: Minimizing Risk and Maximizing Collaboration* (Session F). Chicago: AHLA.

Ambulatory Surgery Center Association. n.d. Medicare Certification. https://www.ascassociation.org/federalregulations/medicarecertification.

American Academy of Family Physicians. 2019. Hospital Credentialing and Privileging FAQs. https://www.aafp.org/practice-management/administration/privileging/credentialing-privileging-faqs.html#privileging.

American Academy of Professional Coders. 2015. http://www.aapc.com.

American Health Information Management Association. 2017. *Pocket Glossary of Health Information Management and Technology*, 5th ed. Chicago: AHIMA.

American Health Information Management Association. 2014. Information Governance Offers a Strategic Approach for Healthcare. *Journal of AHIMA* 85(10):70–75.

American Health Information Management Association. 2013. Integrity of the healthcare record: Best practices for EHR documentation. *Journal of AHIMA* 84(1):58–62.

American Society for Health Care Engineering of the American Hospital Association. n.d. Deemed Status.

http://www.ashe.org/advocacy/orgs/deemedstatus.shtml.

Association for Information and Image Management. 2019. https://www.aiim.org/What-is-Imaging.

Centers for Medicare and Medicaid Services. 2019. Fact Sheet: MDS Changes. https://www.cms.gov/Medicare/Medicare-Fee-for-Service-Payment/SNFPPS/Downloads/PDPM_Fact_Sheet_MDS_Changes_Final.pdf.

Centers for Medicare and Medicaid Services. 2018. CMS-Approved Accrediting Organization Contacts for Prospective Clients. https://www.cms.gov/Medicare/Provider-Enrollment-and-Certification/SurveyCertificationGenInfo/Downloads/Accrediting-Organization-Contacts-for-Prospective-Clients-.pdf.

Centers for Medicare and Medicaid Services. 2017. Medicare Fraud & Abuse: Prevention, Detection, and Reporting. https://www.cms.gov/Outreach-and-Education/Medicare-Learning-Network-MLN/MLNProducts/downloads/fraud_and_abuse.pdf.

Commission on Accreditation of Rehabilitation Facilities. 2016. http://www.carf.org/Documentation_and_Time_Lines.

Health Information and Management Systems Society. n.d. The Legal Electronic Health Record. https://www.himss.org/sites/himssorg/files/HIMSSorg/Content/files/LegalEMR_Flyer3.pdf.

Health Information and Management Systems Society, HIMAA Practice Leadership Task Force and the HIMSS Knowledge Resources Task Force. 2011. *The Legal Electronic Health Record*. Chicago: HIMSS.

The Joint Commission. 2016a. About the Joint Commission. http://www.jointcommission.org/about_us/about_the_joint_commission_main.aspx.

The Joint Commission. 2016b. DSC Cardiovascular. http://www.jointcommission.org/certification/dsc_cardiovascular.aspx.

The Joint Commission. 2016c. DSC Endocrine. http://www.jointcommission.org/certification/dsc_endocrine.aspx.

The Joint Commission. 2016d. DSC Pulmonary. http://www.jointcommission.org/certification/dsc_pulmonary.aspx.

The Joint Commission. 2016e. Standards FAQs. http://www.jointcommission.org/standards_information/jcfaq.aspx.

Kassi, D. and M. Keiter. 2019. Patient Driven Payment Model (PDPM) and the MDS: T Total Evoluation of the SNF Payment Model. https://gravityhealthcareconsulting.com/assets/pdpm---mds---whitepaper-6.5.18.pdf.

Petterson, B. 2013. Content and Structure of the Health Record. Chapter 3 in *Health Information Management Technology: An Applied Approach*, 4th ed. Edited by N. B. Sayles. Chicago: AHIMA.

Smith, C.M. 2001. Practice Brief: Documentation requirements for the acute care inpatient record. *Journal of AHIMA* 72(3):56A–G.

Wiedemann, L.A. 2010. Deleting errors in the EHR. *Journal of AHIMA* 81(9):52–53.

42 CFR 482.22(c): Medical staff bylaws. 2015 (April 1).

42 CFR 482.24(c)(1): Interpretive guidelines. 2009 (June 5).

Clinical Terminologies, Classifications, and Code Systems

Kathy Giannangelo, MA, RHIA, CCS, CPHIMS, FAHIMA

Learning Objectives

- Identify the importance of clinical terminologies, classifications, and code systems to healthcare
- Examine the content of SNOMED CT, Current Procedural Terminology, and terminologies used in nursing practice
- Analyze the different classification systems and their purposes
- Identify code systems for laboratory and clinical observations; professional services, procedures, and supplies; and drugs
- Differentiate among clinical terminologies, classifications, and code systems found in health data and information sets
- Justify the need to have a database of clinical terminologies, classifications, and code systems

Key Terms

Axioms
Classification
Clinical terminology
Code set
Code system
Common Clinical Data Set (CCDS)
Concepts
Data set
Derived classification
Disability
Extension codes
Fully specified name (FSN)
Functioning
Granular level
Health information exchange (HIE)
International Classification of Diseases 11th Revision for Mortality and Morbidity Statistics (ICD-11-MMS)
International Classification of Functioning, Disability, and Health (ICF)
Linearization
Morbidity
Nomenclature
Preferred term (PT)
Reference terminology
RxNorm concept unique identifier (RXCUI)
Semantic interoperability
SNOMED CT identifier (SCTID)
Stem codes
Unified Medical Language System (UMLS)
Vocabulary

Health information management (HIM) professionals play a crucial role in capturing and organizing clinical data. With the adoption of electronic health records (EHRs), organizing clinical data may involve several labels. For example, the Office of the National Coordinator for Health Information Technology (ONC) uses vocabulary (a list of collection of clinical words or phrases with their meanings), terminology, or code set to describe standards to support interoperability (ONC 2018a). Vocabulary is a list or collection of clinical words or phrases with their meanings. Standards organizations may also use the label nomenclature (a recognized system of terms that follows pre-established naming conventions), classification (a clinical vocabulary, terminology, or nomenclature that lists words or phrases with their meanings), or code system (an accumulation of terms and codes for exchanging or storing information). See table 5.1 for general definitions of each label. Nomenclature is a recognized system of terms that follows pre-established naming conventions. Classification is a clinical vocabulary, terminology, or nomenclature that lists words or phrases with their meanings and facilitates mapping standardized terms to broader classifications or administrative, regulatory, oversight, and fiscal requirements. A code is an identifier of data. A code set is any set of codes used to encode data elements, such as tables of terms, medical concepts, medical diagnostic or procedure codes, and includes the descriptors of the codes. A code system is the accumulation of terms and codes for the exchange or storing of information.

Table 5.1 General definitions

Label	Definition
Vocabulary/ Terminology	A set of terms specific to a domain
Nomenclature	A system of names that follows pre-established conventions
Classification	A mono-hierarchical method of organizing related terms together
Code	An identifier
Code set	An accumulation of numeric or alphanumeric codes
Code system	An accumulation of terms and codes for exchanging or storing information

Source: © AHIMA.

This chapter discusses clinical terminologies, classifications, and code systems used in the healthcare industry to encode clinical data in a standardized manner. Clinical terminologies are sets of standardized terms and their synonyms that record patient findings, circumstances, events, and interventions with sufficient detail to support clinical care, decision support, outcomes research, and quality improvement. They contain terms and codes just as a code system does. As this chapter will explain, certain clinical terminologies are more appropriate for the collection of clinical data at a granular level (data consisting of small components or details at the lowest level) such as SNOMED CT. Others are best utilized for the aggregation of clinical data for secondary data purposes; for example, ICD-10-CM.

In addition, terminologies, classifications, and code systems are a key type of data managed by the data governance function. Understanding their purpose and use is necessary to succeed in managing the usability of the data employed by the healthcare organization.

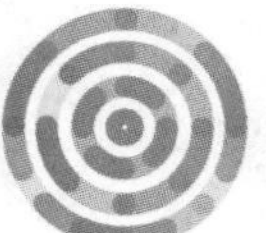

History and Importance of Clinical Terminologies, Classifications, and Code Systems

Clinical terminologies, classifications, and code systems exist to name and arrange medical content so it can be used for patient care, measuring patient outcomes, research, and administrative activities such as reimbursement. What started as a way to identify causes of death for statistical purposes, expanded to reporting diagnoses and procedures on claims for reimbursement. Today, the electronic health record (EHR) can capture the detail of diagnostic studies, history and physical examinations, visit notes, ancillary department information, nursing notes, vital signs, outcome measures,

Figure 5.1 What lies beneath?

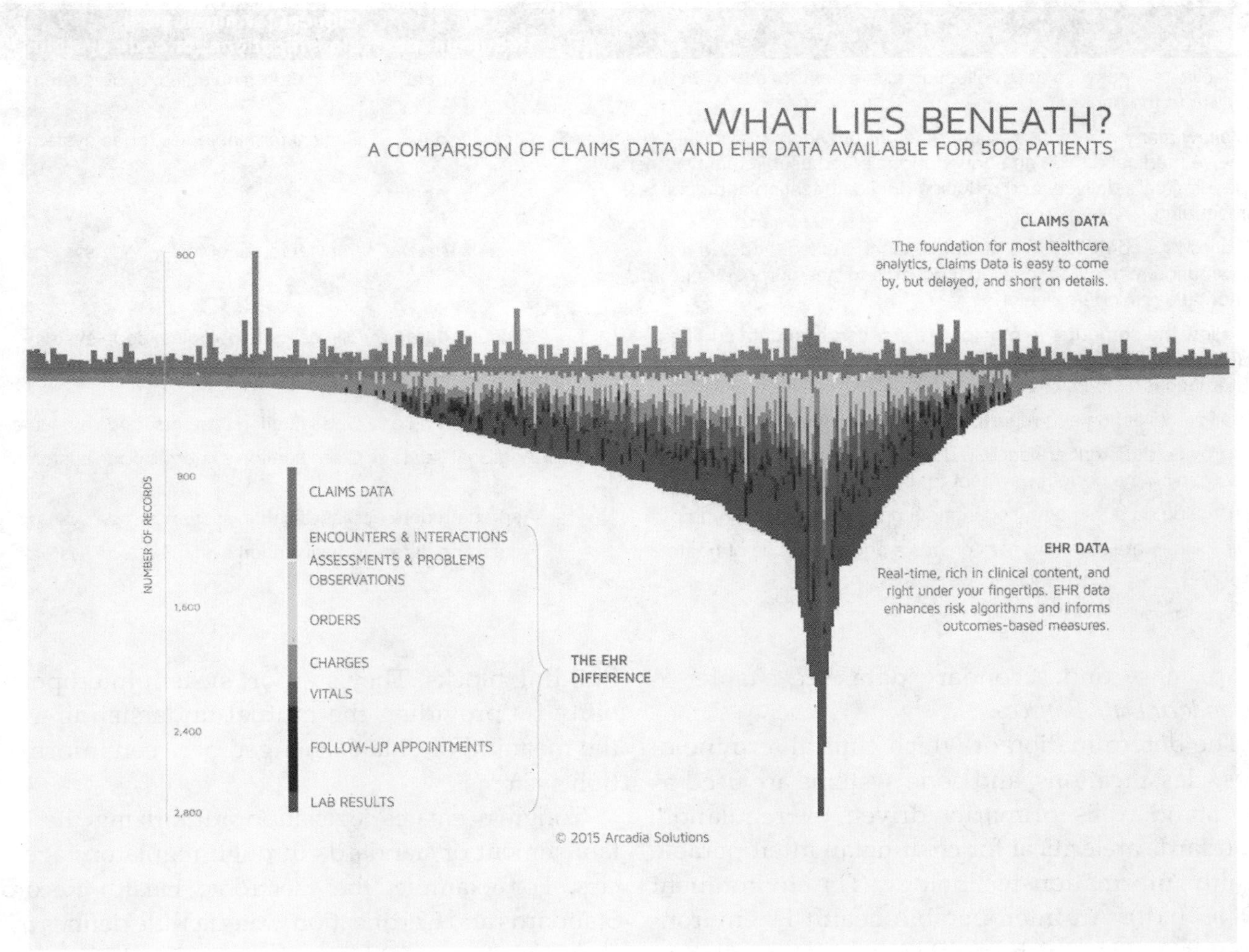

Source: Shulman and Stepro 2015. Used with permission.

and any other clinically relevant observations about the patient. Figure 5.1 illustrates a comparison of claims data and EHR data and the vast difference in clinical content.

Investigating the reasons for collecting data illustrates the importance of clinical terminologies, classifications, and code systems. If data granularity, or detail, is the goal, then clinical terminologies are the best option. On the other hand, if the objective is aggregate data, then classifications are the better choice. Aggregate data is data extracted from individual health records and may be combined to form deidentified information about groups of patients that can be compared and analyzed. With regards to code systems, some are for the collection of clinical data at a granular level while others are for aggregation. Table 5.2 lists examples of data uses and their data requirements. As the table shows, granular data is needed when the details are key to use whereas aggregate data suits when the combination of data provides information about related entities that is sufficient.

Additionally, primary and secondary data uses are relevant to understanding clinical terminologies, classifications, and code systems. A terminology that allows for the collection of clinical data at a granular level is needed for primary data use such as for clinical decision support. One that aggregates the data will work for secondary data use. An example of secondary data use is the identification of diagnoses and procedures for the purpose of billing and payment. For more information

Table 5.2 Examples of data uses and the requirements

Data use	Requirement	Clinical terminologies, classifications, or code systems
To facilitate electronic data collection at the point of care with terms familiar to the user	Granular data	Clinical terminologies, code systems
To allow many different sites and different providers the ability to send and receive medical data in an understandable and usable manner, thereby speeding care delivery and reducing duplicate testing and duplicate prescribing	Granular data	Clinical terminologies, code systems
To allow the computer to manipulate standardized data and find information relevant to individual patients for the purpose of producing automatic reminders or alerts	Granular data	Clinical terminologies, code systems
To allow the computer to manipulate standardized data and find information relevant to individual patients for the purpose of producing automatic reminders or alerts	Granular data	Clinical terminologies, code systems
To allow collection and reporting of basic health statistics	Aggregate data	Classification systems, code systems
To provide data that are used in designing payment systems and determining the correct payment for healthcare services	Aggregate data	Classification systems, code systems
To provide data that are used in monitoring public health and risks	Aggregate data	Classification systems, code systems
To provide data to consumers on costs and outcomes of treatment options	Aggregate data	Classification systems, code systems

Source: Giannangelo 2015.

on primary and secondary data, see chapter 7, *Secondary Data Sources.*

The determination of which clinical terminologies, classifications, and code systems are used as the standard is primarily driven by regulation. Standards are critical for creating an interoperable health information technology (IT) environment (ONC n.d.). An interoperable health IT environment is one in which seamless health information exchange is possible across different EHR systems and the information is understood and shared with those in need of it at the time it is needed. Clinical terminologies, classifications, and code system standards are one of the ONC's interoperability building blocks. They support system interoperability by providing the mutual understanding of the meaning of data exchanged between information systems.

Congress creates legislation authorizing the establishment of standards through regulatory agencies. For example, the Electronic Health Record Standards and Certification Criteria Rule defines the standards that must be used for EHR technology to be certified by the authorized Certification Bodies. Included in this rule are the content standards for representing electronic health information such as SNOMED CT for problems and RxNorm for clinical drugs, which will be discussed later in this chapter.

Clinical Terminologies

A clinical terminology is a set of standardized terms and codes for the healthcare industry for use in encoding clinical data. Examples of clinical terminologies include SNOMED CT, Current Procedural Terminology, and various nursing terminologies. Clinical terminologies form the basis of coded data and provide the data structure required for **semantic interoperability** and **health information exchange**. Semantic interoperability is the mutual understanding of the meaning of data exchanged between information systems. Health information exchange is when health information is electronically traded between providers and others with the same level of interoperability. Clinical terminologies may also be reference terminologies. A **reference terminology** in the health information technology (HIT) domain is "a terminology designed to provide common semantics for diverse implementations" (CIMI 2013).

SNOMED Clinical Terms

SNOMED Clinical Terms, or SNOMED CT, is the most comprehensive, multilingual clinical healthcare terminology in the world (SNOMED International 2017a). There is no book of SNOMED CT codes and no coding professional assigns a SNOMED CT identifier. The terminology instead is implemented in software applications where healthcare providers record clinical information using identifiers that refer to concepts that are formally defined as part of the terminology during the process of care (SNOMED International 2017b). It allows for the collection of clinical data at a granular level. For example, at the point of care a physician using an EHR uses a drop-down list to view the clinical terms relevant to their practice and the patient's problem. While not seen by the physician, the clinical terms have SNOMED CT identifiers attached to them. By selecting the clinical term, the identifier is captured and thereby provides the primary source of information about the patient.

SNOMED CT Purpose and Use

SNOMED CT's overall purpose is to standardize clinical phrases, making it easier to produce accurate electronic health information. Doing so enables automatic interpretation and sharing of clinical information. Semantic interoperability is also possible. (Semantic interoperability is discussed in more detail in chapter 11, *Health Information Systems*.)

With the consistent, reliable, and comprehensive capture of clinical phrases with SNOMED CT, its uses and benefits are many.

With the SNOMED CT encoded data sent securely during the transfer of care to other providers or to patients, the barriers to the electronic exchange are reduced resulting in improved quality of the information. SNOMED CT coded data combined with other encoded data, such as medication and lab results, have a number of uses including clinical decision support, clinical quality measures, and registries (Helwig 2013). For more information on registries, see chapter 7, *Secondary Data Sources*. Quality measures are discussed in chapter 18, *Performance Improvement*.

SNOMED CT is also one of several standards chosen for the entry of structured data in certified EHR systems (ONC 2015). This includes patient problems, encounter diagnosis, procedures, family health history, and smoking status. The National Library of Medicine (NLM) produces the Clinical Observations Recording and Encoding (CORE) problem list subset of SNOMED CT. This subset includes SNOMED CT concepts commonly used for encoding clinical information at a summary level, such as the problem list.

SNOMED CT Content and Structure

SNOMED CT is made up of three main components—concepts, descriptions, and relationships. Each component is assigned a unique, numeric, and machine-readable **SNOMED CT identifier (SCTID)**. The SCTID identifier is a unique integer that includes an item identifier, a partition identifier, and a check-digit. It may also include a namespace identifier when the component originates in an extension. SNOMED International issues a namespace identifier to an organization with the responsibility of creating, distributing, and maintaining a SNOMED CT extension. An extension occurs when the SNOMED CT International release does not contain content needed at the national, local, or organizational level.

The SCTID is nonsemantic; therefore, no meaning is inferable from the numerical value of the identifier or from the sequence of digits. Figure 5.2 provides an example of the SCTID for the concept nosocomial pneumonia found in the international edition and Figure 5.3 shows the SCTID for disorder of right lower extremity found in the US national extension. The partition identifier of 00 and 10 indicates the nature of the component identified is a concept.

Concepts are a unique unit of knowledge or thought created by a unique combination of characteristics. SNOMED CT defines a concept as "a clinical idea to which a unique concept identifier has been assigned" (SNOMED International 2018).

Figure 5.2 SCTID for the concept nosocomial pneumonia SNOMED CT International Edition 20180731 release

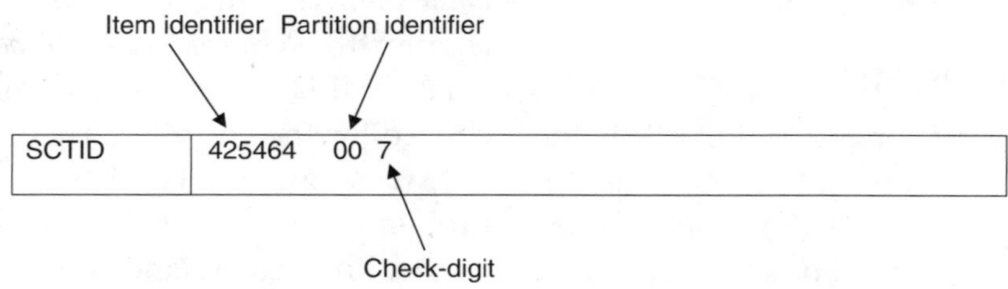

Source: © AHIMA.

Figure 5.3 SCTID for the concept disorder of right lower extremity US national extension 20180901 release

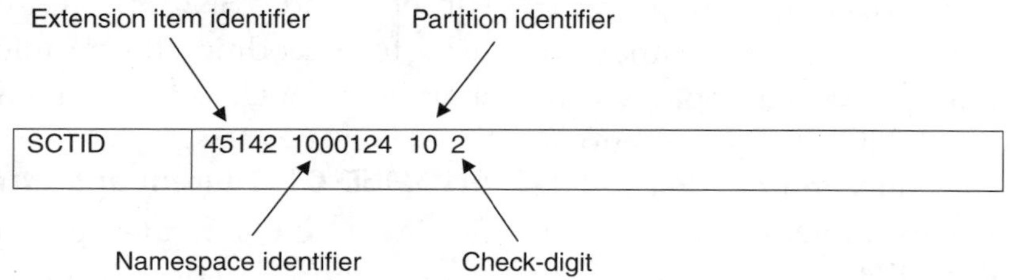

Source: © AHIMA.

Examples of clinical concepts are diagnoses (for example, coronary arteriosclerosis) and procedures (for example, coronary artery bypass grafting). A concept has only a single meaning even though more than one term may be associated with a concept. The SNOMED CT concept definition is a set of one or more **axioms**, or true statements, that serve as a starting point for further reasoning and arguments (SNOMED International 2017a). The axioms may either partially or sufficiently specify the SNOMED CT concept's meaning. When the defining characteristics are enough to define the concept in the context of its hierarchy, it is sufficiently defined. In the case of a concept that does not have the required characteristics to distinguish it from similar concepts, it is partially defined; that is, it is a primitive concept. The concept nosocomial pneumonia is sufficiently defined by the following characteristics:

- Nosocomial pneumonia is a healthcare-associated infectious disease
- Nosocomial pneumonia is an infective pneumonia
- Nosocomial pneumonia has the following attributes:
  - Pathological process: infectious process
  - Associated morphology: inflammation and consolidation
  - Finding site: lung structure

An example of a primitive concept is unsolved lobar pneumonia. Its characteristics are:

- Unsolved lobar pneumonia is a lobar pneumonia
- Unsolved lobar pneumonia is an unsolved pneumonia
- Unsolved lobar pneumonia has the following attributes:
  - Associated morphology: inflammation and consolidation
  - Finding site: structure of lobe of lung

Descriptions are human-readable representations of concepts. A SNOMED CT concept may have multiple descriptions. Each is designated a description type: a fully specified name or a synonym. In SNOMED CT the **fully specified name (FSN)** is the unique text assigned to a concept that completely describes it, and the synonym is an alternative way to describe the meaning of the concept in a specific language or dialect. More than one synonym may exist. One of the synonyms is noted as the **preferred term** and is the description or name assigned to a concept that is used most commonly in a clinical record or in literature for a specific language or dialect. In the example of transient cerebral ischemia, the fully specified name is transient ischemic attack (disorder). The term enclosed in parentheses at the end is called the semantic tag. It allows differentiation among concept domains such as ulcer (disorder) from ulcer (morphologic abnormality). Examples of synonyms for transient ischemic attack (disorder) are transient cerebral ischemia, temporary cerebral vascular dysfunction, and transient ischemic attack. In the case of transient ischemic attack (disorder) the preferred term is *transient cerebral ischemia* for the English language, US dialect.

Relationships are a type of connection between two concepts; for example, a source concept and a destination concept. These relationships between SNOMED CT concepts define them. Structured according to logic-based representation of meanings, they form the poly-hierarchical structure of SNOMED CT. At the top of the hierarchy is the root concept. Descended from the root concept are specific domain hierarchies. For example, coronary arteriosclerosis belongs to the clinical finding domain hierarchy while coronary artery bypass grafting belongs to the procedure domain hierarchy. Figure 5.4 shows how the concept arthritis of the knee belongs only to the clinical finding domain hierarchy.

Values of a range of relevant attributes make up the defining characteristics of a concept (SNOMED International 2018). Defining characteristics include the "is a" relationship and defining attribute relationships. The "is a" relationship type indicates the source concept is a subtype of the destination concept. For example, figure 5.4 shows the "is a" relationship type indicating arthritis of knee is a subtype of arthropathy of knee joint. The defining attribute relationship is not found in all domain hierarchies. For example, the defining attribute relationships for rheumatoid arthritis of hand joint, associated morphology and finding site, are used to associate the source concept rheumatoid arthritis of hand joint to the target concepts of inflammation (associated morphology) and hand joint structure (finding site).

Current Procedural Terminology

The American Medical Association (AMA) owns the copyrights to Current Procedural Terminology (CPT). According to the AMA, "CPT is the most widely accepted nomenclature for the reporting of physician procedures and services under government and private health insurance programs" (AMA 2018). The CPT Editorial Panel in consultation with medical specialty societies represented by the CPT Advisory Committee is responsible for maintaining the terminology.

CPT identifies the services rendered rather than the diagnosis on the claim. The International Classification of Diseases (ICD), which identifies the diagnosis, is discussed later in this chapter. CPT and ICD form units of information about a patient visit in that the diagnosis represented by ICD supports the medical necessity of the service represented by CPT.

CPT is published annually as a print and e-book. It is also available in software applications such as physician practice management systems. Assignment of the CPT code is most often the responsibility of a professional coder based on the healthcare provider's documentation of the medical services or procedures provided.

CPT Purpose and Use

The purpose of CPT is to provide a uniform language that allows for accurate descriptions of medical, surgical, and diagnostic services. It is designed to communicate consistent information about medical services and procedures among physicians, clinical staff, patients, accreditation organizations, and payers for administrative, financial, and analytical purposes.

Despite being copyrighted by the AMA, the Health Insurance Portability and Accountability Act (HIPAA) mandates the use of the CPT in healthcare data electronic transactions. HIPAA named CPT (including codes and modifiers) as the procedure code set for all but hospital inpatient procedures. CPT codes are the five-character identifiers that represent the service or procedure

Figure 5.4 SNOMED CT design

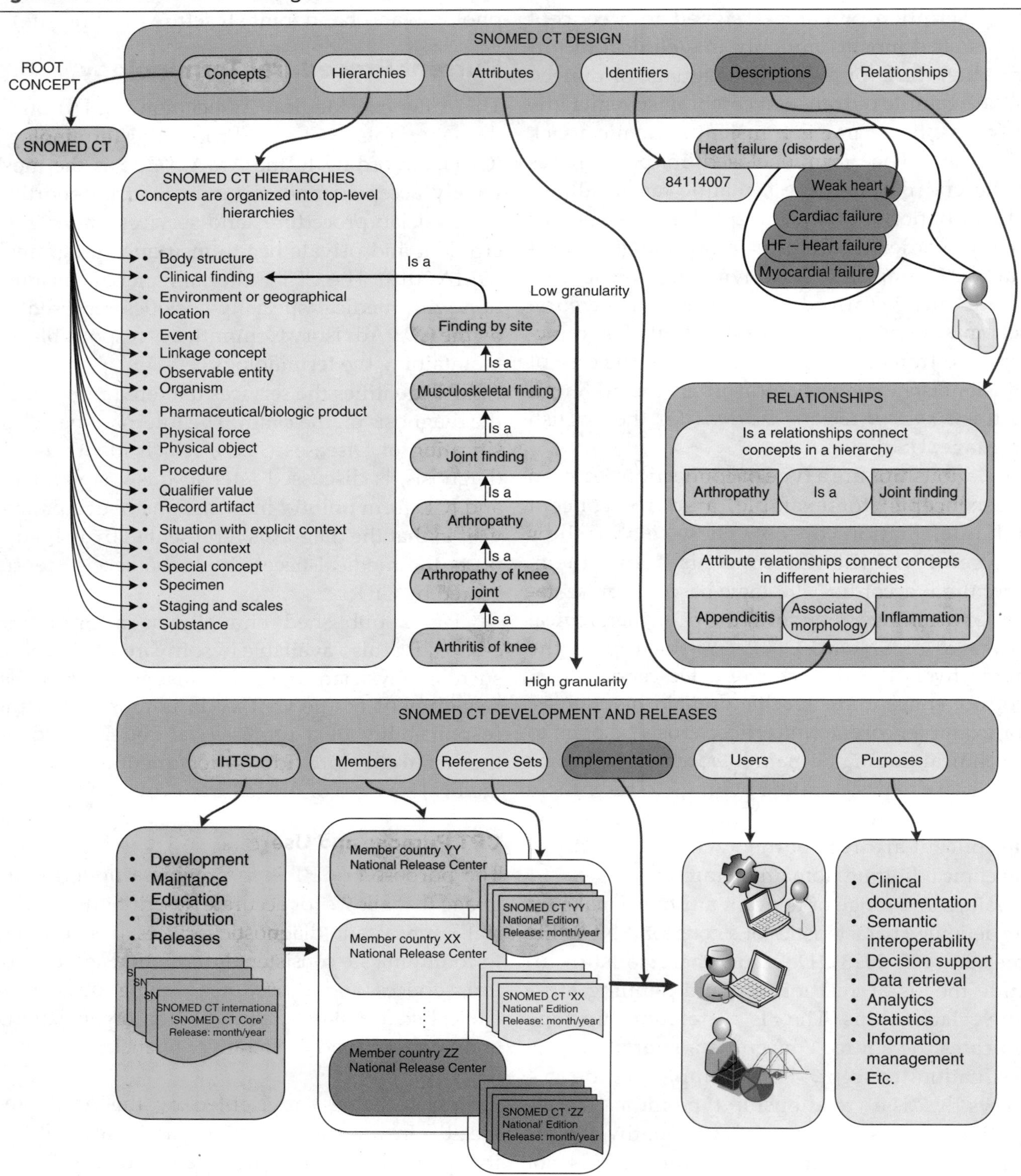

Source: SNOMED International 2017b. Used with permission.

the individual receives from a healthcare provider. Two-character modifiers indicate the service or procedure performed has been altered by some circumstance but not changed in its definition. Thus, physicians and hospitals must use CPT to report medical and procedure services performed by physicians and other healthcare professionals to public as well as private insurers.

CPT Content and Structure

CPT includes codes, descriptions, and guidelines and covers the breadth of health services physicians provide. Descriptions for evaluation and management services such as a new patient office visit, anesthetic services, surgical procedures, radiology services, pathology and laboratory tests, and medical care are all found in CPT. The Centers for Medicare and Medicaid Services (CMS) categorizes CPT as Level I of the Health Care Common Procedure Coding System (HCPCS) discussed later in this chapter.

CPT is divided into categories: Category I, Category II, and Category III. Category I is the major terminology. It contains a description along with a five-digit code for each service or procedure. Two-digit modifiers are available to qualify the service or procedure. For example, the modifier 50 is used to indicate a bilateral procedure. Criteria for inclusion in Category I include the US Food and Drug Administration has approved the service or procedure, many providers in different locations perform it, and it is clinically effective.

Category I CPT includes the following six main sections:

1. Evaluation and Management (E/M)
2. Anesthesia
3. Surgery
4. Radiology
5. Pathology and Laboratory
6. Medicine

The following are examples of Category I CPT services along with their identifiers:

33511 Coronary artery bypass, vein only: 2 coronary arteries

71046 Radiologic examination, chest; 2 views

82951 Glucose; tolerance test (GTT), 3 specimens (includes glucose)

90839 Psychotherapy for crisis; first 60 minutes

Category II CPT is used for performance measurement. This category was created to support data collection about the quality of care rendered by coding certain services and test results that support nationally established performance measures and have an evidence base as contributing to quality patient care. They represent clinical findings or services where there is strong evidence of contribution to health outcomes and high-quality care. The Level II codes are alphanumeric, consisting of four numbers followed by the letter F. The following is an example of a Category II CPT service along with its identifier:

1065F Ischemic stroke symptom onset of less than 3 hours prior to arrival

Category III CPT is for emerging technologies, services, and procedures. They are considered temporary and they may or may not eventually be moved to Category I. Category III codes are alphanumeric, consisting of four numbers followed by the letter T. The following is an example of a Category III CPT procedure along with its identifier:

0345T Transcatheter mitral valve repair percutaneous approach via the coronary sinus

CPT also includes an introduction, an index, and appendices. Within the introduction are section numbers and their sequences and instructions for use of CPT. The index is used to locate a code or code range and is organized by main and modifying terms. Appendices provide information to supplement the main portion of CPT. For example, Appendix A, Modifiers, describes all the modifiers available for use with a CPT code.

Nursing Terminologies

Just as the field of nursing covers a wide range of services, so do the terminologies available to identify those services. The choice of terminology depends on the nursing care documented. In addition, some are location specific. For example, the Nursing Outcomes Classification (NOC) may be used to represent the outcomes of nursing interventions in all settings and the Omaha System is used in the home health setting.

Nursing Terminologies Purpose and Use

Nursing terms provide an effective basis for use in contemporary data systems (Warren 2015, 218). The American Nursing Association (ANA) has specific criteria nursing terminologies must meet to be approved. This includes support of all or part of the nursing process such as assessment and diagnosis. Several organizations, including universities and associations, are responsible for nursing terminology development and maintenance.

The purpose of nursing terminologies is to represent clinical information generated and used by nursing staff (Warren 2015, 207). Nursing terminologies are designed to communicate consistent information about nursing services for a variety of reasons including directing patient care, measuring progress of treatment, as well as for administrative functions, education, and analytical purposes.

Although there is no mandate to use nursing terminologies, the ANA's board of directors published a position statement regarding the inclusion of recognized terminologies within EHRs as well as other HIT applications. The ANA indicated support for the following recommendations:

- Plan implementation of terminologies
- Obtain consensus on which terminology to use
- Make education and guidance available to assist with choosing the terminology
- Use SNOMED CT and LOINC for problems and care plans when exchanging data among settings
- An exchange between providers using the same terminology requires no conversion to SNOMED CT or LOINC
- A clinical data repository involving multiple terminologies draws from national recognized terminologies of ICD-10, CPT, RxNorm, SNOMED CT, and LOINC (ANA 2018)

Table 5.3 Content coverage of ANA-recognized nursing terminologies

ANA-recognized nursing terminology	Content coverage
NANDA International	Thirteen domains: **1.** Health promotion **2.** Nutrition **3.** Elimination/exchange **4.** Activity/rest **5.** Perception/cognition **6.** Self-perception **7.** Role relationship **8.** Sexuality **9.** Coping/stress tolerance **10.** Life principles **11.** Safety/protection **12.** Comfort **13.** Growth/development
Nursing Interventions Classification (NIC)	Seven domains: **1.** Physiological: Basic **2.** Physiological: Complex **3.** Behavioral **4.** Safety **5.** Family **6.** Health system **7.** Community
Nursing Outcomes Classification (NOC)	Seven domains: **1.** Functional health **2.** Physiologic health **3.** Psychosocial health **4.** Health knowledge and behavior **5.** Perceived health **6.** Family health **7.** Community health
Clinical Care Classification (CCC)	Two taxonomies: **1.** CCC of nursing diagnoses and outcomes **2.** CCC of nursing interventions and actions
Omaha System	Three components: **1.** Assessment **2.** Intervention **3.** Outcomes
International Classification for Nursing Practice (ICNP)	Multiaxial representation with seven axes: **1.** Focus **2.** Judgment **3.** Means **4.** Action **5.** Time **6.** Location **7.** Client

Source: Matney 2019, TK.

Nursing Terminologies Content and Structure

Each nursing terminology covers content specific to its use. Table 5.3 lists the content coverage of some of the ANA-recognized nursing terminologies.

The structure also varies among terminologies. For example, each nursing intervention in the Nursing Interventions Classification (NIC) includes a label name, definition, unique number (code), set of activities to carry out the intervention, and background readings, whereas each nursing outcome in the Nursing Outcomes Classification (NOC) includes a definition, list of indicators for evaluating patient status in relation to outcome, a target outcome rating, a place to identify the source of the data, a scale to measure patient status, and a short list of references used in developing the outcome (Matney 2019, TK).

Check Your Understanding 5.1

Answer the following questions.

1. True or false: Category I CPT includes E/M, anesthesia, surgery, radiology, pathology and laboratory, and medicine.
2. True or false: The three main core components of SNOMED CT are the SNOMED CT identifier, concepts, and descriptions.
3. True or false: The SNOMED CT preferred term includes the semantic tag.
4. True or false: Nursing terminologies are used for reimbursement of nursing care for Medicare patients.
5. True or false: If data granularity is the goal of colleting the data, clinical terminologies are the best choice.

Classifications

Classifications are key to secondary data use because they aggregate clinical data for healthcare statistics, design payment systems, and determine the correct payment for healthcare services. They also provide data that are used in monitoring public health risks. Information can be obtained from data encoded with a classification to improve clinical, financial, and administrative performance. Some of these classification systems are discussed in the following sections.

International Classification of Diseases, Tenth Revision, Clinical Modification

The National Center for Health Statistics (NCHS) is the governmental body responsible for the maintenance of ICD-10-CM. It originates from the World Health Organization's *International Statistical Classification of Diseases and Related Health Problems, Tenth Revision* (ICD-10). However, ICD-10-CM greatly expands the classification, resulting in greater specificity and clinical detail.

ICD-10-CM identifies the diagnosis established by the provider. An example is the ICD-10-CM code and the CPT code result (diagnosis of patient and procedure performed) in a package of information about a patient visit performed in the physician's office. This bundle is an example of aggregate data that can be used for many purposes.

ICD-10-CM can be updated twice a year, in October and April, by NCHS. The October update always occurs; the April update occurs when it is necessary for improving the timelessness of data collection. Twice a year the ICD-10 Coordination and Maintenance (C&M) Committee holds public meetings to review proposals for ICD-10-CM revisions. Representatives from NCHS are members of this committee and, based on their advice, the director of NCHS makes the final decisions on ICD-10-CM revisions.

Assignment of the ICD-10-CM code is most often the responsibility of a professional coder based on the healthcare provider's documentation of the patient's diagnosis.

ICD-10-CM Purpose and Use

The purpose of ICD-10-CM is to provide a classification of diseases for morbidity. Morbidity is the state of being diseased including illness, injury, or deviation from normal health. It is intended to classify diagnoses established by physicians at the conclusion of a patient encounter.

ICD-10-CM has many uses. All of those identified previously for classifications apply to ICD-10-CM. One use is mandated by HIPAA, which specifies the use of national standards for electronic healthcare transactions. ICD-10-CM (including the official ICD-10-CM guidelines for coding and reporting) is named as the standard for diseases, injuries, impairments, other health-related problems, their manifestations, and causes of injury, disease, impairment, or other health-related problems.

Thus, healthcare providers must report diagnoses to public as well as private insurers using ICD-10-CM.

ICD-10-CM Content and Structure

ICD-10-CM contains three to seven-character codes and descriptions for patient conditions. This includes symptoms, syndromes, diseases, and other reasons for patients requiring healthcare services. Instructions, referred to as conventions, are also a part of the classification. These are general rules to apply when using ICD-10-CM.

ICD-10-CM is divided into 21 chapters. Many are based on a body system; others are for certain types of conditions such as pregnancy. Within each chapter are blocks of conditions related in some manner, such as a single disease entity, categories, subcategories and, when appropriate, subclassifications. Figure 5.5 displays the blocks for Chapter 4, Endocrine, Nutritional, and Metabolic Diseases, category E11, subcategory E11.2, and subclassification E11.21.

Another component of ICD-10-CM is the alphabetic index. There are two major sections to the alphabetic index—the Index to Diseases and Injuries and the Index to External Causes. Two tables—one for neoplasm and the other for drugs and chemicals—are also included in the index. All content in the index is organized by main and modifying terms. Main terms represent the condition of the patient and modifying terms further explain the condition. For example, failure is the main term and congestive heart the modifying terms for the diagnosis of congestive heart failure.

ICD-10-Procedure Coding System

The Centers for Medicare and Medicaid Services (CMS) is the federal agency responsible for the ICD-10-Procedure Coding System (ICD-10-PCS). It was developed through a contract with 3M Health Information Systems and is being maintained by CMS.

Like CPT ICD-10-PCS identifies the procedure performed by the provider. However, ICD-10-PCS was created as the companion to ICD-10-CM and not as a replacement for CPT. A diagnosis coded in ICD-10-CM code combined with a procedure coded in ICD-10-PCS would be used by a hospital to explain the reason for a patient being admitted and discharged for care and the inpatient procedures performed during the stay. The aggregated data are used to determine hospital payment under the inpatient prospective payment system discussed in chapter 15, *Revenue Management and Reimbursement*.

Updates are possible for ICD-10-PCS twice a year on April 1 and October 1. The April update is

Figure 5.5 Chapter 4, Endocrine, Nutritional, and Metabolic Diseases blocks, category, subcategory, and subclassification

Blocks
E00-E07 Disorders of thyroid gland
E08-E13 Diabetes mellitus
E15-E16 Other disorders of glucose regulation and pancreatic internal secretion
E20-E35 Disorders of other endocrine glands
E36-E36 Intraoperative complications of endocrine system
E40-E46 Malnutrition
E50-E64 Other nutritional deficiencies
E65-E68 Overweight, obesity and other hyperalimentation
E70-E88 Metabolic disorders
E89-E89 Postprocedural endocrine and metabolic complications and disorders, not elsewhere classified

Category E11
E11 Type 2 diabetes mellitus

Subcategory E11.2
E11.2 Type 2 diabetes mellitus with kidney complications

Subclassification E11.21
E11.21 Type 2 diabetes mellitus with diabetic nephropathy

Source: NCHS 2018.

available to address new technologies whereas the October 1st update happens yearly. CMS representatives on the ICD-10 Coordination and Maintenance (C&M) Committee provide advice to the administrator of CMS who makes the final decisions on ICD-10-PCS revisions. CMS makes data files for software vendors and publishers to produce online and print ICD-10-PCS products available on their website.

Upon discharge of the patient from the hospital, a professional coder assigns the ICD-10-PCS code based on the physician documentation.

ICD-10-PCS Purpose and Use

The purpose of ICD-10-PCS is to provide a system for classifying procedures performed on hospital inpatients. It provides a unique code for all substantially different procedures, both currently known and those that may be identified at some future date in time.

Uses for ICD-10-PCS include those identified for classifications in general. Just as HIPAA mandates ICD-10-CM, there is also a requirement for ICD-10-PCS. ICD-10-PCS (including the official ICD-10-PCS guidelines for coding and reporting) is the standard for preventive, diagnostic, therapeutic, or other management procedures or other actions taken for diseases, injuries, and impairments on hospital inpatients reported by hospitals. Hospitals are required to use ICD-10-PCS to report procedures to public as well as private insurers.

ICD-10-PCS Content and Structure

ICD-10-PCS contains seven-character codes and descriptions for procedures. Most of ICD-10-PCS describes medical and surgical procedures. The other sections are divided into the following groups:

Medical and surgical-related sections

- Obstetrics
- Placement
- Administration
- Measurement and monitoring
- Extracorporeal or systemic assistance and performance
- Extracorporeal or systemic therapies
- Osteopathic
- Other procedures
- Chiropractic

Ancillary sections

- Imaging
- Nuclear medicine
- Radiation therapy
- Physical rehabilitation and diagnostic audiology
- Mental health
- Substance abuse treatment
- New technology

ICD-10-PCS is made up of a number of parts including tables, an index, and definitions. The tables are arranged in alphanumeric order and are formatted as a grid that lays out the valid combinations of character values for a procedure code. There are two parts to the table. The upper portion lists the first three characters and their definition, and the lower portion contains columns for the remaining four characters. Each column lists the possible options for completing the seven-character code. Figure 5.6 shows an ICD-10-PCS table.

ICD-10-PCS has an alphabetic index organized by two types of main terms. One type is based on common procedure names such as cholecystectomy and the other type on the value of the third character of the seven-character ICD-10-PCS code. The meaning of the third character varies depending on the section. For example, the third character value for the medical and surgical procedure section is root operation or the objective of the procedure. Resection, as shown in table 5.4, is one of the root operations and is listed as a main term in the index.

Another part of ICD-10-PCS is the definitions. Arranged in section order, definitions are tied to the values of characters 3 through 7 of the seven-character code. Explanations and examples may also be included with the definitions to aid in understanding how the character value is to be applied. To illustrate, the definitions and any associated explanation and examples for the third through fifth characters are shown for T, 0, and 0 in table 5.4.

Figure 5.6 Example of an ICD-10-PCS table

OFT

Section 0 Medical And Surgical *Body System* F Hepatobiliary System and Pancreas *Operation* T Resection: Cutting out or off, without replacement, all of a body part			
Body Part	*Approach*	*Device*	*Qualifier*
0 Liver 1 Liver, Right Lobe 2 Liver, Left Lobe 4 Gallbladder G Pancreas	0 Open 4 Percutaneous Endoscopic	Z No Device	Z No Qualifier
5 Hepatic Duct, Right 6 Hepatic Duct, Left 8 Cystic Duct 9 Common Bile Duct C Ampulla of Vater D Pancreatic Duct F Pancreatic Duct, Accessory	0 Open 4 Percutaneous Endoscopic 7 Via Natural or Artificial Opening 8 Via Natural or Artificial Opening Endoscopic	Z No Device	Z No Qualifier

Source: CMS 2018.

Table 5.4 Example of ICD-10-PCS characters

Character 3 - Operation T Resection	
ICD-10-PCS Value	**Definition**
Resection	Definition: Cutting out or off, without replacement, all of a body part Includes/examples: Total nephrectomy, total lobectomy of lung
Character 4 - Body Part O Liver	
ICD-10-PCS Value	**Definition**
Liver	Includes: Quadrate lobe
Character 5 - Approach O Open	
ICD-10-PCS Value	**Definition**
Open	Definition: Cutting through the skin or mucous membrane and any other body layers necessary to expose the site of the procedure

Source: CMS 2018. Created from publicly available data from the Centers for Medicare and Medicaid Services.

International Classification of Diseases 11th Revision

The foundation component of the *International Classification of Diseases 11th Revision* (ICD-11) is a network of knowledge placed into a database. It is from the foundation component that a linearization and country-specific modifications are built. A linearization is a subset of the foundation component; once created the subset becomes the Tabular list. The Tabular list is built for a use case, such as reporting mortality and morbidity or primary care. The entities selected from the foundation become categories that are jointly exhaustive and mutually exclusive of each other. Each category has a single parent and residual categories (other and unspecified) are generated. For example, the International Classification of Diseases 11th Revision for Mortality and Morbidity Statistics (ICD-11-MMS) is a linearization of the ICD-11 foundation component. ICD-11-MMS will replace the World Health Organization (WHO)'s ICD-10. NCHS has not yet decided if a US specific linearization will be created as a possible replacement for ICD-10-CM.

The establishment of a collaborative open development and maintenance process results in the ICD development version being continuously updated. However, WHO plans to produce an annual official release for international mortality and morbidity use. The first version of ICD-11-MMS was made available on June 18, 2018, and is meant to be used in preparation for implementation. The WHO member states agreed to adopt the eleventh revision of ICD-11 at their world assembly in May of 2019 with reporting using ICD-11 to come into effect on January 1, 2022 (WHO 2019).

The advancements in the information technology field and WHO's intent with ICD-11 to make better use of the digital world may mean the process for ICD-11 code assignment evolves as well. Technology advancements occurring in areas such as artificial intelligence (AI), specifically natural language processing and machine learning, may result in the initial assignment of the ICD-11 code "automatically" based on the healthcare provider's documentation of the patient's condition by the time ICD-11 is implemented. An OptumIQ survey of healthcare senior executives on AI concluded three-quarters of healthcare facilities are actively implementing or have plans to execute an AI strategy (Optum 2018).

ICD-11 Foundation Component and ICD-11-MMS Purpose and Use

WHO embarked on the revision of ICD-11 in 2000 with the goal to produce a classification that reflects scientific and medical advances, can be integrated with electronic health applications and information systems, and makes it significantly easier for healthcare organizations to implement. Accessibility and ease of use were important considerations as was instituting a collaborative open development and maintenance process. In addition, WHO wanted to improve links to terminologies such as SNOMED CT and derived and related classifications such as the International Classification of Functioning, Disability, and Health and International Classification of Diseases for Oncology, both of which are discussed the following section.

While ICD's primary purpose is to classify diseases and injuries, the ICD-11 foundation component's entities also include external causes, signs, symptoms, abnormal findings, complaints, and social factors found in a wide range of health records. ICD use includes mortality, morbidity, epidemiology, case mix, quality and safety, and primary care (WHO 2018a).

ICD-11 Foundation Component and ICD-11-MMS Content and Structure

ICD-11-MMS has 26 chapters, one supplemental section, and an extension code chapter. Many of the 26 chapters are the same as in ICD-10. However, new content expands the classification into areas not covered in the past. For the first time WHO includes ancient Chinese Medicine disorders and patterns, which allows for the recording of epidemiological data about these conditions. The supplementary section for functioning assessment is available as well. There are also new chapters for sleep-wake disorders, conditions related to sexual health, and extension codes.

The ICD-11 foundation component includes a uniform resource identifier (URI). This identifier is a unique character string for each entity. For example, the foundation URI for combined diastolic and systolic hypertension is http://id.who.int/icd/entity/1917449952. The foundation component allows for an entity to be classified in more than one place, that is an entity may have more than one parent. In the case of influenza, certain infectious or parasitic diseases, lung infections, and infections due to influenza virus are its parents.

ICD-11-MMS contains stem codes and extension codes. A **stem code** is a standalone code and can be a single entity or a combination of clinical detail (WHO 2018b). An **extension code** starts with a X, adds detail to the stem code, and must be used with it. Combinations of stem codes or a stem code and extension code(s) result in a string of codes. WHO requires a forward slash (/) or an ampersand (&) and a syntax showing what codes belong together. Code CA40.0Y&XN9YS is the string for Pneumonia due to Legionella pneumophila where the stem code CA40.0Y identifies pneumonia due to other specified bacteria and the extension code XN9YS identifies Legionella pneumophila. The ampersand (&) combines the two. Code BD54/5A11 is an example of two stem codes. This string is for diabetic foot ulcer (BD54) where the cause of the foot ulcer is type 2 diabetes (5A11). A forward slash (/) separates two stem codes.

A code has a minimum of four characters. The first character, either a number or letter, signifies the chapter number. To not confuse an ICD-11-MMS code with one in ICD-10, the second character is a letter. The third character is a number to prohibit the spelling of "undesirable words." For any character where a letter is an option, the letters "O" and "I" are not allowed to avoid confusion with the numbers "0" and "1." Some examples of ICD-11-MMS codes and descriptions are MC18 Ocular pain, BA40.0 Unstable angina, and NC72.20 Fracture of neck of femur, subcapital.

Conventions are also a part of ICD-11-MMS. These include instructions such as code also or use additional code. The ICD-11-MMS Reference Guide contains information on the conventions and instructions on how to apply them. Another component of ICD-11-MMS is the alphabetic index, a list of clinical terms (including synonyms or phrases) used to locate the codes or code combinations for conditions.

International Classification of Functioning, Disability, and Health

International Classification of Functioning, Disability, and Health (ICF) is one of the three reference classifications approved by the WHO Family of International Classification (WHO-FIC) Network. A WHO reference classification is a product of international agreements, is broadly accepted for international reporting on health, and may be used as a model for the development or revision of other classifications (Madden et al. 2012). According to WHO, "ICF is the WHO framework for measuring health and disability at both individual and population levels" (WHO 2018c).

ICD is also a WHO-FIC Network reference classification. ICD classifies heath conditions, whereas ICF classifies states of functioning, disability, and health. For example, a patient with a spinal cord injury with moderate impairment with control of voluntary movement would be represented with an ICD code for condition of the patient, spinal cord injury, and an ICF code for the level of functioning, moderate impairment with control of voluntary movement. ICF provides a standard language, terms, and concepts and an organized data structure for health and disability information (WHO 2013).

WHO updates ICF once a year in October. While the application of the ICF concepts and framework in clinical practice is the responsibility of health professionals such as physical therapists, the individual or the individual's advocate is an integral part of the assessment.

ICF Purpose and Use

WHO specifies four primary ICF purposes:

1. To provide a scientific basis for understanding and studying health and health-related states, outcomes, and determinants
2. To establish a common language for describing health and health-related states to improve communication between different users, such as healthcare workers, researchers, policy makers and the public, including people with disabilities
3. To permit comparison of data across countries, healthcare disciplines, services, and time
4. To provide a systematic coding scheme for health information systems (WHO 2018d)

ICF has a variety of uses including clinical practice, for population-based census or survey data, in educational systems, policy making, and advocacy. Although considered during clinical data content standards discussions, the US has no federal mandate that requires ICF be used.

ICF Content and Structure

ICF is both a model and a classification. The ICF model is a nonlinear, systemic, biopsychosocial model consisting of multiple components including Health Condition, Body Functions and Structures, Activities and Participation, Contextual Factors (that is, Environmental and Personal Factors), and Umbrella Terms. Functioning is the umbrella term for Body Functions, Body Structures, Activities and Participation. It denotes the positive or neutral aspects of the interaction between the health condition and contextual factors; for example, completing the daily routine. Disability is the umbrella term for impairments, activity limitations, and participation restrictions. It denotes the negative aspects of the interaction between an individual and that individual's contextual factors. An example is a person with a panic disorder has anxiety, which limits their ability to go out alone, leading to no social relationships.

As a classification, ICF includes four code components—Body Structures, Body Functions, Activities and Participation, and Environmental Factors. The ICF model component health condition is described by ICD-10.

The first level of classification is the chapter and branches are the tiered levels of the classification (Porter 2019, 305). An example of this structure is shown as follows.

- Body Structures (code component)
  - 7 Chapter 7 Structures related to movement (chapter = first-level classification)
    - 730 Structure of the upper extremity (first branch = second-level classification)
      - 7301 Structure of forearm (second branch = third-level classification)
        - 73010 Bones of forearm (third branch = fourth level of classification) (WHO 2017)

International Classification of Diseases for Oncology, Third Edition

International Classification of Diseases for Oncology, Third Edition (ICD-O-3) is a derived classification of the WHO Family of International Classifications and is based on ICD. A derived classification is one based on a reference classification such as ICD or ICF by adopting the reference classification structure and categories and providing additional detail or through rearrangement or aggregation of items from one or more reference classifications.

Tumor or cancer registries regard ICD-O-3 as their system for classifying the topography and morphology of neoplasms. Topography refers to the anatomical site of a neoplasm's origin and morphology refers to the structure and form. Specifically, morphology pertains to cell type or histology and the neoplasm's biological activity or behavior. The common source for the clinical content to be classified with ICD-O-3 is the pathology report.

ICD-O-3 was published in 2000 with corrections added in 2001 and 2003. WHO produced an additional update—ICD-O-3.1—in 2011. Both ICD-O-3 and ICD-O-3.1 are searchable online through WHO's International Agency for Research on Cancer web page.

ICD-O-3 Purpose and Use

The purpose of ICD-O-3 is to classify diseases for oncology, a branch of medicine that focuses on tumors. Data collected via ICD-O-3 is reported to state, national, and North American cancer registries.

The ICD-O-3 data have uses including the following:

- Planning and evaluating the patient's case management
- Administrative information for facility planners, cancer committees, and practitioners
- Developing and evaluating cancer control programs
- Cancer research (NCI n.d.)

ICD-O-3 Content and Structure

ICD-O-3 is a dual classification. It contains a set of codes for topography and morphology of tumors. The site of origin of the neoplasm is captured by the topography code. This code is the same four-character category as in the malignant neoplasm section of the second chapter of ICD-10. The exceptions are those categories that relate to secondary neoplasms and to specified morphological types of tumors. In addition, ICD-O-3 includes a topography for specific types of tumors such as reticuloendothelial tumors.

With very few histological types available in ICD-10, ICD-O-3 provides greater detail of the histological classification. The morphology code describes the characteristics of the tumor itself, including cell type and biologic activity. For example, code M8170/3 is a hepatocellular carcinoma where the first four digits indicate the histological term (hepatocellular), and the fifth digit after the slash is the behavior code (malignant). A separate single digit indicates the histological grading or

Figure 5.7 Example of the structure of a complete ICD-O-3 code

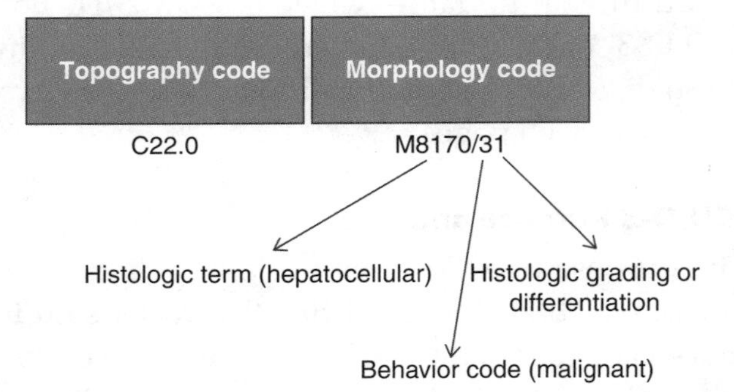

Source: ©AHIMA

differentiation. Figure 5.7 shows the structure of a complete ICD-O-3 code.

There are five main sections of ICD-O-3 are the following:

1. Instructions for Use
2. Topography-Numerical List
3. Morphology-Numerical List
4. Alphabetic Index
5. Differences in Morphology Codes between the second and third editions.

The Alphabetic Index is used for searching for a noun or adjective to locate the code for topography identified with a leading C and morphology identified with a leading M.

Diagnostic and Statistical Manual of Mental Disorders, Fifth Edition

The American Psychiatric Association (APA) developed the Diagnostic and Statistical Manual of Mental Disorders (DSM). As the standard medical classification for mental disorders, the fifth edition provides a reliable source of clinical criteria for mental health and medical professionals when establishing a diagnosis. For example, contained within DSM-5 are diagnostic criteria for depressive, anxiety, feeding and eating, and personality disorders.

A clinician with the appropriate clinical training and experience uses DSM-5 to identify mental disorders. ICD-10-CM codes are incorporated into the classification.

APA updates the ICD-10-CM codes for DSM-5 diagnoses yearly and issues other revisions as needed to address advances in the science of mental disorders. Changes are posted when approved on the APA website. Accessible via a link, the documents list updates to reflect changes or corrections, and other information relevant to mental health. The clinician is responsible for diagnosing the mental disorder using DSM-5, while most often a professional coder is responsible for assigning the ICD-10-CM code based on the documentation of the patient's diagnosis.

DSM-5 Purpose and Use

DSM-5 fills the need for "a clear and concise description of each mental disorder" (APA 2013, 5). It standardizes the clinician's diagnostic process for patients with mental disorders.

By including the ICD-10-CM codes, the clinician can document mental health disorders for administrative requirements such as requesting payment for psychiatric services or to report public health statistics.

DSM-5 may be used to conduct clinical assessments and to develop a comprehensive treatment plan. It is also used as a standard language for communicating between healthcare providers about mental disorders for a variety of purposes such as research. Although DSM-5 has forensic use, the APA warns there are risks and limitations to using it in this setting, as a clinical diagnosis of a DSM-5 mental disorder does not necessarily meet legal criteria for the presence of a mental disorder. It also does not determine a status such as competency or criminal responsibility.

DSM-5 Content and Structure

DSM-5 contains three sections, an Appendix, and an Index. The first section, DSM-5 Basics, provides an introduction along with instructions on how to use the manual. The APA's statement regarding forensic use is also a part of this section. Section II, Diagnostic Criteria and Codes, contains the diagnostic criteria, descriptive text, and ICD-10-CM codes.

Section III, Emerging Measures and Models, provides supplemental content that is not required for clinical use but could be helpful to the clinician. Included in this section are proposed mental disorders, which require further research.

Check Your Understanding 5.2

Match each classification with what it classifies.

1. ________ ICD-10-CM
2. ________ ICD-10-PCS
3. ________ ICF
4. ________ ICD-O-3
5. ________ ICD-11-MMS

a. External causes
b. States of disability
c. Inpatient procedures
d. Chinese Medicine disorders
e. Morphology of tumors

Code Systems

Code system is a very broad term. Given its definition at the beginning of this chapter, some of the terminologies and classifications previously covered could also be called code systems. Thus, a code system may have characteristics of a terminology or a classification. Depending on the system, it may be used at the point of care or for secondary data use. Common healthcare code systems are addressed in the following sections.

Logical Observation Identifiers, Names, and Codes

LOINC is "a is a common language (set of identifiers, names, and codes) for identifying health measurements, observations, and documents" (Regenstrief Institute n.d.). An observation is a measurement, test, or simple assertion and observation identifiers are the universal identifiers (names and codes) for the observation. An observation may be a test ordered or reported, a survey question, or a clinical document. LOINC provides names and codes for identifying laboratory and clinical variables. For example, the LOINC code 24356-8 and its long text name, Urinalysis complete panel—Urine, describes what was observed. Regenstrief Institute is the organization responsible for the development and maintenance of LOINC. The LOINC Committee, a group of experts organized by the Regenstrief Institute to study available standards, determined no code system available was granular enough for observation identifiers. Thus, LOINC was created to fill this gap.

Regenstrief Institute updates LOINC twice a year in June and December. No book of LOINC codes is produced. Regenstrief Institute releases a number of file formats on its website for downloading. Regenstrief Institute also provides several tools for the industry. For example, it offers a web-based LOINC search application used to explore LOINC and a more extensive resource, Regenstrief LOINC Mapping Assistant (RELMA). The purpose of RELMA is to assist in the mapping of local terms to the universal LOINC codes.

LOINC Purpose and Use

The purpose of LOINC is to standardize names and codes for the identification of laboratory and clinical variables. Settings where LOINC is used include clinical institutions to health systems, information technology vendors, research projects, government agencies, and international e-Health projects (McDonald et al. 2018). Professional societies and insurance companies also use LOINC.

LOINC facilitates the exchange of data between diverse electronic systems including the clinical laboratory information management and the EHR. This clinical data can then be used for clinical care and research. Another use is in outcomes management where the clinical data are examined to study the outcome and improve care.

LOINC is also one of several standards chosen for the entry of structured data in certified EHR systems (ONC 2015). This includes using LOINC in a number of situations such as reporting clinical lab test results and vital signs per the Common Clinical Data Set discussed later in this chapter. Other requirements include exchanging patient summaries at transitions of care, using and exchanging social, psychological, and behavioral data, and reporting results to cancer registries and public health agencies for electronic quality measure reporting, patient assessment instruments required in post-acute care settings (Vreeman 2019). Having a structured format for laboratory test information in certified EHRs enables the exchange of data for use in clinical care and research.

LOINC Content and Structure

There are two major groups of LOINC content—laboratory and clinical. The laboratory piece includes just as the name suggests: laboratory tests such as chemistry, urinalysis, serology, and toxicology. For the clinical piece LOINC, the scope is broad. Names and codes are available for observations like vital signs, obstetric ultrasound, radiology studies, respiratory therapy, nursing, clinical documents, and patient assessment instruments to name a few.

The fully specified name of an observation is consists of the following five or six main parts:

1. Component analyte
2. Kind of property
3. Time aspect
4. System
5. Scale
6. Method (only used when different methodologies significantly change the interpretation of the results) (McDonald et al. 2018)

For example, a 12-hour creatinine clearance test breaks down into the following parts:

- Component/analyte: creatinine renal clearance
- Kind of property: Volume rate (VRat)
- Time: 12 hours
- System: Urine and serum/plasma
- Scale: Quantitative

This test can be described formally with the following syntax:

Creatinine renal clearance:VRat:12H:
Ur+Ser/Plas:Qn

In LOINC, each lab test is assigned a unique permanent code. The code identifies the test results in electronic reports in clinical laboratory information management and EHR systems, thereby facilitating data exchange for use in clinical care, quality measurement, and research. The code for a 12-hour creatinine clearance test is 2163-4.

Healthcare Common Procedure Coding System Level II

HCPCS consists of two code systems: Level I and Level II. Level I includes CPT, discussed previously. HCPCS Level II standardizes the reporting of professional services, procedures, products, and supplies. CMS publishes and maintains HCPCS Level II. One section within HCPCS Level II, the Dental Codes, or D codes, are a separate category and are published by the American Dental Association, not CMS.

CMS requires physicians to use HCPCS Level II to report services provided to Medicare and Medicaid patients. Hospitals must report ambulatory surgery services, radiology, and other diagnostic services using HCPCS Level II.

CMS updates HCPCS Level II quarterly on January 1, April 1, July 1, and October 1. A professional coder assigns the HCPCS Level II code based on the physician documentation.

HCPCS Purpose and Use

The primary purpose of HCPCS Level II is to meet the operational needs of Medicare and

Medicaid reimbursement programs. Thus, as expected, HCPCS Level II is required for reimbursement of ambulatory services provided in healthcare settings. This includes physician and hospital outpatient reimbursement. Other uses of the code system include benchmarking, trending, planning, and measurement of quality of care.

HIPAA mandates HCPCS Level II as the standardized coding system for describing and identifying healthcare equipment and supplies in healthcare transactions that are not identified by the HCPCS Level I, CPT codes. Thus, healthcare providers must report these services to public as well as private insurers, using HCPCS Level II.

HCPCS Content and Structure

Level II of HCPCS contains products, supplies, and services. Included in HCPCS Level II are ambulance services, drugs, and durable medical equipment, prosthetics, orthotics, and supplies. Modifiers are used with HCPCS Level II codes to explain various circumstances of procedures and services. Modifiers are also used to enhance a code narrative to describe the circumstances of each procedure or service and how it applies to an individual patient. In some situations, insurers instruct providers and suppliers to add a modifier to provide additional information regarding the service or item identified by the HCPCS Level II code.

HCPCS Level II is divided into the following chapters:

- A Codes: Transportation Services including Ambulance, Medical and Surgical Supplies, Radiopharmaceuticals, and Miscellaneous
- B Codes: External and Parental Therapy
- C Codes: Outpatient Prospective Payment System (Temporary)
- D Codes: Dental Procedures
- E Codes: Durable Medical Equipment
- G Codes: Procedures/Professional Services (Temporary)
- H Codes: Alcohol and Drug Abuse Treatment Services
- J Codes: Drugs Administered Other than by Oral Method
- K Codes: (Temporary Codes)
- L Codes: Orthotic and Prosthetic Procedures and Devices
- M Codes: Medical Services
- P Codes: Pathology and Laboratory Services
- Q Codes: (Temporary)
- R Codes: Diagnostic Radiology Services
- S Codes: Temporary National Codes (Non-Medicare)
- T Codes: Temporary National Codes
- V Codes: Vision and Hearing Services

The index for Level II codes lists terms alphabetically. Drugs are not included in the index but are found in their own table.

RxNorm

RxNorm is both a standardized nomenclature for clinical drugs and a semantic interoperability tool. The NLM, an institute of the National Institutes of Medicine, is responsible for the maintenance of RxNorm. The nomenclature is recognized as a standard for exchanging clinical drug information.

RxNorm normalizes names and unique identifiers for clinical drugs and links its names to the varying names of drugs present in many different vocabularies within the Unified Medical Language System (UMLS) Metathesaurus (NLM 2018a). A normalized name in RxNorm is the ingredient, strength, and dose form for a drug.

RxNorm is updated weekly and there is a monthly full release update. The package includes the standardized nomenclature for clinical drugs and a tool for supporting semantic interoperation between drug terminologies and pharmacy knowledge base systems (Meredith 2019, 237-238). NLM also provides several tools for the industry including a web-based RxNorm browser application called RxNav.

RxNorm Purpose and Use

RxNorm's purpose is to allow computer systems to efficiently and unambiguously communicate drug-related information between hospitals, pharmacies, and other organizations (NLM 2018b). Its objective is to normalize names of generic and branded drugs and attach a unique identifier to that name.

Common RxNorm uses include the following:

- Support interoperability during e-prescribing and formulary management
- Communication between hospital, pharmacy, and other organizations' computer systems, for order entry and analytics and for managing a medication list
- Development of an allergy value set to support effective and interoperable health information exchange (Meredith 2019, 237-238)

RxNorm has been named as the standard for a number of governmental programs. This includes medications for the entry of structured data in certified EHR systems under the Meaningful Use (now called the promoting interoperability program) (ONC 2015). RxNorm is also the standard for medication and medication allergy reporting per the Common Clinical Data Set discussed later in this chapter. The Merit-Based Incentive Payment System e-prescribing measure lists RxNorm as the standard for medications.

RxNorm Content and Structure

The drug name and all of its synonyms represent a single concept, which is assigned an RxNorm concept unique identifier (RXCUI). Figure 5.8 shows the RxNorm graph for an amoxicillin 400 mg chewable tablet. This display shows a text string search using the classic view. At the top after the description is the RxCUI, 308188. On the left is the ingredient (amoxicillin), ingredient plus strength (amoxicillin 400 mg), and ingredient plus strength plus dose form (amoxicillin 400 mg chewable tablet). The combination of ingredient plus strength plus dose form is known as a semantic clinical drug term type. At the bottom are windows displaying the clinical dose form group (bottom left) and dose form group (bottom middle).

Figure 5.8 RxNorm graph for amoxicillin 400 mg chewable tablet

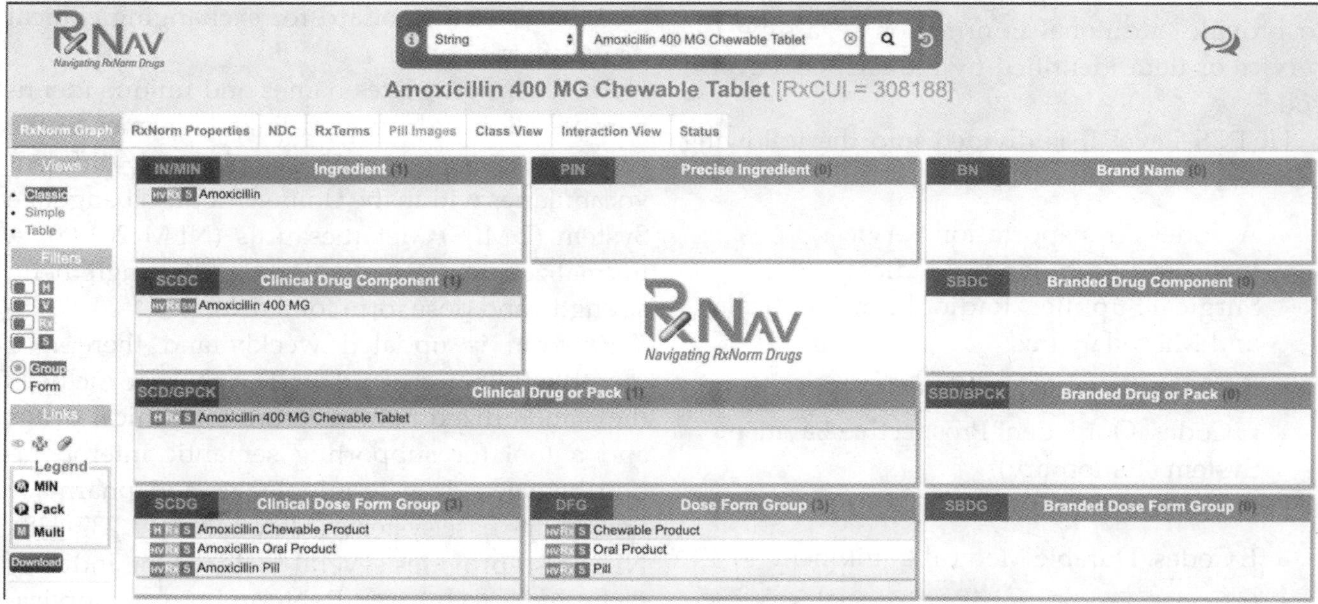

Source: NLM 2019. Created from publicly available data from the U.S. National Library of Medicine (NLM), National Institutes of Health, Department of Health and Human Services.

Check Your Understanding 5.3

Answer the following questions.

1. The standard for clinical lab observations is __________.
2. The RxNorm semantic clinical drug term type contains information on which of the following?
   a. Manufactured drug
   b. Route
   c. Ingredients
   d. Packaged product
3. True or false: HCPCS Level II is standard for supplies under HIPAA.
4. True or false: LOINC is standard for drugs under the promoting interoperability program.
5. Which type of HCPCS Level II code is not published by CMS?
   a. Dental Procedures
   b. Durable Medical Equipment
   c. Vision and Hearing Services
   d. Drugs Administered Other than by Oral Method

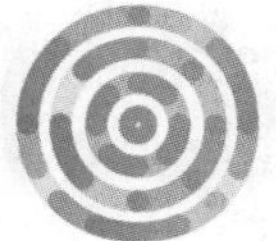

Clinical Terminologies, Classifications, and Code Systems Found in Health Data and Information Sets

There are many reasons for forming a **data set**, a list of recommended data elements with uniform definitions. One reason might be to collect statistical data for reporting to national and state registries (discussed in more detail in chapter 7, *Secondary Data Sources*). Other purposes of data and information sets are to gather data for clinical decision support and for computation and reporting of clinical quality measures (discussed in more detail in chapter 18, *Performance Improvement*). Many of the data elements contained in a data and information set are now captured electronically when data documentation is done at the time of care.

Data and information sets may come from federal data reporting requirements, such as Meaningful Use (now called the promoting interoperability program), and others from public initiatives related to standardized performance measures. (Meaningful use is discussed in chapter 16, *Fraud and Abuse Compliance.*) Data sets may be formed for such activities as research, clinical trials, quality and safety improvement, reimbursement, accreditation, and exchanging clinical information (Giannangelo 2007). Some of these data sets are listed as follows.

Outcomes and Assessment Information Set

The Outcomes and Assessment Information Set (OASIS) is a standardized data set designed to provide the necessary data items to measure outcomes and patient risk factors of Medicare beneficiaries who are receiving skilled services from a Medicare-certified home health agency. According to CMS, "OASIS data items address sociodemographic, environmental, support system, health status, functional status, and health service utilization characteristics of the patient" (CMS 2012).

OASIS has undergone several updates and refinements. OASIS-D version is the version of the OASIS data set that went into effect on January 1, 2019. It is the core data item set for collection on all adult home health patients whose skilled care is reimbursed by Medicare and Medicaid with the exception of patients receiving pre- or postnatal services only. Only a registered nurse (RN) or any of the therapies (physical therapist [PT], speech-language pathologist/speech therapist [SLP/ST], occupational therapist [OT]) can conduct the comprehensive assessment and OASIS data collection (CMS 2019).

A data collection instrument containing the data elements is used by those qualified to do so at various times such as the start of care or upon discharge from home care services. Submission of OASIS data is a CMS requirement if the agency participates in the Medicare program. The data are used in a variety of ways such as the assessment of the patient's ability to be discharged or transferred from home care services or the creation of patient case mix profile reports used by state survey staff in the certification process. The CMS Home Health Compare website's information on home health agency process and improvement outcome measures is based on OASIS data submitted by home health agencies to state repositories. Medicare provides this information to anyone who may have an interest in comparing home health agency performance.

Healthcare Effectiveness Data and Information Set

The Healthcare Effectiveness Data and Information Set (HEDIS), sponsored by the National Committee for Quality Assurance (NCQA), is designed to collect administrative, claims, and health record review data. HEDIS contains more than 90 standard performance measures. Included are data related to patient outcomes and data about the treatment process.

NCQA collects the data from health plans, healthcare organizations, and government agencies. HEDIS survey data and protocols standardize data about specific health-related conditions or issues to evaluate and compare the success of various treatment plans. These data form the basis of performance improvement (PI) efforts for health plans. HEDIS data also are important in the creation of physician profiles for use in positively shaping physician practice patterns by showing comparative clinical performance information to encourage quality improvement or utilization adjustments.

Once the standardized HEDIS data elements from health records are gathered, these data are combined with enrollment and claims data and analyzed according to HEDIS specifications. Healthcare purchasers and consumers can use the information to compare the performance of managed healthcare plans to help decide which plan to contract with or enroll in.

Uniform Hospital Discharge Data Set

The Uniform Hospital Discharge Data Set (UHDDS) is required by Department of Health and Human Services (HHS). This core set of data elements is collected by acute-care, short-term stay (usually less than 30 days) hospitals to report inpatient data elements in a standardized manner. It was developed through the National Committee on Vital and Health Statistics (NCVHS).

The 837I, the institutional standard healthcare claim format for electronic healthcare transactions, and Form CMS-1450, also known as the Uniform Bill UB-04, for paper claims, are the instruments for collecting UHDDS data elements. When diagnosis-related groups (DRGs) were implemented, UHDDS definitions were incorporated into the inpatient prospective payment system (PPS) regulations. For additional information on DRGs and the inpatient PPS, see chapter 15, *Revenue Management and Reimbursement*.

The UHDDS lists and defines a set of common data elements for the purpose of facilitating the collection of uniform and comparable health information from hospitals. Contained in the UHDDS's data dictionary are the definitions of the core data elements to be collected along with each data element's guidelines for use. For example, the UHDDS data element principal diagnosis is defined in the data dictionary as the condition, after study, to be chiefly responsible for occasioning the admission of the patient to the hospital for care. This element and its definition are used to determine a DRG.

Common Clinical Data Set

The Office of the National Coordinator for Health Information Technology (ONC) established a common

Table 5.5 USCDI version 1 data classes

1. Patient name	**2.** Sex (birth sex)
3. Date of birth	**4.** Preferred language
5. Race	**6.** Ethnicity
7. Smoking status	**8.** Laboratory tests
9. Laboratory values/results	**10.** Vital signs
11. Problems	**12.** Medications
13. Medication allergies	**14.** Health concerns
15. Care team members	**16.** Assessment and plan of treatment
17. Immunizations	**18.** Procedures
19. Unique device identifier(s) for a patient's implantable device(s)	**20.** Goals
21. Provenance	**22.** Clinical notes

Source: © AHIMA

set of data types and elements and associated standards for use across several certification criteria. The Common Clinical Data Set (CCDS) is the combination of these common sets of data types and elements and associated standards used across several certification criteria. The CCDS is used across inpatient and ambulatory care settings. Some but not all data types or elements have a standard attached to them. An example of a data element with a specified standard is smoking status. It must be reported with one of the following SNOMED CT identifiers:

- Current everyday smoker. 449868002
- Current some day smoker. 428041000124106
- Former smoker. 8517006
- Never smoker. 266919005
- Smoker, current status unknown. 77176002
- Unknown if ever smoked. 266927001
- Heavy tobacco smoker. 428071000124103
- Light tobacco smoker. 428061000124105

Released as a draft, the U.S. Core Data for Interoperability (USCDI) in meant to help achieve the goals in the 21st Century Cures Act. The USCDI takes the CCDS and adds clinical notes and provenance to the list of data classes. Table 5.5 lists the draft USCDI data classes, which include the CCDS.

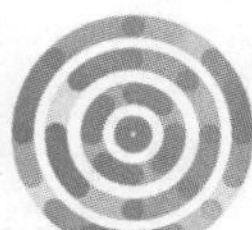

Database of Clinical Terminologies, Classifications, and Code Systems

The number of clinical terminologies, classifications, and code systems in healthcare has grown substantially over the past few decades and some that have been around for several years have undergone revisions and updates expanding their size. Although consolidation in some instances may occur in the future, requirements for use are not limited to just one. With so many available and some of them being quite large, a centralized location is needed to maintain consistent terminology for implementation and use. One such centralized location of health and biomedical terminologies and standards is the Unified Medical Language System (UMLS).

Having access to terminologies, classifications, and code systems from a single source is made possible through the efforts of the NLM via the UMLS. According to the NLM, "the UMLS integrates and distributes key terminology, classification and coding standards, and associated resources to promote creation of more effective and interoperable biomedical information systems and services, including electronic health records" (NLM 2016a).

The UMLS is a multipurpose resource. It contains the Metathesaurus, Semantic Network, and SPECIALIST Lexicon and Lexical Tools, which make up the UMLS Knowledge Resources. In addition, the UMLS Terminology Services (UTS) provides UMLS access. The Metathesaurus contains the codes and terms from over 200 terminology, classification, and coding standards. Those found include terminologies designed for use in EHR systems (for example, SNOMED CT), disease and procedure classifications used for statistical reporting and billing (such as ICD-10-CM and HCPCS), and code systems such as LOINC. The UTS is a set of web-based applications that serves as the gateway to the UMLS Knowledge Sources and the site to download the UMLS data files.

The uses of UMLS are the following:

- Linking health information, medical terms, drug names, and billing codes across different computer systems such as between the physician, pharmacy, and insurance company
- Coordinating patient care among different hospital departments
- Searching engine retrieval
- Data mining
- Reporting public health statistics
- Researching terminology (NLM 2016b)

Check Your Understanding 5.4

Answer the following questions.

1. True or false: Data elements specified in OASIS-D are collected on long-term care patients.
2. True or false: The Common Clinical Data Set definitions are incorporated into the inpatient prospective payment system.
3. LOINC would be found in the UMLS ____________.
   a. Value Set Authority Center
   b. SPECIALIST Lexicon
   c. Semantic Network
   d. Metathesaurus
4. The ____________ is a core component of SNOMED CT.
   a. Identifier
   b. Hierarchy
   c. Concept
   d. Definition
5. The ________ in SNOMED CT is the description assigned to a concept that is used most commonly in a clinical record or in literature for a specific language or dialect.
   a. Main term
   b. Preferred term
   c. Customary term
   d. Fully specified name

Real-World Case 5.1

The 2015 Edition EHR technology certification criteria state the following:

Smoking status: Enable a user to electronically record, change, and access the smoking status of a patient in accordance with the standard specified.

45 CFR 170.315(a)(11). Coded to one of the following SNOMED CT codes:

- Current everyday smoker. 449868002
- Current some day smoker. 428041000124106
- Former smoker. 8517006
- Never smoker. 266919005
- Smoker, current status unknown. 77176002
- Unknown if ever smoked. 266927001
- Heavy tobacco smoker. 428071000124103
- Light tobacco smoker. 428061000124105

Objective: Record smoking status for patients 13 years or older.

Measure: More than 85 percent of all unique patients 13 years old or older seen by the eligible professional or admitted to the eligible hospital's or critical care hospital's inpatient or emergency department during the EHR reporting period have smoking status records as structured data.

A quick reference for meeting the smoking status promoting interoperability requirement is included in the American Academy of Family Physicians (AAFP) Tobacco and Nicotine Cessation Toolkit. The AAFP supports the incorporation of tobacco cessation into EHR templates (AAFP 2015). The quick reference provides guidance on what should be included in a tobacco cessation EHR template.

Real-World Case 5.2

Opioid use is a major concern for healthcare professionals and organizations worldwide. Even governmental agencies are becoming involved. For example, the National Institutes of Health launched the Helping to End Addiction Long-term as a way to speed scientific solutions to curtail the national opioid public health crisis. The accurate identification of opioid use disorder is important to the success of the research that will take place. DSM-5, ICD-10-CM, SNOMED CT, and in the future ICD-11-MMS are all possible ways to identify cases for research.

References

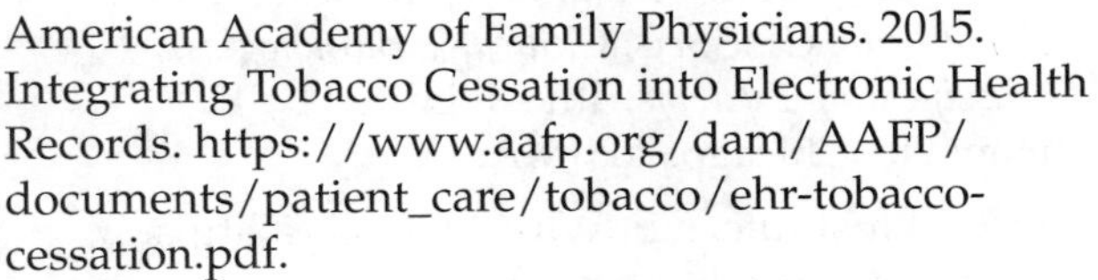

American Academy of Family Physicians. 2015. Integrating Tobacco Cessation into Electronic Health Records. https://www.aafp.org/dam/AAFP/documents/patient_care/tobacco/ehr-tobacco-cessation.pdf.

American Health Information Management Association. 2017. *Pocket Glossary of Health Information Management and Technology*, 5th ed. Chicago: AHIMA.

American Medical Association. 2018. *Current Procedural Terminology*, 4th ed. Chicago: AMA.

American Nursing Association. 2018 (April 19). Inclusion of Recognized Terminologies Supporting Nursing Practice within Electronic Health Records and Other Health Information Technology Solutions. https://www.nursingworld.org/practice-policy/nursing-excellence/official-position-statements/id/Inclusion-of-Recognized-Terminologies-Supporting-Nursing-Practice-within-Electronic-Health-Records/.

American Psychiatric Association. 2013. *Diagnostic and Statistical Manual of Mental Disorders*, 5th ed. Arlington, VA: APA.

Centers for Medicare and Medicaid Services. 2019. OASIS-D Guidance Manual. https://www.cms.gov/Medicare/Quality-Initiatives-Patient-Assessment-Instruments/HomeHealthQualityInits/HHQIOASISUserManual.html.

Centers for Medicare and Medicaid Services. 2018. ICD-10-PCS. http://www.cms.gov/Medicare/Coding/ICD10/2016-ICD-10-PCS-and-GEMs.html.

Centers for Medicare and Medicaid Services. 2012 (August 21). Outcomes and Assessment Information Set (OASIS): Data Set. https://www.cms.gov/Medicare/Quality-Initiatives-Patient-Assessment-Instruments/OASIS/DataSet.html.

Clinical Information Modeling Initiative. 2013. Category: Reference Terminology. http://informatics.mayo.edu/CIMI/index.php/Category:Reference_Terminology.

Giannangelo, K., ed. 2019. Introduction. *Healthcare Code Sets, Clinical Terminologies, and Classification Systems*, 4th ed. Chicago: AHIMA.

Giannangelo, K. 2007. Unraveling the data set, an e-HIM essential. *Journal of AHIMA* 78(2):60–61.

Helwig, A. 2013 (October 29). EHR Certification Criteria for SNOMED CT Will Help Doctors Transition to ICD-10. http://www.healthit.gov/buzz-blog/electronic-health-and-medical-records/ehr-certification-criteria-snomed-ct-doctors-transition-icd10/.

Madden, R., C. Sykes, and T. B. Ustun. 2012. World Health Organization Family of International Classifications: Definition, scope and purpose. https://www.who.int/classifications/en/FamilyDocument2007.pdf?ua=1.

Matney, S. 2019. Terminologies Used in Nursing Practice. Chapter 12 in *Healthcare Code Sets, Clinical Terminologies, and Classification Systems*, 4th ed. Edited by K. Giannangelo. Chicago: AHIMA.

McDonald, C.J., S. Huff, J. Deckard, S. Armson, S. Abhyankar, and D. Vreeman, eds. 2018. Logical Observation Identifiers Names and Codes (LOINC) Users' Guide. https://loinc.org/downloads/loinc/#users-guide.

Meredith, T. 2019. RxNorm. Chapter 8 in *Healthcare Code Sets, Clinical Terminologies, and Classification Systems*, 4th ed. Edited by K. Giannangelo. Chicago: AHIMA.

National Cancer Institute. n.d. SEER Training Modules: Data Standards. http://training.seer.cancer.gov/operations/standards/.

National Center for Health Statistics. 2018. ICD-10-CM. http://www.cdc.gov/nchs/icd/icd10cm.htm.

National Library of Medicine. 2019. RxNav, Version 07-Jan-2019. https://mor.nlm.nih.gov/RxNav/.

National Library of Medicine. 2018a. RxNorm Technical Documentation, Version 2018-1. https://www.nlm.nih.gov/research/umls/rxnorm/docs/index.html.

National Library of Medicine. 2018b. RxNorm Overview. https://www.nlm.nih.gov/research/umls/rxnorm/overview.html.

National Library of Medicine. 2016a. Unified Medical Language System. https://www.nlm.nih.gov/research/umls/.

National Library of Medicine. 2016b. UMLS Quick Start Guide. https://www.nlm.nih.gov/research/umls/quickstart.html.

Office of the National Coordinator for Health Information Technology. n.d. What is EHR interoperability and why is it important? https://www.healthit.gov/faq/what-ehr-interoperability-and-why-it-important.

Office of the National Coordinator for Health Information Technology. 2018a. 2018 Interoperability standards advisory. https://www.healthit.gov/isa/sites/isa/files/2018%20ISA%20Reference%20Edition.pdf.

Office of the National Coordinator for Health Information Technology. 2018b. Draft U.S. Core Data for Interoperability (USCDI) and proposed expansion process. https://www.healthit.gov/sites/default/files/draft-uscdi.pdf.

Office of the National Coordinator for Health Information Technology. 2015 (October 16). 2015 edition health information technology (Health IT) certification criteria, 2015 edition base electronic health record (EHR) definition, and ONC health IT certification program modifications. *Federal Register*. https://www.federalregister.gov/articles/2015/10/16/2015-25597/2015-edition-health-information-technology-health-it-certification-criteria-2015-edition-base.

Optum. 2018. OptumIQ annual survey on AI in health care fact sheet. https://www.optum.com/content/dam/optum3/optum/en/resources/PDFs/OptumIQ_AI%20Survey%20Data%20Points_Media%20Fact%20Sheet.pdf.

Porter, H.R. 2019. International Classification of Functioning, Disability, and Health. Chapter 11 in *Healthcare Code Sets, Clinical Terminologies, and Classification Systems*, 4th ed. Edited by K. Giannangelo. Chicago: AHIMA.

Regenstrief Institute. n.d. What LOINC is. https://loinc.org/get-started/what-loinc-is/.

Shulman, L. and N. Stepro. 2015 (June 3). What Lies Beneath. Arcadia Healthcare Solutions. http://arcadiasolutions.com/lies-beneath/.

SNOMED International. 2018 (July 26). SNOMED CT Editorial Guide. https://confluence.ihtsdotools.org/display/DOCEG/SNOMED+CT+Editorial+Guide.

SNOMED International. 2017a (December 21). SNOMED CT Glossary. https://confluence.ihtsdotools.org/display/DOCGLOSS/SNOMED+Glossary.

SNOMED International. 2017b (July 28). SNOMED CT Starter Guide. https://confluence.ihtsdotools.org/display/DOCSTART.

Vreeman, D. 2019. Logical Observation Identifiers, Names, and Codes. Chapter 10 in *Healthcare Code Sets, Clinical Terminologies, and Classification Systems*, 4th ed. Edited by K. Giannangelo. Chicago: AHIMA.

Warren, J. 2015. Terminologies Used in Nursing Practice. Chapter 12 in *Healthcare Code Sets, Clinical Terminologies, and Classification Systems*, 3rd ed. Edited by K. Giannangelo. Chicago: AHIMA.

World Health Organization. 2019. International Statistical Classification of Diseases and Related Health Problems (ICD-11).

World Health Organization. 2018a (December 18). ICD-11-MMS Reference guide. https://icd.who.int/icd11refguide/en/index.html.

World Health Organization. 2018b. Classifications: The International Classification of Functioning, Disability and Health. http://www.who.int/classifications/icf/en/.

World Health Organization. 2019. World Health Assembly Update, 25, May 2019. https://www.who.int/news-room/detail/25-05-2019-world-health-assembly-update

World Health Organization. 2018d. ICF e-learning tool. https://www.icf-elearning.com/.

World Health Organization. 2017. ICF Browser. http://apps.who.int/classifications/icfbrowser/.

World Health Organization. 2013. A Practical Manual for using the International Classification of Functioning, Disability and Health (ICF). http://www.who.int/classifications/drafticfpracticalmanual.pdf.

Data Management

Danika E. Brinda, PhD, RHIA, CHPS, HCISPP

Learning Objectives

- Identify the different sources where data are created, stored, or transmitted
- Distinguish among data elements, data sets, databases, indices, data mapping, and data warehousing
- Distinguish among information governance, data governance, data stewardship, data integrity, data sharing, and data interchange standards
- Explain the principles of information governance
- Illustrate the impact of data quality on the healthcare organization as it relates to patient care, reimbursement, and healthcare operations
- Examine the purpose of clinical documentation integrity and how it relates to data quality
- Identify the basics of clinical documentation integrity query processes
- Describe the reasons for establishing data quality and data management requirements in provider contracts, medical staff bylaws, and hospital bylaws

Key Terms

Business intelligence (BI)
Bylaws
Clinical documentation
Clinical documentation integrity (CDI)
Critical thinking
Data
Data dictionary
Data element
Data governance
Data integrity
Data interchange standards
Data management
Data mapping
Data mining
Data quality
Data quality management
Data quality management model
Data sets
Data Steward
Data stewardship
Data visualization
Data warehouse
Data warehousing
Database
Database life cycle (DBLC)
Enterprise information management (EIM)
Hospital bylaws
Index
Information
Information assets
Information governance (IG)

Information Governance Principles of Healthcare
Interoperability
Object-oriented database (OODB)
Query
Relational database
Situation, background, assessment, and recommendation (SBAR)
Source data
Standards
Standards development organization (SDO)
Structured data
System characterization
Target data
Unstructured data
Use case

With the advancement of technology in the US healthcare system, most healthcare organizations are inundated with data from multiple sources, which are stored and maintained in a variety of locations. Data are representations of basic facts and observations about people, processes, measurements, and conditions. An example of data is 50 patients were discharged yesterday. Healthcare-specific data focus on patients and include demographic, financial, and clinical data. Data management is the combined practices of HIM, IT, and HI that affect how data and documentation combine to create a single business record for an organization. Effective oversight and management of the data is an essential part of the day-to-day operations of a healthcare organization. Knowing and understanding how data are produced, why certain types and formats of data are produced, how data are stored and managed, and how data integrity is maintained become foundational steps to ensuring the data within healthcare organizations are properly managed.

Data Sources

A foundational step to the management of data within a healthcare organization is to understand the basic sources of data generated and stored by the healthcare organization. Data includes both clinical and administrative elements. The data elements stored in the electronic health record are an example of clinical data. Administrative data includes the data elements required for billing and quality improvement. The common data sources in healthcare: are the following:

- Electronic health records (EHR) (discussed in chapter 11, *Health Information Systems*)
- Practice management systems (discussed in chapter 11, *Health Information Systems*)
- Lab information systems (discussed in chapter 11, *Health Information Systems*)
- Radiology information systems (discussed in chapter 11, *Health Information Systems*)
- Picture archival and communications (PACs) (discussed in chapter 11, *Health Information Systems*)
- Other clinical documentation systems (home health, therapy, long-term care) (discussed in chapter 11, *Health Information Systems*)
- Master patient index (discussed in chapter 3, *Health Information Functions, Purpose, and Users*)
- Other patient index (indices) (discussed in chapter 7, *Secondary Data Sources*)
- Databases (discussed later in this chapter)
- Registries (discussed in chapter 7, *Secondary Data Sources*)

To manage the different aspects of data effectively, the healthcare organization should conduct system characterization. System characterization is the process of creating an inventory of all systems that contain data, including documenting where the data are stored, what types of data are created or stored, how they are managed, with what hardware and software they interact, and providing basic security measures for the systems (Walsh 2013). This process helps identify all sources of data that exist within a healthcare organization, which supports effective oversight over all the data created and maintained by an organization.

Data Management

Managing the data that healthcare organizations create and produce is challenging. Data can exist in an information system, on a file on an employee's computer or file server, in an email, and in many other formats and locations. Healthcare organizations are challenged with how to properly manage all the data that exist and how to effectively use and preserve that data.

The process of data collection has evolved over the years as healthcare organizations migrate from paper-based recordkeeping systems to electronic health records (EHR). For additional information on EHRs, refer to chapter 11, *Health Information Systems.* Additionally, healthcare organizations are collecting more patient data and using the data to support patient care and healthcare operations. The ability to properly collect, analyze, and utilize patient data is more important now than ever before. Third-party payers, government agencies, accreditation organizations, and others also use data to support the healthcare delivery system and improve patient care. One of the challenges for healthcare systems that are managing data in an electronic environment is the vast differences in the collection of healthcare data throughout the organization's electronic information systems, such as EHRs, lab information systems, radiology information systems, and billing systems (discussed in chapter 11, *Health Information Systems*). Many methods, formats, and processes are used for the collection and storage of patient information, such as direct entry into an electronic system, scanning of documents, and uploading of transcribed documentation. Data management is further complicated because data are collected and stored in many locations in the healthcare organization. Given the various methodologies that exist for data collection, understanding data and data collection is important. Data management focuses on understanding data elements, data sets, databases, indices, data mapping, and data warehousing.

Data Elements

The term *data* is actually the plural format of *datum*; however, it is more common to hear the term *data element* to describe one fact or measurement. A **data element** can be a single or individual fact that represents the smallest unique subset of a larger database. Data elements are sometimes referred to as the raw facts and figures. Examples of data elements include age, gender, blood pressure, temperature, test results, and date of birth. Data elements create a measure for progress to be determined and the future to be calculated and planned for. Data elements are entered into different formats through the EHR and other supporting patient systems. **Information** is different from data in that it refers to data elements that have been combined and then manipulated into something meaningful regarding a patient or a group of patients. For example, a healthcare organization can create a report on the data element's most recent A1C test result and diagnosis of a heart attack and analyze and determine if there is a relationship between the A1C test score and the heart attack diagnosis. By taking the specific data elements of the heart attack diagnosis and the most current A1C result, the healthcare organization can create best practices to enhance patient care based on the findings (Davoudi et al. 2015). For more on data and information, see chapter 3, *Health Information Functions, Purpose, and Users.*

To help support and manage data elements within an EHR, the use of a data dictionary is implemented to support standardized input and understanding of all data elements. A **data dictionary** is a listing of all the data elements within a specific information system that defines each individual data element, standard input of the data element, and specific data length. The following are the common data elements within a data dictionary:

- Data field (such as date of birth)
- Definition
- Data type (date, text, number, and so forth)

- Format (such as MM-DD-YYYY)
- Field size (such as 10 digits for phone number)
- Data values (such as M and F for gender)
- Data source (where data are collected)
- Data first entered (when the data element is first used)
- Why item is included (justification for collection of the data element) (AHIMA 2017)

Defining a data dictionary can help with accuracy of patient data and create support for data comparison and data sharing (AHIMA 2016a). (Additional information on the sharing of data is found in chapter 12, *Healthcare Information.*) Table 6.1 provides a sample of a data dictionary defining the data elements in an EHR.

Defining a data dictionary is a fundamental step to understanding data elements and their meaning and usage. It also supports the creation of well-structured and defined data sets by creating standardized definitions of data elements to help ensure consistency of collection and use of the data. For example, the time of discharge could be the time the discharge order was written, the time the order was entered into the information system, or the time the patient actually left the unit. These times could vary widely so it is important that the data dictionary defines which time should be used.

Data Sets

The concept of comparing data and the need for standardization became a common theme for healthcare organizations in the 1960s as a result of the work of the National Center for Health Statistics (NCHS) and the National Committee on Vital and Health Statistics (NCVHS). It became evident that common structure and collection of data elements was needed to collect consistent data to allow for comparison across all healthcare organizations. As a result, the concept of data sets was created. **Data sets** are a recommended list of data elements that have defined and uniform definitions that are relevant for a particular use or are specific to a type of healthcare industry. One of the first defined and used data sets across the US healthcare industry was the Uniform Hospital Discharge Data Set (UHDDS), implemented in the mid-1970s. Created by NCHS, the National Center for Health Services Research and Development, and Johns Hopkins University, UHDDS collects uniform data elements from the health records of every hospital inpatient (Brinda 2016). The main data elements defined in the UHDDS data set are listed in figure 6.1.

Each of the data elements defined within the UHDDS has specific criteria for data collection. For example, the data of birth are defined as the month, day, and year of birth, with a recommendation to collect all four digits of the birth year. Another example is the definition of type of admission. There are two choices—unscheduled or scheduled admission. Each of the types of admission is defined in the data set for use of the UHDDS (Brinda 2016).

Shortly after the UHDDS was created and implemented, the need to expand uniform data sets across other healthcare settings became evident with the continuing movement from an inpatient, acute setting to outpatient care including surgical centers and emergency care settings. A standardized data set for the ambulatory setting, known as the Uniform Ambulatory Care Data Set (UACDS), was created. With fewer data elements than the UHDDS, the UACDS collects data specific to ambulatory care settings with an intent to improve data comparison across different settings of healthcare (see figure 6.2). After the success of the standardization of data elements with the UHDDS and UACDS, the standardization of data sets across healthcare settings commenced. Another key data set is Data Elements for Emergency Department Systems (DEEDS), which collects data for hospital-based emergency departments. The following are other data sets that are defined within healthcare settings:

- Minimum Data Set (MDS)—Long-term care setting
- Outcomes and Assessment Information Set (OASIS)—Home healthcare setting
- Essential Medical Data Set (EMDS)—Emergency care setting

Table 6.1 Sample data dictionary

DATA FIELD	NAME	DEFINITION	DATA TYPE	FORMAT	FIELD SIZE	VALUES	SOURCE SYSTEM	DATE FIRST ENTERED	WHY ITEM IS INCLUDED
Admission Date	ADMIT_DATE	The date the patient is admitted to the facility as an inpatient	date	mmddyyyy	8	Admission date cannot precede birth date or 2007 No hyphens or slashes	Patient Census	2/23/2008	Allows analysis of patients and services within a specific period that can be compared with other periods or trended
Census	CENSUS	The number of inpatients present in the facility at any given time	numeric	x to xx	3	Any whole number from 0 to 999	Patient Census	2/23/2008	Provides analysis of budget variances, aids future budgetary decisions, and allows quicker response to negative trends
Ethnicity	PT_ETHNIC	Patient's ethnicity Must be reported according to official Office of Management and Budget categories	alphanumeric	Ex; letter must be uppercase	2	E1 = Hispanic or Latino Ethnicity E2 = Non- Hispanic or Latino Ethnicity	Patient Census; Practice Management	2/23/2008	Patient demographics aid marketing and planning future budgets and services
Infant Patient	INFANT_PT	A patient who has not reached 1 year of age at the time of discharge	alphanumeric	Age in months = xD to xxD OR xM to xxM	3	Must be > 0 AND < 1 year	Patient Census; Practice Management	2/23/2008	Patient age affects types of services required and payer sources
Inpatient Daily Census	IP_DAY_CENSUS	The number of inpatients present at census-taking time each day, plus any inpatients who were both admitted and discharged after the previous day's census-taking time	numeric	x to xx	3	Any whole number from 0 to 999	Patient Census	2/23/2008	Provides analysis of budget variances, aids future budgetary decisions, and allows quicker response to negative trends
Medical Record Number	MR_NUM	The unique number assigned to a patient's medical record The medical record is filed under this number	alphanumeric	xxxxxx: requires leading zeros	6	000001 to 999999	Patient Census; Practice Management		Provides analysis of services, resource utilization, and patient outcomes at the physician level
Patient Age	PT_AGE	Age of patient calculated by using most recent birthday attained before or on same day as discharge	numeric or alphanumeric	Age in days = xD to xxD OR Age in months = xM to xxM OR Age in years = x to xxx	3	Age must be > 0, and < OR = 124 years; children less than 1 year must be > 0 M AND < 1 year	Patient Census; Practice Management	2/23/2008	Patient age impacts the services utilized and payer sources

continued

Table 6.1 Sample data dictionary (*concluded*)

DATA FIELD	NAME	DEFINITION	DATA TYPE	FORMAT	FIELD SIZE	VALUES	SOURCE SYSTEM	DATE FIRST ENTERED	WHY ITEM IS INCLUDED
Patient Sex	PT_SEX	Patient sex	alphanumeric	letter; must be uppercase	1	M = Male F = Female U = Unknown	Patient Census; Practice Management	2/23/2008	Patient sex impacts the services and specialties utilized
Patient Zip Code	PT_ZIP_CODE	Zip code of patient's residence	alphanumeric	xxxxx-xxxx	11	00000 to 99999; 00000 = Unknown 99999 = Foreign	Patient Census; Practice Management	2/23/2008	Patient demographics aid marketing and planning future budgets/services
Pediatric Patient	PED_PT	A patient who has not reached 18 years of age at the time of discharge	numeric	Age in days = xD to xxD OR Age in months = xM to xxM OR Age in years = x to xxx	3	Age must be > 0 AND < 18 years; children less than 1 year must be > 0 M AND < 1 year	Patient Census; Practice Management	2/23/2008	Patient age impacts the services utilized and payer sources

Source: AHIMA 2017.

With the success of these data sets and the shift toward the ability to share data that are consistent across the healthcare spectrum, the need for additional standards to support standardized data sets continues to be a focus in the healthcare industry.

Databases

Databases are commonly used throughout the healthcare industry to support and store patient information entered into an EHR or maintained on a paper record. A **database** is a collection of data organized in such a way that its contents can be easily accessed, managed, reported, and updated. For proper management of data within a healthcare organization it is important to understand what databases exist, the purposes of the databases, the storage and backup of the databases, and who accesses and uses the

Figure 6.1 UHDDS data elements

Data Element	Definition/Descriptor
01. Personal identification	The unique number assigned to each patient within a hospital that distinguishes the patient and his or her hospital record from all others in that institution.
02. Date of birth	Month, day, and year of birth. Capture of the full four-digit year of birth is recommended.
03. Sex	Male or female
04. Race and ethnicity	04a. Race American Indian/Eskimo/Aleut Asian or Pacific Islander Black White Other race Unknown 04b. Ethnicity Spanish origin/Hispanic Non-Spanish origin/Non-Hispanic Unknown
05. Residence	Full address of usual residence Zip code (nine digits, if available) Code for foreign residence
06. Hospital identification	A unique institutional number across data collection systems. The Medicare provider number is the preferred hospital identifier.
07. Admission date	Month, day, and year of admission
08. Type of admission	Scheduled: Arranged with admissions office at least 24 hours prior to admission Unscheduled: All other admissions
09. Discharge date	Month, day, and year of discharge
10. Physician identification 11. • Attending physician • Operating physician	The Medicare unique physician identification number (UPIN) is the preferred method of identifying the attending physician and operating physician(s) because it is uniform across all data systems.
12. Principal diagnosis	The condition established after study to be chiefly responsible for occasioning the admission of the patient to the hospital for care.
13. Other diagnoses	All conditions that coexist at the time of admission or that develop subsequently or that affect the treatment received and/or the length of stay. Diagnoses that relate to an earlier episode and have no bearing on the current hospital stay are to be excluded.

continued

Figure 6.1 UHDDS data elements (*concluded*)

Data Element	Definition/Descriptor
14. Qualifier for other diagnoses	A qualifier is given for each diagnosis coded under "other diagnoses" to indicate whether the onset of the diagnosis preceded or followed admission to the hospital. The option "uncertain" is permitted.
15. External cause-of-injury code	The ICD-10-CM code for the external cause of an injury, poisoning, or adverse effect. Hospitals should complete this item whenever there is a diagnosis of an injury, poisoning, or adverse effect.
16. Birth weight of neonate	The specific birth weight of a newborn, preferably recorded in grams
17. Procedures and dates	All significant procedures are to be reported. A significant procedure is one that is: • Surgical in nature, or • Carries a procedural risk, or • Carries an anesthetic risk, or • Requires specialized training The date of each significant procedure must be reported. When more than one procedure is reported, the principal procedure must be designated. The principal procedure is one that is performed for definitive treatment rather than one performed for diagnostic or exploratory purposes or was necessary to take care of a complication. If there appear to be two procedures that are principal, then the one most closely related to the principal diagnosis should be selected as the principal procedure. The UPIN must be reported for the person performing the principal procedure.
18. Disposition of the patient	• Discharged to home (excludes those patients referred to home health service) • Discharged to acute care hospital • Discharged to nursing facility • Discharged home to be under the care of a home health service (including a hospice) • Discharged to other healthcare facility • Left against medical advice • Alive, other; or alive, not stated • Died
19. Patient's expected source of payment	Primary source Other sources All categories for primary and other sources are: • Blue Cross/Blue Shield • Other health insurance companies • Other liability insurance • Medicare • Medicaid • Worker's Compensation • Self-insured employer plan • Health maintenance organization (HMO) • CHAMPUS • CHAMPVA • Other government payers • Self-pay • No charge (free, charity, special research, teaching) • Other
20. Total charges	All charges billed by the hospital for this hospitalization. Professional charges for individual patient care by physicians are excluded.

Source: Brinda 2016.

databases. Common databases found in healthcare include Medicare Provider Analysis and Review File, National Practitioner Data Bank, and National Health Care Survey (Sharp 2016). Refer to chapter 7, *Secondary Data Sources*, for specifics on these databases.

The database design and structure impacts how it can be used. A poorly designed database will

Figure 6.2 UACDS data elements

Data Element	Definition/Descriptor
Provider identification, address, type of practice	Provider identification: Include the full name of the provider as well as the unique physician identification number (UPIN). Address: The complete address of the provider's office. In cases where the provider has multiple offices, the location of the usual or principal place of practice should be given. Profession: • Physician including specialty or field of practice • Other (specify)
Place of encounter	Specify the location of the encounter: • Private office • Clinic or health center • Hospital outpatient department • Hospital emergency department • Other (specify)
Reason for encounter	Includes, but is not limited to, the patient's complaints and symptoms reflecting his or her own perception of needs, provided verbally or in writing by the patient at the point of entry into the healthcare system, or the patient's own words recorded by an intermediary or provider at that time.
Diagnostic services	Includes all diagnostic services of any type.
Problem, diagnosis, or assessment	Describes the provider's level of understanding and the interpretation of the patient's reasons for the encounter and all conditions requiring treatment or management at the time of the encounter.
Therapeutic services	List by name all services done or ordered: • Medical (including drug therapy) • Surgical • Patient education
Preventive services	List by name all preventive services and procedures performed at the time of the encounter.
Disposition	The provider's statement of the next step(s) in the care of the patient. At a minimum, the following classification is suggested: 1. No follow-up planned 2. Follow-up planned • Return when necessary • Return to the current provider at a specified time • Telephone follow-up • Returned to referring provider • Referred to other provider • Admit to hospital • Other

Source: Brinda 2016.

result in redundant collection of data and data information errors. Understanding the **database life cycle (DBLC)** is an important step in the proper execution, implementation, and management of databases within healthcare. The following are the six basic steps in the database life cycle:

1. Initial study (determining need for database)
2. Design (identifying data fields, structure, and so forth)
3. Implementation (developing database)
4. Testing and evaluation (ensuring system works as expected)
5. Operation (using database)
6. Database maintenance and evaluation (updating and backing up database and ensuring that it still meets needs)

Health information management (HIM) professionals should be involved in all stages of the database life cycle as they have the knowledge and skills needed to understand the essential steps of data collection privacy and security, and data integrity (Coronel and Morris 2015).

The two most common types of databases used in healthcare are relational databases and object-oriented databases. A **relational database** stores data in tables that are predefined and contain rows and columns of information. Typically, a relational database is two-dimensional as it contains rows and columns. Relational databases are used frequently in the healthcare industry because they are easy to build, use, and query within the application. For example, a healthcare organization might choose to use a relational database to document the number of health record deficiencies a physician has at the time of evaluation for reporting to the organization's board (Sharp 2016). Table 6.2 provides a sample of a relational database for physician deficiency status.

An **object-oriented database (OODB)** is designed to store different types of data including images, audio files, documents, videos, and data elements. OODBs are useful for storing fetal monitoring strips, electrocardiograms, PACs, and more. The OODB is dynamic because it provides the data as well as the object (image and document). Table 6.3 provides an example of an OODB. Using an OODB for the storage of fetal heart monitors allows a healthcare organization to query the database to retrieve an image for a specific person. Another potential use is to produce a report based on the date of the fetal heart monitor for retention and destruction of the images. When this type of database is used, the data are provided with the additional ability to retrieve the file when the link to the image is selected.

Indices

An **index** is a report or list from a database that provides guidance, indication, or other references to the data contained in the database. An index serves as a guide or indicator to locate something within a database or in other systems storing data. For example, an index of a book will provide key terms and where to find each term within a book; the reader is able to find more information and detail regarding a specific topic. The indices used in healthcare identify where the desired information can be found, making it easier to aggregate and analyze data. There are many types of indices used within the healthcare industry. The following are the most common indices:

- *Master patient index*. A guide to locating specific demographic information about a patient such as the patient name, health

Table 6.2 Relational database: physician deficiency status

Provider ID	Total # of deficiencies	History and physical deficiencies	Discharge summary deficiencies	Deficiencies greater than 30 days past due
1285	14	2	5	3
1965	2	1	1	0
8914	35	13	15	25
9462	6	3	2	2
3651	17	11	2	2

Source: ©AHIMA.

Table 6.3 Object-oriented database: fetal heart monitors (FHMs)

Patient ID	FHM start date	FHM end date	FHM image
110011	6/30/15	7/1/15	Link to FHM image
123023	7/1/15	7/3/15	Link to FHM image
154623	7/2/15	7/2/15	Link to FHM image
948513	7/2/15	7/3/15	Link to FHM image

Source: ©AHIMA.

record number, date of birth, gender, and dates of service. For more details, refer to chapter 3, *Health Information Functions, Purpose, and Users*.

- *Disease index*. A listing of specific codes such as *International Classification of Diseases, Tenth Revision, Clinical Modification* (ICD-10-CM) codes that link a disease or diagnosis to a patient. (ICD-10-CM is explained later in this chapter.) Common data in a disease index would include diagnosis codes, health record number, gender, age, race, attending physician, hospital service, patient outcomes, and dates of encounter. A disease index can be used to query a specific diagnosis to determine other attributes of patients with the disease. For example, if a healthcare organization wanted to know the age range and gender of all patients diagnosed with a myocardial infarction, the disease index could be queried to get a listing of patients with that specific diagnosis code(s).
- *Operation or procedure index*. A listing of specific codes such as Current Procedural Terminology (CPT) for procedures or operations performed within the healthcare organization. (CPT is explained later in this chapter.) An operation or procedure code would include information similar to the disease index but would also include the specific code numbers as well as the operating physician. An operation or procedure index can be used to query specific information regarding procedures or operations done within the facility. For example, if a healthcare organization wanted to know the age range of patients who had an appendectomy in the past year, the operation or procedure index could be queried to generate a listing of patients based on the procedure code.
- *Physician index*. A listing of all physicians within a healthcare organization with all the diagnosis and procedure codes linked to each provider within the index. The data collected in this index include physician's identification (code or name), health record number, diagnosis, operations, dates of service, patient gender, patient age, and patient outcome from encounter. A provider index can be used to produce information regarding the work of the provider within a healthcare organization, which can be useful for certification and credentialing purposes. For example, a healthcare organization may need to produce a report for administration detailing the treatment of patients and diagnoses and procedures performed in the past year by a specific provider (Sharp 2016). More information on indexes is found in chapter 7 *Secondary Data Sources*.

Indices support daily operations for healthcare organizations and are tools used to gather specific information quickly.

Data Mapping

Data mapping is a process that allows for connections between two systems. For example, mapping two different coding systems to show the equivalent codes allows for data initially captured for one purpose to be translated and used for another purpose. For example, the ICD-10 code of E10.11, type 1 diabetes mellitus with ketoacidosis can be mapped to SNOMED-CT Code 371055001, type 1 diabetes mellitus with ketoacidosis. This allows for comparison between two different coding systems based on one code. One system in a map is identified as the source while the other is the target. **Source data** is the location from which the data originate, such as a database or a data set; whereas **target data** is the location from which the data are mapped or to where the data are sent. A data map creates a process to evaluate the disparity between the two systems and links the data being collected together. Data mapping is conducted to ensure the data exchange from one database to another is done in a meaningful way and maintains the integrity of the data (Maimone 2016).

During the process of data mapping, each data map should have a defined purpose that specifies why the data map is created and what purpose it serves. The purpose should describe why the data map is needed, what it represents, and how it will be used within the healthcare organization. For example, a healthcare organization may create a data map to show the relationship of the types of ambulatory services such as emergency department or ambulatory surgery and map them directly to the ambulatory services.

Data mapping should be completed carefully to evaluate where the data come from and the relationships of the source data to data in other systems. The process helps to ensure the integrity of the data in all systems. When conducting data mapping within a healthcare organization, evaluating the relationship of the data is fundamental to understanding the equivalence between the data. Equivalence of data is the relationship between the source data and target data in regard to how close or distant the data from the two systems are linked. The three common types of relationships are no match, approximate match, and exact match (Maimone 2016). Table 6.4 shows the differences between the three types of relationships.

When creating data maps, healthcare organizations should create a common format for the output of the map to create consistency and ease the end user's ability to interpret the data map. Table 6.5 is an example of a data map that shows the relationship between ICD-10-CM codes and SNOMED CT codes, both explained later in this chapter.

Data mapping can be a long and tedious task for a healthcare organization; however, it is important from a data management perspective. To properly manage the data and ensure data integrity between systems, data maps serve as the tool to define the meaning and history of data elements within systems. Inaccurate data mapping can result in misinterpretation of data and inaccuracy of information stored and maintained in systems. For example, if the ICD-10-CM code was mapped to the incorrect SNOMED CT code, data used and reported from the SNOMED system could show incorrect information regarding patients diagnosed with cholera, unspecified. Data map creators need to understand the data to be mapped between systems and the reasons for the data mapping. One way of doing this is to create a use case. A **use case** describes how the users will interact with the data map in a specific scenario. Some general data mapping steps are found in table 6.6.

Data Warehousing

Data warehousing is the process of collecting the data from different data sources within a healthcare organization and storing it in a single database that can be used for decision-making.

Table 6.4 Types of relationships used in mapping

Type of Relationship	Description	Example Terms Used (Terms May Vary by Category)
No match	A code (concept) exists in one coding system without a similar concept in the other coding system. No possible connection between source and target system.	No match No map No code
Approximate match	A code (concept) that exists in one coding system may have a direct relationship to the other coding system. Possible direct connection between source and target system.	Approximate match Approximate map Approximate code Related
Exact match	A code (concept) exists in one coding system with a direct relationship to the other coding system. Direct connection between source and target system.	Exact match Equivalent map Equivalent code Equal

Source: Maimone 2016.

Table 6.5 Data map

ICD-10-CM code	ICD-10-CM name	Equivalence	SNOMED CT code	SNOMED CT name
A00.0	Cholera, unspecified	Equal	63650001	Cholera

Source: © AHIMA.

Table 6.6 AHIMA practice brief data mapping best practices: general data mapping steps

Develop a business case first. Questions to ask include: • What is the reason for the project? • What is the expected business benefit? • What are the expected costs of the project? • What are the expected risks?
Define a use case for how the content will be used within applications. Questions to ask include: • Who will use the maps? • Is the mapping between standard terminologies or between proprietary (local) terminologies? • Are there delivery constraints or licensing issues? • What systems will rely on the map as a data source?
Develop rules (heuristics) to be implemented within the project. Questions to ask when developing the rules include: • What is the version of source and target schema to be used? • What is included or excluded? • How will the relationship between source and target be defined (such as are maps equivalent or related)? • What mapping methodologies will be utilized? • What procedures will be used for ensuring intercoder or interrater reliability (reproducibility) in the map development phase? • What parameters will be used to ensure usefulness? (For example, a map from the SNOMED CT concept "procedure on head" could be mapped to hundreds of CPT codes, making the map virtually useless.) • What tools will be used to develop and maintain the map?
Plan a pilot phase to test the rules. Maps must be tested and deemed "fit for purpose," meaning they are performing as desired. This may be done using random samples of statistically significant size. Additional pilot phases may be needed until variance from the expected result are resolved. Reproducibility is a fundamental best practice when mapping.
Develop full content with periodic testing throughout the process. Organizations should perform a final quality assurance test for the maps and review those data items unable to be mapped to complete the mapping phase. Any modifications from the review process should be retested to assure accuracy. Organizations should release the map results to software configuration management where software and content are integrated. They should then perform quality assurance testing on the content within the software application (done in a development environment). They can then deploy the content to the production environment, or go-live.
Communicate with source and target system owners when issues are identified with the systems that require attention or additional documentation for clarity.

Source: Maimone 2016.

A data warehouse is a database that makes it possible to access data that exist in multiple databases through a single query and reporting interface.

Data warehouses allow healthcare organizations to obtain information needed to streamline processes and simplify access to the information that is stored among different databases within a healthcare system. If a user had to query each information system, the amount of time needed to combine the data manually and then analyze the data would serve as a barrier to properly reporting and analyzing the data. With the use of a data warehouse, the data can be consolidated by pulling the data from multiple information systems into a single database that allows for ease in reporting and analysis of the information.

Data mining is the processing of extracting from a database or data warehouse information stored in discrete, structured data format—that is, data that have a specific value. Examples of discrete data are a lab value or a diagnosis code. The following are the advantages to the use of data warehouses:

- One consistent data storage area for reporting, forecasting, and analysis
- Easier and timely access to data
- Improved end-user productivity
- Improved information services productivity
- Reduced costs
- Scalability
- Flexibility
- Reliability (HIMSS 2009)

Since large amounts of data are being captured electronically within healthcare organizations, data warehousing will become a foundational aspect of healthcare operations due to its ability to gather data from multiple databases, incorporate the data, and then produce meaningful information.

Check Your Understanding 6.1

Answer the following questions.

1. True or false: A data element is a single or individual fact that represents the smallest unique subset of larger data.
2. Critique each statement to determine the one that demonstrates the intent of a data set.
   a. A clearly defined data dictionary for the electronic health record
   b. A recommended list of data elements that support a specific healthcare industry
   c. One element within an electronic health record
   d. A database where data are compiled from many sources into one central location
3. The intent and purpose of the creation of a data dictionary is to:
   a. Identify the data elements that you want to collect
   b. Create support for structured data collection
   c. Create use case
   d. Control security
4. The two most commonly used databases in healthcare are:
   a. Relational and object-relational databases
   b. Object-relational and object-linking databases
   c. Relational and object-oriented databases
   d. Object-linking and object-oriented databases
5. True or false: An index creates a definition for data elements within a database.
6. True or false: There is usually only one source of data within a healthcare organization.

Information Governance

Information assets are becoming an essential strategic and operational part of a healthcare organization, requiring a rigorous process that will protect information from unauthorized access, use, disclosure, modification, and destruction. For example, prevent hackers from accessing health information from outside the healthcare organization. Information assets refer to the information collected during the day-to-day operations of a healthcare organization that has value within the healthcare organization. An example is patient data collected to support patient care for the healthcare organization. Without patient data, the healthcare organization would not be able to support the continuity of patient care or the billing of services provided to the patient.

Information governance (IG) is an "organization-wide framework for managing information throughout its lifecycle and supporting the organization's strategy, operations, regulatory, legal, risk, and environmental requirements" (Dickey 2018, p. 38). One of the main goals of IG is to provide trustworthiness of a healthcare organization's information. Having trustworthy information is essential to improving patient care and safety, reducing or mitigating risks to the information, improving operational efficiency, and achieving and maintaining a competitive advantage in healthcare (Fahy et al. 2018). The implementation of an IG framework in a healthcare organization assists in the establishment of policies and procedures that govern the oversight, aligning it to the strategic vision of the organization. In addition, IG helps to prioritize a healthcare organization's investments, establishes the value of information assets, establishes a process to protect information assets, and creates accountability for managing information over the entire healthcare spectrum (Dickey 2018).

Valued Strategic Asset

Information should be treated as a valued strategic asset. A valued strategic asset is a resource that is used in a way that will improve the healthcare organization today and into the future. For example, a healthcare organization needs information (financial projections, cost of services, and so forth) that can assist in the negotiation of contracts that can run for years. A successful IG initiative must have support from the healthcare organization's executive leadership and align directly to the healthcare organization's strategic plan. To ensure the success of an IG initiative, it needs to be "driven from the board of directors and C-Suite level down to the rest of the organization while simultaneously being driven up from the grassroots and recognizing the needs of the end-users of data and information" (Fahey et al. 2018, p 4). One of the initial steps in the IG initiative is to secure an executive sponsor at the C-Suite level of the organization. Some common sponsors of an IG initiative are a Chief Financial Officer, Chief Data or Health Information Officer, Chief Financial Officer, Chief Innovation Officer, Chief Strategy Officer, Chief Medical and Information Officer, and Chief Executive Officer. The executive sponsor will ensure the IG initiative has the appropriate resources such as budget, personnel, and tools; that the goals of the IG initiative align with the healthcare organization's strategy; that the importance of the IG initiative is communicated to the executive team as well as the workforce; and that the appropriate controls and accountability are established to meet the intended goals of the IG initiative (Fahey et al. 2018).

An IG framework can help a company with competing strategic priorities. One of the main ways that an IG initiative can support the strategy of the healthcare organization is by aligning the needs of the leadership with the organizational business strategy and goals. It helps to create the valuation of information and assign resources to the proper areas within an organization. This helps to avoid unnecessary costs with inappropriate assignment of resources to support the organization's information assets (Fahey et al. 2018). Aligning the IG initiative with the healthcare organization's strategic priorities with the support of an executive sponsor is the foundation of a successful IG initiative.

Business Intelligence

An effective IG initiative will support the information that the healthcare organization needs to make good decisions for the organization as well as the population it serves. One of the benefits of IG is the ability to support business intelligence. **Business intelligence** (BI)is the end product or goal of knowledge management. In other words, it is what you can do with what you know about your healthcare organization, your community, and so forth. With data being produced at a rapid rate, IG helps the healthcare organization manage and use the information. Using the information to create and support business intelligence is an essential component of IG. With an effective IG initiative, reliable information will be available to support the compliance efforts, benchmarks, and comparisons of an organization in areas such as population health, quality of care, public reporting, financial performance, and regulatory compliance (Warner 2013a). For example, the ability to analyze the top trends in diagnoses in a healthcare organization will enable the organization to expand service lines or enhance patient outcomes in a specific area.

Situation, Background, Assessment, Recommendation (SBAR)

As a healthcare organization begins to implement IG, the reason and intent of the process must be effectively communicated within the organization. The **situation, background, assessment, and recommendation (SBAR)** tool is an easy to use and understand tool that can help define the intent of the IG program and clearly articulate the entire process to gain organizational and executive support. SBAR uses four distinct components to describe the issues, provide background information, conduct a current state analysis, and define the recommended steps to fix the issue (Glondys 2016; Kadlec 2015). Figure 6.3 describes each component of the SBAR tool.

When using SBAR to support an IG initiative, it is important to be specific about the issue and directly link it to the specific IG principle. If necessary, include information such as accreditation requirements and federal and state regulations to help support the background information. In addition, special considerations should be documented linking the specific issue to the organization's strategic plan (Glondys 2016). Figure 6.4 demonstrates SBAR linked to the IG principle of availability.

Enterprise Information Management

Enterprise information management (EIM) is the set of functions created by a healthcare organization to plan, organize, and coordinate the people, processes, technology, and content needed to manage information for the purposes of data quality, patient safety, and ease of use (Johns 2015). As part of the creation of an IG strategy, healthcare organizations should establish EIM policies and procedures to address the collaboration and integrative efforts used across the system to protect the healthcare organization's enterprise information assets (Warner 2013b).

Information Governance Principles for Healthcare

In 2014, AHIMA established Information Governance Principles of Healthcare (IGPHC), which were aligned with ARMA's Generally Accepted Recordkeeping (GARP) Principles. The IGPHC were intended to be comprehensive and broad to allow for scalability based on the healthcare organization's type, size, role, mission, sophistication, legal environment, and resources. AHIMA intended to offer a framework to help organizations leverage information as an asset, while ensuring compliance with legal requirements and

Figure 6.3 Situation, Background, Assessment, and Recommendation

The SBAR Elements
- **S** = Situation (a concise statement of the problem)
- **B** = Background (pertinent and brief information related to the situation)
- **A** = Assessment (analysis and consideration of options—what you found/think)
- **R** = Recommendation (action requested/recommended—what you want)

Situation
This section of the SBAR process helps determine what is going on and why. In this section, the relevant parties identify the problem and why it is a concern for the organization and then provide a brief description of it.

Background
The goal of the background section is to be able to identify and provide the reason for the problem.

Assessment
At this stage, the situation is analyzed to determine the most appropriate course of action. Include any data that have been gathered and spell out the pros and cons of each option being considered.

Recommendation
Possible solutions that could correct the situation at hand are considered. In this section, a recommendation is provided based on the data presented in the assessment section.

Source: Glondys, 2016, 35.

Figure 6.4 Example: the principle of availability

Situation: New fields are being added to EHRs but are not communicated throughout the organization. Output (for release of information) does not include these data, resulting in incomplete information being released.

Background: No control mechanism exists for altering new fields in the EHR. There is no documented standardized process for changing and adding fields. It follows, then, that there is no education for this practice. There has been no audit of input-to-output flow.

Assessment: Survey IT and clinical areas that frequently request template and data field changes. Audit critical content (that is, core measures) that is not part of standard output. Identify examples of adverse impacts of incomplete data on clinical care (resulting in legal action), coding (resulting in a loss of revenue), and reporting (resulting in low performance). List pros and cons for each approach and identify any associated costs.

Recommendation: Formalize the process and approval procedures for changes to the EHR. Educate the workforce about the approved process for EHR changes.

Special Considerations for IG
This example clearly shows the importance of organization-wide communication, collaboration, and commitment to govern the quality of information. People, processes, and technology in every department should be involved in this effort. Everyone is a stakeholder in information quality.

Source: Glondys, 2016.

other duties and responsibilities. Whether used in whole or in part, the IGPHC were developed to inform an organization's information governance strategy (Datskovsky et. al, 2015a).
The eight principles included:

- *Principle of accountability*. This principle recommended that one person, preferably someone in senior leadership, oversee and implement an IG program within an organization. This individual could help approve policies and procedures to guide implementation of an IG program and remediate identified issues (Datskovsky et. al, 2015a).
- *Principle of transparency*. This stipulates that documentation related to an organization's IG initiatives be available to its workforce and other appropriate interested parties, according to the principle. Records demonstrating transparency of the information governance program should: Document the principles and processes that govern the program; accurately and completely record the activities undertaken to implement the program; and be available to interested parties (Datskovsky et. al, 2015a).
- *Principle of integrity*. According to the principles an (IG) program should be arranged such that "the organization has a reasonable and suitable guarantee of authenticity and reliability." This includes elements such as appropriate workforce training and adherence to the organization's policies and procedures, as well as acceptable audit trails and admissibility of records for litigation purposes.
- *Principle of protection*. An IG program must ensure the appropriate levels of protection from breach, corruption, and loss are provided for information that is private, confidential, secret, classified, and essential to business continuity. This facilitates the protection of sensitive healthcare information.
- *Principle of compliance*. Achieving compliance through IG ensures healthcare entities comply with applicable laws, regulations, standards, and organizational policies, and maintains its information in the manner and for the time prescribed by law or organizational policy (Datskovsky et. al, 2015b). (Compliance is defined in more detail in chapters 9 *Data Privacy and Confidentiality* and 16 *Fraud and Abuse Compliance*.)
- *Principle of availability*. The principle states an organization should maintain information in a manner that ensures timely, accurate, and efficient retrieval. This applies to healthcare teams (patients, caregivers) as well as legal and compliance authorities (Datskovsky et. al, 2015b).
- *Principle of retention*. This helps organizations create processes for proper retention of information based on requirements from regulations, accrediting organizations, and company policy. According to the principle, "[t]he ability to properly and consistently retain all relevant information is especially important, as organizations create and store large quantities—most of it in electronic form." (Datskovsky et. al, 2015c). (Chapter 8, *Health Law*, contains more information regarding retention of information within an organization.)
- *Principle of disposition*. This principle applies to all information in the custody of an organization and encourages them to "secure and appropriate disposition for information no longer required to be maintained by applicable laws and the organization's policies." (Datskovsky et. al, 2015c).
  See chapter 8 for information regarding disposition of information.

AHIMA's Information Governance Adoption Model Competencies

AHIMA's Information Governance Adoption Model (IGAM) consists of 10 competencies that were intended to assist a healthcare organization in applying appropriate IG concepts. The adoption model permitted an organization to focus on those areas of IG that it deemed important. This type of scalability promotes a natural progression of IG improvement in terms of expectations and, more importantly, resources, according to AHIMA's Information Governance Toolkit 3.0 (AHIMA n.d.).

The 10 key organization competencies promoted by the IGAM included:

1. IG Structure
2. Strategic Alignment
3. Enterprise Information Management (EIM)
4. Data Governance
5. IT Governance
6. Analytics
7. Privacy and Security
8. Regulatory and Legal
9. Awareness and Adherence
10. IG Performance

Figure 6.5 summarizes the 10 IGAM Competencies

Figure 6.5 AHIMA's 10 IGAM Competencies

IG STRUCTURE	Creates the information governance program including executive sponsorship, IG committee, and policies and procedures to support the program.
STRATEGIC ALIGNMENT	Ensures the information goverance program strategy aligns with the organization's strategy, mission, vision, and goals.
PRIVACY AND SECURITY	Protects information across all types of media, throughout the life cycle.
LEGAL AND REGULATORY	Verifies a proper, accurate, reliable, efficient response to regulatory audits, information requests, and eDiscovery.
DATA GOVERNANCE	Ensures usable and reliable data through comprehensive and proven data management practices.
IT GOVERNANCE	Strives for risk reduction through an integrated approach to technology selection, evaluation, and use.
ANALYTICS	Proves the value of information governance and contributes to a data-driven decision-making culture in the organization through use of advanced tools and technologies.
ENTERPRISE INFORMATION MANAGEMENT	Guides practice for information through the information lifecycle across the healthcare ecosystem.
IG PERFORMANCE	Measures the performance and impact of the IG program.
AWARENESS AND ADHERENCE	Creates a path for trusted information and safe use of health IT throught consistent behavior with respect to information use, sharing, handling, access, storage, retention, and disposition.

Source: Iron Mountain Advisory Services.

Check Your Understanding 6.2

Answer the following questions.

1. Which term is defined as principles and oversight to manage the information that is produced by the different systems within a healthcare organization?
    a. Information governance
    b. Data governance
    c. Data assets
    d. Information assets

2. Select the process that can help organizations evaluate the current state of best practices with data management, gaps, and areas of opportunity based on risk, strategy, and operations of the organization.
   a. Data governance
   b. Information Governance Adoption Model
   c. Enterprise information management
   d. Business intelligence
3. Define the principle of integrity.
   a. Create a process for ensuring that all the information complies with appropriate laws, regulations, standards, and organizational policies
   b. Create assurances that the data generated and maintained by an organization maintains authenticity and reliability
   c. Create protections to safeguard data and information from improper use and disclosure to avoid data breaches
   d. Create a clear and open documentation process for the information governance strategy and activities within an organization
4. True or false: An information governance initiative is a project within a healthcare organization led by middle level leadership.

Data Governance

Data governance is "enterprise authority that ensures control and accountability for enterprise data through the establishment of decision rights and data policies and standards that are implemented and monitored through a formal structure of assigned roles, responsibilities, and accountabilities" (Johns 2015, 81). Data governance focuses on how healthcare organizations create processes, policies, and procedures for keeping information that is relevant to patient care and healthcare operations. The goal of data governance is maintaining data accuracy and removing unnecessary data from the health record. Commonly, data governance is confused with the term *information governance*, even though there is a clear distinction between the two terms. Data governance focuses on managing the data as they are created within an information system. Simply stated, data governance manages the data put into the different information systems used in healthcare and information governance manages the information output from those systems. The core processes of data governance within a healthcare organization are to establish policies and procedures on how data will be connected, who is responsible for the data, how the data will be stored, and how the data will be distributed within the healthcare organization.

HIM professionals play a key role in the success of implementing information and data governance programs in healthcare organizations. Their training provides them with an understanding of healthcare's clinical, financial, regulatory, and technology environments, which allows them to lead the information governance within an organization and be the liaison between executive leadership and clinical leadership (AHIMA 2011; AHIMA 2014a).

Data Stewardship

Data stewardship is an important component of the data governance process. **Data stewardship** creates responsibility for data through principles and practices to "ensure the knowledgeable and appropriate use of data derived from individuals' personal health information" (Kanaan and Carr

2009, 1). Data stewardship is important due to the increase in availability of health data, the use of the health data within the healthcare industry, the use of health information for population management, and the legal and financial risks associated with health data. Data stewardship is created to establish common and essential practices and principles for the management of health data. Benefits of data stewardship are the following:

- Improved patient safety
- Increased efficiencies
- Decreased cost of care provided
- Improved patient care and outcomes
- Facilitated coordination of care
- Structured data collection
- Comprehensive data collection (Noreen 2017)

Oversight and data stewardship are essential for proper management of information and data. This helps ensure the data and information meet the needs of the healthcare organization. One of the emerging roles in healthcare is the data steward. **Data stewards** are the people within an organization who are responsible for either a specific system or a specific set of data within the organization (Downing 2016). The data steward serves as the subject matter expert for data governance for the healthcare organization, business unit, or data set that they represent. For example, a heart clinic may have a data steward that oversees imaging and EKGs in the clinic, leads data quality initiatives to evaluate potential issues and risks, and leads the remediation process to ensure the accuracy and integrity of the data. The data steward's roles are to establish policies, procedures, and processing for the system, data set, or business unit they support as they relate to data management. In an IG framework, the data steward acts as the liaison between the workforce (users of the systems or data) and the information governance committee to help both sides create priorities, identify specific issues, and create plans for resolving the identified issues. Other common job titles for the data steward in healthcare are business analyst or data analyst (Downing 2016).

The National Committee on Vital and Health Statistics (NCVHS) recommends that the creation of principles for data stewardship fall into four categories: (1) individual's rights, (2) responsibilities of the data steward, (3) needed security safeguards and controls, and (4) accountability, enforcement, and remedies for data stewardship. Individual rights should be analyzed to ensure the following:

- The individual has proper access to their protected health information
- The individual has a right to review and amend their health information
- The individual is provided transparency of information allowing them to understand what information will exist and how it will be used
- The individual must provide consent and authorization for use and disclosure of health information
- Adequate information and education are provided regarding the rights and responsibilities of health information (Kanaan and Carr 2009)

The data steward's responsibilities should be clearly defined to support adherence to the privacy and security of health information including requirements for uses and disclosures and guarantees for gaining access to what is needed to perform job responsibilities. Data security safeguards and controls should be established to define what technical and nontechnical mechanisms are being used to protect the confidentiality, integrity, and accessibility of protected health information. Data stewardship should express accountability of appropriate use as well as sanctions in the event of noncompliance to the requirements (Downing 2016). The goal is to create and build trust and transparency through the entire healthcare organization as it pertains to the use of health data.

Data Integrity

Many tools and functionalities of information systems are available to assist with the quality, completeness, and timeliness of clinical documentation. While these tools and functionalities of information systems create efficiencies in a healthcare organization, they have also been shown to create data integrity issues when not properly implemented and managed (AHIMA 2013; Vimalachandran et al. 2016). **Data integrity** is the assurance that the data entered into an information system or maintained on paper are only accessed and amended by individuals with the authority to do so. Integrity of the documentation within the patient's records includes information governance, data governance, patient identification, authorship validation, amendments and record corrections, and audits of documentation validity for reimbursement (AHIMA 2013; Vimalachandran et al. 2016). A healthcare organization needs to establish proper safeguards with the use of technology, including policies and procedures to help manage the integrity of the data in the health record. The Health Insurance Portability and Accountability Act (HIPAA) requires covered entities (defined in chapter 9, *Data Privacy and Confidentiality*) to implement policies and procedures to protect electronic protected health information from improper alteration or destruction and to establish security measures to ensure electronically transmitted protected health information is not improperly modified (chapter 10, *Data Security,* covers this topic in more detail). AHIMA recommends healthcare organizations institute policies and procedures for the management of data integrity. Some key topics to be included in data integrity policies are the documentation requirements, identification of who can document and the scope of that documentation, timeliness of documentation, and safeguards regarding changing and deleting documentation. Guidelines a healthcare organization establishes to reduce the likelihood of issues or damages to the patient data include the following:

- Committing to comply with laws and regulations in an ethical manner
- Requiring accurate data
- Holding individuals accountable for errors as per medical staff bylaws or rules and regulations
- Identifying penalties for the falsification of information
- Requiring periodic training
- Defining management responsibility (AHIMA 2013)

Specific HIM department policies and procedures should also be established to address the administrative documentation requirements, clinical documentation requirements, entering information into the EHR, correcting and amending the health record, and time frames for correcting the health record (Maimone 2016). HIM professionals need to be a part of establishing proper integrity throughout the health record as they are the custodians of the health record. It is common practice that the HIM department and HIM professionals ensure the health record is complete and accurate, so it is available for the purposes of patient care and healthcare operations.

Data Sharing

Electronic health information systems were implemented to create a foundation for data sharing across healthcare organizations regardless of the information system(s) used. Data sharing allows information to be exchanged via electronic formats to help support and deliver quality healthcare. Also known as health information exchange, data sharing is the electronic exchange of information between providers' electronic systems. Data sharing, or health information exchange, has two basic components: (1) the ability of two or more information systems to communicate and exchange patient information and (2) the ability of two or more information systems to effectively collect and use the information that has been exchanged (Dean 2018). When implemented correctly, a proper data sharing process can assist with coordinating patient information, analyzing patient information across multiple healthcare organizations, and reducing unnecessary repeated tests to support improvement in patient outcomes and patient satisfaction. For example, if a CT scan is performed on a patient prior to referral to another healthcare organization, the results of the CT scan can be shared electronically to prevent the patient from having the same test replicated (Dean 2018). See chapter 12, *Healthcare Information,* for more information regarding health information exchange.

Data Interchange Standards

To help support and drive interoperability and data sharing between healthcare organizations, standards development organizations have created standards for the sharing of information in electronic formats. **Interoperability** is the capability of two or more information systems and software applications to communicate and exchange information. **Standards development organizations (SDOs)** are private or government agencies that are involved in the creation and implementation of healthcare standards. In this case, SDOs define standards to support the process of electronic exchange of data. **Data interchange standards** are developed in order to support and create structure with data exchanges to sustain interoperability. The goal of the data interchange standards is to facilitate consistent, accurate, and reproducible capture of clinical data. Data interchange standards help support data integrity and safeguard data quality when sharing between organizations. Using data interchange standards for interoperability helps to do the following:

- Create a basis to enable the electronic exchange of data between two or more information systems or applications by creating consistent formats and sequences of data that are applied during data transmission
- Reflect the existing clinical and administrative data contained in both paper and electronic information systems to maintain patient data consistency in growing EHRs
- Transfer health data using appropriate business processes and necessary ethical and regulatory demands and guidance
- Foster electronic transmission as a business strategy to support patient care and better patient outcomes
- Promote efficient information sharing among individual computer systems and institutions (AHIMA 2006; Murphy and Brandt 2001)

In the US, SDOs are managed by the American National Standards Institute (ANSI). ANSI is the organization that oversees the creation of data standards from a variety of business sectors, including healthcare. The following are some common SDOs:

- *Health Level 7 (HL7)*. An ANSI-accredited SDO, HL7 established the creation of standards to support the exchange of clinical information in multiple formats
- *Institute of Electrical and Electronics Engineers (IEEE)*. A national organization that creates and develops different standards for hospital information systems that need communication between bedside instruments and clinical information systems (for example, cardiac monitoring performed in the intensive care unit being integrated with the EHR); IEEE currently has standards that allow providers and hospitals to achieve interoperability between medical instrumentation and a computer healthcare information system, and though used in multiple types of systems, it is most often used within acute-care settings
- *National Council for Prescription Drug Programs (NCPDP)*. A committee within the Designated and Standard Maintenance Organization focused on the development of standards regarding exchanging prescription information and payment information; NCPDP created multiple standards including a standardized data dictionary for pharmacy data, standards for transactions of file submissions between pharmacies and processors, standards for common billing unit language for submission of prescription claims, and standards to communicate formulary and benefit information to prescribers (Orlova et al. 2016).

Information and Data Strategy Methods and Techniques

With the implementation of data and information governance, healthcare organizations must evaluate and implement strategies focused on the oversight and management of the information and data in their healthcare organization. Information and data

Figure 6.6 Characteristics of a successful information governance strategy

A successful IG strategy incorporates the following characteristics:

- **Business-led and Business-driven:** Accountability and responsibility for data and information rests with the business owners who lead the departments or business units that create or generate the data and information, as opposed to IT
- **Measurable:** Clear goals and objectives and related metrics are established for performance improvements, reduction of risk, and optimization of data and information
- **Achievable:** A realistic level of resources (funding, staffing, and so on) is provided to develop and sustain IG efforts
- **Avoids complexity:** Initial goals and objectives should be focused and targeted to specific issues or problem areas
- **Communicable:** Communications explain and educate employees and clinicians about their information management responsibilities
- **Copes with uncertainty:** Standardization of processes leads to a more consistent approach and response to threats that can help the organization cope with ambiguity or uncertainties
- **Flexible:** Information management functions provide adequate controls but are designed to allow for flexibility where required to carry out job duties

Source: Washington 2015.

strategies are the steps taken to manage the data and information. The information and data strategies should align to the healthcare organization's overall strategy and support the broader business goals of the organization. The information and data strategies help to promote the collection of quality healthcare data, support decision-making, define proper use of information, and manage the compliance risk of an organization (Washington 2015). Figure 6.6 describes the characteristics of a successful information governance strategy.

Data strategy should be a clear, concise method created to support proper collection and use of healthcare data within an organization that is approved by executive leadership. A data strategy will clearly define the healthcare organization's data policies and procedures, roles and responsibilities for data governance, business rules for data governance, process for controlling data redundancy, management of key master data, use of structured and unstructured data, storage for all healthcare data, and safeguards and protections of the data. The strategy must define the following:

- *Data standardization and integration*. Focus on how the data is being entered into the information system, where the same data might exist in multiple areas, and how it is being integrated into other information systems. For example, review where data of birth is being entered into the information system and if it is always in the same format such as MM/DD/YYYY. Also, evaluate if the information system can pull data from one field to another to avoid re-entering information that has already been entered. The intent of data standardization is to document the location of data collection and ensure standardized formats and meaning of the data.
- *Data quality*. Data quality focuses on entering data that is true, accurate, and relevant to patient care and business operation into the information system. Data quality is discussed in detail later in this chapter.
- *Metadata management*. Refers to managing and defining the metadata within the information system. Metadata refers to the data that characterizes other data such as creation date of data, date sent, date received, last accessed date, and last modification date. It is important to clearly define what metadata will be collected and why it will be collected.
- *Data modeling*. Refers to the creation of documentation to justify business decisions made based on the different data collection and storage systems that are used within an organization. Creating data models and defining the use of data in relation to business mission and vision allow for the support of data standardization across the organization.
- *Data ownership*. Refers to the creation of business leaders, or owners, of specific

areas of the data. For example, the Director of Radiology can be assigned as the business leader, or owner, of the radiology information system. Based on the business need, the business owners are responsible for creating business rules and definitions when collecting specific data to support patient care and their business operations.

- *Data stewardship*. Data stewardship is the evaluation of the data collection based on business need and strategy to ensure the data meets the requirements of patient care and organizational needs (AHIMA 2011; Downing 2016).

A clearly defined data strategy approved by executive leadership is necessary to manage the most important healthcare assets—patient data.

Data Visualization and Presentation

It is important to properly organize and visualize data used for business purposes. Data visualization creates a visual context for data to help people better understand the data and the significance of the data. Data visualization can take a large volume of data and provide key aspects and insights to the data in a visual format (Meyer 2017). Many tools such as graphs, charts, and tables exist to present data. It is easy to create different charts and graphs that provide information and detail regarding data, but it is important to present the data in ways that are appropriate to the healthcare organization and the data being analyzed. For example, to present the frequency of a specific diagnosis by gender, a pie chart—meant to show the percentages of a total—would not be a good selection. A table could provide that information in a better format. Chapter 13, *Research and Data Analysis,* provides specific information regarding data visualization and presentation methods.

Another important aspect for the management and presentation of data is that the data and information need to be meaningful and useful to the organization. Presenting data that do not support an initiative of the organization can be an unproductive use of company resources and time. It is important to define a clear strategy regarding the type of information to be reported to support business strategy. In other words, the focus should be on presenting data that will help the healthcare organization reach its goals. Additionally, the data may provide information and detail that elicit negative feedback. For example, if a healthcare organization is trying to determine if it wants to add an additional cardiac catheterization room, it may choose to evaluate and create data presentations for individuals within a specific geographic area who have been diagnosed with cardiac conditions. Graphs with data pertaining to emergency department visits would not be useful in evaluating the expansion of a cardiac catheterization room. Understanding the data and properly managing it becomes an essential part of handling data assets appropriately.

Critical Thinking Skills

Another key aspect in the management of data assets in the organization is critical thinking skills. Critical thinking refers to the process of analyzing, assessing, and reconstructing a situation to provide enhanced solutions and outcomes to a problem (The Critical Thinking Community n.d.). It is estimated that in the coming years, new technology advancement, including the use of technology in healthcare, will occur every 30 seconds (Humbert 2018). The skill of critical thinking is essential in healthcare. Humbert (2018) stated: "A critical thinker is able to deduce consequences from what he knows, and he knows how to make use of information to solve problems, and to seek relevant sources of information to inform himself....Critical thinking can help us acquire knowledge, improve our theories, and strengthen arguments. We can use critical thinking to enhance work processes and improve social institutions" (p. 56).

The issues and challenges that face healthcare organizations and the healthcare industry continue to become more complex and require the effective evaluation of data to help support the change in the healthcare environment (Meyer 2017; Sharp et al. 2013). Many individuals can effectively utilize critical thinking to analyze a situation and generate solutions to an issue. During the critical thinking process, it is common for data to be analyzed to effectively evaluate the current state and future solution in addition to generating a solution to the current issue. For example, a healthcare organization is currently evaluating a new line of service to add to an outpatient clinic being built in a small community where they currently only have family practice providers. Without critical thinking, an individual may evaluate only common types of care associated with family practice and add that new line of service to the outpatient clinic. From a critical thinking perspective, a healthcare organization may evaluate common referrals to other clinics for the patients seen and treated at the clinic. In addition, they may profile the community in which the clinic exists to understand the population and the care potentially needed. Based on this gathering and analysis of data, an enhanced decision on the nature of care can be made to support the community and its care needs.

With the implementation of EHRs, new roles such as data analysts or EHR analysts are being established for the oversight and management of data collection within a healthcare organization as well as how information is used. While principles of information governance have been established by AHIMA and data governance is an essential component of daily operations, the ability to understand, evaluate, and apply the different principles becomes an essential part of a successful information and data governance program.

Check Your Understanding 6.3

Answer the following questions.

1. True or false: Information governance and data governance are the same concept and can be used interchangeably.
2. Distinguish which of the following are components of AHIMA's principles of information governance.
   a. Accountability and accessibility
   b. Integrity and safeguards
   c. Safeguards and accessibility
   d. Accountability and integrity
3. True or false: Data stewardship is principles and practices established to ensure the knowledgeable and appropriate use of data derived from individuals' personal health information.
4. True or false: Data sharing is needed regardless of the information system used.
5. Identify which of the following describes what information assets are:
   a. Information considered to add value to an organization
   b. Data entered into a patient's health record by a provider
   c. Clearly defined elements required to be documented in the health record
   d. Information collected by a healthcare organization that has value

Data Quality

Data quality is the reliability and effectiveness of data for its intended uses in healthcare operations, decision-making, planning, and patient care. Data quality management is "business processes that ensure the integrity of an organization's data during collection, application (including aggregation), warehousing, and analysis" (Davoudi et al. 2015, 8). Data quality has always been a focus for HIM professionals; with the implementation of the EHR, the need for more complete and accurate information is critical to support proper patient care and corresponding reimbursement.

Data quality serves as one of the most important elements of healthcare operations and patient care. "All data must be accurate, timely, relevant, valid, and complete to ensure the reliability of the information" (Davoudi et al. 2015, 8). This is because the data support patient care and patient safety, provide evidence for reimbursement and accreditation, and afford documentation needed for quality initiatives and research (AHIMA 2015). Without complete and accurate data in a health record, a healthcare organization is at risk for patient safety issues. For example, if a provider does not document what medications were administered to a patient and the exact dosages, the patient may be prescribed another medication that could have adverse effects when combined with the first medication. In addition, there are risks such as having to return payment if the documentation does not support the healthcare organization's billing and reimbursement request. For example, if a physician billed that they performed a procedure, but the documentation does not support the procedure, the physician may have to return the money and rebill the services.

Clinical documentation is "any manual or electronic notation (or recording) made by a physician or other healthcare clinician related to a patient's medical condition or treatment" (Hess 2015). Clinical documentation is the foundation of every health record in that it supports the care the patient received and the reimbursement that should be received for the care. Inaccurate information and poor documentation negatively impact patient care and reimbursement, which can drive up the cost of healthcare (AHIMA 2015), creating a need for data quality and data quality management over healthcare data.

Many accrediting organizations such as the Joint Commission require evidence of clinical care based on the data that is documented in the health record. If the accrediting organization has basic requirements for documentation in the health record, and the healthcare organization does not meet those requirements, it runs the risk of losing accreditation. Data quality is critical to both clinical care and administrative processes. AHIMA's Data Quality Model is an important tool in ensuring the quality of the data collected.

AHIMA's Data Quality Management Model

AHIMA created the data quality management model to support the need for true and accurate data. Data quality management is "the business process that ensures integrity of an organization's data during collection, application, warehousing, and analysis" (Davoudi 2015). Many areas such as patient care, patient outcomes, reimbursement, process improvement, and daily healthcare operations depend on detailed quality of information. Core functions of enterprise information management must be established to create the ability to collect high-quality data from the health record. The goal of EIM is to make sure that information being used for business decisions and patient care is reliable and trustworthy. The data quality management model can help set up policies, processes, and expectations to support EIM within an organization.

The data quality management model defines four domains that link and support data quality. The first domain is application, which is focused on understanding the purpose of data collection. Since the amount of patient data collected through a patient encounter is immense, it is important to evaluate and understand why the data is being gathered and the purpose it serves for the healthcare organization. The second domain is collection, which concentrates on how the data elements are being collected throughout the encounter. Understanding where data is being entered and how it is being entered is an essential part of basic data quality management. This focus allows a healthcare organization to understand if duplicate or redundant information is being collected. The third domain is warehousing, which describes the processes as well as systems a healthcare organization uses to archive data; it also includes understanding where the data is being stored, and how it is being archived and managed. The last domain is analysis, which centers on how the data collected throughout the patient encounter is transformed into meaningful data for use throughout the entire spectrum of the healthcare setting (Davoudi 2015).

Ten characteristics of quality data defined within the AHIMA data quality model are accuracy, accessibility, comprehensiveness, consistency, currency, definition, granularity, precision, relevancy, and timeliness. Understanding and applying each of these characteristics to the data quality management domains is an essential part of effective oversight and management of data quality (Davoudi 2015).

Accuracy

Accuracy focuses on the data being free of errors. It is important that the data within the health record are accurate across the entire health record (that is, the data are valid with the appropriate test results and placed into the proper health record). An example of monitoring the health record for data accuracy is the analysis of patient notes in the health record to ensure they support the diagnosis throughout the entire health record (Davoudi 2015). For instance, the information in an operative report should be compared to information in the discharge summary to confirm the operation performed and findings are accurate (the same) in both documents.

Accessibility

Proper safeguards must be established and employed to ensure the data are available when needed while implementing proper precautions and safeguards to protect the information. An example of data accessibility is ensuring that nurses have access to the health records of patients that they are treating (Davoudi 2015). (See chapters 9, *Data Privacy and Confidentiality,* and 10, *Data Security,* for additional information on access to health records.)

Comprehensiveness

Data comprehensiveness certifies that all required data elements that should be collected throughout the health record are documented. One way to ensure this is happening in the EHR is to use required fields. Required fields allow for the information system to force a response in a specific data element within an information system. For example, the EHR will require at a minimum the user's name, date of birth, address, telephone number, and gender on a specific screen collecting patient information. The information system can require information to be entered into all these fields before the user is able to move to the next screen, which supports comprehensiveness. Training and education should be conducted across the healthcare organization to ensure the staff members collect all the required data elements in the health record (Davoudi 2015).

Consistency

Consistency means ensuring the patient data are reliable and the same across the entire patient encounter. In other words, patient data within the health record should be the same and should not contradict other data also in the health record; for example, a test result and diagnosis should be the same throughout the health record (Davoudi 2015).

Currency

The data within the health record need to be current and up to date. EHRs present information across a broad spectrum of care, including data that may be outdated. Specific procedures should be established for updating data elements used for each patient encounter, including the discontinuation of collected data elements that are no longer current. An example of data currency is reviewing and updating patient medications at each patient encounter to remove medications that are no longer being taken and add any new medications (Davoudi 2015).

Definition

All data elements should be clearly defined to guarantee that all individuals using and collecting the data will understand the meaning of that data element. An example of data definition is defining date of birth as the date the individual was born by month, day, and four-digit year (Davoudi 2015).

Granularity

The data collected for patient care must be at the appropriate level of detail. An example of data granularity is documenting the results of a lab test with the appropriate number of characters after a decimal point in the lab value (Davoudi 2015).

Precision

Data should be precise and collected in their exact form within the course of patient care; for example, documenting the exact measurement, such as the height or temperature of the patient. When information is entered precisely, there should be little to no variability of the data (Davoudi 2015).

Relevancy

Data relevancy is the extent to which the data elements being collected are useful for the purposes for which they are collected. If a healthcare organization collects data that are not relevant in supporting patient care and administration, it adds additional, unnecessary information in the health record. For example, if a patient presents with pain during urination, data collection should be focused around the symptoms, testing, and treatment. Collecting additional data or data not relevant to support treatment, payment, and healthcare operations adds superfluous data to the record. An example of relevancy is the creation of templates to collect the correct information during an emergency department visit for a patient, as this can help assemble accurate and relevant data to support the visit and help prevent additional, nonrelevant information from being collected (Davoudi 2015).

Timeliness

Patient documentation should be entered promptly, ensuring up-to-date information is available within specified and required time frames. Timeliness may vary throughout the health record depending on what the data are being used for and how the data are supporting patient care. An example of timeliness is specifying when notes such as discharge summaries or operative reports should be entered in the information system. Healthcare organizations frequently require specific forms such as orders or admitting evaluations to be entered within a defined period.

HIM professionals work in a variety of roles to support and manage the quality of data, especially as the implementation of the EHR continues. Some common HIM roles include clinical data manager, health data analysis, terminology asset manager, clinical documentation integrity specialist, data collection specialist, and EHR documentation specialist (Davoudi 2015). The HIM professional understands the need for quality data and can bring that knowledge and expertise into many different areas of the healthcare delivery system.

Data Collection Tools

The management of data quality depends on how the data are collected during the patient encounter. With data created, stored, and maintained on paper as well as in electronic format, it is important to ensure the data collection tools—such as forms and computer screens—used throughout a healthcare organization are effective and efficient. HIM professionals should be involved in the creation of data collection tools for both electronic and paper-based tools.

In addition to data collection tools, standardization of the collection of patient data is essential to collect the proper information and reach data quality levels needed to support the enhancement of patient care and the healthcare industry. The two major ways to collect data elements are through the use of electronic templates and paper-based forms. Not all paper forms will convert easily to an electronic format, so it is important to evaluate each of the different screens to ensure the data capture is correct. There are standards for both screen design and paper forms to facilitate data collection.

Screen Design

Most EHRs come with prebuilt forms and templates for use within the information system. For example, a template would contain all the information required for inclusion in the discharge summary such as discharge diagnosis, discharge medications, and follow-up. Usually, prebuilt forms and templates do not match the healthcare organization's specific needs. One reason for this is that a screen typically holds approximately a third of what is contained on a form. In addition, the prebuilt forms may not be constructed to collect the information needed to support the healthcare organization's patient care and payment processes. The Department of Health and Human Services Office of National Coordinator for Health Information Technology (ONC) discusses the need to evaluate workflow and customize patient data collection functions. They recommend the following for patient data collection functions:

- Create templates for common types of notes, visits, and procedures
- Configure patient data lists with multiple choices for diagnoses, medications, and orders
- Develop flow sheets for common vital signs and blood tests, allowing for trending across a period of time
- Confirm that the EHR being used meets basic standards for interoperability and data sharing across systems (HHS 2015).

In addition, analysts who are assisting with building the EHR within the healthcare organization should meet with each department that enters data into the health record to evaluate current data collection processes within the EHR and evaluate additional forms or tools necessary to support current workflow. Some key elements when evaluating forms design is deciding what should be in structured data format and what should be in unstructured data format. Structured data are data that can be read and interpreted by an information system. An example of structured data is a diagnosis code entered in the proper format into the information system, such as an ICD-10-CM code format of XXX.XXXX. If the data element is in the proper format and in the proper location, the information system will read and perform analysis on that data. Other methods to collect structured data include check boxes, drop-down boxes, and radio buttons. Check boxes allow the user to select multiple values. For example, murmurs, gallops, and rubs can be chosen under the cardiac section of the physical exam. Drop-down boxes list the appropriate options, such as states, from which the user can choose. Radio buttons are used when there are few options, such as only male or female, from which the user should choose. Unstructured data, also known as free text, are data entered into the information system with no format specified. An example of unstructured data is a narrative discharge summary that does not follow a specific format or use a template. Unstructured data cannot be interpreted by an information system and usually are not used in structured reports. When choosing how to collect data within an EHR, it is important to evaluate and make decisions based on how data are reported.

Since many healthcare organizations are unsure of what data they need, especially as they transition to the EHR, it is important to have a standardizing committee or process to evaluate data collection within information systems. This individual or group is responsible for assuring that quality data are entered into the information system and proper data reporting is obtained from the information system. The documentation should be used to support decisions for future evaluation.

Forms Design

Forms design is a major part of assuring data quality within a healthcare organization. Forms design is the oversight process in which paper forms are created to make sure that they are easily understood and to collect the correct amount of information necessary. Forms design helps to make sure there is a consistent process to determine if a form is necessary and how it will be developed (Pyramid Solutions 2017). With any new creation of a form, the following questions should be asked:

- What is the purpose of this form?
- Can the data be collected in electronic format versus paper format?
- When will this form be used during the patient encounter and in which type of patient encounters?
- Who will use this form within the healthcare organization?
- What will be done with the paper once it is created (scanned into system, stored in a paper health record)?

Answering these questions during the assessment of a new form will help the form be appropriate and direct whether it is created in paper or electronic format. The disadvantage of paper forms used to support patient care is that they have to be entered into an EHR manually or by scanning the paper documents, which does not allow for reporting. In some cases, paper forms that do not collect patient information, such as productivity forms or staff vacation requests, will not be entered into the EHR, but may be entered into a human resources management system. It is important to evaluate each form to determine if it will remain on paper or be entered into an electronic system.

The following are the recommended steps for controlling, tracking, and managing paper forms:

- Establishing data collection standards within the healthcare organization
- Establishing testing and evaluation process
- Evaluating the quality of new paper and electronic forms
- Systemizing storage, inventory, and distribution of forms
- Numbering, tracking, and using bar codes to manage paper forms
- Establishing a documentation system that supports decisions that are made by the forms committee

Proper and effective management of data collection requires quality data regardless of the media type. HIM professionals play a vital role in this process to verify that proper data is being collected in the best format and to confirm that forms are designed properly to ensure efficient processing of the information.

There is typically a clinical forms committee that manages both paper and electronic forms design. The clinical forms committee should be comprised of a multidisciplinary team and led by the HIM department. Some common recommended committee members are medical staff, nursing staff, purchasing, information services, performance improvement, support and ancillary departments, EHR support, and forms vendor liaison. In addition, anyone directly affected by the new form or computer view should be invited to attend the forms committee meeting. For example, when a form is being redesigned for use in the intensive care unit, nurses and physicians from that clinical area should be invited to give their input.

Forms control, tracking, and management are important issues. At a minimum, an effective forms control program includes the following activities:

- *Establishing standards*. Written standards and guidelines are essential to ensure the appropriate design and production practices are followed. **Standards** are fixed rules that must be followed for every form (for example, where the form title should be located). A guideline, on the other hand, provides general direction about the design of a form (for example, usual size of the font used).
- *Establishing a numbering and tracking system*. A unique numbering system should be developed to identify all organizational forms. A master form index should be established, and copies of all forms should be maintained for easy retrieval. At a minimum, information in the master form index should include form title, form number, origination date, revision dates, form purpose, and legal requirements. Ideally, the tracking system should be automated.
- *Establishing a testing and evaluation plan*. No new or revised form should be put into production or use without a field test and evaluation. Mechanisms should be in place to ensure appropriate testing of any new or revised form.
- *Checking the quality of new forms*. A mechanism should be in place to check all newly printed forms prior to distribution. This should be a quality check to confirm that the new form conforms to the original procurement order.
- *Systematizing storage, inventory, and distribution*. Processes should be in place to ensure the forms are stored appropriately. Paper forms should be stored in safe and

environmentally appropriate environments. Inventory should be maintained at a cost-effective level, and distribution should be timely.

- *Establishing a forms database*. In an electronic system that supports document imaging, a forms database may be used to store and facilitate updating of forms. Such a database can provide information on utilization rates, obsolescence, and replacement of individual forms or documentation templates (Barnett 1996; Pyramid Solutions 2017).

Check Your Understanding 6.4

Answer the following questions.

1. True or false: Healthcare organizations do not need to evaluate the purpose of data collection for assuring data quality.
2. Identify which of the following are the four data quality management domains.
   a. Accessibility, accuracy, consistency, and precision
   b. Application, collection, warehousing, and relevancy
   c. Accessibility, collection, warehousing, and precision
   d. Application, collection, warehousing, and analysis
3. Which of the following data quality characteristics means all data items are included in the information collected?
   a. Accuracy
   b. Consistency
   c. Comprehensiveness
   d. Relevancy
4. True or false: Data granularity is where the data collected is collected at a level of detail that meets the needs of the healthcare organization.
5. Recommend a guideline for maintaining integrity in the health record.
   a. Removing the consequences for the falsification of information
   b. Requiring training that covers the falsification of information and information security only at hire
   c. Assuring documentation that is being changed is permanently deleted from the record
   d. Prohibiting the entry of false information into any of the healthcare organization's health records

Clinical Documentation Integrity

Clinical documentation relates to the quality and integrity of patient data while supporting other functions such as timely coding and reimbursement. Clinical documentation integrity (CDI) is defined as the process of reviewing medical information to verify that documentation is clinical specific, is appropriate, and supports the medical codes assigned (AHIMA 2016c). Historically, CDI programs were created to support reimbursement; however, with the implementation of EHRs and the expanded uses of clinically coded data, CDI programs have shifted to facilitate an accurate representation of healthcare services through complete and accurate patient documentation within the record. The following are some basic goals of a CDI program:

- Obtain specific documentation that can be used to identify the patient's severity of illness
- Identify and clarify missing, conflicting, or nonspecific provider documentation related to diagnoses and procedures
- Support accurate diagnostic and procedural coding, and Medicare Severity

Diagnosis Related Group (MS-DRG) assignment, leading to appropriate reimbursement
- Promote health record completion during the patient's course of care, which promotes patient safety
- Improve communication between physicians and other members of the healthcare team
- Provide awareness and education
- Improve documentation to reflect quality and outcome scores
- Improve coding professionals' clinical knowledge (AHIMA 2016c)

CDI programs can help healthcare organizations enhance patient documentation, reduce errors within the health record, and improve the quality of the patient data entered in the system while supporting patient care and reimbursement for the organization. Figure 6.7 provides an example of how CDI impacts the patient.

CDI programs should be established with the initial review of the health record to verify all necessary components of the health record. The following areas should be evaluated during the initial CDI review process:

- Legibility – documentation should be easy to decipher and understand
- Reliability – documentation should be trustworthy
- Precision – documentation should follow strict medical terminology and be as accurate and exact as possible
- Completeness – documentation should contain all details that are necessary to support continuity of care between caregivers and support billing and reimbursement
- Consistency – documentation should be consistent throughout the entire record
- Clarity – documentation should describe all details regarding the patient's medical care to the highest level of specificity
- Timeliness – documentation must be completed in a timely manner (Barnette et al. 2017; Combs 2016b)

Another impact on CDI is the evaluation of present on admission (POA) reporting requirements. POA refers to the conditions that are present in a patient at the time of ordering the

Figure 6.7 How does CDI impact the patient?

Example Scenario:

This is a 48 y/o male that has hypertensive end-stage renal disease (ESRD) and is on home peritoneal dialysis. He recently had knee replacement surgery. Two days after being discharged home, he went into respiratory failure and was rushed back to the hospital. It was determined he was in fluid overload secondary to a blockage in the peritoneal dialysis catheter from fibrin. This was treated with heparin and returned to normal function. He was discharged home with home health nursing and physical therapy.

After being discharged home, the wife and home health nurse noticed the patient's oxygen level would continue to drop to the low 80s to upper 70s every time he fell asleep. The primary care physician was called and home oxygen was ordered for a decrease in oxygen saturations. A sleep study was also scheduled. The patient then received a call from the home oxygen vendor and was told his insurance would not cover home oxygen for his condition. He was told the only way it could be delivered was if he paid for it out of pocket. It is now 5:00 pm on a Friday evening and the physician's office is closed.

This would be of great concern to a patient in this situation. He knows he needs the oxygen but does he have the money to pay for it? The patient is sick enough to need the oxygen but unfortunately the clinical documentation doesn't have the specificity needed to reflect the true condition of the patient. Home oxygen has a specific set of requirements under the National Coverage Determinations (NCDs) for Medicare that must be met before the treatment will be approved. Some other payers also use these criteria to support medical necessity of certain treatments.

It is important for providers to be aware of National Coverage Determinations and Local Coverage Determinations (LCDs). The Centers for Medicare and Medicaid Services has a website where providers can look at the NCD and LCD requirements (https://www.cms.gov/medicare-coverage-database/indexes/national-and-local-indexes.aspx). In the hospital, patients have case managers who ensure these requirements are met before discharge. But this is not the case in many outpatient settings.

Source: Combs 2016a.

inpatient admission. The goal of the POA reporting is to document which conditions are present in a patient at the time of admission into an acute-care facility versus the conditions that may develop during the patient's stay in the facility (AHIMA 2009; Garrett 2009). A condition acquired during a hospital stay is referred to as a hospital-acquired condition (HAC). If a patient acquires a HAC that increases the cost of the patient care, it may not be paid under Medicare if it is considered preventable. It is important for a CDI program to evaluate these two requirements and make sure proper documentation is in place at the time of the inpatient admission order to prevent loss of reimbursement (AHIMA 2009; Garrett 2009). Chapter 15, *Revenue Management and Reimbursement*, offers more information regarding POA and HACs.

A CDI program usually has dedicated staff that may include HIM professionals, physicians, nurses, and other healthcare professionals. CDI programs impact quality of care and finances within a healthcare organization along with other key stakeholders such as case management, utilization review, medical staff, physician leadership, executive leadership, patient financial services, revenue cycle management, quality and risk management, nursing, and compliance (AHIMA 2018). The CDI program must have clear goals and strategies that align with the healthcare organization's requirement for clear and precise clinical documentation. There are several CDI tools that can be used to enhance the quality of documentation. Clinical documentation specialists use these tools.

One of the successes of a CDI program is to have a physician advisor who will not only participate with the CDI program but also has the clinical respect of his or her peers. The CDI physician advisor serves as a liaison between the CDI specialists, the coding professionals, the quality department, and the providers at the organization, supporting the needs of the CDI program (AHIMA 2016c). The primary responsibilities of the CDI physician advisor are to educate physicians on clinical language and coding guidelines, help providers document and reflect the true severity of the patient's illness, properly capture all the services and treatments performed by the healthcare organization, ensure the documentation supports the code assignments, understand the coded data in quality measures and reporting, and know how documentation impacts payment methodologies. The physician also works closely with the HIM coding department and CDI specialists to review health record documentation, discuss clinical issues that may have been identified during the health record reviews, discuss clinical criteria for disease processes, assist in the development of appropriate, compliant, and ethical provider queries, and review HACs and treatment complications (AHIMA 2016c).

CDI Tools

There are different ways to conduct the CDI review within a healthcare organization. CDI tools help manage and document the work of CDI professionals. A variety of tools can be used to help support CDI processes within an organization. One tool is computer-assisted coding (CAC). CAC is software that can search and evaluate clinical documentation to produce information regarding potential areas for documentation integrity. Electronic documentation is passed through the CAC software application, which analyzes the information and produces a report of procedure and diagnosis codes based on the electronic documentation evaluated. The codes are then manually evaluated for accuracy and completeness. The use of CAC software can speed up the coding process as it allows for evaluation of electronic assigned codes rather than having an individual analyze the entire electronic record and manually assign codes. While CAC is mainly used for the coding of the health record for reimbursement purposes, it can be used to automate part of the CDI process as well as provide an electronic evaluation of documentation (AHIMA 2018). Other CDI tools include audits, tip sheets, educational materials, and queries.

Audits Audits are an essential part of a CDI program. For more on audits refer to chapter 16, *Fraud and Abuse Compliance*. Audits can help an organization determine where there are areas that are missing proper documentation. Audits can also help an organization create a plan on the type of health records and services to focus on for CDI efforts (AHIMA 2018). A healthcare organization can select a specific number of health records from the healthcare organization and perform an audit to determine if the documentation in the health records meets the expectation of the codes being billed to the insurance company. The findings from the audit can provide the healthcare organization with specific details on what areas of the healthcare organization may be at risk due to missing or incomplete documentation. A successful CDI audit program will evaluate all areas of the healthcare organization to determine the areas that are most out of compliance. Additionally, a healthcare organization may decide to increase the number of audits in high-risk billing areas, such as the focus of any federal government billing audits (AHIMA 2018). For example, if the federal government's Medicare program is focusing on recovery audits for inpatient psychiatry, a healthcare organization may want to increase the audits in that area to uncover any areas of concern. After audits are completed, the CDI department can start working with departments and physicians to make sure proper documentation exists to support the billing.

Queries The most common tool used for CDI is a query. A **query** is a communication tool for CDI staff to communicate with providers to obtain clinical clarification, provide a documentation alert, clarify documentation, or ask additional questions regarding documentation. Traditionally, queries have been used to support coding and reimbursement; however, queries are expanding to the process of CDI outside the coding department. Queries may be used to help clarify a complex diagnosis within a health record that does not have proper documentation or clarify procedures that may not be specific enough to support patient care or add a valid code. Queries are used to obtain appropriate reimbursement for the care and services provided to the patient, request more detail regarding the documentation that exists, or clarify contradictory documentation. Contradictory information exists when two parts of a patient's health record provide conflicting information. For example, if an operative report states that the patient had surgery on the right leg, but in the progress notes there is information regarding the surgical wound on the left leg, a query may be requested to confirm which leg was operated on. There are two formats of queries for CDI: electronic query and paper query. Both queries contain the same demographic information such as the patient name, admission date or date of service, health record number, account number, date query initiated, name and contact of the person who created the query, and a statement of issues to be resolved (AHIMA 2018). For additional information on demographic information, refer to chapter 3, *Health Information Functions, Purpose, and Users.*

An electronic query is conducted through an EHR and allows the healthcare provider to offer more clarification or specific information regarding the patient's treatment and diagnosis. The typical process for an electronic query is usually the same format as for a written query, however, the information will be sent electronically and will allow the provider to respond electronically or add an additional clarification note in the health record. A paper query uses a standardized physical document to request clarification or further specify a diagnosis. With the use of paper queries, the health record must be made available to the healthcare provider to review and document the clarification in it. Additionally, the response of the query will be documented on paper and the coder or CDI professional will need access to the entire paper health record after the query is completed. The paper query is retained by the healthcare organization and can be stored within the paper health record or scanned into the EHR. Since the query will support patient care and reimbursement, the healthcare organization must create policies and procedures to manage how the query response will be incorporated into the health record and if it will become part of the legal health record or designated record set (AHIMA 2018b). For additional information on the legal health record, refer to chapter 8, *Health Law.* See chapter 9, *Data Privacy and Confidentiality,* for information on the designated record set.

Rules for Writing Queries When writing queries, regardless of the medium, healthcare organizations must ensure they are not leading physicians to document a particular response, but rather requesting clarification or additional specification. Policies and procedures should delineate who to query, when to query, when not to query, the query format, and the management of the query response. In general, a query should be created when health record documentation meets one of the following criteria: "[it] is conflicting, imprecise, incomplete, illegible, ambiguous, or inconsistent; describes or is associated with clinical indicators without a definitive relationship to an underlying diagnosis; includes clinical indicators, diagnostic evaluation, and/or treatment not related to a specific condition or procedure; provides a diagnosis without underlying clinical validation; or is unclear for present on admission indicator assignment" (AHIMA 2016c).

There are multiple types of data queries: further specificity of a diagnosis, inconsistency in documentation, and missing clinical indicators. Figure 6.8 provides examples of two different types of queries with leading and nonleading questions.

The CDI process needs professional, objective communication. CDI specialists must have strong written and oral communication skills and have basic knowledge of clinical coding guidelines as well as clinical knowledge and knowledge of documentation requirements. All communication, verbal or written, between the CDI professional and the provider needs to be conducted in a professional manner. Most of the information and detail that will be discussed and concluded based on the findings from the CDI process or query process will need to be documented in the health record and may become part of the health record.

Figure 6.8 Examples of queries with leading and nonleading queries

Example Open-Ended Query
A patient is admitted with pneumonia. The admitting H&P examination reveals white blood count of 14,000; a respiratory rate of 24; a temperature of 102 degrees; heart rate of 120; hypotension; and altered mental status. The patient is administered an IV antibiotic and IV fluid resuscitation.

Leading: The patient has elevated WBCs, tachycardia, and is given an IV antibiotic for Pseudomonas cultured from the blood. Are you treating for sepsis?

Nonleading: Based on your clinical judgment, can you provide a diagnosis that represents the below-listed clinical indicators? In this patient admitted with pneumonia, the admitting H&P examination reveals the following:

- WBC 14,000
- Respiratory rate 24
- Temperature 102°F
- Heart rate 120
- Hypotension
- Altered mental status
- IV antibiotic administration
- IV fluid resuscitation

Please document the condition and the causative organism (if known) in the health record.

Example Multiple-Choice Query
A patient is admitted for a right hip fracture. The H&P notes that the patient has a history of chronic congestive heart failure. A recent echocardiogram showed left ventricular ejection fraction (EF) of 25 percent. The patient's home medications include metoprolol XL, lisinopril, and furosemide.

Leading: Please document if you agree the patient has chronic diastolic heart failure.

Nonleading: It is noted in the impression of the H&P that this patient has chronic congestive heart failure and a recent echocardiogram noted under the cardiac review of systems reveals an EF of 25 percent. Can the chronic heart failure be further specified as:

- Chronic systolic heart failure ____________________
- Chronic diastolic heart failure
- Chronic systolic and diastolic heart failure
- Some other type of heart failure
- Undetermined ________________

Source: AHIMA 2016b, 2.

Both providers and CDI professionals must ensure communication is professional and appropriate to support patient care and reimbursement (AHIMA 2016c).

Reporting To help support the need for and successes of the CDI program, it is important to establish reporting tools with key performance indicators (KPIs) to provide to leadership and providers. Key performance indicators are measures that can be used over time to determine if a structure, process, or outcome supports high-quality performance measures against best practices. KPIs must align with an organization's strategy and must be measurable (Malmgren and Solberg 2016). A best practice is to establish a dashboard that is updated on a consistent basis and reviewed for opportunities to expand on areas of concern. Some common reporting areas for a CDI program may include the following:

- Discharges available/Discharges reviewed for CDI
- Number of queries by provider and impact on diagnosis related group
- Number of queries resulting in severity of illness changes
- Provider response to queries and turnaround time by provider
- Outcomes of CDI queries by physician (agree or disagree with CDI specialist)
- Case mix index (CMI) impact by services line
- Reimbursement impact by queries (AHIMA 2016c)

The most important part of leading a CDI program is to establish the reporting dashboard and process to make sure that leadership within the healthcare organization understands the need and impact of the program. It allows providers to see and understand the impact of appropriateness of documentation on reimbursement and case mix index (AHIMA 2016c). Figure 6.9 provides an example of a monthly query repost rate report.

Education One of the major goals of a CDI program is to provide education based on the findings throughout the CDI process. CDI education programs should bring knowledge and information back to the healthcare provider to enhance the quality and completeness of documentation to support the severity of illness. In addition, a CDI education program can be brought back to the HIM coders to help support the accurate assignment of codes based on the documentation. A CDI education component provides usable, efficient, compliant, and meaningful documentation findings to help enhance the patient care workflow, collect complete and accurate data in a timelier fashion, and improve healthcare reimbursement (AHIMA 2016c).

Check Your Understanding 6.5

Answer the following questions.

1. Identify the two types of queries used in clinical documentation integrity.
   a. Manual and electronic
   b. Paper and electronic
   c. Manual and computer-assisted coding
   d. Electronic and computer-assisted coding
2. True or false: The response from a query will never go into the health record as it is just communication between the CDI professional and the provider.
3. Distinguish which of the following is a goal of a CDI program.
   a. Identify the providers who are not performing properly
   b. Ensure documentation is meeting minimum requirements of the medical staff bylaws
   c. Identify and clarify missing, conflicting, or nonspecific physician documentation related to diagnoses and procedures
   d. Analyze the records after the patient is discharged to document missing pieces of information

Figure 6.9 Example of monthly query repost rate report

CHF Monthly Physician Response to Query Process Report							
1st quarter				**2nd quarter**			
Mo.	# CHF Queries	# Answers	% Response	Mo.	# CHF Queries	# Answers	% Response
JAN	150	92	61%	APR	180	110	61%
FEB	89	61	69%	MAY	160	104	65%
MAR	110	79	72%	JUN	98	75	77%
3rd quarter				**4th quarter**			
Mo.	# CHF Queries	# Answers	% Response	Mo.	# CHF Queries	# Answers	% Response
JUL	172	133	77%	OCT	99	53	54%
AUG	132	87	66%	NOV	186	141	76%
SEP	169	115	68%	DEC	201	159	79%

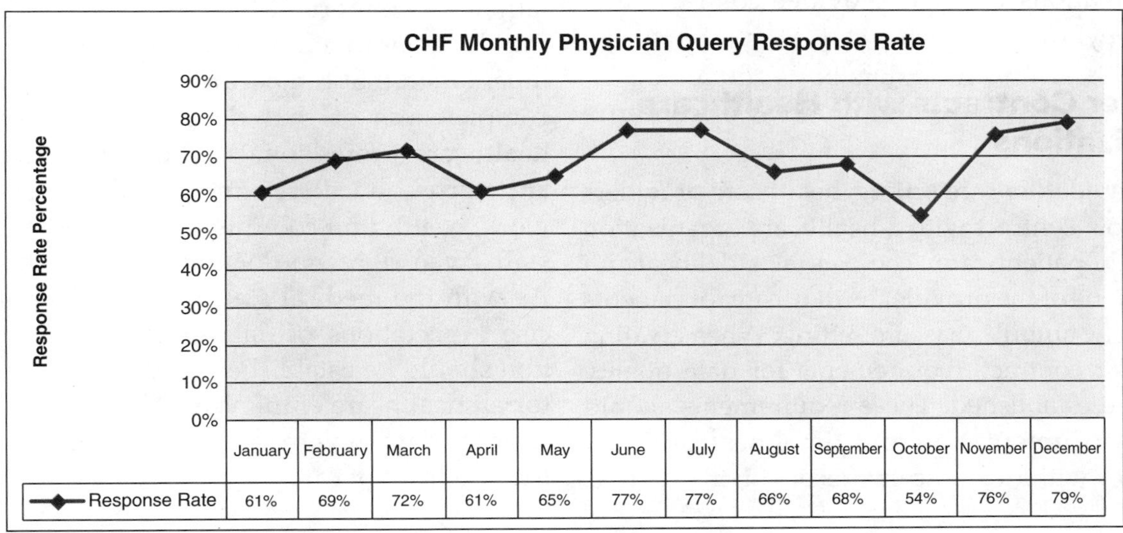

Source: AHIMA 2016c, p. 37.

Data Management and Bylaws

To help with the facilitation of the collection and assurance of quality data within a healthcare organization, bylaws should be created. **Bylaws** are written documents that provide details and information regarding the rules and regulations established by a healthcare organization to help support healthcare operations. Part of the bylaws set the expectations of the medical staff for documentation and timeliness of documentation, which directly impacts an organization's data and information governance. Among the concerns with healthcare operations is ensuring that the information documented in the health record supports patient care as well as quality improvement initiatives and accreditation activities. Additionally, the bylaws should define the processes that align with the organization's data and information governance strategy regarding the completeness and accuracy of health information within a health record, including expectations of timeliness. Data quality is a common area to analyze for the purposes of healthcare operations and creates a need for healthcare organizations to define minimum standards of clinical documentation. The minimum clinical documentation requirements are most often defined in the bylaws of the healthcare organization. By defining the expectations for documentation and data management in the bylaws, the healthcare organization can hold providers accountable if they are not meeting the expectations and impacting the information governance and data governance processes. Additionally, the establishment of data collection and data quality requirements in bylaws can help support and ensure proper documentation as required by the healthcare organization to support the data management processes. Another area commonly addressed in bylaws is ensuring compliance with federal and state laws and regulations through provider contracts and hospital bylaws.

Provider Contracts with Healthcare Organizations

In the ambulatory care setting, healthcare providers enter into a contract with a healthcare organization to provide patient care. The contracts delineate all expectations of the provider as they care for patients in a specific ambulatory care setting. When creating a provider contract, requirements for data quality should be established. These requirements should include documentation and timeliness of documentation within the health record. For example, a provider contract will state that all labs must be reviewed and signed within 24 hours of completion of the lab test. The contract will also include consequences if minimal requirements are not met, such as the cancellation of the contract in the event of a breach.

Hospital Bylaws

Hospital bylaws are written documents that govern the staff members, both medical providers and non-physician providers, who create data within the health record for additional support of patient care and reimbursement. Since medical providers are not the sole authors of clinical documentation, it is important for hospitals to define who can document within the record, the type of documentation that can occur, and the timeliness and completeness of that documentation. Common healthcare professionals who enter information are nurses, ancillary support, therapists, social work, health unit coordinators, and other support staff given rights to document within the record. As with the medical staff bylaws, clear and concise expectations of data entry and documentation should be established, and training provided for all healthcare employees. The hospital bylaws support data governance and data quality across the spectrum of care.

Data Management and Technology

Currently, most of the work supporting data management within healthcare happens in an electronic manner. This is due to the implementation of EHRs and other electronic information systems used to support patient care. Because of the amount of data available in healthcare organizations, data have become valuable assets. While this causes some concern with the amount of data collected by the healthcare organization, it also allows healthcare organizations to use the data to make decisions based on information derived from the data. One of the powerful aspects of having data in electronic format is the ability to use technology to assist in the management of the data.

There are many benefits to using technology in a healthcare organization. Technology can be used to support data management and the implementation of information governance and data governance. Technology can also be used to facilitate working across teams. With advances in technology and the increase in data created, the need for new forms of data management through technology will continue to be a priority in healthcare to ensure standardization in the collection and management of data.

HIM Roles

Many different roles exist for HIM professionals in data management. These roles may exist within a healthcare system, a physician clinic, an insurance company, or a vendor that supports a healthcare organization. HIM professionals can lead an organization's IG initiative as an Information Governance Program Director, support the IG initiative as a data steward or business analyst, support the information systems and data collection as a database administrator, or take on the role of data analyst. HIM roles require the ability to gather information, analyze the information, and transform data into powerful information the healthcare organization can use for strategic, regulatory, quality, and reimbursement purposes.

HIM professionals have always advocated for clear, accurate, and complete documentation in the health record. HIM professionals fit perfectly in the CDI role as they understand medical coding including guidelines, documentation requirements, the need for complete and accurate information, and billing and reimbursement requirements. The clinical documentation specialist is a new role established to improve work processes related to documentation by communicating with providers, improving clinical documentation design, and ensuring accurate documentation to support code assignment. The clinical documentation specialist must have a strong working relationship with the providers and feel comfortable requesting additional information via query processes.

Check Your Understanding 6.6 

Answer the following questions.

1. True or false: When creating bylaws for the medical staff, expectations of data quality should be established and documented within the bylaws.
2. True or false: Without proper definition and requirements of data quality and data collection, it is challenging for healthcare organizations to hold healthcare providers accountable for documentation.
3. When creating requirements of documentation for hospital bylaws, which of the following should be evaluated?
   a. The personal preferences of the healthcare practitioner
   b. The documentation needs based on accrediting bodies
   c. Information taught in the local nursing programs
   d. The wants of the department chairs in a hospital
4. True or false: When creating provider contracts, healthcare organizations should not define disciplinary actions in the event that the contract requirements are not met.

Real-World Case 6.1

A large urban children's hospital in Dallas, Texas, is leading in the delivery of care provided to children from birth through age 18. After implementing an electronic health record, the hospital identified operations in need of improvement. It found that individual business units were working in their own silos with little interdepartmental communication occurring, and the individual business units had different policies, procedures, and processes for information governance and data management. The hospital quickly realized the need to standardize processes and create an effective information governance program to help streamline and manage the vast amount of data being collected across the organization.

Using tools that are available through AHIMA's Information Governance Adoption Model (IGAM), the hospital evaluated the current state of information governance at the organization. This was done through the evaluation and review of information-related policies and procedures throughout the system. It also created the foundation necessary to implement a process to review, edit, and update all those information policies and procedures to create a consistent and standardized process across all business units of the organization. Most important, it showed the need to educate workforce members on the importance of having a consistent format for data collection across the entire organization.

The outcome of implementing an information governance program at the children's hospital produced many benefits. The hospital was able to create a consistent process for training and educating all workforce members to support the transparency of data management to use the information to its competitive advantage. It created a platform to have open and transparent conversations throughout the healthcare organization, supporting the mission of the organization. By streamlining all the policies and procedures across the organization, the hospital was able to break down department silos that existed within the organization and implement an organization-wide culture supporting the information governance program. (Fahy and Hermann 2017.)

Real-World Case 6.2

A medium-sized hospital had been using an electronic health record (EHR) for 12 months. It was having great success in getting the providers to document within a timely fashion; however, many of the notes did not provide enough information to code the record or key components to adequately code diagnoses and procedures were missing. The hospital had a process for physician query, as follows:

- Electronically flag the record for physician query
- Create a paper query form for the provider
- Send the electronic query to the HIM operations department to put in a physician completion folder
- HIM operations adds a deficiency to the patient health record to flag the provider that a coding query needs to be completed
- The provider comes to the HIM department to complete the query
- The deficiency is removed, and the query is scanned into the health record
- HIM operations notifies the coder via e-mail that the query was answered
- The health record is coded and the codes are sent to billing

While it was a strong process and the providers did answer the questions, it caused a spike in the amount of time it took to get the health record coded and billed, as providers usually came into the department once every 20 to 25 days. In some cases, providers would leave the coding queries unanswered for up to 60 days. The average turnaround time for a coding query was 28 days. The hospital needed to accelerate the query process and reduce the physicians' frustrations with having to come to the HIM department.

New functionality within the EHR was used to send an electronic query that automatically assigned the deficiency and sent a note to the provider's inbox alerting them that there was a coding query. The new process had fewer steps and involved fewer people; however, the physicians were concerned that the additional time required to learn the new process and system was impacting time spent with their patients. With careful training and education, the new process was implemented and reduced the steps, which made the physician query process easier for coding,

HIM operations, and the providers. The following are the new process steps:

- Electronically flag the record for physician query
- Create the electronic physician query through predesigned templates and assign the correct physician (this would automatically assign the deficiency and send the coding query to the inbox)
- The physician electronically completes the coding query through the EHR
- The electronic deficiency is automatically removed, and the coding query is electronically submitted to the physician and retained and the health record then automatically flagged to complete coding
- The health record is coded and sent to billing

With the change in the process, the HIM operations department has little involvement unless it is supporting the physician in completing the query. The turnaround time for completion of coding queries was reduced from 28 days to 15 days within the first 60 days of completion. The process was a success and the hospital has significantly reduced the time it takes to code and bill all patient encounters.

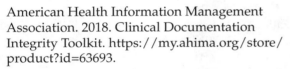

References

American Health Information Management Association. 2018. Clinical Documentation Integrity Toolkit. https://my.ahima.org/store/product?id=63693.

American Health Information Management Association. 2017. Health Data Analysis Toolkit. http://bok.ahima.org/PdfView?oid=302359.

American Health Information Management Association. 2016a. Managing a data dictionary (2016 update). http://library.ahima.org/doc?oid=302014#.XDiyrM9KhTY.

American Health Information Management Association. 2016b. Guidelines for achieving a compliant query practice (2016 update). *Journal of AHIMA*. http://library.ahima.org/doc?oid=301357#.XDjwX89KhTY.

American Health Information Management Association. 2016c. Clinical Documentation Integrity Toolkit. http://bok.ahima.org/PdfView?oid=301829.

American Health Information Management Association. 2015a. Assessing and improving EHR data quality (updated). [expanded online version]. http://library.ahima.org/PB/EHRDataQuality#.Vw55HfkrK9I.

American Health Information Management Association. 2017. *Pocket Glossary of Health Information Management and Technology*, 5th ed. Chicago: AHIMA.

American Health Information Management Association. 2013. Integrity of the healthcare record: Best practices for EHR documentation (2013 update). *Journal of AHIMA* 84(8): 58–62 [extended web version]. http://library.ahima.org/doc?oid=300257#.XDj-Z89KhTY.

American Health Information Management Association. 2011. HIM functions in healthcare quality and patient safety. Appendix B: HIM's role in data governance. *Journal of AHIMA* 82(8). http://library.ahima.org/doc?oid=104977#.Vw581fkrK9I.

American Health Information Management Association. 2009. Understanding HACs and SREs for quality reporting and reimbursement. *Journal of AHIMA* 80(9). http://library.ahima.org/doc?oid=106266#.XDkI3c9KhTY.

American Health Information Management Association. 2006. Data standard time: Data content standardization and the HIM role. *Journal of AHIMA* 77(2). http://library.ahima.org/doc?oid=65894#.XGQ4ys9KjSc.

American Health Information Management Association. n.d. AHIMA's IG Adoption Model for Healthcare. http://www.ahima.org/~/media/ahima/files/him-trends/ig/ighealthrateflyerfinal.ashx.

Barnett, R. 1996. *Managing Business Forms.* Canberra, Australia: Robert Narnett and Associates.

Barnette, E., M. Endicott, C.E. Ericson, M.M. Wieczorek. 2017. Evolving Roles in Clinical Documentation Improvement: Physician Practice Opportunities. *Journal of AHIMA* 88(5): 54-58.

Brinda, D. 2016. Data Management. Chapter 6 in *Health Information Management: An Applied Approach,* 5th ed. Edited by N. Sayles and L. Gordon. Chicago: AHIMA.

Combs, T. 2016a. How do CDI programs impact the patient? http://bok.ahima.org/doc?oid=301975#.XDkEcM9KhTY.

Combs, T. 2016b. Recognizing the characteristics of quality documentation. *Journal of AHIMA* 87(5):32–33. http://bok.ahima.org/doc?oid=301440#.XDkc5M9KhTY.

Coronel, C. and S. Morris. 2015. *Database Systems: Design, Implementation, and, Management*, 11th ed. Stamford, CT: Cengage Learning.

Datskovsky, Galina; Hedges, Ron; Empel, Sofia. 2015a. "Evaluating the Information Governance Principles for Healthcare: Accountability and Transparency." *Journal of AHIMA*. 86:2. 52–53.

Datskovsky, Galina; Hedges, Ron; Empel, Sofia; Washington, Lydia. 2015b. "Evaluating the Information Governance Principles for Healthcare: Compliance and Availability." *Journal of AHIMA*. 86:6. 54–55.

Datskovsky, Galina; Hedges, Ron; Empel, Sofia; Washington, Lydia. 2015c. "Evaluating the Information Governance Principles for Healthcare: Retention and Disposition." *Journal of AHIMA*. 86:9. 50–51.

Davoudi, S., J. Dooling, B. Glondys, T. Jones, L. Kadlec, S. Overgaard, K. Ruben, and A. Wendicke. 2015. Data quality management model (2015 update). http://bok.ahima.org/doc?oid=107773#.XDjq689KhTY.

Dean, A. 2018. The future of healthcare data exchange. *Journal of AHIMA.* https://journal.ahima.org/2018/09/01/the-future-of-healthcare-data-exchange/.

Dickey, J. 2018. Enterprise information management and information strategy: A brief how-to guide. *Journal of AHIMA* 89(9):38–39. http://bok.ahima.org/doc?oid=302595#.XDj6Kc9KjIE.

Downing, K. 2016. The importance of data stewards in information governance. *Journal of AHIMA.* http://journal.ahima.org/2016/05/26/the-importance-of-data-stewards-in-information-governance/.

Fahy, K. and M. Hermann. 2017. Updating organizational policies and procedures for information governance. Case study #6: Enterprise information management at Children's Health System of Texas. *Journal of AHIMA* 88(6):46–47. http://bok.ahima.org/doc?oid=302160#.XGWnh89KjOY

Garrett, G.S. 2009. Present on Admission: Where We Are Now *Journal of AHIMA* 80(7): 22-26.

Glondys, B. 2016. Getting Started with Information Governance: Applying SBAR to IG. *Journal of AHIMA* 87(2): 34-36.

Healthcare Information and Management Systems Society. 2009. Data Warehousing: A New Focus in Healthcare Data Management. http://s3.amazonaws.com/rdcms-himss/files/production/public/HIMSSorg/Content/files/EHR/DataWarehousing.pdf.

Hess, P. 2015. *Clinical Documentation Improvement: Principles and Practices*. Chicago: AHIMA.

Humbert, S. 2018. Tackling touch cases: How to empower critical thinking and temper productivity goals. *Journal of AHIMA* 89(1):56–57.

Johns, M. 2015. *Enterprise Health Information Management and Data Governance*. Chicago: AHIMA.

Kadlec, L. 2015. Getting Started with IG: No Time to Sit and Relax. http://bok.ahima.org/doc?oid=301497#.XTtnP3spCUk.

Kanaan, S.B. and M.M. Carr. 2009. Health Data Stewardship: What, Why, Who, How. AN NCVHS Primer. http://library.ahima.org/PdfView?oid=94786.

Maimone, C. 2016. Data mapping best practices (2016 update). http://bok.ahima.org/doc?oid=302009#.XTuQJ3spCUk.

Meyer, M. 2017. The Rise of Healthcare Data Visualization. *Data Revolution, A Journal of AHIMA blog*. December 21, 2017. http://journal.ahima.org/2017/12/21/the-rise-of-healthcare-data-visualization/.

Malmgren, C. and C.J. Solberg. 2016. Revenue Cycle Management in *Health Information Management: Concepts, Principles, and Practice*, 5th ed. Edited by P,K. Oachs and A.L. Watters. Chicago: AHIMA Press.

Murphy, G. and M. Brandt. 2001. Practice Brief: Health informatics standards and information transfer: Exploring the HIM Role. *Journal of AHIMA* 72(1):68A–68D. http://library.ahima.org/doc?oid=57544#.Vw59VfkrK9I.

Noreen, N. 2017. Data Stewards Play an Important Role in the Future of Healthcare. *IGIQ: A Journal of AHIMA Blog.* November 17, 2017. http://journal.ahima.org/2017/11/17/data-stewards-play-an-important-role-in-the-future-of-healthcare/.

Orlova, A., H. Rhodes, and D. Warner. 2016. Standardizing data and HIM practices for interoperability [expanded web version]. *Journal of AHIMA* 87(11):54-58. http://bok.ahima.org/doc?oid=301924#.XDixDs9KhTY.

Pyramid Solutions. 2017 (September). Best Practices for Paper-Based Form Design. https://pyramidsolutions.com/wp-content/uploads/2017/09/Best-Practices-for-Paper-Based-Form-Design.pdf.

Sharp, M. 2016. Secondary Data Sources. Chapter 7 in *Health Information Management: An Applied Approach,* 5th ed. Edited by N. Sayles and L. Gordon. Chicago: AHIMA.

Sharp, M., R. Reynolds, and K. Brooks. 2013. Critical thinking skills of allied health science students: A structured inquiry. *Educational Perspectives in Health Informatics and Information Management* Summer 2013:1–13.

The Critical Thinking Community. n.d. Our Concept of Critical Thinking. http://www.criticalthinking.org/pages/our-concept-of-critical-thinking/411.

US Department of Health and Human Services Health Information Technology (HHS). 2015. How to Implement Your EHR System. http://www.hrsa.gov/healthit/toolbox/healthitimplementation/implementationtopics/implementsystem/.implementsystem_4.html#Customize Patient Data Collection Functions.

Vimalachandran, P., H. Wang, Y. Zhang, B. Heyward, and F. Whittaker. 2016. 2016 International Conference on Orange Technologies (ICOT). https://arxiv.org/pdf/1802.00577.pdf.

Walsh, T. 2013. Security risk analysis and management: An overview (2013 update). *Journal of AHIMA* 84(11). http://library.ahima.org/doc?oid=300266.

Warner, D. 2013a. (December 18). IG101: Developing Clinical Business Intelligence. https://journal.ahima.org/2013/12/18/ig-101-developing-clinical-business-intelligence/.

Warner, D. 2013b. (December 11). IG 101: Enterprise Information Governance. http://journal.ahima.org/2013/12/11/ig-101-enterprise-information-governance/.

Washington, L. 2015. Information Governance Offers a Strategic Approach for Healthcare (2015 update) – Retired. *Journal of AHIMA* 86(11):56–59. http://bok.ahima.org/doc?oid=107796#.XGRBLM9KjSc.

Secondary Data Sources

Marcia Y. Sharp, EdD, MBA, RHIA

Learning Objectives

- Distinguish between primary and secondary data and between patient-identifiable and aggregate data
- Differentiate between internal and external users of secondary data
- Compare the facility-specific indexes commonly found in hospitals
- Describe the registries used in hospitals according to purpose, methods of case definition and case finding, data collection methods, reporting and follow-up, and pertinent laws and regulations affecting registry operations
- Explain the terms associated with each type of secondary record or database
- Discuss the agencies for approval, education, and certification for cancer, immunization, and trauma registries
- Distinguish between healthcare databases in terms of purpose and content

Key Terms

Abbreviated Injury Scale (AIS)
Accession number
Accession registry
Agency for Healthcare Research and Quality (AHRQ)
Aggregate data
American College of Surgeons (ACS) Commission on Cancer
Case definition
Case finding
Centers for Disease Control and Prevention (CDC)
Certified tumor registrar (CTR)
Clinical trial
Collaborative Stage Data Set
Disease index
Disease registry
Facility-based registry
Health Services Research
Healthcare Cost and Utilization Project (HCUP)
Incident
Index
Injury Severity Score (ISS)
Medical Literature, Analysis, and Retrieval System Online (MEDLINE)
Medicare Provider Analysis and Review (MEDPAR) File
National Cancer Registrars Association (NCRA)
National Center for Health Statistics (NCHS)
National Library of Medicine (NLM)
National Practitioner Data Bank (NPDB)
North American Association of Central Cancer Registries (NAACCR)
Operation index
Patient-identifiable data
Physician index
Population-based registry

Primary data source
Protocol
Public health
Secondary data source
Stage of the neoplasm
Traumatic injury
Unified Medical Language System (UMLS)
Vital statistics

As a rich source of data about an individual patient, the health record's primary purpose is in patient care and reimbursement for individual encounters. (Chapter 3, *Health Information Functions, Purpose, and Users,* discusses the purpose of the health record in more detail). It is difficult to see trends in a population of patients by looking at individual health records. For this purpose, data must be extracted from individual health records and entered into databases. These data may be used in a facility-specific or population-based registry for research and improvement of patient care (explained later in this chapter). Data may be reported to the state and become part of state- and federal-level databases used to set health policy and improve healthcare. With the electronic health record (EHR), it is possible for data to be collected once in the EHR and used many times (secondary records) for a variety of purposes as outlined in this chapter.

The health information management (HIM) professional can play a variety of roles in managing secondary data and databases. The HIM professional plays a key role in database setup. The HIM professional's role includes determining the content of the database and ensuring compliance with the laws, regulations, and accreditation standards that affect its content and use. All data elements included in the database or registry must be defined in a data dictionary. A data dictionary is a descriptive list of names, definitions, and attributes of data elements to be collected in an information system or database (AHIMA 2014a). For more on the data dictionary, see chapter 6, *Data Management.* The HIM professional serves as a data steward to oversee the completeness and accuracy of the data abstracted for inclusion in the database or registry. "Data stewardship is a responsibility guided by principles and practices to ensure the knowledgeable and appropriate use of data derived from individuals' personal health information" (NCVHS 2009, 1). Data stewardship and the role of the data steward are also discussed in chapter 6.

This chapter explains the difference between primary and secondary data and its users. It offers an in-depth look at the types of secondary databases, including indexes and registries, and their functions. Finally, this chapter discusses how secondary databases are processed and maintained.

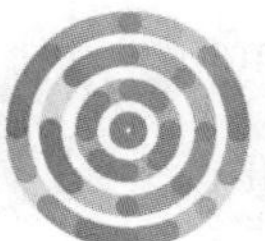

Differences between Primary and Secondary Data Sources

The health record is considered a **primary data source** because it contains information about a patient that has been documented by the professionals who provided care or services to that patient. A primary data source is an original data source where the data are documented or collected by the provider of care. Data derived from the primary health record, such as an index or a database, are considered **secondary data sources**. These data are known as secondary data.

Data are categorized as either patient-identifiable data or aggregate data. With **patient-identifiable data**, the patient is identified within the data either by name, address, date of birth, or social security number or other government issued identification. The health record consists entirely of patient-identifiable data. In other words, every fact in the health record relates to a particular patient identified by name. Secondary data also may be patient identifiable. In some instances, data are entered into a database along with information such as the patient's name maintained in an identifiable form. Registries are an example of patient-identifiable data in a secondary data source.

Data are patient-identifiable if the identity of the patient is linked via address, age, or another identifier. For example, if an individual can be identified by using a combination of elements such as date of birth, zip code, gender, marital status, and phone number, this would be considered patient-identifiable data.

More often, however, secondary data are considered aggregate data. **Aggregate data** include data on groups of people or patients without identifying any patient individually. Examples of aggregate data are statistics on the average length of stay (ALOS) for patients discharged within a particular diagnosis-related group (DRG).

Purposes and Users of Secondary Data Sources

There are four major purposes for collecting secondary data. They are the following:

1. **Quality, performance, and patient safety.** Healthcare organizations, for example, collect core measure information from the health record for the Centers for Medicare and Medicaid Services (CMS) to evaluate the quality of care within the healthcare organization.
2. **Research.** Data taken from health records and entered into databases help researchers determine the effectiveness of alternate treatment methods. An example of this type of secondary data use is a disease database that cross-references an index of human diseases, medications, signs, abnormal findings, and more (Diseases Database 2019). Another example is the secondary data collected from the Patient-Centered Outcomes Research Institute (PCORI) used to help patients, families, and clinicians make better healthcare choices (PCORI 2019).
3. **Population health.** Population health is an "interdisciplinary, customized approach that allows health departments to connect practice to policy for change to happen locally" (CDC 2019a). For example, states require information be reported to them on certain diseases so the extent of the disease can be determined, and steps taken to prevent the spread of that disease.
4. **Administrative.** In credentialing physicians, healthcare organizations are required to access a national database for information on previous malpractice or other adverse decisions against a physician. This information is used to evaluate the qualifications, skills, and performance history of a physician.

In healthcare, the health record is a source for various types of data and serves many purposes. The various users of healthcare data are discussed in the following sections.

Internal Users

Internal users of secondary data are individuals located within the healthcare organization. For example, internal users include medical staff and administrative and management staff. Secondary data enable these users to identify patterns and trends that are helpful to inpatient care, long-range planning, budgeting, and benchmarking with other healthcare organizations.

External Users

External users of patient data are individuals and institutions outside the healthcare organization. Examples of external users are state data banks (discussed later in this chapter) and federal agencies. States have laws mandating that cases of patients with diseases such as tuberculosis, sexually transmitted diseases, and other communicable diseases be reported to the state department. The federal government collects data from the states on vital events such as births and deaths.

The secondary data provided to external users are generally aggregate data, not patient-identifiable data. Thus, these data can be used as needed without risking breaches of confidentiality.

Check Your Understanding 7.1

Answer the following questions.

1. Identify an instance of patient-identifiable data.
   a. The patient was born on March 10 and lives at 123 Main Street
   b. The patient has both cancer and end-stage renal disease and has dialysis three times a week.
   c. There were 50 Medicare patients treated today.
   d. Of all our patients 50 percent have commercial insurance.
2. Identify when an internal user might utilize secondary data.
   a. State infectious disease reporting
   b. Birth certificates
   c. Death certificates
   d. Benchmarking with other healthcare organizations
3. Secondary data are used for multiple reasons including:
   a. Assisting researchers in determining effectiveness of treatments
   b. Assisting nurses in providing patient care
   c. Billing for services provided to the patient
   d. Coding diagnoses and procedures treated
4. True or false: A patient health record is a secondary data source.
5. True or false: A patient health record contains aggregate data.
6. True or false: HIM supervisors and managers are internal users of secondary data.
7. True or false: Secondary data may be used to improve the health of an entire human population.

Types of Secondary Data Sources

Secondary data sources consist of facility-specific indexes; registries, either facility or population based; or other healthcare databases.

Facility-Specific Indexes

The most long-standing secondary data sources are those developed within healthcare organizations to meet their individual needs. These indexes enable health records to be located by diagnosis, procedure, or physician. Prior to extensive computerization in healthcare, these indexes were kept on cards. Today, most indexes are maintained as computerized reports based on data from databases routinely developed in the healthcare organization.

Disease and Operation Indexes

The disease index is a listing in diagnosis code number order of patients discharged from the healthcare organization during a specific time period. Each patient's diagnoses are converted from a verbal description to a numerical code, usually using the *International Classification of Diseases, Tenth Revision, Clinical Modification* (ICD-10-CM). The patient's diagnosis codes are entered into the healthcare organization's health information system as part of the discharge processing of the patient's health record. The index always includes the patient's health record number as well as the diagnosis codes so health records can be retrieved by diagnosis. Because each patient is listed with the health record number, which may be linked to the patient's name and other information, the disease index is considered patient-identifiable data. The disease index also may include information such as the date of discharge and the attending physician's name.

The operation index is similar to the disease index except that it is arranged in numerical order by the patient's procedure code(s) using *International Classification of Diseases, Tenth Revision, Procedure Coding System* (ICD-10-PCS) or Current Procedural Terminology (CPT) codes. For specifics on ICD-10-PCS and CPT, refer to chapter 15, *Revenue Management and Reimbursement*. The other information listed in the operation index is generally the same as that listed in the disease index except that the surgeon may be listed in addition to, or instead of, the attending physician. For additional information on coding systems, see chapter 5, *Clinical Terminologies, Classifications, and Code Systems.*

Physician Index

The physician index is a listing of cases organized by physician name or physician identification number. It also includes the patient's health record number and may include other information, such as date of discharge. The physician index enables users to retrieve information about a particular physician, including the number of cases seen during a specific time period.

Registries

Disease registries are collections of secondary data related to patients with a specific diagnosis, condition, or procedure. Examples of disease registries may include, but are not limited to, Alzheimer's Prevention Registry, Colon Cancer Family Registry, National and State Cancer Registries, and Rare Disease Registry. Registries are different from indexes because they contain more extensive data. Index reports are usually produced using data from the healthcare organization's existing databases. Registries often require more extensive entry of data from the health record. Each registry must define the cases that are to be included; this process is called case definition. In a trauma registry, for example, the case definition might be all patients admitted with a diagnosis that includes the ICD-10-CM trauma diagnosis codes.

After the cases to be included have been determined, the next step is usually case finding. Case finding is a method used to identify the patients who have been seen or treated in the healthcare organization for the specific disease or condition of interest to the registry. After cases have been identified, extensive information is abstracted from the patients' health records into the registry database or extracted from other databases and automatically entered into the registry database.

The sole purpose of some registries is to collect data from health records and make them available for users. Other registries take further steps to enter additional information in the registry database, such as routine follow-up of patients at specified intervals. Follow-up information might include rate and duration of survival and quality of life over time. General terminology associated with registries is defined in figure 7.1 and a list of major registries is displayed in table 7.1.

Figure 7.1 Terminology associated with registries

Accession number: A number assigned to each case as it is entered in a cancer registry
Accession registry: A list of cases in a cancer registry in the order in which they were entered
Demographic information: Information used to identify an individual, such as name, address, gender, age, and other information linked to a specific person
Facility-based registry: A registry that includes only cases from a particular type of healthcare facility, such as a hospital or clinic
Incident: An occurrence in a medical facility that is inconsistent with accepted standards of care
Population-based registry: A type of registry that includes information from more than one facility in a specific geopolitical area, such as a state or region

Source: ©AHIMA.

Table 7.1 Major registries

Registry	Definition
Cancer registry	Tracks the incidence (new cases) of cancer
Trauma registry	Tracks patients with traumatic injuries from the initial trauma treatment to death
Birth defects registry	Collects information on newborns with birth defects
Diabetes registry	Collects cases of patients with diabetes to assist in managing care as well as for research
Implant registry	Tracks the performance of implants including complications, deaths, and defects resulting from implants, as well as implant longevity
Transplant registry	Maintains databases of cases of patients who need organ transplants
Immunization registry	Collects information within a particular geographic area on children and their immunization status and maintains a central source of information for a particular child's immunization history, even when the child has received immunizations from a variety of providers

Source: ©AHIMA.

Cancer Registries

According to the National Cancer Registrars Association (NCRA), the first hospital cancer registry was founded in 1926 at Yale–New Haven Hospital (NCRA 2018a). It has long been recognized that information is needed to improve the diagnosis and treatment of cancer. Cancer registries were developed as an organized method to collect these data. The data may be facility based (for example, within a hospital or clinic) or population based (for example, from more than one healthcare organization within a state or region).

Facility-based registries include cases from a particular type of healthcare organization such as a hospital or clinic. The data from facility-based registries are used to provide information for the improved understanding of cancer, including its causes and methods of diagnosis and treatment. The data collected also may provide comparisons in survival rates and quality of life for patients with different treatments and at different stages of cancer at the time of diagnosis. Population-based registries include information from more than one healthcare organization in a specific geographical area such as a state or region. In population-based registries, the emphasis is on identifying trends and changes in the incidence (new cases) of cancer within the area covered by the registry.

The Cancer Registries Amendment Act of 1992 provided funding for a national program of cancer registries with population-based registries in each state. According to the law, these registries were mandated to collect data such as the following:

- Demographic data about each case of cancer; demographic data describing the individual, including the patient's name, age, gender, race, ethnicity, and birthplace
- Information on the industrial or occupational history of the individuals with the cancers (to the extent such information is available from the same health record)
- Administrative information, including date of diagnosis and source of information
- Pathological data characterizing the cancer, including site, stage of the neoplasm (specifies the amount of metastasis, if any), incidence, and type of treatment (Public Law 102-515 1992)

Case Definition and Case Finding in Cancer Registries As defined previously, case definition is the process of deciding which cases should be entered in the registry. For example, in a cancer registry all cancer cases except skin cancer might meet the definition for the cases to be included. Information on malignant neoplasms, data on benign and borderline brain or central nervous system tumors must be collected by the National Program of Cancer Registries (CDC 2018a).

In the facility-based cancer registry, the first step is case finding. One way to find cases is through the discharge process in the HIM department. During the discharge procedure, coders or discharge analysts can easily earmark cases of patients with cancer for inclusion in the registry. Another case-finding method is using the facility-specific disease indexes to identify patients with diagnoses of cancer. Additional methods may include reviews of pathology reports and lists of patients receiving radiation therapy or other cancer treatments to determine cases that have not been found by other methods.

Population-based registries usually depend on hospitals, physician offices, radiation facilities, ambulatory surgery centers (ASCs), and pathology laboratories to identify and report cases to the central registry. The administrators of a population-based registry have a responsibility to ensure all cases of cancer have been identified and reported to the central registry.

Data Collection for Cancer Registries Data collection methods vary between facility-based and population-based registries. When a case is first entered in the registry, it is assigned an accession number, a number unique to the patient. This number consists of the first digits of the year the patient was first seen at the healthcare organization, and the remaining digits are assigned sequentially throughout the year. For example, the first case in the year might be 21-0001. The 21 indicates that the person was seen in the year 2021. An accession registry is a list of cases in a cancer registry in the order in which they were entered. An accession registry of all cases can be kept manually or provided as a report by the database software. This listing of patients in accession number order provides a way to ensure all the cases have been entered into the registry.

In a facility-based registry, data are initially reviewed and collected from the patient's health record. In addition to demographic information, data in the registry about the patient include the following:

- Type and site of the cancer
- Diagnostic methodologies
- Treatment methodologies
- Stage at the time of diagnosis

The stage provides information on the size and extent of spread of the tumor throughout the body. There are currently several staging systems. The American Joint Committee on Cancer (AJCC) has worked through its Collaborative Stage Task Force with other organizations with staging systems to develop a new standardized staging system—the Collaborative Stage Data Set. This staging system uses computer algorithms to describe how far a cancer has spread (Collaborative Stage Data Collection System 2019). After the initial information is collected at the patient's first encounter, data in the registry are updated periodically through the follow-up process, which is discussed in the section that follows.

Frequently, the population-based registry only collects information when the patient is diagnosed. Sometimes, however, it receives follow-up information from its local, state, or national entities. These entities usually submit information to the central registry electronically.

Reporting and Follow-up for Cancer Registries Formal reporting of cancer registry data is done annually. The annual report includes aggregate data on the number of cases in the past year by site and type of cancer. It also may include information on patients by gender, age, and ethnic group. Often a particular site or type of cancer is featured with more in-depth data provided.

Other reports are provided as needed. Data from the cancer registry are frequently used in the quality assessment process for a healthcare organization as well as in research. Data on survival rates by site of cancer and methods of treatment, for instance, would be helpful in researching the most effective treatment for a type of cancer.

Another activity of the cancer registry is patient follow-up. On an annual basis, the registry attempts to obtain information about each patient in the registry, including whether they are still alive, status of the cancer, and treatment received during the period. Various methods are used to obtain this information. For a facility-based registry, the healthcare organization's patient health records may be checked for return hospitalizations or visits for treatment. Additionally, the patient's physician may be contacted to determine whether the patient is still living and to obtain information about the cancer.

When patient status cannot be determined through these methods, an attempt may be made to contact the patient directly using information in the registry such as the patient's address and telephone number. In addition, contact information from the patient's health record may be used to request information from the patient's relatives. Other methods used include reading newspaper obituaries for deaths and using the Internet to locate patients through sites such as the Social Security Death Index. The information obtained through follow-up is important and allows the registry to develop statistics on survival rates for specific cancers and different treatment methodologies.

Population-based registries do not always include follow-up information on the patients in their databases. However, those who follow up usually receive the information from the reporting entities such as hospitals, physician offices, and other healthcare organizations providing follow-up care.

Standards and Approval Processes for Cancer Registries Several organizations have developed standards or approval processes for cancer programs. The American College of Surgeons (ACS) Commission on Cancer has an approval process for cancer programs. One of the requirements of this process is the existence of a cancer registry as part of the program. The ACS standards are published in the Cancer Program Standards (ACS 2019a). When the ACS surveys the cancer program, part of the survey process is a review of cancer registry activities.

The North American Association of Central Cancer Registries (NAACCR) has a certification program for state population-based registries. Certification is based on the quality of data collected and reported by the state registry. NAACCR has developed standards for data quality and format and works with other cancer organizations to align their various standards sets.

The Centers for Disease Control and Prevention (CDC) also has national standards regarding the completeness, timeliness, and quality of cancer registry data from state registries through the National Program of Cancer Registries (NPCR). The NPCR was developed as a result of the Cancer Registries Amendment Act of 1992. The CDC collects data from the NPCR state registries.

Education and Certification for Cancer Registrars
Traditionally, cancer registrars have been trained through on-the-job training and professional workshops and seminars. The National Cancer Registrars Association (NCRA) has worked with colleges to develop formal educational programs for cancer registrars. A cancer registrar may become credentialed as a certified tumor registrar (CTR) by passing an examination provided by the National Board for Certification of Registrars (NBCR). Eligibility requirements for the certification examination include a combination of experience and education (NCRA 2018b).

Trauma Registries

Trauma registries maintain databases on patients with severe traumatic injuries. A traumatic injury is a wound or other injury caused by an external physical force such as a motor vehicle crash, a gunshot wound, a stabbing, or a fall. Information in the trauma registry may be used for performance improvement and research in the area of trauma care. Trauma registries may be facility based or may include data for a region or state.

Case Definition and Case Finding for Trauma Registries The case definition for the trauma registry varies but frequently involves inclusion of cases with diagnoses from the trauma diagnosis codes in the ICD-10-CM. To find cases with trauma diagnoses, the trauma registrar can access the disease indexes looking for cases with codes from this section of ICD-10-CM. In addition, the registrar may look at deaths in services with frequent trauma diagnoses—such as trauma, neurosurgery, orthopedics, and plastic surgery—to find additional cases.

Data Collection for Trauma Registries After the cases have been identified, information is abstracted from the health records of the injured patients and entered into the trauma registry database. The data elements collected in the abstracting process vary from registry to registry. Abstracting can be either the process of extracting information from a document to create a brief summary of a patient's illness, treatment, and outcome, or extracting elements of data from a source document or database and entering them into an automated system. Data elements in the abstracting process include the following:

- Demographic information on the patient
- Information on the injury
- Care the patient received before hospitalization (such as care at another transferring hospital or care from an emergency medical technician who provided care at the scene of the crash or in transport from the crash site to the hospital)
- Status of the patient at the time of admission
- Patient's course in the hospital
- Diagnosis and procedure codes
- Abbreviated Injury Scale
- Injury Severity Score

The Abbreviated Injury Scale (AIS) reflects the nature of the injury and its threat to life by each body system. It may be assigned manually by the registrar or generated as part of the database from data entered by the registrar. The Injury Severity Score (ISS) is an overall severity measurement calculated from the AIS scores for patients with multiple injuries (Agency for Clinical Innovation 2019).

Reporting and Follow-up for Trauma Registries Reporting varies among trauma registries. An annual report is often developed to show the activity of the trauma registry. Other reports may be generated as part of the performance improvement process, such as self-extubation (patients removing their own tubes) and delays in abdominal surgery or patient complications. Some hospitals report data to the National Trauma Data Bank (ACS 2019b).

Trauma registries may or may not follow up on the patients entered in the registry. When a follow-up is done, the emphasis is frequently on the patient's quality of life after a period of time. Unlike cancer, where physician follow-up is crucial to detect recurrence, many traumatic injuries do not require continued patient care over time. Thus, follow-up is often not given the emphasis it receives in cancer registries.

Standards and Approval Process for Trauma Registries The ACS certifies levels I, II, III, IV, and V trauma centers. As part of its requirements, the ACS states that the level I trauma center must have a trauma registry (ACS 2019c). As part of its certification requirements, the ACS states that the level I trauma center, the type of center receiving the most serious cases and providing the highest level of trauma service, must have a trauma registry (ACS 2019c). See table 7.2 for a description of each trauma center level.

Education and Certification of Trauma Registrars Trauma registrars may be registered health information technicians (RHITs), registered health

Table 7.2 Trauma center levels and definitions

Trauma center level	Description
Level I	Able to provide total care for every aspect of injury from prevention through rehabilitation
Level II	Able to initiate definitive care for all injured patients
Level III	Able to provide prompt assessment, resuscitation, surgery intensive care and stabilization of injured patients, and emergency operations
Level IV	Able to provide advanced trauma life support (ATLS) prior to transfer of patients to a higher-level trauma center; provides evaluation, stabilization, and diagnostic capabilities for injured patients
Level V	Able to provide initial evaluation, stabilization, and diagnostic capabilities, and prepares patients for transfer to higher levels of care

Source: ATS 2018.

information administrators (RHIAs), registered nurses (RNs), licensed practical nurses (LPNs), emergency medical technicians (EMTs), or other health professionals. Training for trauma registrars is through workshops and on-the-job training. The American Trauma Society (ATS) provides core and advanced workshops for trauma registrars and a certification examination for trauma registrars who meet its education and experience requirements through its Registrar Certification Board. Certified trauma registrars have earned the certified specialist in trauma registry (CSTR) credential.

Birth Defects Registries

Birth defects registries collect information on newborns with birth defects. Often population based, these registries serve a variety of purposes. For example, birth defects registries provide information on the incidence of birth defects to study causes and prevention; monitor trends in birth defects; improve medical care for children with birth defects; and target interventions for preventable birth defects.

Case Definition and Case Finding for Birth Defects Registries Birth defects registries use a variety of criteria to determine which cases to include in the registry. Some registries limit cases to those with defects found within the first year of life. Others include those children with a major defect that occurred in the first year of life and was discovered within the first five years of life. Still other registries include only children who were live born or stillborn babies with obvious birth defects.

Cases may be detected in a variety of ways, including review of disease indexes, labor and delivery logs, pathology and autopsy reports, ultrasound reports, and cytogenetic reports. In addition to information from hospitals and physicians, cases may be identified from rehabilitation centers and children's hospitals and from vital records such as birth, death, and fetal death certificates.

Data Collection for Birth Defects Registries A variety of information is abstracted for the birth defects registry, including the following:

- Demographic information
- Codes for diagnoses
- Birth weight
- Status at birth, including live born, stillborn, aborted
- Autopsy
- Cytogenetics results
- Whether the infant was a single birth or one in a multiple birth
- Mother's use of alcohol, tobacco, or illicit drugs
- Father's use of drugs and alcohol
- Family history of birth defects

Diabetes Registries

Diabetes registries include cases of patients with diabetes for the purpose of assistance in managing care as well as for research. Patients whose diabetes is not kept under control frequently have numerous complications. The diabetes registry can keep up with whether the patient has been seen by a physician to prevent complications.

Case Definition and Case Finding for Diabetes Registries There are two types of diabetes mellitus: type 1 and type 2 diabetes. Registries sometimes limit their cases by type of diabetes. In some instances, there may be further definition by age. Some diabetes registries, for example, only include children with diabetes.

Case finding includes the review of health records of patients with diabetes. Other case-finding methods include review of the following:

- Diagnostic codes
- Billing data
- Medication lists
- Physician identification
- Health plans

Although facility-based registries for cancer and trauma are usually hospital based, facility-based diabetes registries are often found in physician offices or clinics. The office or clinic is the main location for diabetes care. Thus, data about the patient to be entered into the registry are available at these sites rather than at the hospital. The health records of diabetes patients treated in physician practices may be identified through diagnosis code numbers for diabetes, billing data for diabetes-related services, medication lists for patients on diabetic medications, or identification of patients as the physician treats them.

Health plans are interested in optimal care for their enrollees because diabetes can have serious complications when not managed correctly. The plans can provide information to the office or clinic on enrollees who are diabetics.

Data Collection for Diabetes Registries In addition to demographic information about the cases, other data collected may include laboratory values such as glycated hemoglobin, also known as HbA1c. This test is used to determine the patient's blood glucose for a period of approximately 60 days prior to the time of the test. Moreover, facility registries may track patient visits to follow up with patients who have not been seen in the past year.

Reporting and Follow-up for Diabetes Registries A variety of reports can be developed from the diabetes registry. For facility-based registries, one report might keep up with laboratory monitoring of the patient's diabetes to allow intensive intervention with patients whose diabetes is not well controlled. Another report might concern patients who have not been tested within a year or have not had a primary care provider visit within a year.

Population-based diabetes registries might provide reporting on the incidence of diabetes for the geographic area covered by the registry. Registry data also might be used to investigate risk factors for diabetes.

Follow-up is aimed primarily at ensuring that the patient with diabetes is seen by the physician at appropriate intervals to prevent complications.

Implant Registries

An implant is a material or substance inserted into the body, such as breast implants, heart valves, and pacemakers. Implant registries have been developed for the purpose of tracking the performance of implants including complications, deaths, and defects resulting from implants, as well as implant longevity. In the recent past, the safety of implants has been questioned. For example, there have been questions about the safety of silicone breast implants and temporomandibular joint implants. When such cases arise, it has often been difficult to ensure all the patients with the implants have been notified of safety concerns. A number of federal laws have been enacted to regulate medical devices, including implants. These devices were first covered under Section 15 of the Food, Drug, and Cosmetic Act. The Safe Medical Devices Act of 1990 was passed (GPO 1990). It was amended through the Medical Device Amendments of 1992 (GPO 1992). These acts required a sample of healthcare organizations to report deaths and severe complications thought to be due to a device to the manufacturer and the Food and Drug Administration (FDA) through its MedWatch reporting system. The MedWatch reporting system alerts health professionals and the public of safety alerts and medical device recalls (FDA 2018). Implant registries may help ensure compliance with legal reporting requirements for device-related deaths and complications.

Case Definition and Case Finding for Implant Registries Implant registries sometimes include all types of implants but often are restricted to a specific type of implant. Examples of specific types of implants may be cochlear, silicone, or temporomandibular joint.

Data Collection for Implant Registries Demographic data on patients receiving implants are included in the registry. The FDA requires that all reportable events involving medical devices include the following information: "User facility report number; name and address of the device manufacturer; device brand name and common name; product model, catalog, serial, and lot numbers; brief description of the event reported to the manufacturer or the FDA; where the report was submitted (for example, to the FDA, manufacturer, or distributor)" (FDA 2018).

Thus, these data items should be included in the implant registry to facilitate reporting.

Transplant Registries

Transplant registries may have varied purposes. Some organ transplant registries maintain databases of patients who need organs. When an organ becomes available, allocation of the organ to the patient is based on a prioritization method. In other cases, the purpose of the registry is to provide a database of potential donors for transplants using live donors, such as bone marrow transplants. Post-transplant information also is kept on organ recipients and donors.

Because transplant registries are used to try to match donor organs with recipients, they are often national or even international in scope. Examples of national registries include the UNet of the United Network for Organ Sharing (UNOS) and the registry of the National Marrow Donor Program (NMDP).

Data collected in the transplant registry may be used for research, policy analysis, and quality control.

Case Definition and Case Finding for Transplant Registries A physician will identify patients needing transplants. Information about the patient is provided to the registry. When an organ becomes available, the patient's information is matched with potential donors. For donor registries, donors are solicited through community information efforts similar to those carried out by blood banks to encourage blood donations.

Data Collection for Transplant Registries The type of information collected varies according to the type of registry. Pre-transplant data about the recipient include the following:

- Demographic data
- Patient's diagnosis
- Patient's status codes regarding medical urgency
- Patient's functional status
- Whether the patient is on life support
- Previous transplantations
- Histocompatibility (compatibility of donor and recipient tissues)

Information on donors varies according to whether the donor is living. For organs harvested from patients who have died, the following information is collected:

- Cause and circumstances of the death
- Organ procurement and consent process
- Medications the donor was taking
- Other donor history

For a living donor, information includes the following:

- Relationship of the donor to the recipient (if any)
- Clinical information
- Information on organ recovery
- Histocompatibility

Reporting and Follow-up for Transplant Registries Reporting includes information on donors and recipients as well as survival rates, length of time on the waiting list for an organ, and death rates.

Follow-up information is collected for recipients as well as living donors. For living donors, the information collected might include complications of the procedure and length of stay in the hospital. Follow-up on recipients includes information on status at the time of follow-up (for example, living, expired, lost to follow-up), functional status, graft status, and treatment, such as immunosuppressive drugs. Follow-up is carried out at intervals throughout the first year after the transplant and then annually after that.

Immunization Registries

There is a scheduled list of immunizations children are supposed to receive during the first six years of life. These immunizations are so important that the federal government has set several objectives related to immunizations in Healthy People 2020, a set of health goals for the nation. These include increasing the proportion of children and adolescents that are fully immunized and increasing the proportion of children in population-based immunization registries (HHS 2019).

Immunization registries usually have the purpose of increasing the number of infants and children who receive the required immunizations at the proper intervals. To accomplish this goal, registries collect information within a specific geographic area on children and their immunization status. They help by maintaining a central source of information for a child's immunization history, even when the child has received immunizations from a variety of providers. This central location for immunization data relieves parents of the responsibility of maintaining immunization records for their children. This helps to ensure there is immunization data on children.

Case Definition and Case Finding for Immunization Registries All children in the population area served by the registry should be included in the registry. Some registries limit their inclusion of patients to only those seen at public clinics. Although children are usually targeted in immunization registries, some registries include information on adults for influenza and pneumonia vaccines.

Children are often entered in the registry at birth. Registry personnel may review birth and death certificates and adoption records to determine which children to include and which children to exclude because they died after birth. In some cases, children are entered electronically through a connection with an electronic birth record system.

Data Collection for Immunization Registries The National Immunization Program at the CDC has worked with the National Vaccine Advisory Committee (NVAC) to develop a core set of immunization data elements to be included in all immunization registries. These data elements include the following:

- Patient name (first, middle, and last)
- Patient birth date
- Patient gender
- Patient race
- Patient ethnicity
- Patient birth order
- Patient birth state and country
- Mother's name (first, middle, last, and maiden)
- Vaccine product
- Vaccine manufacturer
- Vaccination expiration date
- Vaccine lot number (CDC 2018b)

Other elements may be included as needed by the individual registry.

Reporting and Follow-up for Immunization Registries Because the purpose of the immunization registry is to increase the number of children who receive immunizations in a timely manner, reporting should emphasize immunization rates. Immunization registries also can provide automatic reporting of children's immunization to schools to check the immunization status of their students.

Follow-ups are done to remind parents when it is time for immunizations as well as to identify parents who fail to bring the child in for the immunization after a reminder. Reminders may include a letter, email, automatic reminder generated from the EHR, or a telephone call. Autodialing systems may be used to call parents and deliver a prerecorded reminder. Moreover, registries must decide how frequently to follow up with parents who do not bring their children in for immunization. Maintaining up-to-date addresses and telephone numbers is important for providing follow-up. In some states, registries may allow parents to opt out of the registry if they prefer not to be reminded.

Standards and Approval Processes for Immunization Registries The CDC provides funding for some population-based immunization registries. In recognition of the growing importance of an Immunization Information System (IIS) to the broader health information technology landscape, the 2001 IIS Minimum Functional Standards have been revised. The new standards are an attempt to lay the framework for the development of IIS through 2018 (CDC 2018c). The new program goals and standards include objectives from Healthy People 2020 and are listed in figure 7.2.

Figure 7.2 Functional Standards 2013 to 2018 for Healthy People 2020

1. Support the delivery of clinical immunization services at the point of immunization administration, regardless of setting.

1.1 The IIS provides individual immunization records accessible to authorized users at the point and time where immunization services are being delivered.
1.2 The IIS has an automated function that determines vaccines due, past due, or coming due ("vaccine forecast") in a manner consistent with current ACIP recommendations. Any deficiency is visible to the clinical user each time an individual's record is viewed.
1.3 The IIS automatically identifies individuals due or past due for immunization(s), to enable the production of reminder and recall notifications from within the IIS itself or from interoperable systems.
1.4 When the IIS receives queries from other health information systems, it can generate an automatic response in accordance with interoperability standards endorsed by CDC for message content and format and transport.
1.5 The IIS can receive submissions in accordance with interoperability standards endorsed by CDC for message content and format and transport.

2. Support the activities and requirements for publicly purchased vaccine, including the Vaccines For Children (VFC) and state purchase programs.

2.1 The IIS has a vaccine inventory function that tracks and decrements inventory at the provider site level according to VFC program requirements.
2.2 The IIS vaccine inventory function is available to direct data entry users and can interoperate with EHR or other inventory systems.
2.3 The IIS vaccine inventory function automatically decrements as vaccine doses are recorded.
2.4 Eligibility is tracked at the dose level for all doses administered.
2.5 The IIS interfaces with the national vaccine ordering, inventory, and distribution system (currently VTrckS).
2.6 The IIS can provide data and produce management reports for VFC and other public vaccine programs.

3. Maintain data quality (accurate, complete, timely data) on all immunization and demographic information in the IIS.

3.1 The IIS provides consolidated demographic and immunization records for persons of all ages in its geopolitical area, except where prohibited by law, regulation, or policy.
3.2 The IIS can regularly evaluate incoming and existing patient records to identify, prevent, and resolve duplicate and fragmented records.
3.3 The IIS can regularly evaluate incoming and existing immunization information to identify, prevent, and resolve duplicate vaccination events.
3.4 The IIS can store all IIS Core Data Elements.
3.5 The IIS can establish a record in a timely manner from sources such as Vital Records for each newborn child born and residing at the date of birth in its geopolitical area.
3.6 The IIS records and makes available all submitted vaccination and demographic information in a timely manner.
3.7 The IIS documents active or inactive status of individuals at both the provider organization or site and geographic levels.

4. Preserve the integrity, security, availability and privacy of all personally identifiable health and demographic data in the IIS.

4.1 The IIS program has written confidentiality and privacy practices and policies based on applicable law or regulation that protect all individuals whose data are contained in the system.
4.2 The IIS has user access controls and logging, including distinct credentials for each user, least-privilege access, and routine maintenance of access privileges.
4.3 The IIS is operated or hosted on secure hardware and software in accordance with industry standards for protected health information, including standards for security and encryption, uptime, and disaster recovery.

5. Provide immunization information to all authorized stakeholders.

5.1 The IIS can provide immunization data access to healthcare providers, public health, and other authorized stakeholders (for example, schools, public programs, payers) according to law, regulation, or policy.
5.2 The IIS can generate predefined or ad hoc reports (for example, immunization coverage, vaccine usage, and other important indicators by geographic, demographic, provider, or provider groups) for authorized users without assistance from IIS personnel.
5.3 With appropriate levels of authentication, IIS can provide copies of immunization records to individuals or parents and guardians with custodial rights.
5.4 The IIS can produce an immunization record acceptable for official purposes (for example, school, childcare, camp).

6. Promote vaccine safety in public and private provider settings.

6.1 Provide the necessary reports and functionality to facilitate vaccine recalls when necessary, including the identification of recipients by vaccine lot, manufacturer, provider, and time frame.
6.2 Facilitate reporting and/or investigation of adverse events following immunization.

Source: CDC 2018c.

Other Registries

Registries may be developed for any type of disease or condition. Other commonly kept types of registries are cystic fibrosis, cardiac, and registries for chronic disease management and gastroenterology.

A registry can be developed for administrative purposes. The National Provider Identifier (NPI) Registry is an example of an administrative registry. The NPI Registry enables users to search for a provider's national plan and provider enumeration system information, including the national provider identification number. The NPI number is a 10-digit unique identification number assigned to healthcare providers in the US (CMS 2018). There is no charge to use the registry and it is updated daily (National Plan and Provider Enumeration System 2018).

Healthcare Databases

Databases are developed for a variety of purposes. For example, the federal government developed databases to carry out surveillance, improvement, and prevention duties. HIM managers may provide information for these databases through data abstraction or from data reported by a healthcare organization to state and local entities. They also may use these data to perform research or work with other researchers on issues related to reimbursement and health status.

National and State Administrative Databases

Some databases are established for administrative rather than disease-oriented reasons. For example, a database may be developed for claims data submitted on Medicare claims. Other administrative databases assist in the credentialing and privileging of health practitioners. Some of these are discussed next.

Medicare Provider Analysis and Review File The Medicare Provider Analysis and Review (MEDPAR) File is made up of acute-care hospital and skilled nursing facility (SNF) claims data for all Medicare claims. It consists of the following types of data:

- Demographic data on the patient
- Data on the provider
- Information on Medicare coverage for the claim
- Total charges
- Covered charges
- Charges broken down by specific type of service, such as operating room, physical therapy, and pharmacy charges
- ICD diagnosis and procedure codes
- Medicare severity diagnosis-related groups (MS-DRGs)

The MEDPAR file is frequently used for research on topics such as charges for particular types of care and MS-DRGs. The limitation of the MEDPAR data for research purposes is that the file contains only Medicare patients (RPC Health Data Store 2019).

National Practitioner Data Bank The National Practitioner Data Bank (NPDB) was mandated under the Health Care Quality Improvement Act of 1986 to provide a database of medical malpractice payments, adverse licensure actions, and certain professional review actions (such as denial of medical staff privileges) taken by healthcare organizations such as hospitals against physicians, dentists, suppliers, and other healthcare providers (NPDB 2018). The NPDB was developed to alleviate the lack of information about malpractice decisions, denial of medical staff privileges, and loss of medical license. Because these data were not widely available, physicians whose license to practice was revoked in one state or healthcare organization could easily move to another state or healthcare organization and begin practicing again with the current state or healthcare organization being unaware of previous actions against the physician.

Information in the NPDB is provided through a required reporting mechanism. Entities making malpractice payments, including insurance companies, boards of medical examiners, and entities such as hospitals and professional societies, must report to the NPDB. The information reported includes information about the practitioner, the reporting entity, and the judgment or settlement. Information about physicians and other healthcare providers must be provided (NPDB 2018). Entities such as private accrediting organizations and quality improvement organizations are required to report adverse actions to the data bank. In addition, adverse licensure and other actions against any healthcare organization, not just physicians and dentists, must be reported. Adverse actions may include reporting incidents of license suspensions or revocations. An incident is an occurrence in a healthcare organization that is inconsistent with acceptable standards of care. It may also include issues related to professional competence, and malpractice payments. Monetary penalties may be assessed for failure to report.

The law requires healthcare organizations to query the NPDB as part of the credentialing process when a physician initially applies for medical staff privileges and every two years thereafter.

State Administrative Data Banks States frequently have health-related administrative databases. For example, many states collect either Uniform Hospital Discharge Data Set or UB-04/837 institutional data on patients discharged from hospitals located within their area.

National, State, and County Public Health Databases

Public health is the area of healthcare dealing with the health of populations in geographic areas such as states or counties. Publicly reported healthcare data vary from quality and patient safety measurement data to patient satisfaction results. The aggregated data range from a local to national perspective, such as state-specific public health conditions to national morbidity and mortality statistics. In addition, consumers are becoming more actively involved in their healthcare. Publicly reported data may be presented for consumer use through various star ratings on different quality measures via organizations such as The Leapfrog Group, HealthGrades, or Hospital Compare. The Leapfrog Group and Hospital Compare allow users to select various hospitals to compare data such as specific medical conditions, surgical procedures, or overall patient safety ratings. Based on the selections made, data are compared to the hospitals selected as well as to state and national averages.

One of the duties of public health agencies is surveillance of the health status of the population within their jurisdiction. The databases developed by public health departments provide information on the incidence and prevalence of diseases, possible high-risk populations, survival statistics, and trends over time. Data for the databases may be collected using a variety of methods, including interviews, physical examinations of individuals, and reviews of health records. Thus, the HIM manager may have input in these databases through data provided from health records. At the national level, the National Center for Health Statistics (NCHS) has responsibility for these databases. The NCHS provides statistical, accurate, relevant, and timely data that help guide actions and policies to improve the health of the American people. The information or data obtained may be gathered through surveys.

National Health Care Survey One of the major national public health surveys is the National Health Care Survey. To a large extent, it relies on data from patients' health records. It consists of a number of parts, including the following:

- National Hospital Care Survey
- National Hospital Ambulatory Medical Care Surgery
- National Ambulatory Medical Care Survey
- National Survey of Long-Term Care Providers

Data in the National Hospital Care Survey is information on the utilization of healthcare provided in inpatient settings, emergency departments, and outpatient departments. The survey collects data from a nationally representative sample of entities and aims to provide hospital utilization statistics for the nation.

Data for the National Hospital Ambulatory Medical Care Survey are collected on a representative sample of hospital-based and freestanding ambulatory surgery centers. Data include patient demographic characteristics, source of payment, and information on anesthesia given, diagnoses, and surgical and nonsurgical procedures on patient visits.

The National Study of Long-Term Care Providers collects data on the residential care community and adult day services sectors, and administrative data on the home health, nursing home, and hospice sectors.

Because of bioterrorism scares, the CDC developed the National Electronic Disease Surveillance System (NEDSS) that serves as a major part of the Public Health Information Network (PHIN). This system provides a national surveillance system by connecting the CDC with local and state public health partners. It allows the CDC to monitor trends from disease reporting at the local and state levels to look for possible bioterrorism incidents.

Another national public health database is the National Health Interview Survey used to monitor the health status of the civilian, non-institutionalized population of the US. The National Health Interview Survey data are collected through personal household interviews. Interviewers from the U.S. Census Bureau visit American homes to ask about a broad range of health topics. The National Survey of Family Growth collects information on family life, marriage and divorce, pregnancy, infertility, use of contraception, and men's and women's health. Information is collected from personal interviews, from men and women between 15 and 44 years of age.

State and local public health departments develop databases, as needed, to perform their duties of health surveillance, disease prevention, and research. An example of state databases is infectious or notifiable disease databases. Each state has a list of diseases that must be reported to the state—such as measles, and syphilis—so that containment and prevention measures can be taken to avoid large outbreaks of these diseases. As mentioned previously, state and local reporting systems connect with the CDC through NEDSS to evaluate trends in disease outbreaks. There also may be statewide databases or registries that collect extensive information on particular diseases and conditions such as birth defects, immunizations, and cancer.

Vital Statistics Vital statistics include data on births, deaths, fetal deaths, marriages, and divorces. Responsibility for the collection of vital statistics rests with the states. The states share the information with the NCHS. The actual collection of the information is carried out at the local level. For example, birth certificates are completed at the healthcare organization where the birth occurred and then are sent to the state. The state serves as the official repository for the certificate and provides vital statistics information to the NCHS. From the vital statistics collected, states and the national government develop a variety of databases.

One vital statistics database at the national level is the Linked Birth and Infant Death Data Set. In this database, the data from birth certificates are compared to death certificates for infants less than one year of age. This database provides data to conduct analyses for patterns of infant death. Other national programs that use vital statistics data include the National Mortality Followback Survey, the National Maternal and Infant Health Survey, the National Survey of Family Growth, and the National Death Index (CDC 2018d). In some of these databases, such as the National Maternal and Infant Health Survey and the National Mortality Followback Survey, additional information is collected on deaths originally identified through the vital statistics system.

Similar databases based on vital statistics data are found at the state level. Birth defects registries, for example, frequently use vital records data with information on the birth defect as part of their data collection process. For additional information on vital statistics, see chapter 14, *Healthcare Statistics*.

Clinical Trials A clinical trial is a research project in which new treatments and tests are investigated to determine whether they are safe and effective. The trial proceeds according to a protocol, which is the list of rules and procedures to be followed. Clinical trial databases have been developed to allow physicians and patients to find clinical trials. A patient with cancer or AIDS, for example, might be interested in participating in a clinical trial but not know how to locate one applicable to their type of disease. Clinical trial databases provide the data that enable patients and practitioners to determine what clinical trials are available and applicable to the patient.

The Food and Drug Administration Modernization Act of 1997 mandated that a clinical trial database be developed. The National Library of Medicine (NLM) has developed the database, available on the Internet for use by patients and practitioners. The NLM is a biomedical library that maintains and makes available a vast amount of print collections and produces electronic information resources on a wide range of topics (NLM 2019).

Health Services Research Databases Health services research is research concerning healthcare delivery systems, including organization and delivery and care effectiveness and efficiency. Within the federal government, the organization most involved in health services research is the Agency for Healthcare Research and Quality (AHRQ). AHRQ looks at issues related to the efficiency and effectiveness of the healthcare delivery system, disease protocols, and guidelines for improved disease outcomes.

A major initiative for AHRQ has been the Healthcare Cost and Utilization Project (HCUP). HCUP uses data collected at the state level from either claims data or discharge-abstracted data, including the UHDDS items reported by individual hospitals and, in some cases, by freestanding ambulatory care centers. Which data are reported depends on the individual state. Data may be reported by healthcare organizations to a state agency or to the state hospital association, depending on state regulations. The data then are reported from the state to AHRQ, where they become part of the HCUP databases (AHRQ 2018).

HCUP consists of a set of databases, including the following:

- Nationwide inpatient sample (NIS): inpatient database from a sample of hospitals
- State inpatient database (SID): hospital discharge database
- Nationwide emergency department sample (NEDS): database on emergency departments (EDs)
- State emergency department databases (SEDD): database on hospital emergency departments (EDs)
- Kids inpatient database (KID): database of inpatient discharge data on children (AHRQ 2018)

These databases are unique because they include data on inpatients whose care is paid for by all types of payers, including Medicare, Medicaid, private insurance, self-paying, and uninsured patients. Data elements include demographic information, diagnoses and procedures information, admission and discharge status, payment sources, total charges, length of stay, and information on the hospital or freestanding ambulatory surgery center. Researchers may use these databases to look at issues such as those related to the costs of treating particular diseases, the extent to which treatments are used, and differences in outcomes and cost for alternative treatments.

National Library of Medicine The National Library of Medicine (NLM) produces two databases of special interest to the HIM manager—MEDLINE and UMLS.

Medical Literature, Analysis, and Retrieval System Online (MEDLINE) is the best-known database from the NLM. It includes bibliographic listings for publications in the areas of medicine, dentistry, nursing, pharmacy, allied health, and veterinary medicine. HIM managers use MEDLINE to locate articles on HIM issues as well as articles on medical topics necessary to carry out quality improvement and medical research activities.

The Unified Medical Language System (UMLS) provides a way to integrate biomedical concepts from a variety of sources to show their relationships. This process allows links to be made between different information systems for purposes such as the electronic health record. UMLS is of particular interest to the HIM manager because of medical vocabularies such as ICD-10-CM, CPT, and the Healthcare Common Procedure Coding System (HCPCS).

Health Information Exchange Health information exchange (HIE) initiatives were developed to move toward a longitudinal patient record with complete information about the patient available at the point of care. The data are patient-specific rather than aggregate and are used primarily for patient care. Some researchers have looked at the amount of data available through the HIEs as a possible source of data to aggregate for research. Aggregated data can be deidentified to add another layer of protection for the patient's identity. (Chapter 12, *Healthcare Information,* covers HIEs in more detail.)

Data for Performance Measurement The Joint Commission, CMS, and some health plans require healthcare organizations to collect data on core performance measures. Core performance measures are a set of national standardized processes and best practices used to render and improve patient care. These measures are secondary data because they are taken from patients' health records. Whether a healthcare organization reports such measures will be used as a basis for pay-for-performance systems. The goal is to link performance measures to provider payment (for example, helping the healthcare system move away from paying providers based on quantity to a system based on the quality of care rendered). Therefore, it is extremely important that the data accurately reflect the quality of care provided by the healthcare organization (see chapter 3, *Health Information Functions, Purpose, and Users*, for more information).

HIM Roles

Health information management professionals are often involved in various roles using secondary data. These roles may include gathering information from secondary data sources, analyzing data from the data source, or assisting in maintaining the privacy and security of data sources. Healthcare job titles for individuals working with registries may vary from entity to entity. Most of the registry titles include, but are not limited to, cancer registry specialist, certified tumor registrar, HIM technician birth registry, registry coordinator, manager registry services, or trauma registry coordinator or data analyst. Likewise, many HIM professionals may work with healthcare databases. Those job titles may include, but are not limited to, database manager, database specialist, database administrator, data abstractor, or HIM administrative assistant. As the healthcare environment continues to rely on accurate and reliable information, HIM professionals may find themselves working in the world of healthcare secondary data in new and emerging ways.

Check Your Understanding 7.2

Answer the following questions.

1. Which of the following indexes would be used if a physician wanted to conduct a study on patients who have had a C-section?
   a. Physician index
   b. Master patient index
   c. Operation index
   d. Disease index

2. The healthcare organization would like to get approval for their cancer program. They should contact the:
   a. American College of Surgeon's Commission on Cancer
   b. Centers for Disease Control and Prevention
   c. North American Association of Central Cancer Registries
   d. National Committee on Vital Health Statistics

3. After several visits to the hospital, a 75-year-old female has just been diagnosed with cancer. What is the first thing you would do to get this patient entered in the cancer registry?
   a. Assign a patient number
   b. Assign an accession number
   c. Assign a financial record number
   d. Assign a health number

4. Patient data such as name, age, and address are known as:
   a. Primary data
   b. Secondary data
   c. Aggregate data
   d. Identification data

5. What type of registry maintains a database on patients injured by external forces in events out of their control?
   a. Implant registry
   b. Birth defects registry
   c. Trauma registry
   d. Transplant registry

6. Why is the MEDPAR File limited in terms of being used for research purposes?
   a. It only provides demographic data about patients.
   b. It only contains Medicare patients.
   c. It uses ICD-10-CM diagnoses and procedure codes.
   d. It breaks charges down by specific type of service.

7. Which of the following acts mandated establishment of the National Practitioner Data Bank?
   a. Health Care Quality Improvement Act of 1986
   b. Health Insurance Portability and Accountability Act of 1996
   c. Safe Medical Devices Act of 1990
   d. Food and Drug Administration Modernization Act of 1997

8. I started work today on a clinical trial and need to familiarize myself with the rules and procedures to be followed. This information is called the:
   a. Protocol
   b. MEDPAR
   c. UMLS
   d. HCUP

9. An advantage of HCUP is that it:
   a. Contains only Medicare data
   b. Helps determine pay for performance
   c. Contains data on all payer types
   d. Contains bibliographic listings from medical journals

Real-World Case 7.1

Remember, databases are used for a variety of reasons and contain large amounts of secondary data. One significant issue that healthcare professionals face is ensuring the data are kept safe and secure. The digitization of healthcare data has created many benefits, but it has also created challenges. A research report from IntSights, "Chronic (Cyber) Pain: Exposed and Misconfigured Databases in the Healthcare Industry," reveals how hackers are obtaining personally identified information from exposed databases. It is not only old or outdated databases that get breached, some newly established platforms are vulnerable due to misconfiguration or open access. The researchers found that hackers were able to access sensitive data in databases through such simple methods as Google searches (Landi 2018).

Most cybercriminals usually attack for money, but since hospitals don't hold currency, these attackers target the industry for one of three reasons:

1. State-sponsored APTs Targeting Critical Infrastructure: An attempt to infiltrate a network to test tools and techniques to set the stage for larger, future hacks, or to obtain information on a specific individual's medical condition.
2. Attackers Seeking Personal Data: Attackers seek personal data to use in multiple ways such as sell electronic protected health information, blackmail individuals, or use it as a basis for future fraud like phishing or scam calls.
3. Attackers Taking Control of Medical Devices for Ransom: Attackers target medial IT equipment to spread malware that exploits specific vulnerabilities and demands a ransom to release the infected devices (Ainhoren 2018).

Many healthcare organizations are working diligently to protect themselves from cyber-attacks and threats. It is important to constantly evaluate for gaps in the IT infrastructure and implement strategies such as assessing what needs to be secured, mastering identity and mobile device management, testing and re-testing tools, detecting and continuously monitoring threats, and training employees (Davis 2017).

While secondary data such as databases makes it a powerful tool for data collection, it is important for healthcare professionals to be aware of the threats and challenges presented which include privacy, security, data quality, and more.

Real-World Case 7.2

As mentioned before, many databases are maintained at the state and national level for public use. The National Youth Tobacco Survey (NYTS) serves this purpose and others. The NYTS is used to help provide researchers with information to explore in detail. It also is used as part of a public initiative (Healthy People 2020) for surveillance of trends of adolescent tobacco use (CDC 2019b). Evidence of current topics of secondary data (in other words, databases) is all around us.

A recent report from CDC's 2018 NYTS indicates that the use of electronic cigarettes (e-cigarettes) is on the rise. The use of e-cigarettes spiked almost 80 percent among high school students and 50 percent among middle school students in the past year. The recent increase is largely due to the popularity of one e-cigarette brand, which looks like a USB flash drive (Boyles 2018).

Vaping, the act of inhaling the vapors of e-cigarettes, by US teenagers has reached epidemic levels, threatening to hook a new generation of young people on nicotine. "We have never seen use of any substance by America's young people rise this rapidly," HHS Secretary Alex Azar explains. Vaping is ingrained in the high school culture with kids using e-cigarettes in school bathrooms and even during class. Kids don't realize many e-cigarettes contain nicotine. Among younger students, candy-flavored e-cigarettes are the most popular, while fruit-flavored products are popular with older students (Finnegan 2018).

Numerous efforts are underway to prevent and reduce tobacco use among young people. The NYTS was designed to provide national data on long-term, intermediate, and short-term indicators to serve as a baseline for data comparison toward meeting the Healthy People 2020 goal of reducing tobacco use among youth (CDC 2018d).

References

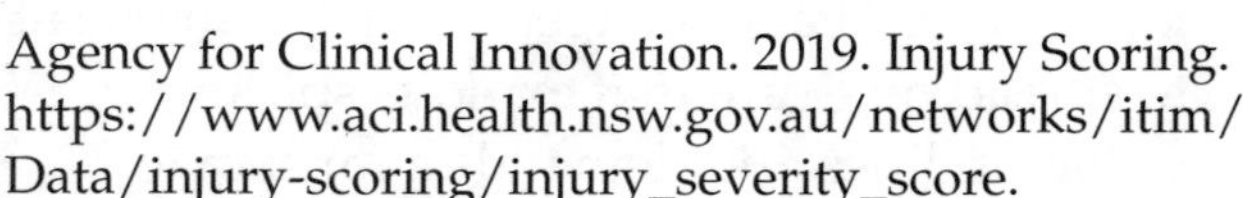

Agency for Clinical Innovation. 2019. Injury Scoring. https://www.aci.health.nsw.gov.au/networks/itim/Data/injury-scoring/injury_severity_score.

Agency for Healthcare Research and Quality. 2018. Healthcare Cost and Utilization Project (HCUP). http://www.ahrq.gov/research/data/hcup/index.html.

Ainhoren, A. 2018. Exposed and Misconfigured Databases in the Healthcare Industry. https://intsights.com/resources/chronic-cyber-pain-exposed-misconfigured-databases-in-the-healthcare-industry.

American College of Surgeons. 2019a. Commission on Cancer. https://www.facs.org/quality-programs/cancer.

American College of Surgeons. 2019b. National Trauma Data Bank. https://www.facs.org/quality-programs/trauma/tqp/center-programs/ntdb.

American College of Surgeons. 2019c. The Committee on Trauma. https://www.facs.org/quality-programs/trauma/tqp/center-programs/vrc.

American Health Information Management Association. 2014a. Health Data Analysis Toolkit. http://http://library.ahima.org/Toolkit/DataAnalysis#.XjGlXGhKg2w.

American Health Information Management Association. 2017. *Pocket Glossary of Health Information Management and Technology*, 5th ed. Chicago: AHIMA.

American Health Information Management Association. 2008. Statement on Data Stewardship. http://library.ahima.org/doc?oid=100307#.Vw_QDPkrLDc.

American Trauma Society. 2018. Trauma Center Levels Explained. https://www.amtrauma.org/page/TraumaLevels.

Boyles, S. 2018. CDC: 3.6 Million Teens Using E-Cigarettes in 2018. https://www.medpagetoday.com/pulmonology/smoking/76396.

Centers for Disease Control. 2019a. Population Health Training in Place Program. https://www.cdc.gov/pophealthtraining/whatis.html.

Centers for Disease Control. 2019b. National Youth Tobacco Survey (NYTS). https://www.cdc.gov/tobacco/data_statistics/surveys/nyts/index.htm.

Centers for Disease Control. 2018a. National Program of Cancer Registries. https://www.cdc.gov/cancer/npcr/index.htm.

Centers for Disease Control. 2018b. Core Data Elements for IIS Functional Standards v4.0. https://www.cdc.gov/vaccines/programs/iis/core-data-elements/iis-func-stds.html.

Centers for Disease Control. 2018c. Immunization Information System Functional Standards. http://www.cdc.gov/vaccines/programs/iis/func-stds.html.

Centers for Disease Control. 2018d. National Notifiable Disease Surveillance System. https://wwwn.cdc.gov/nndss.

Centers for Medicare and Medicaid Services. 2018. National Provider Identifier Standard (NPI). https://www.cms.gov/Regulations-and-Guidance/Administrative-Simplification/NationalProvIdentStand/.

Collaborative Stage Data Collection System. 2019. Collaborative Stage Transition Newsletter. https://cancerstaging.org/cstage/about/Pages/default.aspx.

Davis, J. 2017. Checklist: These 5 Steps Will Future-Proof Your Hospital's Cybersecurity Program. https://www.healthcareitnews.com/news/checklist-these-5-steps-will-future-proof-your-hospitals-cybersecurity-program.

Department of Health and Human Services. 2019. Healthy People 2020. http://www.healthypeople.gov/2020/topics-objectives/topic/immunization-and-infectious-diseases.

Diseases Database. 2019. What is in the Diseases Database? http://www.diseasesdatabase.com/content.asp.

Finnegan, J. 2018. Surgeon General to Healthcare Professionals: Ask Kids About E-cigarette Use. https://www.fiercehealthcare.com/practices/surgeon-general-to-healthcare-professionals-ask-kids-about-e-cig-use.

Food and Drug Administration. 2018. Mandatory Reporting Requirements. http://www.fda.gov/MedicalDevices/DeviceRegulationandGuidance/PostmarketRequirements/ReportingAdverseEvents/ucm2005737.htm#3.

Food and Drug Administration. 2016. Reporting by Health Professionals. http://www.fda.gov/Safety/MedWatch/HowToReport/ucm085568.htm.

Government Publishing Office. 1992. Medical Device Amendments of 1992. http://www.gpo.gov/fdsys/pkg/STATUTE-106/pdf/STATUTE-106-Pg238.pdf.

Government Publishing Office. 1990. Safe Medical Devices Act of 1990. http://www.gpo.gov/fdsys/pkg/STATUTE-104/pdf/STATUTE-104-Pg4511.pdf.

Landi, H. 2018. Report: 30 Percent of Healthcare Databases Exposed Online. https://www.healthcare-informatics.com/news-item/cybersecurity/report-30-percent-healthcare-databases-exposed-online.

National Cancer Registrars Association. 2018a. History. http://www.ncra-usa.org/About/History.

National Cancer Registrars Association. 2018b. Education. http://www.ncra-usa.org/About/Become-a-Cancer-Registrar.

National Committee on Vital and Health Statistics. 2009. Health Data Stewardship: What, Why, Who, How. https://bok.ahima.org/PdfView?oid=94786.

National Library of Medicine. 2019. About the National Library of Medicine. https://www.nlm.nih.gov/about/index.html#.

National Plan and Provider Enumeration System. 2018. https://npiregistry.cms.hhs.gov/.

National Practitioner Data Bank. 2018. https://www.npdb.hrsa.gov/topNavigation/aboutUs.jsp.

Office of the Surgeon General. 2018. https://e-cigarettes.surgeongeneral.gov/documents/surgeon-generals-advisory-on-e-cigarette-use-among-youth-2018.pdf.

Patient-Centered Outcomes Research Institute. 2019. About Us. https://www.pcori.org/about-us.

Public Law 102-515. 1992. Cancer Registries Amendment Act. http://www.cdc.gov/cancer/npcr/pdf/publaw.pdf.

RPC Health Data Store. 2019. MedPAR File. https://healthdatastore.com/data/national-medicare-data/medpar-file/.

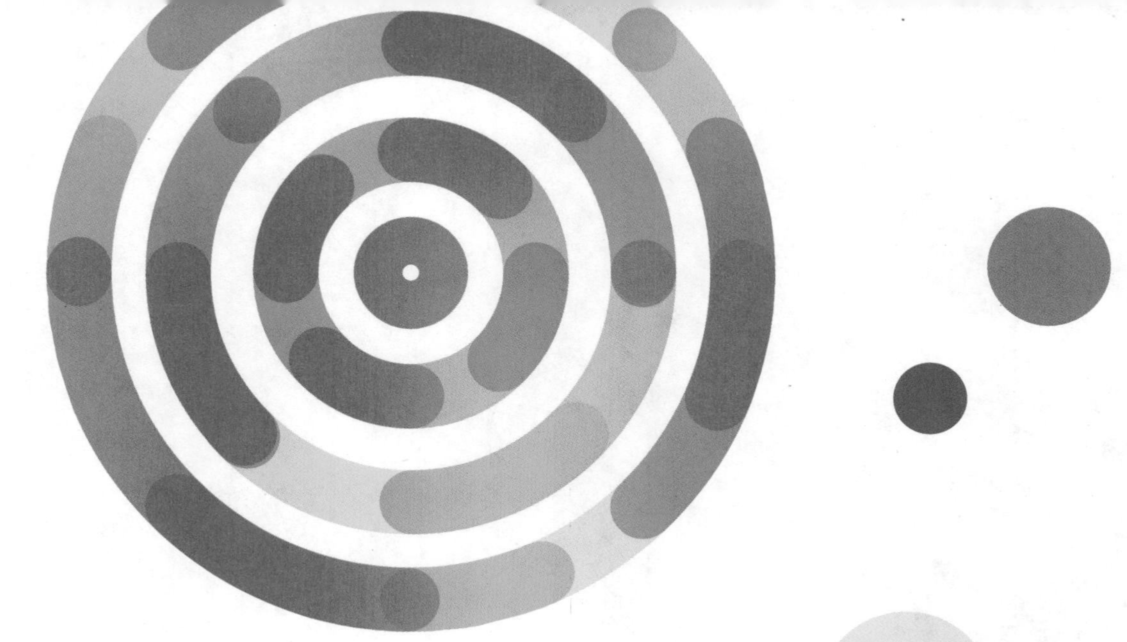

Information Protection: Access, Discloure and Archival, Privacy and Security

Health Law

Laurie A. Rinehart-Thompson, JD, RHIA, CHP, FAHIMA

Learning Objectives

- Compare the types and sources of laws that govern the healthcare industry
- Identify the steps in the legal process
- Apply professional liability theories to situations of wrongdoing
- Articulate patient rights regarding healthcare decisions, including the purpose and types of consents and advance directives
- Identify legal issues in health information management, including factors that govern the creation and maintenance of the health record
- Analyze the content of the legal health record
- Apply legally sound health record retention and destruction principles
- Identify the purpose of medical staff credentialing
- Demonstrate the differences among licensure, certification, and accreditation

Key Terms

Accreditation
Administrative law
Admissibility
Alternative dispute resolution
Appeals
Appellate courts
Arbitration
Authentication
Authorization
Bench trial
Breach
Breach of contract
Business records exception
Causation
Causes of action
Certification
Circuit courts
Civil law
Clinical privileges
Complaint
Consent
Constitutional law
Counterclaim
Court order
Courts of appeal
Credentialing
Criminal law
Cross-claim
Default
Defendant
DepositionDestruction of records
Discovery
District court
Do-not-resuscitate (DNR) order
Durable power of attorney for healthcare decisions (DPOA-HCD)
Duty
E-discovery
Express contract
False Claims Act
Federal Rules of Civil Procedure (FRCP)
Federal Rules of Evidence (FRE)
General consent
General jurisdiction
Health Care Quality Improvement Act of 1986
Hearsay
Implied contract
Informed consent
Injury
Intentional tort
Interrogatories
Joinder
Judicial law
Jurisdiction
Legal health record
Legal hold
Licensure

Limited jurisdiction
Litigation
Living will
Malfeasance
Mediation
Medical malpractice
Metadata
Misfeasance
National Practitioner Data Bank (NPDB)
Negligence
Nonfeasance
Personal health record (PHR)
Plaintiff
Private law
Privileged communication
Public law
Requests for production
Retention
Rules and regulations
Spoliation
Standard of care
Statute of limitations
Statutory law
Subpoena
Subpoena ad testificandum
Subpoena duces tecum
Summons
Supreme courts
Tort
Trial court
Voir dire
Warrant

The most important purpose of the health record is to document patient treatment and provide a means for a patient's healthcare providers to communicate among each other. However, the health record also plays an important role as a legal document. It provides critical evidence in the legal process, including medical malpractice and other personal injury lawsuits, criminal cases, healthcare fraud and abuse investigations and actions, and quasi-judicial proceedings such as workers' compensation determinations.

This chapter discusses legal issues associated with health information and includes an overview of basic legal concepts such as types and sources of law and the court system; legal process and causes of action that form the basis of professional liability; patient healthcare decision making; health record creation and maintenance; ownership and control of the health record; content and retention of the legal health record including content, retention, and destruction; medical staff credentialing; licensure and certification of healthcare professionals; and licensure, certification, and accreditation of healthcare organizations.

Basic Legal Concepts

There are many federal and state statutes and regulations that provide a protective framework around the health record and form its content. The most well-known laws are the federal Privacy Rule of the Health Insurance Portability and Accountability Act (HIPAA) and the American Recovery and Reinvestment Act (ARRA), which are discussed in chapter 9, *Data Privacy and Confidentiality*. However, those are only two of the laws with which the health information management (HIM) professional must be familiar.

In addition to federal and state laws, healthcare organizations may be subject to the standards of accrediting bodies such as the Joint Commission or the Healthcare Facilities Accreditation Program (HFAP), which also contain requirements related to the protection and content of health records.

Types and Sources of Laws

Laws are classified as public or private. Public law involves the government at any level and its relationship with individuals and organizations. Its purpose is to define, regulate, and enforce rights where any part of a government agency is a party (Showalter 2017). The most familiar type of public law is criminal law, where the government is a party against an accused who has been charged with violating a criminal statute. In healthcare, the Medicare Conditions of Participation (COP)—the requirements set forth for healthcare providers who accept Medicare patients—are public law. Public law includes both criminal and civil law (non-criminal law).

Private law involves rights and duties among private entities or individuals. For example, private law applies when a contract for the purchase of a house is written between two parties. Normally, private law encompasses issues related to contracts, property, and torts (injuries). In the medical arena, it often applies when there is a breach of contract or when a tort occurs in malpractice. Private law is also civil law. Table 8.1 depicts the relationship of public and private law to civil and criminal law.

There are four sources of public and private law: constitutions, statutes, administrative law, and judicial decisions, also known as common law or case law.

Constitutions

Constitutional law defines the amount and types of power and authority governments are given. The US Constitution defines and sets forth the powers of the three branches of the federal government. The legislative branch, which is the US Congress and is comprised of the House of Representatives and the Senate, creates statutory law (statutes). Examples of statutory law include Medicare and HIPAA. The executive branch (the president and staff, namely cabinet-level agencies) enforces the law. For example, the Centers for Medicare and Medicaid Services (CMS), an agency within the cabinet-level Department of Health and Human Services (HHS), enforces the Medicare laws. The judicial branch (the court system) interprets laws passed by the legislative branch. This three-branch government structure is also found in state governments. Each state's constitution is the supreme law of that state, but it is subordinate to the US Constitution, the supreme law of the nation (Rinehart-Thompson 2017a). Figure 8.1 illustrates each branch of the US government.

Table 8.1 Relationship of public and private law to civil and criminal law

	Civil Law	Criminal Law
Public Law	X	X
Private Law	X	

Source: Rinehart-Thompson 2017a.

Statutes

Statutes (which form statutory law) are enacted by legislative bodies. The US Congress and state legislatures are legislative bodies. Local bodies, such as municipalities, can also enact statutes, sometimes

Figure 8.1. Branches of the US government

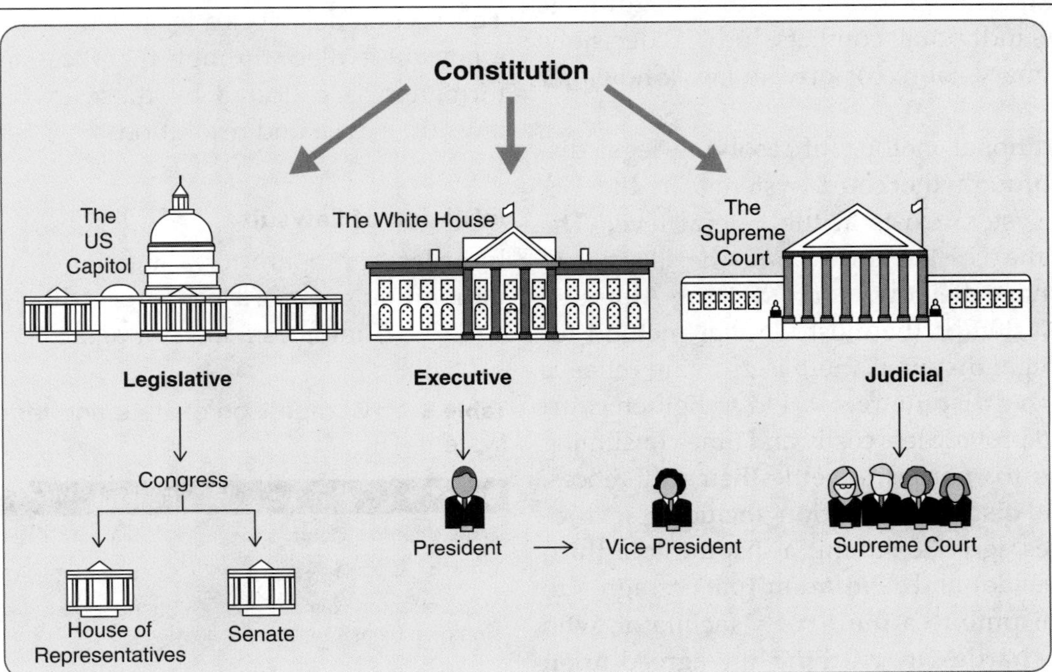

Source: ©AHIMA

referred to as ordinances (Rinehart-Thompson 2017a).

Administrative Law

Administrative law is a type of public law. As previously noted, the executive branch of government is responsible for enforcing laws enacted by the legislative branch. Administrative agencies, which are part of the executive branch, develop and enforce rules and regulations that carry out the intent of statutes. For example, HHS developed rules and regulations to carry out the intent of the HIPAA statute, and it has the power to enforce them. These rules and regulations are administrative law. Another example is the federal Food and Drug Administration (FDA), an agency within HHS, which has the power to develop rules that control the manufacture of drugs. The legislative branch of the federal government has given a number of administrative agencies the power to establish regulations (Rinehart-Thompson 2017a).

Judicial Decisions

The fourth major source of law is judicial law (that is, common law or case law), which is law created from court (judicial) decisions. Courts interpret statutes, regulations, and constitutions, and resolve individual conflicts. Judicial decisions are the primary source of private law (Showalter 2017).

The traditional method of resolving legal disputes is through the court systems. In the US, one court system exists at the federal level. The 50 states, the US territories, and the District of Columbia have their own court systems. Although the court system is the most familiar method for resolving legal disputes, there is growing reliance on alternative dispute resolution to lighten court dockets and provide less costly and time-consuming alternatives for parties to settle their differences. Alternative dispute resolution includes arbitration (parties agree to submit a dispute to a third party to decide) and mediation (parties agree to submit a dispute to a third-party facilitator, who assists the parties in reaching an agreed-upon resolution).

The US court system consists of state and federal courts. Both federal and state court systems have a three-tier structure: trial courts (called district courts in the federal system); courts of appeal or appellate courts (called circuit courts in the federal system) that hear appeals on final judgments of the trial courts; and supreme courts, the highest courts in a court system that hear final appeals from intermediate courts of appeal. Appeals are designed nearly exclusively to address legal errors or problems alleged to have occurred at the lower court, but they are not meant to address the facts of the case again. Table 8.2 compares the nomenclatures of state and federal court systems. In many states, trial courts are divided into courts of limited jurisdiction which hear cases pertaining to a particular subject (for example, landlord and tenant or juvenile) or involve crimes of lesser severity or civil matters of lower dollar amounts. Courts of general jurisdiction hear more serious criminal cases or civil cases involving larger sums of money. Cases presented to courts of appeal or supreme courts are not trial reenactments. Legal documents are prepared by each party's attorney(s), who argue the merits of the case before a panel of appellate judges.

Legal Process

This section describes a legal action from the time a lawsuit is filed, through the phase in which information is collected by those involved in the lawsuit, to trial and resolution.

Initiation of Lawsuit

In order to prepare for a judicial decision as the ultimate outcome of a legal proceeding (litigation), a plaintiff initiates a lawsuit against a defendant

Table 8.2 Comparison of state and federal court systems

State*	Federal
State Supreme Court	US Supreme Court
Court of Appeals	Circuit Court
Trial Court (for example, Common Pleas Court)	District Court

**Terminology* may vary from state to state.
Source: Rinehart-Thompson 2017a.

by filing a complaint in court, which outlines the defendant's alleged wrongdoing. After it is filed, a copy of the complaint is served to the defendant along with a summons. The summons and complaint give the defendant notice of the lawsuit and to what it pertains and informs the defendant that the complaint must be answered or some other action taken. If the defendant fails to answer the complaint or take other action, the court grants the plaintiff a judgment by default.

Usually, the defendant answers the complaint in one of four ways: denying, admitting, pleading ignorance to the allegations, or bringing a countersuit (counterclaim) against the plaintiff by filing a complaint. A defendant may file a complaint (joinder) against a third party or against another defendant (cross-claim). The defendant can ask the court to dismiss the plaintiff's complaint, but not without substantial reason such as lack of evidence.

Discovery

The next stage of litigation is discovery, a pretrial process and a time period in which parties to a lawsuit use various strategies to discover or obtain information about a case, held by other parties, prior to trial. Discovery is encouraged in order to determine the strengths and weaknesses of the other parties' cases. This knowledge helps avoid surprises at trial and perhaps encourages pretrial settlement (Rinehart-Thompson 2017b). Thus, evidentiary rules and court decisions addressing discovery are broad, favoring discovery when it is in doubt. There are several types of discovery methods, but most likely to be encountered are the deposition, which obtains the parties' and other witnesses' out-of-court testimony under oath; interrogatories, which are written questions to the parties in order to obtain information; and requests for production of documents or other pertinent items (Rinehart-Thompson 2017b).

Although it is not a discovery method, an important discovery tool is the subpoena. Initiated on behalf of one of the parties and issued through the court, it is a legal document that facilitates discovery by instructing someone to do something (such as compelling attendance at a deposition or court proceeding) or bring something, such as a document. There are two types of subpoenas: the ***subpoena ad testificandum*** seeks one's testimony and the ***subpoena duces tecum*** seeks documents and other records one can bring with him or her (Rinehart-Thompson 2017b). Subpoenas may direct that originals or copies of health records, laboratory reports, x-rays, or other records be brought to a deposition or to court. In most instances, a subpoena for the disclosure of an individual's health information must be accompanied by an authorization, or permission from that individual for the information to be disclosed. HIM professionals can be subpoenaed to testify as to the authenticity of the health records by confirming the records were compiled in the usual course of business and have not been altered in any way. Because the attorney who subpoenas a HIM professional is most interested in the health record, the information is likely to be compelled via *subpoena duces tecum*.

Another type of discovery tool is the court order. A court order is a document issued by a judge. At times, a court order will be issued to compel the production of health records. If the recipient does not comply with the court order, he or she risks contempt-of-court (namely, failure to comply) sanctions, possibly including jail time. Although both are issued through the court, any legal document that requests a patient's health information must be reviewed carefully to determine whether it is a court order or subpoena. This is because, as noted previously, a subpoena often requires an individual's authorization if health information is being sought (Rinehart-Thompson 2017b).

If health records are relevant to a criminal case, they may be obtained via a warrant. A specialized type of court order, a warrant, is a judge's order that authorizes law enforcement to seize evidence and, often, to conduct a search as well. Criminal cases in which health records are most likely to be obtained via warrant involve healthcare fraud and abuse investigations (Rinehart-Thompson 2017b).

E-Discovery

The concept of discovery as defined earlier seems relatively straightforward with paper health records. However, it is vastly different with electronic health records. E-discovery maintains the same pretrial process as discovery, but parties now obtain and review electronically stored data. The Federal Rules of Civil Procedure (FRCP) incorporated electronic information through the creation of e-discovery rules. The FRCP applies only to cases in federal district courts, but many states have adopted similar e-discovery rules that apply to both civil and criminal cases. While the role of the HIM professional in paper-based discovery was often limited to responding to a subpoena for health records or testifying as to a health record's authenticity, involvement begins much earlier with e-discovery. For example, attorneys for the parties in a lawsuit must agree on matters such as document discovery. Early interaction among a healthcare organization's health information professionals, information technology (IT) professionals, and legal counsel is very important. Electronic health records (EHRs) allow massive volumes of information to be created and stored, subjecting much greater amounts of information to discovery than paper health records. Not all information is discoverable. For example, an incident report is generally not discoverable. An incident report is a quality or performance management tool used to collect data and information about potentially compensable events (events that may result in death or serious injury). Whether it is discoverable or not depends on legal protections (such as a state statute that specifically protects quality assurance records) or the lack thereof. Any electronically stored evidence may potentially be compelled as evidence. Discoverable data includes not only the EHR, but also emails, texts, voicemails that may exist on smartphones, drafts of documents, and information on flash drives. Other information that must be considered as potentially discoverable includes information housed on ancillary systems and other databases throughout a healthcare organization because they may be relevant to a particular case. Discoverable data also include metadata, which are data about data, a concept that was unheard of in paper documents. Metadata includes information that tracks actions such as who accessed or attempted to access a document or an information system, when this occurred, which parts of the document or information system were affected, and what operations or changes (for example, creating, viewing, printing, editing) took place (Rinehart-Thompson 2018). Because the e-discovery rule affects retention and destruction of health information, HIM professionals must be involved in those ongoing processes. To protect discoverable data, they must also ensure records involved in litigation or potential litigation are safeguarded through a legal hold, which is generally a court order to preserve a health record if there is concern about destruction. A legal hold supersedes routine destruction procedures. It also prevents spoliation—the act of destroying, changing, or hiding evidence intentionally (Klaver 2017a).

Trial

After discovery is complete, the trial begins. A jury is selected through a process called voir dire or, if a jury is waived, a judge hears the case (bench trial). Evidence is then presented. The plaintiff's attorney is the first to call witnesses and present evidence. In turn, the defendant's attorney calls witnesses and presents evidence. Typically, in both health-related and non–health-related cases that involve health records as evidence, the record custodian is called as a witness by one party or the other to testify as to the authenticity of a health record sought as evidence. Testifying as to a health record's authenticity means the records custodian is verifying that it contains information about the individual in question, was compiled in the usual course of business, and is reliable and truthful as evidence. Because individuals who document in a health record do not typically falsify their entries, the truthfulness of a health record is generally not questioned. Parties to litigation often agree (stipulate) as to a health record's authenticity and allow it to be entered into evidence without requiring the records custodian to appear in court and testify. The parties may also agree to allow a photocopy of the health record or a printed version of the EHR to be introduced into evidence rather than the original. This generally requires the records custodian to certify in writing that the copy is an exact duplicate of the original. State laws vary on the degree to which courts will consider EHR printouts as evidence.

Many times, a case is settled before it reaches trial. This saves time, money, and emotional hardship on the parties. A settlement may be reached between or among parties and their attorneys with or without intervention from a third party.

After the court (either a jury or the judge) has rendered a verdict, the next stage in litigation is the appeal. If at least one of the parties disagrees with the verdict and has a legal argument on which to base its disagreement (for example, evidence was wrongfully considered at trial), a case may be appealed to the next court for review. The final stage of noncriminal litigation is collection of the judgment, which is a monetary award or in equity (that is, the defendant is required to do, or refrain from doing, something). Examples of collection of monetary judgments include single payments, garnishment of wages (by court order), seizure of property, or a lien on property. Examples of judgments in equity include ordering the completion of a construction project (requiring the defendant to do something) or requiring that a construction project be stopped (requiring the defendant to refrain from doing something). The final stage of criminal proceedings is sentencing, which may include confinement and monetary penalties.

Evidence

An individual may be compelled to testify in court. This may occur after an individual has provided testimony at a deposition, or it may be the first time an individual testifies in a particular case. Rules regarding admissibility, or the court allowing consideration of evidence, are much more stringent than discovery rules (Rinehart-Thompson 2017b). Thus, much information can be shared during pretrial discovery that is not permitted to be admitted as evidence at trial. The Federal Rules of Evidence (FRE) govern admissibility in the federal court system. Separate rules of evidence that often mirror the federal rules govern admissibility in each state.

Generally, only relevant evidence—that which makes a supposed fact either more or less probable—may be admitted at trial. However, even relevant evidence with probative value (that is, significant in providing information) may be deemed nonadmissible if it is outweighed as unfairly prejudicial or if presenting the evidence would cause undue delay. Evidence may also be excluded if it is misleading (for example, providing statistics that do not accurately depict death rates associated with a particular disease) or redundant (for example, an answer from a witness that an attorney attempts more than once to belabor a point, such as a patient's death) (Klaver 2017a). Hearsay is also often excluded. Hearsay is an out-of-court statement used to prove the truth of a matter, and it is inherently deemed untrustworthy because the maker of the statement was not cross-examined at the time the statement was made. Hearsay can be admitted into evidence if it meets one of the hearsay exceptions. The exception most common to the health record is the business records exception. This exception exists because business records are deemed inherently trustworthy and are admissible as long as they are made at or near the time of the event being recorded, are kept in the regular courses of business, and the record was created through the regular practice of business (Klaver 2017a).

Testimony by HIM professionals is often focused on the authenticity of the health record and refers to the document's baseline trustworthiness (Klaver 2017a). HIM professionals must take care to present a professional decorum when testifying by dressing professionally, answering questions honestly and without becoming defensive, and responding to the questions asked rather than unnecessarily elaborating. If the questioning attorney poses a question that is outside the scope of the individual's expertise as a HIM professional (for example, eliciting information about a patient's condition or reason that medical treatment was provided), the HIM professional should respectfully decline to answer the question by stating that it is beyond his or her area of professional expertise.

Causes of Action in Professional Liability

Professionals in many fields, including healthcare, face potential liability for allegedly failing to meet the standards established in their fields of practice.

Medical malpractice is the professional liability of healthcare providers—physicians, nurses, therapists, or others involved in the delivery of patient care. Breach of contract, intentional tort, and negligence are all **causes of action**, or elements under which lawsuits are brought that are related to professional liability. To understand how these causes of action apply, examine the elements of the physician-patient relationship.

A physician-patient relationship is established by either an **implied contract**, also referred to as *consent*, or an **express contract**. Implied contracts are created by the parties' behaviors (for example, a patient's arrival at a physician's office). Express contracts are articulated, either in writing or verbally (a patient's written or verbal agreement to treatment). A contract is usually created by the mutual agreement of the parties involved—in this case, the patient and the physician or another healthcare provider. Termination of the contract usually occurs when the patient either gets well or dies, the patient and physician mutually agree to contract termination, the patient dismisses the physician, or the physician withdraws from providing care for the patient.

No medical liability for breach of contract can exist without a physician-patient relationship. However, when this relationship does exist, the physician's failure to diagnose and treat the patient with reasonable skill and care may cause the patient to sue the physician for **breach of contract**.

Healthcare providers also can be held responsible for professional tort liability when they harm another person. A **tort** is a wrongful civil act that results in injury to another. Tort law is broad and includes non–healthcare-related acts (for example, a driver runs a red light and strikes another vehicle) and healthcare-related acts (a nurse administers the wrong medication). An **intentional tort** is where an individual purposely commits a wrongful act that results in injury. Usually, however, professional liability actions are brought against healthcare providers because of the tort of **negligence**, or unintentional wrongdoing.

Negligence occurs when a healthcare provider does not do what a prudent person would normally do in similar circumstances. The three types of negligence are the following:

1. **Nonfeasance** is the failure to act as a prudent person would, such as not ordering a standard diagnostic test
2. **Malfeasance** is a wrong or improper act that may be unlawful, such as removal of the wrong body part or use of a joint replacement that is known to be problematic (Rinehart-Thompson 2017c)
3. **Misfeasance** is the improper performance during an otherwise correct act, such as nicking the bladder during an otherwise appropriately performed gallbladder surgery

For a negligence lawsuit to be successful, the plaintiff must prove the following four elements:

1. The existence of a **duty** (an obligation established by a relationship) to meet a **standard of care** (degree of caution expected of an ordinary and reasonable person under given circumstances)
2. **Breach** or deviation from that duty
3. **Causation**, the relationship between the defendant's conduct and the harm that was suffered
4. **Injury** (harm) that may be economic (medical expenses and loss of wages) or noneconomic (pain and suffering)

The causes of actions mentioned are not the only ones that can be brought against an individual healthcare provider or a healthcare organization. Other tort actions applicable to healthcare include battery (intentional and nonconsensual contact), assault (intentional contact that causes apprehension of harmful or offensive contact), false imprisonment (intentional confinement against that person's will), infliction of emotional distress (intentional conduct resulting in extreme emotional suffering such as anxiety, sleeplessness, and inability to perform activities), defamation (false communication that injures a person's reputation), invasion of privacy (violation of a person's right for his or her person and information to be left alone), and wrongful disclosure of confidential information by a person with which an individual has a relationship protected by law (for example, physician-patient) (Brodnik et al. 2017).

Patient Rights Regarding Healthcare Decisions

It is an established right in the US that individuals generally have autonomy over their own bodies. Included in this right is the right of individuals to make their own healthcare decisions provided they are not legally incompetent (namely, incompetent by virtue of a mental disability or status as a minor). Consents play an important role in documenting individuals' wishes regarding the healthcare they will receive. Similarly, advance directives are important in documenting individuals' end-of-life decisions.

Consent is one's agreement to receive medical treatment. It can be written (preferable because it offers greater proof) or spoken; further, it can be express (communicated through words) or implied (communicated through conduct or a mechanism other than words, such as an unconscious person who is brought to the emergency department). As a matter of practice, healthcare organizations obtain a general consent from a patient for routine treatment and failure to do so can result in a legal action; generally, for battery, or harmful or offensive contact. When a treatment or procedure becomes progressively more risky or invasive, it is important that informed consent be completed to ensure the patient has a basic understanding of the diagnosis and the nature of the treatment or procedure, along with the risks, benefits, alternatives (including opting out of treatment), and individuals who will perform the treatment or procedure. Informed consent is a process and it is the responsibility of the provider who will be rendering the treatment or performing the procedure to obtain the patient's informed consent and answer the patient's questions such as risks associated with the treatment or procedure, alternatives, and likely consequences if the treatment or procedure is not chosen. Failure to obtain informed consent can result in legal action generally based on negligence (Klaver 2017b). This informed consent must be documented in the health record.

Advance Directives

An advance directive is a special type of consent that communicates an individual's wishes to be treated—or not—should the individual become unable to communicate on his or her own behalf. Once created, it is important that advance directives become a part of an individual's health record.

By creating a durable power of attorney for healthcare decisions (DPOA-HCD) an individual, while still competent, designates another person (proxy) to make healthcare decisions consistent with the individual's wishes on his or her behalf. *Durable* means that the document is in effect when the individual is no longer competent.

A living will is executed by a competent adult, expressing the individual's wishes regarding treatment should the individual become afflicted with certain conditions (for example, a persistent vegetative state or a terminal condition) and no longer be able to communicate on his or her own behalf. Living wills often address extraordinary lifesaving measures such as ventilator support and either the continuation or removal of nutrition and hydration.

A third type of document that always specifies an individual's wish *not* to receive treatment (specifically, cardiopulmonary resuscitation [CPR]) is the do-not-resuscitate (DNR) order. Most often used by individuals who are elderly or in chronically ill health, it directs healthcare providers to refrain from performing the otherwise standing order of CPR should the individual experience cardiac or respiratory arrest. Prior to executing a DNR, the patient and physician should have a discussion and the patient should sign a consent form for DNR. The physician then writes an order in the patient's health record. State law provides the framework for completing DNR orders and forms. Joint Commission-accredited organizations are required to implement policies regarding advance directives and DNR orders (Klaver 2017b).

The lack of advance directives can result in legal battles regarding the undocumented wishes of individuals who become legally incompetent. Highly publicized end-of-life cases regarding individuals and whether they would have wanted continued life-sustaining measures in light of their vegetative state include Karen Ann Quinlan (dispute between family and custodial facility regarding respirator support), Nancy Cruzan (dispute between family and custodial facility regarding continuation of artificially administered nutrition and hydration), and Terri Schiavo (dispute between husband and parents and siblings regarding continuation of artificially administered nutrition and hydration) (Klaver 2017b). In each of these cases, the courts eventually determined that lifesaving measures could be removed. These cases have had significant legal and ethical implications on how healthcare providers handle right-to-die situations, prompting more providers to discuss a patient's end-of-life decisions and encourage the creation of advance directives that will state a patient's wishes or name a decision-maker for the patient.

Check Your Understanding 8.1

Answer the following questions.

1. Laws are classified as:
   a. Public or criminal
   b. Public or private
   c. Criminal or medical malpractice
   d. Trial or appeal
2. Administrative law is a type of:
   a. Criminal law
   b. Private law
   c. Public law
   d. Statutory law
3. Arbitration is the submission of a dispute to a:
   a. Mediator
   b. Third party
   c. Judge, without a jury
   d. Judge, with a jury
4. Medical malpractice
   a. Refers to the professional liability of healthcare providers:
   b. Is related to breach of contract actions only
   c. Excludes intentional torts
   d. Is synonymous with negligence
5. Mrs. Campbell has filed a medical malpractice lawsuit against Dr. Hall. She accomplished this by:
   a. Counterclaim
   b. Voir dire
   c. Cross-claim
   d. Complaint
6. If a defendant fails to answer a complaint or take other action, the court grants the plaintiff a judgment by:
   a. Joinder
   b. Deposition
   c. Default
   d. Oral testimony

7. A tort is:
   a. A wrongful act that results in injury to another
   b. A purposeful wrongful act against another
   c. Mutual consent between two parties
   d. The professional liability of healthcare providers
8. Identify an element of negligence.
   a. Consent
   b. Duty
   c. Summons
   d. Joinder
9. Private law:
   a. Defines, regulates, and enforces rights where any government agency is a party
   b. Involves rights and duties among private parties
   c. Creates statutes
   d. Convicts individuals charged with crimes
10. Identify a source of law.
   a. Standard
   b. Statute
   c. Accrediting body
   d. Guideline
11. Statutes are laws created:
   a. By an administrative body
   b. Between private parties
   c. By trial and appellate courts
   d. By legislative bodies
12. Identify a type of advance directive.
   a. Tort
   b. Jurisdiction
   c. District court
   d. Living will
13. A physician-patient relationship:
   a. Is established by contract
   b. Is temporary
   c. Is permanent
   d. Cannot be subject to a breach of contract legal action
14. Identify consent.
   a. It is one's agreement to receive medical treatment.
   b. It must only be obtained for invasive procedures.
   c. It must be in writing to be legally valid.
   d. It is an element of negligence.
15. A lawsuit by a defendant against a plaintiff is a:
   a. Cross-claim
   b. Joinder
   c. Counterclaim
   d. Summons

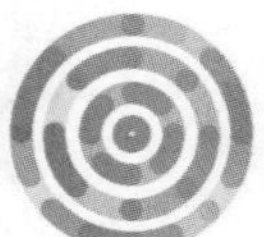

Overview of Legal Issues in Health Information Management

For the HIM professional, legal aspects of health records and health information include the topics addressed in the following sections:

- Creation and maintenance of health records
- Ownership and control of health records, including use and disclosure
- The legal health record including content, retention, and destruction

Additionally, the HIM professional may be involved in the medical staff credentialing process as well as healthcare organization licensure, certification, and accreditation.

Creation and Maintenance of Health Records

Requirements for creating and maintaining health records are usually found in state rules and regulations, typically developed by state administrative agencies responsible for licensing healthcare organizations. Requirements often specify only that health records be complete and accurate. However, other requirements specify categories of information to be kept or outline the detailed contents of the health record.

In some circumstances, the federal government stipulates specific requirements for maintaining health records. For example, the Medicare Conditions of Participation contain specific requirements that must be satisfied by healthcare organizations that seek reimbursement to treat Medicare or Medicaid patients.

In addition to state and federal requirements, accrediting bodies have established standards for maintaining health records. Specifically, the Joint Commission's relevant standards are set forth in the Information Management (IM) and Record of Care, Treatment, and Services (RC) chapters. Acute care, long-term care, home health, and behavioral health providers, among others, must follow these standards if they are to be accredited by the Joint Commission. Private third-party payers play an important role in the maintenance and content of health records. In addition to regulations that specify requirements for Medicare and Medicaid providers, private payers often have specific requirements about content that must be present in the health record for them to reimburse for treatment. Depending on the nature of the external entity that imposes requirements on the healthcare provider, failure to comply with requirements will likely result in some type of penalty such as loss of licensure or accreditation, nonpayment of claims, or fines imposed on the healthcare organization. Thus, health information must be created and maintained appropriately and in compliance with all applicable requirements.

Finally, in addition to governmental, accrediting body, and private payer requirements, professional organizations such as the American Health Information Management Association (AHIMA) publish best practice information. Best practice states that health record entries and health records in their entirety must be complete, accurate, and timely. These characteristics contribute to high-quality patient care and contribute toward a legally defensible health record that can protect a healthcare organization in malpractice litigation. Because health records are frequently admitted into evidence in medical malpractice lawsuits, the absence of complete, accurate, and timely documentation can result in a verdict against the healthcare organization.

Healthcare organizations take all previously mentioned external factors, as well as their unique internal factors, into consideration when establishing their own requirements regarding health record format and content. This is done by incorporating them in organizational policies and procedures and medical staff bylaws.

In general, health record form and content should conform to the guidelines outlined in table 8.3.

Ownership and Control of Health Records, Including Use and Disclosure

HIM professionals must understand the concepts of health record ownership and control. The health record and its contents are owned by the healthcare organization that created and maintains it.

Table 8.3 Documentation guidelines

• Policies should be based on applicable standards, including accreditation, state and local licensure, federal and state regulations, reimbursement requirements, and professional practice standards.
• Content and format of health records should be uniform.
• Entries must be legible, complete, and authenticated by the person responsible for providing or evaluating the service provided.
• Only authorized individuals, as defined by organizational policies and procedures, shall document in the health record. Further, authorship of entries should be clearly defined in the documentation.
• The definition of a legally authenticated entry should be established, with rules for prompt authentication of every entry by the author responsible for ordering, providing, or evaluating the service. Health records must be accurately written, promptly completed, properly filed and retained, and accessible. The system must consist of author identification and record maintenance that ensures the integrity of the authentication and protects the security of the entries.
• Entries should be made as soon as possible after the event or observation is made at the point of care. Entries shall never be made in advance.
• Entries should include the complete date and time. Narrative documentation should reflect the actual time the entry was created.
• The record should reflect facts, using specific language. Avoid using vague or generalized language.
• For patient safety, policies must address standardized terminology, definitions, abbreviations, acronyms, symbols, and dose designations. Prohibited abbreviations, acronyms, symbols, and dose designations should be published.
• Policies should specify who is authorized and responsible to receive and transcribe physician verbal and telephone orders.
• Health record entries must be permanent. Because they are evidence in a legal action, policies and procedures must be established to prevent alteration, tampering, and loss.
• Documentation errors should not be obliterated or changed and should be corrected per procedure. There should be an option for "corrected final" in addition to "preliminary" and "final."
• Policy should address how the patient or patient representative requests corrections and amendments to the record. The amendment should refer to the information questioned and include date and time. Documentation in question should never be removed from the record or obliterated. Per HIPAA, the patient has the right to request an amendment; however, the organization has discretion whether to grant the request.
• Quantitative and qualitative analyses of documents should be conducted according to procedure.
• Policies should differentiate whether research records are part of the legal health record or maintained separately, with the decision verified with the organization's institutional review board.

Source: Fahrenholz 2017.

As the legal custodian, the healthcare organization is responsible to ensure its integrity and security. This is true regardless of whether the health record is paper, imaged, or electronic. Although patients do own the information in the health record, ultimate responsibility for the physical health record still rests with the healthcare organization.

Control of the health record encompasses its *use* (how health information is used internally) and *disclosure* (how health information is disseminated externally). Related to disclosure is patient access to one's own health records. Although health records and other documents (for example, radiologic images) that relate to the delivery of patient care are owned by the healthcare organization, patients and other legitimately interested third parties have the right to access them. The federal HIPAA Privacy Rule grants individuals the right to access their protected health information, with some exceptions that will be discussed in more detail in chapter 9, *Data Privacy and Confidentiality*. As patient portals become more available and encouraged by providers, this right is becoming a patient expectation as well.

Use and Disclosure Under State and Federal Law

Most states have laws that protect patient confidentiality (Brodnik 2017). Known as **privileged communication** statutes, the laws generally prohibit medical practitioners from disclosing information during litigation if that information arises from the parties' professional relationship and relates to the patient's care and treatment. An example is the protection of information shared by a patient with his or her physician during an office visit (Showalter 2017). If patients waive their privilege, the medical provider is no longer prohibited from making disclosures.

State law may specifically provide a patient with the right to access his or her health information. Even if it does not, as previously noted, HIPAA grants an individual the right to access his or her health information for as long as it is maintained, with limited situations where access may be denied. The HIM professional should always follow the stricter law (HIPAA or state). HIPAA also establishes standards by which others may access an individual's health information.

Disclosure of health information without patient authorization may be required under specific state statutes. Examples include reporting vital statistics (for example, births and deaths) and other public health, safety, or welfare situations. For example, healthcare providers may be required to provide information to the appropriate state agency about patients diagnosed with sexually transmitted and other communicable diseases, injured by knives or firearms, or exhibiting wounds that suggest some type of violent criminal activity. The treatment of suspected victims of child abuse or neglect must also be reported. Because requirements vary by state, HIM professionals must know the reporting requirements for the states in which they practice.

Health information has a variety of purposes—from the provision of direct patient care to use by outside entities such as insurance and pharmaceutical companies—and those uses and disclosures must be appropriate. Compliance with legal requirements for appropriate use and disclosure must be ensured, as must adherence to the profession's ethical principles.

Use of Health Records in Judicial Proceedings

The health record of an individual who is a party to a legal proceeding is usually admissible in litigation or judicial proceedings provided it is material or relevant to the issue (Showalter 2017). Either a court order or subpoena is used to obtain health information for a court that has **jurisdiction** (legal authority to make decisions) over the pending litigation. These are discussed in more detail in chapter 9, *Data Privacy and Confidentiality*.

Responses to court orders and subpoenas depend on state regulations. In some instances, states allow copies of health records to be certified and mailed to the clerk of the court or to other designated individuals. In other instances, however, original health records must be produced in person and the records custodian is required to authenticate them. **Authentication** affirms a health record's legitimacy through testimony or written validation that it is indeed the record of the subject individual and the information in it is valid.

Legal Health Record

The **legal health record** is the record used for legal purposes and is the "record released upon a valid request" (Rinehart-Thompson 2017d, 171). The legal health record can exist on any medium (paper, electronic or imaged, or a hybrid). Its content is defined by the healthcare organization that maintains it rather than by law.

Importance of the Legal Health Record

The legal health record distinction is important for several reasons. First, it is important to a healthcare organization's business and legal processes (Rinehart-Thompson 2017d). Second, because the legal health record is the record that must be produced upon request, including legal request, it becomes important to ensure the legal health record is legally sound and defensible as a valid document in legal situations (Rinehart-Thompson 2017d).

It is also important to differentiate the legal health record from other types of records that are integral to health information. These include the designated record set, the EHR, and the personal health record. The designated record set (DRS), which is a term specific to HIPAA and described further in chapter 9, *Data Privacy and Confidentiality*, also includes other records (for example, billing records) and, as such, is more expansive than the legal health record. The EHR is also more expansive because it contains components (such as metadata) that are not ordinarily included in legal health record content. The **personal health record (PHR)** is owned and managed by the individual who is the subject of the health record. As such, it is not the legal business record of the healthcare organization. The PHR is discussed in chapter 3, *Health Information Functions, Purpose, and Users*.

Content of the Legal Health Record

Determining the content of the legal health record can be challenging because of the myriad of documents that exist, the presence of documentation in multiple locations, and—for the EHR—the existence of documentation that does not exist in paper health records. Healthcare organizations should develop and maintain an inventory of all documents and data that could comprise the legal health record, considering all locations in the healthcare organization where such information could exist (for example, separate departments or servers). Electronic document considerations include emails, text messages, electronic fetal monitoring strips, diagnostic images, digital photography, voice files, and video (AHIMA 2011a). Healthcare organizations should also carefully consider whether to include data such as pop-up reminders, alerts, and metadata.

Retention of the Legal Health Record

Retention includes mechanisms for storing records, providing for timely retrieval, and establishing the length of times various types of records will be retained by the healthcare organization. The HIM professional must consider multiple factors when developing health record retention policies to determine how long health records are to be kept. These factors include applicable federal and state statutes and regulations; accreditation standards; operational needs of the healthcare organization; and the type of healthcare organization (for example, hospital or clinic).

Some state laws designate how long health records must be retained in their original form and specify whether they can be stored on media other than that on which they were initially created. Additionally, state and local laws that require information to be maintained for reporting to public authorities (for example, vital statistics and public health data) must be adhered to.

The health record must be available as evidence in legal actions, as governed by statutes and regulations. Health records should be retained for at least the period specified by the state's **statute of limitations**, which is the period of time in which a lawsuit (such as medical malpractice) must be filed. In particular, the health record of a minor should be retained until the patient reaches the age of majority (as defined by state law) plus the period of statute of limitations, unless otherwise provided by state law. For example, if state law defines the age of majority as 18 and the statute of limitations is two years, then the health record would need to be retained until the patient is 20 years old. A longer retention period is necessary because the statute may not begin to run until a potential plaintiff learns of the causal relationship between an injury and the care received. Other claims must also be taken into consideration when determining how long to retain health records as evidence. For example, under the **False Claims Act**, claims of fraud may be brought for up to 10 years after the incident (31 USC 3729). Payer requirements must also be considered; for example, the Medicare Conditions of Participation, which is federal regulation, require five-year retention for hospital health records.

The standards of accreditation bodies such as the Joint Commission and the HFAP must be followed in developing a health record retention policy. The Joint Commission defers to state law by specifying that records are to be retained in compliance with applicable law.

Health record retention also depends on how the healthcare organization uses the information in the health record. For example, an acute-care hospital may have very different retention policies than a long-term-care organization providing geriatric nursing care. Further, a healthcare organization providing care exclusively to children may have different retention policies than a home health agency. Healthcare organizations with significant educational and research activities may need to retain health records for longer periods than other healthcare organizations because existing health records can be useful for these purposes. For example, information may be extracted from health records for research studies.

Governing boards and medical staffs of every healthcare organization must analyze their medical and administrative needs to ensure health records are available for peer review, quality assessment, and other activities. These needs must be considered in conjunction with legal and accreditation requirements. In many instances, healthcare organizations retain health records longer than the law requires to accommodate research or other needs of the healthcare organization.

AHIMA Retention Recommendations

AHIMA routinely publishes recommendations for the retention of health records (AHIMA 2013). HIM professionals should use these to determine how their healthcare organizations compare with industry-wide best practices. AHIMA recommends, at a minimum, that health record retention schedules do the following:

- Be designed to meet a healthcare organization's needs so that health information is available not only for patient care, but also for research, education, and to meet the legal requirements that apply to the healthcare organization
- Be specific about the retention of information, including a description of what information is to be kept, how long it is to be kept, and the medium on which it will stored (for example, electronic or imaged, paper, or hybrid)
- Clearly specify in the policies and procedures the destruction method that is to be used for each medium on which health information is housed (AHIMA 2013).

Table 8.4 shows AHIMA's retention recommendations for various types of health information.

Destruction

Not all information must, or should, be retained forever. Whereas space has historically been a challenge with paper health records, it is easy to presume indefinite or permanent retention of electronic health records because they require little space. However, space can become an issue for electronic health records. Further, from a legal perspective, because a health record can be retained permanently does not mean it should be if it no longer serves a purpose but occupies space.

Just as the HIM professional must consider multiple factors when determining retention, many factors must also be taken into consideration regarding health record destruction. **Destruction of records** is the act of breaking down the components of a health record into pieces that can no longer be recognized as parts of the original health record. The factors to be considered include applicable federal and state statutes and regulations, accreditation standards, pending or ongoing litigation, storage capabilities, and cost.

Any health record involved in investigations, audits, or litigation should not be destroyed, even if the record retention schedule would provide

Table 8.4 AHIMA retention standards

Health information	Recommended retention period
Diagnostic images (such as x-ray film) (adults)	5 years
Diagnostic images (such as x-ray film) (minors)	5 years after the age of majority
Disease index	10 years
Fetal heart monitor records	10 years after the age of majority
Master patient/person index	Permanently
Operative index	10 years
Patient health records (adults)	10 years after the most recent encounter
Patient health records (minors)	Age of majority plus statute of limitations
Physician index	10 years
Register of births	Permanently
Register of deaths	Permanently
Register of surgical procedures	Permanently

Source: AHIMA 2011b.

for destruction otherwise. This is because health records contain valuable evidence and, further, destruction of this important evidence may be indicative of the provider's bad faith. When health records are slated for destruction, procedures must ensure the information is not inappropriately disclosed in the process. For paper health records, common destruction methods include shredding, burning, pulping, or pulverizing (Rinehart-Thompson 2017d). Care should be taken to actually destroy electronic health records rather than merely deleting the pathway to access them. Destruction methods for electronic health records include overwriting; magnetic degaussing or demagnetizing (neutralizing the magnetic field to erase data); and physical destruction of the medium on which the health record resides, including pulverizing (laser discs) and shredding or cutting (DVDs) (AHIMA 2013). With electronic health records, there is the risk of duplicate records remaining in circulation (Rinehart-Thompson 2017d).

Health record destruction may be accomplished by the healthcare organization that owns the records, or the process may be outsourced. In either case, a list of all destroyed health records and the manner of destruction must be documented. A certificate of destruction and an agreement that ensures the protection of the information should both be obtained (AHIMA 2013; Rinehart-Thompson 2017d).

Medical Staff Credentialing

Another area with significant legal implications that the HIM professional may become involved in is medical staff appointments, also referred to as **credentialing**. A basic understanding of the legal issues and some of the functions in the credentialing process are important because the health information professional may be involved in this activity.

The healthcare organization is ultimately responsible for the quality of care it provides. This includes the quality of the medical staff, which consists primarily of the physicians who have been given permission to provide the healthcare organization's clinical services. Depending on the healthcare organization, other providers such as dentists, podiatrists, advance practice nurses, and physician assistants may also serve on a healthcare organization's medical staff.

A healthcare organization's governing board (board of directors) is accountable to establish policies and procedures that ensure reasonable care in the appointment of medical practitioners to the healthcare organization's medical staff and the granting of clinical privileges. **Clinical privileges** are the defined set of services a qualified physician is permitted to perform in that organization such as admitting patients, performing surgeries, or delivering infants.

Credentialing includes both the initial appointment and reappointment of individuals to the medical staff and determination of the extent of their privileges. The customary process by which an application for medical staff appointment and privileges involves review at several levels. These include the appropriate clinical departments, credentials committee, medical staff executive committee, and board of directors. Although the board of directors relies on the advice and recommendations of the medical staff, ultimate responsibility for making appointments and reappointments and for ensuring the medical staff members are qualified to perform the functions for which they have been granted privileges rests with the board (Pozgar 2016).

An important part of the credentialing process is querying the **National Practitioner Data Bank (NPDB)**, which was established by the federal **Health Care Quality Improvement Act of 1986**. One goal of the NPDB is to limit the movement of physicians throughout the US where their negative histories such as medical malpractice liability and loss of privileges at other healthcare organizations may go undetected. NPDB regulations include requirements for reporting information to the NPDB and querying information from the NPDB prior to granting medical staff privileges (Pozgar 2016).

Penalties and liability can result from failure to use the NPDB.

The HIM professional may serve as the medical staff coordinator, involving the collection, organization, verification, and storage of all information associated with credentialing. This includes information about the individual staff member's professional background, credentials, previous professional experience, and quality profiles. All this information, including that obtained from the NPDB, is confidential. Therefore, policies and procedures must be in place to specify who may have access to what information and under what circumstances.

Licensure

Licensure is a designation given to an individual or an organization by a governmental agency or board that gives the individual permission to practice, or the healthcare organization to operate, within a certain field of practice. For example, physicians, nurses, and physical therapists must be licensed to practice. In many states, hospitals must be licensed in order to treat patients. Where licensure exists for a practice area, it is mandatory. Once an individual or healthcare organization becomes licensed, it is subject to further regulation by the relevant governmental body to ensure it is maintaining at least a minimal level of competence. For individuals, further regulation may include required continuing education. The legal significance of licensure in healthcare is that a government entity has deemed the individual or healthcare organization qualified to provide competent and safe patient care. HIM professionals are not licensed, but can be certified, meaning they are officially recognized by a private entity as meeting certain qualifications in the field. However, they may take part in or coordinate licensure maintenance for their healthcare organization. They may also assume the role of ensuring that licensure records of individual practitioners are updated and maintained by the healthcare organization in which they work.

Certification

Certification of individuals is a designation given by a private organization to acknowledge a requisite level of knowledge, competencies, and skills. Whether or not certification is required for an individual to practice (as is licensure) is an employer decision. Certification may either be entry level or mastery level. In the HIM profession, RHIA (Registered Health Information Administrator) and RHIT (Registered Health Information Technician) credentials signify entry-level generalist competency. AHIMA also offers mastery-level specialty certifications such as the CHPS (Certified in Healthcare Privacy and Security), CCS (Certified Coding Specialist), and CHDA (Certified Health Data Analyst). For information on these credentials, see chapter 1, *Health Information Management Profession*. In healthcare organizations, certification is a designation by HHS that its Conditions of Participation have been met. Although certification is not required for a healthcare organization to operate, it is required for the organization to participate in (and thus be reimbursed by) the Medicare and Medicaid programs.

Accreditation

The HIM professional will likely find herself or himself in a role that involves compliance with accreditation standards. This role may involve compliance with standards relating to health information or coordinating a healthcare organization's overall compliance with the standards of the body by which it is accredited. **Accreditation** is a designation given to a healthcare organization by an accrediting body, demonstrating that the healthcare organization has met the accrediting body's requirements for excellence. Accreditation is generally viewed as the highest level of competence or validation that a healthcare organization can demonstrate. In acute care, Joint Commission is the most prevalent accrediting body. Other accreditors include the HFAP, DNV GL Healthcare, and Center for Improvement in Healthcare Quality (CIHQ). There are accrediting bodies in other care settings as well, such as the Accreditation Association for Ambulatory Health Care (AAAHC) and the Commission on Accreditation of Rehabilitation Facilities (CARF), a prevalent accreditor in rehabilitation. By successfully completing an acute care–deemed status survey by The Joint Commission, HFAP, DNV GL Healthcare, or CIHQ, a healthcare organization that is accredited by one of these healthcare organizations is also deemed to have met Medicare and Medicaid requirements and thus holds concurrent accreditation and Medicare and Medicaid certification.

HIM Roles

With familiarity in health law and a deep knowledge of the health record, HIM professionals can fill nontraditional roles. Many of these positions require advanced training to have the skill set needed to apply for and be accepted into the following dynamic positions:

- *Medical malpractice health record analyst*. This position is dedicated to facilitating health record review for either plaintiff or defense attorneys in the medical malpractice claims and litigation management process. HIM professionals can assist parties and their legal counsel by developing case summaries and preparing chronologies of medical events that are pertinent to a legal case.
- *Patient advocate*. HIM professionals can serve as patient advocates in many roles, including assistance with health literacy and medical bill interpretation. Included in this role is assisting patients toward a greater understanding about healthcare decision-making, including consents and advance directive options.
- *Risk Management*. Identifying, monitoring, and preventing risks are key initiatives in any healthcare organization. Although the risk management function is often reserved for attorneys, in smaller healthcare organizations it may be an ideal role for HIM professionals due to their familiarity with and understanding of the health record, incident reporting, and the analysis and monitoring of trends.
- *Credentialing*. A long-standing position for HIM professionals in some healthcare organizations, credentialing and re-credentialing medical staff members requires organizational and investigative skills. Familiarity with medical staff requirements also makes the HIM professional a qualified person for this role.
- *Accreditation*. Because of the complexity associated with preparation for and compliance with accrediting body standards, healthcare organizations both large and small have positions for individuals who are responsible to manage the accreditation process. Because of their organizational skills and the relationship between health information and many accreditation standards, HIM professionals are suited to fill these roles.
- *Medical Scribe*. Some HIM professionals work with physicians as a medical scribe. The medical scribe takes on some of the clerical responsibilities of retrieving test results, navigating the EHR, and documenting in the health record as instructed by the physician (Gooch 2016).

Check Your Understanding 8.2

Answer the following questions.

1. A health record is owned by the:
   a. Patient who is the subject of the record
   b. Healthcare organization that created and maintains it
   c. Staff members who document in it
   d. Insurance company that pays for the patient's care
2. A court's legal authority to make decisions is called:
   a. Joinder
   b. Judicial law
   c. Jurisdiction
   d. Litigation
3. Identify the action of a health records custodian to affirm the legitimacy of a health record.
   a. Testimony
   b. Authentication
   c. Jurisdiction
   d. Certification
4. Identify a characteristic of the legal health record.
   a. It must be electronic
   b. It includes the designated record set
   c. It is the record disclosed upon request
   d. It includes a patient's personal health record
5. The health record content is defined by a number of standards including:
   a. Constitutional amendments
   b. Nursing licensure laws
   c. Accrediting body standards
   d. Record retention policies
6. The principal purpose of the health record is to:
   a. Serve as evidence in litigation
   b. Support statistical analysis and research
   c. Document patient treatment and allow providers to communicate
   d. Provide a record for reimbursement purposes
7. The National Practitioner Data Bank:
   a. Allows a healthcare organization to be reimbursed by Medicare and Medicaid
   b. Is a type of certification for healthcare providers
   c. Limits movement of physicians with negative histories
   d. Was repealed by Congress
8. AHIMA recommends that the operative index be retained for:
   a. 5 years
   b. 7 years
   c. 10 years
   d. Permanently
9. Identify the true statement regarding health information retention.
   a. Retention depends only on accreditation requirements.
   b. Retention periods differ among healthcare organizations.

c. The operational needs of a healthcare organization cannot be considered.
d. Retention periods are frequently shorter for health information about minors.

10. Identify the true statement regarding the development of health record destruction policies.
    a. All applicable laws must be considered.
    b. The healthcare organization must find a way not to destroy any health records.
    c. Health records involved in pending or ongoing litigation may be destroyed.
    d. Only state laws must be considered.

11. Identify a characteristic of credentialing.
    a. It is ultimately the responsibility of the medical staff.
    b. It is the hiring of qualified nurses in a hospital.
    c. It applies to the granting of specific clinical privileges to medical staff members.
    d. It grants one level of privileges to all medical staff members.

12. Medical staff credentialing refers to:
    a. Rewarding physicians who have treated the most patients
    b. Appointing and granting clinical privileges to physicians
    c. Renewing physicians' medical licenses
    d. Establishing physicians' medical malpractice premiums

13. Defining what a physician can do is known as:
    a. Accreditation
    b. Licensure
    c. Credentialing
    d. Clinical privileges

14. ____ gives an individual permission to practice or a healthcare organization permission to operate within a certain field of practice.
    a. Licensure
    b. Certification
    c. Accreditation
    d. Medicare Conditions of Participation

15. Electronic health data should be destroyed by:
    a. Pulverizing
    b. Degaussing
    c. Shredding
    d. Burning

Real-World Case 8.1

In October 2018, Cook County (Illinois) commissioners voted to approve a nearly $4 million settlement of a medical malpractice lawsuit at Stroger Hospital, a healthcare organization that is part of the Cook County Health and Hospital Systems (CCHHS). The lawsuit stemmed from a 2013 bedside pericardiocentesis that, plaintiff's attorneys argued, should have been performed in a cardiac catheterization lab. Despite the large settlement, CCHHS CEO noted that the settlement was neither an admission of malpractice or of wrongdoing by the providers or the health system. Although it is not known how much a jury would have awarded the plaintiff, a jury verdict would have been a declaration of malpractice, which was avoided through the settlement (Pratt 2018).

Real-World Case 8.2

Healthcare organizations develop record retention guidelines in accordance with applicable laws (for example, a state's statute of limitations for medical malpractice and Medicare Conditions of Participation retention requirements) and operation needs (for example, research, education, and strategic planning). If a healthcare organization follows its guidelines, and those guidelines conform to applicable laws, the healthcare organization is legally compliant. There is generally not a requirement that patients be notified of a healthcare organization's health record retention periods. This, however, has not been the case in California, which has had a notification requirement in place for several years. Additionally, Senate Bill 1238 was presented in the California Senate in 2018 to amend Section 123106(e) and 123107 of the California Health and Safety Code, to require healthcare providers, by the date that service is first delivered or as soon possible after emergency care, to inform the patient or patient's representative of the intended retention period for the patient's health records (California Senate Bill 1238 2018). Providers are also required to notify the patient at least 60 days before the record is to be destroyed.

References

American Health Information Management Association. 2017. *Pocket Glossary of Health Information Management and Technology*, 5th ed. Chicago: AHIMA.

American Health Information Management Association. 2013. Retention and Destruction of Health Information (updated October 2013). http://library.ahima.org/doc?oid=300217#.XBm0c_ZFw2w.

American Health Information Management Association. 2011a. Fundamentals of the legal health record and designated record set. *Journal of AHIMA* 82(2): expanded online version. http://library.ahima.org/doc?oid=104008#.Vw_Ty_krLDc.

American Health Information Management Association. 2011b. Retention and Destruction of Health Information. Appendix D: AHIMA's Recommended Retention Standards (2011 update). http://bok.ahima.org/Doc/2/0/C/105018#.XBqf0WhKh9M.

Brodnik, M.S. 2017. Access, Use, and Disclosure and Release of Health Information. Chapter 15 in *Fundamentals of Law for Health Informatics and Information Management.* Edited by M.S. Brodnik, L.A. Rinehart-Thompson, and R.B. Reynolds. Chicago: AHIMA.

Brodnik, M.S. 2017. Glossary in *Fundamentals of Law for Health Informatics and Information Management.* Edited by M.S. Brodnik, L.A. Rinehart-Thompson, and R.B. Reynolds. Chicago: AHIMA.

California Senate Bill 1238. 2018. Patient Records: Maintenance and Storage. http://leginfo.legislature.ca.gov/faces/billTextClient.xhtml?bill_id=201720180SB1238.

Fahrenholz, C.G. 2017. Clinical Documentation and the Health Record. Chapter 2 in *Documentation for Medical Records*. Edited by C.G. Fahrenholz. Chicago: AHIMA.

Gooch, K. 2016. 17 Things to Know About Medical Scribes. https://www.beckershospitalreview.com/hospital-physician-relationships/17-things-to-know-about-medical-scribes.html.

Klaver, J.C. 2017a. Evidence. Chapter 5 in *Fundamentals of Law for Health Informatics and Information Management*. Edited by M.S. Brodnik, L.A. Rinehart-Thompson, and R.B. Reynolds. Chicago: AHIMA.

Klaver, J.C. 2017b. Consent to Treatment. Chapter 8 in *Fundamentals of Law for Health Informatics and Information Management*. Edited by M.S. Brodnik, L.A. Rinehart-Thompson, and R.B. Reynolds. Chicago: AHIMA.

Pozgar, G.D. 2016. *Legal Aspects of Health Care Administration.* Burlington, MA: Jones & Bartlett Learning.

Pratt, G. 2018 (October 17). Cook County Board votes in favor of $4 million settlement in Stroger medical malpractice case. *Chicago Tribune.* https://chicagotribune.com/news/local/politics/ct-met-cook-county-lawsuit-settlement-20181017-story.html.

Rinehart-Thompson, L.A. 2018. *Introduction to Health Information Privacy and Security.* Chicago: AHIMA.

Rinehart-Thompson, L.A. 2017a. The Legal System in the United States. Chapter 3 in *Fundamentals of Law for Health Informatics and Information Management.* Edited by M.S. Brodnik, L.A. Rinehart-Thompson, and R.B. Reynolds. Chicago: AHIMA.

Rinehart-Thompson, L.A. 2017b. Legal Proceedings. Chapter 4 in *Fundamentals of Law for Health Informatics and Information Management.* Edited by M.S. Brodnik, L.A. Rinehart-Thompson, and R.B. Reynolds. Chicago: AHIMA.

Rinehart-Thompson, L.A. 2017c. Tort Law. Chapter 6 in *Fundamentals of Law for Health Informatics and Information Management.* Edited by M.S. Brodnik, L.A. Rinehart-Thompson, and R.B. Reynolds. Chicago: AHIMA.

Rinehart-Thompson, L.A. 2017d. The Legal Health Record: Maintenance, Content, Documentation, and Disposition. Chapter 9 in *Fundamentals of Law for Health Informatics and Information Management.* Edited by M.S. Brodnik, L.A. Rinehart-Thompson, and R.B. Reynolds. Chicago: AHIMA.

Showalter, J.S. 2017. *The Law of Healthcare Administration.* Chicago: Health Administration Press.

31 USC 3729: False Claims Act. 1986.

Data Privacy and Confidentiality

Laurie A. Rinehart-Thompson, JD, RHIA, CHP, FAHIMA

Learning Objectives

- Differentiate between disclosure and use
- Apply the HIPAA Privacy Rule, including American Recovery and Reinvestment Act (ARRA) requirements such as breach notification, with regard to health information use and disclosure
- Educate individuals regarding to whom and to what the HIPAA Privacy Rule applies
- Analyze the respective requirements of the individual rights provided by the HIPAA Privacy Rule
- Distinguish the key HIPAA Privacy Rule documents: Notice of Privacy Practices, HIPAA consent, and authorization
- Differentiate authorization and right of access
- Assess the requirements associated with each type of commercial use of Protected health information (PHI): marketing; sale of information; and fundraising
- Recommend appropriate enforcement actions due to HIPAA Privacy Rule violations
- Protect health information through use of disclosure policies and procedures that apply to both state law and HIPAA regulations
- Apply authorization requirements to the valid disclosure of health information
- Identify types of medical identity theft as well as fraud detection activities required by the Red Flags Rule
- Explain role of patient advocate

Key Terms

Administrative simplification
American Recovery and Reinvestment Act (ARRA)
Authorization
Breach
Breach notification
Business associate (BA)
Business associate agreement (BAA)
Clinical Laboratory Improvement Amendments (CLIA) of 1988
Complaint
Confidentiality
Covered entity (CE)
Deidentified information
Department of Health and Human Services (HHS)
Designated record set (DRS)
Disclosure
Disclosure of health information
Facility directory
Fair and Accurate Credit Transactions Act (FACTA)
Federal Trade Commission (FTC)
Fundraising
Health Information Technology for Economic and Clinical Health Act (HITECH)
Health Insurance Portability and Accountability Act (HIPAA)
Health plans

Healthcare clearinghouses
Healthcare providers
HIPAA consent
Individual
Individually identifiable health information
Marketing
Medical identity theft
Minimum necessary standard
Notice of privacy practices
Office for Civil Rights (OCR)
Office of the National Coordinator for Health Information Technology (ONC)
Personal representative
Preemption
Privacy
Privacy officer
Privacy Rule
Protected health information (PHI)
Psychotherapy notes
Red Flags Rule
Right of access
Right to request accounting of disclosures
Right to request amendment
Right to request confidential communications
Right to request restrictions of PHI
Sale of information
Treatment, payment, and operations (TPO)
Unsecured PHI
Use
Workforce

Privacy is a social value and is the right "to be let alone" (Rinehart-Thompson and Harman 2017). The US Constitution does not grant a right of privacy, but courts have interpreted it to give privacy rights in certain areas such as religion and child-rearing. Patients have a right to their privacy. Although there is no constitutional right of privacy to one's health information, the health record is not a public document and – further – privacy protections to health information have been established through court cases as well as laws such as the Health Insurance Portability and Accountability Act (HIPAA), discussed in great detail in this chapter.

Confidentiality is similar to privacy, but it stems from the sharing of private thoughts in confidence with someone else. Legally, such sharing is protected when the communication is between parties such as physician and patient, attorney and client, or clergy and parishioner. Laws define those communications that are protected (Brodnik 2017a).

Use and Disclosure

Use is how a healthcare organization avails itself of health information internally, such as a nurse reviewing a patient's health record. Disclosure is how health information is disseminated outside a healthcare organization. An example of disclosure is providing patient information to an insurance company. Use and disclosure are usually associated with the concepts of ownership and control of the health record because the organization that owns and controls the health record is also able to control the use and disclosure of its contents. Compliance with all applicable privacy and confidentiality laws and standards is important to avoid inappropriate use and disclosure of health information. Disclosure becomes very important when a healthcare organization is involved in litigation and health information becomes key evidence necessary for fact-finding during the discovery process and at trial, as described in chapter 8, *Health Law.*

State Laws—Privacy

Laws protecting the privacy of health information vary significantly from state to state. Some states have laws that are very specific while others are general or even absent. Every person or organization that is subject to HIPAA (federal law) must abide by the state law. State laws supersede HIPAA if the state law is stricter. This is the concept of preemption, which is discussed later in this chapter.

In addition to state laws that protect health information privacy, all states have laws that require the disclosure of health information, even without patient authorization. These include the reporting of vital statistics (births and deaths) and other public health, safety, or welfare situations. For example, healthcare providers may be required to provide information to the appropriate state agency about patients who suffer from sexually transmitted and other communicable diseases, have been injured by knives or firearms, or have wounds that suggest some type of violent criminal activity. The treatment of suspected victims of child abuse or neglect also must be reported. These purposes are permitted by HIPAA and described later in the chapter.

HIPAA Privacy Rule and ARRA

The HIPAA Privacy Rule is one of the key federal regulations that governs the protection of protected health information (PHI). This chapter provides an overview of HIPAA legislation (namely, the Privacy Rule) and the accompanying American Recovery and Reinvestment Act (ARRA) of 2009.

HIPAA and ARRA Overview

As shown in figure 9.1, HIPAA contains five titles. Title II is the most relevant title to the health information management (HIM) professional. It contains provisions relating to the prevention of healthcare fraud and abuse and medical liability (medical malpractice) reform, as well as administrative simplification. The HIPAA Privacy Rule resides in the administrative simplification provision of Title II along with the HIPAA security standards, national provider identifiers, and transaction and code set standardization requirements. Administrative simplification is HIPAA's attempt to streamline and standardize the healthcare industry's non-uniform business practices, such as billing, to include the electronic transmission of data.

Before HIPAA was enacted, no federal statutes or regulations generally protected the confidentiality of health information. Specific laws applied only in particular circumstances, such as to providers of Medicare services or to those receiving federal funds to provide substance abuse treatment.

Patient privacy protection laws governing access, use, and disclosure had largely resided with the individual states. They varied considerably, creating a patchwork of laws across the United States. Many states had passed laws to protect highly sensitive health records such as mental health and HIV/AIDS, but many states had no statutes or regulations to protect health information generally. If health information was wrongfully disclosed, individuals had to resort to lawsuits, often alleging negligence. With the Privacy Rule, protection was achieved uniformly across all the states through a consistent set of standards affecting providers, healthcare clearinghouses, and health plans.

The legal doctrine of preemption means that federal law (for example, the HIPAA Privacy Rule) may supersede state law. However, the HIPAA Privacy Rule is only a federal floor, or minimum, of privacy requirements so it does not preempt or supersede stricter state statutes (or other federal statutes). *Stricter* means that a state or federal statute provides an individual with greater privacy protections or gives individuals greater rights with respect to their PHI. If a question arises, it is important to consult with legal counsel to determine whether federal or state law prevails.

The American Recovery and Reinvestment Act (ARRA) provided significant funding for health information technology and other economic stimulus funding, and it also made important changes to the HIPAA Privacy and Security Rules. These changes are located in the Health Information Technology for Economic and Clinical Health Act (HITECH), which is a part of ARRA.

Office of the National Coordinator for Health Information Technology (ONC)

The Office of the National Coordinator for Health Information Technology (ONC) was

Figure 9.1 HIPAA structure

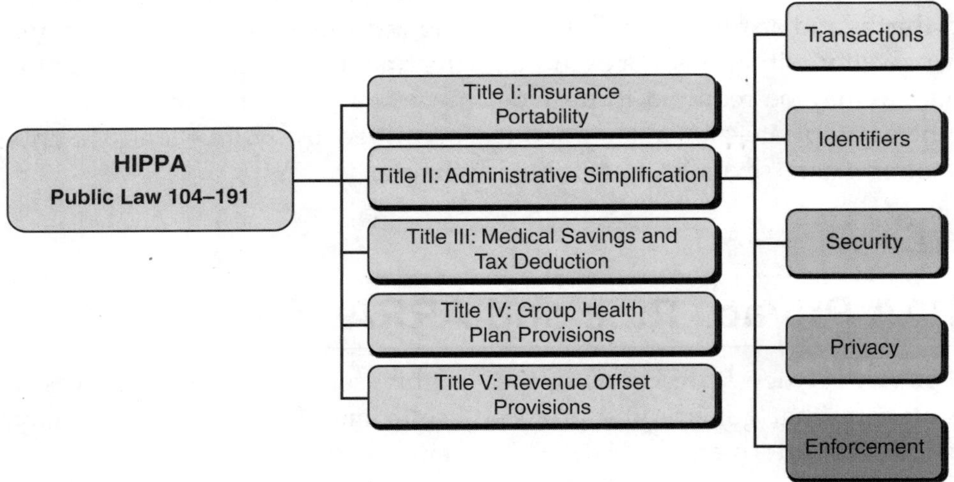

Source: Walsh 2016. Reprinted with permission.

first established by presidential executive order. It is now recognized by statute as an entity within the Department of Health and Human Services (HHS). It has been the primary federal entity responsible for coordinating national efforts to implement and use health information technology, and to promote the exchange of electronic health information. HHS currently includes a number of offices and agencies including the Office of Policy, Office of Standards and Technology, and Office of the Chief Privacy Officer, which plays an important role in promoting electronic health information privacy and security (ONC 2018).

Applicability of the Privacy Rule

The Privacy Rule does not apply to every person or every organization. It also does not apply to all types of information. This section identifies, first, *to whom* the Privacy Rule applies: persons or organizations identified as covered entities, business associates, and workforce. This section also discusses *what* the Privacy Rule protects: protected health information (PHI).

Covered Entities

A covered entity (CE) is a person or organization that must comply with the HIPAA Privacy Rule. The three types of covered entities are the following:

1. Healthcare providers, but only those that conduct certain transactions (financial or administrative) electronically. Healthcare providers include hospitals, long-term care facilities, physicians, and pharmacies.
2. Health plans, which pay for the cost of medical care (for example, a health insurance company).
3. Healthcare clearinghouses, which process claims between a healthcare provider and payer (for example, an intermediary that processes a hospital's claim to Medicare to facilitate payment).

Electronic transactions specified in the act include but are not limited to health claims and encounter information, health plan enrollment and disenrollment, healthcare payment and remittance advice, health plan premium payments, referral certification, and coordination of benefits.

Business Associates

The Privacy Rule also applies to entities that are business associates of HIPAA-covered entities. A business associate (BA) is a person or organization other than a member of a CE's workforce that performs functions or activities on behalf of or for a CE that involves the use or disclosure of PHI. Common BAs include consultants, billing companies, transcription companies, accounting firms, and law firms. ARRA also included in the BA definition patient safety organizations (PSOs), which utilize information to improve the safety and quality of patient care; health information organizations (HIOs); e-prescribing gateways and persons who facilitate data transmissions; as well as personal health record (PHR) vendors who, by contract, enable CEs to offer PHRs to their patients as part of the CE electronic health record (EHR) (HHS 2010, 40872).

A BA's subcontractors are also BAs if they require access to an individual's PHI, regardless of whether an agreement has actually been signed (HHS 2010, 40873). BAs and their subcontractors must comply with certain HIPAA provisions and are subject to the same civil and criminal penalties that CEs face for violating the law. In addition to the Privacy Rule, BAs and their subcontractors must also comply with the HIPAA security provision, which is covered in more detail in chapter 10, *Data Security*.

The Privacy Rule does not allow CEs to disclose PHI to BAs unless the two enter into a written contract, or business associate agreement (BAA), that meets HIPAA and ARRA requirements. However, if a person or organization meets the definition of a BA, they are a BA by law (even if the required agreement has not been signed) and are subject to penalties if they violate HIPAA. The BA may use or disclose PHI once it agrees to the CE's requirements to protect the information's security and confidentiality. The CEs must respond to BA noncompliance, and ARRA requires BAs to respond to CE noncompliance. The BA does this by corrective action or by severing the relationship with the CE.

The BAAs must be HIPAA- and ARRA-compliant. There are components that an agreement between a CE and BA should contain. These are outlined in figure 9.2.

Figure 9.2 Components of a business associate agreement

- Parties to the BAA (CE and BA; BA and subcontractor of BA)
- Purpose of the BAA (compliance with HIPAA and ARRA)
- Definitions (breach; electronic PHI; individual; PHI; law; Secretary of HHS; security incident)
- Obligations and activities of the BA
- Permitted uses and disclosures by BA (or subcontractor)
- Obligations of the CE
- Term and termination
- Indemnity for both parties
- Limitation of liability
- Miscellaneous
- Signatures, titles, contact information

Source: ©AHIMA 2016.

Workforce Members

Both CEs and BAs (including their subcontractors) are responsible under the Privacy Rule for their workforce members. A workforce consists not only of employees, but also volunteers, student interns, trainees, board of directors, and even employees of outsourced vendors who routinely work on-site in the CE's facility.

To illustrate this, examine the following scenario. Tidy Team, a company that contracts with Mercy Hospital to provide janitorial services, employs Ted as a custodial worker. Ted has been assigned to Mercy Hospital. As part of his duties, he routinely cleans the floors and empties the trash in the HIM department. What is Tidy Team's relationship with Mercy Hospital? What is Ted's relationship with Mercy Hospital? Does a BA relationship exist here?

In this example, the hospital contracted Tidy Team to clean, not to use or disclose individually identifiable health information. The fact that Ted is in close proximity to such information on a regular basis does not make him (or Tidy Team) a BA. Because he routinely works in Mercy Hospital's HIM department, however, he should be treated as a workforce member and trained as such.

Protected Health Information

The Privacy Rule safeguards protected health information (PHI). The PHI either identifies an individual or provides a reasonable basis to believe the person could be identified from the information given. PHI can be in any form including electronic, paper, and oral. Determining whether information is PHI or not requires meeting all parts of a three-part test. First, the information must be held or transmitted by a CE or a BA in any of the forms listed previously. Second, it must be individually identifiable health information. To be individually identifiable, the information must either identify the person or provide a reasonable basis to believe the person could be identified from the information. Third, it must relate to a person's past, present, or future physical or mental health condition, the provision of healthcare, or payment for the provision of healthcare. The PHI of deceased persons loses PHI status and is no longer protected by HIPAA after the individual has been deceased more than 50 years.

Deidentified Information

Deidentified information does not identify an individual because personal characteristics have been stripped from it in such a way that it cannot be later constituted or combined to reidentify an individual. Not all patient information is PHI. Deidentified information is not protected by the HIPAA Privacy Rule. Deidentified information is commonly used in research.

Information technology is powerful in assisting with the collection and analysis of data, so it is possible to identify individuals by combining specific data. Therefore, the HIPAA Privacy Rule requires the CE to do one of the following to ensure deidentification:

- The CE can strip certain elements to ensure the patient's information is truly deidentified. These elements are listed in figure 9.3 (Rinehart-Thompson 2018)
- The CE can have an expert apply generally accepted statistical and scientific principles and methods to minimize the risk that the information might be used to identify an individual (Rinehart-Thompson 2018)

Figure 9.4 identifies methods of deidentification that can be used to remove the data elements found in figure 9.3.

Other Basic Concepts

In addition to understanding *to whom* the Privacy Rule applies and *what* it protects, it is important to understand other basic HIPAA concepts, which are discussed in the sections that follow.

Individual

The Privacy Rule defines an individual as the person who is the subject of the PHI (45 CFR 160.103).

Figure 9.3 Data elements to be removed for deidentification of information

Eighteen identifiers must be removed for deidentification. They pertain to the individual, relatives, employers, and household members:	
• Names	• Health plan beneficiary numbers
• Geographic subdivisions smaller than a state, including street addresses, city, county, precinct, and zip code if the geographic unit contains fewer than 20,000 people; the initial three digits of the zip code must be changed to 000 or zip codes with the same three initial digits may be combined to form a unit of more than 20,000 people	• Account numbers • Certificate and license numbers • Vehicle identifiers and serial numbers, including license plate numbers • Device identifiers and serial numbers
• All elements of dates, except the year, directly related to an individual including birth, admission, discharge, and death dates; in addition, all ages over 89 and all elements of dates (including the year) that would identify such age cannot be used, however individuals over 89 can be aggregated into a single category of 90 and over	• Web universal resource locators (URLs) • Internet protocol (IP) address numbers • Biometric identifiers, including fingerprints and voiceprints • Full-face photographic images and any comparable images
• Telephone numbers • Fax numbers • E-mail addresses • Social Security numbers • Health record numbers	• Any other unique identifying number, characteristic, or code except for permissible reidentification to match information back to the person (code must not be derived from or related to information about the individual, cannot be translated to her or her identity, may not be used for any other purpose, and may not disclose the reidentification mechanism)

Source: 45 CFR 164.514(b)(2)(i).

Figure 9.4 HIPAA Privacy Rule De-Identification Methods

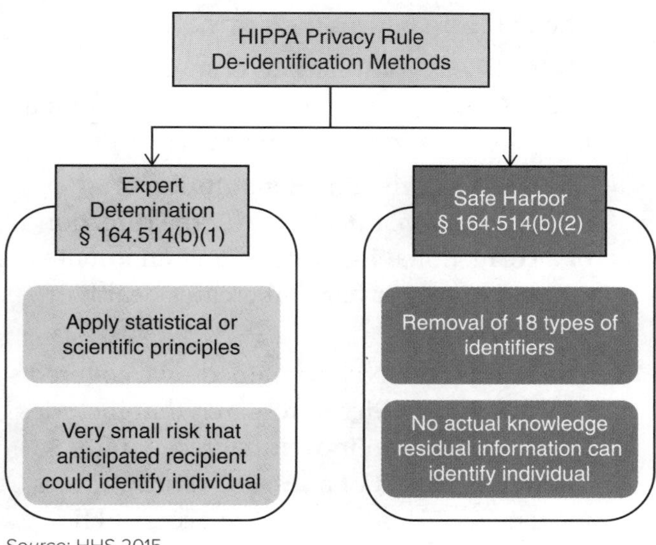

Source: HHS 2015.

Personal Representative

A personal representative is a person who has legal authority to act on another's behalf. Per the Privacy Rule, a personal representative must be treated the same as an individual regarding use and disclosure of the individual's PHI.

Designated Record Set

A designated record set (DRS) includes the health records, billing records, and various claims records that are used to make decisions about an individual (45 CFR 164.501). HIPAA provisions apply to the DRS. The DRS is broader than the legal health record, which was discussed in chapter 8, *Health Law*, because it contains more components than those that would ordinarily be produced upon request.

Minimum Necessary

The minimum necessary standard requires that uses, disclosures, and requests be limited to only the amount needed to accomplish an intended purpose. For example, for payment purposes, only the minimum amount of information necessary to substantiate a claim for payment should be disclosed. The minimum necessary standard does not apply to PHI used, disclosed, or requested for treatment, payment, or operation purposes.

To ensure compliance with the minimum necessary standard, policies and procedures should identify those persons or classes of persons who work for the CE and who need to access PHI to perform their duties. They should further identify what PHI is needed to perform their jobs. For example, employees working in the housekeeping department would not have the same level of access to PHI as a nurse working in critical care.

ARRA has specified that, without final clarification of *minimum necessary*, CEs are to use the limited data set (PHI with certain specified direct identifiers removed) for using or disclosing only minimum necessary information, while reverting back to the *amount needed to accomplish the intended purpose* definition when the limited data set definition is inadequate (AHIMA 2009). For example, decision-making is specific to the CE, which must determine what PHI is reasonably needed to accomplish that particular purpose, given the nature of its business (HHS 2006; reviewed 2013).

Treatment, Payment, and Operations

Treatment, payment, and operations (TPO) is an important concept because the Privacy Rule provides a number of exceptions for PHI that is being used or disclosed for TPO purposes. *Treatment* means providing, coordinating, or managing healthcare or healthcare-related services by one or more healthcare providers. For example, treatment includes caring for patients admitted to the hospital or coming for an appointment with a physician. Treatment also includes healthcare provider consultations and referrals of the patient from one provider to another.

Payment includes activities by a health plan to obtain premiums, billing by healthcare providers or health plans to obtain reimbursement, claims management, claims collection, review of the medical necessity of care, and utilization review.

The Privacy Rule provides a broad list of activities that are healthcare *operations.* They include quality assessment and improvement, case management, review of healthcare professionals' qualifications, insurance contracting, legal and auditing functions, and general business management functions such as providing customer service and conducting due diligence. Operations do not include marketing or fundraising activities.

Individual Rights

There are two key goals to the Privacy Rule: (1) to provide greater privacy protections for one's health information (this also serves to limit access by others) and (2) to provide an individual with greater rights with respect to his or her health information. The Privacy Rule's individual rights further the second goal. The individual rights include right of access, right to request amendment of PHI, right to accounting of disclosures, right to request restrictions of PHI, right to request confidential communications, and right to complain of Privacy Rule violations. These rights are described as follows.

Right of Access

The Privacy Rule's **right of access** allows an individual to inspect and obtain a copy of his or her own PHI contained within a designated record set, such as a health record (45 CFR 164.524). The right of access extends as long as the PHI is maintained, although the Privacy Rule does not require health records be retained for a specified period. There are exceptions to the right of access. For example, **psychotherapy notes**, which are behavioral health notes that document a mental health professional's impressions from private counseling sessions; information compiled in reasonable anticipation of a civil, criminal, or administrative action or proceeding; or PHI subject to the Clinical Laboratory Improvements Act (CLIA) are all exceptions to the right of access. Covered entities with EHRs must make PHI available electronically per individual request if it is readily producible or if the individual requests to send PHI to a designated person or entity electronically (Rinehart-Thompson 2018).

Per the Privacy Rule, there are times when a CE can deny an individual access to PHI. These are described as follows and are generally categorized as *no opportunity to review* or *opportunity to review*.

No Opportunity to Review A CE can deny an individual access to PHI without providing him or her an opportunity to review or appeal the denial in the following situations:

- The PHI is in psychotherapy notes
- The PHI was compiled in reasonable anticipation of, or for use in, civil or criminal litigation or administrative action
- The CE is a correctional institution or provider that has acted under the direction of a correctional institution, and an inmate's request for his or her PHI creates health or safety concerns
- The PHI is created or obtained by a covered healthcare provider in research that includes treatment, and an individual receiving treatment as part of a research study agrees to suspend his or her right to access PHI temporarily, while the study is in progress
- The PHI was obtained from someone other than a healthcare provider under a promise of confidentiality and the access requested would be reasonably likely to reveal the source of the information
- The PHI is contained in records that are subject to the federal Privacy Act (5 USC 552a) if the denial of access under the Privacy Act would meet the requirements of that law
- The PHI is maintained by a CE that is subject to the **Clinical Laboratory Improvement Amendments (CLIA) of 1988**, which regulates the quality of laboratory testing, and CLIA would prohibit access
- The PHI is maintained by a CE exempt from CLIA requirements (Rinehart-Thompson 2018)

The PHI refers to another individual who is not a healthcare provider, and a licensed healthcare professional has concluded from the documentation that the access requested is likely to cause significant harm to that other individual (45 CFR 164.524)

Opportunity to Review In two instances, the Privacy Rule requires a CE to give an individual the right to review a denial of access. These are situations where a licensed healthcare professional determines that access to requested PHI would likely endanger the life or physical safety of the individual or another person or would reasonably endanger the life or physical safety of another person mentioned in the PHI.

When a denial is made, the CE must write the denial in plain language and include a reason. Second, it must explain that the individual has the right to request a review of the denial. Third, it must describe how the individual can complain to the CE and must include the name or title and phone number of the person or office to contact. Finally, it must explain how the individual can lodge a complaint with the secretary of HHS.

The individual has the right to have the denial reviewed by a licensed healthcare professional who did not participate in the original denial and is designated by the CE to act as the reviewing official. The CE must grant or deny access in accordance with the reviewing official's decision.

The Privacy Rule gives individuals the right to request access to their PHI, but the CE may require that requests be in writing. An individual's request for review of PHI must be acted on no later than 30 days after the request is made (or 60 days if the PHI is not on-site). This may be extended once by a maximum of 30 additional days if the individual is given a written statement (within the 30 days) explaining the reasons for the delay and the date by which the CE will respond. A CE must arrange a convenient time and place for an individual to inspect his or her PHI; otherwise, a copy of the PHI must be mailed if requested. The Privacy Rule allows a reasonable cost-based fee when the individual requests a copy of PHI or agrees to accept summary or explanatory information. The fee may include the cost of the following:

- Copying, including supplies and labor of copying
- Postage, when the individual has requested that the PHI be mailed
- Preparing an explanation or summary, if agreed to by the individual (45 CFR 164.524)

The HIPAA does not permit retrieval fees to be charged to patients. However, they are permitted for non-patient requests. If a CE does not wish to calculate actual or average costs for electronic PHI, the **Office for Civil Rights (OCR)**, the federal agency within HHS that is responsible for enforcing the Privacy Rule, recommends a flat fee up to $6.50. Fees cannot be assessed to individuals who access their PHI via a View, Download, and Transmit function of a certified electronic health record (Rinehart-Thompson 2018).

A CE must provide access to the PHI in the format requested if it is readily producible in such form or format. If not, it must be produced in a readable hard-copy form or other format agreed to by the CE and the individual.

The right of access gives the individual the right to obtain his or her own PHI, or to direct a CE to transmit PHI about that individual to a third party without barriers or unreasonable delays. Disclosure to a patient does not require patient authorization using the HIPAA authorization form that is described later in this chapter; however, for validation and record-keeping purposes the CE may require that the request be in writing (Rinehart-Thompson 2018). Certain limits cannot be placed on individuals exercising the right of access. For example, the patient cannot be limited to patient portal information only and cannot be required to physically appear at the CE to receive their PHI (HHS 2016).

The right of access becomes more complex when an individual directs a CE to transmit PHI about the individual to a third party. Oftentimes, these access requests appear to have been initiated by a third party instead of from the individual. As a result, seemingly identical requests may be handled differently (one as a patient access request and one as a third-party request requiring authorization) and fees assessed differently.

Right to Request Amendment of PHI

The Privacy Rule allows an individual the **right to request amendment**. With this right, one may request that a CE amend PHI or a record about the individual in a designated record set (45 CFR 164.526). The CE may deny the request when it determines that the PHI or the health record did not comply with the following:

- Was not created by the CE
- Is not part of the designated record set
- Is not available for inspection as noted in the regulation of access (for example, psychotherapy notes, inmate of a correctional institution, and so on)
- Is accurate or complete as is (45 CFR 164.526)

A CE may require that the amendment request be in writing. The CE may also require the requester to include a rationale for the amendment, as long as the requester was notified in advance that a rationale would be required (usually in the Notice of Privacy Practices, discussed later in this chapter).

An individual's amendment request must be acted on no later than 60 days after receipt by allowing it or denying it in writing. The CE may extend its response once, by 30 days, if it explains the reasons for the delay in a written statement and gives a date by which it will act. If an amendment is granted, the Privacy Rule requires a CE to do the following:

- Identify the documentation in the designated record set that is affected by the amendment, append the information, and supply a link to the amendment's location where applicable. For example, if the diagnosis is incorrect, the amendment will have to appear or be linked to each report in the designated record set
- Inform the individual that the amendment was accepted and have him or her identify the persons with whom the amendment needs to be shared and then obtain his or her agreement to notify those persons. The CE must make reasonable efforts to provide the amendment within a reasonable amount of time to anyone who has received the PHI (45 CFR 164.526)

Denials must be made within 60 days of the request, be written in plain language, and contain the following:

- The basis for the denial
- The individual's right to submit a written statement disagreeing with the denial
- The process by which the individual can submit his or her disagreement
- A statement explaining how, when the individual does not submit a disagreement, he or she may request that both the original amendment request and the CE's denial accompany any future disclosures of the PHI that is the subject of the amendment
- A description of how the individual may complain to the CE, including the name or title and telephone number of the contact person or office (45 CFR 164.526)

The CE can prepare a written rebuttal if the individual submits a disagreement statement, and it must provide the individual with a copy of the rebuttal.

All requests for amendments, denials, the individual's statement of disagreement, and the CE's rebuttal (if one was created) must be appended or linked to the record or PHI that is the subject of the amendment request. Future disclosures of the subject information must include this material or a summary. If a request for amendment was denied and the individual did not write a statement of disagreement, the request for amendment and denial must accompany future disclosures only if the individual requests such action.

Right to Request Accounting of Disclosures

Maintaining some type of accounting procedure for monitoring and tracking PHI disclosures has been a common practice in HIM departments. However, the Privacy Rule has a specific standard with respect to such recordkeeping. Per the right to request accounting of disclosures, an individual has the right to receive an accounting of certain disclosures made by a CE (45 CFR 164.528). The Privacy Rule requires an accounting of all disclosures within the six years prior to the date on which the accounting was requested. A CE may either account for the disclosures of its BAs or require the BAs to make their own accounting.

BAs must respond to accounting requests that are made directly to them.

The types of disclosures that must be accounted for are limited, but include those made erroneously (that is, breaches, which are discussed later in the chapter), for public interest and benefit activities (discussed later in this chapter) where patient authorization is not obtained, and pursuant to a court order. Disclosures for which an accounting is *not* required (that is, exceptions) are the following disclosures:

- For TPO (this exception only applies to CEs without EHRs)
- To individuals to whom the information pertains, or the individual's personal representative
- Incidental to an otherwise permitted or required use or disclosure (for example, a patient's name appears on a sign-in sheet at a physician office; this is a permitted use that may be seen by [disclosed to] the next patient who signs in)
- Pursuant to an authorization
- For use in the facility directory, to persons involved in the individual's care, or for other notification purposes
- To meet national security or intelligence requirements
- To correctional institutions or law enforcement officials
- As part of a limited data set
- That occurred before the compliance date for the CE (45 CFR 164.528) (Rinehart-Thompson 2018)

The definition of healthcare operations is broad, but the Privacy Rule has carved out exceptions to this definition so the following must be included in an accounting of disclosures. For example, mandatory public health reporting is not part of a CE's operations (this includes state requirements to report births [birth certificates]; communicable diseases; and incidents of abuse or suspected abuse of children, mentally disabled individuals, and the elderly). As a result, these must be included in an accounting of disclosures. For example, if a physician's office reports a case of tuberculosis to a public health authority, that disclosure must be included if the patient requests an accounting. If a CE provides PHI to a third-party public health authority to review, but the third party does not actually review it, the third-party's access must be included in an accounting of disclosures.

Disclosure pursuant to a court order (if without a patient's written authorization) is also subject to an accounting of disclosure. However, disclosure pursuant to a subpoena that is accompanied by a patient's written authorization is not subject to an accounting of disclosure because the authorization exempts the disclosure from the accounting of disclosure requirement. The accounting of disclosure requirement includes disclosures made in writing, by telephone, or orally. In some situations, an individual's right to an accounting of disclosure may be suspended at the written request of a health oversight agency or law enforcement official indicating that an accounting of disclosure would impede its activities. This request should specify how long such a suspension is required. The Privacy Rule provides a list of exceptions to the accounting of disclosure requirement, but not disclosures that must be accounted for. An accounting of disclosure must include the following items:

- Date of disclosure
- Name and address (when known) of the entity or person who received the information
- Brief description of the PHI disclosed
- Brief statement of the purpose of the disclosure or a copy of the individual's written authorization or request (45 CFR 164.528)

A CE must act on a request for an accounting of disclosures no later than 60 days after receipt (extended by no more than 30 days if the CE notifies the individual in writing of the reasons for the delay and the date by which the accounting of disclosure will be made available).

The first accounting of disclosure within any 12-month period must be provided to the patient without charge. Additional requests within a 12-month period may be assessed a reasonable, cost-based fee if the individual is informed in advance and given an opportunity to withdraw or modify the request or avoid or reduce the fee.

The Privacy Rule requires that documentation be maintained on all accounting of disclosure requests, including information included in the accounting of disclosure, the written accounting that was provided to the individual, and the titles of persons or offices responsible for receiving and processing requests for an accounting of disclosure. Policies and procedures must be developed to ensure the PHI disclosed from all areas of the CE, likely including departments outside HIM, can be tracked and compiled when an accounting of disclosure request is received.

Right to Request Restrictions of PHI

An individual can request that a CE restrict the uses and disclosures of PHI to carry out TPO (45 CFR 164.522(a)(1)). This is the right to request restrictions of PHI. In almost all cases, a CE can decline a restriction request. However, restriction requests must be complied with (unless otherwise required by law) if the disclosure would be made to a health plan for payment or operations purposes and the individual had paid for the healthcare service or item completely out of pocket (Rinehart-Thompson 2018).

When a CE agrees to a restriction, whether voluntarily or mandated, it must live up to the agreement. To illustrate how difficult this can be, examine the following scenario. A patient, Mr. Smith, agrees to allow a hospital to tell callers that he has been admitted to the hospital and therefore is in the facility directory. Such notification is a hospital operation. However, he requests that this information be restricted and withheld only from his Aunt Mary and Uncle Jack, if they should call. Should the hospital agree to this restriction request? In this scenario, the hospital is not required to agree. In fact, the hospital probably should not agree to this request because of the administrative difficulty of informing certain individuals, but not others, of Mr. Smith's status. There is also the risk of accidentally violating the request. It would be difficult for every receptionist to recall this small restriction, particularly if other patients had similar restrictions on their information. The risk of violation simply becomes too great.

The individual or the CE can terminate a restriction that was agreed upon. When the CE entity initiates termination of the agreement, it must inform the individual that it is doing so. However, the termination is only effective with respect to the PHI created or received after the individual has been informed (45 CFR 164.522(a)(1)).

Right to Request Confidential Communications

Healthcare providers and health plans must give individuals the opportunity to request that communications of PHI be routed to an alternative location or by an alternative method (45 CFR 164.522(b)(1)). This is the right to request confidential communications. Healthcare providers must honor such a request without requiring a reason if it is reasonable. Health plans must honor such a request if it is reasonable and if the requesting individual states that disclosure could pose a safety risk. However, providers and health plans may refuse to accommodate requests if the individual does not provide information as to how payment will be handled or an alternative address or method by which he or she can be contacted.

An example of a request for confidential communications would be a woman who requests that billing information from her psychiatrist, from whom she is seeking treatment because of a domestic violence situation, be sent to her work address instead of to her home.

Right to Complain of Privacy Rule Violations

A CE must provide a process for an individual to file a complaint or allegation about the entity's policies and procedures, its noncompliance with them, or its noncompliance with the Privacy Rule (45 CFR 164.530(d)(1)). The CE's notice of privacy practices, described later in this chapter, must contain contact information at the CE level and inform individuals of the ability to submit complaints to HHS. All complaints must be documented along with corresponding dispositions.

Check Your Understanding 9.1

Answer the following questions

1. The right of privacy:
   a. Has been granted by the US Constitution
   b. Has been granted via court decisions
   c. Does not apply to health information
   d. Does not exist
2. One state's law protects the privacy of health information to a greater extent than HIPAA does.
   a. The state law will be preempted by HIPAA
   b. The state law is invalid because it does not provide the same level of protection as HIPAA
   c. The state law may supersede HIPAA
   d. The state's law must be consistent with HIPAA
3. Julie wants to review her health records, but she is asking about the Privacy Rule's requirements pertaining to record retention. HIPAA establishes that a patient has the right of access to inspect and obtain a copy of her PHI:
   a. For as long as it is maintained
   b. For six years
   c. Forever
   d. For 12 months
4. HIPAA regulations:
   a. Never preempt state statutes
   b. Always preempt state statutes
   c. Preempt less strict state statutes where they exist
   d. Preempt stricter state statutes where they exist
5. The Privacy Rule applies to:
   a. Healthcare providers only
   b. Only healthcare providers that receive Medicare reimbursement
   c. Only entities funded by the federal government
   d. Covered entities and their business associates
6. The Privacy Rule extends to protected health information:
   a. In any form or medium, except paper and oral forms
   b. In any form or medium, including paper and oral forms
   c. That pertains to mental health treatment only
   d. That exists in electronic form only
7. Bob is exercising his HIPAA right to request confidential communications of both Memorial Hospital and TruePlus, his health plan. When asked by both entities how he will handle payments, he declines to provide them with any information. As a result:
   a. TruePlus must still honor the request
   b. Only Memorial Hospital may deny the request
   c. Memorial Hospital must still honor the request
   d. Both Memorial Hospital and TruePlus may deny his request
8. Elizabeth has requested a copy of her PHI from Memorial Hospital. Which of the following is acceptable for Memorial Hospital to charge Elizabeth?
   a. A reasonable cost-based fee
   b. It may not charge Elizabeth at all
   c. It may impose any fee authorized by state statute
   d. It can charge only for the cost of the paper on which the information is printed

9. Business associate agreements are developed to cover the use of PHI by:
   a. The covered entity's employees
   b. Organizations outside the covered entity's workforce that use PHI to perform functions on behalf of the covered entity
   c. The covered entity's entire workforce
   d. The covered entity's janitorial staff
10. The term *minimum necessary* means that healthcare providers and other covered entities must limit use, access, and disclosure to the least amount to:
   a. Retain records needed for patient care
   b. Accomplish the intended purpose
   c. Treat an individual
   d. Perform research
11. DataSource is a business associate of Davis Health System. An individual who was a patient in the Davis Health System contacts DataSource, requesting an accounting of disclosures and stating that this is his right per the HIPAA Privacy Rule. DataSource:
   a. Does not have to respond to the patient because it is not a covered entity
   b. May refer the request to Davis Health System
   c. Does not have to respond to the patient because this is not a HIPAA individual right
   d. Must respond to the patient and provide an accounting of disclosures
12. Deidentified information:
   a. Does not identify an individual
   b. Is information from which only a person's name has been stripped
   c. Can be constituted later or combined to reidentify an individual
   d. Is subject to the HIPAA Privacy Rule

HIPAA Privacy Rule Documents

The Privacy Rule outlines three key documents that inform patients and give them a degree of control over their PHI. The notice of privacy practices and the authorization—are required, whereas the HIPAA consent to use or disclose PHI is optional.

Notice of Privacy Practices

Except for certain exceptions for health plans and inmates in correctional facilities, an individual has the right to a notice explaining how his or her PHI will be used and disclosed (45 CFR 164.520). This **notice of privacy practices** must also explain in plain language the patient's rights and the CE's legal duties with respect to PHI.

Healthcare providers with a direct treatment relationship with an individual must provide the notice of privacy practices by the first service delivery date (for example, first visit to a physician's office, first admission to a hospital, or first encounter at a clinic), including service delivered electronically. Notices must be available at the site where the individual is treated and must be posted in a prominent place where patients can reasonably be expected to read them. If the CE has a website with information about their services and benefits, the notice of privacy practices must be prominently posted to it. The notice of privacy practices must be updated to reflect material changes. It must state that uses and disclosures not described in the notice will require an authorization. It must also address marketing and the right to opt out of fundraising communications (both of which are explained later in this chapter). A CE's obligation to comply with a restriction request if the item or service is paid in full out-of-pocket must also be included in the notice. AHIMA outlines the requirements for the content of the notice of privacy practices (McLendon and Rose 2013). In general, the notice is to include the following:

1. A header such as: "this notice describes how information about you may be used and disclosed and how you can get access to this information. Please review it carefully"
2. A description, including at least one example of the types of uses and disclosures that the CE is permitted to make for treatment, payment, and healthcare operations
3. A description of each of the other purposes for which the CE is permitted or required to use or disclose PHI without the individual's written consent or authorization
4. A statement that other uses and disclosures will be made only with the individual's written authorization and that the individual may revoke such authorization
5. When applicable, separate statements that the CE may contact the individual to provide appointment reminders or information about treatment alternatives and other health-related benefits and services that may be of interest to the individual
6. A statement indicating that most uses and disclosures of psychotherapy notes (where appropriate), uses and disclosures of protected health information for marketing purposes, and disclosures that constitute a sale of protected health information require authorization. CEs that do not record or maintain psychotherapy notes are not required to include a statement
7. A statement regarding fundraising communications and an individual's right to opt out of receiving such communications, if a CE intends to contact an individual to raise funds for the CE. If a CE does not make fundraising communications, then this statement does not need to be included
8. For health plans that perform underwriting activities only, a statement must be included indicating the health plan is prohibited from using or disclosing genetic information for underwriting purposes
9. A statement of the individual's rights with respect to PHI and a brief description of how the individual may exercise these rights including:
   a. The right to request restrictions on certain uses and disclosures as provided by 45 CFR 164.522(a)(1), including a statement that the CE is not required to agree to a requested restriction
   b. For healthcare providers only, a statement indicating the right to restrict certain disclosures of PHI to a health plan when the individual pays out of pocket in full for the healthcare item or service
   c. The right to receive confidential communications of PHI
   d. The right to access, inspect, and receive a copy of PHI on paper, including the right to have electronic copies if kept in electronic form
   e. The right to request electronic copies of PHI be forwarded to a third party
   f. The right to request an amendment of PHI
   g. The right to receive an accounting of disclosures
   h. The right to be notified of the CE's privacy practices
   i. The right to control PHI use for marketing, sales, and research
   j. The right to be notified of a breach to PHI
   k. The right to file complaints with the Office for Civil Rights
10. A statement that the CE is required by law to maintain the privacy of PHI and to provide individuals with a notice of its legal duties and privacy practices with respect to PHI
11. A statement that the CE is required to abide by the terms of the notice currently in effect
12. A statement that the CE reserves the right to change the terms of its notice and to make the new notice provisions effective for all PHI that it maintains
13. A statement describing how the CE will provide individuals with a revised notice
14. A statement that individuals may complain to the CE and to the Secretary of Health and Human Services if they believe their privacy rights have been violated; a brief description of how one files a complaint with the CE; and a statement that the individual will not

be retaliated against for filing a complaint. Include contact information

15. The name or title and the telephone number of a person or office to contact for further information
16. An effective date, which may not be earlier than the date on which the notice is printed or otherwise published

Consent to Use or Disclose PHI

Under the Privacy Rule healthcare providers are not required to obtain **HIPAA consent**, which is the patient's agreement to use or disclose individually identifiable information for TPO (45 CFR 164.506(b)). However, some healthcare providers obtain consents as a matter of policy. Except for special circumstances such as emergencies (discussed in this section), the HIPAA consent is usually obtained at the time care is provided and has no expiration date. However, the individual can revoke the HIPAA consent as long as the revocation is in writing. HIPAA consents should be written in plain language. The CE must document and retain signed HIPAA consents and revocations. A sample HIPAA consent is provided in figure 9.5.

Figure 9.5 Sample HIPAA consent for the use or disclosure of individually identifiable health information

Consent to the Use and Disclosure of Health Information
for Treatment, Payment, or Healthcare Operations

I understand that as part of my healthcare, this organization originates and maintains health records describing my health history, symptoms, examination and test results, diagnoses, treatment, and any plans for future care or treatment. I understand that this information serves as:

- A basis for planning my care and treatment
- A means of communication among the many health professionals who contribute to my care
- A source of information for applying my diagnosis and surgical information to my bill
- A means by which a third-party payer can verify that services billed were actually provided
- A tool for routine healthcare operations such as assessing quality and reviewing the competence of healthcare professionals

I understand and have been provided with a Notice of Information Practices that provides a more complete description of information uses and disclosures. I understand that I have the right to review the notice prior to signing this consent. I understand that the organization reserves the right to change its notice and practices and prior to implementation will mail a copy of any revised notice to the address I've provided. I understand that I have the right to object to the use of my health information for directory purposes. I understand that I have the right to request restrictions as to how my health information may be used or disclosed to carry out treatment, payment, or healthcare operations and that the organization is not required to agree to the restrictions requested. I understand that I may revoke this consent in writing, except to the extent that the organization has already taken action in reliance thereon. Therefore, I consent to the use and disclosure of my healthcare information.

☐ I request the following restrictions to the use or disclosure of my health information.

Signature of Patient or Legal Representative

____

Witness ______________________________

Date Notice Effective ______________________________

Date or Version ______________________________

☐ **Accepted** ☐ **Denied**

Signature ______________________________

Title ______________________________

Date ______________________________

Source: HHS 2000. 82818.

Authorization

Written authorization by an individual, granting permission for a specific use or disclosure of his or her health information, is a longstanding legal requirement and health information practice. However, the authorization is a key component of the Privacy Rule. As a general requirement, the Privacy Rule states that an authorization for uses and disclosures must be obtained from an individual (45 CFR 164.508). However, there are a number of exceptions, outlined later in this chapter.

Authorizations are always required for the use or disclosure of psychotherapy notes except to carry out TPO; for treatment by the originator of the notes; in mental health training programs by the CE; to defend a legal action or other proceeding brought by the individual; or for oversight of the originator of the notes (45 CFR 164.508(a)). The Privacy Rule also provides other specifications for authorization, including those requested by a CE for its own uses and disclosures and those requested for disclosures by others. This section of the Privacy Rule also generally prohibits requiring an authorization as a condition of treatment and allows authorizations to be combined only in certain situations (45 CFR 164.508).

The Privacy Rule requires that authorizations be obtained for uses and disclosures of PHI in research unless the CE obtains documentation that an Institutional Review Board (IRB) or privacy board has approved an alteration or waiver. Where authorizations are required, the Privacy Rule requires that the authorization contain the required core elements, which are described later in this chapter.

An individual may revoke an authorization at any time if it is in writing. However, revocation does not apply to disclosures that have already been made. CEs must document and retain signed authorizations and revocations and must permit individuals to review what was disclosed pursuant to authorizations.

Table 9.1 outlines differences among the three key Privacy Rule documents discussed in this section.

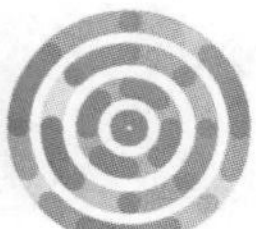

Uses and Disclosures of Health Information: Authorization and Patient Right of Access

As table 9.2 shows, PHI may not be used or disclosed by a CE unless the individual who is the subject of the information authorizes the use or disclosure in writing or the Privacy Rule *requires or permits* such use or disclosure without the individual's written authorization. The Privacy

Table 9.1 Differences among notice of privacy practices, consent, and authorization

	Notice of privacy practices	Consent	Authorization
Required?	Required by HIPAA	Optional	Required by HIPAA
Requirements regarding TPO	Must explain TPO uses and disclosures, along with other types of uses and disclosures	Only obtains patient permission to use or disclose PHI for TPO purposes	Is used to obtain for a number of types of uses and disclosures, although it not required for TPO uses and disclosures
PHI this document addresses	Provides prospective and general information about how PHI might be used or disclosed in the future (and includes information that may not have been created yet)	Provides prospective and general information about how PHI might be used or disclosed in the future for TPO purposes (and includes information that may not have been created yet)	Obtains patient permission to use or disclose specific information that generally has already been created and for which there is a specific need
Required for treatment?	May not refuse to treat an individual because he or she declines to sign this form	May condition treatment on individual signing this form	May not refuse to treat an individual because he or she declines to sign this form
Time limit on document validity	No time limit on validity of the document	No time limit on validity of the document	Time limit on validity of document (specified by an expiration date or event)

Source: Adapted from Rinehart-Thompson 2018.

Table 9.2. Authorization requirements for use and disclosure of PHI

I. Patient authorization required:
All situations except those listed in Part II

II. Patient authorization not required:

A. When use or disclosure is required, even without patient authorization

- When the individual/patient or individual's/patient's personal representative requests access or accounting of disclosures (with exceptions)
- HHS investigation, review, or enforcement action

B. When use or disclosure is permitted, even without patient authorization

- Patient has opportunity to informally agree or object
  - Facility directory
  - Notification of relatives and friends
- Patient does not have opportunity to agree or object
  - Public interest and benefit
    1. As required by law
    2. For public health activities
    3. To disclose PHI regarding victims of abuse, neglect, domestic violence
    4. For health oversight activities
    5. For judicial and administrative proceedings
    6. For law enforcement purposes (six specific situations)
    7. Regarding decedents
    8. For cadaveric organ, eye, or tissue donation
    9. For research, with limitations
    10. To prevent or lessen serious threat to health or safety
    11. For essential government functions
    12. For workmen's compensation
  - Situations other than public interest and benefit
    13. TPO
    14. To the individual/patient
    15. Incidental disclosures
    16. Limited data set

Source: Rinehart-Thompson 2018.

Rule *requires* such use or disclosure in only two situations: when the individual or individual's personal representative requests access to or an accounting of disclosures of the PHI (with the exceptions detailed earlier in this chapter), and when HHS is conducting an investigation, review, or enforcement action.

In addition to the two situations where use or disclosure is *required* without the individual's written authorization (section II.A of table 9.2), there are many situations where the Privacy Rule *permits* a CE to use or disclose PHI without an individual's written authorization (45 CFR 164.510 and 164.512). These exceptions to the patient authorization requirement are summarized in section B of table 9.2.

Patient Has Opportunity to Agree or Object

As listed in table 9.2 (section II.B), the Privacy Rule lists two circumstances where PHI can be used or disclosed without the individual's written authorization, although the individual must be informed in advance and given an opportunity to informally agree or object (45 CFR 164.510). In both circumstances, the CE may inform the individual verbally and obtain his or her verbal agreement or objection.

The first circumstance is when the healthcare organization maintains a facility directory of patients for persons who ask for individuals by name, and for clergy. The information may include the patient's name, location in the healthcare organization (room number), condition described in general terms (such as critical or stable), and religious affiliation. Disclosure of an individual's religious affiliation is limited to members of the clergy.

The CE must inform the patient of the information to be included in the facility directory and to whom information may be disclosed. The patient must have the opportunity to prohibit all uses or disclosures from the facility directory or request restrictions of some of the uses and disclosures.

When it is not possible to get the patient's agreement (for example, in emergencies), the CE can use and disclose PHI in the facility directory if the disclosure is consistent with the prior expressed preference of the patient or if the CE believes it is in the patient's best interest. When it becomes possible after the emergency situation, the CE must inform the patient and give him or her the opportunity to object to use and disclosure from the facility directory.

The second circumstance is disclosing, to a family member or a close friend, PHI that is directly relevant to his or her involvement in the patient's care or payment. The patient's written authorization is not required but verbal agreement is, if it can be obtained. Likewise, a CE may disclose PHI, including the patient's location, general condition, or death, to notify or assist in the notification of a family member, personal representative, or some other person responsible for the patient's care (45 CFR 164.510(b)). It must be reasonably inferred from the circumstances that the patient does not object to the disclosure.

The CE may also use or disclose PHI to a public or private entity authorized by law or by its charter to assist in disaster relief efforts.

Patient Does Not Have Opportunity to Agree or Object

There are 16 circumstances where PHI can be used or disclosed without an individual's authorization, and the individual does not have the opportunity to agree or object. The first 12 circumstances are sometimes referred to as public interest and benefit circumstances because they are of benefit to society (45 CFR 164.512). Although the Privacy Rule permits the 12 public interest and benefit uses or disclosures without an individual's authorization, if it would violate a state law that otherwise protects the patient's information, the information cannot be legally used or disclosed. This is because, as a general rule, the Privacy Rule does not preempt state laws that provide a greater level of privacy protection.

A use or disclosure may meet more than one of the following 12 public interest and benefit situations:

1. *As required by law*. Disclosures are permitted when required by laws that meet the public-interest requirements of disclosures relating to victims of abuse, neglect, or domestic violence, judicial and administrative proceedings, and law enforcement purposes (45 CFR 164.512(a)).
2. *Public health activities*. These include preventing or controlling diseases, injuries, and disabilities, and reporting disease, injury, and vital events such as births and deaths. Examples include the reporting of adverse events or product defects to comply with US Food and Drug Administration (FDA) regulations and, when authorized by law, reporting a person who may have been exposed to a communicable disease and may be at risk for contracting or spreading it (45 CFR 164.512(b)). Disclosure of students' immunization records may be considered a public health disclosure. Where applicable law requires that a school obtain a student's authorization records prior to enrollment, authorization is not required for the information to be disclosed to the school. An oral agreement from the student's legal guardian or the student (if age of majority has been reached) is, however, still required.
3. *Victims of abuse, neglect, or domestic violence*. An example is the reporting to authorities authorized by law to receive information about child or other abuse or neglect. In non–child abuse situations, the Privacy Rule requires the CE to promptly inform the individual or personal representative that a report has been or will be made unless it believes that doing so would place the individual at risk of serious harm or not be in his or her best interest (such as informing the personal representative, who is believed to be responsible for the abuse, neglect, or other injury) (45 CFR 164.512(c)).
4. *Healthcare oversight activities*. An authorized health oversight agency may receive PHI for activities authorized by law such as audits,

civil or criminal investigations, licensure, and other inspections (45 CFR 164.512(d)).

5. *Judicial and administrative proceedings*. Disclosures of specified PHI are permitted in response to a court order or an administrative agency order. For subpoenas and discovery requests, the party seeking the PHI must assure the CE that it has made reasonable efforts to make the request known to the subject individual. The CE also must be assured that the time for the individual to raise objections to the court or administrative agency has elapsed and that either no objections have been filed, all objections have been resolved, or a qualified protective order has been secured (45 CFR 164.512(e)).
6. *Law enforcement purposes*. The Privacy Rule specifies six instances when disclosures to law enforcement do not require patient authorization or the patient has no opportunity to agree or object:
   - Pursuant to legal process or otherwise required by law: Examples of legal process include a court order, a court-ordered warrant, or a subpoena or a summons issued by a judicial officer. An example of "otherwise required by law" is a state law that requires certain types of wounds or other physical injuries to be reported to law enforcement.
   - In response to a law enforcement official's request for the purpose of identifying or locating a suspect, fugitive, material witness, or missing person. Only the following may be disclosed: name and address, date and place of birth, Social Security number, ABO blood type and Rh factor, type of injury, date and time of treatment, date and time of death (if applicable), and description of distinguishing physical characteristics including height, weight, gender, race, hair and eye color, and presence or absence of facial scars or tattoos.
   - In response to a law enforcement official's request about an individual who is, or is suspected to be, a victim of a crime (when the individual agrees to the disclosure or when the CE is unable to obtain the individual's agreement because of incapacity or other emergency circumstance). The law enforcement official must show the information is needed to determine whether a violation of law has occurred, that immediate law enforcement activity depends on the disclosure, and that disclosure is in the best interest of the individual as determined by the CE.
   - About a deceased individual when the CE suspects that the death may have resulted from criminal conduct.
   - To a law enforcement official when the CE believes in good faith that the information constitutes evidence of criminal conduct that occurred on the CE's premises.
   - To a law enforcement official in response to a medical emergency when the CE believes that disclosure is necessary to alert law enforcement to the commission and nature of a crime, the location or victims of such crime, and the identity, description, and location of the perpetrator of such crime. Further, it is permitted when the CE believes the medical emergency was the result of abuse, neglect, or domestic violence (45 CFR 164.512(f)).
7. *Decedents*. Disclosures to a coroner or medical examiner are permitted to identify a deceased person, determine a cause of death, or for other purposes required by law. In accordance with applicable law, disclosures to funeral directors are permitted, as necessary, to allow them to carry out their duties with respect to the decedent. This type of information also may be disclosed in reasonable anticipation of an individual's death (45 CFR 164.512(g)).
8. *Cadaveric organ, eye, or tissue donation*. PHI may be disclosed to organ procurement agencies or other entities to facilitate procurement, banking, or transplantation of cadaveric organs, eyes, or tissue (45 CFR 164.512(h)).

9. *Research*. Authorizations for the use of PHI in research are required except where an IRB or privacy board alters or waives the authorization requirement (in whole or in part) and documents it (45 CFR 164.512(i)). Table 9.3 provides a detailed analysis of the responsibilities of both the IRB and the researcher under the Privacy Rule requirements. A CE may combine conditioned authorizations (that is, those that condition research-related treatment upon research participation) and unconditioned authorizations (that is, those that do not condition research-related treatment upon research participation) as long as the conditioned and unconditioned components are clearly distinguished and the individual is able to opt in to the unconditioned research

Table 9.3 Actions required for use of PHI in research

Type of Information	IRB	Researcher	Research subject (patient or decedent)
PHI preparatory to research	None*	Representation that use is solely and necessary for research and will not be removed from covered entity	None
Deidentified health information	None*	Removal of safe-harbor data or statistical assurance of deidentification	None
Limited data set	None*	Removal of direct identifiers and data use agreement	None
Individually identifiable health information on decedents	None*	Representation that use is solely and necessary for research on decedents and documentation of death upon request of covered entity	None
PHI of human subjects (whether research is interventional or record review)	Waive authorization requirement if determined that risk to privacy is minimal	Representation that: 1. Privacy risk is minimal based on: • Plan to protect identifiers • Plan to destroy identifiers unless there is a health or research reason to retain • Written assurance that PHI will not be reused or redisclosed 2. Research requires use of specifically described PHI 3. Justify the waiver 4. Obtain IRB approval under normal or expedited review procedures	None
	Approve alteration of authorization (for example, to restrict patient's access during study) if determined that risk to privacy is minimal	Same as above	Sign altered authorization form
	Approve research protocol ensuring that there is an authorization for use either combined with consent for and disclosure of PHI research or separate		Sign authorization combined with consent for research or sign standard authorization for use and disclosure of PHI for research as described in authorization

* There may be requirements imposed by the IRB, but there are none imposed by HIPAA.

Source: Amatayakul 2003.

activities (HHS 2018a). This provision does not apply to psychotherapy notes (Rinehart-Thompson 2018).

10. *Threat to health and safety*: Use or disclosure is allowed if thought necessary to prevent or lessen a serious and imminent threat to the health or safety of an individual or the public. Disclosure must be made to a person who can reasonably prevent or lessen the threat. Disclosures are permissible when law enforcement officials must apprehend an individual who may have caused harm to the victim being treated or when the individual appears to have escaped from a correctional institution or lawful custody. For correctional institutions or a law enforcement official who has lawful custody of an inmate, the Privacy Rule allows disclosures if the institution states that the information is necessary to provide continuing healthcare; to secure the health and safety of the individual or other inmates, officers, employees, transportation personnel, or law enforcement on the premises; or to ensure the administration and maintenance of the institution's safety, security, and good order (45 CFR 164.512(j)).
11. *Specialized government functions*: These include information regarding armed forces personnel for military and veteran's activities, for purposes of national security and intelligence activities, for protective services for the President of the United States and others, and for public benefits and medical suitability determinations (45 CFR 164.512(k)).
12. *Workers' compensation*: The Privacy Rule permits the disclosure of PHI relating to work-related illness or injury or a workplace-related medical surveillance if the disclosure complies with workers' compensation laws (45 CFR section 164.512(l)).

The remaining four types of uses and disclosures that do not require patient authorization or an opportunity for the patient to agree or object are TPO; disclosure to the subject individual; incidental disclosures; and limited data set. The first two were addressed earlier in this chapter; the remaining two are explained as the following:

- *Incidental uses or disclosures* occur as part of a permitted use or disclosure (CFR 164.502(a)(1)(iii)). For example, calling out patients' names in a physician office is an incidental disclosure because it occurs as part of office operations. It is permitted as long as the information disclosed is the minimum necessary (for example, the patient's name with no diagnostic information).
- A *limited data set* is PHI that excludes direct identifiers of the individual, the individual's relatives, employers, or household members without completely deidentifying them (45 CFR 164.514(e)(2)). Restrictions are lifted for items such as ages and dates, and parts of geographic subdivisions that are deemed not too specific (for example, city, state, or zip code) (Rinehart-Thompson 2018). Such PHI may be used or disclosed, provided it is used or disclosed only for research, public health, or healthcare operations.

Table 9.4 outlines the differences between the HIPAA authorization versus the patient's right of access.

Check Your Understanding 9.2

Answer the following questions.

1. Notices of privacy practices must be available at the site where the individual is treated and:
   a. Must be posted next to the entrance
   b. Must be posted in a prominent place where it is reasonable to expect that patients will read them
   c. May be posted anywhere at the site
   d. Do not have to be posted at the site

2. Janice is a well-informed patient. She knows that the Privacy Rule requires that individuals be able to:
   a. Be granted all requested restrictions on uses and disclosures of PHI
   b. Be granted all requested amendments to their PHI
   c. Receive a copy of the notice of privacy practices
   d. Receive free copies of their protected health information

3. Treatment of an individual can be conditioned on the signing of the:
   a. Authorization
   b. HIPAA consent
   c. Notice of privacy practices
   d. Research waiver

4. Which of the following describes HIPAA consents?
   a. They are the same as authorizations.
   b. They expire 60 days after they are executed.
   c. They are required under the Privacy Rule.
   d. They are not required to permit use and disclosure of PHI for treatment, payment, or operations.

5. Jill's information is included in the facility directory. This listing:
   a. Could occur only with Jill's written authorization
   b. Is automatic upon Jill's admission to the hospital
   c. Is present because Jill informally agreed to it
   d. Includes all PHI in Jill's designated record set

6. Per the opportunity to verbally agree or object:
   a. A patient may disallow information to be sent to his or her health plan for payment purposes
   b. A hospital may communicate with family members involved in the patient's care
   c. A patient may verbally revoke an authorization
   d. A hospital may disclose PHI to law enforcement

7. A funeral home is contacted to retrieve a patient's body. This contact and disclosure of information about the decedent is:
   a. A public interest and benefit exception to the authorization requirement
   b. Only permissible if the decedent's next of kin has given written authorization for information about the decedent to be disclosed to the funeral home
   c. A violation of the HIPAA Privacy Rule
   d. Subject to a HIPAA consent by the next of kin

8. Release of birth and death information to public health authorities:
   a. Is prohibited without patient consent
   b. Is prohibited without patient authorization
   c. Is a public interest and benefit disclosure that does not require patient authorization
   d. Requires both patient consent and authorization

9. An individual's authorization for research purposes:
   a. Is always required
   b. Is not required if the research involves a clinical trial
   c. Is never required
   d. Is not required if an IRB or privacy board alters or waives the authorization requirement

10. A nurse called Dee by her first name in a physician's office when Dee was to be seen by the physician. This was:
   a. An incidental disclosure
   b. Not subject to the minimum necessary requirement
   c. A disclosure for payment purposes
   d. An automatic violation of the Privacy Rule

Table 9.4 HIPAA authorization vs. right of access

HIPAA Authorization	Right of Access
Permits, but does not require, a covered entity to disclose PHI	**Requires** a covered entity to disclose PHI, except where an exception applies
Requires a number of elements and statements, which include a description of who is authorized to make the disclosure and receive the PHI, a specific and meaningful description of the PHI, a description of the purpose of the disclosure, an expiration date or event, signature of the individual authorizing the use or disclosure of his or her own PHI and the date, information concerning the individual's right to revoke the authorization, and information about the ability or inability to condition treatment, payment, enrollment, or eligibility for benefits on the authorization.	Must be in writing, signed by the individual, and clearly identify the designated person and where to send the PHI
No timeliness requirement for disclosing the PHI; Reasonable safeguards apply (for example, PHI must be sent securely)	Covered entity must act on request no later than 30 days after the request is received
Reasonable safeguards apply (for example, PHI must be sent securely)	Reasonable safeguards apply, including a requirement to send securely; however, individual can request transmission by unsecure medium
No limitations on fees that may be charged to the person requesting the PHI; however, if the disclosure constitutes a sale of PHI, the authorization must disclose the fact of remuneration	Fees limited as provided in 45 CFR 164.524

Source: HHS 2016.

Breach Notification

As originally implemented, the Privacy Rule required CEs to mitigate (lessen the harmful effect) of the wrongful use or disclosure of PHI as much as possible. However, notification to the individual was optional (Rinehart-Thompson 2018). This changed with ARRA, which defined a breach. ARRA also added **breach notification** requirements that specify victims of breaches be notified and, depending on the number of individuals affected, the federal government and media outlets also be notified. CEs and BAs are subject to HHS-issued breach notification regulations, and non-covered entities and non-BAs (including PHR vendors) are subject to breach notification regulations issued by the **Federal Trade Commission (FTC)**. The FTC is a federal agency that promotes consumer protection.

Definition of Breach

A **breach** is an "unauthorized acquisition, access, use or disclosure of PHI that compromises the security or privacy of such information" (Rinehart-Thompson 2018). There are three exceptions to the breach definition:

1. Unintentional acquisitions made in good faith and within the scope of authority
2. Disclosures where the recipient would not reasonably be able to retain the information
3. Disclosures by a person authorized to access PHI to another authorized person at the CE or BA (Rinehart-Thompson 2018)

A breach should be presumed following an impermissible use or disclosure unless the CE or BA demonstrates a low probability that the PHI has been compromised (Rinehart-Thompson 2018). A four-factor risk assessment is used to determine whether PHI has been compromised:

1. Nature and extent of PHI involved, including types of identifiers involved and how likely it is that reidentification can occur
2. Who the unauthorized recipient of the PHI was
3. Whether the PHI was actually obtained or viewed
4. Degree to which the CE or BA mitigated the risk (for example, immediate destruction of the PHI) (HHS 2013)

Breach notification requirements apply only to unsecured PHI that technology has not made unusable, unreadable, or indecipherable to unauthorized persons (Rinehart-Thompson 2018). This PHI is considered to be most at risk. Using the breach definition, list of exceptions, and four-factor risk assessment, covered entities must identify whether incidents are to be reported. Further, per their agreements, BAs must notify CEs of breaches. Finally, all workforce members must be educated to notify the appropriate contact person within the CE when they learn of a breach so the required notifications can be made.

Notification Requirements

Breaches by CEs and BAs (both are governed by HHS breach notification regulations) are deemed discovered when the breach is first known or reasonably should have been known. All individuals whose information has been breached must be notified without unreasonable delay, and not more than 60 days, by first-class mail or a faster method such as by telephone if there is the potential for imminent misuse. If 500 or more individuals are affected, they must be individually notified immediately, and media outlets must be used as a notification mechanism as well. The Secretary of HHS must specifically be notified of the breach (Rinehart-Thompson 2018). All breaches affecting fewer than 500 people must be logged by the CE in an HHS online reporting system and submitted annually as a report not later than 60 days after the end of the calendar year (Rinehart-Thompson 2018).

Individuals who are notified that their PHI has been breached must be given a description of what occurred (including date of breach and date that breach was discovered); the types of unsecured PHI that were involved (such as name, Social Security number, date of birth, home address, account number); steps that the individual may take to protect himself or herself; what the CE is doing to investigate, mitigate, and prevent future occurrences; and contact information for the individual to ask questions and receive updates.

Companion breach notification regulations by the FTC provide protection to individuals whose information has been breached by non-covered entities and non-BAs that are PHR vendors, third-party service providers of PHR vendors, or other non-HIPAA covered entities or BAs that are affiliated with PHR vendors (Rinehart-Thompson 2018). In addition to notifying the individuals affected by the breach, these entities must also notify the FTC of the breach. Third-party PHR service providers shall notify the PHR vendor or entity of the breach. Other notification requirements, such as the content and nature of breach notices, parallel HHS requirements (Rinehart-Thompson 2018).

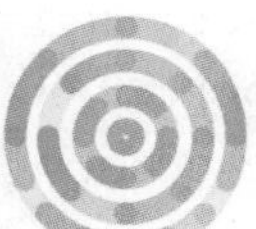

Requirements Related to Commercial Uses: Marketing, Sale of Information, and Fundraising

The Privacy Rule defines marketing as communication about a product or service that encourages the recipient to purchase or use that product or service (45 CFR 164.501). PHI use or disclosure for marketing requires an authorization from the individual except in certain cases. The following marketing activities do not require authorization:

- Occur face to face between the CE and the individual, or
- Concern a promotional gift of nominal value provided by the CE

Some activities look like marketing but do not meet the Privacy Rule's definition of marketing. As a result, no authorization is required for the following:

- Communications to describe health-related products and services provided by, or included in the plan of benefits of, the CE itself or a third party
- Communication for treatment of the individual
- Case management or care coordination for the individual, or to direct or recommend

alternative treatments, therapies, healthcare providers, or care settings (45 CFR 164.501)

Unless a communication fits one of the above categories, authorization is required.

Uses and disclosures for healthcare operations do not require authorization. The categories here are not healthcare operations (even if they otherwise meet the definition) if the CE was paid for making the communication. There are exceptions, however. If a communication describes a currently prescribed drug, if the payment was reasonable (and the CE made the communication and received an authorization from the recipient), or the communication was made by a BA on behalf of a CE and is consistent with a BAA, then the communication will be considered a healthcare operation despite payment (AHIMA 2009). If the CE has received—or will receive—direct or indirect payment in exchange for making a communication to an outside entity, this must be prominently stated.

In addition, when the communication is directed toward a specific target audience (for example, not a broad spectrum or cross-section of patients), it must instruct individuals how to opt out of future communications.

If a CE uses PHI to target an individual or group based on health status or condition, it must determine that the product or service being marketed may benefit the health of the type of individual being targeted before it makes the communication. Then, the communication must explain why the individual has been targeted and how the product or service relates to his or her health.

Related to the concept of marketing is the sale of information. A CE or BA is prohibited from selling (receiving direct or indirect compensation in exchange for) an individual's PHI without that individual's authorization. The authorization must also state whether the individual permits the recipient of the PHI to further exchange the PHI for compensation. Exceptions to this prohibition include public health and research data, treatment, and healthcare operations to a BA pursuant to a BAA, to an individual who is receiving a copy of his or her own PHI, and for other exchanges deemed by the Secretary of HHS to be permissible (Rinehart-Thompson 2018).

For fundraising activities that benefit the CE, the CE entity may use or disclose to a BA or an institutionally related foundation, without authorization, demographic information (name, address or other contact information, age, date of birth, gender); dates of healthcare services provided to the individual; department of service (for example, urology); treating physician; health insurance information; and outcome information (45 CFR 164.514(f)). However, the CE must inform individuals in its notice of privacy practices that PHI may be used for this purpose. It must also include in its fundraising materials instructions on how to opt out of receiving materials in the future. If a fundraising activity targets individual based on diagnosis (for example, patients with kidney disease are solicited in a capital campaign for a new kidney dialysis center), prior authorization is required. Fundraising communications that meet the definition of healthcare operations must clearly and conspicuously provide the opportunity to opt out of future communications. This opt-out is a revocation of authorization (Rinehart-Thompson 2018).

HIPAA Privacy Rule Administrative Requirements

The Privacy Rule provides standards regarding administrative requirements that are important to the health information professional, including the following:

- Designation of a privacy officer and a contact person for receiving complaints
- Standards for policies and procedures and changes to policies and procedures
- Requirements for privacy training
- Requirements for establishing privacy safeguards for handling complaints

Designation of Privacy Officer

The Privacy Rule requires CEs to designate an individual as a chief privacy officer to be responsible for privacy practices within the CE. This position is ideally suited to the background, knowledge, and skills of the health information professional because the role includes developing and implementing privacy policies and procedures, facilitating organizational privacy awareness, performing privacy risk assessments, maintaining appropriate forms, overseeing privacy training, participating in compliance monitoring of BAs, ensuring that patient rights are protected, maintaining knowledge of applicable laws and accreditation standards, and communicating with the Office for Civil Rights (OCR) and other entities in compliance reviews and investigations of alleged privacy violations (AHIMA 2015).

Additionally, the CE must designate a person or office as the responsible party for receiving initial complaints about alleged privacy violations. This individual must be able to provide further information about matters covered by the CE's notice of privacy practices.

Standards for Policies and Procedures

The CE must implement policies and procedures to ensure compliance with the Privacy Rule. This process includes an ongoing review of privacy policies and procedures and ensuring that all policy changes are consistent with changes in the privacy and security regulations. Any regulatory changes that materially affect the CE's notice of privacy practices must be reflected in the notice; thus the notice may have to be updated. All revisions must be noted in the policies, procedures, or notice of privacy practices. Health information professionals are ideally qualified for developing and overseeing policies and procedures.

Privacy Training

Every member of the CE's workforce (as defined earlier in this chapter) must be trained in privacy policies and procedures to include maintaining the privacy of patient information, upholding individual rights guaranteed by the Privacy Rule, and reporting alleged breaches and other Privacy Rule violations. Each new employee must be trained within a reasonable period of time after joining the workforce. When material changes are made to policies or procedures regarding privacy, employees must receive additional training. It is also recommended that refresher training be provided to all workforce members at least annually.

Further, the CE must maintain documentation showing that privacy training has occurred. Although not required, a signed acknowledgment of training by each workforce member is helpful to show compliance.

CEs must have safeguards and mechanisms in place to protect the privacy of PHI. This includes appropriate administrative, technical, and physical safeguards. These safeguards should work hand in hand with those specified in the Privacy Rule. (See chapter 10, *Data Security*, for more additional information on HIPAA security regulations.)

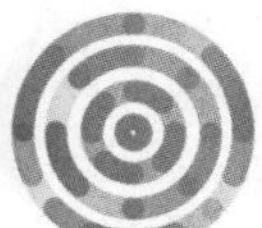

Enforcement of Federal Privacy Legislation and Rules

Legal responsibility for HIPAA privacy *and* security violations is not limited to CEs. Employees or other individuals can be individually prosecuted. Civil and criminal penalties also apply to both BAs and CEs.

Penalties

ARRA/HITECH established tiered penalties, with a range of \$100 to \$50,000 per violation for unknowing violations; \$1,000 to \$50,000 per violation if due to reasonable cause (knew or would have known of violation with reasonable diligence); \$10,000 to \$50,000 per violation for willful neglect that was corrected; and \$50,000 per violation for willful neglect that was uncorrected. There is a \$1.5 million annual cap for identical violations in each category. The nature and extent of both the violation and the harm determine the amount assessed within each statutory range.

Compensation of individuals harmed by a Privacy Rule violation was included in the ARRA provisions, but no further action has been taken for this to occur.

Legal Action by State Attorneys General

State attorneys general may bring civil actions in federal district court on behalf of residents believed to have been negatively affected by a HIPAA violation. To that end, the OCR trained all state attorneys general on this. Previously, only the Office of Civil Rights held this enforcement right; however, it now encourages collaboration with state attorneys general to bring legal action. Individuals still cannot bring lawsuits under a HIPAA cause of action (Rinehart-Thompson 2018).

Audits

HIPAA enforcement does not occur solely based on complaints, as it did originally. Unannounced audits by OCR to detect Privacy and Security Rule violations are mandated for CEs and BAs. Desk and on-site audits determine whether comprehensive policies and procedures are in place and whether they have been implemented to comply with the Privacy and Security Rules.

Disclosure of Health Information

The disclosure of health information process has long been central to the health information professional's responsibilities. **Disclosure of health information** is the process of providing PHI access to individuals or entities that are authorized to either receive or review it (Brodnik 2017b).

Protecting the security and privacy of patient information is one of a healthcare organization's top priorities, and the HIM department is usually responsible for determining appropriate access to and disclosure of health information from patient health records. For example, disclosure of health information may take the form of a patient's request to mail copies of his or her health records to a healthcare provider.

The Disclosure of Health Information Function

Management of the disclosure of health information function includes the following steps:

Step 1: *Enter the request in the disclosure of health information database.* Generally, information such as patient name, date of birth, health record number, name of requester, address of requester, telephone number of requester, purpose of the request, and specific health record information requested is entered in the computer. Figure 9.6 is an example of a computer screen used for entering disclosure of health information data.

Step 2: *Determine the validity of authorization.* The HIM professional will compare the authorization form signed by the patient with organizational requirements for authorization to determine the validity of the authorization form. The healthcare organization's requirements are based on state and federal (for example, HIPAA) regulations. Certain types of information such as substance abuse treatment records, behavioral health records, and HIV records require that specific components be included in the authorization form per state and federal regulations. If the request is valid, the HIM professional proceeds to the next step. If the authorization is invalid, the problem with the authorization is noted in the disclosure of health information database and it is returned to the requester with an explanation.

Step 3: *Verify the patient's identity.* The HIM professional must verify that the patient has been a patient at the healthcare organization. To do this, the HIM professional compares the

Figure 9.6 Disclosure of health information database screen

eSmartlog New Request

NEW REQUEST REQUEST SEARCH REPORTS MAIN MENU ARCHIVE RAC QUEUE ELECTRONIC INSURANCE REQUESTS QUEUE CONTACT US SIGNOUT 2/13/2019 5:17:04 PM(EDT) 32

28838 : Ahima Virtual Lab

Requester Information

				Log Id	204425314
Phone No	800-430-0021	Name	Frank Burns	Type	Attorney
Address	123 Vine St	City	Macklamore	State-Zip	IL-60601
# of Days to Complete:		Request Letter Date:		Due Date:	

Patient Information

Date Format: MM-DD-YYYY

Date Received	02 - 13 - 2019				
Medical Record #		First Name		Last Name	
Claim #		DOB		SSN	
Dates of Service		Patient Account/Control #			
Chart Location	Risk Management	Attention Of			
Complete Date		MR Pages		Delivery Method	Mail
Comments				HIPAA reportable disclosure	
Student ID		Instructor ID		School Logon	

Main Reason for Request: --Please Select--

Additional Request Details: Bill To and Ship To addresses are different

Submit Request | Clear Form | Correspondence Letters 204425314

Source: ©CIOX Health eSmartlog. Used with permission.

information on the authorization form with information in the master patient index. The patient's name, date of birth, Social Security number, address, and phone number are used to verify the identity of the patient whose record is requested. The patient's signature in the health record is compared with the patient's signature on the authorization for disclosure of health information form.

Step 4: *Process the request*: The health record is retrieved (paper or electronic) and only the information authorized for release is copied or printed and released. The patient information may also be faxed or otherwise released directly from the EHR.

To comply with the Privacy Rule, a healthcare organization must maintain an account of disclosures.

Disclosure of health information may also be a response to a *subpoena duces tecum* (discussed in chapter 8, *Health Law*). It is necessary to verify that the subpoena is valid, and the requested information may be released to the court in compliance with applicable state or federal law. In response to a subpoena, a representative from the HIM department may appear in person either in court or at a deposition and give sworn testimony as to the health record's authenticity.

The disclosure of health information function has grown immensely in the past decade, due in part to the Privacy Rule. Staffing has increased in some departments to address this growth. Other HIM departments outsource disclosure of health information to companies that specialize in this function. This may be done to keep pace with requests or to eliminate backlogs. These outsource companies are BAs and therefore must meet all of the requirements of a BA. Even with outsourcing, however, the HIM department remains ultimately responsible for ensuring that proper practices and all laws are followed.

Disclosure of Health Information Quality Control

Quality control in disclosure of health information includes both productivity (that is, turnaround time) and accuracy (namely, that information is released appropriately). The HIM department receives a high volume of requests and must prioritize the processing of disclosure of health information. Continuity of care requests are processed before other types of requests to align with the mission of most healthcare organizations. The HIM department must establish productivity standards to meet the expected turnaround time of various requests. With these standards the average turnaround times for disclosure of health information may be tracked, and delays in responding to requests for information may be addressed. While productivity information may be collected manually, electronic systems offer tools for data manipulation and can provide individual production statistics, departmental request volumes, and information regarding request turnaround times. The accuracy of disclosure of health information must also be monitored. The following examples illustrate how the timeliness and accuracy of disclosure of health information can be monitored.

To monitor timeliness, the date a request is received and the date that health records are sent are entered into a disclosure of health information database. This information can be used to generate a report that will determine whether the health records are being sent in a timely manner.

To monitor accuracy of disclosure of health information, random authorizations are checked to verify their validity and to ensure compliance with federal and state regulations. A validation that the appropriate health records were released is also conducted. The error rate (or, alternatively, the accuracy rate) can be determined and compared against a set standard established by the healthcare organization (Cerrato and Roberts 2013).

Authorizations

Authorizations have long been a key component of the disclosure of health information process, used as a tool to document and validate the legal use and disclosure of health information. While the Privacy Rule generally requires authorization for the use and disclosure of PHI and specifies situations where authorization is not required (discussed earlier in this chapter), it also specifies requirements for a valid authorization form. Elements of the authorization form, such as patient name and signature, dates of service to be released, and names of the entities both disclosing and receiving the information, are well established in health information practice. However, with the passage of the Privacy Rule many established health information practices have also become legal requirements.

Valid Authorization

The Privacy Rule provides specific parameters regarding the content required for a valid authorization. Under the Privacy Rule, an authorization must be written in plain language. A valid authorization is one that contains at least the following elements:

- A description of the information to be used or disclosed that identifies the information in a specific and meaningful fashion
- The name or other specific identification of the person(s), or class of persons, authorized to make the requested use or disclosure
- The name or other specific identification of the person(s), or class of persons, to whom the CE may make the requested use or disclosure
- An expiration date or event that relates to the individual or the purpose of the use or disclosure
- A statement of the individual's right to revoke the authorization in writing and the exceptions to the right to revoke, together with a description of how the individual may revoke
- A statement that information used or disclosed pursuant to the authorization may be subject to redisclosure (subsequent disclosure of health information) by the recipient and no longer protected by this rule
- Signature of the individual and date
- When the authorization is signed by a personal representative of the individual, a description of the representative's authority to act for the individual (45 CFR 164.508(c))

An authorization is considered invalid when any one of the following defects exists:

- The expiration date has passed or the expiration event is known by the CE to have occurred
- The authorization has not been filled out completely
- The authorization is known by the CE to have been revoked
- The authorization lacks a required element (for example, appropriate signature)
- The authorization violates the compound authorization requirements, if applicable
- Any material information in the authorization is known by the CE to be false (45 CFR 164.508(b))

Health information professionals must also ensure the validity of an authorization by confirming that the patient or patient's personal representative actually signed the form (through signature comparisons), the person who signed the form is legally competent, and evidence does not exist indicating the authorization form was signed involuntarily or without the patient's knowledge (Brodnik 2017b). When the patient or other authorized individual picks up the health information, he or she must validate their identity – generally with a drivers license.

Who Can Authorize Release

Legally competent individuals have the right to authorize or refuse to authorize the disclosure of their own health information. As noted previously in this chapter, the Privacy Rule provides many exceptions to the authorization requirement. Additionally, there are situations where an individual is deemed not legally competent, and authority to authorize release of their health information resides with someone else. For example, by law (and with exceptions), minors are deemed legally incompetent and a personal representative (a parent or guardian) will provide the authorization. Minors who are emancipated, given a legal status that gives them full rights to make decisions for themselves, can authorized the release. The requirements for emancipation vary by state but generally apply when the minor is married, is self-supporting, and lives on their own (Brodnik 2017a). In other words, they are not living with or receiving support from their parents. Adults may also be legally incompetent by virtue of a permanent disability (such as a developmental disability) or a temporary condition (for example, incompetent to stand trial until restored to competency). A legal guardian then acts to handle the matters of the incompetent individual, including authorizing the release of health information. Table 9.5 highlights the authority to grant authorization based on the type of individual whose health information is involved. Where highly sensitive information is involved, such as behavioral health, substance abuse, HIV/AIDS, or genetic information, the same principles apply regarding who has the legal authority to authorize the disclosure of health information. However, legal requirements and best practices also dictate that individuals specifically designate their permission and forms denote individuals' awareness that highly sensitive information will be released.

Table 9.5 Authority to grant authorization for disclosure of health information

	Permitted to authorize disclosure?	If no, who can authorize disclosure?
Legally competent adult	Yes	N/A
Legally incompetent adult (permanent)	No	Personal representative (for example, guardian)
Legally incompetent adult (temporary)	No	Personal representative (until competency is restored) (for example, guardian)
Minor	No	Personal representative (for example, parent or guardian)

Source: © AHIMA

Medical Identity Theft

Medical identity theft is a crime that challenges healthcare organizations and the health information profession. A type of healthcare fraud that includes both financial fraud and identity theft involves either (a) the inappropriate or unauthorized misrepresentation of one's identity (for example, the use of one's name and Social Security number) to obtain medical services or goods, or (b) the falsifying of claims for medical services in an attempt to obtain money (Dixon 2006). Regardless of the purpose, the individual's health information is either created under the wrong name or altered, leading to potentially deadly consequences. Medical identity theft does not include the inappropriate change of patient information if the patient's identity has not been assumed or abused by someone else. Likewise, using a patient's financial information to purchase nonmedical goods or service is not medical identity theft because there are financial, but not medical, consequences.

Medical identity theft can be internal or external. Internal medical identity theft is committed by insiders in a healthcare organization, such as clinical or administrative staff with access to vast amounts of patient information. Culprits range from individuals acting alone to sophisticated crime rings that may infiltrate a healthcare organization to commit internal medical identity theft. Individuals outside a healthcare organization who assume a person's identity, perhaps to utilize the victim's health insurance benefits, commit external medical identity theft. As a result, medical information about the culprit is created under the victim's name, and information about the two individuals may be intertwined (Olenik and Reynolds 2017). The addition of information about another patient in the victim's record can result in improper medical treatment. For example, if the perpetrator's blood type is wrongfully entered into the victim's record, the victim could receive a transfusion of the wrong blood type. This is potentially fatal. The World Privacy Forum suggests that internal crimes occur more frequently than external ones (Dixon 2006). Further, there is concern that the evolution of the EHR may assist culprits by granting them broad access to patient information.

Patient Verification

It is important to verify a patient's identity at the beginning of a healthcare encounter by requiring presentation of a driver's license, taking a photograph of the patient for future reference, or even using biometric identifiers such as fingerprints. However, there are two caveats. Patient verification does not hinder internal medical identity theft. Further, the measures listed rely on valid baseline patient verification. If the information the healthcare organization relies upon is the culprit's information (for example, photo, signature, or fingerprint), all future encounters will be based on fraudulent information, decreasing the chances of detecting the fraud or otherwise causing the healthcare organization to wrongfully identify the true patient as the culprit if he or she later presents to that healthcare organization for treatment. Measures to combat internal medical identity theft include performing background checks on new hires and contractors (Olenik and Reynolds 2017). The collection of Social Security numbers should be limited, and staff access to this sensitive information should also be limited. EHR access and access to other business records should only be given to the extent that people need information to complete their jobs. Technical measures also include routinely monitoring access or attempted access through audit trails and using features such as screen savers and automatic logoffs. These technical safeguards are discussed in chapter 10, *Data Security*.

Fair and Accurate Credit Transactions Act (FACTA)

The federal Fair and Accurate Credit Transactions Act (FACTA) requires financial institutions and creditors to develop and implement written identity theft programs that identify, detect, and respond to red flags that may signal the presence of identity theft. Although this law does not specifically address medical identity theft, many healthcare organizations meet the definition of creditor, which is anyone who meets one of the three following criteria:

1. Obtains or uses consumer reports in connection with a credit transaction
2. Furnishes information to consumer reporting agencies in connection with a credit transaction
3. Advances funds to—or on behalf of—someone, except for funds for expenses incidental to a service provided by the creditor to that person

The law includes the Red Flags Rule, which consists of five categories of red flags that are used as triggers to alert the healthcare organization to a potential identity theft (16 CFR Part 681). The following are the five categories are:

1. Alerts, notifications, or warnings from a consumer reporting agency
2. Suspicious documents
3. Suspicious personally identifying information such as a suspicious address
4. Unusual use of, or suspicious activity relating to, a covered account
5. Notices from customers, victims of identity theft, law enforcement authorities, or other businesses about possible identity theft in connection with an account (16 CFR Part 681)

In addition to mandated red flags, healthcare providers must act to prevent, detect, and mitigate activities in an effort to address both external and internal incidents. Employee awareness and training, and implementation of organization-wide policies and procedures, are important.

Patient Advocacy

Over time, the role of the HIM professional has evolved. It continually becomes more multifaceted. Today, it includes the role of patient advocate. As a patient advocate, the HIM professional is a steward of the patient's health record, ensuring not only its integrity but also safeguarding it according to all applicable laws, policies and procedures, and industry best practices. However, as the healthcare industry has placed increasing emphasis on patient-centered healthcare, patient empowerment, and health literacy, health information professionals must also prioritize patient rights to ensure the patients gain needed and legal access to their health records and have the tools to understand the information documented about them.

Compliance

Compliance is an industry concept that means conformance with applicable laws. A culture of compliance within a healthcare organization is critical. Healthcare is a heavily regulated industry and there are many healthcare-specific laws and relevant non–healthcare-specific laws with which healthcare organizations must comply (for example, fair labor standards and environmental regulations). This chapter has focused on laws that regulate the privacy of patient information, most notably the HIPAA Privacy Rule. Compliance with the Privacy Rule is critical to safeguard individuals' health information and preserve their dignity while, at the same time, avoiding penalties that are assessed as the result of noncompliance.

HIM Roles

Health information privacy has always been a core principle of the HIM profession. The HIPAA Privacy Rule has codified that principle, while also making the role of privacy officer a required position. Standard privacy officer responsibilities include the following:

- Development and implementation of privacy policies and procedures
- Promotion of organizational privacy awareness
- Performance of privacy risk assessments
- Maintenance of HIPAA-required forms and records
- Facilitation of privacy training sessions and maintenance of training records
- Compliance monitoring of BAs

- Protection of patient health information rights
- Knowledge of applicable laws and accreditation standards
- Receipt of complaints alleging HIPAA Privacy Rule violations
- Internal investigation of alleged HIPAA Privacy Rule violations
- Participation in breach notification analyses
- Reporting and mitigation of breaches
- Communication with OCR and other entities in compliance reviews and investigations

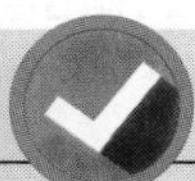

Check Your Understanding 9.3

Answer the following questions.

1. Medical identity theft includes:
   a. Using another person's name to obtain durable medical equipment
   b. Purchasing an EHR
   c. Purchasing surgical equipment
   d. Using another healthcare provider's national provider identifier to submit a claim
2. Per the Fair and Accurate Credit Transactions Act (FACTA), which of the following is not a red flag category?
   a. An account held by a person who is over 80 years old
   b. Warnings from a consumer reporting agency
   c. Unusual activity relating to a covered account
   d. Suspicious documents
3. Misty is the privacy officer for a large physician practice. She is preparing training sessions about HIPAA Privacy policies and procedures that have been recently updated. Misty is working with administration to make some decisions about the training sessions. Which of the following is correct?
   a. Every member of the covered entity's workforce should be trained.
   b. Only individuals employed by the covered entity should be trained.
   c. Training materials, such as PowerPoints, are to be retained for five years.
   d. Training attendance logs do not have to be retained.
4. As a general rule, which of the following is a legally competent individual?
   a. A minor with a developmental disability
   b. An adult with a developmental disability
   c. A minor without a developmental disability
   d. A minor's personal representative
5. The King's Hospital Foundation is reviewing its protocol for an upcoming fundraising appeal. Which of the following is true regarding the HIPAA Privacy Rule and fundraising?
   a. Fundraising materials do not have to include opt-out instructions.
   b. Prior authorization is required if individuals are not targeted based on diagnosis.
   c. Individuals must be informed in the Notice of Privacy Practices that their information may be used for fundraising purposes.
   d. Authorization is always required for fundraising solicitations.
6. The use or disclosure of PHI for marketing:
   a. Always requires written authorization from the patient
   b. Does not require written authorization for face-to-face communications with the individual
   c. Requires written authorization from the patient when products or services of nominal value are introduced
   d. Never requires written authorization from the patient

7. Mary's PHI has been breached. She must be informed of all of the following *except*:
   a. Who committed the breach
   b. Date the breach was discovered
   c. Types of unsecured PHI involved
   d. What she may do to protect herself

8. The privacy officer is responsible for all of the following *except*:
   a. Handling complaints about the covered entity's violations of the Privacy Rule
   b. Developing and implementing privacy policies and procedures
   c. Providing information about the covered entity's privacy practices
   d. Encrypting all electronic PHI

9. Beth is the privacy officer at Kings Hospital. She knows that she must report breaches to the Office for Civil Rights in the Department of Health and Human Services. Which of the following breach notification statements is correct?
   a. She is only required to report breaches when 500 or more individuals are affected.
   b. She must report breaches of both secured and unsecured PHI.
   c. She must report a breach even when only one person's PHI is breached.
   d. Breach notification only applies when 20 or more individuals are affected.

10. A valid authorization must contain all the following *except*:
   a. A description of the information to be used or disclosed
   b. A signature and stamp by a notary
   c. A statement that the information being used or disclosed may be subject to redisclosure by the recipient
   d. An expiration date or event

Real-World Case 9.1

HIPAA privacy breaches are of great concern and they occur too frequently. The Office for Civil Rights (OCR) in the Department of Health and Human Services reported in December 2018 that a critical access hospital in Colorado reached a settlement via a resolution agreement to pay $111,400 to HHS and to adopt a corrective action plan because it allowed a former employee to have continued remote access to ePHI, affecting 557 individuals. No business associate agreement had been signed with the former employee (HHS 2018b).

This case highlights that actions as simple as immediately terminating access to systems upon employment separation can avoid breaches. Procedures that incorporated a routine termination process would have prevented an incident of this nature.

The fact that this incident involved a critical access hospital, which is small by definition and in comparison, to its multi-hospital healthcare system counterparts, demonstrates that breaches and penalties resulting from breaches do not occur in large organizations only. Covered entities and business associates of all types and sizes can commit breaches and be penalized for them.

Real-World Case 9.2

Anndorie Cromar is a medical identity theft victim. A pregnant woman used Cromar's medical identity to pay for maternity care at a nearby hospital. Because the infant was born with drugs in her system, the state's child protective services (CPS) assumed she was Cromar's infant and threatened to take Cromar's four children away. It required a DNA test to get her name off of the infant's birth certificate, but years to get her health records corrected. "That first stage was the most terrifying thing I've ever experienced in my life, getting the call from CPS and having them say, 'We are coming to take your kids'" (Andrews 2016).

Medical identify theft is not detected and stopped readily like financial fraud, where the bank or credit card company calls when they see suspicious charges on a person's account. Consumers therefore need to be particularly vigilant about information that can be stolen to commit medical identity theft: personal, medical, and insurance information. Consumers should do the following:

- Scrutinize insurance company explanation of benefits forms and correspondence from healthcare providers and health insurers
- Be suspicious of inaccurate statements and bills, including documentation relating to services they did not receive
- Routinely review credit reports for debts that do not belong to them
- Treat insurance cards and policy numbers with the same care as Social Security numbers, and not share them readily

Additionally, consumers should not post information about medical treatments on social media. A criminal could use that information, along with other personal data located online, to create a complete and accurate profile by which to exploit the victim. Once the perpetrator's and victim's medical information are intertwined, it is much more difficult to undo than simple financial identity theft cases. Further, because medical identity theft involves a person's health profile, it cannot be shut down as quickly as a credit card number can (Andrews 2016).

References

Amatayakul, M. 2003. HIPAA on the job: Another layer of regulations: Research under HIPAA. *Journal of AHIMA* 74(1):16A–16D.

American Health Information Management Association. 2016. Guidelines for a Compliant Business Associate Agreement. http://library.ahima.org/doc?oid=301918#.XCp2H_ZFw2w.

American Health Information Management Association. 2015. Sample (Chief) Privacy Officer Job Description. http://library.ahima.org/doc?oid=107672#.Vw_3FPkrLDc.

American Health Information Management Association. 2017. *Pocket Glossary of Health Information Management and Technology*, 5th ed. Chicago: AHIMA.

American Health Information Management Association. 2009. Analysis of health care confidentiality, privacy, and security provisions of the American Recovery and Reinvestment Act of 2009, Public Law 111-5. http://library.ahima.org/PdfView?oid=91955.

Andrews, M. 2016 (August 25). The rise of medical identity theft. *Consumer Reports*. https://www.consumerreports.org/medical-identity-theft/medical-identity-theft/.

Brodnik, M.S. 2017a. Introduction to the Fundamentals of Law for Health Informatics and Information Management. Chapter 1 in *Fundamentals of Law for Health Informatics and Information Management.* Edited by M.S. Brodnik, L.A. Rinehart-Thompson, and R.B. Reynolds. Chicago: AHIMA.

Brodnik, M. 2017b. Access, Use, and Disclosure and Release of Health Information. Chapter 15 in *Fundamentals of Law for Health Informatics and Information Management.* Edited by M.S. Brodnik, L.A. Rinehart-Thompson, and R.B. Reynolds. Chicago: AHIMA.

Cerrato, L. and J. Roberts. 2013. Health Information Functions. Chapter 7 in *Health Information Management Technology: An Applied Approach.* Edited by N. Sayles. Chicago: AHIMA.

Dixon, P. 2006 (May 3). Medical identity theft: The information crime that can kill you. *World Privacy Forum.* http://www.worldprivacyforum.org.

Department of Health and Human Services. 2018a. Research. https://www.hhs.gov/hipaa/for-professionals/special-topics/research/index.html.

Department of Health and Human Services. 2018b. Colorado hospital failed to terminate former employee's access to electronic protected health information. U.S. Department of Health and Human Services. Resolution Agreements. https://www.hhs.gov/hipaa/for-professionals/compliance-enforcement/agreements/index.html.

Department of Health and Human Services. 2016. Individuals' Right under HIPAA to Access their Health Information 45 CFR 164.524. https://www.hhs.gov/hipaa/for-professionals/privacy/guidance/access/index.html.

Department of Health and Human Services. 2015. Guidance Regarding Methods for De-identification of Protected Health Information in Accordance with the Health Insurance Portability and Accountability Act (HIPAA) Privacy Rule. https://www.hhs.gov/hipaa/for-professionals/privacy/special-topics/de-identification/index.html.

Department of Health and Human Services. 2013. Breach Notification Rule. https://www.hhs.gov/hipaa/for-professionals/breach-notification/index.html.

Department of Health and Human Services. 2011. HIPAA Privacy Rule accounting of disclosures under the Health Information Technology for Economic and Clinical Health Act. 45 CFR Part 164. *Federal Register* 76(104):31426–31449.

Department of Health and Human Services. 2010. Modifications to the HIPAA Privacy, Security, and Enforcement Rules under the Health Information Technology for Economic and Clinical Health Act; Proposed Rule. 45 CFR Parts 160 and 164. *Federal Register* 75(134):40868–40924.

Department of Health and Human Services. 2006 (last reviewed 2013). How are covered entities expected to determine what is the minimum necessary information that can be used, disclosed or requested for a particular purpose? https://www.hhs.gov/hipaa/for-professionals/faq/207/how-are-covered-entities-to-determine-what-is-minimum-necessary/index.html.

Department of Health and Human Services. 2000. *Federal Register* 65(250):82818.

McLendon, K. and A. D. Rose. 2013. Notice of Privacy Practices (2013 update). AHIMA Practice Brief. http://bok.ahima.org/doc?oid=107006#.Vtn_b_krJQI.

Office of the National Coordinator for Health Information Technology. 2018. Healthit.gov.

Olenik, K. and R.B. Reynolds. 2017. Security Threats and Controls. Chapter 13 in *Fundamentals of Law for Health Informatics and Information Management.* Edited by M.S. Brodnik, L.A. Rinehart-Thompson, and R.B. Reynolds. Chicago: AHIMA.

Rinehart-Thompson, L.A. 2018. *Introduction to Health Information Privacy and Security.* Chicago: AHIMA.

Rinehart-Thompson, L. and L. Harman. 2017. Privacy and Confidentiality. Chapter 3 in *Ethical Health Informatics: Challenges and Opportunities*, 3rd ed. Edited by L. Harman and J. Glover. Burlington, MA: Jones & Bartlett Learning.

Walsh, T. 2016 (February 23). E-mail exchange with author. tw-Security. http://www.tw-security.com/.

5 USC 552a: Privacy Act. 1974.

16 CFR Part 681: Identity Theft Rules. 2012.

45 CFR 160.103: Definitions. 2013.

45 CFR 164.501: Definitions. 2013.

45 CFR 164.502(a)(1)(iii): Uses and disclosures of protected health information: general rules. 2013.

45 CFR 164.506(b): Consent for uses and disclosures permitted. 2013.

45 CFR 164.508: Uses and disclosures for which an authorization is required. 2013.

45 CFR 164.508(a): Authorizations for uses and disclosures. 2013.

45 CFR 164.508(b): Implementation specifications: General requirements. 2013.

45 CFR 164.508(c): Implementation specifications: Core elements and requirements. 2013.

45 CFR 164.510: Uses and disclosures requiring an opportunity for the individual to agree or to object. 2013.

45 CFR 164.510(b): Uses and disclosures for involvement in the individual's care and notification purposes. 2013.

45 CFR 164.512: Uses and disclosures for which an authorization or opportunity to agree or object is not required. 2013.

45 CFR 164.512(a): Uses and disclosures required by law. 2013.

45 CFR 164.512(b): Uses and disclosures for public health activities. 2013.

45 CFR 164.512(c): Disclosures about victims of abuse, neglect or domestic violence. 2013.

45 CFR 164.512(d): Uses and disclosures for health oversight activities. 2013.

45 CFR 164.512(e): Disclosures for judicial and administrative proceedings. 2013.

45 CFR 164.512(f): Disclosures for law enforcement purposes. 2013.

45 CFR 164.512(g): Uses and disclosures about decedents. 2013.

45 CFR 164.512(h): Uses and disclosures for cadaveric organ, eye or tissue donation purposes. 2013.

45 CFR 164.512(i): Uses and disclosures for research purposes. 2013.

45 CFR 164.512(j): Uses and disclosures to avert a serious threat to health or safety. 2013.

45 CFR 164.512(k): Uses and disclosures for specialized government functions. 2013.

45 CFR 164.512(l): Disclosures for workers' compensation. 2013.

45 CFR 164.514(b)(2)(i): Implementation specifications: Requirements for de-identification of protected health information

45 CFR 164.514(e)(2): Implementation specification: Limited data set. 2013.

45 CFR 164.514(f): Standard: uses and disclosures for fundraising. 2013.

45 CFR 164.520: Notice of privacy practices for protected health information. 2013.

45 CFR 164.522(a)(1): Right of an individual to request restriction of uses and disclosures. 2013.

45 CFR 164.522(b)(1): Confidential communications requirements. 2013.

45 CFR 164.524: Access of individuals to protected health information. 2013.

45 CFR 164.526: Amendment of protected health information. 2013.

45 CFR 164.528: Accounting of disclosures of protected health information. 2013.

45 CFR 164.530(d)(1): Complaints to the covered entity. 2013.

Data Security

Megan R. Brickner, MSA RHIA

Learning Objectives

- Identify threats to the security of data
- Demonstrate the elements of a data security program
- Demonstrate methods of incident detection
- Identify methods to safeguard data from inappropriate access
- Apply disaster planning and disaster recovery mechanisms to a situation where data availability has been disrupted
- Identify the primary components of the security provisions of the Health Insurance Portability and Accountability Act and extensions by the HITECH Act and American Recovery and Reinvestment Act
- Recommend methods of ensuring the availability of data
- Recommend methods of forensics

Key Terms

Access control
Access safeguards
Administrative safeguards
Application control
Application safeguards
Audit control
Audit trail
Authentication
Authorization
Automatic logout
Backdoor program
Baiting
Biometrics
Business continuity plan (BCP)
Chief security officer (CSO)
Computer virus
Computer worm
Context-based access control (CBAC)
Contingency plan
Cryptography
Data availability
Data consistency
Data definition
Data integrity
Data loss prevention
Data security
Decryption
Digital certificates
Digital signatures
Disaster recovery plan
Edit check
Electronic protected health information (ePHI)
Emergency mode of operations
Encryption
External threats
Firewall
Forensics
HIPAA Security Rule
Impact analysis
Implementation specifications
Incident
Incident detection
Information technology

Information Technology Asset Disposition (ITAD)
Internal threats
Intrusion detection
Intrusion detection system (IDS)
Likelihood determination
Malware
Network controls
Password
Phishing
Physical safeguards
Private key infrastructure
Public key infrastructure (PKI)
Ransomware
Risk analysis
Risk management
Role-based access control (RBAC)
Rootkit
Security
Security breach
Single-key encryption
Single sign-on
Smart card
Sniffers
Social engineering
Spear phishing
Spyware
Tailgating
Technical safeguards
Token
Trigger events
Trojan horse
Two-factor authentication
Unsecured electronic protected health information
User-based access control (UBAC)

Privacy, as described in chapter 9, *Data Privacy and Confidentiality*, is a fundamental right to be undisturbed by intrusion. Privacy, within the context of one's own personal data or the sensitive data belonging to an organization, is the ability and the right of an individual or organization to control the collection, use (how a healthcare organization avails itself of health information), and disclosure (how information is disseminated) of that personal and sensitive data. Use and disclosure are also defined in chapter 9. **Security** is the practice or means by which privacy is preserved and protected. **Data security**, on the other hand, is the process of keeping data, both in transit and at rest, safe from unauthorized access (access to data by individuals who should not have access), alteration (unauthorized modification), or unauthorized destruction (destroying data without permission). Very often, the terms *data security* and *data privacy* are used interchangeably, although they have very different meanings. Protecting the privacy of data starts with addressing the following questions:

- What, if any, data should be collected?
- How can it be used?
- Who can have access to it?
- How long should the data kept?
- How does one control the access to data once it is obtained?

Once those questions are answered and standards and thresholds are put into place, security controls can be used. Security controls protect the privacy of data by limiting the access to personal and sensitive information and protecting the data from unauthorized access, use, and disclosure as well as protect the data from unauthorized alteration and destruction. Security controls include administrative, physical, and technical safeguards that will be addressed in this chapter. It is important to note that it is impossible to establish and maintain data privacy without data security. Data security ensures that the data are kept confidential and maintains data integrity and availability.

Ensuring the Integrity of Data

Data integrity means that data are complete, accurate, consistent, and up to date so the data are reliable. Reliability is a measure of consistency of data items based on their reproducibility and an estimation of their error of measurement. In other words, data are always the same. Data integrity must be maintained over the data life cycle, beginning with the design and implementation of the information systems that collect and store the data to the retrieval and, if applicable, the destruction of the data. Data integrity also ensures data recoverability and searchability by ensuring the accuracy and consistency of stored data. For example, with a database, automated error checking and data validation ensure data integrity. Data integrity is the extent to which healthcare data are complete, accurate, consistent, and timely. Data integrity ensures the data are of the best quality and accuracy throughout their life cycle. Data integrity is a part of data governance and information governance, which are covered in chapter 6, *Data Management*. Within the healthcare setting, data integrity ensures the completeness and accuracy of health record documentation maintained within an electronic health record (EHR) as described in chapter 1, *Health Information Management Profession*. Ensuring the integrity of healthcare data is important because healthcare providers use it when making decisions about patient care. Human error, software bugs, viruses, hardware malfunctions, storage media and server crashes, and natural disasters such as water and fire can compromise the integrity of data. Robust security programs will be able to respond to such incidences to ensure the data are recovered and data integrity is maintained.

Ensuring the Availability of Data

Ensuring **data availability** means making sure the organization can depend on the information system to perform as expected, and to provide information when and where it is needed.

In healthcare, it is important that patient data are accessible and available at all times. Retrieval and access problems occur when the information system is unreliable or unavailable (for example, either planned or unplanned downtime). Patient data should be available seven days a week, 24 hours a day to facilitate patient care. To keep the data available, hardware must be maintained and replaced when necessary. Software also must be updated to ensure any issues and security vulnerabilities are corrected. Healthcare organizations must have backup and downtime procedures in place to ensure patient care and business operations can continue in the event of a disruption; for example, if the computer network goes down and data cannot be accessed electronically. Backup procedures are also necessary to be in compliance with federal and state regulations. Data backup procedures may involve server redundancy (duplicate information on one or more servers) and sending data to off-site contracted vendors or data warehouses for safe and secure storage and access.

Backup policies and procedures should specify what files and programs require backup, what type of backup should be performed, how frequently it should occur, and how it is to be conducted. For example, a backup policy and procedure may require that all data operating systems, which consist of software that run the basic functions of a computer, and utility files, which are small programs that provide additional support for the operating systems, be adequately and systematically backed up, including all updates to the software which address any vulnerabilities that occur with the information system. The policy may also indicate whether a full procedure (all data at one time) or incremental procedure (only the data since the last backup) is performed and the frequency with which it should occur (such as daily or weekly).

Documentation should record what is backed up and where the backed-up data are stored. Copies of backup media and records of backups should be stored at a secure location away from the site where the original records are stored. For example, the healthcare organization located in Alabama might back their data up at a location in Kansas. This action is taken so that if a disaster such as a fire or flood occurs at the main site, backup copies will be unaffected. There are many companies that specialize in digital off-site storage.

To ensure the backups are working properly, regular tests of restoring data and software from backed-up copies should be performed to ensure the data can be restored if the data are lost. This loss can be due to hardware failure or other destruction of data or other failure.

Information systems have both planned and unplanned downtimes that affect information system availability. For example, planned downtime may occur when system upgrades are scheduled. Unplanned downtime may occur due to an unforeseen disruption such as an electrical outage or hardware failure. In either case, protocols should be developed to maintain data availability to the greatest extent possible. These protocols should be part of the regular information technology infrastructure and incorporated into the security program of the healthcare organization.

Every healthcare organization is subject to security breaches, or unauthorized data or system access, by people from both inside and outside the healthcare organization. It is essential to recognize the scope of the data security needs of the healthcare organization and to develop a systematic and comprehensive program to deal with them. Security breaches also can occur through hardware or software failures and when an intruder hacks into the information system. More often, however, the security breach occurs when an employee within a healthcare organization either accesses information without authorization or deliberately alters or destroys information. Therefore, the healthcare organization's security program must have protections in place to monitor its employees and to keep outsiders from harming or accessing information resources. These protections will be addressed later in this chapter. A data loss prevention strategy, which assists organizations with controlling and limiting what (sensitive) data are moved or transferred outside of an organization's information technology infrastructure by individuals, is also an essential element of data availability and contributes to the overall effectiveness of a data security program. Effective data security does not just happen. It requires planning, training, and the implementation of realistic policies and procedures that address both internal and external threats.

Data Security Threats

Before implementing a data security program, it is important to understand the potential threats to data security. Threats from a number of sources can cause the loss of data privacy, and compromise data integrity or the availability of data. All threats can be categorized as either internal threats (threats that originate within an organization) or external threats (threats that originate outside an organization) (Rinehart-Thompson 2018). Both internal threats and external threats can be caused by people or by environmental and hardware and software factors.

Threats Caused by People

Humans are the greatest threat to electronic health information. Threats to data security from people can be classified into the following five general categories:

1. *Threats from insiders who make unintentional errors.* Examples include employees who accidentally make a typographical error, inadvertently delete files on a computer disk, or unknowingly disclose confidential information. Unintentional error is one of the major causes of security breaches.
2. *Threats from insiders who abuse their access privileges to information.* Examples include employees who knowingly disclose information about a patient to individuals who do not have proper authorization; employees with access to computer files who purposefully snoop for information they do not need to perform their jobs; and employees who store information on a thumb or flash drive, remove it from the organization on a laptop or other storage device, and subsequently lose the device or have it stolen.
3. *Threats from insiders who access information or computer systems for spite or profit.* Generally, such employees seek information to commit fraud or theft. Identity theft—stealing information from patients, their families, or other employees—is on the rise and can result in prosecution of those employees who obtained that information unlawfully.
4. *Threats from intruders who attempt to access information or steal physical resources.* Individuals may physically come onto the organization's property to access information or steal

equipment such as laptop computers or printers. They also may loiter in the organization's buildings hoping to access information from unprotected computer terminals or to read or take paper documents, computer disks, or other information.

5. *Threats from vengeful employees or outsiders who mount attacks on the organization's information systems.* Disgruntled employees might destroy computer hardware or software, delete or change data, or enter data incorrectly into the information system. Outsiders might mount attacks that can harm the organization's information resources. For example, malicious hackers can plant viruses in a computer system or break into telecommunications systems to degrade or disrupt information system availability (Olenik and Reynolds 2017).

Four of the threats listed can involve an organization's employees; therefore, it is important for an organization to remain vigilant to ensure their employees and others with routine access to patient data appropriately use this data.

Social Engineering

Although sophisticated technological breaches of data security occur and are discussed in the media, the most common way that hackers (unauthorized individuals) breach the security of data is through the deployment of social engineering. **Social engineering**, within the context of data security, is the manipulation of individuals (or targets) to freely disclose personal information or account credentials to hackers. The hackers pose as someone or something that the target is familiar with to gain access to information that would otherwise be private and secure. Hackers can deploy a variety of social engineering techniques. Some of these techniques are more sophisticated in nature than others, but all of them can be highly effective when used on an unsuspecting target. Some hackers will go so far as to research and impersonate an unsuspecting target to gain access to sensitive and valuable information; for example, a hacker might pretend to be the target's boss. Social engineering techniques will be discussed further in this chapter.

The four main types of social engineering (phishing, spear phishing, baiting, and tailgating) are the following:

1. *Phishing*. This is the most common type of social engineering technique. **Phishing** is accomplished using email. The hackers send a target what appears to be a legitimate email correspondence from a legitimate company or organization requesting that the target click a link within the email and provide, typically, log-in and password credentials to an information system or application. For example, a target may receive a phishing email from what appears to be his or her bank. The hacker develops an email that looks very similar to legitimate correspondence from the target's bank. The hacker then would alert the target that there is something wrong with his or her account and the target must click a link and provide his or her credentials to have the matter resolved.
2. *Spear Phishing*. **Spear phishing** is similar to *phishing* but requires a little more work on the part of the hacker. When the hacker engages in spear phishing, the hacker researches the individual whose identity the hacker will assume by looking up social media accounts and researching the individual's activity on the web. The hacker will typically assume the identity of an individual in a high-level leadership position of an organization. While assuming this online identity, the hacker will then target other individuals within the organization to try to obtain personal information from them.
3. *Baiting*. **Baiting** involves hackers leaving an infected USB or flash drive in a public area in the hope that someone will come by, pick it up, and use it out of curiosity. If it is used, the individual's computer will become infected with whatever virus was loaded onto the USB or flash drive. Another version of baiting involves the hacker sending out emails with embedded links to random

recipients. When the link is clicked, it loads malicious software that can then transfer sensitive data to the hacker without the individual's knowledge.

4. *Tailgating*. Tailgating is a social engineering technique that allows a hacker, imposter, or other unauthorized individual to use an authorized individual's access privileges to gain access to a restricted physical area. For example, an imposter, hacker, or other unauthorized individual wants to gain access to a building that requires badge access. This unauthorized individual follows closely behind an individual who just swiped his or her badge and gains access by simply following the other individual inside the building. It is human nature for a person to hold a door open for someone behind him or her and not let the door close on that person. The unauthorized person knows this and exploits the good nature of another individual.

Threats Caused by Environmental and Hardware or Software Factors

People are not the only threats to data security. Natural disasters such as earthquakes, tornadoes, floods, forest fires, and hurricanes can demolish physical facilities and electrical utilities.

In 2017, Hurricane Harvey devastated Texas. Hurricane Harvey affected a very large geographic area, impacting that area with tremendous flooding. Although the loss of life and property was enormous, the hospitals there were appropriately prepared and were able, for the most part to continue to care for the influx of patients from the surrounding areas due to their robust disaster recovery preparedness.

Further, a devastating tornado ripped through Florida in 2018, literally decimating many hospitals there. Despite careful disaster planning, many hospitals were terribly underprepared for the devastation and had to turn away patients in their time of need. In many cases, the hospitals were not able to access their electronic health records, possibly because they did not have backups offsite.

While this kind of devastation is not ordinary, healthcare organizations must protect themselves against the loss caused by environmental factors. Healthcare organizations across the nation should send backup information to vaults that are located many miles off-site, perhaps in a distant state, to assist in the recovery of data should a natural disaster or other catastrophic event destroy on-site computer systems. To recover from the devastation caused by nature, healthcare organizations must have backup and recovery procedures in place for both paper and electronic health records and other important organizational data.

Other causes of security breaches are operating system, software, and hardware failures. These include hardware breakdowns and software failures that cause information systems to shut down or malfunction unexpectedly. Examples include a hard-disk crash that destroys or corrupts data, and a program that has not been updated, which may make it vulnerable to attack. Another example is a failed, weak, or poorly configured firewall.

Electrical outages and power surges also can cause problems. When an electrical outage occurs, information is unavailable to the end user. Data might be corrupted or even lost. Power surges also can destroy or corrupt information. Thus, healthcare organizations must have the appropriate equipment to protect information systems from power surges and backup equipment to keep them operating during an outage.

Yet another type of threat is a hardware or software malfunction. Security breaches may be introduced when new software or hardware is added to the information system or when it is not properly tested.

While malfunctions of various software applications can corrupt data, another type of threat is caused by intentional software intrusions known as malicious software or malware. Malware is any type of software attack designed to disrupt mobile or computer operations. Malware can take partial or full control of a computer and can compromise data security and corrupt both data and hard drives. Examples of malware include the following:

- *Phishing*. Phishing is accomplished using email. The hackers send a target what appears to be a legitimate email correspondence from a legitimate company or organization requesting that the target click a link within the email and provide, typically, log-in and password credentials to an information system or application. Phishing is also considered to be social engineering, which was discussed earlier in this chapter.
- *Computer virus*. A **computer virus** is a program that reproduces itself and attaches itself to legitimate programs on a computer. A virus can be programmed to change or corrupt data. Frequently viruses can slow down the performance of a computer system.
- *Computer worm*. A **computer worm** is a program that copies itself and spreads throughout a network. Unlike a computer virus, a computer worm does not need to attach itself to a legitimate program. It can execute and run itself.
- *Trojan horse*. A **Trojan horse** is a program that gains unauthorized access to a computer and masquerades as a useful function. A Trojan horse virus is capable of compromising data by copying confidential files to unprotected areas of the computer system. Trojan horses may also copy and send themselves to email addresses in a user's computer.
- *Spyware*. **Spyware** is a computer program that tracks an individual's activity on a computer system. Cookies are a type of spyware. These programs can capture private information such as an individual's password, credit card numbers, usernames, or account numbers. The following information can then be used for identity theft.
- *Backdoor program*. A **backdoor program** is a computer program that bypasses normal authentication processes and allows access to computer resources, such as programs, computer networks, or entire computer systems.
- *Rootkit*. A **rootkit** is a computer program designed to gain unauthorized access to a computer and assume control of and modify the operating system.
- *Ransomware*. **Ransomware** is malicious software that hackers employ to block access to a computer system or particular computer files. The victim of a ransomware attack will know that his or her computer has been attacked because an electronic ransom note will appear in the computer screen. Typically, the hacker will give the victim a code to gain access to the computer or computer files once a ransom is paid. The hacker will ask for the ransom to be paid in bitcoin, which is electronic currency.

Malware usually gains access to computers via the internet as attachments in emails or through browsing a website that installs the software after the user clicks on a pop-up window. To prevent the intrusion of malware, organizations establish antivirus policies and procedures that establish the use of antivirus software and specify: (1) what devices should be scanned, such as file servers, mail servers, desktop computers; (2) what programs, documents, and files should be scanned; (3) how often scans should be scheduled; (4) who is responsible for ensuring that scans are completed; and (5) what action should be taken when malware is detected. In addition, filters can be used to filter both incoming and outgoing email so that malware is quarantined.

In addition to an antivirus policy, healthcare organizations should have security awareness policies and training that deal with prevention of and identification of malware in place.

Strategies for Minimizing Security Threats

The first and most fundamental strategy in minimizing security threats is to establish a secure organization that is responsible for managing all aspects of computer security. This involves appointing someone in the organization to coordinate the development of security policies and to make certain that they are followed. Generally, this individual is called the **chief security officer (CSO)**.

In addition to appointing someone to the CSO position, the healthcare organization appoints an advisory or policy-making group. This group is called the information security committee or a similar title. It works with the CSO to evaluate the healthcare organization's security needs, establish a security program, develop associated policies and procedures, including monitoring and sanction policies, and ensures the policies are followed. The development and enforcement of sanction policies and procedures, which impose penalties, are important so employees understand the consequences for noncompliance with security rules.

The **HIPAA Security Rule** established a national standard for the protection of individually identifiable electronic health records that are created, received, and used by a covered entity. The rule does not specify the roles and composition of an information security committee, but the responsibilities extend well beyond the protection of data and involve human resources, which typically assists in workforce clearances (that is, granting appropriate data access levels to individuals), employee termination procedures (for example, eliminating an employee's access to data immediately upon severance or notice of severance from the healthcare organization), and application of sanctions to employees who violate established policies (Miaoulis 2011). Other roles include executive-level managers who should have a high-level understanding of the data security policies and procedures and approve security budgets. In addition, the health information management (HIM) director or designee should sit on the information security committee to assist in determining levels of system access, authorization (access rights and privileges based upon policy), and audit trail reviews. Access is the ability of a subject to view, change, or communicate with an object in a computer system. Authorizations and audit trails are discussed later in this chapter. Other management positions involved in the information security committee are the chief information officer (CIO), information technology system directors, network engineers, and representatives from clinical departments (lab, nursing, pharmacy, radiology) as appropriate.

Another strategy for minimizing security threats is helping employees within a healthcare organization to be more aware of their data security environment. Specifically, from a social engineering perspective, employees need to be better equipped to identify potential data security threats. As described earlier, social engineering, specifically phishing, has become a problem across all industries. Since most people have either a business or personal email address, would-be hackers have numerous opportunities to attempt to trick someone into giving them their personal information.

Too often healthcare organizations have a data security incident. A security incident is the "attempted or successful unauthorized access, use, disclosure, modification, or destruction of information or interference with system operations in an information system" (45 CFR Parts 160, 162, and 164 2013, 62). An example is when one employee uses another employee's password. Prevention is key to averting data security incidences. Educating employees regarding what is at stake if a data security incident occurs and arming them with knowledge to identify a potential threat is of the utmost importance. Red flags that indicate an email might be a phish include the use of gmail.com rather than .org for an email from the administrator of the healthcare organization.

One of the easiest ways to identify a potential threat is to verify the sender of the email. When hackers send a phishing email to a target, they often conceal the true identity of the sender for good reason. The hacker wants to trick the target into thinking the email is coming from a legitimate sender. One way to confirm that the sender of an email is legitimate is to hover the pointer over the *From* display name to see what email address appears. Figure 10.1 shows a sample of a phishing attempt. In a phishing email, the display name is vastly different from the actual sender's email address.

Figure 10.1 Sample phishing email

Important news

Jane Doe <jane.doe@email.com
To john.smith @email.com

1:49 PM

Quick reply Reply all Forward Delete

Click on the link to get some important news.

http://hcktxwzz.com

Source: © AHIMA.

Check Your Understanding 10.1

Answer the following questions.

1. External security threats can be caused by:
   a. Employees who steal data during work time
   b. A facility's water pipes bursting
   c. Tornadoes
   d. The failure of a healthcare organization's software
2. A data loss prevention strategy is an essential element to:
   a. Data availability
   b. Data integrity
   c. Data infrastructure
   d. Data reliability
3. Employees who seek information to commit fraud or theft are included in what category of insider threat?
   a. Abuse privileges
   b. Access systems for spite or profit
   c. Steal physical resources
   d. Vengeful employees
4. What is the term used to indicate that data is complete, accurate, consistent, and up to date?
   a. Availability
   b. Confidentiality
   c. Integrity
   d. Security
5. Critique each option to determine the true statement related to internal security threats.
   a. They are caused by people.
   b. They are caused by disgruntled employees.
   c. They originate within a healthcare organization.
   d. They are natural disasters.

6. Identify the type of malware that can copy and run itself without attaching itself to a legitimate program.
   a. Computer worm
   b. Backdoor program
   c. Trojan horse
   d. Spyware
7. This method of social engineering involves hackers leaving an infected USB or flash drive in a public area in the hope that someone will pick it up and use it.
   a. Tailgating
   b. Phishing
   c. Spear phishing
   d. Baiting
8. Data backup policies and procedures may include:
   a. Server redundancy
   b. Ensuring all data is maintained on-site
   c. Maintaining one copy of all data
   d. Avoiding the use of power generators
9. A healthcare organization's data privacy efforts should encompass:
   a. Patient information only
   b. Employee information only
   c. Patient and organizational information only
   d. Patient, employee, and organizational information
10. The categories of security threats by people demonstrate an organization's greatest potential liability group consists of:
   a. Patients
   b. Visitors
   c. Employees
   d. Hackers outside the organization
11. What is the most common social engineering technique?
   a. Tailgating
   b. Phishing
   c. Baiting
   d. Trojan horse

Components of a Security Program

The HIPAA Security Rule went into effect in April 2005. The Security Rule focuses on administrative, physical, and technical safeguards (defined later in the chapter) as they relate to the protection of electronic protected health information (ePHI). Electronic protected health information is protected health information that is "created, received, or transmitted" electronically (45 CFR Parts 160, 162, and 164 2013, 61). All covered entities (CEs), as defined in chapter 9, *Data Privacy and Confidentiality,* have electronic data that needs to be protected from unauthorized access, disclosure, loss, and destruction. The authors of the HIPAA Security Rule made the requirements and obligations of the rule flexible to allow each CE to meet the obligations and requirements in ways that are suitable and appropriate for the size and structure of the organization. For example, more sophisticated information technology will be expected of a 1,000-bed hospital than a two-physician practice.

Information technology is computer technology (hardware and software) combined with telecommunications technology (data, image, and voice networks).

The HIPAA Security Rule provisions and requirements will be addressed at length later in the chapter. To implement those requirements, a CE must establish a security program that meets the requirements of the Security Rule and is effective in doing so. Information security professionals developed the Confidentiality, Integrity and Availability (CIA) Triad of Information Security to determine if a security program is effective. The CIA Triad, presented in figure 10.2, is a baseline standard for determining whether a security program is effective. The triad allows for the implementation and evaluation of a security program based upon three goals that are guaranteed if an information system is secured. Those goals are the following:

1. Confidentiality: Only authorized and appropriate individuals access the data within an information system.
2. Integrity: The data within the system can be trusted. This was discussed at the beginning of the chapter.
3. Availability: The data within the system is available to the end user wherever and whenever it is needed.

Figure 10.2 Effective security program guarantee – CIA triad.

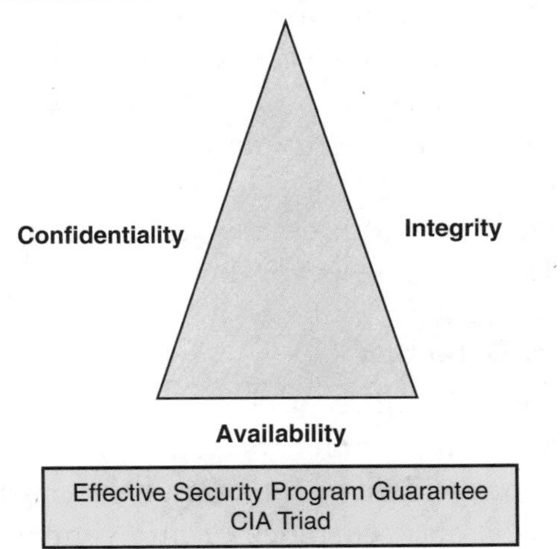

Source: © AHIMA.

An effective security program will be able to guarantee the triad at any given moment, even in times of disaster recovery.

An effective security program also contains the following components:

- Employee awareness including ongoing education and training
- Risk management program
- Access safeguards
- Physical and administrative safeguards
- Software application safeguards
- Network safeguards
- Disaster planning and recovery
- Data quality control processes (Carlon 2013)

Each component of the security program will be discussed as it relates to the establishment of a CE's security program. Some of these same elements will also be discussed in relation to the provisions of the Security Rule later in this chapter.

Employee Awareness

As discussed previously, employees are often responsible for threats to data security. Consequently, employee awareness is a particularly important tool to reduce security breaches by wrongdoers (either intentional or unintentional) and to make employees mindful of security breaches so they can recognize them, respond to them, and report them appropriately.

The CE should offer a formal security awareness training that educates every new employee on the confidential nature of protected health information (discussed more in chapter 9, *Data Privacy and Confidentiality*). The program should inform employees about the CE's security policies and the consequences of failing to comply with them. The CE should give each employee a copy of its security policies as they relate to the employee's job function. The CE also should require every employee to sign a yearly confidentiality statement. Finally, because data security is such an important part of everyone's job, employees should receive periodic and ongoing security reminders. The security reminders can include policy and procedure refreshers, tips on how to identify suspicious emails, or general information about the employees' obligations from a data security perspective.

Included in the employee awareness program should be policies and procedures regarding mobile devices, the use of email, faxing, and scanned information, and appropriate and inappropriate use of social media.

Risk Management Program

Another strategy in protecting the CE's data is to establish a risk management program. **Risk management** is a comprehensive program of activities intended to minimize the potential for injuries to occur in a facility and to anticipate and respond to ensuring liabilities for those injuries that do occur. Risk management includes the processes in place to identify, evaluate, and control risk, defined as the organization's risk of accidental financial liability. CEs must take steps to prevent, detect, and mitigate both external and internal incidents. Mitigation is the steps taken to reduce the impact that a violation of the HIPAA Security Rule has on a patient. For example, the CE may purchase a year's monitoring of a patient's credit in the event of a security violation. A well-conceived risk management program can aid prevention, detection, and mitigation of security breaches including identity theft.

Risk Analysis

The Security Rule requires a CE to implement security measures that are sufficient to reduce risk and vulnerabilities. Risk management begins with a **risk analysis**, which involves assessing security threats and vulnerabilities, and the likely impact of any vulnerability.

A security threat is a situation that has the potential to damage a healthcare organization's information system. In addition to threats and vulnerabilities, a CE should also identify how ePHI is created, managed, stored, and transmitted within the CE and whether vendors or consultants use or maintain ePHI. Of increasing importance is the threat created by the use of mobile devices (phones, tablets, laptops, and so forth). These devices are particularly at risk as they are easily lost or stolen.

Once security threats are identified, it is important for a CE to make a **likelihood determination**, which is an estimate of the probability of threats occurring, and an **impact analysis**, which is an estimate of the impact of threats on information assets. For example, a CE may be located in a region with frequent tornadoes (high likelihood). It is known that tornadoes can be extremely destructive (high impact). For this CE, it would make sense to implement expensive safeguards to protect and back up its information assets against tornadoes. If a threat is low likelihood and low impact (for example, a tornado on the Pacific coast), expenditure of time and money to protect against the threat is not a wise use of resources. CEs on the Pacific coast would have to address mudslides, earthquakes, and wildfires. The CE must conduct this type of analysis on every identified threat—manmade, environmental, and those caused by hardware and software factors—in order to prioritize those that should be addressed first and to which resources should be allocated.

It is essential to determine the value of information to the CE and the consequences of its loss when establishing a risk management program. For example, the CE would have to determine what impact a security breach would have on quality of care, revenue, service, and other aspects of the CE's operations. Identification of a CE's information assets includes an inventory of application software, hardware, networks, and other information assets. Once information assets have been identified, their value to the CE is determined. Value is determined based on a number of factors such as criticality of the asset in daily operations, degree of harm resulting if the asset is not available, legal and regulatory requirements, and loss of revenue should the asset be lost or damaged.

Incident Detection

Once possible threats and vulnerabilities are known, it is important to be able to detect whether a threat or incident or intrusion has occurred. An **incident** is an occurrence or an event. **Incident detection** methods should be used to identify both accidental and malicious events. Detection programs monitor the information systems for abnormalities or a series of events that might indicate that a security breach is occurring or has occurred. Intrusion detection systems can be used for this purpose. An intrusion detection system monitors the CE's network and information systems to "detect and identify" suspicious activity (Dowling 2017, 5). The CE can customize the intrusion detection system to a monitoring level that is at the appropriate level for the CE (Dowling 2017). In other words, it can be made stronger or weaker depending on the needs of the CE.

Incident Response Plan and Procedures

Once a security incident has been identified, there must be a coordinated response from the CE to mitigate the incident. An incident response plan includes management procedures and responsibilities to ensure a quick response is effectively implemented for specific types of incidents. For example, in some instances the plan may call for a "watch and warn" response that includes monitoring and notification of an incident but takes no immediate action. In other instances, a "repair and report" response may be instituted, whereby immediate mitigation and repair of the issue is initiated and reported to the team of individuals responsible for responding to the issue. This type of response may be used in the case of a virus attack. A third type of response is "pursue and prosecute," which includes monitoring an attack, minimizing the attack, collecting evidence, and involving a law enforcement agency. This last example might be used in instances of suspected identity theft. Under the Health Information Technology for Economic and Clinical Health (HITECH) Act, breach notification requirements provide for those situations when affected individuals must be notified about an information security breach affecting their PHI.

The HIPAA Security Rule requires that security incidents be identified, reported to the appropriate persons (which will include the Information Security Officer, leadership, and IT technicians), and documented. Responses to an incident include workforce notification, preserving evidence, mitigating harmful effects caused by the breach, and evaluating the incident as a part of the CE's risk management process (Rinehart-Thompson 2018).

Access Safeguards

Establishing **access safeguards** is a fundamental security strategy. This is the identification of which employees should have access to what data. The general practice is that employees should have access only to data they need to do their respective jobs. For example, a registrar in the admitting office and a nurse would not have access to the same kinds of data. By establishing access safeguards, a CE is taking steps to lessen its vulnerabilities, although it cannot prevent them altogether because of the security threats that humans present.

Determining what data to make available to an employee usually involves identifying classes of information based on the employee's role in the CE. So, the CE would determine what information a registrar, for example, would need to know to do his or her job. Subsequently, every individual who works as a registrar would have access to the same information.

Every role in the CE should be identified, along with the type of information required to perform it. This is **role-based access control (RBAC)** and is the one used most often in healthcare organizations. Additionally, **user-based access control (UBAC)** grants access based on a user's individual identity. For example, every employee in the quality improvement department could potentially have a different degree of access if they have unique responsibilities in that department. **Context-based access control (CBAC)** limits a user's access based not only on identity and role, but also on a person's location and time of access (Rinehart-Thompson 2018). For example, two respiratory therapists may be given the same access based on their identical roles. However, with CBAC access, their access will be further refined (and may differ) based on the units to which they are assigned and the respective shifts they work.

Access control is the restriction of access to information and information resources (such as computers) to only those who are authorized, by role or other means. For access control to be effective, mechanisms that restrict access must be in place. There are a number of access control mechanisms that can be used (discussed later in this chapter). However, the sophistication of the method used should correspond with the value of the information being protected. In other words, the more sensitive or valuable the information, the stronger the control mechanisms need to be. For example, access to health information about patients in a behavioral health unit will only be granted to staff who work in that unit. Identification, authentication, and authorization are the foundation upon which access control mechanisms are based.

Identification

The basic building block of access control is identification of an individual who is accessing the information system. Usually identification is performed through the username or user number. Identification methods must be robust so that an imposter cannot successfully pose as a legitimate user and enter a system illegitimately.

Authentication

The second element of access control is authentication. Authentication is the act of verifying a claim of identity. There are three different types of information that can be used for authentication—something you know, something you have, or something you are. The next section will discuss methods of authentication that fall into these three categories.

- ***Passwords*** Examples of *something you know* include such things as a personal identification number (PIN), a password, or your mother's maiden name. Passwords are frequently used in conjunction with username. Policies and procedures should be in place to ensure passwords cannot be easily compromised. For example, passwords should be of a specific length, include special characters and numbers, should be case sensitive, and should not be words that are included in a dictionary or related to the user's identification or personal information. For example, "password" and "12345" are weak yet popular passwords if they are allowed by the information system in which they are used. Password policies should include mandatory changes of passwords at specified intervals. These types of restrictions help to limit the chance of an intruder guessing a password or using a program called a password cracker to identify passwords. To help increase security, many information systems will lock out a user after a specified number of unsuccessful attempts to gain access to an information system. In addition, password policies should prohibit users from sharing passwords or writing or displaying passwords. While passwords provide the least amount of security compared to other methods, if properly managed and used, they can be an effective security strategy.
    - o *Strengths*: Long passwords are harder to compromise.
    - o *Weaknesses*: Passwords are easy to search and easily stolen if written down. Passwords are easily forgotten if long. Hackers can "sniff" or intercept passwords at various stages of input.
- ***Smart Cards and Tokens*** Smart cards and token cards are examples of *something you have.* A smart card is a small plastic card with an embedded microchip that can store multiple identification factors for a specific user. Usually a smart card is used in combination with a user identification or password. A one-time password (OTP) token is a small electronic device programmed to generate and display new passwords at certain intervals. An OTP token is usually used in combination with user identification or a password. To access a system, a user puts in an identification code and the OTP token generates a one-time password that is displayed on the token.
    - o *Strengths*: Smart cards or tokens only require a pin to be remembered versus a password. Because there is no password, smart cards and tokens prevent dictionary attacks whereby the hacker electronically and repeatedly inputs

different passwords in the hopes of guessing the correct password.

- o *Weaknesses*: Smart cards and tokens can be stolen and access can be compromised if a static pin number is assigned to a specific smart card, and the user writes the static pin on the back of the smart card.

- ***Biometrics*** *Something you are* refers to biometrics. Biometrics is identity verification based upon measurements of a person's physical characteristics. Examples of biometrics include palm prints, fingerprints, voiceprints, and retinal (eye) scans.
  - o ***Strengths***: Biometrics require no passwords and are very hard to replicate.
  - o *Weaknesses*: Biometrics can cause false rejection or false acceptance due to the technology still being somewhat new. Also, there are people who are very reluctant to have their fingerprints taken due to privacy concerns.

Strong authentication requires providing information from two of the three different types of authentication information. For example, an individual provides something he knows and something he has. This is called two-factor authentication. Examples of two-factor authentication include the use of smart cards or tokens with user identification. Two-factor authentication is a stronger method of protecting data access than user identification with passwords. An example of two-factor identification is being used at Walt Disney World in Florida. Guests insert their park tickets and have their index finger scanned.

Single sign-on is another authorization strategy that allows a user to log in to many separate, although related, information systems. Single sign-on allows a user to log in one time and be able to access many information systems. This prevents the user from having to log in to each information system individually; for example, an encoder and an electronic health record.

Different information systems have different requirements for usernames and passwords. This requires the single sign-on to translate and store the username and password for all of the information systems involved. When the user is finished, the single sign-off is used to log out of all of the information systems with one action.

Authorization

The third element of access control is authorization. Authorization is a right or permission given to an individual to use a computer resource, such as a computer, or to use specific applications and access specific data. It is also a set of actions that gives permission to an individual to perform specific functions such as read, write, or execute tasks.

Authorization to use an information system is usually addressed through identification and authentication as described previously. Authorization to use specific applications (for example, order entry, coding, and registration) and specific data would be different for different individuals in a CE. For example, employees in the admitting and registration department would not be given the same authorization to information systems and data as nurses.

Usually authorization is managed through special authorization software that uses various criteria to determine if an individual has authorization for access, sometimes referred to as an access control matrix. For example, authorization may be based on not only the individual's identity but also the individual's role (role-based) and physical location of the resource (that is, access to only certain computers), and time of day (context-based) as described earlier in this chapter.

Information systems may require verification that a human, not a computer, is accessing a website or storage portal. A Completely Automated Public Turing test to tell Computers and Humans Apart (CAPTCHA) requires the user to respond to a question that it is assumed could not be answered by a machine. A typical example of a CAPTCHA is when access to a site requires the user to type in a string of characters that appears skewed or distorted. Another common CAPTCHA is to identify images that contain a specified item such as a sign or a vehicle.

Physical Safeguards

Physical safeguards refer to the physical protection of information resources from physical damage, loss from natural or other disasters, and theft. This includes protection and monitoring of the workplace, data center (computer room), and any type of hardware or supporting information system infrastructure such as wiring closets, cables, and telephone and data lines.

This equipment should be in secure locations and protected from natural and environmental hazards and intrusion. Environmental hazards include such things as fire, floods, moisture, temperature variations, and loss of electricity. To protect it from natural or environmental hazards, equipment should be housed in structurally sound and safe areas. There should be smoke and fire alarms, fire suppression systems, heat sensors, and appropriate monitored heating and cooling systems in place. Appropriate backup power sources such as uninterruptable power supply (UPS) devices or power generators should be available if a power outage occurs.

To protect from intrusion, there should be proper physical separation from the public. Doors, locks, audible alarms, and cameras should be installed to protect particularly sensitive areas such as data centers. Identification procedures such as the use of badges to identify employees should be in place. Processes should be established for logging into and out of computer hardware or media. For example, if a data disk or device is being transported or removed from one location to another, there should be a sign-out and sign-in procedure to track access and removal. Furthermore, sign-in and sign-out logs should be in place to track access to sensitive areas such as data centers.

Backup and recovery procedures are also a part of physical security. Backup and recovery procedures should specifically include server, data, and network policies and procedures.

Provisions must also be made to protect workstations that are more exposed to the public. For example, locking devices can be used to prevent removal of hardware and other devices. Automatic logouts, which are simply timed logouts that reduce the chances that one's account will be used by someone else, can be used to prevent access by unauthorized individuals. For example, a user may be automatically logged out if there has been no activity within five minutes. Laptops and other mobile devices such as personal digital assistants (PDAs) pose significant threats because they can be easily lost or stolen. Documentation of the custody of such devices must be addressed. One such method is maintaining a custody log that documents who has had custody of the device, the time period of custody, and what files and data were on the device during the custody period. Policies and procedures that cover laptop or mobile device use should be in place. Other security mechanisms such as two-factor authentication (discussed previously) and full disk encryption should be used (discussed later in this chapter.) Global positioning systems (GPS) can also be installed on laptops as well as information systems to remotely locate a computer to retrieve and delete data from it, should a computer be lost or stolen. With these features, a computer can be located quickly and appropriate law enforcement officials notified.

In any security program, employee education is one of the best defenses for protection of data and computer resources. Training programs on data security should be conducted at least annually for all employees and cover applicable security responsibilities, policies, and procedures.

Administrative Safeguards

Administrative safeguards include policies and procedures that address the management of computer resources. For example, one such policy might direct users to log off the information system when they are not using it or employ automatic log-offs after a period of inactivity. Other policies include password security (inappropriate sharing, minimum password requirements, changing the frequency of updating passwords, and failed log-in monitoring) and timely removal of terminated employees' system access. Another policy might prohibit employees from accessing the internet for purposes that are not work related. Finally, a CE should have a policy on Information Technology Asset Disposition (ITAD) that identifies how all data storage devices are destroyed and purged of data prior to repurposing or disposal.

Software Application Safeguards

Another security strategy is to implement application safeguards. Application safeguards are controls contained in application software or information systems to protect the security and integrity of information. One common application control is authentication, as previously described. Through the use of passwords, tokens, or biometrics, an information system keeps a record of end users' identifications and authentication mechanisms and then matches the authentication mechanism to each end user's privileges. This ensures that end users can access only the information they have permission to access.

Another application control is the audit trail. The audit trail is a software program that tracks every single access or attempted access of data in the information system. It logs the name of the individual who accessed the data, terminal location or IP address (internet protocol address which identifies the computer used), the date and time accessed, the type of data, and the action taken (for example, modifying, reading, or deleting data). System administrators examine audit trails using special analysis software to identify suspicious or abnormal system events or behavior. Because the audit trail maintains a complete log of system activity, it can also be used to help reconstruct how and when an incident or failure occurred. This information helps to identify ways to avoid similar problems in the future. Depending on the CE's policy, audit trails are reviewed periodically, on predetermined schedules or relative to highly sensitive information.

Yet another application control is the edit check. Edit checks help to ensure data integrity by allowing only reasonable and predetermined values to be entered into the computer. For example, an information system using this feature would disallow an *International Classification of Diseases, Tenth Revision, Clinical Modification* (ICD-10-CM) code that does not exist. Application controls are important because they are automatic checks that help preserve data confidentiality and integrity.

Network Safeguards

Another important strategy used to guard against security breaches is to implement network safeguards. Many networks are used to transmit healthcare data today, and the data must be protected from intruders and corruption during transmission within and external to the organization. With the widespread use of the internet, network controls also are essential to prevent the threat of hackers. The following are some common safeguards.

Firewalls

A firewall (also called a secure gateway) is a part of an information system or network that is designed to block unauthorized access while permitting authorized communications. It is a software program or device that filters information and serves as a buffer between two networks, usually between a private (trusted) network like an intranet (within the organization and not accessible outside) and a public (untrusted) network like the internet. Firewalls allow internal users access to an external network while blocking malicious hackers from damaging internal systems. All messages entering or leaving the private network pass through the firewall, which examines and evaluates each message and blocks those that do not meet predefined security criteria. For example, an email message that is believed to contain a Social Security number may be prohibited from leaving the private network. An email believed to contain a virus may be prohibited from entering the private network. It may control the size of the file that is allowed through the firewall. A firewall is configured to permit, deny, encrypt, or decrypt computer traffic.

Cryptographic Technologies

Cryptography is a branch of mathematics that is based on the transformation of data by developing ciphers, which are codes that are to be kept secret. Cryptography is used as a tool for data security. Strong cryptography improves the security of information systems and their data. There are several types of cryptographic technologies. Cryptographic technologies—such as encryption, digital signatures, and digital certificates—are used to protect information in a variety of situations. This includes protecting data when they are in storage (data at rest), on portable devices such as laptops and flash drives, and while they are being transmitted across networks. Three of these technologies used in healthcare are discussed as follows.

Encryption Encryption is a method of encoding data, converting them to a jumble of unreadable scrambled characters and symbols as they are transmitted through a telecommunication network so that they are not understood by persons who do not have a key to transform the data into their original form. Data are usually encrypted using some type of algorithm, or a standard set of operating rules. Upon receipt, data can only be decoded and restored back to their original readable form (decryption) by using a special algorithm. Encryption takes the message from one computer and encodes it in a form that only the receiving computer can decode. For example, an email containing ePHI can be encrypted whereby as the message is moving from one inbox to another, the message itself is scrambled so as not to be intercepted by a would-be hacker.

One type of encryption is called private key infrastructure, or single-key encryption. In this method, two or more computers share the same secret key and that key is used both to encrypt and decrypt a message. However, the key must be kept secret. If it is compromised in any way, the security of the data is likely to be eliminated. Because the key that decodes the information is transmitted with the data, it could be intercepted (Rinehart-Thompson 2018). The best-known secret key security is called the data encryption standard (DES) published by the National Institute of Standards and Technology (NIST).

A common encryption method used over the internet is a system called Pretty Good Privacy (PGP), or public key infrastructure (PKI). This method uses both a public and a private key, which form a key pair. The sending computer uses a key to encrypt the data and it gives a key to the recipient computer to decrypt the data. With this type of encryption there is a registry of public keys, called a certificate authority. If one user wants to send an encrypted message to another, the registry is consulted, and the receiving user's public key is used to encrypt the data. Only the recipient, who knows the private key, can decrypt the message into its original form.

Digital Signatures A digital signature or digital signature scheme is a public key cryptography method that ensures that an electronic document such as an email message or text file is authentic. This means that the receiver knows who created the document and is assured the document has not been altered in any way since it was created.

In this method data are electronically signed by applying the sender's private key to the data. The digital signature can be stored or transmitted in the data. The receiving party can then verify the signature by using the public key of the signer.

Digital signatures are sometimes confused with e-signatures. E-signature usually means a system for signing or authenticating electronic documents by entering a unique code or password that verifies the identity of the person and creates an individual signature on a document. E-signatures do not necessarily use cryptography.

Digital Certificates Digital certificates are used to implement public key encryption on a large scale. A digital certificate is an electronic document that uses a digital signature to bind together a public key with an identity such as the name of a person or an organization, address, and so forth. The certificate can be used to verify that a public key belongs to an individual. An independent source called a certificate authority (CA) acts as the middleman who the sending and receiving computer trusts. It confirms that each computer is who it says it is and provides the public keys of each computer to the other.

Web Security Protocols

Transmission protocols that allow devices to speak to one another when on a network are another method of data security. Transport Layer Security (TLS) and its predecessor Secure Sockets Layer (SSL) are based on public key cryptography. These protocols are the most common protocols used to secure communications on the internet between a web browser and a web server. Versions of these protocols can be used for almost any application but are frequently used for electronic mail, internet faxing, instant messaging, e-commerce transactions, and voice communications over the Internet (VoIP).

These protocols allow authentication of the server. Once authentication of the server is established, secure communication can begin using symmetric encryption keys. The user's message is encrypted in the user's web browser using an encryption key from the host website. The message is then transported to the host website in encrypted format. Once received by the website, the message is decrypted.

Intrusion Detection Systems

Intrusion detection is the process of identifying attempts or actions to penetrate an information system and gain unauthorized access. Intrusion detection can either be performed in real time or after the occurrence of an intrusion. The purpose of intrusion detection is to prevent the compromise of the confidentiality, integrity, or availability of a resource.

Intrusion detection can be performed manually or automatically. Manual intrusion detection might take place by examining log files, audit trails, or other evidence for signs of intrusions. A system that performs automated intrusion detection is called an **intrusion detection system (IDS)**. Procedures should be outlined in the CE's data security plan to determine what actions should be taken in response to a probable intrusion. For example, typical actions to be taken might include notification of appropriate individuals, generating an email alert, and so on. Penetration testing may be conducted. Penetration testing is when the CE hires a hacker to try to break into their information systems in order to test the quality of the security measures in place.

Disaster Planning and Recovery

As discussed, CEs must prepare for emergencies such as natural disasters. Further, CEs must prepare both for events that cause minimal disruption (for example, short-term power outages) and for large-scale events such as tornadoes. A contingency plan and its component disaster recovery plan will guide a CE through undesirable non-routine events. In CEs, the continuation of medical services to patients is the highest priority. An important element of medical services is the protection and continued availability of health information (Rinehart-Thompson 2018).

Risk Analysis

According to the Security Rule requirements, the CE must assess the internal and external data security risk environment and evaluate vulnerabilities (internal weaknesses) the CE has with respect to ePHI. Conducting **risk analysis**, which allows for the identification and prioritization of those risks, helps the CE ensure it is maintaining the confidentiality, integrity, and availability of ePHI. Ongoing risk analysis allows a CE to keep up with the ever-changing threats and vulnerabilities as they happen.

When a CE prepares to conduct a risk analysis, it is important to keep in mind that the Security Rule does not stipulate or require that a particular approach be used for such an analysis. The CE is required, through the risk analysis, to identify potential threats compared to its identified vulnerabilities to determine the level of risk. Risk itself can take many forms including disruption in business, loss of privacy, and legal and financial penalties. Based on the risk analysis, CEs can implement policies, procedures, and other safeguards to counteract the risk.

Disaster Planning

Disaster planning occurs through a **contingency plan**—a set of procedures, documented by the CE, to be followed when responding to emergencies. The disaster plan identifies what a CE and its personnel need to do during and after security incidences and other events, like natural disasters, that limit or prevent access to the CE and patient information. Disaster planning typically includes policies and procedures to help the business continue operations during an unexpected shutdown or disaster. It also includes procedures the business can implement to restore its information systems and resume normal operation after the disaster.

The contingency plan is based on information gathered during the risk assessment and analysis discussed previously. The risk assessment includes the probability that an unexpected shutdown will occur. Using this information, the contingency plan is developed based on the following steps:

Step 1: Identify the minimum allowable time for system disruption

Step 2: Identify alternatives for system continuation

Step 3: Evaluate the cost and feasibility of each alternative

Step 4: Develop procedures required for activating the plan (Johns 2008)

Disaster Recovery

An immediate component of a contingency plan is the disaster recovery plan, which addresses the resources, actions, tasks, and data necessary to restore those services identified as critical, such as the EHR, as soon as possible, and to manage business recovery processes. The business continuity plan (BCP) is a set of policies and procedures that direct the CE how to continue its business operations during an information system shutdown. Similarly, an emergency mode of operations prescribes processes and controls to be followed until operations are fully restored. For health information, an important part of the disaster recovery plan is ensuring the availability and accuracy of data as soon as possible after a disaster. As described earlier in the chapter, ongoing data backup is critical for this reason. Restoring system integrity and ensuring that all data are recovered requires that all parts of the information system be verified after the disaster has occurred. Usually one information system or one component of an information system is brought up at a time and processes are verified to ensure they are working correctly.

A plan is only as good as its implementation. The disaster recovery plan must be tested periodically to ensure all the parts of the plan—from disaster identification to backup and recovery—work as expected (Johns 2008).

Data Quality Control Processes

Ensuring data quality is an essential part of any data security program. Responsibility for ensuring data quality is shared by many organization stakeholders. For example, data accuracy begins with any individual who enters or documents data or systems that capture and provide data such as intensive care unit monitoring systems. Monitoring and tracking systems that ensure data quality are part of a data security program.

Data availability, consistency, and definition are three data quality dimensions that are often addressed using computer tools. As described earlier, data availability means that data are easily obtainable. Chapter 6, *Data Management*, covers data quality characteristics in more detail. Computer tools are used to monitor unscheduled computer downtime, determine why failures occurred, and provide data to help minimize future problems. Data consistency, a component of data integrity, means that data do not change no matter how often or in how many ways they are stored, processed, or displayed. Data values are consistent when the value of any given data element is the same across applications and information systems. Procedures are usually developed to monitor data periodically to ensure they are consistent across information systems.

Data definition is describing the data. Every data element should have a clear meaning and a range of acceptable values. For example, gender should have male and female as the only acceptable values. Data definitions and their values are usually stored in a data dictionary, which is discussed in chapter 6, *Data Management*.

Check Your Understanding 10.2

Answer the following questions.

1. An HIM professional using her password can access and change data in the hospital's master patient index. A patient accounting representative, using his password, cannot perform the same function. Limiting the class of information and functions that can be performed by these two employees is managed by:
   a. Network controls
   b. Audit trails
   c. Administrative controls
   d. Access controls
2. Data that has been converted into unintelligible format that must be decoded before it is legible is:
   a. An audit trail
   b. Encryption
   c. A password
   d. A physical safeguard
3. Identification of an organization's security threats and vulnerabilities is conducted during:
   a. Risk analysis
   b. Likelihood determination
   c. Impact analysis
   d. Authentication
4. Identify a threat to data security.
   a. Cryptographic technologies
   b. People
   c. Intrusion detection systems
   d. Access controls
5. Password policies should:
   a. Include mandatory scheduled password changes
   b. Permit password sharing only between good friends
   c. Require that passwords consist of numbers only
   d. Require that passwords be changed every 30 days
6. Identify an example of an administrative safeguard.
   a. Placing heat sensors near computer equipment
   b. Writing a policy regarding automatic computer log-offs
   c. Locking data center doors
   d. Placing computer monitors to face away from public areas
7. A firewall:
   a. Is an administrative safeguard
   b. Filters information between networks
   c. Only limits incoming information
   d. Only limits outgoing information
8. The CIA triad includes:
   a. Coordination, Integrity, and Accountability
   b. Confidentiality, Intrusion, and Availability
   c. Confidentiality, Integrity, and Accountability
   d. Confidentiality, Integrity, and Availability

Coordinated Security Program

A CE employee with responsibility for data security can manage threats to data security with a coordinated security program. This individual should be someone at the middle or senior management level. As mentioned earlier, he or she is frequently called the CSO. Figure 10.3 lists some of the CSO's functions.

When the data security program with policies and procedures is in place, the CSO is responsible for ensuring that everyone follows them. This is done using monitoring and evaluation systems, typically on an annual basis. Many CEs use outside information system auditing firms to conduct their security policy evaluations. In addition to the yearly audit, the CSO will establish procedures to audit and evaluate current processes randomly.

All data security policies and procedures should be reviewed and evaluated at least yearly to make sure they are up-to-date and still relevant to the organization.

HIPAA Security Provisions

The HIPAA Security Rule established standards to protect ePHI. The Department of Health and Human Services established the HIPAA Privacy Rule (discussed in chapter 9, *Data Privacy and Confidentiality*) and the HIPAA Security Rule. These standards apply to every health plan, healthcare clearinghouse, and healthcare provider processing financial or administrative transactions electronically. Additional changes to the Privacy and Security Rules were created as a result of the American Recovery and Reinvestment Act (ARRA) of 2009.

ARRA moved the enforcement for HIPAA security compliance from the Centers for Medicare and Medicaid Services' Office of Electronic Standards and Security to the Department of Health and Human Services Office for Civil Rights (OCR). The HITECH Act under ARRA increased enforcement of the provisions of the Privacy Rule and Security Rule through tougher penalties and greater breach reporting requirements. Prior to ARRA, audits were only conducted when there was a complaint. ARRA allowed random audits to be conducted. Enforcement of the HIPAA Security Rule must be taken seriously by CEs because penalties are severe and include both financial penalties and prison.

Security Rule standards are grouped into five categories. These categories are the following:

1. Administrative safeguards
2. Physical safeguards
3. Technical safeguards
4. Organizational requirements

Figure 10.3 Common functions of the chief security officer

- Conduct strategic planning for information system security
- Develop a data and information systems security policy
- Develop data security and information systems procedures
- Manage confidentiality agreements for employees and contractors
- Create mechanisms to ensure that data security policies and procedures are followed
- Coordinate employee security training
- Monitor audit trails to identify security violations
- Conduct risk assessment of enterprise information systems
- Develop a business continuity plan

Source: © AHIMA

5. Policies and procedures and documentation requirements

Essentially, the HIPAA Security Rule provisions follow the established best practices for the development and implementation of effective security policy. The requirements of the HIPAA Security Rule enforce the protection of information and access by authorized individuals only.

General Rules

The General Rules provide the objective and scope for the HIPAA Security Rule as a whole. They specify that CEs must develop a security program that includes a range of security safeguards to protect individually identifiable health information maintained (defined in chapter 9, *Data Privacy and Confidentiality*) or transmitted in electronic form. The General Rules include the following:

- CEs must demonstrate and document that they have done the following:
  - Ensured the confidentiality, integrity, and availability of all ePHI that is created, received, maintained, or transmitted by the covered entity
  - Protected ePHI against any reasonably anticipated threats or hazards to the security or integrity of ePHI
  - Protected ePHI against any reasonable or anticipated uses or disclosures that are not permitted under the HIPAA Privacy Rule
  - Ensured compliance with the HIPAA Security Rule by workforce members
- The Security Rule is flexible, scalable, and technology neutral. Regarding flexibility, HIPAA allows a CE to adopt security protection measures that are appropriate and reasonable for it. For example, security mechanisms will be more complex in a large hospital than in a small group practice. In determining which security measures to use, the following must be taken into account:
  - Size, complexity, and capabilities of the CE
  - Technical infrastructure, hardware, and software capabilities
  - Security measure costs
  - Probability and criticality of the potential risks to ePHI
- Scalable means that the Security Rule is written so that it accommodates CEs of any size. Technology neutral means that specific technologies are not prescribed, allowing organizations to develop as their technological capabilities evolve (Rinehart-Thompson 2018).
- The HIPAA Security Rule identifies standards that CEs must comply with. Business associates, hybrid entities, and other related entities (discussed in chapter 9, *Data Privacy and Confidentiality*) are also required to comply with these standards.
- **Implementation specifications** define how standards are to be implemented. Implementation specifications are either required or addressable. CEs must apply all implementation specifications that are required. Addressable does not mean optional. For those implementation specifications that are labeled addressable, the CE must conduct a risk assessment and evaluate whether the specification is appropriate to its environment. After conducting a risk assessment, if the CE finds that the specification is not a reasonable and appropriate safeguard for its environment (for example, a small CE may decide not to encrypt PHI because it deems it too expensive to do so), then the CE must do the following:
  1. Document why it is not reasonable and appropriate to implement the specification as written.
  2. Implement an equivalent alternative method if reasonable and appropriate.
- Maintenance: HIPAA requires CEs and business associates to maintain their security measures. Maintenance requires review and modification, as needed, to comply with

the provision of reasonable and appropriate protection of ePHI (45 CFR 164.306).

Administrative Safeguards

Administrative safeguards, as introduced earlier in the chapter, are documented, formal practices to manage data security measures throughout the CE. They require the CE to establish a security management process similar to the concepts discussed earlier in this chapter.

The administrative safeguards detail how the security program should be managed from the CE's perspective. Policies and procedures should be written and formalized in a policy manual. The CE should issue a statement of its philosophy (why security is important) on data security. Further, it should outline data security authority and responsibilities throughout the CE. There are a number of ways that a CE can control the use of terminals, including user limitations such as maximum allowed log-in attempts, screen savers, and the timing out of terminals when a determined period of inactivity has been reached. Physically, computers should be able to be locked when not in use, and a CE should maintain an inventory such that all computers used within the CE can be identified.

The administrative safeguards include the following standards that CEs must implement:

- *Security management process*. A CE must have a defined security management process. This means that there is a process in place for creating, maintaining, and overseeing the development of security policies and procedures; identifying vulnerabilities and conducting risk analyses; establishing a risk management program; developing a sanction policy; and reviewing information system activity.
- *Assigned security responsibility*. Each CE must designate a security official to assume the role described earlier in this chapter.
- *Workforce security*. The CE must ensure appropriate clearance procedures to grant access to individually identifiable information to workforce members who need to use ePHI to perform their job duties and must maintain appropriate oversight of authorization and access. Likewise, the CE must prevent access to information to those who do not need it and have clear procedures of access termination for employees who leave the CE. These individuals must be removed from the information systems immediately to prevent disgruntled former employees from altering or otherwise harming the data. Sanction policies must also be in place. These sanction policies outline how employees are penalized when they violate the CE's security policy and procedures.
- *Information access management*. This standard requires the CE to implement a program of information access management. It includes specific policies and procedures to determine who should have access to what information.
- *Security awareness and training*. This standard requires the CE to provide security training for all members of the workforce as described above.
- *Security incident procedures*. This standard requires the implementation of policies and procedures to address security incidents, including responding to, reporting, and mitigating suspected or known incidents.
- *Contingency plan*. This standard requires the establishment and implementation of policies and procedures for responding to emergencies or failures in systems that contain ePHI. It includes a data backup plan, disaster recovery plan, emergency mode of operation plan, testing and revision procedures, and applications and data criticality analysis to prioritize data and determine what must be maintained or restored first in an emergency.
- *Evaluation*. A periodic evaluation must be performed in response to environmental or operational changes affecting the security of ePHI and appropriate improvements in policies and procedures should follow.

- *Business associate contracts*. This standard requires business associates to appropriately safeguard information in their possession and CEs to receive satisfactory assurances that the business associates will do so (45 CFR 164.308).

Figure 10.4 identifies the HIPAA Security Rule Administrative Safeguards.

Physical Safeguards

Physical safeguards include the protection of hardware, software, and data from natural and

Figure 10.4 HIPAA Security rule administrative safeguards

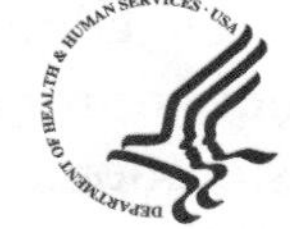

1 Security 101 for Covered Entities

Security Standards Matrix (Appendix A of the Security Rule)

ADMINISTRATIVE SAFEGUARDS			
Standards	Sections	Implementation Specifications (R) = Required, (A)=Addressable	
Security Management Process	164 308(a)(1)	Risk Analysis	(R)
		Risk Management	(R)
		Sanction Policy	(R)
		Information System Activity Review	(R)
Assigned Security Responsiblity	164 308(a)(2)		(R)
Workforce Security	164 308(a)(3)	Authorization and/or Supervision	(A)
		Workforce Clearance Procedure	(A)
		Termination Procedures	(A)
Information Access Management	164 308(a)(4)	Isolating Health Care Clearinghouse functons	(R)
		Access Authorization	(A)
		Access Establishment and Modification	(A)
Security Awareness and Training	164 308(a)(5)	Security Reminders	(A)
		Protection from Mabolous Sofftware	(A)
		Log-in Monitoring	(A)
		Password Management	(A)
Security Incident Procedures	164 308(a)(6)	Response and Reporting	(R)
Contingency Plan	164 308(a)(7)	Data Backup Plan	(R)
		Disaster Recovery Plan	(R)
		Emergency Mode Operation Plan	(R)
		Testing and Revision Procedures	(A)
		Applications and Data Criticality Analysis	(A)
Evaluation	164 308(a)(8)		(R)
Business Associate Contracts and Other Arrangements	164 308(b)(1)	Writting Contract or Other Arrangement	(R)

Source: CMS.2007

environmental hazards and intrusion. Physical safeguards consist of the following:

- *Facility access controls.* Policies and procedures must be implemented to appropriately manage not only the physical security of information systems, but also the buildings that house those information systems. This is accomplished through building infrastructure as well as access management related to the individuals who are and are not permitted to access those facilities. Restoration of data is also required under this provision during and after disaster recovery as well as regular repairs and updating of physical components of the facilities with documentation to demonstrate such maintenance has taken place.
- *Workstation use.* Policies and procedures must relate to workstations that access ePHI and include proper functions to be performed, how they are to be performed, and the physical environment in which those workstations exist.
- *Workstation security.* Provisions under workstation security require that physical safeguards, as described earlier, be implemented for workstations with access to ePHI.
- *Device and media controls.* This standard requires the CE to specify proper receipt and removal of hardware and media with ePHI and to address items as they move within the CE. The entity must also address procedures for removal or disposal including reuse or redeployment of electronic media, data backup, and the identity of persons accountable for the process. ITAD policies are required under this standard. These policies should address end of life cycle hard drives, laptops, servers, and other media that have contained sensitive data. Because such equipment is often redeployed in the CE, all ePHI and any other sensitive data must be removed. Before hard drives, servers, or laptops are disposed of, appropriate data destruction must be carried out (45 CFR 164.310).

Technical Safeguards

Of all the safeguards that are required to be implemented to some degree in compliance with the HIPAA Security Rule, the technical safeguards are

Figure 10.5 HIPAA security rule physical safeguard standards

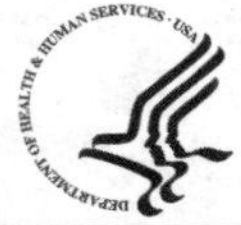

1 Security 101 for Covered Entities

PHYSICAL SAFEGUARDS			
Standards	Sections	Implementation Specifications (R) = Required, (A)=Addressable	
Facility Access Controls	164.310(a)(1)	Contingency Operations	(A)
		Facility Security Plan	(A)
		Access Control and Validation Procedures	(A)
		Maintenance Records	(A)
Workstation Use	164.310(b)		(R)
Workstation Security	164.310(c)		(R)
Device and Media Controls	164.310(d)(1)	Disposal	(R)
		Media Re-use	(R)
		Accountability	(A)
		Data Backup and Storage	(A)

Source: CMS 2007.

the most important aspect to a secure system due to the ever-changing and advancing of technologies across all industries, especially healthcare.

The technical safeguards, which are the technology and the policies and procedures regarding the use and operation of the technology, consist of five broad categories. These provisions include those things that can be implemented from a technical standpoint using computer software, including the following:

- *Access controls*. The access controls standard requires implementation of technical procedures to control or limit access to health information. The procedures would be executed through some type of software program. This requirement ensures that individuals are given authorization to access only the data they need to perform their respective jobs. The implementation specifications include unique user identifications, emergency access procedures (for example, a break-the-glass capability that allows an individual who normally would not have access to the information access to it in an emergency; however the use of this access must be monitored), automatic log-off after a predetermined period of workstation inactivity, and encryption and decryption, discussed earlier in the chapter.
- *Audit controls*. The audit control standard requires that procedural mechanisms be implemented to record activity in systems that contain ePHI and that the output be examined to determine appropriateness of access. Audit trails were discussed earlier in this chapter.
- *Integrity*. The data integrity standard requires CEs to implement policies and procedures to protect ePHI from being improperly altered or destroyed. In other words, this standard requires CEs to provide proof that their data have not been altered in an unauthorized manner. Data authentication can be substantiated through audit trails and system logs that track users who have accessed or modified data via unique identifiers.
- *Person or entity authentication*. This standard requires that those accessing ePHI must be appropriately identified and authenticated as discussed earlier in this chapter.
- *Transmission security*. This standard requires the guarding of data against unauthorized access (interception) or improper modification without detection when they are in transit, whether via open networks such as the internet or private networks such as those internal to an organization. The two implementation specifications—integrity controls and encryption—are addressable. The Security Rule itself does not require encryption unless the CE deems it appropriate, but the security of ePHI transmitted over public networks or communication systems must be accomplished. Data encryption that provides protection for data across transmission lines is important because eavesdropping is easily accomplished using devices called sniffers. Sniffers can be attached to networks for the purpose of diverting transmitted data. A sniffer is a software security product that runs in the background of a network, examining and logging packet traffic and serving as an early warning device against crackers. A hacker is an individual whose job is to identify weaknesses in an information system so that they can be corrected. A cracker is an individual who exploits any weaknesses in an information system (Munson 2017). Protecting data during transmission is only one role of encryption. Data at rest can also be encrypted. Data at rest are data that are in storage such as in a database. Passwords stored in a database may also be encrypted. Thus, if a cracker breaks into the password database, the data will be unusable (45 CFR 164.312). Figure 10.6 is HIPAA Security Rule technical safeguards.

Organizational Requirements

This section includes the following two standards—one addresses business associates (BA)

Figure 10.6 HIPAA Security Rule Technical Safeguards

1 Security 101 for Covered Entities

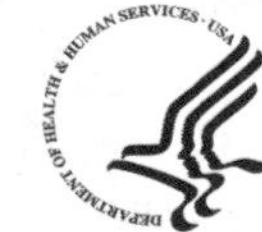

TECHNICAL SAFEGUARDS			
Standards	Sections	Implementation Specifications (R)= Required, (A)=Addressable	
Access Control	164.312(a)(1)	Unique User Identification	(R)
		Emergency Access Procedure	(R)
		Automatic Logoff	(A)
		Encryption and Decryption	(A)
Audit Controls	164.312(b)		(R)
Integrity	164.312(c)(1)	Mechanism to Authenticate Electronic Protected Health Information	(A)
Person or Entity Authentication	164.312(d)		(R)
Transmission Security	164.312(e)(1)	Integrity Controls	(A)
		Encryption	(A)

Source: CMS 2007.

and similar entities and the other addresses group health plan requirements.

1. *Business associate or other contracts*. CEs must obtain a written contract with BAs or other entities (hybrid or other) that handle ePHI. The written contract must stipulate that the BA will implement HIPAA administrative, physical, and technical safeguards and procedures and documentation requirements that safeguard the confidentiality, integrity, and availability of the ePHI that it creates, receives, maintains, or transmits on behalf of the CE. The contract must ensure any agent, including a subcontractor, agrees to implement reasonable and appropriate safeguards. Specifically, HIPAA requires a BA to report to the CE any security incident or breach of ePHI of which it becomes aware. The CE must authorize termination of the contract if it determines that the BA has violated a material term of the contract.
2. *Group health plan requirements*. Group health plans must ensure their plan documents provide that the plan sponsor (an entity that provides a health plan for its employees) will reasonably and appropriately safeguard ePHI that is created, received, maintained, or transmitted by or to plan sponsors on behalf of the health plans (45 CFR 164.314).

Policies and Procedures and Documentation Requirements

The Security Rule requires that CEs and BAs have policies and procedures and that they be documented in writing. The following other information about any actions, assessments, or activities associated with the HIPAA Security Rule also must be in writing.

- *Policies and procedures*. Entities must implement reasonable and appropriate policies and procedures to comply with the HIPAA security standards, implementation specifications, and other requirements. Policies and procedures should be developed and implemented considering the section on flexibility outlined in the rule.
- *Documentation*. Entities must maintain their security policies and procedures in writing (this includes electronic format). Any actions, assessments, or activities related to the HIPAA Security Rule also must be documented in writing. Documentation

must be retained for six years from the date of its creation or the date when it last was in effect, whichever is later. It must be made available to those individuals responsible for implementing security procedures.

Further, it must be reviewed periodically and updated as needed, in response to environmental or organizational changes that affect the security of ePHI (45 CFR 164.316).

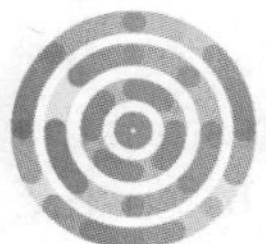

American Recovery and Reinvestment Act of 2009 Provisions

The HITECH Act, a portion of ARRA, broadened privacy and security provisions including greater individual rights and protections when third parties handle individually identifiable health information. These changes had a significant impact on the security provisions.

The single most important change was the requirement that business associates of HIPAA-covered entities must comply with most of the same rules as CEs. As noted in chapter 9, *Data Privacy and Confidentiality,* BAs perform functions or activities on behalf of or for a CE that involve the use or disclosure of PHI. Common BAs include consultants, billing companies, transcription companies, accounting firms, and law firms.

With the implementation of the ARRA, potential BA liability increased. BAs are now held directly responsible for not complying with the administrative, physical, and technical safeguards of the HIPAA Security Rule, as well as the policies and procedures and documentation requirements.

Another important change per the HITECH Act was defining breach and adding breach notification requirements. Breaches only apply to **unsecured electronic protected health information**, which is ePHI that has not been made unusable, unreadable, or indecipherable to unauthorized persons (AHIMA 2013a). Thus, the need for encryption is clear. With regard to security, breach notification has implications for the protection of data in all the following phases:

- Data at rest—for example, data contained in databases, file systems, or flash drives
- Data in motion—for example, data moving through a network or wireless transmission
- Data in use—for example, data in the process of being created, retrieved, updated, or deleted
- Data disposed—for example, discarded paper records or recycled electronic media. It is critical to use appropriate data destruction methods to ensure disposed data cannot be read, retrieved, or reconstructed in any way (AHIMA 2009)

Forensics

Forensics is the process of identifying, analyzing, recovering, and preserving data within an electronic environment. With appropriate policies and procedures in place, it is the responsibility of the CE and its managers, directors, CSO, and employees with audit responsibilities to review access logs, audit trails, failed log-ins, and other reports generated to monitor compliance with the policies and procedures. These types of events are usually called **trigger events** and include the following employees viewing:

- Records of patients with the same last name or address of the employee
- VIP records (celebrities, board members, political figures)

- Records of those involved in high-profile events in the community
- Records with little or no activity for 120 days
- Other employee's records
- Files of minors
- Files of those treated for infectious diseases or sensitive diagnoses such as HIV/AIDS or sexually transmitted diseases
- Records of patients for whom the viewing employee did not provide care
- Records of a spouse (without the same surname)
- Records of terminated employees
- Portions of records of a discipline not consistent with the employee's expertise (Walsh and Miaoulis 2014)

The CE should have specific policies and monitoring procedures in place to track employees' access via sign-on and password and periodically audit all reports, especially when incidents occur or VIPs are treated. HIPAA requires a regular review of system activity such as monitoring new user access, reviewing system access by users in general, and testing the access of recently terminated employees to ensure they have, in fact, been removed from access roles. There have been numerous cases where employees have inappropriately accessed the hospital records of high-profile individuals. These actions have led to discipline, including termination and fines, after audit trails revealed unauthorized access.

Check Your Understanding 10.3

Answer the following questions.

1. According to American Recovery and Reinvestment Act revisions:
   a. No changes were made to the HIPAA standards
   b. Potential business associate liability was increased under HIPAA
   c. Business associate liability was decreased under HIPAA
   d. Breaches apply to both secured and unsecured PHI
2. A covered entity has robust policies and procedures. The government is investigating a security breach. How far back can the government request documentation related to data security policies and procedures?
   a. Six years
   b. Five years
   c. Two years
   d. Ten years
3. The patient's address is the same in the master patient index, electronic health record, laboratory information system, and other information systems. This means that the data values are consistent and therefore indicative of which of the following?
   a. Data availability
   b. Data accessibility
   c. Data privacy
   d. Data integrity
4. Identify an example of a technical safeguard.
   a. A policy that states that passwords cannot be shared
   b. A policy that states that only authorized people can access the data center
   c. Locking the door of the data center
   d. Assigning passwords that limit access to computer-stored information

5. According to HIPAA standards, the designated individual responsible for data security:
   a. Must be identified by every covered entity
   b. Is only required in large facilities
   c. Is only required in hospitals
   d. Is not required in small physician office practices
6. Critique each statement to determine the true statement regarding a coordinated security program.
   a. The CSO must hold a lower level position so as not to create controversy.
   b. All security policies and procedures should be updated every six months.
   c. This type of program should only be established if an organization has sufficient funds to support it.
   d. Someone inside the CE must be responsible for data security.
7. An automated flag just notified us that a VIP's health record was accessed. This might have been as the result of a(n):
   a. Trigger
   b. Audit
   c. Policy and procedure
   d. Monitor of data in use
8. An employee views a patient's electronic health record. It is a trigger event if:
   a. The employee and patient have the same last name
   b. The patient was admitted through the emergency department
   c. The patient is over 89 years old
   d. A dietitian views a patient's nutrition care plan
9. If an implementation specification is addressable:
   a. It is optional
   b. If not implemented, the organization must document why it is not reasonable and appropriate to do so
   c. If not implemented, the organization does not have to account for its absence
   d. It must be carried out as written

HIM Roles

As data continue to proliferate and breaches continue to occur at an alarming rate, HIM professionals will continue to play an increasing and vital role in leading initiatives and efforts to reduce and prevent data breaches. As health information has become more electronic in nature, HIM roles in general have taken more of a technology emphasis. HIM professionals with graduate degrees can assume the role of the Chief Security Officer. HIM professionals can also conduct audits and risk assessments and otherwise participate in the security program of a CE. Additional roles will continue develop within the HIM field to meet the new needs and challenges brought about by new technology.

Real-World Case 10.1

The Department of Health and Human Services reported on its website a $3,000,000 settlement with Touchstone Medical Imaging. One of Touchstone's servers allowed access to ePHI via the internet. More than 300,000 patients were impacted. The ePHI included names, Social Security information, and more. Touchstone did not investigate the matter in a timely manner. The investigation also found that a risk analysis had not been conducted and business associate agreements were not in place (Source: HHS 2019).

Real-World Case 10.2

You are the Chief Security Officer of Anywhere Hospital. You just received a frantic email from one of your help desk employees in the Information Technology department. There is a suspected malware infection that is spreading across your computer network. You ask your staff member whether there has been data loss or corruption. Your team member responds by saying that she does not know yet; the security team has been called and will begin the investigation process, starting with the origin of the malware. A quick and thorough response to this incident is of the utmost importance and is crucial to avoid disrupting patient care systems.

A little while later, you discover that the malware was launched from within the network via email; specifically, the malware was launched on the vice president's workstation in his office when he opened an email containing the malware. The hospital's Network Intrusion Detection System did not pick up abnormal traffic coming through the firewall.

References

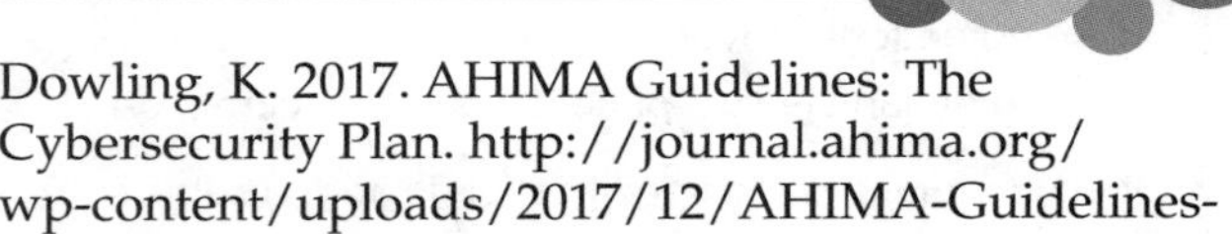

American Health Information Management Association. 2017. *Pocket Glossary of Health Information Management and Technology*, 5th ed. Chicago: AHIMA.

American Health Information Management Association. 2013a. Analysis of Modifications to the HIPAA Privacy, Security, Enforcement, and Breach Notification Rules Under the Health Information Technology for Economic and Clinical Health Act and the Genetic Information Nondiscrimination Act; Other Modifications to the HIPAA Rules. http://library.ahima.org/PdfView?oid=106127.

American Health Information Management Association. 2009. Analysis of the Interim Final Rule, August 24, 2009: Breach Notification for Unsecured Protected Health Information. http://library.ahima.org/PdfView?oid=100232.

Carlon, S. 2013. Information Security. Chapter 17 in *Health Information Management Technology: An Applied Approach*. Edited by N.B. Sayles. Chicago: AHIMA.

Centers for Medicare and Medicaid Services. 2007. Security 101 for Covered Entities. https://www.hhs.gov/sites/default/files/ocr/privacy/hipaa/administrative/securityrule/security101.pdf.

Department of Health and Human Services. 2019. Tennessee diagnostic medical imaging services company pays $3,000,000 to settle breach exposing over 300,000 patients' protected health information. https://www.hhs.gov/about/news/2019/05/06/tennessee-diagnostic-medical-imaging-services-company-pays-3000000-settle-breach.html.

Dowling, K. 2017. AHIMA Guidelines: The Cybersecurity Plan. http://journal.ahima.org/wp-content/uploads/2017/12/AHIMA-Guidelines-Cybersecurity-Plan.pdf.

Institute of Medicine. 2011. Health IT and Patient Safety: Building Safer Systems for Better Care. Consensus Report. http://www.iom.edu/Reports/2011/Health-IT-and-Patient-Safety-Building-Safer-Systems-for-Better-Care.aspx.

Johns, M.L. 2008. Privacy and Security in Health Information. In *Electronic Health Records: A Guide for Clinicians and Administrators*, 2nd ed. Edited by J. Carter. Philadelphia: American College of Physicians.

McCann, E. 2014 (January 2). 4-Year Long HIPAA Breach Uncovered. HealthITNews. http://www.healthcareitnews.com/news/four-year-long-hipaa-data-breach-discovered.

Miaoulis, W.M. 2011. *Preparing for a HIPAA Security Compliance Assessment*. Chicago: AHIMA.

Munson, L. 2017. What are the Main Differences Between Hackers and Crackers? http://www.security-faqs.com/what-are-the-main-differences-between-hackers-and-crackers.html.

National Institute of Standards and Technology. 2008. An Introductory Resource Guide for Implementing the Health Insurance Portability and Accountability Act (HIPAA) Security Rule. http://csrc.nist.gov/publications/nistpubs/800-66-Rev1/SP-800-66-Revision1.pdf.

Olenik, K., and R. Reynolds. 2017. Security Threats and Controls. Chapter 13 in *Fundamentals of Law for Health Informatics and Information Management.* Edited by M.S. Brodnik, L.A. Rinehart-Thompson, and R.B. Reynolds. Chicago: AHIMA.

Rinehart-Thompson, L.A. 2018. *Introduction to Health Information Privacy and Security.* Chicago: AHIMA.

Walsh, T, and W. M. Miaoulis. 2014. Privacy and Security Audits of Electronic Health Information (2014 Update). *Journal of AHIMA* 85(3):54-59.

45 CFR 160, 162, and 164. HIPAA administrative simplification regulation text. 2013 (unofficial version, as amended through March 26). https://www.hhs.gov/sites/default/files/ocr/privacy/hipaa/administrative/combined/hipaa-simplification-201303.pdf.

45 CFR 164.306: Security standards: General rules. 2006.

45 CFR 164.308: Administrative safeguards. 2006.

45 CFR 164.310: Physical safeguards. 2006.

45 CFR 164.312: Technical safeguards. 2006.

45 CFR 164.314: Organizational requirements. 2006.

45 CFR 164.316: Policies and procedures and documentation requirements. 2006.

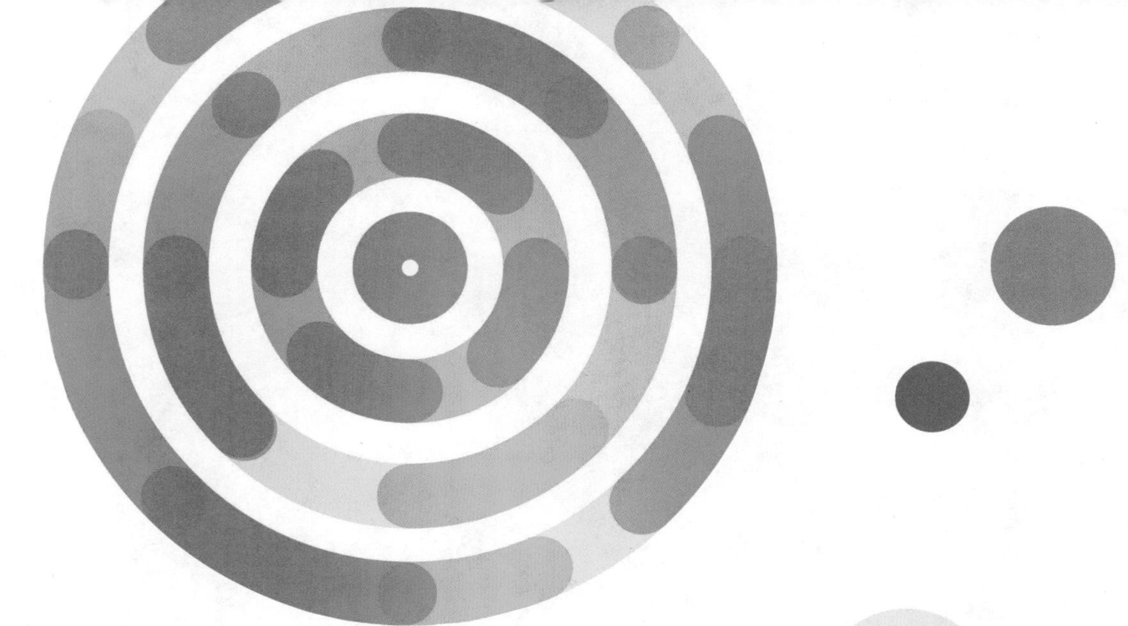

PART IV

Informatics, Analytics, and Data Use

Health Information Systems

Margret K. Amatayakul, MBA, RHIA, CHPS, CPEHR, FHIMSS

Learning Objectives

- Identify the scope of health information systems and how they have evolved to their current state of implementation in hospitals, ambulatory care, and other settings
- Apply the systems development life cycle in the planning, selection, implementation, and ongoing management of health information systems
- Utilize a systems approach to achieve systems integration so health information systems support the national mission to improve health and healthcare, and reduce healthcare costs

Key Terms

3D printing
Accredited Standards Committee X12 (ASC X12)
Adoption
Alert fatigue
Alternative payment models (APMs)
Analytics
Ancillary systems
Application program interface (API)
Application service provider (ASP)
Artificial intelligence (AI)
Auto-analyzer
Automated drug dispensing machines
Bar code medication administration record (BC-MAR)
Best of breed
Best of fit
Big data
Billing system
Biometrics
Business intelligence (BI)
Certificate authority
Certification
Change control program
Chart conversion
Chart tracking
Chief medical informatics officer (CMIO)
Claims data
Clearinghouse
Client/server system
Clinical data repository (CDR)
Clinical data warehouse (CDW)
Clinical decision support (CDS)
Clinical decision support system (CDSS)
Clinical Document Architecture (CDA)
Clinical Laboratory Improvement Amendments (CLIA) of 1988
Clinical transformation
Closed-loop medication management
Cloud computing
Computerized provider order entry (CPOE)
CONNECT
Consent directive
Consent management systems
Consolidated Clinical Document Architecture (C-CDA)

Continuity of care document (CCD)
Contraindication
Customer relationship management (CRM)
Data
Data conversion
Data dictionary
Data governance framework (DGF)
Data model
Data quality
Data Use and Reciprocal Support Agreement (DURSA)
Diagnostic studies
Digital certificate
Digital Imaging and Communications in Medicine (DICOM)
Direct Project
Discrete reportable transcription (DRT)
Document imaging
Drug knowledge database
Due diligence
eHealth Exchange
End user
Enterprise architecture (EA)
e-prescribing (e-Rx)
e-prescribing for controlled substances (EPCS)
Evidence-based medicine (EBM)
e-visits
Fast Healthcare Interoperability Resource (FHIR)
Federal Health IT Strategic Plan 2015–2020
Go-live
Health information exchange (HIE)
Health information organization (HIO)
Health information system
Health Information Technology for Economic and Clinical Health (HITECH)
Health Insurance Portability and Accountability Act of 1996 (HIPAA)
Health IT
Health Level Seven (HL7)
Hospital in the home
Human computer interfaces (HCI)
Identity management (IdM)
Identity matching algorithm
Identity proofing
Implementation
Inference engine
Information
Interface
Interface engine
Interoperability
Issues management
Kiosk
Knowledge
Knowledge sources
Laboratory information system (LIS)
Logical Observations, Identifiers, Names, and Codes (LOINC)
Machine learning
Meaningful Use
Meaningful Use (MU) program
Medication five rights
Medication reconciliation
Message format standards
Metadata
National Council for Prescription Drug Programs (NCPDP)
National Drug Codes (NDC)
Natural language processing (NLP)
Nursing information system
Office of the National Coordinator (ONC) for Health Information Technology
Online analytical processing (OLAP)
Online transaction processing (OLTP)
Operating rules
Optimization
Opt in/opt out
Patient acuity staffing
Patient financial system (PFS)
Patient portal
Patient safety
Personal health record (PHR)
Personalized medicine
Pharmacy information system
Physician champion
Picture archiving and communications system (PACS)
Point-of-care (POC) documentation
Policy interoperability
Population health
Population health management (PHM)
Portals
Power user
Primary care physician (PCP)
Process interoperabilityProject management office (PMO)
Protocol
Provider
Radio-frequency identification (RFID)
Radiology information system (RIS)
Record locator service (RLS)
Registration-admission, discharge, transfer (R-ADT)
Registry
Requirements specification
Results management
Revenue cycle management (RCM)
Rules engine
RxNorm
Scribe
SCRIPT
Semantic interoperability
SMART goals
Smart peripherals
Software as a Service (SaaS)
Source systems
Speech dictation
Steering committee
Storage management
Structured data
Sunsetting
System
System build
System configuration
Systems development life cycle (SDLC)
Technical interoperability
Telehealth
Template
Transaction
Two-factor authentication
Unintended consequence
Unstructured data
Use
Value
Value-based care (VBC)
Vendor selection
Virtual private network (VPN)
Web services architecture (WSA)
Workstations on wheels (WOWs)
XML (eXtensible markup language)

The Office of the National Coordinator (ONC) for Health Information Technology is the agency within the federal government tasked to be the health information technology (typically referenced as health IT) resource to the nation. In 2015, the ONC issued the Federal Health IT Strategic Plan 2015–2020 in which it describes a vision and mission for the United States' use of health information technology (IT):

> Vision: High-quality care, lower costs, healthy population, and engaged people. Mission: Improve the health and well-being of individuals and communities through the use of technology and health information that is accessible when and where it matters most (ONC 2015).

In addition, the Federal Health IT Strategic Plan identified four overarching goals for health IT, which are both sequential as enumerated below, and interdependent as shown in figure 11.1. The following goals ultimately focus on improving the health and well-being of the nation:

- Advance person-centered and self-managed health
- Transform healthcare delivery and community health
- Foster research, scientific knowledge, and innovation
- Enhance the nation's health IT infrastructure

Dissemination of knowledge is stated as a goal in the Federal Health IT Strategic Plan. Knowledge is more than information; knowledge is the application of experience to information that provides value to the information beyond only serving as evidence of actions taken. Data are raw facts and figures without context or meaning; information is data that have been processed in a useful and meaningful manner.

Figure 11.1 Federal Health IT Strategic Plan 2015–2020

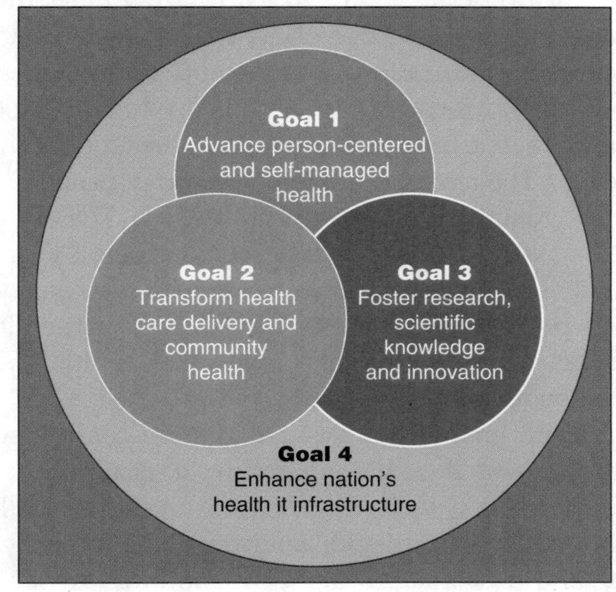

Source: ONC 2015

This chapter discusses the scope of health information systems, the importance of standards, and the need to take a systems approach to planning, selecting, implementing, and managing health information systems so that the ultimate result meets the national vision and mission for healthcare and the goals for each healthcare provider (hospital, physician, nursing home, and others). The role health information management (HIM) professionals play in acquiring, implementing, gaining adoption, and optimizing use of health information systems is also discussed in this chapter.

Health Information Systems

The term health IT, or health information and technology, is used by the ONC because of its focus on information technology for healthcare. Information technology used by healthcare entities includes computer hardware and software to enable the collection and processing of data into useful information. Information technology includes communication and network technologies that enable data and information to be exchanged across various computers. Such technology, however, would apply in any environment. In addition, technology alone does not achieve the ultimate goal of gaining benefits from its use. People, policy, and process elements must be addressed for healthcare professionals to learn how to use and make the most effective use of the hardware, software, communications, and network technologies.

Health information system is used to describe the full scope of adopting health information technology. The term **system** refers to components that work together to accomplish a goal. The term *health information system* may be considered to include technical components and people, policy, and process components that work together to support the goal of improving the health and well-being of the nation.

Health information systems may be considered narrowly or broadly. For example, a laboratory information system (LIS) in a hospital is a health information system with a narrow focus on receiving and processing orders for laboratory testing, collecting and processing specimens, and documenting, delivering, and storing results. LISs also support department management, including staffing, equipment maintenance, supplies, and compliance.

As such, a health information system for a hospital laboratory includes the following:

- Hardware: computers, printers, laboratory devices
- Software: computer programs designed to process orders for lab tests, produce specimen collection lists for hospitalized patients, produce labels for specimen containers, produce test results, and conduct quality assurance on lab testing processes
- Communications and network technologies (connections with a **computerized provider order entry [CPOE] system**), used by providers to enter orders for lab tests as well as medications and other procedures, laboratory testing devices, pharmacy systems to obtain drug information that may impact test results, and destination systems, such as the electronic health record (EHR) system to convey results to providers and billing systems to capture charges for the lab tests
- Operational and cultural adaptations necessary to use the technologies in performing **diagnostic studies** (all diagnostic services of any type, including history, physical examination, laboratory, x-ray and others that are performed or ordered pertinent to the patient's reasons for the encounter) on various specimens collected from patients and applying professional judgment in evaluating the quality of the data representing the results
- Policies and standards from the local healthcare organization in which the information system is housed as well as accrediting and licensing bodies that must be followed for design of the technology and its use. For example, policies and standards for a LIS may include use of certain terminologies, such as the **Logical Observations, Identifiers, Names, and Codes (LOINC)**, which is federally mandated for ordering and reporting lab results. The **Clinical Laboratory Improvement Amendments (CLIA) of 1988** are federal regulatory standards that ensure quality laboratory testing. They were modified in 2014 to ensure patients may have direct access to their test results, even prior to review by their ordering provider (*Federal Register* 2014).
- Workflow and process designs ensure the most efficient and effective use of the technology (chapter 17, *Management*, covers workflow in more detail).

An EHR system is broader in scope than a LIS. An EHR supports physicians, nurses, and other healthcare professionals in their documentation and communications concerning patients within the healthcare enterprise. An EHR has connection points to many focused health information systems in a healthcare organization. These health information systems include the LIS, pharmacy information system, radiology information system, nursing information system, dietary information system, emergency department system, and many others. There are also an increasing number of connections with other healthcare and related organizations, such as physician offices, health plans, public health departments, immunization registries, ambulance services, quality measure registries, vendors, and others. Healthcare organizations are using EHRs to connect with patients in multiple ways. Connections may be available through portals (windows into information systems), personal health records (PHRs), personal medical devices, apps on smart phones, and telehealth services that assist in providing remote diagnosis and treatment through telecommunications technology.

Another health information system that may be either narrow or broad is afforded by health information exchange (HIE) services. HIEs enable sharing of health information across disparate entities. While EHRs are accessible within a given healthcare entity, the primary purpose of an HIE is to support authorized exchange of health data across entities that subscribe to the service. This function extends data sharing more broadly than an EHR but is often relatively narrow in scope. It may serve only to share where an EHR for a patient is located; or it may maintain a repository of limited data, such as lab results and medication lists that can be accessed by subscribers. In this narrow context, the HIE maintains patient and provider directories and provides consent management and security services. To support such basic services at low or no cost to providers, many HIEs provide additional services. These broader services vary by HIE. Some HIEs offer clearinghouse services for revenue cycle management. Others may offer data mapping to reconcile differences between coding systems or versions of coding systems. Increasingly, many HIEs offer data aggregation and analysis, quality measure data collection and reporting, and business intelligence services (HealthIT.gov. 2018; HIMSS 2012a; AHIMA 2013).

Perhaps the broadest possible health information system is one that does not exist, but could be viewed as a virtual system of all EHRs (encompassing all of the narrow systems within an organization), all HIEs (to support exchange across organizations), and potentially other information systems, such as ancestry and genomic systems and others. While such a broad health information system is not likely to exist as a single entity, the goal is to ultimately support the sharing of health information to achieve the best possible healthcare and experience of care at a reasonable cost.

As suggested by the many health information systems that exist and which may continue to be developed or enhanced as new information technology emerges, it is important to recognize that many health information systems need to be periodically updated and expanded, or even phased out and replaced with new technology. The sections that follow will discuss the current state of health information systems and their scope—including source systems, core EHR applications, specialty systems, HIE systems, automated medical devices, supporting infrastructure, and connectivity systems.

Current State of Health Information Systems

Health information systems for lab, pharmacy, and other ancillary services are not new. Physicians and nurses have relied on these information systems as an important means to exchange diagnostic reports, medication, and other information since the early 1970s. EHRs were initially conceived around this time, but did not become a primary focus for healthcare providers until 2009 with the passage of the Health Information Technology for Economic and Clinical Health (HITECH) Act legislation. HITECH provided eligible hospitals and professionals with financial incentives, in terms of healthcare payment adjustments, to make meaningful use of EHRs. This incentive program is commonly referred to as the Meaningful Use (MU) program (now known as promoting interoperability) and describes an EHR that is qualified for earning incentives as one that:

> includes patient demographic and clinical health information, such as medical history and problem lists; and has the capacity to provide clinical decision support, support physician order entry, capture and query information relevant to healthcare quality, and exchange electronic health information

with and integrate such information from other sources (HealthIT.gov. 2016).

While most hospitals and many healthcare professionals have implemented an EHR within their healthcare organizations, the MU program started winding down in 2016. Since then, requirements for using an EHR have been incorporated into **alternative payment models (APMs)**, which are new ways the federal government is paying for care. Such payment models are used in what is now being referred to as **value-based care (VBC)** strategies to improve the quality of care and drive down its cost. In this context, **value** refers to improving the quality of care to achieve a healthier nation, which can result in reducing the cost of care overall. For example, for physicians to be paid under Medicare, they must supply data to the federal government via their EHR for quality measurement. Different payment models are then applied based on provider factors, including the level of risk a provider is willing to assume (QPP,CMS.gov/apms. 2018; Feeley and Mohta 2018). (Reimbursement is discussed in chapter 15, *Revenue Management and Reimbursement.)*

The degree to which EHRs are used by healthcare professionals varies significantly. As a result, EHRs are "never done" (Gue 2018); they require continuous updating and improvement. The terms and definitions that describe the various stages in which any new information system may exist in healthcare, include the following:

- **Implementation** refers to technology having been installed and configured to meet the basic requirements of the healthcare organization. Demonstration to end users has taken place. **End users** are those persons who will use the information system in the course of their daily processes and procedures.
- **Use** refers to the fact that those who are supposed to apply the technology to their daily work have been trained and are starting to apply the technology at a simple level. For example, nurses may enter data into nurse assessment **templates** (a guide for documentation) and document medication administration using the technology. Physicians may use an EHR to review lab results and other information collected by other healthcare professionals. Often "use" has not addressed workflow and process changes that enable intended users to seamlessly incorporate the technology into their everyday operations. Simple usage should begin immediately after implementation, but within a few months users should be moving to adoption.
- **Meaningful Use**, as noted above, is a term used by the federal government for the program designed to incentivize use of EHRs. The term *meaningful* was chosen to reflect the purposeful desire to go beyond simply using the EHR as a search tool. There were two components to the MU program. One component was managed by the ONC and specified the functionality an EHR must have in order for a provider to qualify to earn the incentives. The other component of the MU program was the degree of use providers should make of the qualified EHR as specified by CMS (CMS 2014). CMS supplied monetary incentives through its Medicare and Medicaid reimbursement systems. Three stages were initially planned, with two stages fulfilled and the third stage moved to CMS's VBC programs (QPP.CMS.gov/mips. 2018).
- **Adoption** is a term frequently associated with the intent of MU. Adoption of health information systems reflects that the healthcare organization has implemented all the major components of technology, although there may be some available technology that is more specialized, costly, and time-consuming to implement that has not yet been implemented. Adoption with respect to the EHR requires users to rely on technology to enter and retrieve most information, and where decision support is included to use it when appropriate. Adoption of EHRs demonstrates effective integration into the daily routines of

healthcare. Adoption also should indicate it generally takes no more time to use an EHR than the paper health record, and generally yields greater value to the user than the paper health record. Unfortunately, adoption of EHRs has yet to be fully achieved, as many healthcare professionals find that EHRs are more time-consuming than paper and some find them to be distracting during patient care. In general, hospitals find them more helpful than not, and have supported physicians in using medical scribes (an assistant who gathers information and documents care into the EHR) and other workarounds that enable them to achieve EHR benefits. Some physician offices delayed implementation, others have abandoned the EHRs they implemented, and a number of them are in the process of replacing initially acquired systems with newer and improved systems (Spitzer 2018).

- **Optimization** is the state that demonstrates not only effective adoption of health information systems for routine operations, but also an understanding and appropriate use of the technology's features with workflow and process improvements that can improve clinical efficiency (Monica 2018) and improve a healthcare entity's bottom line (Siwicki 2018). At this state, the healthcare organization implements all or almost all the technology available to it. The user who optimizes health information systems has fully embraced the standard vocabularies supported by the technology, pays attention to alerts and reminders, is able to generate various reports that meet unique needs, frequently tailors the system to further take advantage of documentation aids, and may be considered a power user. **Power users**, people whose expertise in the information system is above others, are able to use technology to significantly improve their productivity and will likely see healthcare quality and cost benefits as well (HIMSS Analytics 2017).

Scope of Health Information Systems

Health information systems have evolved over time to automate an increasing number of information processing functions. Figure 11.2 summarizes health information systems in the sequence in which they have generally been adopted within hospitals. This sequence started with various administrative and financial systems, then departmental clinical systems, and subsequently some or all specialty clinical systems and "smart" peripherals (such as clinical equipment with electronic components that support information collection and alerts). Collectively, these are referred to as source systems because they are the source of basic data for the core clinical systems that comprise the EHR. Many core clinical systems have been implemented with the help of the MU program. Both source systems and core clinical systems depend on supporting infrastructure technology (various types of input/output devices and databases) and connectivity systems (network technology and standards). The major types of health information systems are summarized in more depth and variations between hospitals and physician practices are described after figure 11.2.

Source Systems

Source systems capture and supply the EHR and other broad health information systems with data. Source systems may include administrative and financial applications, ancillary/clinical departmental applications, specialty clinical systems, and "smart" peripherals.

Administrative and Financial Applications

Administrative and financial applications are usually managed by specific departments, such as admitting, patient financial services, revenue cycle management, business intelligence, and health information management. However, they are not considered departmental systems because they manage patient-specific data needed for all other applications, and do not process data that aid in management of the departments as do ancillary, or departmental systems (see the next section).

Figure 11.2 Overview of health IT systems in hospitals

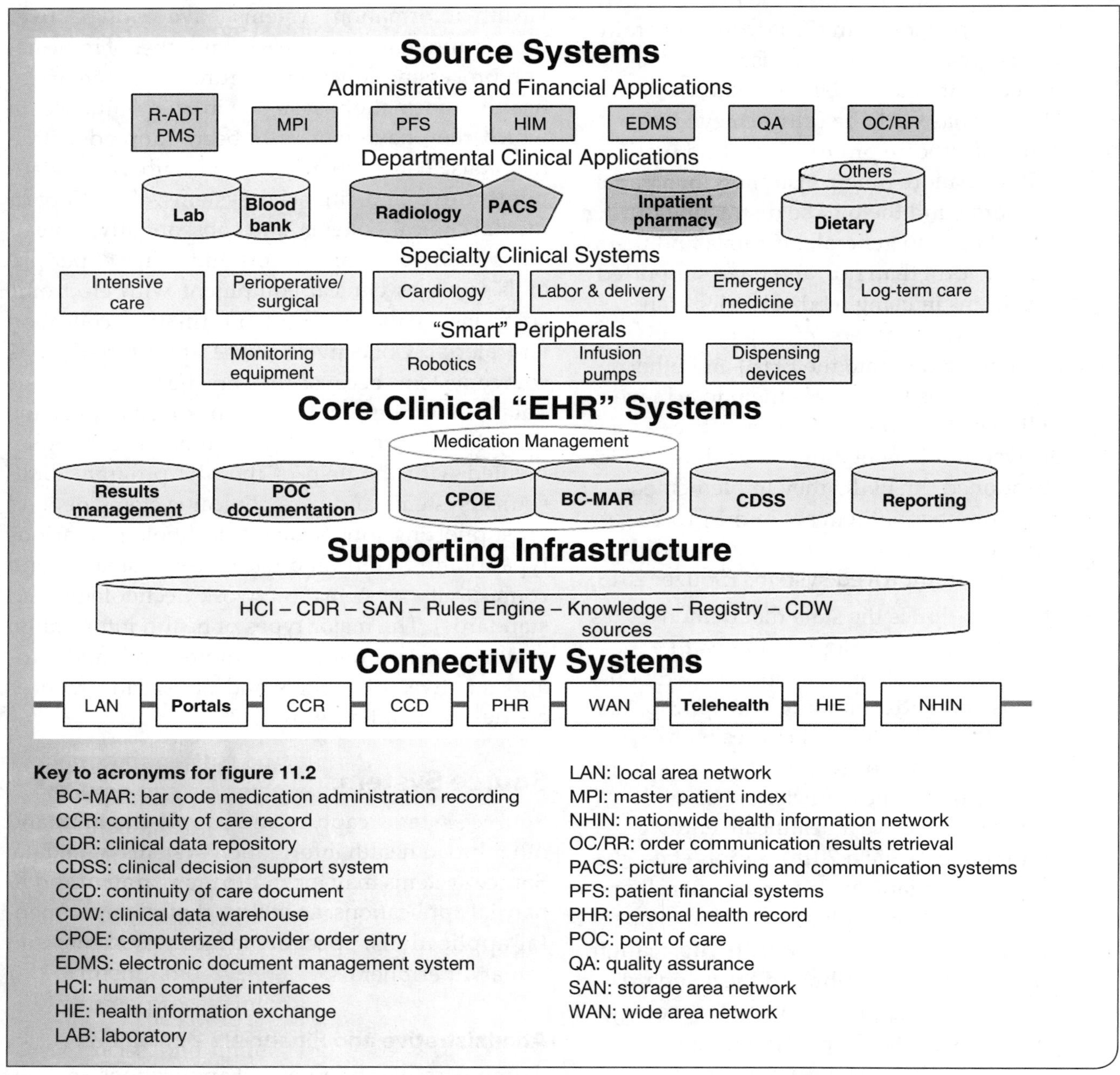

Source: © Margret\A Consulting, LLC. Reprinted with permission.

In general, administrative and financial applications include the following:

- Registration-admission; discharge transfer (R-ADT) systems (in hospitals)
- Practice management systems (PMS) (in physician offices)
- Master patient index (MPI)
- Patient financial systems (PFS)
- Revenue cycle management (RCM) systems
- Quality measurement, reporting, and improvement systems (Quality)
- Health information management (HIM) systems
- Human resources, physician compensation, procurement, and many others

Increasingly, healthcare organizations are adopting business intelligence (BI) systems, which integrate, analyze, and supply financial and clinical data to support both administrative/financial and clinical decision-making. (Chapter 6, *Data Management,* describes the specifics on business intelligence.)

Registration, Admission, Discharge, Transfer Systems Registration-admission, discharge, transfer (R-ADT) systems in hospitals register patients for inpatient admission or outpatient services. The R-ADT captures demographic and insurance data and supplies this data to other applications as needed. An R-ADT system tracks when patients are admitted to the hospital and opens an account for them. It also tracks all patient transfers within the hospital, such as a patient moving from an intensive care unit to a cardiac unit. Finally, the R-ADT system closes the account when a patient is discharged, transferred to another healthcare organization, or dies. Other related information systems keep track of the healthcare organization's census, track who is in what bed, compile length of stay information, and maintain an MPI. In a physician practice, an equivalent system might be a practice management system, although in some cases only a scheduling system is in place.

Patient Financial Systems Patient financial systems (PFSs), frequently called billing systems in a physician practice, serve to check patient insurance eligibility, capture charges for services (including codes for office visits), compile and send claims to payers, receive payment and remittance advice, and identify unpaid or denied claims for which other collections efforts must be made. Revenue cycle management (RCM) system is a term that often refers to the broader process of not only creating, submitting, analyzing, and obtaining payment for healthcare services, but also negotiating contracts with health plans, coding and clinical documentation integrity, conducting utilization review, and other functions. The full scope of RCM is enumerated in figure 11.3 (Amatayakul 2017a). (Chapter 15, *Revenue Management and Reimbursement,* covers the revenue cycle management in more detail.)

The RCM functions that exchange data between providers and health plans are referred to as transactions. Each transaction, such as eligibility verification, claims status inquiry, and so forth have mandated standards for use under the Health Insurance Portability and Accountability Act of 1996 (HIPAA). The standards specify in what format the data should be compiled and what data should be exchanged with payers.

Figure 11.3 Scope of Revenue Cycle Management

- Contract negotiation
- Patient demographics and insurance capture
- Eligibility and benefits verification
- Co-pay collection
- Patient financial counseling
- Prior approval for certain service coverage
- Case management
- Utilization management
- Charge capture and chargemaster maintenance
- Coding and clinical documentation integrity
- Claims review and edits ("cleaning"/scrubbing")
- Claims submission
- Filing for contractual payments and shared risk arrangements
- Claim status determination
- Claim attachments
- Remittance advice and payment posted to accounts receivables
- Audits, denials, and appeals
- Accounts receivables follow-up and collections
- Bad debt/charity management
- Analytics and reports

Source: © Margret\A Consulting, LLC. Reprinted with permission.

These standards are developed by the American National Standards Institute Accredited Standards Committee X12 (ASC X12). For example, the ASC X12 837 standard specifies the data and format for a claim. Also required are standard operating rules that further explain the standards, so their use is consistent across health plans. Figure 11.4 illustrates the HIPAA transactions and their relationship to clinical data.

Capturing, reporting, analyzing, and using clinical quality measure data is an important application to comply with governmental and private health plans. It is becoming increasingly important for information from quality measure reporting to be used at the point of care. Quality measure reporting required by Medicare is aided by CMS providing electronic Clinical Quality Measure (eCQM) specifications. Data required for the eCQMs must be downloadable from an EHR. When data are documented only in narrative form, they cannot be automatically downloaded to the eCQM collection system; these data must be manually abstracted from the EHR. Some health plans may require quality measures data be collected from other source systems, for example healthcare costs, instrumentation, or other elements not typically documented in an EHR. HIM and nursing professionals generally perform quality data capture. Quality data may be sent directly to the entity requiring the data, such as Medicare and other health plans. Many providers also find it valuable to send their quality data to commercial services that can aid in assuring its accuracy and completeness and provide analytical services for comparative information.

Increasingly claims data (data supplied on a claim for reimbursement purposes) are being integrated with clinical data (namely, the data documented about a patient's health status and treatment) for alternative payment initiatives and to aid in strategic planning for the overall healthcare organization. As claims data and clinical/quality data, which is discussed in chapter 4, *Health Record Content and Documentation*, are used together, healthcare quality and cost improvements can be made. This integration of financial and clinical data provides BI that helps support business decisions by both the administrative and clinical leadership of healthcare organizations. For example, with more complete clinical information available at the time of admission, a hospital is better able to verify a patient's eligibility for health plan benefits so that it is not faced with a denied claim later. Information that shows the hospital how many and what type of patients are readmitted within 30 days of discharge for the same condition is another example of BI that will enable a hospital to take proactive measures to monitor these patients more closely after discharge. Physicians are also starting to use integrated claims data and clinical

Figure 11.4 HIPAA transactions and clinical data

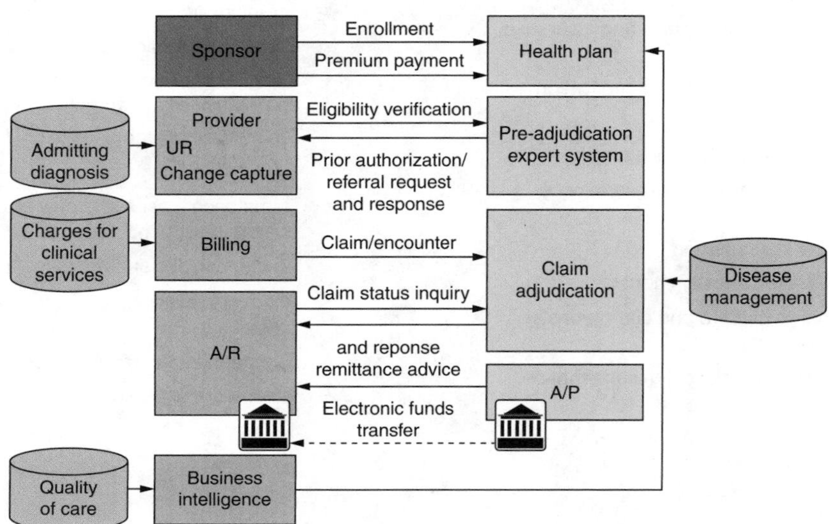

Source: © Margret\A Consulting, LLC. Reprinted with permission.

data to evaluate medical necessity for repeat diagnostic studies, assess the value of costly drugs, and help patients make informed decisions about their healthcare options (Horstmeier 2017).

Health Information Management departments typically do not have a specific departmental information system but do manage and use several separate applications that assist in performing various tasks within the department. As noted above, HIM departments may manage some of the RCM functions such as coding of diagnoses, procedures, and professional services and clinical documentation integrity to ensure the documentation in the EHR supports the diagnoses, procedures, and professional services identified. HIM departments may also support some of the applications that complement the EHR. Complementary systems include document imaging systems (when used only to scan paper forms), electronic document management systems (EDMS) (when scanning is coupled with workflow tools), or electronic document/content management (ED/CM) systems (when both documents and the data in a document have XML [eXtensible markup language] tags applied for ease of searching for content). Also included may be speech dictation systems that enable speech to be translated directly into a narrative document and discrete reportable transcription (DRT) systems that combine speech dictation with natural language processing (namely, the ability for a computer to not only convert speech to words, but apply sophisticated computer processes to put the words into appropriate context). Today, DRT can populate predefined templates with structured data. Consent management systems are those that help maintain patient preferences about who may have access to their health information. These may be managed in conjunction with release of information (ROI) systems, the EHR, and HIE services. HIM applications vary by how far the healthcare organization has progressed in implementing its EHR applications. For example, if the healthcare organization continues to retain some paper health records, the HIM department may have a chart tracking system to manage location of paper records (or to manage archived paper records). HIM systems are discussed in more detail in chapter 3, *Health Information Functions, Purpose, and Users.*

Health Information Technology departments are similar to HIM departments with respect to not necessarily having departmental management systems but having responsibility for supporting the information technology infrastructure and connectivity systems to enable effective use of all of an entity's information systems.

Clinical Departmental Applications

Clinical departmental applications, also called ancillary systems, serve primarily to manage the department in which they exist, while at the same time providing key clinical data for the EHR. There are three main departmental systems that are necessary for an EHR to function in a hospital. They are the following:

- The Laboratory information system (LIS) will receive an order for a lab test; generate a work list for specimen collection, labels for specimen containers, and accession numbers to track specimens; retrieve results from an auto-analyzer (device that analyzes the specimen); perform quality control; maintain an inventory of equipment and supplies needed to perform lab tests; and manage information on departmental staffing and costs. The LIS supplies the lab results to the user, either as a paper copy printout or an electronic print file, which is structured data (data able to be processed by the computer) to an EHR. The blood-banking and clinical pathology systems are often separate from the LIS.
- The Radiology information system (RIS) performs functions similar to the LIS—receiving an order for a procedure; scheduling it; notifying hospital personnel or the patient if performed as an outpatient; tracking the performance of the procedure and its output (that is, images in analog or digital form); tracking preparation of the report; performing quality control; maintaining an inventory of equipment and supplies; and managing departmental staffing and budget. Radiology departments also obtain picture archiving and

communication systems (PACS), which digitize the results of radiological modalities, such as x-rays, computerized tomography (CT) systems, and others, and provide special viewing capabilities of these images via a computer. Standardization for PACS is established by the Digital Imaging and Communications in Medicine (DICOM) organization. Some PACS also can connect directly with a RIS, thereby providing the ability to integrate images with data.
- The Pharmacy information system receives an order for a drug in a hospital; aids the hospital's pharmacist in checking for contraindications (situations that should be avoided as potentially harmful to a patient); directs staff in compounding any drugs requiring special preparation; assists in dispensing the drug in the appropriate dose and for the appropriate route of administration; maintains inventory (documenting medications in stock using the National Drug Codes (NDC), the terminology maintained by the Food and Drug Administration (FDA) for use in identifying FDA-approved drugs; supports staffing and budgeting; and performs other departmental operations.

Other clinical departments in a hospital, such as dietary and nutrition, have information systems that are similar to LIS, RIS, and Pharmacy. They receive orders and supply results (or services) to users, as well as manage the respective department operations.

Specialty Clinical Systems

Specialty clinical systems are acquired to support the unique needs of specialty services. Examples of systems used primarily in hospitals or specialty organizations are intensive care units, perioperative and surgical services, labor and delivery services, and emergency departments. In addition to these information systems that serve to aid in management of a department as well as to support documentation of services provided to patients, various clinical specialties may also have unique functionality, ideally as part of the healthcare organization's EHR (such as cardiology, nephrology, and many others). Other clinical system needs may be unique to the services being provided and those systems are often stand-alone systems. These include long-term and post-acute care (LTPAC), dentistry, behavioral health (BH), and various therapy services (such as physical therapy, respiratory therapy, occupational therapy).

Population health is defined as "the science and art of preventing disease, prolonging life, and promoting health through the organized efforts and informed choices of society, organizations, public and private communities, and individuals" (cited in Health Catalyst 2019). As such, population health management (PHM) is the aggregation of data across multiple health information system resources and the analysis of that data into actions providers can use to improve both clinical and financial outcomes (Phillips 2018). PHM information systems are less a separate system than a repurposing of existing information systems (especially Quality and BI) and use more advanced supporting infrastructure (such as analytics and artificial intelligence) to aid in managing healthcare most effectively in general, and patients in a value-based care environment. The most common functions of PHM systems are those to support care coordination, care transformation, patient engagement, and care analytics to reduce practice variation while accounting for social determinants of health which are believed to account for 80 percent of what affects health outcomes outside of the traditional boundaries of healthcare delivery (Health Catalyst 2019).

"Smart" Peripherals

Automated medical devices (also called smart peripherals), until recently, have generally not been considered information systems, even though they have generated data as well as information—for example a measurement of a person's blood pressure on a display screen is a data point as well as information for the provider and patient. A smart system can also be a continuous feed of data such as a fetal monitoring strip or blood sugar level. Other examples of automated medical devices include vital signs monitors, cardiac output monitors, defibrillators, electrocardiographs, infusion pumps, physiologic monitors, and ventilators (HIMSS Analytics

2010). Increasingly, these medical devices not only collect and report data, but they use the data to provide "smart" services, such as monitoring response to medications and making adjustments, or alerting nursing staff. Many healthcare organizations are also connecting these devices to their EHR via medical device integration (ECRI Institute 2014).

Core Clinical EHR Systems

There are generally five main applications that define an EHR. These include the following and are illustrated in figure 11.5, as a closer look at the EHR section of figure 11.2.

1. Results management
2. Point-of-care (POC) clinical documentation
3. Medication management encompassing CPOE and bar code medication administration recording (BC-MAR) systems
4. Clinical decision support (CDS) systems (CDSS) (of various types)
5. Analytics and reporting

The EHR applications include the basic functionality required for earning incentives in the MU program and now for participation in alternative payment models. To earn MU incentives and to participate in alternative payment models, an EHR application must have certification from an ONC-designated certifying body indicating that the EHR meets all of the required functionality criteria for the program. The criteria, however, do not require all possible EHR functionality that is available, some of which is critical for most providers. For example, program requirements do not include support for charge capture even though most healthcare providers find this an essential part of their EHR that needs to link to their patient financial services and revenue cycle management systems.

It is also important to note that there are some variations in the core EHR applications as they are used in a hospital or in a physician practice. One main difference is that in a hospital, the EHR applications are often implemented separately; whereas in a physician practice, EHR applications tend to be more integrated. Other differences are noted as each of these core applications is described more fully in the following sections.

Results Management

Results management is an EHR application that enables diagnostic study results (such as lab results) to be reviewed in a report format and for the data within the reports to be processed. Users can compare, trend, and graph the results. Depending on their level of sophistication, results management systems may also be able to compare lab results with other clinical data. For example, a graphic display could depict lab results as a function of medications administered or be compared with a patient's vital signs. Lab results can also be extracted directly from the EHR for use in quality measurement studies, clinical research, and BI systems. For a healthcare organization to have results management, all data to be processed must be in structured format and ideally stored within a clinical data repository (see Supporting Infrastructure below).

The importance of results management cannot be emphasized enough, as 70 percent of the ability to reach a diagnosis for a patient depends on lab results (Wians 2009). Similarly, as medications are increasingly powerful in their impact on the human body, monitoring vital signs and lab results in association with medication administration is critical to appropriate medication management.

Point of Care Documentation

Another EHR component is point-of-care (POC) documentation. The intent of these applications is to inform the user what data needs to be recorded

Figure 11.5 Core clinical EHR systems

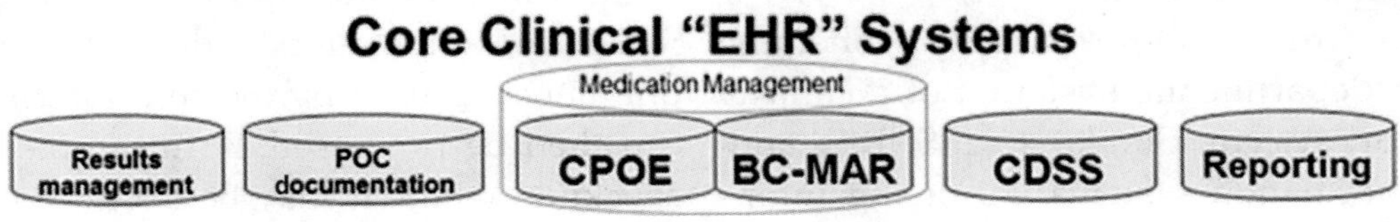

Source: © Margret\A Consulting, LLC. Reprinted with permission.

for the patient and to use that data to supply clinical decision support (CDS), including alerts and reminders, at the time when the clinician is able to be most responsive to alerts and reminders. POC documentation systems supply templates to the user to be completed primarily via point-and-click, drop-down, type-ahead, and other data-entry tools. Usually the EHR has a library of templates. The user may choose the appropriate template, or the user's dashboard may display the appropriate template based on the user's profile as indicated via the log-in or by the patient's admitting diagnosis or chief complaint at the time of a physician's office visit. Some templates are extremely sophisticated and as the user enters data, the data fields adjust accordingly. As a simple example, a template for conducting a history and physical exam for a male patient would not display data fields applicable to females. If the information system detects that the patient's condition involves heart disease, additional data fields may be displayed for associated signs, symptoms, and potential complications. The result is structured data that the computer is essentially processing into clinical documentation. More information on dashboards can be found in chapter 12, *Healthcare Information.*

POC documentation systems include support for documentation of all patient care administered by healthcare professionals. While ideally all such documentation should be integrated, frequently such documentation is compartmentalized, especially in hospitals. This is often the case because the nature of the data to be collected and volume varies considerably. Nursing staff may have separate screens for nurse admission assessments, nursing problem lists, nurses' notes, vital signs (which may also be captured directly from patient monitoring systems), intake and output records, and other nursing documentation. Medication administration is also a nursing documentation requirement, but such systems are typically grouped under medication management systems, as described in the next section.

A **nursing information system** is generally considered a departmental system, not a clinical documentation system. Similar to LIS, RIS, and pharmacy information systems, a nursing information system manages the nursing department, including staffing, credentialing, training, budgeting, and other managerial functions. Clinical data may be combined with department operations data in a nursing information system to provide **patient acuity staffing** levels, where the number of staff needed for any shift or day is determined by how acutely ill the current patients are.

In a hospital, physicians are expected to document a problem list, history and physical exam, consults, operative reports, and a discharge summary. These are largely dictated and electronically fed as an image into the EHR. Physician progress notes may be handwritten and scanned into the EHR. Medical scribes may be used to support direct data entry into the EHR. According to the American Health Information Management Association (AHIMA) (2012), a medical **scribe** is an individual who enters clinical documentation into the EHR to reduce administrative burden. Scribes may also assist providers in navigating EHRs, respond to messages on behalf of physicians as directed, locate information, or perform research. An American Medical Association study has determined that scribes can cut physician documentation time in half, and with their additional roles can increase revenue to offset their cost (AMA 2017). The Joint Commission provides guidelines recognizing scribe usage; and, in 2017 the American Healthcare Documentation Professionals Group announced it would offer a scribe certification (Bresnick 2017).

The problem list is increasingly managed through a combination of sources including the admission order for the admitting diagnosis and directly from a drop-down menu for discharge diagnoses and procedures. The MU program required that the problem list ultimately be automated and coded with either ICD or SNOMED-CT codes. Physician orders are documented in a CPOE system (discussed later in this chapter).

In physician practices, physicians (and their scribes) and nurses often enter clinical documentation directly into the EHR as structured data. Structured data refer to data elements that are uniquely captured by the computer in fields that can then be processed. An example is drug–lab checking, where it may be necessary to have lab data (such as the results of a liver function study) before ordering a certain type of drug that may adversely affect the liver. Drug–lab checking can be performed in a CDS system, however such CDS depends on the selection of a specific drug programmed into the information system and lab data results also programmed into the computer that are available to the CDS system. The CDS system then can compare what drug is ordered against a patient's lab values to determine if there are contraindications. Structured data is contrasted with unstructured data, or narrative information not able to be uniquely processed by a computer. For example, a lab value posted to a specific field can be compared with other such lab values. A lab value simply documented in a note, comment field, or as a scanned image of paper cannot be processed by the computer in the same way as structured data.

Medication Management

Medication management refers to the use of certain information systems that help ensure patient safety, or preventing harm to patients, learning from errors, and building a culture of safety (Hughes 2008). These are often referred to as closed-loop medication management systems because they automate the processes from the point a drug is ordered to the point it is administered. These systems include CPOE, e-prescribing (e-Rx) as a special type of CPOE, BC-MAR, medication reconciliation systems that compare drugs ordered against drugs dispensed and administered, and automated drug dispensing machines, as well as the policies, procedures, and workflows associated with ensuring proper drug ordering, dispensing, administering, and monitoring of reactions. Although there is no recommended sequence for implementing these information systems, many hospitals in the past implemented CPOE last because it is difficult to get physicians to use such information systems in the hospital. This is changing as MU incentives require use of a CPOE system first, then medication administration record systems. In the ambulatory setting, e-Rx has sometimes been implemented as a stand-alone system before an EHR (and its CPOE functionality) because some insurers and Medicare were providing incentives for its use. Physicians also found great value in the CDS for drug choices and in managing prescription refills and renewals.

CPOE Systems CPOE systems can be used for entering all orders such as patient admission, laboratory tests, x-rays and other diagnostic studies, dietary and nutrition, therapies, nursing services, consults, discharge of patient, referrals, and even building personal task lists, as well as entering orders for medications. In the past, these orders were usually handwritten by the physician and were either internally faxed to various departments as applicable or transcribed by nursing personnel (such as ward secretaries or unit clerks) into an order communication system. This type of system, however, included no CDS. While some physicians prefer not to have to enter their own orders or pay attention to CDS alerts, it is believed that such support ultimately will improve the quality of healthcare.

CDS in CPOE systems initially provided many alerts that may not have been specific or relevant to a given patient, resulting in alert fatigue, or the ignoring of alerts due to their volume and irrelevancy. For example, reminding a provider to check for an allergy to a drug should not be necessary if a comprehensive medication history is being obtained and documented by a nurse or pharmacist. Such an allergy alert should only appear if the physician is ordering a contraindicated medication. Appropriate alerting to drug–allergy and drug–drug contraindications (situations that should be avoided as potentially harmful to a patient) is a complex process that requires not only accurate data from the patient and throughout the patient's care, but an up-to-date drug knowledge database (namely, a subscription service that provides current information about drugs and is accessible to users and the CDS).

Another concern with CPOE systems is that they are often based on standard order sets. Standard order sets are lists of specific diagnostic studies and treatments as appropriate for specific diagnoses or procedures to be performed. These order sets reflect the current knowledge about patient care from research, experts, and other sources of evidence-based medicine (EBM). A standard order set is frequently used for patients with common conditions. For example, a standard order set is often used for admissions for normal pregnancies, where the obstetrician only needs to approve of the standard items or make applicable changes rather than having to document the entire set of items normally required. However, although EBM may reflect the best scientific evidence on how to treat a patient with a specific condition, one size does not always fit all human beings. Even a woman with a normal pregnancy may have certain preferences, allergies, or additional conditions that must be taken into account when using the standard order set for normal pregnancy. As a result, most standard order sets need to be modified for each patient. In haste, a physician may accept the standard orders or may make an error in modifying them—which may result in unintended consequences (AHRQ 2011). An unintended consequence is an unanticipated and undesired effect of implementing and using an EHR (Rollins 2012). While these often have been attributed to the EHR software itself as early as in 2006 (Campbell et al. 2006) and continue to be cited today (Vanderhook and Abraham 2017), they often reflect that a user may not have applied professional judgment or due diligence in using the EHR.

CPOE systems also generate the patient's medication list. The medication list is required under the MU program to be coded using one of the code sets standardized under RxNorm, which is a system maintained by the National Library of Medicine to normalize drug names across disparate vocabularies. Caution must be applied here, as the medication list will only be as accurate and complete as all systems contributing information to it. For instance, if a medication is ordered prior to surgery, suspended during surgery, reinstated after surgery but then changed before administration, not only must the CPOE and BC-MAR contribute correct medication information, but the surgery information system may also need to interface with the medication management systems, which is not always the case.

E-Rx E-Rx is a special type of CPOE used exclusively to write a prescription and transmit it electronically to retail pharmacies. The format and content of the prescription transmitted is standardized by the National Council for Prescription Drug Programs (NCPDP), a standards development organization that sets standards for the pharmacy industry. The NCPDP SCRIPT standard is the standard developed for electronically transmitting a prescription. As such, the SCRIPT standard is used in ambulatory settings, including not only the physician practice but when a patient is discharged from the hospital or emergency service with a prescription and in hospital outpatient departments or clinics. The e-Rx system includes medication alerts and reminders just as the hospital-based CPOE system, but also includes formulary information that identifies whether the patient's health plan covers the cost of a drug and what co-pay may be required. Physicians can then work with their patients to find the most cost-effective as well as clinically suitable drug. Because e-Rx systems are able to transmit prescriptions directly to retail pharmacies, physicians benefit from fewer calls from pharmacies not able to read their handwriting or needing to advise the physician that a drug ordered is not going to be covered by the patient's insurance because it is not on the list (formulary) of covered drugs; that is, it is considered "off formulary." Physicians are also able to receive electronic communications from retail pharmacies, such as for renewal approvals that can significantly save time in a practice. In 2010, the Drug Enforcement Administration (DEA), which previously banned use of e-prescribing for controlled substances (EPCS) such as narcotics, set special requirements allowing for use of EPCS. These requirements include use of a product that provides identity proofing (authentication credentials used to electronically sign such prescriptions) and two-factor authentication—a signature type that includes at least two of the following three elements: something known, such as a password; something held, such as a token or digital certificate; and something that is personal, such as biometrics (fingerprints, retinal scan, or other) to enable such use. Digital certificates are issued by a certificate authority, an organization that verifies a person's credentials (such as the provider's DEA number for EPCS) and can revoke the certificate if the credentials are revoked.

BC-MAR Bar code medication administration recording is the documentation of administering medication to a patient and is a function performed by nurses in a hospital. Nurses use a bar code reader to positively identify the patient and the medications to be administered to the patient. Bar codes are parallel arrangements of dark elements, referred to as bars, and light elements, referred to as spaces, that represent information, such as the patient name, drug name, and other data. The frequency and care that must be taken to ensure a nurse administers the right drug, in the right dose, through the right route, at the right time, and to the right patient (the medication five rights) is critical to avoid medication errors. As a result, computerized systems have been created. Early medication administration systems were simply electronically generated paper lists of medications from the pharmacy information system after it processed physician orders. Later, the lists were retained on the computer and nurses were expected to post the date and time of medication administration to the computer. Any exceptions or issues with medication administration, however, were still included in handwritten nurses' notes. Most importantly, these systems, while providing a legible list of medications did not fully address the medication five rights.

BC-MAR systems require the hospital to have each patient identified with a bar code (usually on a wrist band) and to package (or buy prepackaged) drugs in unit dose form, each with a bar code or radio-frequency identification (RFID) tag that identifies the drug, dose, and intended route of administration. (An RFID tag serves the same function as a bar code but enables wireless transmission of the data rather than requiring a bar code to be read with a scanner.) At the time the drug is to be administered to a patient, the nurse logs into the BC-MAR system and scans the patient's wrist band and unit dose package. The information system automatically dates and time stamps the entry made through this process. As a result, the medication five rights have been followed. Most BC-MAR systems also enable notes to describe exceptions; for example, that the patient was in surgery at the time the next dose was to be administered. BC-MAR systems provide some CDS as do CPOE systems, often including links to additional information about drugs. BC-MAR systems also generate reports on timely administration of drugs.

There are some issues with using BC-MAR systems. One is that the bags that are specially compounded with multiple drugs administered intravenously require labels to reflect all the drugs in the compound. Not all hospital pharmacy information systems can produce such labels. In this case, special care must be taken to manually check and enter the medications being administered. The other important issue associated with using BC-MAR systems is bringing the computer, bar-code wand, and medication to the patient bedside. Some hospitals use wireless workstations on wheels (WOWs). Because WOWs can become heavy with their various devices plus a long-life battery, an alternative is to carry (sometimes by wearing a sling) a tablet computer that may be outfitted with a wand device and the medication. Walking around all day with such equipment, however, is also not comfortable. Finally, it is important for the hospital to fully define what constitutes a medication administration error—a wrong time, for instance, may or may not be due to an error but rather the availability of the patient.

Medication Reconciliation The medication reconciliation process can be automated, although not as easily as the other elements of medication management. Each time a patient is transferred across levels of care, such as when admitted, transferred into an intensive care unit, or sent to surgery, the medications the patient should be administered need to be reviewed. Often certain medications must be discontinued, or a dose altered as a result of the change in level of care. Because the clinicians who work with the patient are different at each different level of care, connecting all the information systems at the different levels of care has been a challenge, and only a few hospitals have been successful.

Automated Drug Dispensing Machines Finally with respect to medication management, automated drug dispensing machines, which are technically smart peripherals, are available that both secure and make drugs more readily available to nursing staff. These machines are typically filled by pharmacy department staff based on the physician orders.

Clinical Decision Support

Clinical decision support (CDS) is a key component of the EHR and sets it apart from simply automating paper documents. CDS functionality in the EHR helps physicians, nurses, and other clinical professionals—collectively referred to as clinicians—as well as patients themselves make decisions about patient care. Some examples of CDS as previously discussed include alerts about potential drug contraindications, out-of-range lab results, and standard order sets in CPOE. In addition, CDS templates can help determine what documentation of clinical findings is necessary; provide suggestions for prescribing less expensive but equally effective drugs; supply protocols (specification of appropriate processes, based on expert best practices and clinical research findings) for certain health maintenance procedures; and alert that a duplicate lab test is being ordered. There are countless other decision-making aids for all stakeholders in the care process.

CDS may be built into each of the core EHR applications. However, CDS is also acquired as separate information systems that work in conjunction with the EHR applications. In general, the CDS found in the core EHR applications is rudimentary because it typically can only process data within the given application. More sophisticated CDS requires the convergence of different types of data from the various EHR components. As a result, separate applications are used to help integrate and analyze these data.

Separate CDS applications may be fully integrated with the core EHR applications or employed in a stand-alone fashion. An example of a separate CDS application is one that provides drug–lab checking, such as whether a drug is contraindicated for a patient with poor liver function. This is not a routine function of CPOE or LIS but requires the combination of data from both sources and the ability to deliver the alert back to the appropriate system(s). This is commonly referred to as a separate clinical decision support system (CDSS), even though it may be fully integrated into the core EHR applications through supporting infrastructure. Other examples of separate CDSSs that are integrated into the EHR include the templates used in clinical documentation, standard order sets used in CPOE, and clinical pathways that guide nursing services. While some EHR products build a basic set of templates directly into their clinical documentation systems, others require a separate CDSS to generate the templates, or provide more sophisticated and customizable templates than exist in the basic clinical documentation applications.

CDSSs that are used in a stand-alone fashion are often those specific to a unique function. For example, a CDSS that is used in a stand-alone manner in a hospital includes an information system to alert infection control nurses of a potential hospital-acquired infection. It provides advice on which medication may be most effective in combating the infection given the causative agent. Such an information system compiles data from clinical documentation (such as documentation of a high temperature), lab results (such as the strain of bacteria that is causing the infection), x-ray results (such as a finding of pneumonia), and other sources processed against automated clinical reference information to produce the specific findings.

An example of a CDSS used in a stand-alone fashion by physicians is a differential diagnosis system. This system may compare diagnostic images against a library of images and their known conditions, which is especially useful for radiologists, dermatologists, pathologists, and others. Other differential diagnosis CDS systems compare data from clinical documentation, especially the history of present illness and review of systems, with a library of known signs and symptoms for specific diagnoses. Some of these are used only when the differential diagnosis is obscure. Others may be a routine part of a protocol, such as for assessing a patient presenting to the emergency department with chest pain. Still another CDSS can aid in identifying whether a patient's symptoms are due to a new condition or are the result of an adverse reaction to a medication. Figure 11.6 summarizes the different forms of CDS and CDSS.

Figure 11.6 Types of clinical decision support

Data display
Data always available
Flow sheets (for example, problem list, medication list)
- Maintain longitudinally
- Across continuum

Dynamic displays
- Flow sheet, graphic, table, narrative—helps review data
- Clinical imaging integration
- Search tools
- Query support

Summaries or abstracts
- Quickens access, supports continuity of care
- Flags problems

Workflow
In-basket
- Reminders in support of timeliness, compliance

Schedule and patient list
- Patient status continuously

Workgroup tools
- Easy handoffs

Refills choice lists
Integrated clinical and financial
- Medical necessity checking
- Overcomes inability to pay for treatment

Telephony (the process of connecting a telephone to an electronic device), e-mail and visits, instant messaging
- Quick response

Data retrieval
Single sign-on (for multiple applications)
- Overcomes interface versus integration (through one system or repository) issues

Ease of navigation aids adoption
Density of screen
- "Flip-ability"
- Avoids getting lost in "drill downs"

Specialized formats focus information
Customized screens
- Standards versus personal preference

Data entry
Context-sensitive templates and order sets guide documentation
Provides immediate access to active decision support
- Alerts and reminders
- Clinical calculations
- Therapy critiquing and planning

Patient self-assessment and PHR
Medication list maintenance (by patient or claims consolidator)
Structured data and registry support
- Contributes to downstream knowledge
- Wellness or disease management reminders, interventions due, recalls

Access to reference information
- Context-insensitive, portal
- Context-sensitive, direct links

Source: © Margret\A Consulting, LLC. Reprinted with permission.

CDS is an increasingly important tool in value-based care, as it helps healthcare professionals encourage healthy lifestyles – thereby improving the overall health of the individual and lowering costs. For example, an alert that a patient is a smoker could trigger a suggestion for smoking cessation. Another example might be the ability of the information system to calculate the patient's body mass index (BMI) for recommending weight counseling. Caution must be applied in displaying and using some of these alerts, such that they should be able to be tailored to the patient. This may mean that an alert is turned off or frequency reduced for a given patient. Many ambulatory EHRs include reminders for preventive or chronic care services, such as dates when a vaccine, cancer screening, diabetes care, or other services are due.

Analytics and Reporting

Analytics and reporting are the final core EHR application. **Analytics** refers to statistical processing of data to reveal new information. Reporting is supplying the results of analytics to the intended recipient.

Analytics goes beyond the simple use of descriptive statistics, such as how many patients were seen for a specific condition, to questions such as which form of treatment for the specific condition had the best outcomes. The ability to produce such reports is increasingly important as there is ever more pressure to improve quality and reduce the cost of healthcare. Analytics, however, entail sophisticated processes to be performed on data—such as data mining, forecasting, neural networks (mathematical modeling that makes connections between data to discover relationships).

In healthcare, analytics has been primarily performed in academic and research institutions, by health plans, at pharmaceutical manufacturers, and for public health departments. Analytics has produced many clinical benefits for the healthcare industry, such as in genomic research and **personalized medicine** (also known as precision medicine) that tailors treatment to the individual, given not only comorbidities but genomic characteristics and predispositions (SAS n.d.). Analytics are also used to create BI, such as in predicting prescribing patterns of physicians or the impact of a disaster on local emergency services (Strome 2013). For more specifics on analytics, refer to chapter 12, *Healthcare Information*.

Although most information systems can generate some data for analysis and reporting, there has been strong interest for the EHR to provide more robust analysis of data. Unfortunately, the nature of the type of database required for POC documentation and CDS, referred to as a clinical data repository (CDR), does not support complex analytics and reporting. The purpose of a CDR is primarily online transaction processing (OLTP), where each access, entry, or other process performed on data is a transaction. Often it is necessary to move data from the CDR to a separate database that has been optimized to perform analytics and reporting (online analytical processing [OLAP]). This type of database is referred to as a clinical data warehouse (CDW). In addition, healthcare organizations that want to perform sophisticated analytics need staff highly skilled in such statistical techniques. It may be that a given hospital or physician practice cannot perform the analytics and reporting itself, but it sends data to a vendor who performs the analytics. An increasing number of EHR vendors are supplying such services, often aggregating data from many customers to enlarge the pool of data, making the results of analysis on the data more valid and reliable. When this data pool has a large volume of data, it is referred to as big data. Big data offers greater reliability and validity. Big data analytics implies massive amounts of data that can be analyzed quickly in near real time to return new information to users at the POC. When data are collected from active patient health records, the data reflect current experience and analytics is then able to produce new knowledge as well as new information.

Another trait of big data in addition to its volume and velocity is that all the data do not need to be structured. Unstructured data can be analyzed and parsed into structured data as part of processing big data. It is still important to ensure the quality of unstructured data being captured in health information systems so that the results of analysis can be as accurate as possible. Data quality refers to adherence to standard data definitions and metadata (that is, data about data) requirements. Data models that organize data to depict relationships among data help ensure the quality of data collected by health information systems. Standard vocabularies (the compilation of terms formally adopted for use in health information systems) are used for data exchange across different health information systems. This exchange capability is referred to as semantic interoperability, or the ability to share common meanings for data across systems. Another important element that improves data quality in health information systems is a data dictionary that lists all data elements used in a health information system with their definitions and characteristics. For example, a data dictionary for a given health IT system would include the term *temperature* and specify that it must be documented in centigrade. AHIMA developed a data quality management model to illustrate these characteristics (AHIMA 2015).(The data dictionary and the AHIMA Data Quality Management Model are explained in chapter 6, *Data Management*.)

Health plans have analyzed data from healthcare claims for a long time, and now they are receiving additional data from commercial labs, claims attachments, patient-entered data, and other sources to perform even more sophisticated analytics. Such information may impact whether the hospital or physician practice receives a favorable discount rate on its fees for services. Quality benchmarking depends on analytics. (Benchmarking is discussed in chapter 18, *Performance Improvement.*) Consumers are beginning to look at which hospital excels in cardiac care or has a center of excellence for orthopedics. Having aggregated data to understand why one healthcare organization is ahead in its quality metrics over another can help poorer performers improve. Analytics and reporting are not only used for retrospective quality or research studies; an important set of reports include rule-based lists for patient follow-up. Patient follow-up lists have not been easy to generate in the past, as much of the data had to be manually abstracted from paper records, transcription, or scanned images of documents. However, the ability to identify all patients requiring follow-up after discharge, for chronic disease care, to notify them of a drug or device recall, to send preventive care reminders, or any of many other similar types of reports or lists is integral to quality patient care.

Most analytics implementations are still retrospective. However, it can be anticipated that the use of big data analytics in near real time, especially when coupled with **artificial intelligence (AI)** (which is the application of algorithms that analyze data and make applicable recommendations [Pearl 2018]) will help providers at the POC improve clinical decision-making. Examples of such improved decision-making include the ability to select affordable therapies (Chaiken 2011) and make earlier diagnoses of complex conditions such as rheumatoid arthritis and multiple sclerosis (Kalatzis et al. 2009).

Check Your Understanding 11.1

Answer the following questions.

1. Identify a source system.
   a. Clinical decision support system
   b. Laboratory information system
   c. Results management system
   d. Medication reconciliation system
2. A ________________ is considered a core clinical EHR component.
   a. Computerized provider order entry system
   b. Pharmacy information system
   c. Document imaging
   d. Registration-admission, discharge, transfer system
3. Dr. Smith always orders the same 10 things when a new patient is admitted to the hospital in addition to some patient-specific orders. What would assist in ensuring that the specific patient is not allergic to a drug being ordered?
   a. Clinical decision support
   b. Pharmacy information system
   c. Electronic medication administration record system
   d. Standard order set
4. What provides alerts and reminders to clinicians?
   a. Clinical decision support system
   b. Electronic data interchange
   c. Point-of-care charting system
   d. Workflow system
5. E-prescribing systems are used to:
   a. Inventory and dispense drugs in retail pharmacies
   b. Write orders for drugs to be administered in hospitals
   c. Send prescriptions to retail pharmacies
   d. Report adverse drug events
6. Which factor in a BC-MAR system supports medication five rights?
   a. Bar code reading
   b. Documentation of medication administered
   c. List of medications to be administered to the patient
   d. Reports of accuracy of medication administration

7. Why is medication reconciliation the most difficult function of closed-loop medication management systems to implement?
   a. Bar code systems contain only limited information.
   b. Multiple systems, potentially across healthcare settings, must be connected
   c. Nurses do not have sufficient time to obtain a medication history.
   d. Vendors are reluctant to design such systems due to cost.

8. What stage describes when users are not yet using all the available EHR functionality?
   a. Adoption
   b. Implementation
   c. Optimization
   d. Meaningful use

9. Templates are intended to:
   a. Afford free text entry of narrative information
   b. Provide data entry support consistent with patient type
   c. Require use of a standard set of orders for every patient
   d. Support copy and paste of content from one record to another

10. Which of the following characterizes the current state of EHRs?
   a. EHRs aid in comparing the quality of care rendered across healthcare organizations.
   b. EHRs enable complex analysis of all patient data for the healthcare organization.
   c. EHRs provide data and support for data collection about one patient at a time.
   d. EHRs support the ability to generate lists of patients with similar characteristics.

Supporting Infrastructure

Supporting infrastructure (see figure 11.2) refers to the technology that allows the various applications to work. This includes hardware and software of various forms and sophistication. Hardware includes **human computer interfaces (HCI)**, which are any form of input device used by humans, including monitors, keyboards, printers, scanners, and many other devices that enable human interaction with computing technology. Hardware also includes all the computer servers and associated cabling and other tools for processing and storage.

A key component of supporting infrastructure is the need to provide interoperability. **Interoperability** is the term used to describe the ability of one information system to exchange data with another information system in a way that the data exchanged are usable to each part of the exchange. Interoperability comes in several forms. For example, with semantic interoperability, the terminology used carries the same meaning to all parties to an exchange.

Technical interoperability is the most basic form of interoperability. Technical interoperability refers to the exchange of any data element across information systems. In healthcare, many basic applications were developed before the internet and World Wide Web (WWW) were widely available. As such, application software was written using **message format standards** to structure the format of the data that are processed by the applications and which could only support point-to-point communications. The ASC X12 standard for exchanging claims and other administrative and financial data and the NCPDP standard for exchanging prescriptions between an e-prescribing system and a retail pharmacy previously described are examples of message format standard. Diagnostic study results data, POC documentation, medication management data, and other such clinical documentation are exchanged among applications using similar standards from the **Health Level Seven (HL7)** standards development organization. The HL7 is a not-for-profit, standards-developing organization dedicated to providing a comprehensive framework and related standards for the exchange, integration, sharing, and retrieval of electronic health information that supports clinical practice and the management, delivery, and evaluation of health services.

As a result of the early development of health information systems software, most technical interoperability today requires an **interface**, which is software that serves as a translator between different applications which may have different structures for data or may use different vocabularies to encode data. For example, if the R-ADT system needs to send patient demographic data to the LIS, an interface will identify what data should be sent from what fields in the R-ADT system to the fields in the LIS. In the software used by most health information systems today, interfaces are required because communications may also be used to exchange data between one organization and another, such as between a physician's office and a commercial laboratory. Interfaces, however, are costly to write and maintain. Every exchange between two applications requires an interface. Since there are many applications in any given entity, many interfaces are required. Furthermore, anytime one information system is upgraded or modified in some way, the interface between it and all other applications with which it exchanges data must be adjusted. It also must be noted that each application in any given entity is unique to that entity. As a result, **interface engines** are often required to manage all the interfaces for a given entity, and with a very limited number of external entities.

Because applications, and hence their interfaces, are unique to a given entity, interfacing is not an effective way to exchange data across many different organizations. For example, a physician's office likely needs to exchange prescription information with many different retail pharmacies. Today for such exchanges to occur, a go-between that can manage the translation process is used, for which entities pay a fee each time an exchange takes place. The go-between is a vendor, typically called a **clearinghouse**. Some health information exchange organizations also serve this purpose for other forms of health information (see Connectivity Systems in the next section).

Over time, health information systems software was written or modified to encompass many of the applications needing to exchange data within a given healthcare organization. As such, computer servers were configured to support the larger volume of data across the various applications. (A server is a "master" computer that "serves" the needs of many end-user computers.) The differences between two major server functions were previously described: a CDR (typically used to house and process the broader range of LIS, RIS, EDMS, EHR, and many other applications being brought together) and a CDW (to integrate at least some of the data from the CDR and perform analytics). A **registry** is another type of application that typically houses and performs analysis and data reporting on a subset of clinical data. A common example is a tumor registry. When quality measurement data are submitted to a vendor, the vendor is essentially compiling a registry. The server that supports a registry is something of a cross between these two server functions.

There are also special servers. Examples are the interface engine previously described and an **inference engine** (also called a **rules engine**), which supplies the rules that govern clinical decision support. An example of such a rule might be: If a patient is allergic to penicillin, generate an alert when a physician orders any medication with the same active ingredients as in penicillin. Such servers need to have access to **knowledge sources**, which are resources that provide information about the properties of drugs, the latest research about new surgical procedures, and other information needed to support clinical decision-making. Because knowledge sources must always be kept up to date with new information about drugs, surgical protocols, and much other information, they are generally provided through a vendor that operates through a subscription service.

While this description of many interfaces and unique server types paints a rather bleak picture for interoperability in healthcare, progress is being made to take advantage of **web services architectures (WSA)** that utilize tools to aid in exchanging data in a one-to-many (rather than point-to-point) manner. WSA refers to the use of web-based forms of interfaces—such as XML structures—to enable sharing across multiple parties.

Another important element of supporting infrastructure, however, is management of the infrastructure. As such, a plan describing what technology will be adopted, how the technology will be procured, and how the technology will work together is needed. This plan is often in the form of an enterprise architecture (EA). An EA is needed because large hospitals may have nearly a thousand applications, with hundreds of applications being common in medium-sized hospitals. Physician practices may have only one combined PMS and EHR, but frequently have some ancillary and specialty systems—potentially accumulating 10 to 20 or more information systems. An EA helps keep track of all the applications and how they work together. Drilling down further, a data governance framework (DGF) provides a logical structure for managing all of the healthcare organization's data. A DGF addresses data governance and stewardship, data quality management, specifications of terminologies for data, roles and responsibilities for collection and use of data, metadata management, data storage and warehousing, and data security. The EA and DGF are vital for managing the different applications necessary for today's health information needs.

Infrastructure also must consider the processes and policies for using applications. These are increasingly being referred to as process interoperability and policy interoperability. Process interoperability refers to the use of workflows and procedures that best support use of technology. Some process interoperability can be aided by software. For example, if there are a series of steps to be taken by different people, in different departments, with different information systems, software can be supplied to direct the sharing of data in the appropriate sequence as each person, department, and system completes its work. In other cases, process interoperability may be a human factor to be addressed in training and optimization. Policy interoperability refers to the rules that govern exchange of data. These rules are incorporated into software development. For example, access controls are security rules built into information systems to ensure only the appropriate access is afforded. In fact, virtually every aspect of computer use is impacted by some form of policy.

Acquiring these information systems is also a key part of infrastructure, requiring a strategic plan and project management. A project management office (PMO) (in a larger healthcare organization) or project manager aids in compiling a project's budget, allocating resources, maintaining a task list, identifying dependencies among tasks, establishing timelines, and managing a schedule. The PMO may focus only on health information systems or may be broader in scope to encompass other major projects, such as building construction, mergers and acquisitions, and others.

Supporting infrastructure also must address security. Healthcare is facing increasing security threats – both internal and external. Security processes can take time and attention that is often thought to detract from the primary purpose of healthcare, which is highly time sensitive. Until recently, it has also been thought that healthcare data carry little monetary value and hence are "safer" than other data. This is not true, and theft of healthcare data can carry much more severe ramifications for individuals whose information is compromised. Data security is discussed in chapter 10, *Data Security*.

Connectivity Systems

Connectivity systems (see figure 11.2) help support the exchange of data across separate information systems within a healthcare organization and across organizations, and also with individuals.

To exchange data among health information systems, computers must be networked together. When exchanging data within the organization, the network is referred to as a local area network (LAN), and when exchanging data across organizations, such as from a provider to a payer, the network is referred to as a wide area network (WAN). WANs need a secure connection, which is often a virtual private network (VPN), which is an encrypted private connection over the internet.

Increasingly, both hospitals and physicians not only exchange information among providers and with patients for treatment and payment, but also move data for operational functions, such as for supplying quality data to a registry as previously described, and to store data. Various data storage management (archiving data organized for retrieval) techniques exist. These may include a storage area network (SAN) that supports the ability to retrieve data from any storage location for use in the EHR. Some SANs may be local to the healthcare organization. Others may use **cloud computing**, which refers to using computing services remotely over the internet, often through a vendor or vendors to archive data and in some cases to provide application software, including an EHR (Knorr 2018).

In addition to operational needs for connectivity systems, there is also a growing need to exchange health information with disparate providers and patients for care purposes. There are essentially three general forms of connectivity processes used today in healthcare—telehealth, patient-exchanged information, and health information exchange.

Telehealth and Newer Forms of Healthcare Delivery

The oldest form of exchanging health information is telehealth—a process that uses telecommunications to send voice, still pictures, and video between a remote location (where the patient is) and a base location (such as a hospital) for the purposes of diagnosis and, in some cases, treatment. Some might not consider telehealth to be a form of health information system because its primary purpose in providing remote healthcare is so often conveyed in sound or picture, though most telehealth conducted today does include the exchange of health information.

Telehealth, however, has many challenges, some of which are only now being addressed. For example, connectivity is a challenge because telehealth is so often used to reach remote parts of the country, on a battlefield, and across the world. Telecommunications technology is not always the best in such areas. Broadband, for example, is still not available, or at least reliable, in all parts of the US. Physician licensure has been another major challenge, where a physician may not be licensed to practice in another state, hence precluding the ability to cross state lines when conducting telehealth. Reimbursement for telehealth is not always provided by health plans, or only under certain, limited conditions. Specialized equipment must also be brought to the site where the patient is located. All these challenges are being addressed where there is high need. For example, robots have been developed to reach injured soldiers. The Veterans Administration (VA) has constructed all its telehealth services to rely solely on dial-up telephone connections because many veterans needing telehealth are in remote areas. Telehealth is experiencing increasing interest to reach prison inmates, inner city communities where there are safety issues, and in various care coordination activities where patients have transportation limitations. Medicare reimbursement for telehealth services continues to expand.

In addition to telehealth, new forms of healthcare delivery are being adopted. Some are very "low-tech" such as **e-visits** (telephone communications between patient and provider) and others such as **hospital-in-the-home** (where new connectivity mechanisms help monitor patients at home) have more technology requirements (Carollo 2018). What is also new relating to these technologies is the level of reimbursement for such services, the recognition that keeping people outside of a physician's office waiting room or even a hospital bed may reduce spread of infection, and make people more comfortable and happier which can also contribute to health improvement.

New technologies that have an information system component to them include new medical procedures, prosthetics, and machine learning. New medical procedures include techniques such as liquid biopsies that monitor tumors noninvasively. **3D printing** is creating new prosthetics and ways to improve organ and tissue repairs (Das 2016). It was previously described that AI is the ability for software algorithms to analyze data and make applicable recommendations (including to 3D printers). Extending beyond AI is **machine learning**, in which AI applications adjust the algorithms supplied in the software based on additional data, potentially providing ever more sophisticated clinical decision support (Garbade 2018).

Patient-Exchanged Health Information

Another form of exchanging health information is to use the patient as the go-between. This might be considered even older than telehealth when considering the patient—or patient's family member or caregiver—has always been the knowledge base for history of present illness and other information. However, from a technology perspective, portals, electronic personal health records, and the continuity of care document are technologies that are newer than telehealth.

A **patient portal** is special software that enables patients to log on to a website from home or a **kiosk** (special form of input device geared to people less familiar with computers) in a provider's waiting room to have access to some of their health information and other services. In many cases, the portal is used primarily for administrative functions, such as to request an appointment and even directly schedule an appointment, pay bills, obtain patient educational material, sign informed consents, exchange email with a provider, and request release of information. Under the MU program, the portal has been a common way for patients to access their health summary information. In some cases; the portal only provides health summary information. In other cases, it may provide a view into parts of the EHR or even the entire EHR. A portal may also be a way to access a personal health record supplied by a provider. (However, the MU program does not require a PHR.) In some cases, patients are starting to enter their own health history using a template that directs them to enter specific information via the portal that is then available to providers during the visit. Some providers are supporting e-visits through a portal, where existing patients can exchange email in lieu of visiting the physician's office for follow-up or recurring care needs. E-visits are now reimbursable by some insurance companies. Portals are also used by providers to connect from their office to a hospital or other healthcare organization, and to health plans, such as for eligibility verification or for submitting prior authorization requests.

The **personal health record (PHR)** has been defined by AHIMA as an electronic or paper health record maintained and updated by an individual for himself or herself; a tool that individuals can use to collect, track, and share past and current information about their health or the health of someone in their care. Although use of an electronic system for PHRs is encouraged by AHIMA, many more patients use a paper-based file folder as their PHR rather than an electronic offering. Whether electronic or paper-based, patients are expected to own and manage the information in the PHR, which comes from both healthcare providers and the individual. The PHR is maintained in a secure and private environment, with the patient determining rights of access. It is separate from and does not replace the legal health record of any provider or their EHR.

Today, PHRs are in a state of transition. The PHR may be provided through a portal offered by a provider or may be a stand-alone system offered via a vendor, employer, or affinity group that may be managed by the stand-alone entity or by the patient. A PHR offered by a healthcare provider is an excellent tool if there is only one PHR for all who treat the patient, and especially if it enables more than minimal functionality. If a patient has multiple healthcare providers, however, it is likely that the patient will also have multiple PHRs. Today, there is little connectivity between the PHRs. The patient might as well have a paper-based record system of their own if they wish to have any integration of data across these PHRs. PHRs offered by many healthcare providers also do not allow patients to enter data, rather they can only view lab results and other summary health information. This somewhat defeats the purpose of having a centralized place that can be used to document changes in personal health status or communicate in real time with providers about changes in a patient's health status, such as high blood sugars or weight gain in a patient with congestive heart failure.

PHRs have been most popular with patients who have chronic illnesses or with caretakers of elderly patients having to manage multiple providers, many drugs, and other data.

The **continuity of care document (CCD)** is yet another effort to supply patients with more information about their healthcare. The CCD is essentially a set of summary data about an episode of care. It uses the **Clinical Document Architecture (CDA)** standard developed by HL7 that aids in the creation and exchange of XML documents between health information systems. When the CCD is rendered as an XML document, the CDA provides structure (including a description of document content for users and discrete data for computer processing), vocabulary standards, and codes for sharing clinical documents in XML format. Subsequently, HL7 has created a transport mechanism not only for the CCD, but for a number of other healthcare documents. These document templates are collectively referred to as the Consolidated Clinical Document Architecture (C-CDA).

The C-CDA may be transmitted electronically via HL7 standard messages, in attachments to emails, or via standard internet file transfer protocols, such as file transfer protocol (FTP).

Because the traditional HL7 (and other healthcare information standards) only enable point-to-point exchange of data rather than seamless, on-demand information exchange such as is performed on the WWW, HL7 has created a new standard it is calling the Fast Healthcare Interoperability Resource (FHIR). FHIR is a set of resources that address common use cases in exchanging health information. They are based on application program interface (API) technology, which provides a set of tools for building software applications. FHIR resources each have a tag that acts as a unique identifier, much like the URL of a web page. A FHIR resource can support the exchange of text (including documents from the C-CDA), structured data elements, and metadata across a wide variety of devices from computers to cell phones (Bresnick 2016).

Another set of technologies that are supporting patient-exchanged health information are those from other industries. Non-healthcare companies merging with healthcare organizations or even planning to offer new forms of support for patients are lending considerable knowledge and skills to healthcare, including new applications for typically non-healthcare information systems. Something as simple as customer relationship management (CRM) systems (which serve as a database of customers [patients] and relationships they may or could have with service providers, such as transportation companies, home health agencies, meals-on-wheels, and others) can be helpful. For example, care coordinators and patient navigators could use a CRM system as they attempt to arrange transportation services for patients to get to their physician offices for follow-up visits (Auer 2015). CRM systems can also aid in provider networking tasks and patient engagement.

Health Information Exchange

Health information exchange (HIE) is another way to exchange information across multiple organizations and individuals. HIE is most often managed by an organization referred to as a health information organization (HIO). The HIO typically provides governance, fee structure, and policies and procedures for exchanging health information; it is a business associate under HIPAA. HIOs have struggled financially, as paying for exchanging health information when generally provider-to-provider exchange has been free of charge—albeit a slow process—has not been accepted as well as expected.

In general, an HIO provides several key services, shown in figure 11.7. These include:

- Patient identification, usually using an identity matching algorithm in which specified patient demographic information is compared to select the patient for whom information is to be exchanged. The algorithmic process is determined by the vendor supplying the service but uses sophisticated probability equations to identify patients.
- The record locator service (RLS) is a process that seeks information about where a patient, once identified, may have a health record available to the HIO.
- Identity management (IdM) (not to be confused with patient identification) provides security functionality, including determining who (or what information system) is authorized to access information, authentication services, audit logging, encryption, and transmission controls.
- Consent management is yet another HIO service. In consent management, patients have opt in/opt out privileges for having their health information exchanged. As noted previously, the patient will often provide a consent directive for this purpose.

Figure 11.7 HIO services

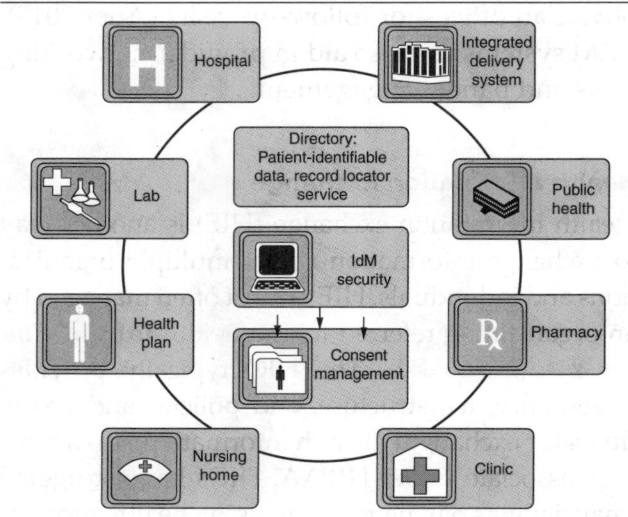

Source: © Margret\A Consulting, LLC. Reprinted with permission.

In addition to these basic services, each HIO establishes what type of data exchange it will support. For example, there are some that only conduct e-prescribing—exchanging prescriptions between providers who write prescriptions and retail pharmacies. Some states sponsor an HIO; if so, the HIO helps support public health activities (for example, immunization registry reporting) and often some basic exchange of emergency information. Because such HIOs must help exchange information across many disparate types of health information systems, usually only a limited amount of information is able to be exchanged. To exchange more comprehensive information (and perhaps also to gain market share), EHR vendors have started to support exchange of health information across all organizations using the same EHR vendor.

HIE is developing across the nation. Initially referred to as the nationwide health information network (NHIN), the federal government wants such a network to be grounded in both federal and private sector needs. Today this is referred to as the eHealth Exchange. It includes federal agencies involved in healthcare and nonfederal organizations coming together (with assistance from a federal contractor) to offer a secure, trusted, and interoperable health information exchange service (The Sequoia Project 2018). Today, the eHealth Exchange connects all 50 states and is used by the Department of Defense, VA, CMS, and Social Security Administration as well as 30 percent of all US hospitals, 10,000 medical groups, 8,200 pharmacies, and more than 900 dialysis centers—essentially connecting more than 100 million patients. Participants sign a Data Use and Reciprocal Support Agreement (DURSA), participant agreement, and testing agreement. There are both testing and exchange fees for use.

There are two ways to connect using the eHealth Exchange. They are the following:

1. Direct exchange uses an initiative called the Direct Project for securely *pushing* patient health information to a known, trusted receiver using secure email technology (HIMSS 2013).
2. CONNECT is an alternative way to connect with the eHealth Exchange. CONNECT is open-source software that implements health exchange specifications. It enables discovery of where there may be information as well as directly retrieving it from the source (HIMSS 2012b).

Check Your Understanding 11.2

Answer the following questions.

1. Software that is written to help exchange data between two applications is:
   a. Interoperability
   b. Interface
   c. e-Health Exchange
   d. Systems integration

2. Which of the following describes telehealth?
   a. It is the diagnosis or treatment of a patient who is not physically present with the provider.
   b. It is an exchange of email for routine clinic visits.
   c. It is call center services for disease management.
   d. It is remote monitoring.
3. The Consolidated Clinical Document Architecture (C-CDA) is a:
   a. Summary health record
   b. Collection of healthcare document templates in XML format
   c. Standard for formatting structured data in healthcare
   d. Specification for the content of an EHR
4. An HIO provides identity management to:
   a. Help locate a specific patient
   b. Assure appropriate security services
   c. Validate a patient's consent for sharing information
   d. List all providers participating in the exchange
5. True or false: Cloud computing is a process where data (and software) are housed on remote servers accessible through the internet.
6. True or false: The HL7 FHIR standard brings interoperability into the world of web-based connectivity.
7. True or false: In order to locate where a patient has health information, the Direct Project is used in a health information exchange environment.
8. True or false: A patient must access a PHR via a portal.
9. True or false: The eHealth Exchange is a free service available to all healthcare providers.

Systems Development Life Cycle

As described, health information systems include both technology (hardware and software) and operational elements addressing the needs of people (users), required policies, and process improvement. Health information systems also reflect a life cycle. This life cycle demonstrates the need to manage changes so the system continues to produce the desired results.

The **systems development life cycle (SDLC)** refers to the steps taken from an initial point of recognizing the need for a desired result, through the steps taken to ensure all components needed for the system to achieve the desired result are addressed. This cycle is repeated whenever the system fails to continue to produce the desired result (NIST 2008). Failure of an information system to produce the desired result may be due to internal or external changes. For example, if a health information system was acquired a number of years ago and there is a new federal mandate for adoption of new standards, the healthcare organization must address needed changes in the system, or obtain a replacement, to continue to produce desired results. The general nature of an SDLC is illustrated in figure 11.8.

There may be variations in how the steps in the SDLC are described depending on the context in which it is used. For example, a hardware or software developer may go through an SDLC when creating a new product. The vendor may identify the need for a new product, then determine the feasibility of creating the new product with specifications that would satisfy the new product needs, design the product, develop it for mass production, maintain the product as small changes in the environment impact it, and monitor sales to justify continued maintenance or **sunsetting** (that is, no longer selling or supporting) the product. In a healthcare provider setting, the SDLC helps identify a need for health information systems support. The healthcare provider will then specify requirements needed to achieve the need, acquire a new information system, implement the new information system, maintain it, and monitor that it continues to meet needs over time. Sometimes a health information system may need to be replaced, in which case the SDLC of acquiring a new product is repeated.

While the SDLC is most often applied when information systems are being developed or acquired, it can be applied as part of a continuous improvement process to ensure that any system meets ongoing and new needs. For example, taking a systems view and applying the SDLC can be a useful process when planning any new service offerings. A hospital may be considering developing a center of excellence in orthopedics or acquiring small community hospitals. A physician's office may be considering a merger or expansion of services into retail offerings. An integrated delivery network may be evaluating the usefulness of spinning off long-term care facilities it operates. The key value of the SDLC is to apply a formal logical process to ensure all components needed for a system to optimally achieve its value are in place. Each of the components in the SDLC is discussed next.

Identify Needs

Needs for a healthcare organization that a health information system should address arise from various activities conducted by the healthcare organization or may be mandated by the federal government, health plans with which the healthcare organization contracts, or other external sources. Commonly referred to as needs identification, a healthcare organization may periodically conduct strategic planning that identifies a need; for example, more timely data available to infection control nurses, or that the surgical suite needs to improve communications with other departments. A hospital may find that its major commercial health plan has decided to promote VBC, wherein access, price, quality, efficiency, and alignment of incentives, rather than volume alone factor into payment for care. Negotiating a VBC contract will necessitate significantly more integration of financial and clinical data.

Needs are most commonly expressed as goals. Goals for what and how health information systems will achieve desired results reflect current and anticipated needs and should drive all elements of planning for the systems. Ideally, these should be written as **SMART goals**, or statements that identify results that reflect the following:

- **S**pecific
- **M**easurable
- **A**ttainable
- **R**elevant
- **T**ime-based

Figure 11.9 is an example of a SMART goal for a hospital performing strategic planning for a health information system.

Figure 11.8 Systems development life cycle

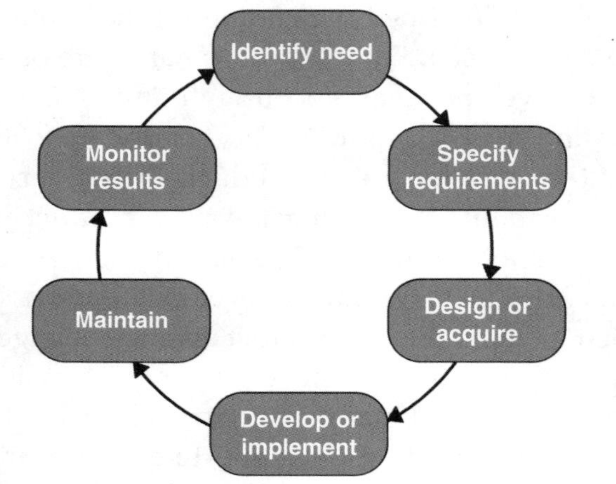

Source: © Margret\A Consulting, LLC. Reprinted with permission.

Figure 11.9 Example of a SMART goal

Example of a SMART goal	
(Note: SMART goals must contain all S-M-A-R-T components, but to read the goal statement easily, the comporents do not have to be in a S-M-A-R-T sequence.) Goal: Improve the near-miss medication error rate by 80 percent using a BCMAR system that is implemented with adequate training and process improvement over a period of one year.	
Specific:	Improve the near-miss medication error rate
Measurables:	by 80 percent
Relevant:	using a BCMAR system
Attainable:	that is implemented with adequate training and process improvement
Time-based:	over a period of one year

Source: © Margret\A Consulting, LLC. Reprinted with permission.

Any given organization will have several SMART goals for its health information system. For example, a clinic may include the following goal in its planning:

> Physicians will reduce unnecessary diagnostic studies tests by 10 percent (measurable) over the next two years (time-based) using the interoperability capability of the system (realistic) that, when a test order is placed, makes available (attainable) the results from previous tests performed across the continuum of care for the patient specific to type of test and patient needs (specific).

SMART goals should address all system components, including desired functionality, specific technology requirements to support the desired functions, and the expectations for people to adopt new policies and processes to ensure achievement of goals and, therefore, provide value back to the organization for its investment (Amatayakul 2017b).

Specify Requirements

Once needs are identified, a healthcare organization will want to specify detailed requirements for how the needs can be met. For health information systems, most healthcare organizations convene a steering committee that will identify and document a detailed set of specifications, often referred to as a requirements specification.

A steering committee may be an overarching committee comprised of key stakeholders to health information systems in general, or, less commonly, a steering committee will be convened for each specific health information system project and include only stakeholders associated with that project. The latter is normally not advisable because of the systems nature of health IT. For example, a BC-MAR will be impacted by CPOE and a pharmacy information system. Ultimately, it will also need to be integrated with a medication reconciliation system and may need to interoperate in the future with a home medication administration system.

The broadest possible set of stakeholders in a steering committee will ensure that all needs for a specific health information system are met. Members of the steering committee for health information systems should include heavy representation from physicians, nurses, and other health professionals, including a physician champion. The physician champion is a well-respected physician who can informally help the physician community adapt to and ultimately adopt health information systems. The position of chief medical informatics officer (CMIO) is being created in hospitals and large clinics. The CMIO is a salaried physician (most often part time so that he or she retains credibility with other practicing physicians) who is heavily involved in policy development, workflow and process improvement, and ongoing maintenance of CDS and other systems requiring significant physician input. Both the physician champion and CMIO help achieve a clinical transformation—a fundamental change in how medicine is practiced using health information systems to aid in diagnosis and treatment.

In addition to the healthcare professional representation, IT representatives, the health information management professional, key operational staff, the procurement officer, and potentially others will round out the steering committee membership.

Guided by the SMART goals that define the overall need, the steering committee will seek input from the specific health information system's key stakeholders to enumerate specific requirements. For example, when planning for a BC-MAR system, nurses, pharmacists, IT staff, physicians, and quality assurance professionals may be the key stakeholders. They will review the literature, consult with peers in other healthcare organizations, and perhaps attend a trade show or visit another healthcare organization with a BC-MAR system to understand more about it and what users like and do not like.

Design or Acquire

Today, most healthcare organizations acquire health information systems from a commercial vendor. There are few healthcare organizations left in the US that have and continue to support a homegrown, or self-designed information system—these are gradually being discarded in favor of commercial systems.

Commercial systems have several important advantages. First, they are generally cheaper in the long term because they offer economies of scale by selling the same product to many others. Second, they can be more interoperable. Vendors know they will have to do some integration with systems from other vendors in any given healthcare organization. In addition, with federal goals for interoperability (including changing the name of the program requiring an EHR from MU to Promoting Interoperability in its alternative payment models [CMS 2019]), vendors know they will not survive in the marketplace if their systems do not support interoperability. Third, the unique configurations that are often the hallmark of homegrown systems are feasible with many commercial products. These products offer toolkits that allow a user organization to tailor the information systems to their needs, while not impacting the underlying product's architecture—thus assuring both customization for users and interoperability with other information systems. Finally, vendor longevity in the marketplace is more assured than that of the custom programmer hired for a specific job for one organization who then moves on to another custom job for another organization—leaving the first organization without ongoing support for maintenance of the system.

Acquiring a health information system may be performed in one of two ways. If a healthcare organization already has many health information system components from one vendor (often described as a best-of-fit environment), the healthcare organization likely will acquire additional components from the same vendor. A small amount of due diligence (steps taken to confirm various facts about the product) may be performed to ensure the healthcare organization that it does not need to go to another vendor to acquire the product, thus moving toward a best-of-breed environment where different components are acquired from different vendors. Much like home-grown systems, best-of-breed environments started disappearing during the MU program era, but may be returning as a result of the HL7 FHIR standard that supports much easier interoperability, thus enabling acquisition of more specialty products.

Whatever their status, healthcare organizations should acquire health information systems through a formal vendor selection process. The steps in vendor selection are the following:

1. *Needs identification.* This step entails understanding and documenting the goals for the information system being acquired.
2. *Requirements specification.* This involves determining and documenting the detailed features and functions desired in the information system in order to meet the healthcare organization's specific goals.

   Requirements specification must also describe the way the healthcare organization will acquire the health information system. Client/server systems are those where commercial software is installed on servers housed and maintained within the healthcare organization itself, housed within the healthcare organization and managed by an outsourced company, or housed and maintained by a contractor for the healthcare organization. The benefit to client/server systems is the extent to which the software can be configured to meet the special needs of the healthcare organization. The primary disadvantage is that the healthcare organization must manage the IT infrastructure or hire a contractor to do so. An alternative is an application service provider (ASP) or Software as a Service (SaaS) arrangement. There are both similarities and differences between these two. Both essentially offer health information systems on a subscription basis, with the software and servers housed remotely. In an ASP arrangement, only a moderate amount of custom configuration is feasible, and the healthcare organization pays for 100 percent usage time, but it does not have responsibility for managing the technology infrastructure. Functionality is delivered to the user via dedicated communications technology. The SaaS arrangement is similar to the ASP, but there is generally less custom configuration ability. The SaaS offers a pay as you go model, where you only pay for the actual time using the information system. This may work well for physician offices, but generally not for hospitals that have 24-hours a day, 7-days a week, 365-days a year use requirements. The SaaS model may be delivered via dedicated communications technology or cloud computing.

3. *Request for Proposal (RFP).* An RFP includes developing and disseminating a description of the healthcare organization, its goals for the information system, its requirements specification, and a statement of how the vendor should respond to the request for proposal. In recent years, an RFP was considered too much work both for organizations to compile and vendors to respond to. Many healthcare organizations were so new to health information systems that they did not know what requirements they wanted met. However, with more experience, many are realizing that it is probably the only way to ensure a comprehensive understanding of requirements and their availability in a product. Dissemination of the RFP was also challenging in the past with so many vendors. Small providers often relied on their specialty society recommendations or "friends," who may have been biased and too narrow in scope should the practice expand beyond the one specialty. Today, the consumer is more informed and has had an opportunity to learn about a variety of vendors. Sending the RFP to four to six vendors is realistic and doable.
4. *Analysis of RFP responses.* This is a formal review of the responses to the RFPs against the requirements specification. This process should be done as objectively as possible. Often the requirements analysis is used as a score sheet to help identify gaps or potential issues. While it cannot be expected that any one vendor will be able to fully address every requirement, prioritizing the requirements and determining which vendors should be further considered is a key step. At this point the four to six vendors should be narrowed to three or four at the most.
5. *Due diligence.* This involves requesting a product demonstration, checking references, and potentially conducting site visits to see the product in actual use. Depending on the size and location of the healthcare organization, a product demonstration might be conducted on-site or via a webinar. However, it is conducted, there should be plenty of time set aside to fully put the product through its paces. Because most vendors will spend a lot of time before the actual product demonstration discussing the values and history of the company, the healthcare organization needs to take charge of the demonstration and set timelines for how much time should be spent on such introductory information, how much should be spent with the vendor conducting a demonstration, and how much time should be allowed for further discussion and even more in-depth review of certain features and functions. Demonstrations may range from a two-hour webinar to a full day or even longer on-site for large organizations. At least half of the time allotted should be spent on a detailed review of features and functions. At the conclusion of all forms of due diligence, a vendor and one backup should be chosen.
6. *Contract negotiation.* This may be the most critical, and often not well-performed, step in the vendor selection process. If money is to be spent on the vendor selection process, a consultant who knows the marketplace should be hired and legal counsel should be involved. Vendor contract offerings are notoriously one-sided. Recently, many small providers have realized that they did not negotiate that federally regulated updates to information systems must occur on a timely basis and at no cost to the healthcare organization. Many contracts also include payment schedules that require between 50 percent and 90 percent of the cost upfront—which should be far less. Contracts must also recognize the responsibilities of the vendor under HIPAA. The best form of contract negotiation is for the healthcare organization or organization representative to prepare a list of issues to be addressed, present it to the vendor, and then hold a series of conversations to address each issue. Price should

be the final negotiation step. An important caveat in contract negotiation, however, is that the result should be a win-win situation, not a win-loss, where the vendor loses so much money on the deal that they are unwilling or become unable to deliver on their promises. Implementation should not begin with an adversarial relationship between the vendor and the organization.

Develop and Implement

Once a commercial product has been acquired, there are development and implementation steps to be taken by the healthcare organization and vendor. A large part of acquiring a commercial product is associated with the implementation of the product. The vendor installs the software on specified hardware. Usually the vendor is also contracted for managing the implementation and appoints a project manager to do so. During implementation, **system configuration** (sometimes called **system build**) is conducted. This process provides customization of templates, review and customization of decision support, and other functions; in addition, master files and directories are loaded, and potentially some **data conversion** is performed. For example, a physician's office would want to have their logo displayed on the system, a list of all their patients made available to the application, fee schedules loaded, and data conversion to move their current accounts receivables to the new information system. Depending on whether there was a previous EHR, either EHR data must be moved to the new information system (data conversion), typically by a vendor or other contractor; or key parts of the paper health record content must be entered (**chart conversion**). This entry may be done by staff, a contractor, or new users as patients are seen. While new users usually do not want to do this, it is an excellent way to learn the information system and reduce unnecessary chart conversion steps.

Training is also a critical element of implementation. Some vendors will include, or sell for a separate price, training on using the information system, and may use a contractor for this. Other vendors supply a CD or webinar as their training option. This is usually insufficient for most new users, even when the user has experience with a different vendor's information system. In addition, training is not a one-time event—there needs to ongoing orientation, introduction to principles, training, reinforcement, sometimes certification of users, and re-training or focused training. When the system is upgraded, modified, or enhanced, training is needed again. Most of such training is left to the healthcare organization. For additional information on training, see chapter 20, *Human Resources Management and Professional Development*.

Other implementation steps for which the healthcare organization is responsible are management of the vendor and elements of implementation related to people, policy, and processes. Most healthcare organizations find it necessary to also appoint a project manager who is responsible for managing vendor relations, including **issues management** where any issues that arise during the implementation are documented, brought to the attention of the vendor, and hopefully resolved or escalated so that resolution is accomplished. Most (but not all) vendors typically do not perform change management that helps new users become acclimated to the significant change in not only documentation but the practice of medicine that results from using health IT, (additional) training, **go-live** (first use of the information system in actual practice) support, monitoring usage post implementation, workflow and process analysis and redesign, and policy development. Experience has shown that these elements may be more critical to the success of a health information system than the hardware and software. Change management is discussed in chapter 17, *Management*.

Workflow, process analysis, and redesign are often acknowledged by a vendor as important, but most vendors do not have time to provide such services. Those vendors who are at the top of the pricing scale do provide workflow and process analysis and redesign—and their results demonstrate the value of this. Unfortunately, many healthcare organizations are so overwhelmed by the amount of effort required in an implementation that they either do not have the energy or overlook this critical step. As noted previously, unintended consequences can occur from use of health IT and most have been related to lack of training, lack of policy surrounding appropriate use of the information systems, and lack of attention to workflow and process changes (Amatayakul 2011).

Testing of the software to guarantee it works with the hardware selected, has been configured properly, and users understand how to use the information system is also challenging. Many vendors will claim that their system has already been tested by virtue of their numerous customers, but each customer will have a unique information system build so this argument is not fully valid. Testing is often left to either super users using the information system in advance of go-live and finding issues the vendor must address, or by the end users themselves as they start to use the information system. The latter is not desirable, as the end users are already fearful of the change. Unfortunately, time often runs out and users want to begin using the system before it can be fully tested by super users.

Maintain

System maintenance refers to numerous tasks that keep the health information system running smoothly. Some tasks are routine in nature, such as preventive maintenance including the application of security patches or upgrades as delivered by vendors; others are corrective, modifying, or enhancing and performed based on calls to the help desk with issues or change requests for a modification or enhancement. Any changes to the fundamental system should be documented in a formal **change control program**. A change control program ensures there is documented approval for the change to be made and evidence that all elements of implementation, testing, rollout, training, and such are performed.

In a client/server environment, routine and some corrective system maintenance is left to the healthcare organization's staff or contractors; while other corrective, modifying, or enhancing maintenance may require consultation or direct work performed by the original vendor. Whoever performs system maintenance should provide regular reports on what maintenance has been done and this should be compared with policy, issues logs, and change requests. In an ASP or SaaS environment, most system maintenance will be performed by the vendor except for maintenance on local hardware and any software not covered by the ASP or SaaS vendor. Healthcare organizations are advised to keep track of issues they report to the ASP or SaaS vendor and confirm they are appropriately addressed.

Monitor Results

To complete the SDLC, monitoring results is an essential element that ensures health information systems continue to meet the healthcare organization's goals and identify when there are new needs. A formal monitoring program should begin immediately after go-live. The project manager or a compliance officer (or both) may be responsible for monitoring. The monitoring program should include formal processes such as user surveys, observations, benefits realization studies, and results analysis, as well as informal processes like the proverbial bagel breakfasts, pizza lunches, or milk and cookie breaks. During and immediately after go-live, it is helpful to have a break room set up where new users can unwind and talk about the system. Food is always inviting and often eases tensions when there are issues. Other forms of celebration for getting through the go-live day and reaching other milestones are also helpful. As time passes to more routine use, informal feedback mechanisms may move to weekly, monthly, or quarterly opportunities, but should continue indefinitely. Feedback from both formal and informal methods should be documented and addressed. Users must see that their concerns are given attention.

Although results monitoring is improving, many healthcare organizations do not monitor results well. Staff complaints, technology issues, and low levels of use are often known, but not tracked in any formal manner. Often changes are not made until a crisis occurs or the next federal mandate is enforced. Monitoring use, however, can result in achieving full adoption and even optimization, which leads to goals being achieved more quickly and comprehensively.

HIM Roles

Health information professionals' roles will continue to evolve as health information systems enhancements occur. Health information systems is very dynamic today. Constantly, new information technologies are being developed and new applications are being adopted for use in healthcare. In addition, there are many changes in regulations, standards, accreditation requirements, and practices that can significantly alter the course of health information systems. HIM professionals are able to identify new applications that are coming about as a result of new technology in general and in particular from mergers, acquisitions, and ventures of non-healthcare businesses (such Amazon, JPMorgan, and Berkshire Hathaway). It can be anticipated that in the next few years, significantly more changes will come about that impact healthcare. Examples of those changes may include the following:

- Use of CRM applications for care coordination
- Just-in-time delivery of services
- Increasing number of retail clinics and other delivery mechanisms to overcome access issues
- Consumer (patient) empowerment
- Analytics and artificial intelligence

Check Your Understanding 11.3

Answer the following questions.

1. Which of the following is a characteristic of the systems development life cycle?
   a. It lists the components of a health information system so that organizations do not have gaps in their strategic planning.
   b. It describes the steps to ensure all components needed for a system to achieve its desired results are addressed.
   c. It is a roadmap for vendor selection of any products needed to meet an organization's vision, mission, and goals.
   d. It serves as a guide to vendors on health information system requirements.
2. The systems development life cycle is cyclical because:
   a. There are six steps that are repeated continuously
   b. Feedback from monitoring results initiates repetition of the steps in the cycle
   c. It varies with the stages in which an organization has adopted health IT
   d. System theory reinvents itself periodically
3. In the systems development life cycle, desired outcomes may be best specified as:
   a. Requirements specifications
   b. Steps in product selection
   c. SMART goals
   d. Request for proposal
4. A health information system steering committee that best guides an organization's technology plans includes:
   a. Physician leadership
   b. All information technology staff that will work on the project
   c. Legal counsel
   d. EHR vendor
5. Steps taken to confirm various facts about a product are referred to as:
   a. Vendor selection
   b. Systems development life cycle
   c. Certification
   d. Due diligence

6. Which of the following is true in contract negotiation?
    a. Price is the most important thing to negotiate.
    b. It is best to use an attorney who can ensure the product acquired will work.
    c. All issues with terms of the contract can and should be negotiated.
    d. Vendors should take charge of payment schedules to ensure payback.
7. Moving data from an old system to a new system requires which of the following?
    a. Data conversion
    b. Chart conversion
    c. Loading master files
    d. System build
8. An approach to help new users acclimate to the new technology is:
    a. Change control
    b. Change management
    c. Training
    d. Testing
9. A situation in which a healthcare organization has multiple vendors represented in its applications is referred to as:
    a. Best of breed
    b. Best of fit
    c. Application service provider
    d. Legacy environment
10. During implementation of health IT, the step most often not performed or not performed well is:
    a. Contract negotiation
    b. Issues management
    c. Maintenance
    d. Workflow and process analysis and design

Real-World Case 11.1

A diabetic patient, John, moves to a new city and uses the internet to select a local primary care physician (PCP), who is a generalist physician and will coordinate his overall care. He can select a PCP who appears to have strong outcomes in diabetes and positive patient satisfaction scores. John schedules an appointment via the physician's website and is set up with a user ID and password to link the PCP with John's PHR, which is a record he maintains himself by uploading copies of records from various providers he has seen over the years. This enables the PCP to view and retrieve pertinent information from other providers and information John has recorded about his diet, over-the-counter medications taken, and other information related to compliance with his diabetic treatment regimen.

John asks his former hometown physician to send information to his new PCP. The physician does so using standard content and format specifications for exchanging referral information between providers. With the information supplied by the PHR and his former PCP, the new PCP's EHR is prepopulated with a current problem list, recent laboratory results, and other data. Additionally, the new PCP can add John's medication history to the EHR by linking to information available from John's health plan.

When John visits the new PCP, information from these various sources will be validated and updated. The new PCP can document all components of John's visit at the time of the visit, including demonstrating medical necessity for lab work by applying ICD diagnosis codes and generating appropriate evaluation and management (E/M) codes for the level of service provided. The PCP decides to put John on a strict smoking-cessation program and exercise routine, with plans to adjust medications according to John's vital signs and blood sugar levels, which will be monitored remotely through a medical device.

All is going well until John has an accident at work that requires a visit to the emergency department, subsequent admission to the hospital, and outpatient physical therapy. All his providers, however, are members of a health information organization (HIO). As a result, each provider has immediate access to the specific information needed to treat John throughout his care and for which John has provided a consent directive enabling him to opt in to the sharing of such information with all participants in the HIO.

At the hospital, the physician providing care can reconcile all of John's medications in accordance with the Joint Commission requirements and select medications that have been screened against John's known allergies. The hospital is also part of a health reform mechanism that ties reimbursement to quality metrics. This improves the quality of healthcare and reduces costs in an assigned population of patients. As a result, the hospital has access to John's previous lab and x-ray results, so repeating these lab tests is not necessary—saving John time and potential health risks and reducing overall costs. In selecting the physical therapy referral, the hospitalist has access to John's health plan benefits information, so no time is wasted in arranging for physical therapy to begin.

John's PCP also continuously monitors the impact of the accident on John's diabetes during his hospitalization and makes appropriate adjustments. After John is discharged and in physical therapy, the health plan can monitor whether he is following the prescribed exercise routine and can notify the PCP to follow up if necessary. John can access tailored discharge instructions that superimpose his picture on the exercise instructions so that it is clear how to avoid further injury. In addition, each provider John encountered throughout this episode of care follows up with him on the smoking-cessation program he started with his PCP, motivating him to stop smoking.

Real-World Case 11.2

Clinic for Kids is a provider practice with three pediatricians, two nurse practitioners, three licensed practical nurses, a half-time behavioral health therapist, and a part-time office manager. It earned initial certification as a patient-centered medical home and acquired an EHR over 10 years ago from a small, start-up company which provided the EHR via a subscription service and which also maintained the clinic's computers. One of the pediatricians refused to use the EHR but agreed to allow a nurse practitioner to scribe. Another pediatrician reviews the EHR at the point of care, but documents notes on scraps of paper and takes them home at the end of the day to enter into the EHR. The third pediatrician and the nurse practitioners are power users of the EHR, although the pediatrician is often frustrated with the lack of analytics support, especially as the clinic wants to participate in alternative payment models. The nurse practitioners, who are also taking on the role of care coordinators to further the VBC initiatives, find the EHR limiting in "customer relationship management" tools and the lack of interoperability with their patients, other providers, schools, and social service agencies. The behavioral health therapist, as a contractor, maintains separate paper-based records. At the time of the conversion to ICD-10-CM a few years ago, the EHR company went out of business. As a result, the clinic's office manager hired a part-time medical coder and IT support person who created a small registry on an Access database and documented ICD-10-CM data therein, which a healthcare claims clearinghouse then merged with claims data.

All members of the clinic recognize they need a new EHR, but they are now frustrated with the affordable offerings that do not incorporate the latest of technologies. Their primary hospital affiliation has one of the major EHR vended systems. The hospital has offered to supply a small-office version of the product to the clinic. The clinic is evaluating the cost differential, as the product costs more but the cost could be outweighed by cost reductions in compiling the coding database and clearinghouse fees. They also believe their nurse practitioners could be put to better patient care use with a better EHR and hence see more patients. At least two of the physicians are convinced that in a VBC environment, they would gain more than they would lose because their quality of care has always been outstanding. One of the clinic's health plans and the local school are also looking into ways to support the clinic in its IT management needs.

References

Agency for Healthcare Research and Quality. 2011 (August). Guide to Reducing Unintended Consequences of Electronic Health Records. http://psnet.ahrq.gov/resource.aspx?resourceID=23191.

Amatayakul, M. 2017a. Revenue Cycle Management. Chapter 19 in *Health IT and EHRs,* 6th ed. Chicago: AHIMA.

Amatayakul, M. 2017b. Health IT Goal Setting and Measuring the Impact on Healthcare Value. Chapter 4 in *Health IT and EHRs,* 6th ed. Chicago: AHIMA.

Amatayakul, M. 2011. *A Stepwise Approach to Workflow and Process Management for Health Information Technology and Electronic Health Records*. Boca Raton, FL: Productivity Press.

American Health Information Management Association. 2015 (update). Data quality management model. *Journal of AHIMA* 86(10): expanded web version. http://bok.ahima.org/PB/DataQualityModel#.Vje-S53nZkh.

American Health Information Management Association. 2017. *Pocket Glossary of Health Information Management and Technology*, 5th ed. Chicago: AHIMA.

American Health Information Management Association. 2013 (January). Understanding the HIE landscape. *Journal of AHIMA* 84(1):56–63.

American Health Information Management Association. 2012 (November). Using medical scribes in a physician practice. *Journal of AHIMA* 83(11):64–69.

American Medical Association. 2017 (December 21). EHR Scribes Cut Physician Documentation Time in Half, Study Says. https://www.ama-assn.org/practice-management/digital/ehr-scribes-cut-physician-documentation-time-half-study-says.

Auer, D. 2015 (April 8). Care coordination in a post-EHR world: How CRM and mobile tools are enabling change. *Becker's Hospital Review*. https://www.beckershospitalreview.com/healthcare-information-technology/care-coordination-in-a-post-ehr-world-how-crm-and-mobile-tools-are-enabling-change.html.

Bresnick, J. 2017 (May 2). New medical scribe exam keeps an eye on EHR data integrity. *Health IT Analytics*. https://healthitanalytics.com/news/new-medical-scribe-exam-keeps-an-eye-on-ehr-data-integrity.

Bresnick, J. 2016 (March 22). 4 basics to know about the role of FHIR in interoperability. *Health IT Analytics*. https://healthitanalytics.com/news/4-basics-to-know-about-the-role-of-fhir-in-interoperability.

Campbell, E.M., D.F. Sittig, J.S. Ash, K.P. Guappone, and R.H. Dykstra. 2006. Types of unintended consequences related to computerized provider order entry. *Journal of the American Medical Informatics Association* 13(5):547–556.

Carollo, K. 2018 (November 18). Healing at home: Hospital-at-home model takes care to patients. *Cardiovascular Business*. https://www.cardiovascularbusiness.com/topics/healthcare-economics/healing-home-hospital-home-model-takes-care-patients.

Centers for Medicare and Medicaid Services. 2019. Promoting Interoperability (PI) https://www.cms.gov/Regulations-and-Guidance/Legislation/EHRIncentivePrograms/index.html?redirect=/EHRIncentivePrograms.

Centers for Medicare and Medicaid Services. 2014. EHR Incentive Programs. *Federal Register*. https://www.federalregister.gov/articles/2014/09/04/2014-21021/medicare-and-medicaid-programs-modifications-to-the-medicare-and-medicaid-electronic-health-record. 79 FR 52909 page 52909-52933.

Chaiken, B.P. 2011. Web 3.0 data-mining for comparative effectiveness and CDS. *Patient Safety & Healthcare Quality* 8(5):10–11.

ECRI Institute. 2014 (January). EMR Integration Vendors and You: Hearing Each Other Loud and Clear. The Bench: ECRI Institute. http://www.ecri.org.

Das, R. 2016 (March 30). Five Technologies That Will Disrupt Healthcare by 2020. *Forbes*. https://www.forbes.com/sites/reenitadas/2016/03/30/top-5-technologies-disrupting-healthcare-by-2020/#53e0ca9b6826.

Feeley, T.W. and N.S. Mohta. 2018 (November). Transitioning Payment Models: Fee-for-Service to Value-Based Care. *NEJM Catalyst Insights Report*. https://catalyst.nejm.org/transitioning-fee-for-service-value-based-care/.

Garbade, M.J. 2018 (September 14). Clearing the Confusion: AI vs Machine Learning vs Deep Learning Differences. Towards Data Science. https://towardsdatascience.com/clearing-the-confusion-ai-vs-machine-learning-vs-deep-learning-differences-fce69b21d5eb.

Gue, D.G. 2018. EHR Optimization: Necessary Because EHRs Are Never "Done." Phoenix Health Systems. https://www.phoenixhealth.com/future-of-health-it/ehr-optimization-ehrs-never-done/.

Health Catalyst. 2019. Population Health Management: Systems and Success. https://www.healthcatalyst.com/population-health/.

HealthIT.gov. 2018 (March 21). What Are the Different Types of Health Information Exchanges? https://www.healthit.gov/faq/what-are-different-types-health-information-exchange.

HealthIT.gov. 2016. Glossary. https://www.healthit.gov/policy-researchers-implementers/about-onc-health-it-certification-program.

HealthIT.gov. 2014 (March 20). Step 3: Select or Upgrade to a Certified EHR. https://www.healthit.gov/providers-professionals/ehr-implementation-steps/step-3-select-or-upgrade-certified-ehr.

Healthcare Information and Management Systems Society. 2013. HIMSS HIE in Practice Series, Frequently Asked Questions: eHealth Exchange, the Direct Project, and CONNECT. http://www.himss.org/ResourceLibrary/ResourceDetail.aspx?ItemNumber=11657.

Healthcare Information and Management Systems Society. 2012a. Health Information Exchanges Part 2: Putting the HIE into Practice. https://www.himss.org/sites/himssorg/files/HIMSSorg/Content/files/HIMSS_HIE_Presentation_PuttingHIEPractice.pdf.

Healthcare Information and Management Systems Society. 2012b. The eHealth Exchange and CONNECT Overview. http://www.himss.org/ResourceLibrary/ResourceDetail.aspx?ItemNumber=10555.

HIMSS Analytics. 2017. Electronic Medical Record Adoption Model (EMRAM). https://www.himssanalytics.org/emram.

HIMSS Analytics. 2010 (December 1). Medical Devices Landscape: Current and Future Adoption, Integration with EMRs, and Connectivity. A HIMSS Analytics White Paper. http://www.lantronix.com/wp-content/uploads/pdf/Medical-Devices-Landscape_Lantonix_HIMMS_WP.pdf.

Horstmeier, P. 2017. Why Your Healthcare Business Intelligence Strategy Can't Win Without a Data Warehouse. *Health Catalyst*. http://www.healthcatalyst.com/wp-content/uploads/2014/08/Why-Your-Healthcare-Business-Intelligence-Strategy-Can%E2%80%99t-Win-without-a-Data-Warehouse.pdf.

Hughes, R.G., ed. 2008 (April). *Patient Safety and Quality: An Evidence-Based Handbook for Nurses*. Rockville, MD: Agency for Healthcare Research and Quality.

Kalatzis, F.G., N. Giannakeas, T.P. Exarchos, L. Lorenzelli, A. Adami, M. Decarli, S. Lupoli, F. Macciardi, S. Markoula, I. Georgiou, and D.I. Fotiadis. 2009. Developing a genomic-based point-of-care diagnostic system for rheumatoid arthritis and multiple sclerosis. *Proceedings for Engineering in Medicine and Biology Society (EMBC), Annual International Conference of the IEEE*, pp. 827–830.

Knorr, E. 2018 (October 2). What is Cloud Computing? Everything You Need to Know Now. *InfoWorld*. https://www.infoworld.com/article/2683784/cloud-computing/what-is-cloud-computing.html.

Monica, K. 2018 (September 5). 5 EHR Optimization Activities for Improving Clinical Efficiency. *EHR Intelligence*. https://ehrintelligence.com/news/5-ehr-optimization-activities-for-improving-clinical-efficiency.

National Institute of Standards and Technology. 2008. Special Publication (SP) 800-64, Revision 2, Security Considerations in the System Development Life Cycle. http://csrc.nist.gov/publications/PubsSPs.html.

Office of the National Coordinator for Health Information Technology. 2015a. Federal Health IT Strategic Plan: 2015–2020. https://www.healthit.gov/sites/default/files/9-5-federalhealthitstratplanfinal_0.pdf.

Pearl, R. 2018 (March 13). Artificial Intelligence in Healthcare: Separating Reality from Hype. *Forbes*. https://www.forbes.com/sites/robertpearl/2018/03/13/artificial-intelligence-in-healthcare/#747231471d75.

Philips. 2018. What is Population Health Management? https://www.usa.philips.com/healthcare/medical-specialties/population-health/what-is-population-health-management.

Quality Payment Program, CMS.gov/apms. 2018. APMs Overview. https://qpp.cms.gov/apms/overview.

Quality Payment Program, CMS/mips. 2018. MIPS Overview. https://qpp.cms.gov/mips/overview.

Rollins, G. 2012. Unintended consequences: Identifying and mitigating unanticipated issues in EHR use. *Journal of AHIMA* 83(1):28–32.

SAS. n.d. Analytics in Healthcare. SAS White Paper. http://www.sas.com/en_us/whitepapers/analytics-healthcare-102465.html.

Siwicki, B. 2018 (October 25). EHR optimization leads to 53% increase in cash collections at rangely hospital. *Healthcare IT News*. https://www.healthcareitnews.com/news/ehr-optimization-leads-53-increase-cash-collections-rangely-hospital.

Spitzer, J. 2018 (April 16). 30% of physician practices plan to replace EHR by 2021: 4 things to know. *Becker's Hospital Review*. https://www.beckershospitalreview.com/ehrs/30-of-physician-practices-plan-to-replace-ehr-by-2021-4-things-to-know.html.

Strome, T.L. 2013. Chapter 1"Toward Healthcare Improvement Using Analytics": in *Healthcare Analytics for Quality and Performance Improvement*. Hoboken, NJ: Wiley & Sons, Inc.

The Sequoia Project. 2018. What's the Difference Between eHealth Exchange, Carequality, and The Sequoia Project? https://sequoiaproject.org/about-us/whats-difference-ehealth-exchange-carequality-sequoia-project/.

Vanderhook, S. and J. Abraham. 2017 (May 15). Unintended consequences of EHR systems: A narrative review. *Proceedings of the International Symposium on Human Factors and Ergonomics in Health Care*. 6(1):218–225. https://journals.sagepub.com/doi/abs/10.1177/2327857917061048.

Wians, F.H. 2009. Clinical laboratory tests: which, why, and what do the results mean? *Laboratory Medicine* 40(2):105–113. http://labmed.ascpjournals.org/content/40/2/105.full.

Healthcare Information

Hertencia Bowe, EdD, MSA, RHIA, FAHIMA
Lynette M. Williamson, EdD, RHIA, CCS, CPC, FAHIMA

Learning Objectives

- Justify the importance of healthcare information to the healthcare industry
- Explain the role of data analytics in healthcare information
- State the strategic uses of healthcare information
- Define consumer informatics
- Explain the connection between consumer information access, health literacy, telehealth, navigational tools, and healthcare information
- Differentiate between the benefits and challenges of sharing healthcare information

Key Terms

Clinical data analytics
Clinical data repository
Clinical data warehouse
Clinical decision support system (CDSS)
Dashboard
Database
Data abstraction
Data analytics
Data capture
Data mining
Data standards
Data visualization
Decision support system (DSS)
Discrete data
eHealth Exchange
Executive information system (EIS)
Healthcare data analytics
Health informatics
Health information exchange (HIE)
Health literacy
Key indicator
Natural language processing (NLP)
Patient portal
Patient safety
Personal health record (PHR)
Point-of-care charting
Scorecard
Social media
Structured data
Telehealth
Unstructured data

Healthcare information is used to monitor the quality of patient care, conduct medical research, and accurately reimburse healthcare organizations. Healthcare information is based on personal health data about individuals primarily for provider use in the management of patient care. Data collection techniques include traditional methods such as paper health records as well as eHealth tools such as templates. "A template is an EHR documentation tool utilized for the collection, presentation, and organization of clinical data elements" (Buttner et al. 2015). The sources of health information include the healthcare provider through documentation in the health record and the individual through the use of a personal health record. A personal health record (PHR) is a record created and managed by an individual in a private, secure, and confidential environment. The personal health record will be covered later in this chapter. In addition, the federal incentives for the adoption of the electronic heath record (EHR) have progressed healthcare information exchange, including returning a patient care summary to the patient. Databases of healthcare information collected or maintained by healthcare providers, institutions, payers, and government agencies are of great importance to those who use them; for example, researchers or public health agencies. These databases are used for administrative purposes, including determination of payment for services provided, measurement of quality performance indicators, and research.

Per the Federal Health IT Strategic Plan for 2015-2020, the benefits of electronic health information include lower healthcare cost, increased healthcare quality, improved population health, and an improvement in consumer engagement. The Federal Health IT Strategic Plan is illustrated in figure 12.1.

With the implementation of the EHR and the changes that result, the roles and career options for health information management (HIM) professionals is growing. Some of the new roles include data analytics, consumer engagement, and health information exchange (HIE). This chapter discusses HIE information from the perspective of data analytics and explores the strategic uses of health information. In addition, the consumer's link to healthcare information—specifically their needs for information, ease of access, navigational tools, telehealth, and PHRs—is described. The various aspects of sharing and exchanging healthcare information are also addressed.

Figure 12.1 Strategies to achieve health IT goals

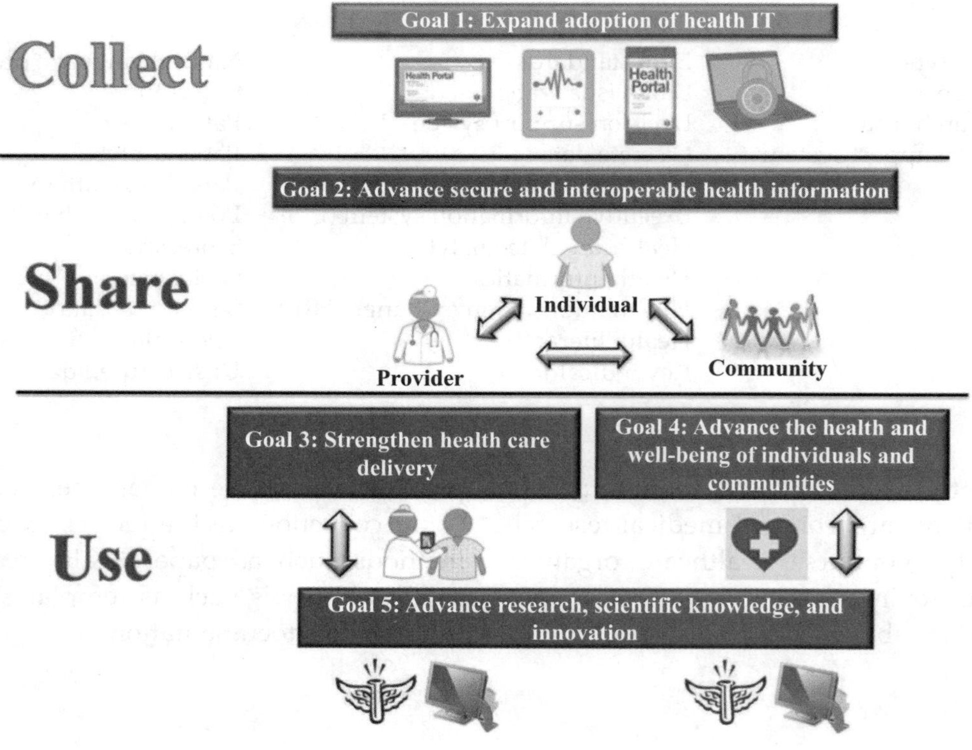

Source: ONC 2014a

Role of Data Analytics in Healthcare Information

Data are needed to arrive at information. Health data are not health information until they are interpreted, evaluated, and appropriately displayed (RWJF 2015). The difference between data and information is described in chapter 3, *Health Information Functions, Purpose, and Users.* Data analytics is the science of examining raw data with the purpose of drawing conclusions about that information. For example, data analytics can help hospitals with staffing by predicting the number of patients treated at a healthcare organization each month. The raw data examined in this example are admissions data, such as admissions records, rates, and patterns, which are analyzed over a period of time. Data analytics of admissions data can lead to the development of a web-based interface that enables physicians, nurses, and hospital administrators to forecast visits and admission rates for the future (Sreenivasan 2018).

The role of data analytics depends on the type of data being captured, reviewed, and used for the purpose of turning them into healthcare information. Multiple types of data exist, two of which—administrative and clinical—are further explained in the next section. If the data are of a clinical nature, then the analytics revolve around the contents of the health record. Clinical data could include elements such as lab values, number of patients with pneumonia, and so on. Administrative data are focused on other components such as financial data. A type of data analytics that uses clinical data is a clinical decision support (CDS) system. A CDS is a type of data analysis since it takes information from more than one source and provides an avenue for clinicians to make observations and decisions. "Clinical decision support provides clinicians, staff, patients or other individuals with knowledge and person-specific information, intelligently filtered or presented at appropriate times, to enhance health and healthcare" (ONC 2013).

Clinical data about an individual can also be combined with clinical data from other individuals to form population-based healthcare data. The resulting information may be used to improve the health of the public. For example, the occurrence of measles in one town could be combined with measles occurrence in a state or a region and that information could then be communicated on a national level if the rate of measles in children has increased from previous years. Analytics has the potential to play a role in leveraging data to improve healthcare quality and patient outcomes. For example, the data compare the health of a group from one region or state to another. The following is an introduction to analytics, its tools, and the knowledge areas for HIM professionals in data analytics.

Introduction to Analytics

There are different types of analytics. Descriptive analytics answers the question "what happened," diagnostic analytics answers the question "why did it happen," predictive analytics answers "what will happen," and prescriptive analytics answers "how can we make it happen" (Laney et al. 2012). To further illustrate for clinical data analytics, descriptive analytics could be centered on the increase in the incidence of Legionnaires' disease in individuals 65 years and older in a specific state over a five-year period of time. Diagnostic analytics would review the why of increased rates of Legionnaires' disease. For predictive analytics, once the why is found, it could be extrapolated that an increase will be seen in other states if certain conditions are found. Using this same situation, prescriptive analytics would examine ways to reduce the potential rate of increase of Legionnaires' disease in individuals over age 65 even if certain conditions (as found in the diagnostic phase) occur.

Analytics involves acquiring, managing, studying, interpreting, and transforming data into useful information. Types of data include clinical, financial, and operational data and the types of analytics include healthcare data analytics and clinical data analytics. Healthcare data analytics is the practice of using data to make business decisions in healthcare, whereas clinical data analytics is the process by which health information is captured, reviewed, and used to measure quality of care provided. What data are involved, the consumer of the information, and the decision the analysis supports influences the analytic process and choice of tools. However, there are certain steps that occur to prepare healthcare data for data analysis. The first step is data capture, which helps ensure the data needed are available and that the data are correct. Data collection is discussed later in this chapter. The second is data provisioning, which ensures that the data are in a format that can be manipulated for data analysis. For example, in the data field gender, male might be "1" and female "2." Data analysis, where data are interpreted, is the final stage of transforming raw data into meaningful analytics.

Analytics Tools

The amount and types of data available for analysis have increased as more data are available electronically. In addition, as technology advances, the various tools available to perform analytics allow for new ways to study and present the data. A few of the more common tools are those used for visualization, to report on process measures, to capture the data, and for extracting and examining data from a database.

Data Visualization

Data visualization is the presentation of data using a graph, diagram, or chart. The graphic display of data can help the viewer understand the data trend. For example, it can identify areas that need action, such as addressing a decline in the number of patients or an increase in the infection rate. Types of data visualization tools include tables, charts, and graphs. Choosing one visualization method over another can mean the difference between correct or incorrect data representation and drawing an accurate or erroneous conclusion. For example, tables display exact values whereas graphs show trends.

Following established guidelines for data visualization results in the delivery of a clear message. Those overall guidelines for creating any visual presentation, including the following:

- Understand the data
- Evaluate the information to communicate and the way it should be visualized
- Define your audience and examine how they process visual information
- Display the intended information to the appropriate audience in the clearest, simplest form (SAS 2018)

Tables are used to organize quantitative data or data expressed as numbers. Charts (such as pie charts and bar charts) and graphs (such as line graphs) are appropriate when presenting relationships. For example, in figure 12.2 the first pie chart shows percentages that add up to more than 100 percent, while percentages in the second chart are a part of the whole and add up to 100 percent. Each tool has specific features to keep in mind when depicting the data. For more information on presenting statistical data using tables, charts, and graphs, see chapter 13, *Research and Data Analysis.*

Figure 12.2 provides an example of a poor and an improved pie chart display.

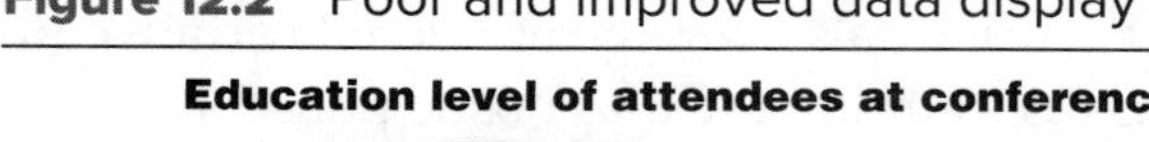

Figure 12.2 Poor and improved data display

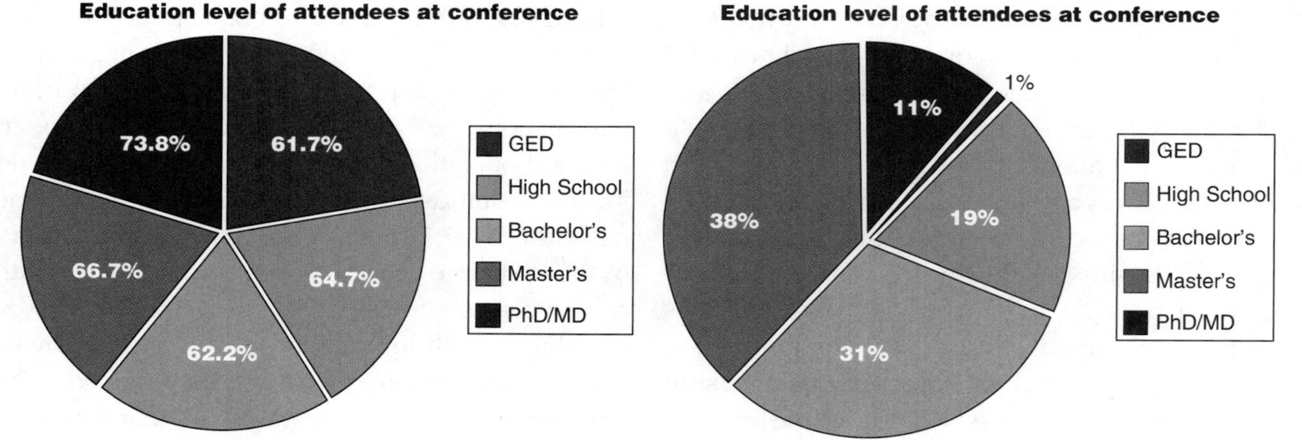

Source: ©AHIMA.

Dashboard

The dashboard is a data analytics tool that is a computerized visual display of specific data points. Typically, a dashboard focuses on a process and the rate of achievement. A dashboard is different from a scorecard. A scorecard, which can also be a computerized visual display, focuses on outcome or goal achieved, such as money raised for an event or cause. Both a dashboard and a scorecard can involve key indicators. A key indicator is a quantifiable measure used over time to determine whether some structure, process, or outcome in the provision of care to a patient supports high-quality performance measured against best practice criteria. For example, a key indicator could monitor death rates or infections. Chapter 18, *Performance Improvement*, discusses scorecards in more detail.

Health information management professionals use dashboards to monitor a number of indicators to improve performance and meet quality goals such as reducing the infection rate. To track the process measure over time, metrics (way to measure something) or benchmarks are established. Information is displayed on a dashboard to show the status of predetermined benchmarks. Often dashboards use color such as red, yellow, and green in a stoplight scheme. Similar to a traffic light, red means stop and go back, yellow means caution, and green means all good. Dashboards provide early warning signals and alert the manager to areas in need of attention.

For example, a recent HIM trend is instituting a clinical documentation integrity (CDI) program. Since this is not a small undertaking, dashboards can assist in measuring whether the program is successful. A monthly dashboard might show the number of clarifications requested by a CDI specialist that impacted a diagnosis-related group based on a benchmark. The dashboard would show green if the metric is met, yellow if it is in progress or halfway met, and red if the metric is below standard.

Dashboards are also used to manage revenue cycle management performance. For example, the Healthcare Financial Management Association (HFMA) has a web-based application called MAP App for use by healthcare providers to check revenue cycle performance and evaluate against provider peer groups (HFMA 2019). The HFMA's key performance indicators can be used to track, monitor, and improve revenue cycle performance.

Data Capture Tools

Data capture is the process of recording data in a health record system or database. A database is an organized collection of data, text, references, or pictures in a standardized format, typically stored in an information system for multiple applications. A database contains a large amount of data, often from multiple sources. Additionally, a database can provide comparisons using tools from within the database software. One of the most common healthcare databases is the relational database, which stores data in predefined tables consisting of rows and columns. Healthcare providers as well as patients may be the source of the data. There are several tools available for acquiring health-related data. Historically, data capture into a health record was via written notes or traditional voice dictation that was transcribed and typed into a paper report. Another method for data capture is scanning documents into electronic document management systems that create a picture of the scanned document, making it accessible electronically. Devices also include traditional keyboard or touch screen handheld computers or patient-generated health data devices (discussed later in this chapter). When the software application is run on a mobile platform such as a tablet or cellular phone, system and application software (often referred to as apps) is needed for the device to function and perform the desired tasks.

Electronic healthcare data capture is a fundamental function of the EHR (HealthIT 2018). The EHR is an information system with several components and data capture is an element in each component. The components include source systems (such as the laboratory information system), core clinical EHR systems (such as point-of-care charting), supporting infrastructure such as human–computer interfaces, and connectivity systems such as personal health records (Amatayakul 2013, 16–19). In point-of-care charting, the information is entered into the health record at the time and location of service. Nurses entering data using a tablet as they conduct patient assessments at the bedside is an example of point-of-care charting.

A human–computer interface is the device used by humans to access and enter data into an information system. A number of mobile devices are used for data entry into point-of-care charting systems. These handheld devices include tablet computers, laptop computers, and smartphones. These devices often contain built-in methods to facilitate the capture of structured data such as predefined or custom-built templates or forms with drop-down menus and point and click fields and word macros. These devices exist to make data collection easier.

The outcome of point-of-care charting can be unstructured or structured data. Unstructured data are nonbinary, human-readable data, whereas structured data are binary, machine-readable data in discrete fields. An example of unstructured data is free text that describes the patient's description of his or her condition. An example of structured data is using checkboxes to indicate patient symptoms. Structured data has many advantages over unstructured data when it comes to data analytics and health information exchange. Structured and unstructured data are covered in more detail in chapter 6, *Data Management.*

The structured data's entry fields and the potential entries in those fields are controlled, defined, and limited, resulting in discrete data. Discrete data represent separate and distinct values or observations; that is, data that contain only finite numbers and have only specified values. Stored in databases and data warehouses, these standardized data are available in a usable and accessible form. However, physicians and other healthcare providers may express frustration when limited to recording only certain data in specific fields. While a set format ensures consistency and provides standard meaning, it may limit details considered important by clinicians.

When considering methods for EHR data capture, follow these best practices:

- Collect data at the point of care directly from the patient
- Facilitate data accuracy using guidelines for documentation per governmental and other stakeholder standards
- Create and evaluate data integrity policies
- Establish information governance guidelines (AHIMA 2019)

Additionally, key areas such as patient identification, the use of documentation templates, copy and paste functionality, making amendments and corrections, and the incorporation of data captured in other areas of a healthcare organization not networked to the EHR such as outpatient services should be part of the role of HIM (AHIMA 2019).

Data capture may also occur with word processing software. The word processing copy and paste functionality in an EHR system must be carefully monitored and limited or prohibited to prevent data quality issues. Examples of data quality issues include copying outdated information or copying content from one patient to another that does not apply. Measures for preventing data quality problems include the following:

- Clearly label the information as copied from another source
- Limit the ability for data to be copied and pasted from other information systems
- Limit the ability of one author to copy from another author's documentation
- Allow a provider to mark specific results as reviewed
- Allow only key, predefined elements of reports and results to be copied or imported
- Monitor a clinician's use of copy and paste (AHIMA Work Group 2015)

For additional information on the copy and paste function and risks associated with it, refer to chapter 3, *Health Information Functions, Purpose, and Users.*

Two other technologies—speech recognition (speech-to-text) and natural language processing (NLP)—provide yet another way to acquire health data. NLP is a technology that converts human language (structured or unstructured) into data that can be translated and then manipulated by computer systems. Integration of these technologies within the EHR can result in the provision of clinical information needed by providers to inform decision-making.

Back-end speech recognition (BESR) is a specific use of speech recognition technology (SRT) in an environment where the recognition process occurs after the completion of dictation by sending voice files through a server. In BESR, an employee edits or corrects the dictation. Front-end speech recognition (FESR) is a process where the provider speaks into a microphone or headset attached to a PC and upon speaking, the words are displayed as they are recognized. The physician corrects misrecognitions at the time of dictation. Use of FESR integrated with an EHR provides the best outcome, as the provider is able to respond to prompts from the EHR resulting in more complete, accurate, and timely documentation (AHIMA 2013). Templates and macros are also tools used with SRT to capture data. Macros are used by transcriptionists to insert content into a transcribed document with just a few keystrokes. For example, the transcriptionist might create shortcuts to insert commonly used phrases or other content. As the output of SRT is digital text, combining it with NLP results in the conversion of the text or any free text narrative into data that can be translated and then manipulated by computer systems. Once transformed, it becomes searchable along with other structured data.

Data Mining

Data mining is the process of extracting and analyzing large volumes of data from a database for the purpose of identifying hidden and sometimes subtle relationships or patterns and using those relationships to predict behaviors. It is a key piece of analytics and of the knowledge discovery process. There are several knowledge discovery process models such as the Knowledge Discovery in Databases (KDD), Sample, Explore, Modify, Model, Assess (SEMMA), and Cross-Industry Standard Process for Data Mining (CRISP-DM) as well as hybrid models. Each has defined steps, with data mining being one of them.

The available data for analytics strategy and mining can come from EHRs and various databases such as a clinical data repository and clinical data warehouse. A clinical data repository is a central database that focuses on clinical information. The clinical data warehouse allows access to data from multiple databases and combines the results into a single query and reporting interface. Specific applications of data mining methods are customized for certain uses of the extracted data. For example, data mining may be used to extract clinical data directly from the EHR for the purpose of compiling content for reporting clinical quality measures. The clinical data warehouse lends itself to data mining as it encompasses multiple sources of data. The varying sources of data that feed a clinical data warehouse may include data sets, clinical data repositories, a case-mix system, laboratory information systems, or a health plans database. The data in the clinical data warehouse depends on how they will be used. For example, if the clinical data warehouse is going to be used to determine what treatment is most effective, then data would need to include data that would support that research. In this case, the clinical data warehouse might include blood pressure, test results, symptoms, treatments, and more. In the clinical data warehouse, the data from these sources can be "mined" to identify and implement better evidence-based solutions.

Systematically analyzing the data uncovers hidden patterns or trends for use in predicting behaviors. The information discovered from data mining databases aids clinical research. For example, data mining could be used to detect early signals of potential adverse drug events. Other data mining applications are used for the evaluation of treatment effectiveness, management of healthcare, customer relationship management, and detection of fraud and abuse (Koh and Tan 2005).

HIM Professionals and Analytics

Analytics start with data and HIM professionals, with their understanding of healthcare data, help ensure correct and accurate data are captured. HIM professionals are also proficient in business operations and clinical processes. However, data analytics require going beyond these into competencies such as business intelligence (see chapter 6,

Data Management), database administration, inferential and descriptive statistics (see chapter 13, *Research and Data Analysis*), health information technology (see chapter 11, *Health Information Systems*), and project management (see chapter 17, *Management*) (Sandefer et al. 2015).

AHIMA lists the following knowledge topics as important for data analytics:

- Clinical, financial, and operational data
- Understanding of database queries (such as structured query language [SQL])
- Understanding statistical software
- Data mining
- Quality standards, processes, and outcome measures
- Risk adjustment
- Business practices (for example, workflow or payer guidelines)
- Medical terminology
- Healthcare reimbursement methodologies
- Classification systems
- Source data
- Qualitative and quantitative analysis (AHIMA 2015a)

Strategic Uses of Healthcare Information

There are many reasons to collect data and turn it into information, including administrative uses such as claims submission, revenue cycle management, meeting quality measurement reporting requirements, assessing health status and outcomes, and performing clinical research. As health information technology (IT) systems evolve, the ability to aggregate the collected data improves and the information from it better supports strategic analytics and organizational decision-making. Through interpretation and evaluation of aggregated data from a variety of sources, development of strategies to improve patient care outcomes, reduce costs, and plan the future are possible through decision support, quality measurement, and clinical research, which are addressed in the following sections.

Decision Support

Information systems in healthcare are adopted for a variety of reasons. One of these is to improve the outcome in decision-making tasks. A **decision support system (DSS)** is an information system that gathers data from a variety of sources and assists in providing structure to the data by using various analytical models and visual tools to facilitate and improve the ultimate outcome in decision-making tasks associated with nonroutine and nonrepetitive problems. For example, the DSS can help administration decide whether to add an additional operating room. Management is the primary user of a DSS for operational as well as strategic decisions. It is not used for day-to-day decisions such as scheduling staff. A **clinical decision support system (CDSS)** is a "special subcategory of clinical information systems designated to help healthcare providers make knowledge-based clinical decisions" (Fenton and Biedermann 2014, 39). (Clinical information systems are discussed in more detail in chapter 11, *Health Information Systems.*) In DSS and CDSS, typically the problem in need of solving is unstructured or the circumstances are unknown. A CDSS could deliver targeted clinical decision support by supplying clinical reminders and alerts impacting the quality and efficiency of care. For example, within an EHR the clinician may receive a reminder that it is time for the patient's annual gynecological exam.

With data, analytical models, and visual tools at their disposal, the user can perform simulations of patterns based on various assumptions, monitor and assess key indicators, or perform data comparisons to look for trends. For example, to evaluate the success or failure of interventions, track trends, and identify opportunities for improvement, a manager may monitor readmission rates using a scorecard generated by the DSS.

An **executive information system (EIS)**, a type of DSS, facilitates and supports senior managerial decisions. Given that information is an enterprise strategic asset, an EIS is required to consider the broad needs of the healthcare organization. An EIS can transcend the organizational structure, transform the business by standardizing and describing solutions throughout the enterprise, and drive information-centric decision-making (3e Services LLC 2015).

The EIS is the source for identifying high-level strategic, operational, financial, or clinical issues. Rather than managing at the individual departmental level, an EIS can pull together financial, operational, and clinical information, with enterprise-wide policies and guidelines, to help the executive find actionable insights to drive enterprise performance. Organization-wide operational and informational processes improve with an EIS because business problems can be exposed, or business opportunities discovered. Examples of organization-wide operational and informational process key indicators executives may monitor include surgical volume and patient satisfaction. Figure 12.3 provides an example of a dashboard.

Quality Measurement

Using healthcare information to improve the quality of healthcare is not a new strategic initiative. What has changed, however, is the health IT available

Figure 12.3 Example of dashboard

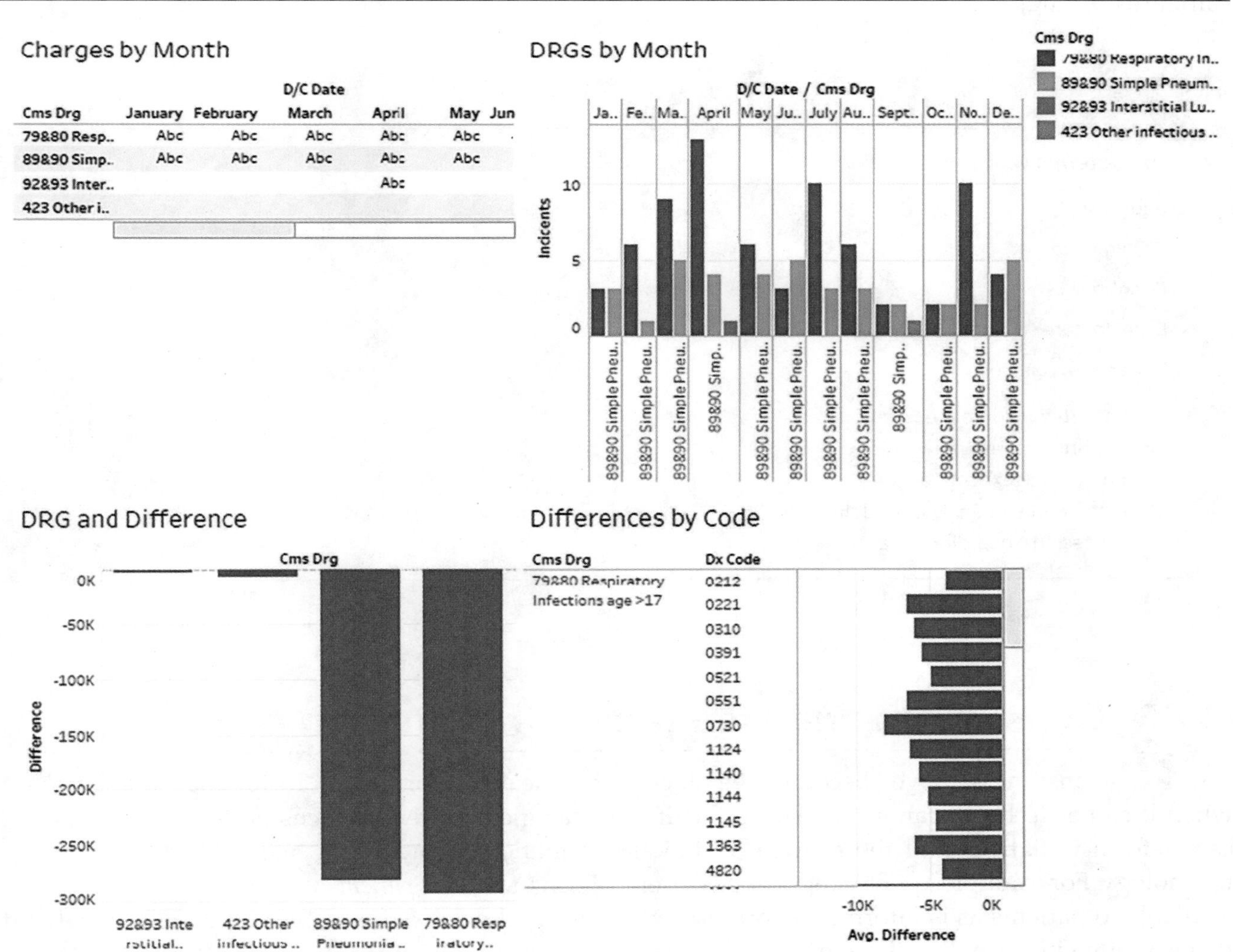

Source: © AHIMA Virtual Lab dashboard created with Tableau Software. Used with permission.

to collect and analyze the data for the purpose of turning it into healthcare information. For example, instead of manual data abstraction, which is the identification of data elements by an individual through health record review, data mining can extract clinical data directly from the EHR using standards and guidelines. Then the mined data can be compiled and used to report clinical quality measures. Healthcare information can also be used to improve care effectiveness; for example, alerts can be sent to administrators and physicians when measures related to quality and patient safety fall outside a normal range along with notifications of what may be causing these abnormalities. Also, health system effectiveness (for example, knowing which intervention was ineffective) could result in better healthcare outcomes for patients based on standards of care.

Clinical Research

Besides patient care, one of the original reasons for collecting data and analyzing its information is to research and study diseases and interventions. Information systems can support research by supplying the health data needed to inform clinical research programs and population and public health surveillance. In these cases, multiple sources of data are integrated into a central repository where it is possible to find early markers of disease, and historical data can be used to simulate and model trends in long-term care needs. For example, healthcare information such as an individual's genetic profile and local trends in disease prevalence may be used in patient-centered outcomes research. (Chapter 13, *Research and Data Analysis*, covers research in more detail.)

Check Your Understanding 12.1

Match the terms with the definitions.

1. Scorecard
2. Data mining
3. Dashboard
4. Data capture
5. Speech recognition

a. Reports outcome measures
b. Reports process measures
c. Speech-to-text conversion
d. Extraction and analysis of data
e. Process of recording data

Consumers and Healthcare Information

Consumers have become the focus when it comes to healthcare as a result of healthcare reform initiatives and the growth of digital technology. For example, quality reporting is often available to patients as is information on diseases that is written in a way that the average person can understand. The Office of the National Coordinator for Health Information Technology (ONC) has a strategic initiative to focus on technology and information to provide a higher quality of health. Terms such as *patient-centered care*, *patient-centric care*, and even *person at the center* are utilized and indicate the shift to the individual as the focal point when it comes to healthcare. The stated mission of the ONC is to make a positive impact on health at the community level and individual level by engaging consumers and making health information accessible (Executive Summary, n.d.).

What follows is a brief introduction to consumer health informatics, and an overview of information access and navigation tools such as patient portals. Social media in relation to health information is discussed. Information sharing specific to personal health records (PHRs) is then discussed.

Introduction to Consumer Health Informatics

Health informatics is the field of information science concerned with the management of all aspects of health data and information through the application of computers and computer technologies (Fenton and Biedermann 2014, 2). Adding consumers to health informatics makes them the focus for the technology that acquires, manages, maintains, and uses the data and information. Thus, "consumer informatics is the field devoted to informatics from multiple consumer or patient views" (AMIA n.d.). Consumer health informatics is a subtype of health informatics. A patient portal to a provider's website where a PHR can be developed and maintained is an example of consumer health informatics. Clinical email communication, such as a physician reviewing lab results with a patient by sending the patient an email is another example of consumer health informatics.

With any number of computer technologies available to the consumer, such as mobile health (mhealth), health information is only a click away. Mobile health includes applications available for smartphones that provide health information. For example, wearable devices that show how many steps a person takes in a day or the distance they walk is a type of mhealth device. The focus of a mhealth tool is on patient self-care. Patients can engage in their care through numerous health IT technologies designed for information access and navigation as well as those that allow the sharing of information. These health IT technologies improve patient–provider communication, allow for closer patient monitoring, and increase information access, all of which facilitate patient involvement with care providers. For example, through social networking sites consumers can connect with others who have the same condition and learn about their experiences.

Health Literacy

An important piece of patient-centered healthcare is health literacy. Over the years, the definition of health literacy has evolved. Previously health literacy was thought of as merely a person's ability to read health information (Cutilli and Bennett 2009). Current definitions of health literacy focus on specific skills needed to navigate the healthcare system and the importance of clear communication between healthcare providers and their patients. **Health literacy** is "the degree to which individuals have the capacity to obtain, process, and understand basic health information and services needed to make appropriate health decisions" (HHS 2010). People's ability to navigate, share, and engage in their own healthcare is impacted by health literacy skills. Second to privacy and security concerns, health literacy is the leading barrier to lack of consumer use of patient portals and mhealth technologies (Arcury et al. 2017).

Today's healthcare consumers are empowered to take part in managing their own health by becoming more health literate. However, many adults may not be proficient in health literacy and may lack the skills needed to manage their health and prevent disease (USDHHS 2008). Many factors contribute to the current state of inadequate health literacy, including "lack of coordination among health care providers, confusing forms and instructions, limited use of multimedia to convey information, insufficient time and incentives for patient education, differences in language and cultural preferences and expectations between physicians and patients, overuse of medical and technical terms to explain vital information" (HHS 2010, 25).

Health information management professionals support health literacy by ensuring patients' ability to understand and act on health information (JC 2010). According to the National Action Plan to Improve Health Literacy, strategies that health information professionals can endorse to improve health information, communication, informed decision-making, and access to clinical and public health services include the following:

- "Help to train all health care staff in the principles of health literacy and plain language
- Create collections or repositories of materials (for example, insurance forms and instructions, informed consent and other legal documents, aftercare and medication instruction, and patient education materials) in several languages and review the materials with members of the target population
- Help to disseminate existing communication tools and resources for patients" (HHS 2010, 30)

Health information management professionals support health literacy as they take on the responsibility for encouraging the development of competent healthcare consumers. Health literacy actions that HIM professionals engage in include providing consumers, or their designee, access to their personal health information in "useable standardized electronic form" (Heubusch 2010) or explaining to patients and families what their health information says and how to use it (Czahor et al. 2016). Furthermore, HIM professionals can educate consumers on the importance of compiling and maintaining a PHR, along with what type of information to include and how to obtain the information (Grebner 2015). During a patients' initial navigation on a patient portal, HIM professionals can serve as patient advocates by educating patients on HIPAA compliance with web-based and mobile device PHR applications (Grebner 2015). Health literacy training programs can also be developed by HIM professionals to give healthcare consumers the ability to understand these topics as well as where to find additional reputable information about their health conditions.

Health information can be overwhelming, even for people with advanced literacy skills (HHS 2008). As medical science continues to evolve rapidly, information learned during the school years often becomes outdated or is forgotten. Furthermore, health information provided to patients in a traumatic or unfamiliar situation is not likely to be retained.

Studies have shown that people who are more health literate are less likely to be misinformed about the body and natural causes of disease and their relationships to lifestyle factors. For example, without knowledge, patients may not understand how lifestyle factors such as diet and exercise affect many health outcomes.

Skills necessary to be health literate include reading, listening, analytical and decision-making skills, as well as the ability to apply these skills to various healthcare situations. For example, it includes the ability to know when to seek medical care, understand instructions on prescription drug bottles, appointment information, medical education brochures, physician's directions and consent forms, and the ability to navigate complex healthcare systems (NNLM, n.d.). Another important health literacy skill is numeracy, the ability to understand and use numbers. Examples of numeracy skills include understanding nutrition labels, measuring medications, and calculating cholesterol and blood sugar levels. Each of these tasks requires mathematical skills. Another example is electing a health plan or comparing prescription drug coverage, which requires calculating premiums, co-pays, and deductibles (HHS n.d.a). Figure 12.4 shows the four levels of literacy.

Addressing health literacy issues is not the sole responsibility of those providing healthcare services. Healthcare policymakers, purchasers and payers, regulatory bodies, healthcare consumers, and patients themselves all play important roles in ensuring health literacy. Culture is also a very important part of health literacy. Recognizing the role that culture plays in how people communicate, understand, and respond to health information helps better to understand health literacy (HHS n.d.b).

Telehealth

The use of technology to connect a patient and a clinician across a distance is the chief component of telehealth (see chapter 11, *Health Information*

Figure 12.4 Four levels of Literacy

Four Levels of Literacy

The 2003 National Assessment of Adult Literacy was the first large-scale national survey of ability to read, understand, and apply health-related information. It assigned proficiency to four categories associated with key abilities and sample tasks.

Levels	Key abilities	Sample Tasks
Below Basic A grasp of no more than the simplest, most concrete literacy skills 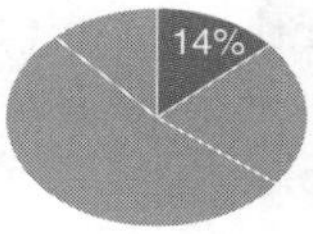 14%	• Locating easily identifiable information in short, commonplace prose texts • Locating easily identifiable information and follwing written insructions in simple documents, such as charts or forms • Locating numbers and using them to perform simple quantitative operations	• Searching a short, simple text to find what a patient may drink before a medical test • Signing a form
Basic Skills needed to perform simple everyday literacy activities 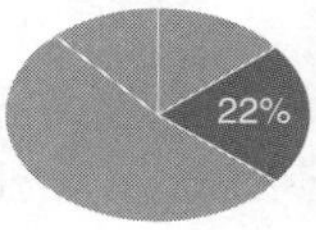 22%	• Reading and understanding information in short, commonplace prose texts • Reading and understanding information in simple documents • Locating easily identifiable quatitative information and using it to solve simple one-step problems	• Giving two reasons a person with no symptoms of a disease should be tested for it • Entering names and birth dates in a health insurance application • Calculating what time to take a medication by combining two pieces of information
Intermediate Skills necessary to perform moderately challenging literacy activities 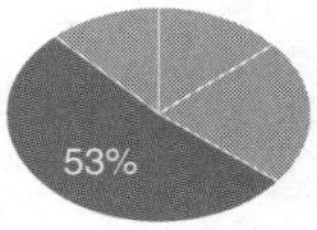 53%	• Reading and understading moderately dense, less commonplace prose texts, making simple interferences, determining cause and effect, and recognizing the author's purpose • Locating information in dense, complex documents and making simple interference about the information • Locating less familier quantitative information and using it to solve problems when the arithmetic operation is not specified or easily inferred	• Consulting reference materials to determine which foods contain a particular vitamin • Finding the age range during which children should receive a particular vaccine by using a chart showing all childhood vaccines and the ages when children should receive them • Determining a healthy weight range for a person of a specified height, based on a graph that relates height and weight to body mass index
Proficient Skills neccssary to perform more complex and challenging literacy activities 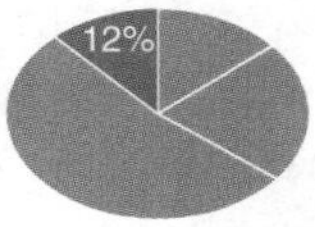 12%	• Reading lengthy, complex, abstract prose texts and synthesizing information and making complex inferences • Integrating, synthesizing, and analyzing multiple pieces of information located in complex docments • Locating more abstract quantitative in formation and using it to solve multistep problems when arithmetic operations are not easily inferred and problems are more complex	• Comparing the power of attorney with a living will and determining the advantages of the power of attorney • Interpreting a table about blood pressure, age, and physical ability • Computing the price per year of an insurance policy

Source: AHIMA 2010.

Systems, for more information.). Telehealth can also be used to send clinical information on the daily status of a patient's health to a physician via technology. In the evolving area of consumer health informatics, telehealth is being focused on to increase access to and provide quality healthcare. Telehealth is an option utilized to monitor chronic disease in patients and to provide access to medical care in locations that are lacking in clinical staff. This allows for patients as consumers to be active in decisions related to their health and to use digital technology to gain access to healthcare (Demiris 2016). Telehealth can be used to track vital signs and monitor other clinical information such as blood sugar. Telehealth provides a way to interact with patients and caregivers and to engage them in short-term and long-term health-related decision-making. Short-term conditions are nonurgent or nonemergency medical situations. For example, a short-term condition might be an ear infection or an upper respiratory infection. Long-term use of telehealth can be focused on more intensive healthcare intervention such as cardiac monitoring. As the consumer, an individual with a chronic condition can be more involved in their healthcare. Another factor of telehealth for the consumer may be the cost. Telehealth medical visits may cost less than an office visit, making them advantageous for the consumer (Wicklund 2018). One barrier is patient adoption of telehealth options. The ONC recognized this barrier in a published white paper, Designing the Consumer-Centered Telehealth & eVisit Experience: Consideration for the Future of Consumer Healthcare (Bobinet and Petito n.d.). With the ability to access urgent care and emergency centers, the role of telehealth is still being examined by stakeholders especially in areas where remote access may not be warranted. In the white paper, the ONC identified nine important principles of consumer-focused telehealth design and incorporation as a part of the healthcare option tools. Several of these principles focus on the technology aspects. For the consumer, the vital principles center on the experience for the patient and ensuring there is a balance between accessibility, data overload, meaningful care, and quality of care (Bobinet and Petito n.d.).

Information Access and Navigational Tools

The Medicare and Medicaid EHR Incentive Programs funded by the American Recovery and Reinvestment Act of 2009 stimulated the healthcare industry to adopt EHRs. One of the objectives to achieve Meaningful Use (MU) (now Promoting Interoperability) for certified EHR technology is to provide patients with the ability to electronically view, download, and transmit their health information within a certain number of days of the information being available to the eligible professionals (physicians and other healthcare professionals identified by the law). By providing patients access to an electronic copy of their health information they and their caregivers can be more engaged in their care. (Promoting Interoperability is explained in more detail in chapter 16, *Fraud and Abuse Compliance.)*

Consumer health IT applications for information access and navigation include hardware, software, and applications accessed via a computer, tablet, or phone. The ability to use mobile devices, patient portals, and social networking websites allows consumers to not only manage their health information electronically but also to participate in their healthcare via electronic means.

Mobile Devices

Portable, wireless computing devices or mobile devices include tablet computers, laptop computers, and smartphones. These devices combined with mobile medical apps can help consumers gain access to useful information wherever they may be and whenever it is needed. Apps for smartphones include pharmaceutical references with information about side effects and dosage amounts, access to licensed healthcare professionals allowing video chats about a medical problem, and guides providing step-by-step first aid instructions.

According to the US Food and Drug Administration (FDA), a mobile medical app is a mobile app that meets the definition of device in the Federal Food, Drug, and Cosmetic Act and either is intended "to be used as an accessory to a regulated medical device; or to transform a mobile platform into a regulated medical device" (FDA 2015).

The FDA considers the mobile app's intended use in determining whether the definition of a device has been met. The FDA guidance states a mobile app intended for use in performing a medical device function (such as for diagnosis of disease or other conditions) is a medical device, regardless of the platform on which it is run (FDA 2015). An example would be mobile apps intended to run on smartphones to analyze and interpret EKG waveforms to detect heart function irregularities.

Patient Portals

A patient portal is an information system that allows consumers to log in to a secure online website to gain access to personal health information and navigate around it once inside the information system. The types of patient portals and the modules implemented will offer the following different functionalities:

- Accessing a subset of the patient's health records (for example, medical history, health issues, medication list, test results, care plans, allergy list)
- Sending a secure message to the patient's healthcare provider(s)
- Uploading clinical information and telemetry (for example, blood pressure, blood glucose values, and weight measured at home)
- Completing forms electronically instead of on paper (e-forms)
- Accessing a child's or elderly parent's records with appropriate authorization (proxy access)
- Scheduling appointments
- Requesting medication refills
- Accessing billing records
- Paying bills online (Carayon et al. 2015)

A patient portal is a way to engage patients by giving them an avenue to access and review their health history (AHIMA 2016). Patient portals are one element in the focus on increasing communication, using technology, and engaging patients (AHIMA 2016). For example, a patient may come to the patient portal to learn more about symptoms he or she is experiencing. An interactive decision tool would help the patient assess the symptoms through a series of questions. If the patient visits the portal to better understand a current diagnosis, a link to educational material about the condition is available. Either scenario may result in communication with the provider via secure messaging about what was learned.

Social Media

Social media is defined as websites or applications that provide an avenue for personal networking and the sharing of information. A number of healthcare-focused social networks are available to consumers as individuals come together to interact and receive support from others with similar interests. Online communities specific to a condition or disease provide the consumer with information about the condition and which treatments may have greater success than others.

Providers use social media to inform consumers about diseases, conditions, and treatments. For example, Mayo Clinic's website contains patient care and health information on many diseases and conditions. In addition, the site has a symptom checker; a list of tests and procedures that includes a definition of each, how the test or procedure is performed, and how to prepare; risks and results; and details about drugs and supplements. Large well-known healthcare institutions such as the Cleveland Clinic and Johns Hopkins Medicine publish photos and videos. For example, the Cleveland Clinic provides patient education videos that contain actual surgery images.

Government agencies also use social media to inform consumers about healthcare. The Centers for Disease Control and Prevention (CDC) lists a number of mobile social activities including apps, a CDC video streaming station, and infographics. The Department of Health and Human Services Office of Disease Prevention and Health Promotion has initiatives aimed at healthcare consumers, which contain evidence-based health information and tools to help consumers make informed health choices along with their healthcare providers.

Personal Health Records

An important piece of patient-centered healthcare is information sharing. Patients generate data outside of provider settings. Sharing it with their providers expands the depth, breadth, and continuity of information resulting in the potential for improved healthcare outcomes.

Health IT tools connect patients and providers and allow them to share information, which strengthens the consumer engagement experience. Patient portals discussed previously are one such tool. Another tool is the personal health record. A PHR is a record created and managed by an individual in a private, secure, and confidential environment. It differs from an EHR, which is created and managed by the healthcare provider. A PHR can be about the individual's health or the health of someone in his or her care and be used as a tool to collect, track, and share past and current information. Sharing the contents of a PHR with providers can enhance existing data, fill in information gaps, and provide a more complete picture of a patient's health. Other benefits of a PHR are improved patient engagement and enhanced provider–patient communication.

Data from a PHR is patient-generated health data (PGHD). ONC identified PGHD as an important issue for advancing patient engagement because patients may become more involved with their care when patient–provider communication includes the use of the patient-generated data as part of healthcare decision-making. According to ONC, PGHD are "health-related data created, recorded, or gathered by or from patients (or family members or other caregivers) to help address a health concern" (ONC 2018a). Examples of PGHD include health and treatment history and data from a wearable monitor, such as an exercise-tracking device

Information in Personal Health Records

PHRs can contain information from several sources including patients and healthcare providers. While there is not a standard set of data and reports to include in a PHR because specific content depends on the type of healthcare received, the following reports are common to most health records:

- *Identification sheet*. Form originated at the time of registration that contains demographic information
- *Problem list*. List of significant illnesses and operations
- *Medication record*. List of medications prescribed or administered
- *History and physical*. Past and current illnesses and surgeries, current medications and family history, as well as a physical exam performed by the physician
- *Progress notes*. Notes made by the physicians, nurses, therapists, and social workers that reflect their observations, the patient's response to treatment, and plans for continued treatment
- *Consultation*. Opinion about the patient's condition made by a physician other than the attending physician
- *Physician's orders*. Physician's directions to nurses and other members of the healthcare team regarding medications, tests, diets, and treatments
- *Imaging and x-ray reports*. Findings of x-rays, mammograms, ultrasounds, and scans
- *Lab reports*. Results of tests conducted on body fluids
- *Immunization record*. Documentation of immunizations given for diseases such as polio, measles, mumps, rubella, and the flu
- *Consent and authorization forms*. Consents for admission, treatment, surgery, and release of information (AHIMA 2015b)

Other health information such as exercise and diet plans, health goals, and home monitoring system results such as blood pressure levels may also be a part of the PHR.

Models of Personal Health Records

A PHRs can be as simple as paper documents placed into a folder. However, an electronic PHR is better because of the accessibility factor and to gather, update, integrate, and manipulate the information more easily.

The two main types of electronic PHRs are the following:

1. *Stand-alone*. Patients fill in information they want to share with their healthcare provider. The information is stored on patients' computers or through an online system. Some stand-alone PHRs accept data from external sources, such as healthcare providers and laboratories. Patients choose with whom they share the information.
2. *Tethered or connected*. A type of PHR that is linked to a specific healthcare organization's EHR. A tethered PHR allows patients to access their records through a secure portal (HealthIT 2014).

There are many sources of PHRs. In addition to those listed, employers and independent vendors offer PHRs. Connecting the PHR to the patient's legal health record protects it under the Health Insurance Portability and Accountability Act (HIPAA) Privacy Rule (ONC n.d.). (Chapter 9, *Data Privacy and Confidentiality*, provides more detail on HIPAA.)

Patient Safety

The World Health Organization (WHO) defines **patient safety** as "the prevention of errors and adverse effects to patients associated with health care" (WHO 2018). Sharing the contents of a PHR with providers can enhance existing data, fill in information gaps, and provide a more complete picture of a patient's health, creating an opportunity to improve patient safety. For example, a PHR with information about allergies, medications, and adverse drug reactions compiled from multiple sources can be used by a provider to reconcile the information against what is contained in the EHR, thus preventing medication errors or adverse events leading to patient harm. PHRs also support telehealth capabilities where access to the health information could impact clinical decision-making. In a medical emergency situation, a PHR may provide information when the patient cannot. Telehealth is covered in more detail in chapter 11, *Health Information Systems*.

Check Your Understanding 12.2

Answer the following questions.

1. True or false: One type of electronic PHR is the tethered PHR.
2. True or false: Scheduling appointments is a required functionality for a patient portal.
3. True or false: Home monitoring system results such as blood pressure levels are part of a PHR.
4. True or false: Consumer health IT applications for information access and navigation include smartphones.
5. True or false: PHRs can contain information from patients but not from healthcare providers.
6. True or false: Telehealth is used to provide patients direct email access to physicians.
7. True or false: Health literacy is required to be able to complete pre-visit online medical questionnaires.
8. True or false: For PHRs there is a data standard.
9. True or false: Telehealth is a way to provide patients more correct information on common diseases such as diabetes and hypertension.
10. True or false: Data found in a PHR can be termed patient-generated health data.

Health Information Exchange

Health information exchange (HIE) is an important part of the healthcare industry. While there are several definitions of HIE, all of them note the exchange of information is done electronically, and the capacity exists for different information systems and software applications to exchange data. These definitions are the following:

- A HIE is the exchange of health information electronically between providers and others with the same level of interoperability, such as labs and pharmacies.
- A HIE "allows physicians, nurses, pharmacists, other healthcare providers, and patients to appropriately access and securely share a patient's vital medical information electronically—improving the speed, quality, safety and cost of patient care" (ONC 2018b).
- A HIE "provides the capability to electronically move clinical information among disparate healthcare information systems and maintain the meaning of the information being exchanged" (HIMSS 2014).

Determining a course of treatment having only the information contained in a single health record or encapsulated by a single provider of care is shortsighted and could result in duplicative treatments. While not an easy task, moving away from an ownership view of health data to a continuity of care perspective facilitates coordinated patient care. Successfully exchanging and integrating the information into clinical work practice fills information gaps and provides a more complete picture of a patient's health situation resulting in more informed clinical decisions by the healthcare team.

The remaining portion of this chapter provides an introduction to HIE, lists its forms, describes the benefits and users of HIE, explains eHealth exchange, states the challenges with sharing healthcare information, and identifies HIE roles for HIM professionals.

Impact of HIE

Health Information Technology for Economic and Clinical Health (HITECH) legislation and MU regulations mandate HIE functionality and its use. A qualified EHR under HITECH includes, as one of the criteria, that the EHR has the capacity to exchange electronic health information with and integrate such information from other sources (45 CFR 170.102). A health information exchange organization is one that supports, oversees, or governs the exchange of health-related information among organizations according to nationally recognized standards. These health information exchange organizations provide the means for HIE to occur. The health information exchange organization compiles data from a number of healthcare providers so that the physician currently treating the patient has a complete picture of the patient's medical history and treatment including all current medications.

With the introduction of the Medicare Access and CHIP Reauthorization Act of 2015 (MACRA), the MU mandate for participating in the Medicare EHR Incentive Program transitioned to become one of four components of a new Merit-Based Incentive Payment System (MIPS) (HealthIT 2019). The focus of the new MIPS remains on quality, cost, and use of certified EHR technology (CEHRT) in a cohesive program that avoids redundancies (HHS 2016). Ultimately the MACRA establishes new ways to pay physicians for caring for Medicare beneficiaries (NRHI n.d.) and further enables data sharing. For details about the MACRA and the MIPS, refer to chapter 11, *Health Information Systems*.

Health information exchanges are achieving national healthcare reform goals of better-quality care, improved population health, and lower costs. Recent studies show when physicians, nurses, pharmacists, and other healthcare providers can share a patient's computerized medical information electronically, decreased duplicated procedures, reduced imaging, lowered healthcare costs, and improved patient safety occur (Landi 2018).

An acronym that is sometimes confused with HIE is HIX, or health insurance exchange. A HIX is a marketplace where patients can choose a health insurance plan based on price. A HIX evolved as a result of the ACA in efforts to assist with the health insurance market reform. While the Affordable Care Act (ACA) itself refers to these entities as exchanges, the endorsed term when referring to Americans using the exchange is *health insurance marketplace*. Health insurance exchanges are also known as marketplaces, health benefits exchange, health care exchange, health insurance marketplace, and affordable insurance exchanges (Karl 2012; Obamacare Facts 2018). Health insurance exchanges are discussed in more detail in chapter 15, *Revenue Management and Reimbursement*.

Interoperability

Health information exchange and health information interoperability are not the same. Interoperability is defined as the ability of computers to share information. An interoperable health IT environment is one in which seamless health information exchange is possible across diverse EHR systems and the information is understood and shared with those in need of it at the time it is needed. There needs to be some exchange for interoperability to occur. What happens to the information after it is exchanged determines whether interoperability occurs. If the information is accepted—for example, an email is sent from one computer to another—then there was an exchange. However, if the information exchanged is understood by both computer systems and no meaning is lost when exchanged resulting in seamless use of it, this series of events meets the definition of interoperability. For additional information on interoperability, see chapter 6, *Data Management*.

Forms of Health Information Exchange

The three key forms of HIE. Standards, policies, and information technology serve as the foundation for the following three forms:

1. *Directed exchange* is the "ability to send and receive secure information electronically between care providers to support coordinated care" (ONC 2018b). Examples of patient information include ancillary test orders and results, patient care summaries, and consultation reports. The encrypted patient information is sent electronically and securely between parties with an established relationship. For example, directed exchange is used to report public health data to the state health department.
2. *Query-based exchange* is the "ability for providers to find and/or request information on a patient from other providers, often used for unplanned care.... Query-based exchange is used to search and discover accessible clinical sources on a patient" (ONC 2018b). For example, a query-based exchange can assist a provider in obtaining a health record on a patient who is visiting from another state, resulting in more informed decisions about the care of the patient.
3. *Consumer-mediated exchange* is the "ability for patients to aggregate and control the use of their health information among providers" (ONC 2018b). For this form of exchange the patient, not the provider, is the driver. For example, a patient portal may allow personal health information to be uploaded for provider access.

Benefits of Health Information Exchange

There are many benefits to HIE. One of the primary benefits is enhanced patient care coordination. Other potential benefits for patients, providers, payers, and communities include the following:

- Reduction of duplicative treatments
- Elimination of redundant or unnecessary testing
- Fewer medication and medical errors, which can be costly and have a negative impact on the patient
- Increased patient safety
- Achievement of a basic level of interoperability
- More informed decision-making for more effective care and treatment
- Improved public health reporting and monitoring
- Improved transitions of care

- Improved population health
- Improved efficiency in the healthcare system
- Reduction in paperwork, allowing more time for discussions about health concerns and treatments

Users of Health Information Exchange

Essential to changing from a fragmented provider-centric healthcare system to a patient-centered one are the users of the health information. Physicians, laboratories, hospitals, pharmacies, consumers, health plans, payers, and communities are all examples of users of electronically exchanged information. For example, a primary care provider electronically sends a clinical summary that includes basic clinical information regarding the care provided such as medications, problems, upcoming appointments, or other instructions to the patient portal.

Health information exchange requires a team effort to be successful. Technologically capable and willing exchange partners need to exist. Functionality within the EHR needs to exist so a conversation with the vendor is necessary to determine HIE capability or the time frame for availability. Even if the functionality is there, a lack of cooperation among EHR vendors can hinder exchange. In addition, how the data are integrated into existing records and workflow can be challenging for providers. There may also be state laws blocking access to patient data. Other barriers to HIE users are competing priorities, financial concerns, issues related to data ownership, and privacy and security. Also, there must be a mechanism to allow patients to opt in or opt out of participating in HIE.

eHealth Exchange

The HIE can occur at the local, state, regional, and national levels. The eHealth Exchange is a nationwide community of exchange partners. The community of federal and state agencies, large provider networks, hospitals, medical groups, pharmacies, technology vendors, payers, and others agree to securely share information via the internet using a common set of standards and specifications. Components of an eHealth Exchange include the following:

- A Legal/Trust Framework, where participants agree to one set of legal/trust documents in order to be able to exchange data with all other participants
- A governance model that incorporates a broad spectrum of perspectives by involving a representative set of participants from industry and government
- Defined operating policies and procedures, so that all participants know what is expected of them and their end users, and in turn, they know what they can expect from other participants
- Technical services, such as a service registry directory of the other Exchange participants, a security layer based upon a public key infrastructure, and interoperability testing
- Operational support, such as interoperability subject matter expertise, convening capabilities and meeting support, governance expertise, technical expertise and services, and outreach (The Sequoia Project 2016)

The eHealth Exchange has been successful in interoperable sharing of clinical information such as care summaries and quality data. In 2012 the eHealth Exchange transitioned its management to The Sequoia Project, a nonprofit 501(c)(3) to advance the implementation of secure, interoperable nationwide health information exchange. The eHealth Exchange has become the nation's largest health data sharing network, supporting 120 million patients (HealthIT n.d.).

Challenges with Sharing Healthcare Information

ONC's principal objective for electronic health information exchange is for "information to follow a patient where and when it is needed, across organizational, health IT developer and geographic boundaries" (ONC n.d.). For example, health information that can follow a patient as they encounter healthcare at a physician office, in an acute-care hospital, and at a skilled nursing facility; all are examples of possible times when health information would cross cities and different types of healthcare organizations. While this is a creditable goal, there are challenges to sharing health information among stakeholder groups from a cultural as well as technical standpoint. Two such challenges are patient identity and data standards.

Patient Identity

When it comes to patient identity and HIE, integrity is of prime importance to linking the patient to the correct information. The ability to match patients and health information begins with complete and accurate data collection. Errors identified should be corrected immediately to prevent issues with patient care that can result in poor data quality. Sophisticated algorithms such as those discussed in chapter 3, *Health Information Functions, Purpose, and Users,* should be used to help confirm a patient's identity (AHIMA 2017).

Matching patient records to the correct person becomes increasingly difficult as organizations share records electronically using diverse information systems, and in a mobile culture where patients seek care in many healthcare settings. Some healthcare organizations use multiple information systems for clinical, administrative, and specialty services, which increases the chances of identity errors occurring when matching health records. Also, many regions experience a high number of individuals who share the exact name and birthdate, leading to the need for additional identifying attributes to be used when matching patient records.

Other issues and circumstances that lead to unmatched or mismatched health records include differences in how names and addresses are formatted in various information systems, the quality of data as it is entered into information systems at patient registration, and the creation of duplicate records for the same patient within an information system (ONC 2014).

There are two ways in which patient records fail to match accurately:

1. "Records for different patients are mistakenly matched. When medical records for different patients are mistakenly matched (known as a "false positive"), it can present safety and privacy concerns for patients. For example, a provider may inadvertently use information about the wrong patient, such as diagnoses or medication lists, to make clinical decisions. In addition, if the wrong patient's medical information is added to a patient's record, it could result in disclosure of that information to a provider or patient who is not authorized to view it" (United States Government Accountability Office 2019).
2. "Records for the same patient are not matched. When medical records for the same patient are not matched (known as a "false negative"), it can affect patient care. For example, providers may not have access to a relevant part of the patient's medical history—such as current allergies or prior diagnostic test results—which could help them avoid adverse events and also provide more efficient care, such as by not repeating laboratory tests already conducted" (United States Government Accountability Office 2019).

Because of its complexity, establishing and maintaining patient identity and integrity is fraught with challenges, some of which include the following:

- Not requiring proof of identification at the time data are collected
- Not making accurate registration a priority in the emergency department
- Data quality issues with patient identification data stored and managed in siloed legacy systems
- Not correcting data errors in a timely and comprehensive manner (AHIMA Work Group 2014)

Data Standards

Data standards are the agreed-upon specifications for the values acceptable for specific data fields.

Data standards allow healthcare organizations to exchange health information in a format that ensures the data remain comparable. A number of different types of data standards are used in healthcare to capture all of the administrative and clinical data that is needed. Some of these include the following:

- Logical Observations Identifiers Names and Codes (LOINC) is a standard that provides the structure for lab tests and clinical observations to be shared electronically.
- Clinical Document Architecture (CDA) creates documents in the health record such as discharge summaries and progress notes so that the information can be shared electronically with other healthcare providers.
- Continuity Care Record identifies key data that is needed as the patient moves from one healthcare provider to another for continued care. The data is what the healthcare provider needs to continue patient care.
- Digital Imaging and Communications in Medicine (DICOM) is the standard used to exchange images used in radiology (Sayles and Kavanaugh-Burke 2018).

ONC is harmonizing the standards utilized in healthcare. Harmonization is reviewing similar standards and working out the differences in the standards through a committee (ASTM International 2005). An example of a specific criterion developed by ONC in the data standard selection process is whether the standard is used by federal agencies to electronically exchange health information with organizations engaging in the eHealth Exchange. An outcome of this work is the publication of best available lists. Table 12.1 shows examples from these lists.

Table 12.1 Best available standards and implementation specifications

	Purpose	Standard(s)	Implementation specification(s)
Vocabulary, code set, and terminology	Lab tests Patient "problems"	LOINC SNOMED CT	
Content and structure	Care plan Data element based on query for clinical health information	HL7 Clinical Document Architecture (CDA) Release 2.0, Normative Edition Fast Healthcare Interoperability Resources (FHIR)	HL7 Implementation Guide for CDA Release 2: Consolidated CDA Templates for Clinical Notes (US Realm) Draft Standards for Trial Use Release 2
Transport	Simple way for participants to push health information directly to known, trusted recipients Data sharing through service-oriented architecture (SOA) that enables two systems to interoperate together	Simple Mail Transfer Protocol (SMTP) RFC 5321 For security, Secure or Multipurpose Internal Mail Extensions (S/MIME) Version 3.2 Message Specification, RFC 5751 Hypertext Transfer Protocol (HTTP) 1.1, RFC 723X (to support RESTful transport approaches) Simple Object Access Protocol (SOAP) 1.2 For security, Transport Layer Security (TLS) Protocol Version 1.2, RFC 5246	
Services	Data element based query for clinical health information Image exchange	Fast Healthcare Interoperability Resources (FHIR) Digital Imaging and Communications in Medicine (DICOM)	

Source: ONC 2015.

Check Your Understanding 12.3

Answer the following questions.

1. Identify which of the following is a form of HIE.
   a. Provider-mediated exchange
   b. Data exchange
   c. Consumer-mediated exchange
   d. Collected exchange
2. Identify the true statement about patient identity issues.
   a. Patients should provide proof of identity.
   b. Identity issues result only from poor quality data.
   c. Identity issues do not include merging two patients' health records together.
   d. Correcting errors is not a priority.
3. All definitions of HIE mention:
   a. The exchange of information is manual or done electronically
   b. The exchange of information is manual
   c. The exchange of information is done electronically
   d. The exchange of information maintains the meaning of the information being exchanged
4. Identify the standard that should be used to share radiological images.
   a. DICOM
   b. LOINC
   c. CDA
   d. CCR
5. Identify which of the following is a benefit of HIE.
   a. A basic level of interoperability is met.
   b. An advanced level of interoperability is met.
   c. Billing records are accessible.
   d. Medication refills can be sent electronically.
6. Per the ONC, HIE capabilities include:
   a. Providing health insurance market reform
   b. Sharing patient health information and e-prescribing
   c. Using mobile devices to engage patients as consumers
   d. Providing health insurance portability both inside and outside of the US
7. HIX provide:
   a. Patient portals and PHR templates
   b. Standards on executive information and clinical decision support systems
   c. Consumers the ability to choose a healthcare plan and reform the health insurance market
   d. Consumers web-based healthcare applications, social networking sites, and a tethered PHR
8. The data standard for representing lab tests is:
   a. HTTP
   b. DICOM
   c. LOINC
   d. ONC
9. True or false: Data integrity is a vital element of HIE.
10. True or false: Query-based exchange is the preferred model of HIE when sharing data with the health department.

HIM Roles

The roles for HIM professionals in healthcare information can be expanded to include positions focused on HIE and consumer informatics. For the area of consumer information, the roles include working within a healthcare organization, physician practice group, or directly with consumers. Specific HIM roles could include patient portal representative, consumer advocate, PHR liaison, or patient information coordinator. Figure 12.5 lists the recommended best practices for HIM practitioners in a consumer or patient engagement role.

The roles for HIM professionals in HIE include defining the data exchange model, developing guidelines for data stewardship and data governance, developing data integrity and quality standards, identifying strategies to ensure accurate patient identity, ensuring that privacy and security requirements are met, and performing provider and patient education about why HIE is important. A study conducted on trends in HIE organizational staffing found the data integration and master patient and client index roles as the primary staffing challenge and top jobs in demand (AHIMA and HIMSS 2012). Figure 12.6 lists additional HIM skills of value to HIE leadership.

Figure 12.5 Recommended best practices for consumer or patient engagement

- Establish or participate in an organizational committee, council, or information governance board whose charge is to address facilitation of patient engagement. This group should review all existing and proposed policies and procedures related to health information access with an eye toward gaps and barriers to patient engagement.
- When health information is accessed electronically by patients through portals, ensure requests for clarifications, corrections, or amendments can be supported by automated workflow that confirms receipt of the request and routes the requests to the appropriate place and person.
- Reach out to community groups as a speaker on patient engagement.
- Work with clinicians to include a comprehensive set of clinical information, including physicians' notes and other forms of documentation, within the patient portal that goes beyond limited information such as appointment dates and lab results.
- Take on a leadership role with the patient portal managing portal processes.
- Establish a central and convenient (to patients) location for receiving and processing requests for all types of health information regardless of media, department, or source. This means establishing a one-stop shop for archived paper records, compact discs, diagnostic imaging media, pathology slides, and such.
- Create policies and design workflows for accepting and managing patient-generated health information.
- Eliminate fees to patients for providing them with electronic copies of their health information.
- Stay up to date with public policy proposals and standards development that addresses and supports consumer engagement.

Source: Washington 2014.

Figure 12.6 HIM contributions to HIE

HIM professionals can bring a variety of much-needed skills to HIEs. HIE leadership can look to HIM principles to provide support and guidance in the following areas:

- Drafting data governance and stewardship policies, including data ownership, data integrity, and data quality
- Managing master patient index and enterprise master patient index data conversions, development, and maintenance
- Developing and implementing HITECH privacy and security rule requirements
- Developing and implementing HIPAA privacy and security rule requirements
- Creating release of information policies, procedures, and practices
- Addressing state and federal requirements for patient confidentiality
- Meeting breach notification requirements
- Integrating data elements from multiple systems, organizations, and providers
- Identifying best practices in information management and records retention

Source: AHIMA 2010.

Real-World Case 12.1

A research project conducted by Geisinger Health System looked at the interaction between patients and their providers and pharmacists with medication lists were made available through a patient portal. For this research project, prior to an upcoming appointment, patients were able to review their medication lists and submit changes if the content was inaccurate. A pharmacist followed up with the patient either by phone or secure online messaging. The pharmacist reviewed the information submitted by the patient via the portal, revised the medication record, and informed the patient's provider. The revision was also documented in the EHR along with the source of the change (Deering 2013).

At McGill University Health Centre, a medication reconciliation research project was conducted using a newly developed web-based software tool, RightRx. The objective of reconciliation at the hospital level was focused on patient safety and to align the community and hospital medication lists (Tamblyn et al. 2018). RightRx provided a way to automate the drug information and to sort drug orders from physicians. This study concluded that "future development should focus on standardization of medication administration data, order sentences to support dose-based prescribing, and patient-friendly information about medication changes" (Tamblyn et al. 2018). Both studies focused on the use of electronic tools in the area of pharmacological management.

Real-World Case 12.2

A local community hospital is planning a health fair. At the event, the clinical staff will provide free blood-pressure screening and basic dental exams. There will also be a 20-minute exercise clinic and information on healthy eating, smoking cessation, and maintaining a healthy lifestyle. Also, information will be presented via brochures on some of the most commonly seen diseases in the United States: diabetes, hypertension, Alzheimer's disease, and chronic kidney disease. The team planning this event includes HIM professionals. When reviewing the planned events at the health fair and brochures, the HIM committee members are concerned about health literacy for this community outreach event.

References

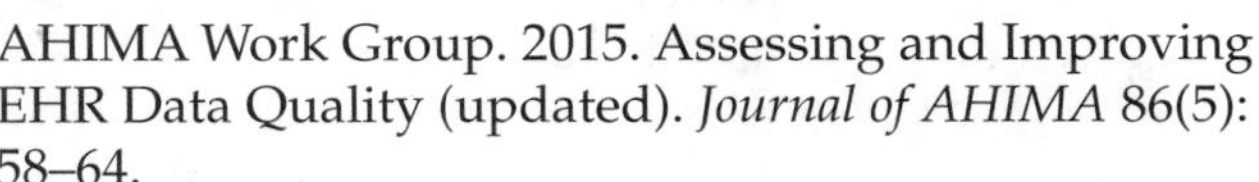

AHIMA Work Group. 2015. Assessing and Improving EHR Data Quality (updated). *Journal of AHIMA* 86(5): 58–64.

AHIMA Work Group. 2014. Managing the Integrity of Patient Identity in Health Information Exchange (updated). http://library.ahima.org/doc?oid=300436#.VxE0rPkrK9I.

Amatayakul, M.K. 2013. *Electronic Health Records: A Practical Guide for Professionals and Organizations*, 5th ed. Chicago: AHIMA.

American Health Information Management Association. 2019. Practice Brief: Ensuring the Integrity of the EHR. http://bok.ahima.org/doc?oid=302635#.XGiUxKJKguU.

American Health Information Management Association. 2016. Consumer Engagement Toolkit. http://bok.ahima.org/PdfView?oid=301404.

American Health Information Management Association. 2015a. Certified Health Data Analyst (CHDA). http://www.ahima.org/certification/chda.

American Health Information Management Association. 2015b. myPHR. https://www.myphr.com/StartaPHR/what_is_a_phr.aspx.

American Health Information Management Association. 2017. *Health Data Analysis Toolkit*. Chicago: AHIMA. http://library.ahima.org/PdfView?oid=302359.

American Health Information Management Association. 2017. *Pocket Glossary of Health Information Management and Technology*, 5th ed. Chicago: AHIMA.

American Health Information Management Association. 2013. Speech recognition in the electronic health record (updated). *Journal of AHIMA* 84(9): expanded web version. http://library.ahima.org/doc?oid=300181#.VxE1Y_krK9I.

American Health Information Management Association. 2012. Ensuring Data Integrity in Health Information Exchange. http://library.ahima.org/PdfView?oid=105612.

American Health Information Management Association. 2010. Understanding the HIE landscape. *Journal of AHIMA* 81(9):60–65.

American Health Information Management Association and Healthcare Information and Management Systems Society. 2012. Trends in Health Information Exchange Organizational Staffing. http://www.himss.org/ResourceLibrary/genResourceDetailPDF.aspx?ItemNumber=31182

American Medical Informatics Association. n.d. Consumer Health Informatics. https://www.amia.org/applications-informatics/consumer-health-informatics.

Arcury, T.A., S.A. Quandt, J.C. Sandberg, D.P. Miller Jr, C. Latulipe, X. Leng, J.W. Talton, K.P. Melius, A. Smith, and A.G. Bertoni. 2017. Patient portal utilization among ethnically diverse low income older adults: Observational study. *JMIR Medical Informatics* 5(4):e47. https://asset.jmir.pub/assets/88b6b27b5c47bea8f8da3ea1c1a4da65.pdf.

ASTM International. 2005. Harmonization. https://www.astm.org/SNEWS/MARCH_2005/plaintalk_mar05.html.

Bobinet, K. and J. Petito. n. d. Designing the Consumer-Centered Telehealth & eVisit Experience: Considerations for the Future of Consumer Healthcare. [White Paper]. https://www.healthit.gov/sites/default/files/DesigningConsumerCenteredTelehealtheVisit-ONC-WHITEPAPER-2015V2edits.pdf.

Buttner, P., S. L. Goodman, T. R. Love, M. McLeod, and M. Stearns. 2015. Practice Brief: Electronic Documentation Templates Support ICD-10-CM/PCS Implementation (2015 update). http://library.ahima.org/doc?oid=107665#.XHSRAKbsbIU.

Carayon P., P. Hoonakker, R. Cartmill, and A. Hassol. 2015. Using Health Information Technology (IT) in Practice Redesign: Impact of Health IT on Workflow. Patient-Reported Health Information Technology and Workflow. (Prepared by Abt Associates under Contract No. 290-2010-00031I). AHRQ Publication No. 15-0043-EF. Rockville, MD: Agency for Healthcare Research and Quality.

Cutilli, C. C. and I. M. Bennett. 2009. Understanding the health literacy of America: Results of the National Assessment of Adult Literacy. *Orthopedic Nursing* 28(1):27–32; quiz 33-4. https://www.ncbi.nlm.nih.gov/pmc/articles/PMC2668931/#R5.

Czahor, A., G. Evans, B. Friedman, and E. Head. 2016. HIM's Role in Value-Based Reimbursement: Three Leaders Weigh in on Impact. http://library.ahima.org/doc?oid=301941#.XUtz93spCUl.

Deering, M.J. 2013. Issue Brief: Patient-Generated Health Data and Health IT. http://www.healthit.gov/sites/default/files/pghd_brief_final122013.pdf.

Demiris, G. 2016. Consumer Health Informatics: Past, Present, and Future of a Rapidly Evolving Domain. Yearbook of Medical Informatics. https://www.ncbi.nlm.nih.gov/pmc/articles/PMC5171509/.

Department of Health and Human Services. 2016. Medicare Program; Merit-based Incentive Payment System (MIPS) and Alternative Payment Model (APM) Incentive under the Physician Fee Schedule, and Criteria for Physician-Focused Payment Models. http://www.nrhi.org/uploads/qpp_executive_summary_of_final_rule.pdf.

Department of Health and Human Services. 2008. America's Health Literacy: Why We Need Accessible Health Information. An Issue Brief. https://health.gov/communication/literacy/issuebrief/#survey.

Department of Health and Human Services. n.d.a. Quick Guide to Health Literacy. https://health.gov/communication/literacy/quickguide/quickguide.pdf.

Department of Health and Human Services. n.d.b. Fact sheet: Health literacy basics. https://health.gov/communication/literacy/quickguide/factsbasic.htm.

Department of Health and Human Services, Office of Disease Prevention and Health Promotion. 2010. National Action Plan to Improve Health Literacy. Washington, DC. https://health.gov/communication/HLActionPlan/pdf/Health_Literacy_Action_Plan.pdf.

Executive Summary. n.d. Health IT Dashboard. https://dashboard.healthit.gov/strategic-plan/federal-health-it-strategic-plan-exec-summary.php.

Fenton, S.H. and S. Biedermann. 2014. *Introduction to Healthcare Informatics*. Chicago: AHIMA.

Food and Drug Administration. 2015 (February 9). Mobile Medical Applications: Guidance for Industry and Food and Drug Administration Staff. http://www.fda.gov/downloads/MedicalDevices

/DeviceRegulationandGuidance /GuidanceDocuments/UCM263366.pdf.

Grebner, Leah A., and Raymound Mikaelian. 2015. "Best Practices in mHealth for Consumer Engagement." *Journal of AHIMA* 86(9): 42–44. http://bok.ahima.org/ doc?oid=107740.

Healthcare Financial Management Association. 2019. HFMA's MAP. http://www.hfma.org /Map/MapApp/.

Healthcare Information and Management Systems Society. 2014. *HIMSS Dictionary of Healthcare Information Technology Terms, Acronyms and Organizations,* 4th ed. Chicago: HIMSS.

HealthIT. 2019. Meaningful Use and the Shift to the Merit-based Incentive Payment System. https://www.healthit.gov/topic/meaningful-use-and-macra /meaningful-use.

HealthIT. 2018. What are the advantages of electronic health records? Retrieved from https://www.healthit.gov/faq/what-are-advantages-electronic-health-records

HealthIT. 2014. Are there different types of personal health records (PHRs)? https://www.healthit.gov/faq/are-there-different-types-personal-health-records-phrs.

HealthIT. n.d. Interoperability Proving Ground. https://www.healthit.gov/techlab/ipg/node/4 /submission/1076.

Heubusch, K. 2010. Access + understanding: The role of health literacy in patient-centric health IT. *Journal of AHIMA* 81(5):32–34. http://library.ahima.org /doc?oid=100034#.XD5J7FVKguV.

Karl, E. S. 2012. What's in a name? Breaking down health information exchange, one definition at a time. *Journal of AHIMA* 83(6):62–63. http://library.ahima.org/doc?oid=105548#.XDP4oVVKguU.

Laney, D., A. Bitterer, R.L. Sallam, and L. Kart. 2012. Predicts 2013: Information Innovation. http://insight.datamaticstech.com/dtlsp/rna_Presales /knowledgeHub/Gartner/predicts_2013 _information_in_246040.pdf.

Koh, H.C. and G. Tan. 2005. Data mining applications in healthcare. *Journal of Healthcare Information Management* 19(2):64–72.

Landi, H. 2018 (June 5). Healthcare Informatics. Study: Health Information Exchanges Improve Care, Reduce Costs. https://www.healthcare-informatics.com /news-item/hie/study-health-information-exchanges-improve-care-reduce-costs.

National Network of Libraries of Medicine. n.d. Health Literacy. https://nnlm.gov/initiative s/topics/health-literacy.

Network for Regional Healthcare Improvement. n.d. What is MACRA, The Medicare Access and CHIP Reauthorization Act of 2015 (MACRA). http://www .nrhi.org/work/what-is-macra/what-is-macra/.

Obamacare Facts. 2018. ObamaCare, Health Insurance Exchange. https://obamacarefacts.com/obamacare-health-insurance-exchange/.

Office of the National Coordinator for Health Information Technology. 2018a. Patient-Generated Health Data. https://www.healthit.gov/topic /scientific-initiatives/patient-generated-health-data.

Office of the National Coordinator for Health Information Technology. 2018b. What are the Different Types of Health Information Exchange? https://www .healthit.gov/faq/what-are-different-types-health-information-exchange.

Office of the National Coordinator for Health Information Technology. n.d. Connecting health and care for the nation: A 10-year Vision to Achieve an Interoperable Health IT Infrastructure. https://www .healthit.gov/sites/default/files /ONC10yearInteroperabilityConceptPaper.pdf.

Office of the National Coordinator for Health Information Technology. 2015. The 2015 Interoperability Standards Advisory. http://www.healthit.gov/policy-researchers-implementers/2015-interoperability-standards-advisory.

Office of the National Coordinator for Health Information Technology. 2014. Federal Health IT Strategic Plan. http://www.healthit.gov/sites /default/files/federal-healthIT-strategic-plan-2014.pdf.

Office of the National Coordinator for Health Information Technology. 2013. Clinical Decision Support. http://www.healthit.gov/policy-researchers-implementers/clinical-decision-support-cds.

Office of the National Coordinator for Health Information Technology. n.d. Personal Health Records: What Providers Need to Know. http://www.healthit.gov/sites/default/files/about-phrs-for-providers-011311.pdf.

Robert Wood Johnson Foundation. 2015. Data for Health: Learning What Works. http://www.rwjf.org/en/library/research/2015/04/data-for-health-initiative.html.

Sandefer, R., D. Marc, D. Mancilla, and D. Hamada. 2015. Survey predicts future HIM workforce shifts: HIM industry estimates the job roles, skills needed in the near future. *Journal of AHIMA* 86(7):32–35.

SAS. 2018. Data Visualization Techniques: From Basics to Big Data with SAS® Visual Analytics. https://www.sas.com/content/dam/SAS/en_us/doc.

/whitepaper1/data-visualization-techniques-106006.pdf.

Sayles, N. B. and L. Kavanaugh-Burke. 2018. Introduction to Information Systems for Health Information Technology. Chicago: AHIMA.

Sreenivasan, S. 2018. Five Examples of How Big Data Analytics in Healthcare Save Lives. https://www.healthworkscollective.com/how-big-data-analytics-in-healthcare-saves-lives/.

Tamblyn, R., N. Winslade, T. Lee, A. Motulsky, A. Meguerditchian, M. Bustillo, S. Elsayed, D.L. Buckeridge, I. Couture, C.J. Qian, T. Moraga, and A. Huang. 2018. Improving patient safety and efficiency of medication reconciliation through the development and adoption of a computer-assisted tool with automated electronic integration of population-based community drug data: The RightRx project. *Journal of the American Medical Informatics Association* 25:482–495. https://psnet.ahrq.gov/resources/resource/31573/improving-patient-safety-and-efficiency-of-medication-reconciliation-through-the-development-and-adoption-of-a-computer-assisted-tool-with-automated-electronic-integration-of-population-based-community-drug-data-the-rightrx-project.

The Joint Commission. 2010. Advancing Effective Communication, Cultural Competence, and Patient- and Family-Centered Care: A Roadmap for Hospitals. https://www.jointcommission.org/assets/1/6/ARoadmapforHospitalsfinalversion727.pdf.

The Sequoia Project. 2016. eHealth Exchange Overview. https://sequoiaproject.org/wp-content/uploads/2016/05/eHealth-Exchange-Overview-Feb-2016-v2.pdf.

3e Services LLC. 2015. Developing an Enterprise Information Strategy: A Pillar of Success in Building the Future of Healthcare. http://static1.squarespace.com/static/53c98477e4b0985ac7917c0d/t/54c13ffce4b0c7e0a73a3be5/1421950972341/3eServices_EIS+HealthCare+Whitepaper_01_21_15.pdf.

United States Government Accountability Office. 2019. Health Information Technology: Approaches and Challenges to Electronically Matching Patient's Records across Providers. https://www.gao.gov/assets/700/696426.pdf.

Washington, L. 2014. Enabling consumer and patient engagement with health information. *Journal of AHIMA* 88(2):56–59.

Wicklund, E. 2018. Telehealth May Save Money, but It's Not Yet a Necessity for Consumers. https://mhealthintelligence.com/news/telehealth-may-save-money-but-its-not-yet-a-necessity-for-consumers.

World Health Organization. 2018. Patient safety. http://www.euro.who.int/en/health-topics/Health-systems/patient-safety.

45 CFR 170.102: Health information technology standards, implementation specifications, and certification criteria and certification programs for health information technology. 2012.

Research and Data Analysis

Lynette M. Williamson, EdD, MBA, RHIA, CCS, CPC, FAHIMA

Learning Objectives

- Apply graphical tools for data presentation
- Utilize descriptive statistics in healthcare decision-making
- Understand the normal distribution and how it affects the use of certain types of statistics
- Determine when to use inferential statistics
- Analyze data to identify trends in quality, safety, and outcomes of care
- Explain common research methodologies
- Explain how research methodologies are used in healthcare
- Explain purpose of randomization
- Differentiate between the roles of various healthcare research organizations

Key Terms

Agency for Healthcare Research and Quality (AHRQ)
Aggregate data
Analysis of variance (ANOVA)
Bar chart
Box-and-whisker plots
Bubble charts
Centers for Disease Control and Prevention (CDC)
Chart
Chi-square test
Comparative data
Confounding factors
Continuous variable
Correlational studies
Descriptive statistics
Descriptive studies
Discrete variable
Ethnography
Experimental study
Frequency
Frequency polygon
Graph
Grounded theory
Healthcare research organizations
Histogram
Incidence rate
Independent variable
Individual data
Inferential statistics
Institutional Review Board (IRB)
Interval variables
Line graph
Mean
Measures of central tendency
Measures of variability
Median
Mixed-methodology
Mode
Nominal variables
Normal distribution
Ordinal variables
Pareto chart
Percentile
Pie chart
Presentation software

Proportion	Randomization	Standard deviation
Prospective study	Range	Statistical packages
Qualitative research	Ratio variables	Stem and leaf plots
Qualitative variables	Regression equations	*t*-tests
Quantitative study	Research methodologies	Table
Quantitative variables	Retrospective study	Variance
Quasi-experimental study	Scatter charts	World Health Organization (WHO)

Data is a part of our lives, it is used in personal dealings and work settings multiple times every day. Data presented via social media, in digital and printed documents (newspapers, magazines, and so on), and in daily newscasts can be abundant and perhaps at times overwhelming. In the area of healthcare, data collection and data use are a vital component to remain competitive. Since healthcare data such as information on admissions, clinical facts, reimbursement figures, and data related to medical coding are so abundant, methods to analyze and present the data in an understandable and useful fashion are needed. Healthcare providers are inundated with healthcare data and struggle to find the meaning of data in a quick and efficient manner. Health information management (HIM) professionals are the bridge between data and information. HIM professionals take data, present it clearly, and provide it to those who will use it to make important decisions. (Data and information are defined and discussed in detail in chapter 3, *Health Information Functions, Purpose, and Users*.)

This chapter discusses the presentation of statistical data and provides information on descriptive and inferential statistics, research methodologies, how to analyze information, healthcare research organizations, and ethics in research. Data presentations include the use of tables, charts, and graphs. Descriptive statistics and the normal distribution are discussed to demonstrate methods of quantifying data using frequencies and percentiles, measures of central tendency (mean, median, mode), and measures of variability (range, variance, standard deviation). Data analysis is described using examples that relate to quality and safety. Quantitative, qualitative, and mixed-methods approaches are discussed in the research methodologies section of this chapter. The Centers for Disease Control, the World Health Organization, and the Agency for Healthcare Research and Quality are described in this chapter. The discussion concludes with ethics and HIM roles as they relate to the research arena.

Presentation of Statistical Data

The key to presenting data is to make it clear, concise, and understandable. Tables, charts, and graphs (discussed later in this chapter) can be used to do this. When deciding whether to use a table, graph, or chart to present data, one must consider the type of data or variables that are being presented. In general, "variables are characteristics that are measured and may take on different values" (Forrestal 2017a). In research, **quantitative variables** are numerical variables that can be classified as discrete or continuous. **Discrete variables** are variables that can take on a finite number of values, usually whole numbers, or numbers that can be counted such as 204, 65, and 534. For example, in a college parking lot there are a finite amount of parking slots; therefore, when counting cars in spaces, the total will be a discrete variable. The opposite of a discrete variable is a continuous variable. **Continuous variables** include any numerical value that goes from one whole number to the next whole number. An example of a continuous variable could be weight; if the athletes on a team weigh between 150 and 200 pounds, then each individual athlete's weight (150, 155, 160, and so forth) would be a continuous variable. Another example of a continuous variable is the cost of a patient's hospital stay ($30,567.32) or a patient's height presented as 62.596 inches. Quantitative variables can be further broken down into interval and ratio variables. Interval variables are those that have equal units with an arbitrary zero point. An example is temperature on the Fahrenheit scale. The temperature difference between 45 degrees and 50 degrees is the same as the temperature difference between 30 degrees and 35 degrees. Zero does not equal absence of temperature. Ratio variables are the most common quantitative variables used in healthcare. These include numbers that can be compared meaningfully with one another (four grapefruits are twice as many as two grapefruits). Zero is truly zero on the ratio scale. Examples include height (inches or meters) and weight (pounds or kilograms).

Qualitative variables are categorical, meaning that the variable is from a specific category or group such as gender or age. Qualitative variables are given or assigned to items that are not numerical. An example is eye color. There are several eye colors, including blue, green, and brown; none of them are numerical. But if a research study is collecting data on eye color, then each possible eye color is assigned a number (brown = 1, green = 2, blue = 3) to allow for a statistical formula to be conducted. All qualitative variables are discrete; qualitative variables can be subdivided into nominal or ordinal type. Nominal variables are those in which a number is assigned to a specific category such as 1 = male and 2 = female. Ordinal variables are ranked variables in which numbers are assigned to rank a category in an ordered series, but the numbers do not indicate the magnitude of the difference between any two data points. An example of a ranked variable is a response for a question on a patient satisfaction questionnaire such as: The wait time to see your physician was appropriate, where 1 = strongly agree, 2 = agree, 3 = disagree, 4 = strongly disagree. Table 13.1 summarizes the different types of variables and gives examples of each. Electronic spreadsheets and spreadsheet software can be used to construct nearly all the charts, graphs, and tables explained in this chapter.

Tables

Tables, which can include both numbers and text, are an excellent way to display data. Tables can be used to organize and categorize data and to examine the detail of a specific concept, category, or response. Table 13.2 demonstrates the demographic characteristics of physicians who participated in a focus group to discuss the effects of the *International Classification of Diseases, Tenth Revision, Clinical Modification* (ICD-10-CM) and the *International Classification of Diseases, Tenth Revision, Procedure Coding System* (ICD-10-PCS) on their physician practices. It can be easily seen from table 13.2 that 75 percent of the physicians in this focus group had no exposure to ICD-10-CM or ICD-10-PCS.

The key to building a table is to make it stand alone so anyone reading it can understand the information displayed. All tables should include the following elements: the table legend or title;

Table 13.1 Examples of types of variables: quantitative and qualitative

Quantitative or numerical variables	
Continuous	**Discrete**
Interval: Temperature	Number of medical records coded
Ratio: Height, weight, costs, charges	Number of patients who receive a colonoscopy
Qualitative or categorical variables	
	All discrete variables
Nominal (discrete categorical variables)	Gender (1 = male, 2 = female), race (1 = Caucasian, 2 = African American, and such), smoking status (1 = nonsmoker, 2 = smoker)
Ordinal (discrete ordered variables)	Patient satisfaction scores (1 = not satisfied to 5 = very satisfied), quality of life scores (1 = not healthy to 5 = very healthy), pain scales (0 = no pain, 5 = moderate pain, 10 = worst pain)

Source: ©AHIMA

column titles; the body of the table, which includes the actual data; lines that divide certain parts of the table; and a footnote or reference citation if the table text was taken from an article or other source.

Some data are better presented in a format other than a table, because it may take readers longer to review and understand a table than another form of presentation. For example, when presenting data for clinicians using patient test results from electronic health records (EHRs), a bar chart or pie chart may be a more effective format than a table (Brewer et al. 2012). Various types of charts and graphs are discussed in the following sections.

Table 13.2 Demographic characteristics of physician participants in a focus group study on the effects of ICD-10-CM/PCS on their practice

Respondents (N = 12) N = number of physicians responding			
Demographics			
	Mean		Standard deviation
Age	54.67		12.71
Years of experience	23.42		12.48
Gender	#	%	
Male	9	75	
Female	3	25	
Setting	#	%	
Hospital (or other facility) only	5	41.6	
Private practice only	2	16.7	
Both	5	41.6	
Medical specialty	#	%	
Emergency medicine	2	16.7	
Ophthalmology	1	8.3	
Internal medicine, geriatrics	1	8.3	
Plastic or reconstructive surgery	1	8.3	
General surgery	1	8.3	
Obstetrics and gynecology	1	8.3	
Psychiatry	2	16.7	
Family medicine	1	8.3	
Hematology and oncology	1	8.3	
Physical medicine	1	8.3	
Previous use of EHR	#	%	
Yes	10	83.3	
No	2	16.7	
Exposure to ICD-10-CM/PCS	#	%	
Yes	3	25	
No	9	75	

Source: Watzlaf et al. 2015.

Charts and Graphs

Charts and graphs provide a picture of the numerical data being processed into information. Charts by definition "generally display nonquantitative information such as the flow of subjects through a process" (APA 2012). Graphs are data presentations that show the relationship of the included variables (APA 2012). Information presented in charts or graphs can be used for data analysis and decision-making. It can be difficult to succinctly describe what is happening with large amounts of data. Charts and graphs can be the perfect choice to present data in part because they are easy to understand and can provide a clear picture of the data being reviewed. There are different types of charts and graphs to use when transforming data into information. Each graph or chart has guides or rules to follow to determine whether it is appropriate for presentation of the data. Bar charts, pie charts, line graphs, histograms, frequency polygons, scatter charts, bubble charts, stem and leaf plots, and box-and-whisker plots are some of the charts and graphs explained in the following sections.

Bar Charts

Bar charts are simple charts used to describe qualitative, categorical, or discrete variables such as nominal or ordinal data. The bars may be drawn vertically in which the value represents the height of the bar drawn or horizontally in which the value represents the length of the bar drawn. There are several types of bar charts. The easiest bar chart to build is the one-variable bar chart, which displays a bar to represent the amount of the specific category. For example, figure 13.1 presents a hypothetical example of a one-variable bar chart for the number of healthcare organizations located in an urban, suburban, or rural setting in a specific region.

Two-variable bar charts can also display an important summary of healthcare data. Figure 13.2 demonstrates a two-variable chart and includes not only the number of healthcare organizations in the region but also the number of trauma units in each of those settings. The two-variable bar chart

Figure 13.1 Example of a one-variable bar chart

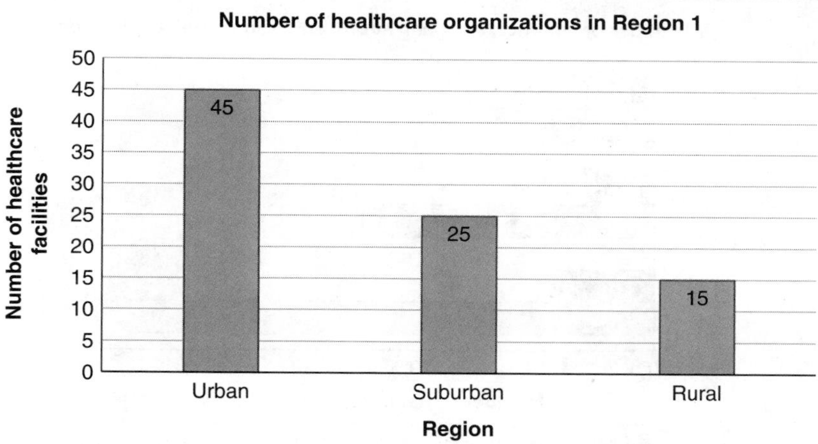

Source: ©AHIMA

Figure 13.2 Example of a two-variable bar chart

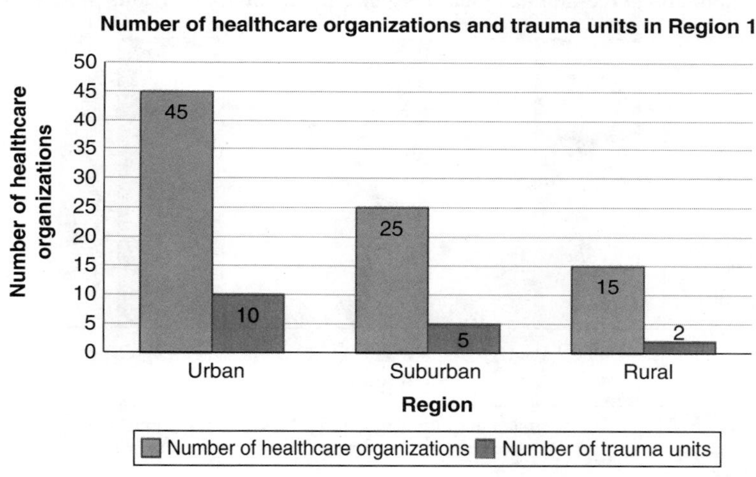

Source: ©AHIMA

can further distinguish or classify additional variables. Figures 13.3 through 13.5 demonstrate other examples of bar charts. The horizontal bar chart is used when label titles are long and therefore more difficult to read and when sorting the data from the smallest amount at the top to the largest amount at the bottom.

The stacked bar chart can also be used when demonstrating a comparison of the proportion of two things. Shown in figure 13.4, the stacked bar chart demonstrates the proportion of the number of trauma units in relation to the number of healthcare organizations. The stacked bar chart can help visualize the proportion.

When titles get longer or if data is shown from the smallest at the top to the largest at the bottom as well as showing proportions of two areas, the horizontal stacked bar chart can be used. Figure 13.5 provides an example of a horizontal stacked bar graph.

When constructing bar charts, it is important to know the audience, keep it simple, and make it clear, colorful, and concise. When using a bar chart, the main goal is to succinctly provide clear and easy to understand data. This includes providing a title, axes labels, legend, a number within or above the bars, percentages if it helps to clarify an aspect of the data, and appropriate colors to distinguish

Figure 13.3 Example of a horizontal bar chart

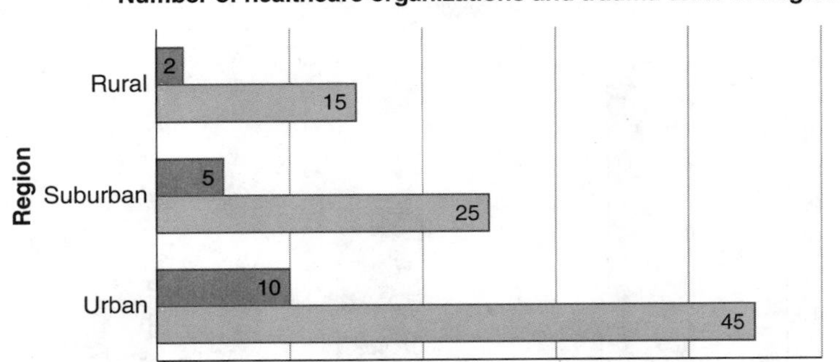

Source: ©AHIMA.

Figure 13.4 Example of a stacked bar chart with percentage of the whole

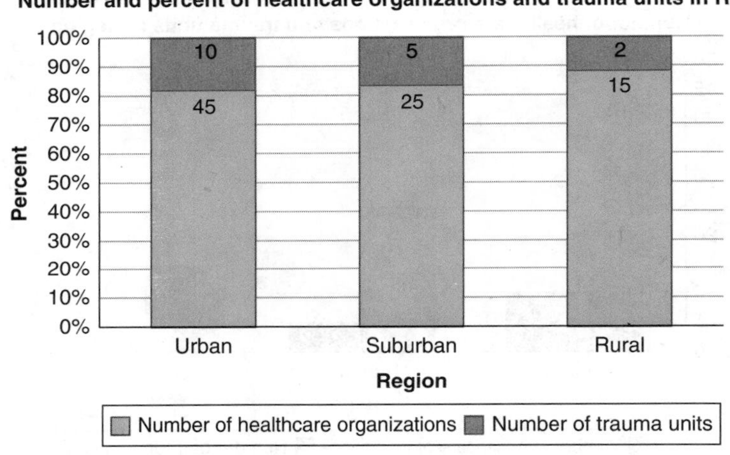

Source: ©AHIMA.

Figure 13.5 Example of a horizontal stacked bar char

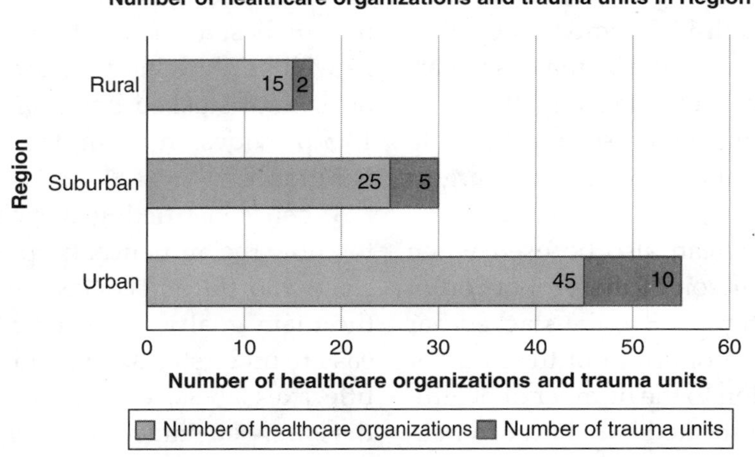

Source: ©AHIMA.

between groups. Everyone is different and sometimes what is clear to one person may not be to another, so knowing the audience ensures the appropriate type of bar chart is constructed to meet the audience's preferences. Review figure 12.3 for examples of a poorly designed and an improved pie chart data representation.

Pareto Charts

A Pareto chart is similar in appearance to a bar chart, but the highest-ranking value is listed as the first column, the next highest ranking is second, and so on, to the lowest ranking. This type of graphical presentation was created by Vilfredo Pareto and is based on his theory that "the significant few things will generally make up 80 percent of the whole, while the trivial many will make up about 20 percent" (Productivity-Quality Systems 2015). In other words, 80 percent of the data is significant while 20 percent is not. Pareto charts show data in terms of arranging it into categories and then ranking each category according to its importance. An example of a Pareto chart is found in figure 13.6. In healthcare, a Pareto chart can help analyze data about the frequency or causes of problems in a process. Pareto charts also display a cumulative line that shows the overall effect of each of the categories that make up the whole. Pareto charts are useful in quality improvement processes. Chapter 18, *Performance Improvement*, covers pareto charts in more detail.

It shows how a billing manager collected data over a period of time to determine the causes for claim denials for Medicare inpatient stays. The chart (figure 13.6) illustrates four categories: coding error, medical necessity, registration error, and other. For each category the number of denials is presented with a bar. After reviewing the chart, the billing manager can determine that coding errors are the largest cause for Medicare denials. Therefore, this could be the first area to review to improve and decrease Medicare denials. The cumulative data line with bullets identifies what the result will be if all four categories are added together moving from left to right for a cumulative effect.

Pie Charts

Pie charts are simple graphs that use the slices of the pie to explain numerical proportion in relation to the whole, or 100 percent. Pie charts are used a great deal in healthcare because they can depict a breakdown of numerical data elements by percentages. Pie charts, as shown in figure 13.7, can be used to provide information on percentages. In figure 13.7 the slices of the pie relate to the percentage of healthcare organizations by regional setting: urban, suburban, rural, and total. Pie charts, however, may not be the best format to use when comparing data elements or when using many data elements because the slices of the pie can become too small to interpret. When explaining simple types of data,

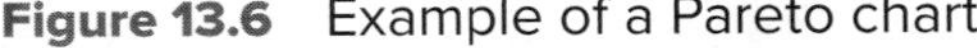

Figure 13.6 Example of a Pareto chart

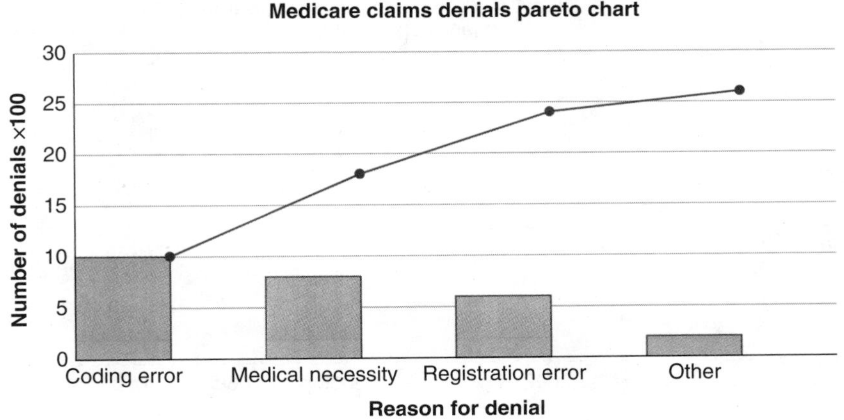

Source: ©AHIMA.

broken down into percentages, the pie graph may be a good statistical graphic to use. Using the same numbers that were used in figure 13.1, figure 13.7 provides not only the slices of the pie but also the individual percentages within each slice for easier reading and interpretation.

Line Graphs

A line graph is a graphical device used to display continuous data and to show changes or trends of the data over time. The x-axis on the line graph, from left to right, designates time (such as month, day, or year) and the y-axis shows the quantity of the plotted data. A line graph could be used as illustrated in figure 13.8 to show the healthcare expenditures for one hospital over the period of 10 years from 2000 to 2011. A line graph looks similar to a frequency polygon although its purpose is different and is explained later in this chapter. A line graph is best to use when there are many different data points or more than one set of data to plot; multiple lines can be put on one graph for very useful comparisons. The data used to create the line graphs in figures 13.8 and 13.9 are shown in table 13.3.

Figure 13.7 Example of pie chart

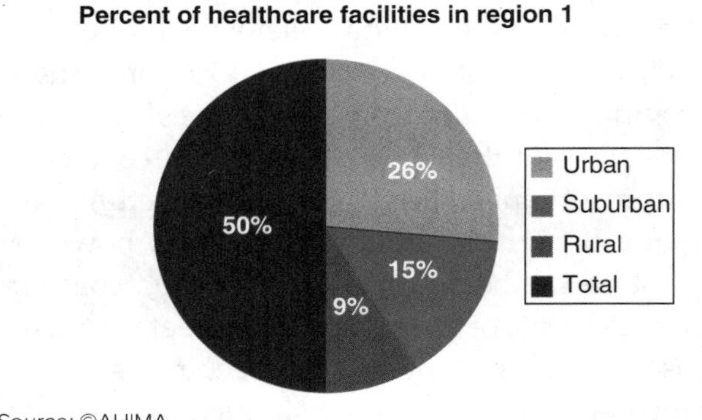

Source: ©AHIMA.

Histograms

A histogram is a graph that represents the frequency distribution of numerical data. A frequency distribution is a visual display of data that demonstrates where data falls. For example, table 13.4 is a frequency distribution table. It provides the number of patients that fall into each of the weight categories listed. It also provides the percent of the total number of patients that fall within each weight category.

A histogram should be used with continuous data that is part of a frequency distribution. It differs from a bar graph because histograms use continuous data, there are no spaces between the bars, and each bar has a class interval at its base and the frequency or percentage of cases in that class interval at its height. See figure 13.10 for an example of a histogram with six groups of body mass index (from underweight to extremely obese) on the x-axis and percentage of population on the y-axis.

Frequency Polygons

A frequency polygon is another graphical means to display a frequency distribution using continuous

Figure 13.8 Example of a line graph

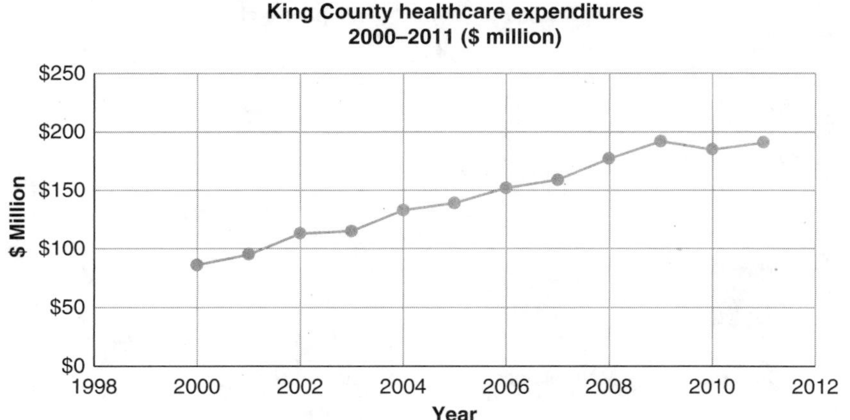

Source: CMS 2016.

Figure 13.9 Example of a line graph comparing two types of data

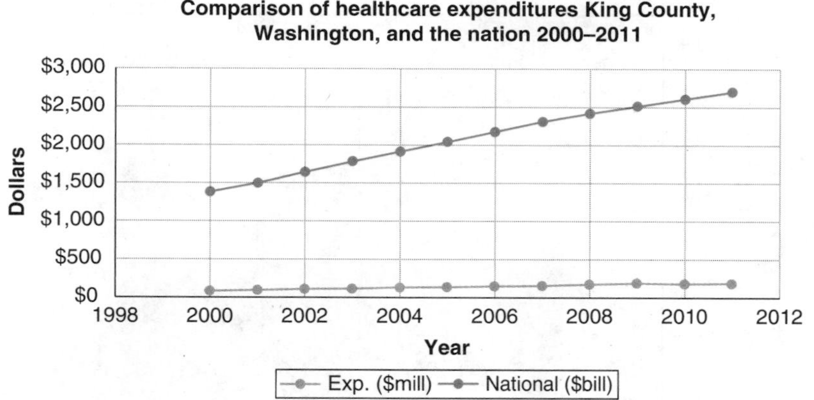

Source: CMS 2016.

Table 13.3 Data used to build line graphs for figures 13.8 and 13.9

Year	Expenditures ($ million)	National ($ billion)
2000	$86	$1,377.20
2001	$95	$1,493.40
2002	$113	$1,638.00
2003	$115	$1,778.00
2004	$133	$1,905.70
2005	$139	$2,035.40
2006	$152	$2,166.70
2007	$159	$2,302.90
2008	$177	$2,411.70
2009	$192	$2,504.20
2010	$185	$2,599.00
2011	$191	$2,692.80

Source: ©AHIMA.

Table 13.4 Example of a frequency distribution table

	Frequency	Percent
Valid 123.00	1	10.0
125.00	1	10.0
145.00	1	10.0
155.00	2	20.0
165.00	1	10.0
176.00	1	10.0
187.00	1	10.0
201.00	1	10.0
233.00	1	10.0
Total	10	100.0

Source: ©AHIMA.

data in a line form. A single data point placed at the midpoint of the interval is used to mark the specific number of observations within that interval. Each point is then connected by a line. Figure 13.11 shows a frequency polygon over an outline of a histogram for the same data. In this example from the Centers for Disease Control and Prevention (CDC), it is easier to see the peak of the epidemic in the frequency polygon. Frequency polygons differ from line graphs in that frequency polygons (and histograms) display the entire frequency distribution (counts) of the continuous variable; a line graph plots only the specific data points over time.

Scatter Charts

A **scatter chart**, scatter plot, scatter diagram, or scatter graph is used to demonstrate a relationship between two variables. For example, if per the researched data a relationship between age and a medical condition such as myocardial infarction has been found, this connection can be shown in a scatter chart. For this type of chart, one of the two variables is plotted on the x-axis, and the other is plotted on the y-axis. A strong relationship between the two variables is seen as the data come closer to forming a straight line. For example, figure 13.12 demonstrates a strong positive relationship between age and income. When both variables increase and decrease at the same time, the scatter chart will show a positive relationship. When one variable increases and the other variable decreases,

Figure 13.10 Example of a histogram that shows the distribution of body mass index in adults with diagnosed diabetes in the United States, 1999–2002

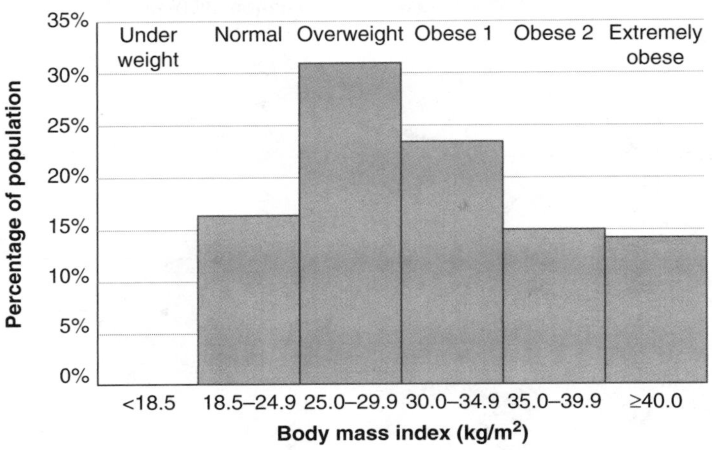

Source: CDC 2004.

Figure 13.11 Example of a frequency polygon and histogram

The histogram shows number of cases as columns. The frequency polygon shows number of cases as data points connected by lines. The midpoints of intervals of the histogram intersect the frequency polygon. For the frequency polygon, the first data point is connected to the midpoint of the previous interval on the x-axis. The last data point is connected the midpoint of the following interval.

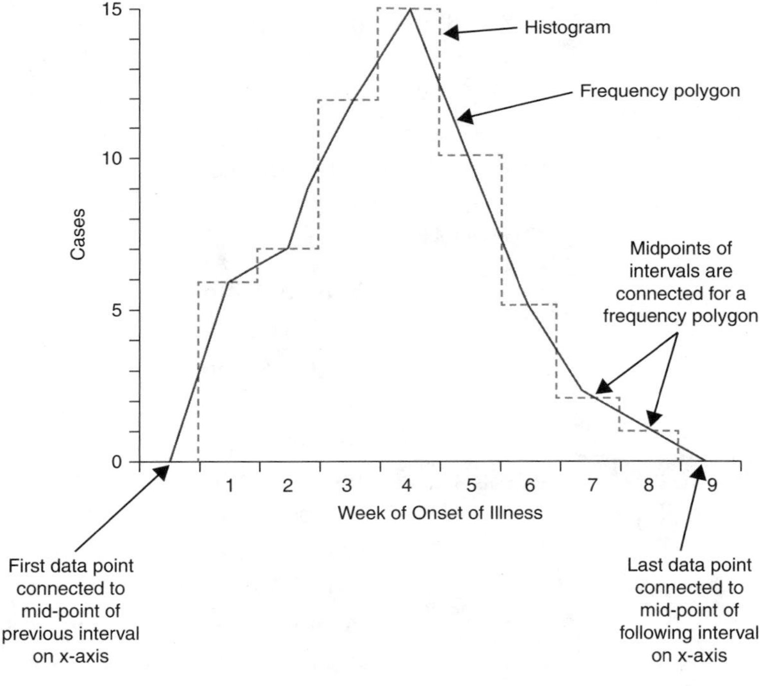

Source: CDC 2012.

the scatter chart will display a negative relationship. In figure 13.13, the scatter chart shows a negative relationship between age and physical activity, demonstrating that as age increases, physical activity decreases. In figure 13.13 physical activity is ranked from 0 = no physical activity to 5 = high level of physical activity. In figure 13.14, a scatter chart shows no relationship between age and the number of pets a person has in their household. As illustrated by figures 13.12, 13.13, and 13.14, scatter charts, or graphs, show the nonlinear relationships between variables. Therefore, researchers can use

Figure 13.12 Scatter chart showing a strong positive relationship between age and income

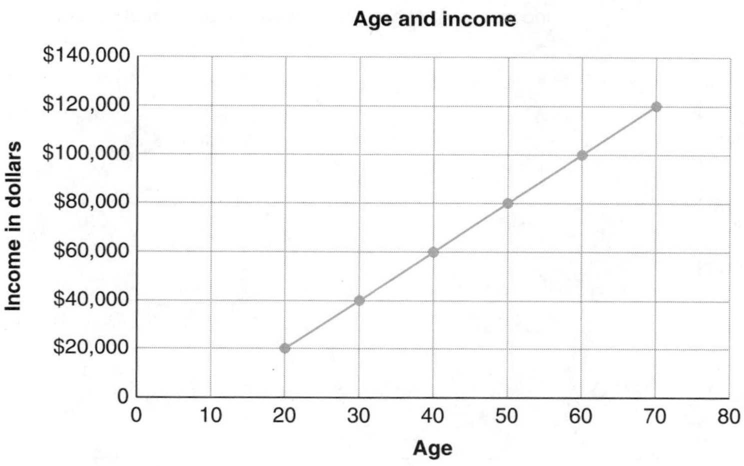

Source: ©AHIMA.

Figure 13.13 Scatter chart showing a strong negative relationship between age and physical ability

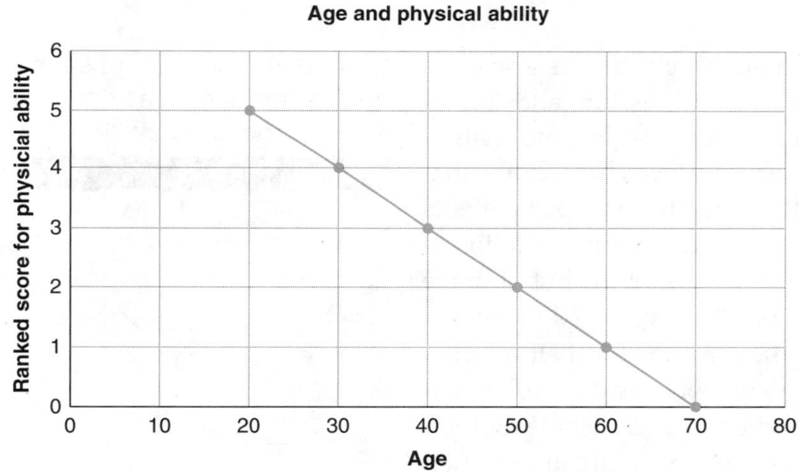

Source: ©AHIMA.

Figure 13.14 Scatter chart showing no relationship between age and number of pets a person has in their household

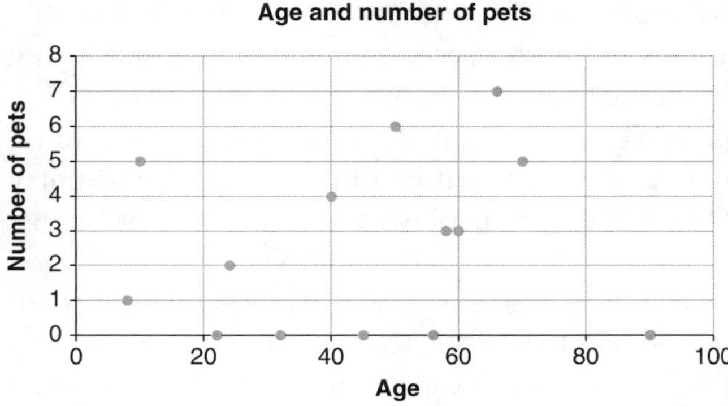

Source: ©AHIMA.

scatter charts to determine quickly whether further calculations are needed—if the scatter chart demonstrates nonlinear relationships, then no further calculations, such as correlation or regression statistics, are needed.

Bubble Charts

A **bubble chart** is like a scatter chart except that it compares three data variables. Therefore, when presenting information, a bubble chart can illustrate more data if that meets the needs and focus of the situation. For example, if a healthcare organization is reviewing the socioeconomic levels of its patients and the cost of their care during

Figure 13.15 Bubble chart showing a relationship of three variables

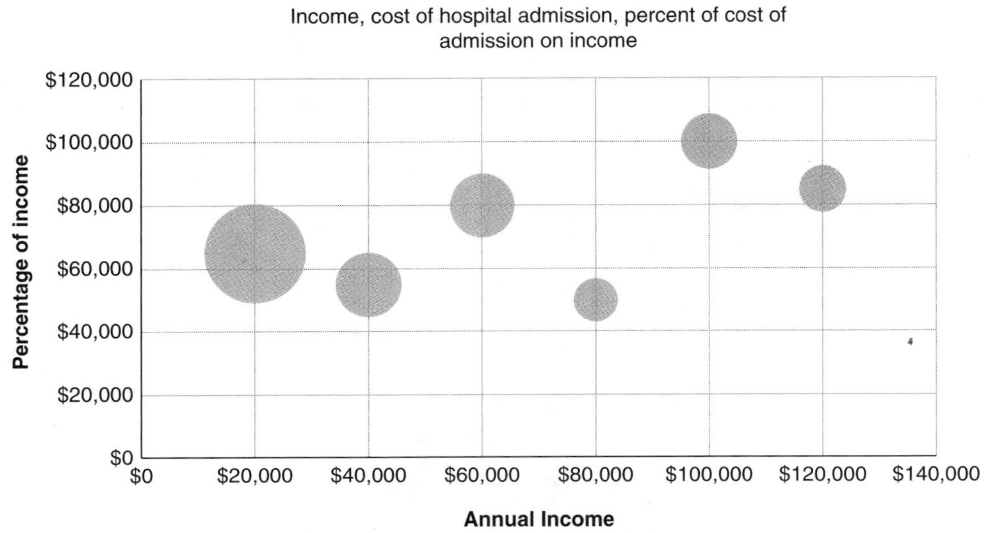

Source: ©AHIMA.

inpatient admissions, a bubble chart can show three data points: income, cost of admission, and the relationship to the patient's personal income. This is shown in figure 13.15. This bubble chart shows that the larger the bubble, the more that group of patients had to pay for their hospital admission in relation to their income. Looking at the size of the bubbles, the patients who earned $20,000 per year had to pay the greatest proportion of their income for their hospital admission, and the patients who made $80,000 had to pay the lowest proportion of their income for their hospital admission. This could be useful information to researchers looking at patients who do not have health insurance and are self-pay upon admission.

Stem and Leaf Plots

In stem and leaf plots, data can be organized so that the shape of a frequency distribution is revealed. As an example, a stem and leaf plot is constructed on the number of discharges across cities in one particular state for Medicare severity diagnosis-related group (MS-DRG) 39, extra-cranial procedures without complication or comorbidity (CC) or major complication or comorbidity (MCC) (CMS 2014). The data are listed as follows and ranked from the smallest to largest number of discharges:

14, 14, 15, 18, 18, 21, 24, 25, 27, 27, 29, 31, 32, 33, 34, 43, 45, 51, 66, 67

Table 13.5 Example of stem and leaf plot using discharges across a state for MS-DRG 39, extra-cranial procedures without CC or MCC

Stem	Leaf
1	44,588
2	145,779
3	1,234
4	35
5	1
6	67

Source: CMS 2014.

To develop the stem and leaf plot, the numbers are separated into two parts. The first digit (in this example, the tens digit) is listed once as per occurrence in the stem column, and the last digit(s) (in this example, the ones digit) are placed in the leaf column. The first number, 14, is separated so that 1 goes in the stem column and 4 is the first listing in the leaf column. In the second 14, the first digit is already in the stem column (1) so the second (4) is placed in the leaf column as the second entry (44). Table 13.5 displays a continuation of the list of numbers in the given example.

The completed stem and leaf plot shows the distribution of the data set. The stem and leaf plot shows that the lowest value in the distribution is 14 (created by using the digit in the first row in the first column [1] and the first digit in the first row of the second column [4]) and the highest is 67 (the digit in the last row in the first column [6] and the second digit in the last row of the second column [7]) and that there are six observations in the 20s group (created by adding the number of digits in the row that displays the tens digits for 2). With this type of display it is easy to see that the largest number of discharges is 67 (the digit in the last row in the first column and the second digit in the last row of the second column).

Box-and-Whisker Plots

Box-and-whisker plots visually summarize several main factors: median, range, and outliers. In this type of data presentation, the box represents quartiles, or quarters. The lines coming from the boxes (or quarters) are termed *whiskers* and illustrate the range of data values. "The median line is in the center of a box formed by the upper and lower quartiles" (Forrestal 2017b 177). Box-and-whisker plots can be used to provide a visual comparison of multiple data sets in a succinct way; for example, the results of a patient satisfaction survey that had questions with a possible scaled response, such as highly agree, agree, neutral, disagree, and highly disagree. The box-and-whisker plot in figure 13.16 shows the proportion of African-American patients and their 30-day mortality rates categorized by amount of hospitals. In general, a box-and-whisker graphical display provides information on the range of data results. If the research focuses on groups of participants (or hospitals as in figure 13.16), then each box on the graph shows the data range for each group.

Statistical Packages and Presentation Software

There are many statistical packages that can be used to facilitate the data collection and analysis processes. These packages simplify the statistical analysis of data and are often used in addition to spreadsheet software. Table 13.6 displays the types of data that can be entered when using statistical software packages as well as the output that can be generated.

Presentation software is software used to build slides when presenting a specific topic, idea, research data, or any type of information. Presentation of data and information is an important function of HIM. For example, key performance indicators such as length of stay or nosocomial infection rates are often reported on a monthly basis. The HIM professional may be asked to present this information in a way that clearly displays the information and identifies trends that may need to be addressed. Different graphic designs, animations, and polls can also be added to slides to enhance and support the data presented. For example, an HIM professional would need to use presentation software when demonstrating how coding productivity changed after the implementation of ICD-10-CM/PCS and the slides would show an increase or decrease in coder productivity.

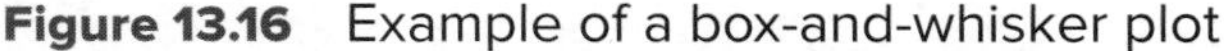

Figure 13.16 Example of a box-and-whisker plot

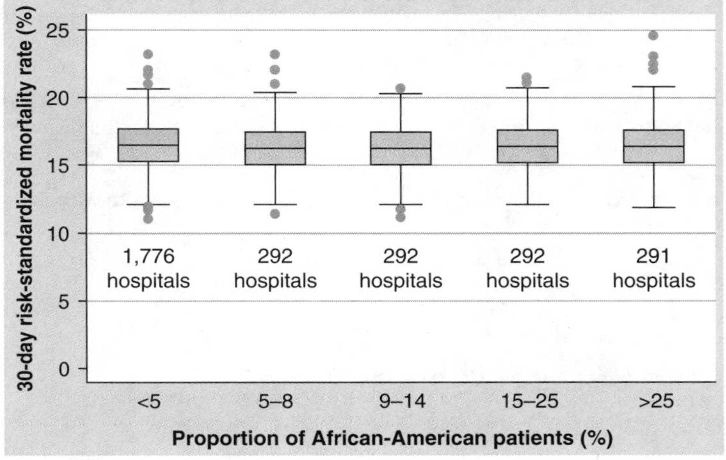

Source: CMS 2010, 14.

Table 13.6 Common data configurations for statistical software

<table>
<tr><th>Data type</th><th>Description</th><th>Example</th></tr>
<tr><td>Data list or input</td><td>Data list or input includes the name of the variable, the type of the variable such as string, numeric, how long the variable is, and how many decimal places to keep in the number</td><td>Name of variable: codingtestscore, coderstatus
Variable type (numeric or string): numeric
Width of variable: 4
Number of decimals: 2</td></tr>
<tr><td>Value labels</td><td>Value labels assign a value to a specific variable and appears in the output for easy interpretation.</td><td>Coder Status
1 = advanced
2 = intermediate
3 = beginner</td></tr>
<tr><td>Missing values</td><td>Missing values are values that do not have a number or value assigned to the variable. Missing values can be displayed in output and can be recoded by the user if necessary. One may need to recode or add a number in case it was missed by the data entry.</td><td>Statistics
<table>
<tr><th></th><th>Variable Name codingtestscore</th><th>Variable Name coderstatus</th></tr>
<tr><td>N Valid</td><td>8</td><td>8</td></tr>
<tr><td>Missing</td><td>2</td><td>2</td></tr>
</table>
Key:
N = population; n = sample
Valid = all variables that have a value assigned to them
Missing = variables that do not have a value assigned to them
The numbers in the first column show the valid number of individuals that have a coding test score and the number of individuals that are missing a coding test score.
The numbers in the second column show the valid number of individuals that have a coder status assigned (advanced, intermediate, beginner) and the number of individuals that are missing a coder status.</td></tr>
<tr><td>Output</td><td>Output includes statistics that can be generated from the data that is collected and entered into the software or spreadsheet. Statistics can be generated such as descriptive statistics (frequency tables, percentiles, graphs, measures of central tendency) as well as advanced statistics</td><td>Report
codingtestscore
<table>
<tr><th>coderstatus</th><th>Mean</th><th>N</th><th>Standard Deviation</th></tr>
<tr><td>advanced</td><td>93.0000</td><td>3</td><td>5.00000</td></tr>
<tr><td>intermediate</td><td>89.5000</td><td>2</td><td>0.70711</td></tr>
<tr><td>beginner</td><td>73.3333</td><td>3</td><td>6.42910</td></tr>
<tr><td>Total</td><td>84.7500</td><td>8</td><td>10.51190</td></tr>
</table></td></tr>
</table>

Source: ©AHIMA.

Check Your Understanding 13.1

Answer the following questions.

1. An HIM professional is creating a data presentation. The data in the presentation is from the Center for Medicare and Medicaid Services website and illustrates the condition of pneumonia and readmission rates for all hospitals in a specific state.

   Of the options provided below, identify the best choice to graphically display data with this type of focus.
   a. Pareto chart
   b. Pie chart
   c. Line graph
   d. Table
2. True or false: The two-variable bar chart cannot be used to display summary data.

3. Identify the two graphs that are the best option for displaying frequency distributions using continuous data.
   a. Histogram and frequency polygon
   b. Bar chart and line graph
   c. Scatter chart and stem and leaf plot
   d. Pie chart and frequency polygon
4. Identify the best chart to compare three data variables (healthcare spending per person, country population, and gross domestic product) of the included countries.
   a. Bar chart
   b. Pie chart
   c. Bubble chart
   d. Scatter chart
5. Identify an example of a value label variable.
   a. Coder status
   b. Coder test score
   c. Weight
   d. Height
6. True or false: A pie chart presents information on range and outliers.
7. A scatter plot is best used to illustrate:
   a. A frequency distribution
   b. Continuous data changes
   c. Numerical percentages
   d. A relationship between two variables
8. True or false: A box-and-whisker plot graphically depicts data set medians.
9. Identify the best graphical form to be used when examining a problem and a process.
   a. Pareto chart
   b. Pie chart
   c. Line graph
   d. Histogram
10. Identify an example of a ratio variable.
   a. 0 to 10 degrees Fahrenheit
   b. A height measurement of 5 feet 11 inches
   c. 1 = female
   d. 5 = strongly agree, 4 = agree, 3 = disagree

Descriptive Statistics

Descriptive statistics include frequencies, percentiles, measures of central tendency (mean, median, and mode) and measures of variability (range, variance, and standard deviation). Descriptive statistics are used to give information on data and for organization and summarization. Generally, descriptive statistics do not provide information on data relationship (such as between groups of data results) or any results focused on cause and effect found by the research. In HIM research, descriptive statistics can be used to show the frequency of the number of HIM professionals that believe they are leaders in information governance or the age of patients for a particular month in a healthcare organization vary. Range, variance, and standard deviation, termed measures of variability, are components of this area of statistics. For example, descriptive statistics such as range could be used to show the physical weights of a group of patients recently diagnosed with diabetes mellitus. Further, measures of variability fall into the 25th, 50th, or 75th percentile, and the mean, median, and mode of DRG can be used to further examine the spread of data and how outliers influence the distribution of the data. Frequency, percentile, measures of central tendency, and measures of variability are discussed in the following sections.

Frequency and Percentile

Frequency is the number of times something occurs in a particular population or sample over a specific period of time. For example, if researchers wanted to determine how often subjects considered themselves a leader in information governance (IG), they could ask the subjects whether they consider themselves a leader in IG and then count how many of the subjects said yes and how many said no.

The researchers could then build a frequency table based on this question and its results. The results could be displayed in a frequency table like table 13.7.

A percentile is a measure used in descriptive statistics that shows the value below which a given percentage of scores in a given group of scores fall. For example, the 40th percentile is the score below which 40 percent of the other scores in a given group of scores fall. Also, if a score is in the 95th percentile, it is higher than 95 percent of the other scores. A percentile can be broken up into quartiles. Quartiles are values that break up a list of numbers into quarters such as the 25th percentile, or first quartile; 50th percentile, or second quartile; and 75th percentile, or third quartile. For example, if a researcher wanted to determine how the age of their subjects were separated based on quartiles, they could collect the age for each subject, create a spreadsheet, and use statistical software to provide percentiles of the data collected.

Table 13.8 demonstrates how the age of 250 individuals is categorized in 25th, 50th, and 75th percentiles. One can see that age 36 is at the 25th percentile, age 45 is at the 50th percentile, and age 53.25 is at the 75th percentile. This shows that age 36 is the age below which 25 percent of the other ages fall, 45 is the age below which 50 percent of the other ages fall, and 53.25 is the age below which 75 percent of the other ages fall within this particular group of subjects. This demonstrates that the majority of the subjects are not considered elderly, since elderly would include those equal to or over the age of 65.

Table 13.7 Example of a frequency table

Do you consider yourself a leader in IG?	Frequency
Yes	150
No	45
No response	5
Total	200

Source: ©AHIMA.

Measures of Central Tendency

Measures of central tendency include the mean, the median, and the mode. These measures are defined as representing "the clustering of the majority of a data set's values around its middle value" (Forrestal 2017b 177). Mean, median, and mode relate to location within a researched or gathered set of numerical data.

Mean

The mean is the average of a group of numerical values. To calculate a mean, first the data group must be obtained. For example, a data group could be patients admitted to the cardiac unit of a hospital. Using the patients' lengths of stay (LOS) for the month of January, a mean LOS could be calculated. The LOS for the six patients was 5, 8, 6, 4, 7, and 3 days. To calculate the mean of these lengths of stay, add the days of stay together:

$$5 + 8 + 6 + 4 + 7 + 3 = 33 \text{ total days}$$

Then divide by 6, the total number of patients:

$$33/6 = 5.5 \text{ days}$$

The mean LOS per cardiac patient is 5.5 days.

Table 13.8 Example of percentiles

Statistics			
Age in years			
N	Valid		250
	Missing		0
Percentiles		25	36.00
		50	45.00
		75	53.25

N = Population

Source: ©AHIMA.

Median

When values are ranked, the median is the value in which there is the same amount of numbers above and below. It is the middlemost value when arranged in numerical order. For an odd number of observations, the median is the middle number in an ordered set of numbers; for an even number of observations it is the mean or average of the middle two numbers.

For example, the systolic blood pressure of five patients is provided as follows.

140, 190, 120, 116, 109

The first step to compute the median is to rank these values from lowest to highest:

109, 116, 120, 140, 190

The median is 120 since it is the middlemost value when counting from left to right and from right to left. If one more systolic blood pressure value were added to this data set, then the median would be determined by counting to the middle from left to right and right to left and then taking the average of the two middle values. For example, if 140 is added to the existing values, then the new data set will include the following:

109, 116, 120, 140, 140, 190

The new median will be:

$$120 + 140 = 260/2 = 130$$

Mode

The mode is the value that occurs most frequently in a given set of observations or values. In the systolic blood pressure scores example, the mode is 140 because it occurs more than any of the other values. Sometimes data sets have two modes and are then called bimodal.

Modes are used mostly with nominal variables, medians are used mainly for ordinal or ranked variables, and the mean is used primarily with continuous or quantitative variables, such as interval or ratio. Continuous and quantitative variables are defined earlier in this chapter.

Measures of Variability

Measures of variability examine the spread of different values around the measures of central tendency. The measures of variability include the range, variance, and standard deviation.

Range

The range is the simplest measure of variation to compute and is calculated by taking the difference between the highest and lowest values. It is quick and easy to do, but not that useful since it only considers extremes and not the entire sample of data values. The range in the systolic blood pressure data set is: 190 – 109 = 81.

Variance

The variance is the average of the squared deviations from the mean. Its symbol is σ^2 for populations and s^2 for samples.

Standard Deviation

The standard deviation is the measure of variability that is used most often and displays how data are related to the mean. The variance and standard deviation can be cumbersome to compute by hand, but statistical applications make it easy to automatically generate results. Using the same array of data for the systolic blood pressure, table 13.9 provides the mean, range, variance, and standard deviation. The interpretation of these measures is what is most important. In table 13.9, the variance and standard deviation are both fairly large values, which means there is great variability of the systolic blood pressure scores around the mean. This makes sense since the mean is 135.8 and the scores range from 109 to 190, which does demonstrate large amounts of variability.

Table 13.9 Example of range, variance, and standard deviation

Statistics		
Systolic blood pressure		
N	Valid	6
	Missing	0
Mean		135.8333
Standard Deviation		29.43750
Variance		866.567
Range		81.00

N = Number

Source: ©AHIMA.

Check Your Understanding 13.2

Answer the following questions.

1. Why are descriptive statistics used?
   a. To illustrate the relationship between age and cause of pneumonia in patients admitted to a hospital from 2015 to 2020
   b. To graph how often patients within a specific age range and gender are being readmitted due to a cardiac condition
   c. To illustrate the frequency of an element such as a hemoglobin rate below 12.0 in a group of patients
   d. To illustrate the relationship between cases of measles and pertussis before and after vaccination
2. Identify which of the following is not a measure of central tendency.
   a. Mean
   b. Mode
   c. Percentile
   d. Z-score
3. Identify which of the following measures examine the spread of different values around the middle value.
   a. Measures of central tendency
   b. Measures of variability
   c. Measures of frequency
   d. Measures of percentile
4. Identify which of the following measures is simple to compute and calculated by taking the difference between the highest and lowest values.
   a. Mean
   b. Median
   c. Range
   d. Standard deviation
5. The measure used in descriptive statistics that shows the value below which a given percentage of scores in a given group of scores fall is called a:
   a. Percentile
   b. Frequency distribution
   c. Standard deviation
   d. Median

Normal Distribution

When presenting data graphically, if the data follows a symmetrical or bell curve, then the data is termed a **normal distribution**. In a normal distribution, the mean, median, and mode are equal. An example of a normal distribution or curve is shown in figure 13.17.

The properties of a standard normal distribution include:

- The appearance of a bell-shaped curve that is symmetrical about the mean and extends infinitely in both directions (positive and negative).
- The total area under the curve equals 1, so the area of one half of the curve is equal to 0.50 and the area of the other half is equal to 0.50. Also, the area under the curve between two points can be interpreted as the relative frequency of the values included between those points. One standard deviation from the mean = 68.26 percent of the area, two

standard deviations = 95.45 percent of the area, and three standard deviations = 99.74 percent of the area under the curve.

- Being defined by two parameters: the mean, m, and the standard deviation.

Figure 13.18 provides an example of a normal curve superimposed on a histogram. The center of the distribution, or mean, is 17. (The median and the mode also are 17.) The standard deviation is 2.595 or, with rounding, 2.6. This means that 68 percent of the observations in the frequency distribution fall within 1 standard deviation from the mean or 2.6 standard deviations from 17 (17 ± 2.6). Thus, approximately 68 percent of the observations fall between 14.4 and 19.6; 95 percent fall between 2 standard deviations from the mean or (2.6 x 2 = 5.2) 5.2 standard deviations from 17 (17 ± 5.2) or

Figure 13.17 Example of a normal curve

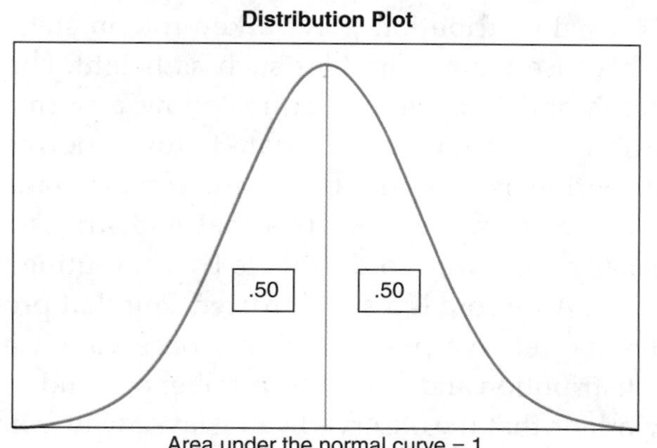

Source: ©AHIMA.

Figure 13.18 Example of a histogram with a normal curve

Statistics

Hospital LOS

N	Valid	100
	Missing	0
Mean		17.25
Median		17.00
Mode		17

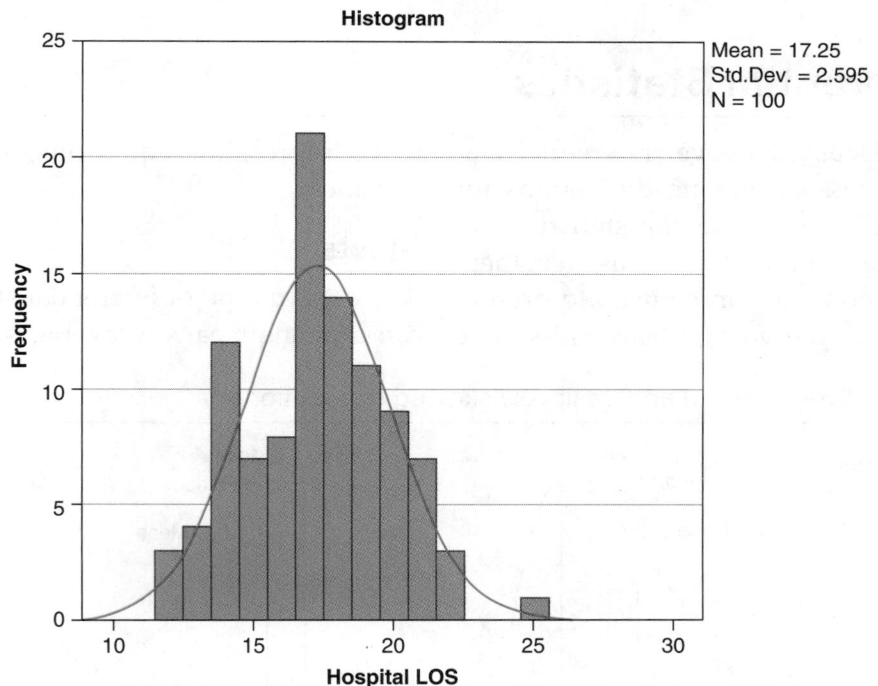

LOS = length of stay

Source: ©AHIMA.

between 11.8 and 22.2; and 99.7 percent fall between 3 standard deviations from the mean or (2.6 x 3 = 7.8) 7.8 standard deviations from 17 (17 ± 7.8) or between 9.2 and 24.8.

Normal distribution plays a key role in statistics because many variables such as height, cholesterol, and body temperature follow a normal distribution. Determining if data follow a normal distribution is important because certain statistics can be computed on data that is distributed normally. One way to do this is by computing a Z-score. A Z-score is a standardized unit that provides the relative position of any observation in the distribution and is also the number of standard deviations that the observed value lays away from the mean. Transforming the raw observations to Z values makes it possible to make comparisons between distributions. Using **inferential statistics** (defined in the next section), researchers can then make inferences about certain types of data. Inferential statistics are techniques that can be used to make deductions based on the evidence of the data and reasoning.

$$\text{Z} - \text{score} = \frac{\text{Observation or x} - \text{Mean}(\mu)}{\text{Standard Deviation}(\sigma)}$$

Z-scores represent the number of standard deviations above or below the mean, so a Z-score of –2.5 represents a score that is 2.5 standard deviations below the mean.

For example, if a prospective employee scores a 95 percent on a billing exam, with an employee average of 80 percent and a standard deviation of 5, using the given formula, the Z-score will be:

$$\frac{95-80}{5} = 3$$

This means that the score of 95 percent is 3 standard deviations above the mean.

Sometimes data do not follow a normal distribution and are pulled toward the tails of the curve. When this occurs, it is referred to as having a skewed distribution. Because the mean is sensitive to extreme values or outliers, it gravitates in the direction of the extreme values, thus making a long tail when a distribution is skewed. When the tail is pulled toward the right side, it is called a positively skewed distribution; when the tail is pulled toward the left side of the curve it is called a negatively skewed distribution. Figure 13.19 shows a positively skewed and negatively skewed curve.

Inferential Statistics

As discussed above, inferential statistics is the process of making deductions for a larger population based on the statistical results taken from a sample. Within this area, there are several methods that can be used to present research judgments including *t*-tests, chi-square tests, regression equations, and analysis of variance.

t-tests

A ***t*-test** is a type of inferential statistical test that can examine means or averages from a group of

Figure 13.19 Negatively skewed and positively skewed distribution

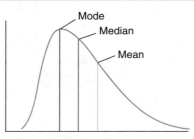

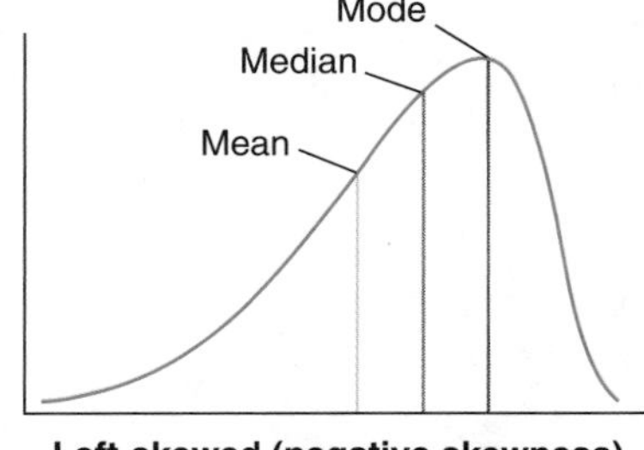

Source: ©AHIMA.

data. The focus of a *t*-test is to use the mean from a research sample group and then infer how that mean would be found in the larger population. A *t*-test can also be conducted when looking at research study groups to determine if the means of two groups are statistically significant. A foundational element of *t*-testing is the establishment of both a null and an alternative hypothesis. The null hypothesis is centered on the prediction that there will be no difference found between the groups of the research study. The alternative hypothesis is just that, a different or opposite statement of the null hypothesis.

An example of null and alternative hypotheses can be seen in a scenario where a researcher is researching health information technology (HIT) graduates' Registered Health Information Technician (RHIT) exam scores and grade point averages (GPA). The research question could be: Do students with a high GPA score above the national average on the RHIT exam? The null hypothesis is that the students with a GPA score of 3.5 or higher score above the national average on the RHIT exam. The alternative hypothesis is that students with a GPA score of 3.5 or higher ***do not*** score above the national average on the RHIT exam.

Then using a one-sample *t*-test, the difference between the population mean and the research sample mean can be determined. To narrow the population, the research sample could be the past two years of graduates of a specific college or university-based HIT program. The mean from their RHIT exam results and their GPAs could then be statistically evaluated. The data from this sample could then be used statistically to form a conclusion for the overall population of students taking the RHIT exam. The goal of the *t*-test is to determine if the averages between the chosen two groups of the research study is statistically significant.

Chi-square Tests

Chi-square tests are a type of inferential statistical testing done to determine and present information on data frequency. There are two general types of chi-square tests: goodness of fit and test for independence. The determining factor in choosing which chi-square test to use is the number of nominal variables. Also, the focus of using this type of test is to examine if there is a difference between data gathered from a sample population.

Number of Variables	Chi-Square Test
One	Chi-square goodness of fit
Two	Chi-square test for independence

Regression Equations

There are several types of regression equations: simple, multiple, logistic, multinominal, and multiple logistic. Regression equations are used to determine if there is a relationship between variables and to identify what type of relationship is present. The two types of relationship are correlation and predictable. In healthcare, regression equations and statistical presentations of these findings can be used to identify trends and make forecasts. An example of the use of regression equations would be to review data on hospital LOS and cost of care during that stay. A regression equation could be applied to data from these elements over a period of three years and the results used to infer or predict what the trends will be for LOS and increased or decreased cost of care in the future.

Analysis of Variance

Another type of inferential statistical testing is analysis of variance (ANOVA). An ANOVA is a test used to find and examine the differences in the determined averages (means) within and between data groups. There are several types of ANOVAs, including one-way ANOVA, two-way ANOVA, and multivariate ANOVA. An example of when and how an ANOVA could be used is provided at the end of this section. In general, if the researcher is seeking to examine the average results of survey responses obtained from two groups of study participants, an ANOVA could be the statistical test to calculate.

In the earlier example, two groups were used for a *t*-test. For an ANOVA test to be applied, three or more groups of data must be used. An ANOVA cannot be done with just two data groups or two sets of responses. Additionally, the configuration of the data variables determines the type of ANOVA. The two possible data variable types are dependent and independent. An independent variable is defined as a research element that is changed or controlled by the research environment or the researcher. The dependent variable is the element being examined by the research or researcher. If there are two independent variables and a continuous dependent variable, then a two-way ANOVA test can be done to show differences.

For example, a research study is being conducted with students enrolled in online courses as the participants. The students participating in the research study must complete a survey. The research is focused on the students' perceived sense of isolation when taking online courses. One group of students participating in the study have recorded video lectures in their online class. The other groups of students do not have any recorded video lectures in their online class. The independent variable is the recorded video lectures. The dependent variable is the students' perception of isolation. In the examination of the results of this study, an ANOVA test would be done and presented. If the study has at least two dependent variables, then a multivariate ANOVA, or MANOVA, is the statistical test used. Using the same example as above, if an additional variable, such as the graduation rates for both groups, were added, then a MANOVA would be used to show results based on having two dependent variables (students' perceived sense of isolation and graduation rates), neither of which are controlled by the researcher.

Check Your Understanding 13.3

Answer the following questions.

1. True or false: In a normal distribution, the mean, median, and mode are not equal.
2. True or false: The total area under the curve of a normal distribution equals 1.
3. True or false: Z-scores represent the number of standard deviations above or below the mean, so a Z-score of –1.5 represents a score that is 1.5 standard deviations above the mean.
4. Determining if data follow a normal distribution is important because certain statistics can be computed on data that are distributed normally. Which of the following is one type of these statistics?
   a. Mean
   b. Median
   c. Z-score
   d. Mode
5. Two standard deviations from the mean in a normal distribution equals what percent of the area?
   a. 68.26 percent
   b. 95.45 percent
   c. 99.74 percent
   d. 100 percent
6. A curve or distribution in which the tail is pulled to the right is called which of the following types of distribution?
   a. Negatively skewed
   b. Positively skewed
   c. Normal
   d. Bimodal
7. If a student scores an 82 percent on an ICD-10-CM/PCS coding exam and the class average is 60 percent with a standard deviation of 4, what is the Z-score and what does this tell us about the student's coding exam score?
   a. Z = 5.5; the score of 82 percent is 5.5 standard deviations above the mean
   b. Z = 5.5; the score of 82 percent is 5.5 standard deviations below the mean
   c. Z = 5; the score of 82 percent is 5 standard deviations above the mean
   d. Z = 7.5; the score of 82 percent is 7.5 standard deviations above the mean

8. True or false: An analysis of variance statistical test would be used to summarize a data sample such as gender or reported job roles.
9. True or false: Regression is used to determine relationships between the variables.
10. True or false: A null hypothesis is an important element that must be done before conducting an ANOVA statistical test.

How to Analyze Information

After data have been collected and reviewed, the statistical test(s) to use can be determined. This determination is based on several elements that include the research goal, the objective of the presentation, and the audience seeking information from the data. Deciding which type of descriptive statistical graphic to present (bar chart, pie chart, histogram, and so on) is part of the analysis process. This is also part of taking the data and transforming it to information. In general, descriptive statistics are used if the intention of the presentation is to describe or summarize. If the goal is to make predictions or judgments based on the data collected, inferential statistical tools can be used (Johnson and Christensen 2017). The steps for information analysis include the following:

1. Determine the objective of the information being presented. What are you trying to say or show with the data? What was the research focused on and how does that relate to the problem?
2. Consider who the information will be presented to. How can you make the information clear and concise for the audience?
3. Review the information on the various statistical tests to determine which one fits the needs of your presentation.
4. Consider a team approach that includes an individual well-versed in statistics. If working with clinical data, a person with a background in that area should be on the team. Also, consider having an editor to review the work before it is finalized.

Figure 13.20 illustrates how data can be analyzed for a presentation. In this example, the focus is on a survey, which is how the data for the project discussed were gathered. After the data have been analyzed, the information will be presented to the board of the corporation. The first part of figure 13.20 presents the background on how the data were gathered. The second portion lists the analysis process steps.

Quality, Safety, and Effectiveness of Healthcare

Using data to assess quality, safety, and healthcare outcomes such as the effectiveness of healthcare is prominent throughout healthcare organizations today. In fact, several federal government agencies such as the Centers for Medicare and Medicaid Services (CMS) provide financial incentives for healthcare organizations that demonstrate high levels of quality, safety, and effectiveness of healthcare services. Quality measures developed by CMS are used in the pay-for-reporting programs for specific healthcare providers. The Joint Commission also uses data analysis to make decisions regarding patient safety and other measures of effectiveness of care. How is this data examined and how can HIM professionals assist? When the healthcare organization wants to measure variations within healthcare units—such as identifying variability across nursing units for the number or percentage of falls that occurred—a line graph would be an appropriate tool. Descriptive statistics in a table can also be used alongside the graph to provide more detail on the percentage of falls in total and by nursing unit across the healthcare organization. Quality, safety, and effectiveness of healthcare are also assessed by many other organizations such

Figure 13.20 Example of how data can be analyzed for presentation

Background:

Greenfield Corporation conducted a survey of healthcare providers in the states of Delaware, Maryland, and Pennsylvania. The focus of the survey was on the adoption of an electronic health record (EHR) or electronic medical record (EMR) in the physician office setting. Those surveyed where internal medicine, family practice, and allergy physicians with private office practices (the physician practices were not owned by a healthcare network, group, or hospital entity). The goal of the survey was to determine if the physicians had adopted an EHR/EMR in their office and if not, what the barriers were to doing so (for example, financial or psychological). Survey questions included demographic information such as age and gender of the physician and basic information on the practice such as number of patients seen daily and monthly.

The health information management (HIM) company of D & A Associates has been hired by Greenfield to review and present the results of the surveys at an upcoming board meeting. The company is reviewing the results of this data as part of a strategic plan to develop an EHR product specifically for the physician practice market that is not part of a larger health network.

Surveys were returned from 150 physicians.

Analysis Process:

1. D & A Associates reviews the objective of the scheduled presentation to the Greenfield board of directors.
2. D & A Associates assigns a team to this project. The team includes a team leader, an HIM professional, a statistician, an HIM assistant, and an editor.
3. D & A Associates reviews the data and determines if descriptive statistics should be used or if inferential statistics could be applied or both. Is it enough to summarize and describe the data collected from the surveys or should judgments be made? The strategic plans of the Greenfield Corporation and its ideas for the EHR/EMR product are considered. The best way to present the data concisely is also considered. Various statistical tests are then conducted based on the team's decision.
4. Once these decisions have been made, drafts of the presentations are created. The team and the editor review the draft proposals before the final board presentation.

as the National Commission for Quality Assurance (NCQA), which has developed Healthcare Effectiveness Data and Information Set (HEDIS) measures; Patient-Centered Outcomes Research Institute (PCORI), which focuses on the patient and engages the patient in the all phases of research related to healthcare outcomes; and the Agency for Healthcare Research and Quality (AHRQ), whose mission is to make healthcare safer, higher quality, more accessible, equitable, and affordable. The American Health Information Management Association (AHIMA) provides examples of publicly reported data by organizations such as the ones previously mentioned (AHIMA 2013). Much of the data collected is considered "big data" since it incorporates multiple sources from not only healthcare data but also financial, geographical, and human resource data. Analysis of big data does not necessarily mean that upper level statistics must be used. One can start with descriptive levels of statistics and then move on to inferential statistics if the problem to be solved needs this higher level of statistics.

Structure and Use of Health Information and Healthcare Outcomes

Data can be structured in many ways. Healthcare organizations collect data that can fall into three different groups—individual, comparative, and aggregate.

Individual Data

Healthcare data that is housed within the EHR, or data collected from a case study, a focus group of individuals, or during an interview or survey are all considered individual data. This data can be helpful in providing direct care to patients, and for quality improvement studies or for larger descriptive studies. However, when using this type of data to make decisions related to a certain area of healthcare by evaluating it against other levels of data, then it becomes comparative data.

Comparative Data

When individual data is organized numerically and collated to evaluate against standards or benchmarks, it is described as comparative data. For example, when a healthcare organization collects individual data on whether a patient acquired a healthcare-associated infection, such as ventilator-associated pneumonia (VAP), it is first documented in the individual patient's EHR. Queries throughout the entire EHR system will provide output on the number of cases of VAP that develops 48 hours or longer after mechanical ventilation is given by means of an endotracheal tube or tracheostomy, in order to designate it as a healthcare-associated infection. This type of infection is referred to as a hospital-acquired infection (HAI). Once this data is gathered and collated, it can then be compared to other rates of VAP across the state, region, or nation.

Aggregate Data

Aggregate data is when individual, comparative, or other multiple sources of data are compiled and analyzed to draw conclusions about a specific topic or area. For example, in a focus group study, data, observation, and interview data were compiled into an aggregate format so that none of the individuals in the multiple healthcare organizations that participated could be identified in any way. Varying methods and skills of leadership among HIM leaders and facilities were compared and contrasted in order to generate conclusions. However, since the focus group sample was small, not all the conclusions could be generalized (Sheridan et al. 2016). In fact, any data compiled from samples of data have limitations since the sample of data may not accurately reflect the characteristics across that entire population. One way to reduce this is to compare the sample's demographic characteristics to the population's demographics (if this information is available); if the characteristics prove similar, it increases the reliability of the sample data.

Check Your Understanding 13.4

Answer the following questions.

1. The first step in information analysis is:
   a. Determining who the information will be presented to
   b. Determining the appropriate statistical test to use
   c. Using a team with members with different skill sets
   d. Determining the objective of the information
2. Individual data can be used to:
   a. Compare two groups
   b. Determine relationship between variables
   c. Provide patient care
   d. Group data together
3. Comparing a healthcare organization's death rate to the death rates of similar healthcare organizations across the country uses ________ data.
   a. Comparative
   b. Individual
   c. Aggregate
   d. Big
4. The research study requires data to be compiled and summarized. This is ________data.
   a. Individual
   b. Comparative
   c. Aggregate
   d. Evaluative

5. Analysis of big data does not necessarily mean that upper level statistics must be used. One can start with levels of _______ statistics and then move on to _______statistics if the problem that needs to be solved requires this higher level of statistics.
   a. Inferential; descriptive
   b. Descriptive; inferential
   c. Random; nonrandom
   d. Social; scientific

Research Methodologies

There are several types of research methodologies that can be used to perform research on healthcare and HIM topics. Research studies can range from exploratory or descriptive studies that strive to generate new hypotheses based on data collected to experimental studies that provide interventions or treatments that can reduce the spread of an existing disease. These research methodologies can be classified as quantitative, qualitative, and mixed methods. Typically, institutional review boards must approve any research study before it is conducted. These methods and the institutional review board will be covered in the next few sections.

Quantitative Studies

Research results that are numerical in nature and can be illustrated with descriptive or inferential statistics are quantitative and would be a quantitative study. Types of quantitative studies include descriptive, correlational, retrospective, prospective, and experimental and quasi-experimental.

Descriptive Studies

Descriptive studies include research that is exploratory in nature and generates new hypotheses from the data collected. For example, a descriptive study approach was used to explore how the use of automated coding software (computer-assisted coding [CAC]) could be used to enhance anti-fraud activities. This study used a traditional descriptive study approach that consisted of the five steps that follow beginning with a review of literature and ending with the reporting of the research results.

1. The literature on CAC software, anti-fraud software within CAC systems, and the extent of fraud and abuse related to CAC systems was reviewed
2. Interviews with federal agencies were conducted to gather information about instances of improper reimbursement or potential fraud involving the use of CAC software
3. A description of products was developed based on a product information form completed by vendors
4. Researchers then interviewed vendors and users about CAC and anti-fraud software to determine how they used these products
5. Descriptive statistical results were reported through matrices, flowcharts, and tables to demonstrate the impact of automated coding tools on coding and billing accuracy. A model was designed that summarized features, processes, and staffing (Garvin et al. 2006)

Correlational Studies

Correlational studies are similar to descriptive studies except that the correlational study determines if a relationship may exist between two variables. This means that the researcher will try to determine if an increase or decrease in one variable corresponds to an increase or decrease in the other variable. The purpose of performing correlational studies is to determine which variables are connected in some way. However, correlation does not equal causation. For example, a researcher may be interested in patterns related to whether the use of electronic cigarettes, or e-cigs, affects school performance in teenagers. To determine a correlation, the researcher will interview teens to determine if and how often they smoke e-cigs and compare this to their grades in the past month. A correlation coefficient is then used to determine how strong the association is between the two variables. The closer the correlation coefficient is to +1 or –1, the stronger the relationship between the variables. A strong positive relationship (closer to +1) means that as one variable increases, the other also increases. A strong negative relationship (closer to –1) means that as one variable decreases, the other variable increases. Hypothetically, if the research team collected data on the number of times a teen smoked an e-cig and on their SAT score, they might find that the correlation coefficient is a –0.845. The correlation coefficient of –0.845 is very close to –1. This indicates a negative correlation, which in this example means that as e-cig use increases, SAT scores decrease. There are two types of correlation coefficients: Pearson correlation coefficient and Spearman correlation coefficient. If the researcher collects continuous variables, then the Pearson correlation coefficient should be used. If ordinal or ranked variables are collected, then the Spearman correlation coefficient should be used.

Retrospective Studies

A retrospective study is one in which the researcher is looking into the past for data; the data is historical and not currently obtained. In epidemiology, researchers conduct retrospective studies (also called case-control studies) by reviewing records and asking the subjects to recall past events in order to determine the presence or absence of the independent variable under study. This is compared in samples of subjects with the disease under study (cases) and without the disease (controls). For example, if a researcher were interested in whether the use of estrogen replacement therapy (ERT) caused colon cancer in postmenopausal women, they would recruit a group of women with colon cancer (cases) and another group of women without colon cancer (controls) as subjects. Controls could be selected by recruiting subjects who also were treated by the same healthcare organization as the cases or were friends or siblings of the cases. The more similar the controls are to the cases for everything except the disease under study (colon cancer), the better. The research team would then review the women's health records to determine if they ever used ERT. The research team might also want to validate the information found in the health records by interviewing the subjects and asking them if they ever took ERT. This type of study is also called an analytic study because it tries to determine causation, or whether an independent variable (ERT) produced the dependent variable (colon cancer). Statistics used to determine causation include the odds ratio or the odds of getting the disease under study if you have the determinant variable or independent variable. Often the odds ratio is displayed in a two-by-two table, as shown in table 13.10.

The formula used to compute the odds ratio is AD/BC = (70 x 80) / (20 x 30) = 5,600/600 = 9.3

The interpretation of this result for the odds ratio is that someone who takes ERT is approximately nine times more likely to get colon cancer than someone who does not take ERT.

Prospective Studies

A prospective study is defined as research that is designed to follow the study participants into the future to see if there is a relationship that develops for the study variables. An example of a prospective study is one in which a cohort of individuals are followed to determine if a particular characteristic or risk factor(s) such as smoking or exposure to a specific substance may be causing the disease or outcome under study. This type of study does something that the retrospective, case-control design does not—it determines whether

Table 13.10 Example of odds ratio for the retrospective (case-control) study

Independent variable ERT	Dependent variable (colon cancer)		
	Colon cancer	No colon cancer	Total
ERT use	70 (A)	30 (B)	100
No ERT use	20 (C)	80 (D)	100
Totals	90	110	200

Source: ©AHIMA.

the characteristic(s) or risk factor(s) under study truly preceded the disease. The prospective study starts with subjects who have the risk factor (exposed group) but are free of the disease and compares them to individuals without the risk factor (unexposed group) who are also free of the disease. The two groups are then followed to determine if and when the subjects develop the disease. To begin, subjects are examined at a baseline to ensure they do not have the disease when the study commences. To do this, the researcher must collect data related to their occupation, medical history, and social habits. Physical exams and lab tests may also be necessary. It is important to collect other general characteristics such as age, sex, race, and such in addition to the characteristic of interest, in order to account for the influence of any factors known to be related to the disease. These are called confounding factors. **Confounding factors** are those characteristics other than the characteristic of interest that may also be related to the disease under study. If subjects cannot be correctly categorized into exposed and unexposed groups, the prospective design should not be used.

It is important to have correct classification of exposure because if participants' exposure to certain elements is not correctly classified, it may lead to invalid study results. The most widely known example of a prospective study is the Framingham Heart Study, which began in 1948, is a project of the National Heart, Lung, and Blood Institute and Boston University, and is still in progress today (FHS 2015). Its original goal was to identify risk factors for cardiovascular disease (CVD) since the causes of heart disease and stroke were not known and the death rates were steadily increasing. The researchers decided to study this over a long period of time using a large group of participants who had not yet developed CVD or had a heart attack or stroke. The researchers recruited 5,209 men and women between the ages of 30 and 62 from Framingham, Massachusetts, and started physical exams and interviews to determine any type of CVD. The participants returned to the study every two years for follow-up physical exams, lab tests, and so forth, and in 1971 the researchers enrolled a second-generation cohort of the participants' adult children and spouses. In 2002, a third generation of participants was recruited, which included the grandchildren of the original cohort. Clinicians use many of the findings from the Framingham Heart Study when treating CVD, since it identified major risk factors of CVD such as high blood pressure, high cholesterol, smoking, lack of physical activity, diabetes, and obesity. It was also instrumental in finding related factors that play a part in the development of CVD, such as triglyceride and HDL cholesterol levels, as well as psychosocial issues, age, and gender (FHS 2015). Prospective studies generate incidence—the number of new cases that occurred during a specific period of time in a population at risk for developing the disease—not the prevalence of a disease. The calculation for the incidence rate is given in table 13.11. **Incidence rates** can then be used to calculate the relative risk (table 13.12). The formula for calculating incidence rate follows. Incidence Rate =

$$\text{Incidence Rate} = \frac{\text{Number of new cases over a time period} \times 1{,}000}{\text{Population at risk}^{*}}$$

**Those free of disease at the start of the study*

An example of computing the incidence rates and relative risk is shown as follows.

Therefore, using this hypothetical data, one can say that the risk of developing CVD with a BMI

Table 13.11 Example computing the incidence rates

	Disease	No Disease
Exposed	(A)	(B)
Not exposed	(C)	(D)
Totals		

Incidence rate of exposed = A/[A + B]
Incidence rate of unexposed = C/[C + D]
Relative risk: [A/(A + B)]/[C/[C + D]]
Source: ©AHIMA.

Table 13.12 Example of computing relative risk

	CVD	No CVD
BMI > 27	50 (A)	20 (B)
BMI < 27	10 (C)	60 (D)
Totals	60	80

Incidence rate of exposed = A/(A+B) = 50/(50+20) = 0.71
Incidence rate of unexposed = C/(C + D) = 10/(10 + 60] = 0.14
Relative risk: [A/(A + B)]/[C/(C + D)] = 0.71/0.14 = 5.1
Source: ©AHIMA.

greater than 27 is approximately 5 times that of developing CVD with a BMI less than 27. The difference between the odds ratio and the relative risk is that the odds ratio is an estimate of the risk since the study from which it was taken is based on retrospective data. The relative risk from a prospective study is considered "true risk" since it demonstrates that the risk factor under study came before the disease since participants were followed to collect the data and, therefore, determine the risk of disease.

Experimental Studies

The **experimental study** design is the most powerful when trying to establish cause and effect. In healthcare, experimental research studies can entail exposing participants to different interventions in order to compare the results of these interventions with the outcome. The intervention may include testing experimental drugs, new approaches to surgery, or other types of interventions such as smoking cessation treatments. Experimental studies can also be referred to as clinical trials. The National Institutes of Health (NIH) has a service that provides a registry and a database of results of clinical trials that have been conducted or are currently being conducted across the world (NIH 2015a). Pretests and posttests are used in observational experimental research. The pretest is performed to determine the baseline level of the independent variable under study and the posttest is determined to measure the same independent variable after the intervention. For example, blood pressure is taken before and after an experimental medication is used as the intervention in a sample of participants that were previously unable to control their blood pressure with other medications. The independent variable is the experimental medication and the dependent variable is the blood pressure. In experimental research studies like clinical trials, researchers must pay attention to many things, but three main areas are extremely important because experiments are a part of this study design. For healthcare, there are several important factors since experimental or clinical trials involve human participants. These factors are the following:

- Eligibility of appropriate participants (inclusion and exclusion criteria)
- Randomization
- Ethical issues

Eligibility of appropriate participants includes the development of certain criteria so that the proper participants are recruited for the experimental study. For example, in a study entitled, "Evaluation of a Stepped Care Approach to Manage Depression in Diabetes" some of the inclusion criteria include the following:

- Age greater than or equal to 18 and less than or equal to 70
- Diabetes mellitus
- Elevated depressive symptoms

Some of the exclusion criteria include the following:

- Severe depressive episode
- Current psychotherapeutic or psychiatric treatment
- Current anti-depressive medication
- Severe physical illness (that is, cancer, multiple sclerosis, dementia)
- Terminal illness (NIH 2015b)

Quasi-Experimental Studies

The **quasi-experimental study** is similar to the experimental study except that randomization of participants is not included in a quasi-experimental study. Also, the researcher may not manipulate the independent variable and there may be no control or comparison group. Quasi-experimental studies can be performed over time and may not include individual participants but whole healthcare systems. For example, researchers performed a quasi-experimental study to examine the association between implementation of a certified outpatient EHR and control of diabetes in patients with the disease. They implemented the EHR across 17 medical centers and then tested the difference in certain lab tests before and after implementation.

They found the EHR improved drug treatment intensity, monitoring, and control for patients with diabetes (Reed et al. 2012).

Qualitative Research

Qualitative research designs involve collecting types of data that reflect a participant's perceptions, feelings, or attitudes about a certain subject. The methods used to collect qualitative data can include observations, focus groups, case studies, informal conversational interviews, and in-depth interviews. An example of observation can be as simple as taking time to observe a physical object on your desk at home or at work. Look at the object in relation to its shape, size, color, material composition, and its purpose and write these observations down. This also can be performed in an HIM department, where the researcher observes how coders react to their first exposure to the use of a clinical documentation improvement software system. The researcher could observe them as they are trained on the information system or as they use the information system and then document their observations. Qualitative research is chosen because it can provide robust data on a new topic or it can provide background for larger studies on the same topic. Grounded theory and ethnography are explained in more detail since HIM professionals may find themselves conducting research in these areas.

Grounded Theory

Grounded theory is a research method that enables the researcher to develop a theory that is substantiated or confirmed by the data. It is a systematic method that can use multiple methods (both quantitative and qualitative findings) and pull it all together to develop a theory. Because it includes data collected through methods such as conversing with subjects on a specific topic, it is usually categorized under qualitative research, but it can also include quantitative information (Grounded Theory Institute 2014). First, the researcher should identify the topic area such as information governance (IG). The researcher will then consult all the previous research and possibly the researchers that have defined and discussed information governance. Data collection may include several types of data—qualitative, quantitative, or a mixture of both—in the particular topic area. Data can be from sources such as articles, news reports, pictures, photographs, videos, recordings, and the like. It can also include conversing with individuals or groups. For example, to learn more about information governance, the researcher may choose leaders in the field of IG and create focus groups of individuals with a background in IG and ask them questions about the topic. In grounded theory, the researcher codes the data as it is collected and makes memos and observations simultaneously so that at the end of this refining process, the research is used to develop a theory. It is also important that the researcher be familiar with literature on the topic so that his or her theory coincides with what is currently published and accepted. The researcher's theory is then published or presented in a model that can be used by others to conduct further research in that area.

Ethnography

Ethnography is a methodology where the researcher delves into a particular culture or organization in great detail in order to learn everything there is to know about them and to develop new hypotheses. Ethnography is not objective and includes opinions of the researcher. No two ethnographers will examine a specific culture or organization the same way. Ethnography's focus is on people, culture, and life. The researcher takes notes while out in the field observing the people and their experiences in a particular culture, so the researcher can create a more thorough and specific description of all interactions, experiences, perceptions, and opinions. In one particular example of an ethnographic study, a researcher examined the social relationship between a physician and patient as the patient is diagnosed with clinical illness. The specific aims of the research were to identify and describe the most important social practices between urologists and patients as they are diagnosed with cancer. The researcher worked in urology offices and hospitals primarily using participant observation to collect his data, which is one of the primary tools of ethnographic research. He found that a healing relationship between the patient and clinician emerged as the diagnosis unfolded (Meza 2013).

Mixed-Methods Approach

A mixed-methodology approach includes using both quantitative and qualitative data in a research study design. According to the published report sponsored by the NIH Office of Behavioral and Social Science Research, mixed-methods research includes the following aspects:

- Using research questions that focus on real-life, multilevel perspectives, across many cultures
- Using multiple methods (for example, intervention trials and in-depth interviews)
- Integrating these multiple methods or combining them to extract the strengths of each
- Focusing the research within philosophical and theoretical positions (Creswell et al. 2011)

According to a report sponsored by the NIH, mixed-methods research is more than collecting qualitative data from interviews or observations or gathering multiple types of quantitative evidence through surveys and diagnostic tests (Creswell et al. 2011). It involves the intentional collection of both quantitative and qualitative data in order to combine the strengths of both to answer the research questions. Mixed-methods research designs are usually performed when qualitative or quantitative data alone are not sufficient to answer the research question. For example, if an HIM professional wanted to explore the underutilization of the cancer registry at one healthcare organization, he or she could first collect quantitative data on the number of requests the cancer registry received. However, more qualitative informal interviews with physicians and other potential users may also be needed. Therefore, a mixed-methods approach would be the best research design in this case.

Randomization

When study participants are randomly chosen to be in the experimental, control, or comparison group using an indiscriminate method, so each participant has an equal chance of being selected for one of the groups, it is called randomization. Randomization is important in effectively testing whether the specific intervention made a difference in the outcome of the disease. For example, if researchers wanted to determine whether an experimental medication made a difference in a person's anxiety level, they would recruit participants who were diagnosed with anxiety and then randomly assign them to a group that will take the experimental drug or a group that will take a placebo or pill that does not include the experimental drug. The researchers would also collect pretest data on participants' anxiety level through interviews before they were randomized into the experimental or control group. They would then provide the medication over a period of time and collect data via interviews on the anxiety levels of participants in both the experimental and control groups. Anxiety level data should provide a score that can be compared pre- and post-intervention. Once this data is collected, the difference in the average anxiety scores can be compared before and after the intervention in both the experimental and control groups. The paired *t*-test is a statistical test that can be used to determine if the differences seen pre- and post-intervention are significantly different statistically and not due to chance. If significant values are found more in the experimental group than in the control group, then the researchers can conclude that the experimental drug was successful.

Check Your Understanding 13.5

Match the research study design with its appropriate description.

1. Uses a combination of quantitative and qualitative data
2. Exploratory, generates new hypotheses
3. Determines if a relationship exists between two variables
4. Another name for case-control study
5. The Framingham Heart Study is an example
6. Uses randomization to determine who receives the medication under study
7. Type of study used when examining the impact of the implementation of an EHR on outcomes of diabetes patients
8. Studies a particular culture in great detail
9. Uses multiple methods to determine a new theory
10. Collect robust types of data

a. Qualitative research
b. Quasi-experimental study
c. Retrospective study
d. Prospective study
e. Mixed-methods approach
f. Ethnography
g. Experimental study
h. Grounded theory
i. Descriptive study
j. Correlational study

Institutional Review Board

The Department of Health and Human Services (HHS) describes the role of the **Institutional Review Board (IRB)** as one that protects human subjects involved in research activities. The IRB determines whether research conducted on human subjects is appropriate and protects the participants' rights. The major focus of the IRB is not whether the research is appropriate for the organization or researcher to conduct, but that it contains all the appropriate protections for human subjects involved in the research (45 CFR 46). There are three major categories for IRB review and approval, and they include exempt, expedited, and full board approval. Exempt research activities that are the most closely related to HIM fall into the following three main categories:

1. Research conducted in an educational setting involving normal education practices such as testing different teaching methods
2. Research that includes using tests, interviews, or observations, unless identifiable and pose risks
3. Collection or study of existing data or specimens as long as it has been deidentified (45 CFR 46)

Expedited research includes those studies that pose only minimal risk to human subjects; examples include those studies that collect identifiable information on human subjects that may include sensitive information such as identifiable health information on subjects that are HIV positive.

Full board approval is required for those studies that do not fall under exempt or expedited. Most of the studies performed by HIM professionals are categorized as exempt or expedited. It is best to meet with a member of the IRB at the healthcare organization to determine under which category the research study would fall. Once the review category is determined, the researcher must then submit their research protocol to the IRB for review and approval. This takes about two weeks and if a decision is made that the research falls under the exempt category, then the researcher does not have to renew the study annually, as they must do under expedited and full board reviews. Also, informed consent is normally not required under exempt research as it is for expedited and full board study reviews (45 CFR 46).

Researchers should always remember that whenever any human subjects are used in research, the IRB should be consulted, and the research protocol should be submitted to the organization's IRB for review and approval. Even if research is conducted on individuals that are not patients—such as interviewing employees, students, or even collecting data on human subjects from existing records—IRB approval should still be obtained.

Healthcare Research Organizations

There are many types of healthcare research organizations that conduct, promote, or support research across the healthcare system. The Centers for Disease Control and Prevention (CDC), the World Health Organization (WHO) and the Agency for Healthcare Research and Quality (AHRQ) are all key healthcare research organizations. Their roles in healthcare research are discussed in the following sections.

Centers for Disease Control and Prevention

The Centers for Disease Control and Prevention (CDC) is a US government agency whose mission is to collaborate with the public to create the expertise, information, and tools people and communities need to protect their health, through health promotion, prevention of disease, injury, and disability, and preparedness for new health threats. The CDC does this by confronting global diseases such as helping to combat the recent Ebola virus outbreak, tracking diseases (like influenza and foodborne outbreaks) to find out what is causing individuals to become ill, helping healthcare organizations, and cultivating public health. The CDC's role extends to public health workforce development and providing processes for monitoring emerging health threats and disparities (CDC 2014). The CDC employs researchers to meet many of these goals, but they also provide funding and support to other researchers who can then use grants to conduct research to meet their objectives. The CDC and the National Center for Health Statistics provides mounds of data, statistical reports, and surveys that can be used to conduct research as well (CDC 2015).

World Health Organization

The World Health Organization (WHO) works to direct and coordinate authorities on international health through the United Nations. WHO's health-related focus areas include the following:

- Health systems
- Noncommunicable diseases such as heart disease, cancer, stroke, diabetes, chronic lung disease, and mental health conditions
- Promoting health throughout the course of life to include environment and social determinants of health as well as gender, equity, and human rights
- Communicable diseases such as HIV, tuberculosis, and malaria

- Preparedness, surveillance, and response through emergencies that occur worldwide
- Corporate services that include all of WHO's tools, functions, and resources

WHO provides data, publications, and funding support to researchers across the world (WHO 2015).

Agency for Healthcare Research and Quality

The Agency for Healthcare Research and Quality (AHRQ) is a federal agency within HHS whose mission is to make healthcare safer, higher quality, more accessible, equitable, and affordable, and to work within HHS and with other partners to make sure that the evidence is understood and used. Its priority areas of focus include the following:

- Improving healthcare quality by accelerating implementation of patient-centered outcomes research (PCOR). This priority is being met through the Patient-Centered Outcomes Research Institute (PCORI), which provides funding to researchers to perform research that is patient-centered and patient-engaged. Every research study funded by PCORI must include patients within all aspects of the research methodology process
- Making healthcare safer by preventing healthcare-associated infections (HAI), accelerating patient safety in healthcare organizations, reducing harm associated with obstetrical care, improving safety and reducing medical liability, and accelerating patient safety in nursing homes
- Increasing accessibility to healthcare
- Improving healthcare affordability, efficiency, and cost transparency through improved data measures and public reporting strategies

Similar to the CDC and WHO, AHRQ also provides multiple sources of data, information, funding, and support to researchers in the healthcare sector (AHRQ 2015).

Ethics in Research

Ethics, as discussed in chapter 21, *Ethical Issues in Health Information Management*, are a set of principles used for both understanding and decision-making. In the arena of research, ethics center on the treatment of research participants and the professional actions of the researcher (Johnson and Christensen 2017). "Treatment of research participants is the most important and fundamental issue that researchers confront. Conduct of research with humans has the potential for creating physical and psychological harm" (Johnson and Christensen 2017 128). A key word in this statement is *potential*. Research can be designed and conducted in a way to reduce participant risk. All researchers should have training in how to conduct ethical research. This training should include how to communicate risk to potential participants and how to reduce the potential of risk.

The American Educational Research Association (AERA) has published a code of ethics that outlines the professional competence and responsibilities of researchers (AERA 2018). The first principle is professional competence, which includes researchers understanding their limits and striving to provide an excellent work product (AERA 2011). Additionally, NIH also provides guidance for ethical research. The seven elements per the NIH include validity, informed consent, respect for participants, review of risk-benefit, subject selection, social/clinical worth, and independent assessment (NIH n.d.). After researcher training, the IRB process is a vital element to ensure the planned research is being created and conducted in an ethical manner.

HIM Roles

The roles for HIM professionals in research are evolving. AHIMA provides a career map (https://my.ahima.org/careermap) that highlights career pathways that include aspects of emerging research roles such as provider reimbursement analyst, informatics researcher, and data analytic mapping specialist. For additional information on the AHIMA Career Map, refer to chapter 1, *Health Information Management Profession*. Research can be part of many jobs and roles. Having a research mindset and skill set can be useful in many capacities that are part of various HIM job functions. Roles such as HIM department manager and coding manager can include data collection and analysis, which is part of research.

This evolving change for HIM professionals is also evidenced by the focus of AHIMA Foundation's research journal, *Perspectives in HIM*. This online journal provides an avenue for publishing research related to the HIM field. The objective of this journal is twofold: to provice a way to connect research to the daily functions of HIM professionals and to provide a method to support interprofessional collaboration that will allow for HIM to be a vital element of the healthcare landscape moving forward (Perspectives in Health Information Management n.d.).

Check Your Understanding 13.6

Answer the following questions.

1. Which of the following examines research study plans to determine appropriateness for human subjects?
   a. AHIMA
   b. IRB
   c. NIH
   d. WHO
2. An HIM researcher would most likely be involved in _________ IRB research.
   a. Exempt
   b. Expedited
   c. Full board approval
   d. HIM does not do IRB research
3. This type of research includes those studies that pose only minimal risk to human subjects.
   a. Exempt
   b. Expedited
   c. Full board approval
   d. Clinical trial research
4. Maria Smallwood is an HIM researcher. Maria is seeking data that will allow her to benchmark her healthcare organizations against others in the prevention of disease and injuries. Identify which of the following organizations listed can provide the data Maria is seeking.
   a. ADRQ
   b. AHIMA
   c. CDC
   d. WHO

5. Identify which of the following organizations provides funding for research that is focused on patient engagement and is patient centered.
   a. CDC
   b. HHS
   c. PCORI
   d. WHO

6. The ___________ strives to improve the quality and accessibility of healthcare.
   a. CDC
   b. AHRQ
   c. WHO
   d. HHS

7. The organization whose primary focus is improving healthcare across the world is the:
   a. CDC
   b. WHO
   c. AHRQ
   d. Joint Commission

8. Patients must be involved in the design of the research study if the researcher is to receive funding from which of the following organizations?
   a. PCORI
   b. CDC
   c. WHO
   d. AHA

Real-World Case 13.1

Researchers were interested in assessing the relationship between obesity and breast cancer recurrence and fatality in postmenopausal African-American and Caucasian women with primary breast cancer. Data was collected on women with primary breast cancer and included the following variables:

- Age
- Age at diagnosis of breast cancer
- Weight
- Height
- Data of diagnosis of breast cancer
- Menopausal status
- Diagnosis and coding of tumor (histopathology and topography)
- Stage of tumor
- Size of tumor
- Number of positive lymph nodes
- Estrogen receptor analysis
- Progesterone receptor analysis
- Site of distant metastasis
- First course of treatment (surgery, radiation, chemotherapy)
- Additional treatment
- Five-year recurrence and survival rates

Recurrence and survival status were determined by reviewing the cancer registry follow-up data and health record information across the multiple healthcare sites involved in this study. The cancer registries were accredited by the American College of Surgeons and used active follow-up on all cancer patients. Postmenopausal status was determined as subjects older than 55 years. In subjects younger than age 55, postmenopausal status was determined by consulting the cancer registry data and health records (hospital and physician office). Premenopausal patients and patients whose menopausal status could not be determined from the data were excluded from the study. Body mass index (BMI) was based on height and weight collected from the health record or cancer registry at the date of diagnosis only. Values greater than 27 were considered to indicate obesity. The effect of weight changes during the follow-up period was not evaluated.

Real-World Case 13.2

An HIM Director for a large healthcare network is seeking to increase the HIM budget and add departmental line items for two areas: the employees' annual HIM membership cost and professional development training. The healthcare network is comprised of 3 acute-care hospitals, 30 physician office practices, and 2 rehabilitation centers. There are HIM employees at each hospital and rehab center, and there is a centralized HIM office for the physician practices. In total, there are 50 HIM employees, all with various levels of certification from CCA to RHIA. Currently, the healthcare network does not pay for the annual AHIMA membership cost. Nor does the network provide in-house professional development opportunities for HIM employees. However, the network will only hire HIM staff with credentials and requires that the employees maintain AHIMA's continuing education unit (CEU) requirements. The director has researched information on the cost, the various credentials within the HIM departments for the network, and the needs in terms of professional development for the next fiscal year. The HIM employee composition is the following:

- 50 HIM employees
- 3 with CHDA credential
- 2 with CDIP credential
- 15 with CCS credential
- 20 with RHIT credential
- 10 with RHIA credential
- 30 with more than one credential

References

Agency for Healthcare Research and Quality. 2015. http://www.ahrq.gov/.

American Educational Research Association. 2018. Research Ethics. https://www.aera.net/About-AERA/Key-Programs/Social-Justice/Research-Ethics.

American Educational Research Association. 2011 (February). Code of Ethics. https://www.aera.net/Portals/38/docs/About_AERA/CodeOfEthics(1).pdf.

American Health Information Management Association. 2017. *Pocket Glossary of Health Information Management and Technology*, 5th ed. Chicago: AHIMA.

American Health Information Management Association. 2013. Understanding publicly available healthcare data. *Journal of AHIMA* 84(9): expanded web version. http://library.ahima.org/doc?oid=300183#.VxE-MvkrK9I.

American Psychological Association. 2012. *Publication Manual of the American Psychological Association*, 6th ed. Washington, DC: APA.

Brewer N.T., M.B. Gilkey, S.E. Lillie, B.W. Hesse, and S.L. Sheridan. 2012. Tables or bar graphs? Presenting test results in electronic medical records. *Medical Decision Making* 32(4):545–553.

Centers for Disease Control and Prevention. 2015. http://www.cdc.gov/about/organization/mission.htm.

Centers for Disease Control and Prevention. 2014 (April). Mission, Role and Pledge. https://www.cdc.gov/about/organization/mission.htm.

Centers for Disease Control and Prevention. 2012. *Principles of Epidemiology in Public Health Practice*, 3rd ed. http://www.cdc.gov/ophss/csels/dsepd/ss1978/ss1978.pdf.

Centers for Disease Control and Prevention. 2004. Prevalence of overweight and obesity among adults with diagnosed diabetes–United States, 1988–1994 and 1999–2002. *MMWR Morbidity and Mortality Weekly Report* 53:1066–1068.

Centers for Medicare and Medicaid Services. 2016. National Health Expenditure Data. https://www.cms.gov/Research-Statistics-Data-and-Systems/Statistics-Trends-and-Reports/NationalHealthExpendData/index.html.

Centers for Medicare and Medicaid Services. 2014. Inpatient Prospective Payment System (IPPS) Provider Summary. https://data.cms.gov/Medicare/Inpatient-Prospective-Payment-System-IPPS-Provider/97k6-zzx3.

Creswell, J.W., A.C. Klassen, V.L. Plano Clark, and K.C. Smith for the Office of Behavioral and Social Sciences Research. 2011 (August). *Best Practices for Mixed-Methods Research in the Health Sciences.* https://www2.jabsom.hawaii.edu/native/docs/tsudocs/Best_Practices_for_Mixed_Methods_Research_Aug2011.pdf.

Forrestal, E. J. 2017a. Research Frame and Designs. Chapter 1 in *Health Informatics Research Methods: Principles and Practice,* 2nd ed. Edited by V. Watzlaf and E. J. Forrestal. Chicago: AHIMA Press.

Forrestal, E. J. 2017b. Applied Statistics. Chapter 9 in *Health Informatics Research Methods: Principles and Practice,* 2nd ed. Edited by V. Watzlaf and E. J. Forrestal. Chicago: AHIMA.

Framingham Heart Study. 2015. A Project of the National Heart, Lung and Blood Institute and Boston University. https://www.framinghamheartstudy.org/.

Garvin, J.H., V. Watzlaf, and S. Moeini. 2006. Development and Use of Automated Coding Software to Enhance Anti-fraud Activities. *Perspectives in Health Information Management*, CAC Proceedings. http://library.ahima.org/PdfView?oid=65240.

Grounded Theory Institute. 2014. http://www.groundedtheory.com/what-is-gt.aspx.

Johnson, R. B. and L. Christensen. 2017. *Educational Research: Quantitative, Qualitative, and Mixed Approaches,* 6th ed. Washington, DC: SAGE Publications.

Meza, J.P. 2013. *The Diagnosis Narratives and the Healing Ritual* [dissertation]. Paper 848. Detroit, MI: Wayne State University.

National Institutes of Health. 2015a. ClinicalTrials.gov. https://clinicaltrials.gov/ct2/home.

National Institutes of Health. 2015b. Evaluation of a Stepped Care Approach to Manage Depression in Diabetes, https://clinicaltrials.gov/ct2/show/NCT01812291.

National Institutes of Health. n.d. Guiding Principles for Ethical Research. https://www.nih.gov/health-information/nih-clinical-research-trials-you/guiding-principles-ethical-research.

Perspectives in Health Information Management, n.d. About. https://perspectives.ahima.org/about-the-journal/.

Productivity-Quality Systems. 2015. Pareto Diagram. http://www.pqsystems.com/qualityadvisor/DataAnalysisTools/pareto_diagram.php.

Reed, M., J. Huang, I. Graetz, R. Brand, J. Hsu, B. Fireman, and M. Jaffe. 2012. Outpatient electronic health records and the clinical care and outcomes of patients with diabetes mellitus. *Annals of Internal Medicine* 157(7):482–489.

Sheridan, P., V. Watzlaf, and L. Fox. 2016. HIM Leaders and the practice of leadership through the lens of Bowen theory. *Perspectives in Health Information Management*. Spring.

Watzlaf, V., Z. Alakrawi, S. Meyers, and P. Sheridan. 2015. Physicians' outlook on ICD-10-CM/PCS and its effect on their practice. *Perspectives in Health Information Management.* Winter:1–23.

World Health Organization. 2015. http://www.who.int/en/.

45 CFR 46: Basic HHS policy for protection of human research subjects. 2009.

Healthcare Statistics

Marjorie H. McNeill, PhD, RHIA, CCS, FAHIMA

Learning Objectives

- Explain the meaning of measurement and the data collection process
- Differentiate among nominal-level, ordinal-level, interval-level, and ratio-level data
- Identify various ways in which statistics are used in healthcare
- Explain hospital-related statistical terms
- Calculate hospital-related inpatient and outpatient statistics
- Differentiate between community-based morbidity and mortality rates
- Calculate community-based morbidity and mortality rates
- Calculate the case-mix index
- Calculate ambulatory care statistical data
- Calculate population-based statistics
- Differentiate between incidence and prevalence rates
- Calculate incidence and prevalence rates
- Identify the use of the National Notifiable Diseases Surveillance System

Key Terms

Ambulatory care
Ambulatory surgery center/ambulatory surgical center (ASC)
Average daily census
Average length of stay (ALOS)
Bed count
Bed count day
Bed turnover rate
Case fatality rate
Case mix
Case-mix index (CMI)
Cause-specific mortality rate
Census
Clinic outpatient
Consultation rate
Continuous data
Coroner
Crude birth rate
Crude death/mortality rate
Daily inpatient census
Discrete data
Emergency patient
Encounter
Fetal autopsy rate
Fetal death (stillborn)
Fetal death rate
Gross autopsy rate
Gross death rate
Hospital-acquired (nosocomial) infection rate
Hospital autopsy
Hospital autopsy rate
Hospital death rate
Hospital inpatient
Hospital inpatient autopsy
Hospital newborn inpatient
Hospital outpatient
Incidence rate
Infant mortality rate
Inpatient admission
Inpatient bed occupancy rate (percentage of occupancy)

Inpatient discharge
Inpatient service day (IPSD)
Interval-level data
Length of stay (LOS)
Maternal death rate (hospital based)
Maternal mortality rate (community based)
Measurement
Medical examiner (ME)
National Vital Statistics System (NVSS)
Neonatal mortality rate
Net autopsy rate
Net death rate
Newborn (NB)
Newborn autopsy rate
Newborn death rate
Nominal-level data
Nosocomial (hospital-acquired) infection
Notifiable disease
Occasion of service
Ordinal-level data
Outpatient
Outpatient visit
Population-based statistics
Postneonatal mortality rate
Postoperative infection rate
Prevalence rate
Proportion
Proportionate mortality rate (PMR)
Rate
Ratio
Ratio-level data
Referred outpatient
Scales of measurement
Surgical operation
Surgical procedure
Total length of stay (discharge days)
Vital statistics

Complete and accurate information is at the heart of good decision-making. The health information management (HIM) professional is responsible for ensuring that data collected are accurate and organized into information that is useful to healthcare decision makers.

The primary source of clinical data in a healthcare organization is the health record. To be useful in decision-making, data taken from the health record must be as timely, complete, and accurate as possible. Secondary sources of data are generated by abstracting data from the health record and placing it into an index, registry, or database. Data are compiled in various ways to help make decisions about patient care, the healthcare organization's financial status, and for planning for the future of the healthcare organization. This chapter discusses common statistical measures and types of data used by organizations in different healthcare settings. A discussion of normal distribution and descriptive statistics is given, chapter 13, *Research and Data Analysis,* also covers these topics in more detail.

Before discussing statistical measures used in healthcare, it is important to define measurement and how collected data are classified. **Measurement** refers to the systematic process of data collection, repeated over time or at a single point in time. The process of collecting the data must be consistent in order to ensure the results are the same no matter who is collecting the data. If there is consistency in the data collection, comparisons can be made within and across organizations.

Data collected falls on one of four **scales of measurement**: nominal, ordinal, interval, or ratio. Furthermore, the data collected is described as either continuous or discrete. **Continuous data** are those that represent measurable quantities but are not restricted to certain specified values while **discrete data** represent separate and distinct values or observations. These characteristics influence the type of graphic technique used to display the data and the types of statistical analyses that can be performed. Weight, height, and temperature are examples of continuous data. The number of students in a class and the number of new cancer cases are examples of discrete data.

Nominal-level data fall into groups or categories. This is a scale that measures data by name only. The groups or categories are mutually exclusive; that is, a data element cannot be classified to more than one group. Some examples of nominal data collected in healthcare are related to patient demographics such as mailing address, race, or gender. There is no order to the data collected within these categories.

Data that fall on the ordinal scale have some inherent order, and higher numbers are usually associated with higher values. In **ordinal-level data**, the order of the numbers is meaningful, not the number itself. Staging of Parkinson's disease is an example of a variable that has order. Parkinson's disease is often classified in five stages—with stage I showing mild symptoms, to stage V that takes over a patient's physical movements. In this example, the higher number is associated with the most severe type of symptoms; however, we cannot measure the difference between the levels in exact numerical terms. A Likert scale is often used in this level of measurement. A Likert, or rating, scale is commonly used in questionnaires to gather data. It primarily has five potential choices (strongly agree, agree, neutral, disagree, strongly disagree) but will sometimes include 10 or more (BusinessDictionary.com 2019).

The most important characteristic of interval-level data is that the intervals between successive values are equal. On the Fahrenheit scale, for example, the interval between 20°F and 21°F is the same as between 21°F and 22°F. But because there is no true zero on this scale, it is not appropriate to say that 40°F is twice as warm as 20°F.

In ratio-level data there is a defined unit of measure and a real zero point, and the intervals between successive values are equal. A real zero point means there is an absolute zero. Only when a zero on a scale truly means the total absence of a value can the scale be described as ratio-level. For example, consider the variable length of stay (referring to the time a patient is in a healthcare organization). Length of stay (LOS) has a defined unit of measurement, day, and a real zero point—0 days. Because there is a real zero point, we can state that a LOS of six days is twice as long as a LOS of three days. Multiplication on the ratio scale by a constant does not change its ratio character, but addition of a constant to a ratio measure does. For example, if two days is added to each LOS so that the stays are eight and five days respectively, the ratio of their stays is no longer 2:1. However, if the respective lengths of stay is multiplied by two (for example, 6 × 2 and 3 ×2), the ratio between the two lengths of stay remains 2:1.

Table 14.1 Scales of measurement

Scale of measurement	Examples
Nominal	Name, gender, race
Ordinal	Likert scale (a rating scale), anything that is ordered
Interval	Temperature
Ratio	Age, height, length of stay

Source: © AHIMA.

This fourfold structure is a useful classification for data and the four levels are hierarchically arranged so that higher levels include the key properties of the levels so that ratio-level data include the three key properties found in nominal, ordinal, and interval level data. Table 14.1 lists the scales of measurement and examples.

Discrete versus Continuous Data

Another way to classify data involves categorizing them as either being discrete or continuous. Data that are nominal or ordinal are also considered discrete. Discrete data are finite numbers; that is, they can have only specified values. The number of children in a family is an example of discrete data. A family can have two or three children but cannot have 2.25 or 3.5 children. The numbers represent actual measurable quantities rather than labels.

Other examples of discrete data include the number of motor vehicle crashes in a particular community, the number of times a woman has given birth, the number of new cases of cancer in a state within the past five years, and the number of beds available in a hospital.

In discrete data, a natural order exists among the possible data values. In the example of the number of times a woman has given birth, a larger number indicates that she has had more children; the difference between one and two births is the same as the difference between four and five; and the number of births is restricted to whole numbers (a woman cannot give birth 2.3 times). For the most part, measurements on the nominal and ordinal scales are discrete (Horton 2017).

Continuous variables are either interval or ratio-level, but some ratio-level variables are discrete. Continuous data represent measurable quantities but are not restricted to certain specified values. A variable that is continuous can take on a fractional value. For example, a patient's temperature may be 102.6°F. Another example is height. One could say that someone is approximately 6 feet tall, refine it to 5 feet 10 inches, and refine it still further to 5 feet 10.5 inches. Age is yet another example. A person may have been 20 years old on his or her last birthday, but now the person would be over 20 years some part of another year. Arithmetic operations—addition, subtraction, multiplication, and division—may be performed on continuous variables (Horton 2017).

Check Your Understanding 14.1

Identify the scale of measurement for each of the following variables and indicate whether each variable is discrete (d) or continuous (c).

1. __________ Gender
2. __________ Height
3. __________ Zip code
4. __________ Blood pressure
5. __________ Heart failure classification I, II, III, IV
6. __________ Age
6. __________ Ethnicity
8. __________ Marital status
9. __________ Length of stay
10. __________ Discharge disposition (home, skilled nursing facility [SNF], and such)
11. __________ Weight
12. __________ Level of education
13. __________ Race
14. __________ Temperature in degrees Fahrenheit
15. __________ Types of third-party payers

Common Statistical Measures Used in Healthcare

Healthcare data are collected to describe the health status of groups or populations. The data reported about healthcare organizations and communities describe the occurrence of illnesses, births, and deaths for specific periods of time. Data that are collected may be either facility based or population based. The sources of facility-based statistics are acute-care facilities, long-term care facilities, and other types of healthcare organizations. The population-based statistics are gathered from cities, counties, states, or specific groups within the population, such as individuals affected by diabetes.

Health statistics assist in improving the quality of patient care. Statistics also provide information for important decision-making in the daily operation of a healthcare organization. Statistical data is used by various healthcare professionals, including providers, administrators, department managers, public health officials, researchers, and more. For example, organizations use health statistics to determine patient outcomes, calculate resource utilization, and provide performance data.

Reporting statistics for a healthcare organization is similar to reporting statistics for a community. Rates for healthcare organizations are reported as per 100 cases or percent; a community rate is reported as per 1,000, 10,000, or 100,000 people. For example, if a hospital experienced 4 deaths in a given month and 100 patients were discharged in the same month, the death rate would be 4 percent ([4 × 100]/100). If there were 400 deaths in a community of 80,000 for a given period of time, the death rate would be reported as 50 deaths per 10,000 population ([400 × 10,000]/80,000) for the same period of time. The following terms are common for the HIM professional to use in determining statistics.

Three Common Examples of Ratio-Level Data: Ratios, Proportions, and Rates

Many healthcare statistics are reported in the form of a ratio, proportion, or rate. A ratio is a calculation that compares two quantities found by dividing one quantity by another. A proportion is the relation of one part to another or to the whole with respect to magnitude, quantity, or degree. A rate is a measure used to compare an event over time.

These measures are used to report morbidity (illness), mortality (death), and natality (birth) at the local, state, national, and international levels. These measures indicate the number of times something happened relative to the number of times it could have happened. All three measures are based on formula 14.1.

Formula 14.1 General formula for calculating rates, proportions, and ratios

The following list of equations differentiates among ratio, proportion, percentage, and rate, where $x = 5$ men and $y = 3$ women.

Ratio: $$\frac{x}{y} = \frac{5}{3}$$

Proportion: $$\frac{x}{(x+y)} = \frac{5}{(5+3)}$$

Rate: $$R = \frac{Part}{Base}, \text{ or } R = \frac{P}{B}$$

Ratio

In a ratio, two quantities are compared, such as patient discharge status (x = alive, y = dead), and may be expressed so that x and y are completely independent of each other, or x may be included in y. For example, the outcomes of patients discharged from Community Hospital are compared in one of two ways:

Alive/dead, or x/y

Alive/(alive + dead), or $x/(x/y)$

In the first example, x is completely independent of y. The ratio represents the number of patients discharged alive compared to the number of patients who died. If 10 patients died and 90 patients were discharged alive, the ratio of deaths to live discharges is written as 10:90 and verbalized as 10 to 90. In the second example, x is part of the whole ($x + y$). The ratio represents the number of patients discharged alive compared to all patients discharged. This is written as 10:100. Both expressions are considered ratios.

Proportion

A proportion is a type of ratio in which x is a portion of the whole ($x + y$). In a proportion, the numerator is always included in the denominator. For example, if 4 males out of a group of 24 have had prostate cancer, where x = 4 (males who have had prostate cancer) and y = 20 (males who have not had prostate cancer), the calculation would be 4 divided by 24 (20 + 4) or 4/24. The proportion of males who have had prostate cancer is 0.1666 = 0.17. Figure 14.1 describes the procedure for calculating ratios and figure 14.2 describes the procedures for calculating proportions.

Rate

Rates are often used to measure events over a period of time. Rates are commonly expressed as a percentage and therefore should include the percent (%) sign after the number value.

Like ratios and proportions, rates may be reported daily, weekly, monthly, or yearly. This allows for trend analysis and comparisons over time. The basic formula for calculating a rate is

$$\frac{\text{number of times something happened}}{\text{number of times it would have happened}} \times 100$$

Figure 14.1 Calculation of a ratio; discharge status of patients discharged in a month

1. Define x and y:
   x = number of patients discharged alive
   y = number of patients who died
2. Identify x and y:
   $x = 250$
   $y = 20$
3. Set up the ratio x/y:
   250/20
4. Reduce the fraction so that either x or y equals 1:
   12.5/1

There were 12.5 live discharges for every patient who died.

Source: © AHIMA.

Figure 14.2 Calculation of a proportion; discharge status of patients discharged in a month

1. Define *x* and *y*:
   x = number of patients discharged alive
   y = number of patients who died
2. Identify *x* and *y*:
   x = 250
   y = 20
3. Set up the ratio *x*/(*x* + *y*):
   250/(250 + 20) = 250/270
4. Reduce the fraction so that either *x* or *y* equals 1:
   0.93/1

The proportion of patients discharged alive was 0.93.

Source: © AHIMA.

When multiplying by 100, the decimal point is in the correct place to be expressed as a percentage. There is a big difference between the values 0.123 percent (not multiplied by 100) and 1.23 percent.

Healthcare organizations calculate many types of morbidity and mortality rates. For example, the cesarean-section (C-section) rate is a measure of the proportion, or percentage, of C-sections performed during a given period of time. C-section rates are closely monitored because they present more risk to the mother and infant and because they are more expensive than vaginal deliveries. In calculating the C-section rate, the number of C-sections performed during the specified period of time is counted and this value is placed in the numerator. The number of cases, or the population at risk, is the number of women who delivered during the same time period. This number is placed in the denominator. By convention, inpatient hospital rates are reported as the rate per 100 cases and are expressed as percentages. The formula for calculating the risk of contracting a disease is shown in formula 14.2.

Formula 14.2 Calculating risk for contracting a disease

$$\text{Risk rate} = \frac{\text{Number of cases occurring during a given time period}}{\text{Total number of cases or population at risk during the same time period}}$$

Figure 14.3 shows the procedure for calculating a rate. In the example, 45 of the 705 deliveries at University Hospital during the month of June were C-sections. In the formula, the numerator is the number of C-sections performed in June (the given period of time) and the denominator is the total number of deliveries including C-sections (the population at risk) performed within the same time frame. In calculating the rate, the numerator is always included in the denominator. Also, when calculating a facility-based rate, the numerator is first multiplied by 100, and then divided by the denominator.

Figure 14.3 Calculation of a rate; C-section rate for June 20XX

During June, 705 women delivered; of these, 45 deliveries were by C-section. What is the C-section rate for June at University Hospital?

1. Define the numerator (number of times an event occurred) and the denominator (number of times an event could have occurred):
   Numerator = total number of C-sections performed during the time period
   Denominator = total number of deliveries, including C-sections, in the same time period
2. Identify the numerator and the denominator:
   Numerator = 45
   Denominator = 705
3. Set up the rate:
   45/705
4. Multiply the numerator by 100 and then divide by the denominator:
   ([45 × 100]/705) = 6.38%

The C-section rate for June is 6.438 percent.

Source: © AHIMA.

Because hospital rates rarely result in a whole number, they are usually rounded. The hospital should set a policy on whether rates are to be reported to one or two decimal places. Before rounding, the division should be carried out to at least one more decimal place than desired.

When rounding, if the last number is five or greater, the preceding number should be increased one digit. In contrast, if the last number is less than five, the preceding number remains the same. For example, in figure 14.3, when rounding 6.38 percent to one decimal place, the rate becomes 6.4 percent because the last number is greater than five. When rounding, for example, 2.563 percent to two places, the rate becomes 2.56 percent because the last digit is less than five. Rates of less than 1 percent are usually carried out to three decimal places and rounded to two. For rates less than 1 percent, a zero should precede the decimal to emphasize that the rate is less than 1 percent; for example, 0.56 percent.

Check Your Understanding 14.2

Indicate if the statement represents a rate, a ratio, or a proportion.

1. In a study of acute myocardial infarction, there were seven males to nine females.
2. In many healthcare insurance policies, the insurance company covers 0.80 of the amount.
3. Medicare admissions outnumber commercial insurance admissions three to two.
4. At the annual state HIM meeting, 85 of the registrants were female and 35 were male. Therefore, 0.71 percent of the registrants were female.
5. Of the 250 patients admitted in the past six months, 36 percent had type 2 diabetes mellitus.

Acute-Care Statistical Data

In the daily operations of any organization, whether in business, industry, or healthcare, data are collected for decision-making. To be effective, the decision makers must have confidence in the data collected. Confidence requires that the data collected be accurate, reliable, and timely. The types of data collected in the acute-care setting are discussed in the following sections.

Administrative Statistical Data

Hospitals collect data on inpatients and outpatients on a daily basis. Hospitals use these statistics to monitor the volume of patients treated daily, weekly, monthly, annually, or within some other specified time frame. The statistics give healthcare decision makers the information needed to plan healthcare organizations and services and to monitor inpatient and outpatient revenue streams. For these reasons, the HIM professional must be well versed in data collection, reporting, and analysis methods.

Standard definitions have been developed to ensure all healthcare providers collect and report data in a consistent manner. The *Pocket Glossary of Health Information Management and Technology*, currently in its 5th edition, developed by the American Health Information Management Association (AHIMA), is a resource commonly used to describe the types of healthcare events for which data are collected. It includes definitions of terms related to healthcare organizations, health maintenance organizations (HMOs), and other health-related programs and facilities and emerging HIM and health information technology (HIT) topics. The following terms and definitions will be used in this chapter:

Term	Description
Hospital inpatient	• A patient who is provided with room, board, and continuous general nursing service in an area of an acute-care hospital where patients generally stay at least overnight
Hospital outpatient	• A hospital patient who receives services in one or more of the hospital's facilities when he or she is not currently an inpatient or home care patient • An outpatient who is classified as either an emergency patient or a clinic outpatient • An emergency patient who is admitted to the emergency services department of a hospital for the diagnosis and treatment of a condition that requires immediate medical, dental, or allied health services to sustain life or to prevent critical consequences • A clinic outpatient who is a patient admitted to a clinical service of a clinic or hospital for diagnosis and treatment on an ambulatory basis

continued

Term	Description
Hospital newborn inpatient	• A patient who is born in the hospital at the beginning of the current inpatient hospitalization • Newborns who are usually counted separately because their care is very different from that of other inpatients • Infants who are born on the way to the hospital or at home and later admitted to a hospital are considered hospital inpatients, not hospital newborn inpatients
Inpatient admission	• An acute-care hospital's formal acceptance of a patient who is to be provided with room, board, and continuous nursing service in an area of the healthcare organization where patients generally stay at least overnight
Inpatient discharge	• The termination of hospitalization through the formal release of an inpatient by the hospital • Patients who are discharged alive (by physician's order) who are discharged against medical advice (AMA), or who died while hospitalized Unless otherwise directed by your healthcare organization's administration, inpatient discharges include deaths

Source: © AHIMA 2017

Inpatient Census Data

The HIM professional is responsible for verifying the census data that are collected daily. The census reports patient activity for a 24-hour reporting period. Included in the census report is the number of inpatients admitted and discharged for the previous 24-hour period as well as the number of intra-hospital transfers. An intra-hospital transfer is a patient who is moved from one patient care unit to another (for example, a patient may be transferred from the intensive care unit [ICU] to the medicine unit). The usual 24-hour reporting period begins at 12:01 a.m. and ends at 12:00 midnight. In the census count, adults and children (A&C) are reported separately from newborns.

Before compiling census data, however, it is important to understand the related terminology. The census is the number of hospital inpatients present in a hospital at any given time. For example, the census in a 300-bed hospital may be 250 patients at 2:00 p.m. on June 1, but 245 patients an hour later. Because the census may change throughout the day as admissions and discharges occur, hospitals designate an official census-taking time. In most healthcare organizations, the official count takes place at midnight. The census-reporting time can be any other time, but it must be consistent throughout the healthcare organization and occur at the same time each day.

The result of the official count taken at midnight is called the daily inpatient census. This is the number of inpatients present at the census-taking time each day plus any patients who were admitted and discharged that same day. For example, if a patient was admitted to the ICU at 1:00 p.m. on June 1 and died at 4.00 p.m. on the same day, he would be counted as a patient who was both admitted and discharged on the same day. Most healthcare organizations have a census-taking policy that outlines the process for census reporting and tracking.

Because patients admitted and discharged on the same day may not be present at the census-taking time, hospitals must account for them separately. If they did not, credit for the services provided to these patients would be lost. The daily inpatient census reflects the total number of patients treated during the 24-hour period. Figure 14.4 displays a sample daily inpatient census report.

A unit of measure that reflects the services received by one inpatient during a 24-hour period is called an inpatient service day (IPSD). The number of IPSDs for a 24-hour period is equal to the daily inpatient census; that is, one service day for each patient treated. In figure 14.4, the total number of inpatient service days for June 2 is 260.

Figure 14.4 Daily inpatient census report—A&C

June 2	
Number of patients in hospital at midnight, June 1	250
+ Number of patients admitted June 2	+40
– Number of patients discharged, including deaths, June 2	–35
Number of patients in hospital at midnight, June 2	255
+ Number of patients both admitted and discharged, including deaths	+5
Daily inpatient census at midnight, June 2	260
Total inpatient service days, June 2	260

Source: © AHIMA.

Table 14.2 Number of IPSDs

Day	Census	Same day admissions and discharges	Inpatient service days
Day 1	250	0	250
Day 2	255	0	255
Day 3	240	2	242
Total			**747**

Source: © AHIMA.

IPSDs are compiled daily, weekly, monthly, and annually. They reflect the volume of services provided by the healthcare organization—the greater the volume of services, the greater the revenues to the healthcare organization. Daily reporting of the number of IPSDs is an indicator of the healthcare organization's financial condition.

As mentioned, the daily inpatient census is equal to the number of IPSDs provided for that day as shown in table 14.2.

The total number of IPSDs for a week, a month, and so on can be divided by the total number of days in the period of interest to obtain the average daily census. Referring to table 14.2, 747 IPSDs is divided by three days to obtain an average daily census of 249. The average daily census is the average number of inpatients treated during a given period of time. The general formula for calculating the average daily census is shown in formula 14.3.

In calculating the average daily census, A&C and newborns (NB) are reported separately. This is because the intensity of services provided to adults and children is greater than it is for newborns. To calculate the A&C average daily census, the general formula is modified as shown in formula 14.4. Many healthcare organizations use a whole number when reporting the census.

Formula 14.3 Calculating the average daily census

$$\text{Average daily census} = \frac{\text{Total number of inpatient service days for a given period}}{\text{Total number of days in the same time period}}$$

Formula 14.4. Calculating the average daily census for adults and children

$$\text{Average daily census for A\&C} = \frac{\text{Total number of inpatient service days for A\&C for a given period}}{\text{Total number of days in the same time period}}$$

The formula for calculating the average daily census for newborns is shown in formula 14.5. For example, the total number of IPSDs provided to adults and children for the week of June 1 is 1,825, and the total for newborns is 125. Using the formulas, the average daily census for adults and children is 261 (1,825/7) and for newborns it is 18 (125/7). Notice that the answer to the newborn average daily census was 17.9 but using the standard practice of reporting census information as a whole number, the figure reported would be 18. The average daily census for all hospital inpatients for the week of June 1 is 278.6 or 279 ([1,825 + 125]/7). Table 14.3 compares the various formulas for calculating the average daily census.

Formula 14.5 Calculating the average daily census for newborns

$$\text{Average daily census for NBs} = \frac{\text{Total number of inpatient service days for NBs for a given period}}{\text{Total number of days in the same time period}}$$

Table 14.3 Calculation of census statistics

Indicator	Numerator	Denominator
Average daily inpatient census	Total number of inpatient service days for a given period	Total number of days for the same period
Average daily inpatient census for adults and children (A&C)	Total number of inpatient service days for A&C for a given period	Total number of days for the same period
Average daily inpatient census for newborns (NBs)	Total number of inpatient service days for NBs for a given period	Total number of days for the same period

Source: © AHIMA.

Check Your Understanding 14.3

Answer the following questions.

1. Community Hospital reported the following statistics for their newborn unit at 12:01 a.m. June 1: Census 10; Births 5; Discharges 3; 1 Newborn born and transferred to University Hospital. Calculate the following for June 2:
   a. Inpatient census
   b. Daily inpatient census
2. Community Hospital reported the following statistics for their intensive care unit at 12:01 a.m. June 1: Census 12; 1 patient admitted directly from the Emergency Services Department (ESD); 1 patient transferred from the surgery unit; 1 patient transferred from the medicine unit; 1 patient transferred to the medicine unit; 1 patient admitted and died the same day. Calculate the following for June 2:
   a. Inpatient census
   b. Daily inpatient census
3. Community Hospital reported the following statistics for adults and children at 12:01 a.m. April 1: Census 160; Admissions 20; Discharges 15; 1 patient admitted and died the same day; 1 patient admitted and discharged alive the same day. Calculate the following for April 2:
   a. Inpatient census
   b. Daily inpatient census
   c. Inpatient service days

Inpatient Bed Occupancy Rate

Another indicator of the hospital's financial position is the **inpatient bed occupancy rate**, also called the percentage of occupancy. The inpatient bed occupancy rate is the percentage of official beds occupied by hospital inpatients for a given period of time. In general, the greater the occupancy rate, the greater the revenues for the hospital. For a bed to be included in the official count, it must be set up, staffed, equipped, and available for patient care. The total number of inpatient service days is used in the numerator because it is equal to the daily inpatient census or the number of patients treated daily. The occupancy rate compares the number of patients treated over a given period of time to the total number of beds available for the same period of time.

For example, if 250 patients occupied 300 beds on June 2, the inpatient bed occupancy rate would be 83.3 percent ([250/{300 × 1}] × 100). If the rate were for more than one day, the number of beds would be multiplied by the number of days within that particular time frame. For example, if 1,830 IPSDs were provided during the week of June 1 in the same hospital, the inpatient bed occupancy rate for that week would be 87.1 percent ([1,830/{300 × 7}] × 100).

The denominator in this formula is actually the total possible number of inpatient service days. That is, if every available bed in the hospital were occupied every single day, this would be the maximum number of IPSDs that could be provided. The IPSDs are based on the bed count. The **bed count** is the number beds available in the hospital that have the staff and resources necessary to care for patients at any given point in time. This is an important concept, especially if the official bed count changes for a given reporting period. For example, if the bed count changed from 300 beds to 310, the bed occupancy rate would reflect the change. The total number of inpatient beds times the total number of days in the period is called the total number of **bed count days**. The general formula for the inpatient bed occupancy rate is shown in formula 14.6.

Formula 14.6 Calculating the inpatient bed occupancy rate

$$\text{Inpatient bed occupancy rate} = \frac{\text{Total number of inpatient service days for a given period}}{\text{Total number of inpatient bed count days for the same period}} \times 10$$

What happens when the bed count changes? For example, the bed count changed on June 20 from 300 beds to 310 beds and the total number of inpatient service days provided was 8,327. To calculate the inpatient bed occupancy rate for June, the total number of bed count days must be determined. There are 30 days in June; therefore, the total number of bed count days is calculated as:

$$\text{Number of beds, June 1-June 19} = 300 \times 19 \text{ days}$$
$$= 5{,}700 \text{ bed count days}$$
$$\text{Number of beds, June 20-June 30} = 310 \times 11 \text{ days}$$
$$= 3{,}410 \text{ bed count days}$$
$$5{,}700 + 3{,}410 = 9{,}110 \text{ bed count days}$$

The inpatient bed occupancy rate for the month of June is 91.4 percent ([8,327/9,110] × 100).

As with the average daily census, the inpatient bed occupancy rate for adults and children is reported separately from that of newborns. To calculate the total number of bed count days for newborns, the official count for newborn bassinets is used. Table 14.4 reviews the formulas for calculating inpatient bed occupancy rates.

It is possible for the inpatient bed occupancy rate to be greater than 100 percent. This occurs when the hospital faces an epidemic or disaster. In this type of situation, hospitals set up temporary beds that usually are not included in the official bed count. As an example, Community Hospital experienced an excessive number of admissions in December because of an outbreak of pneumonia. In December, the official bed count was 125 beds. On December 5, the daily inpatient census was 135. Therefore, the inpatient bed occupancy rate for December 5 was 108 percent ([135/125] × 100).

Table 14.4 Calculation of inpatient bed occupancy

Rate	Numerator	Denominator
Inpatient bed occupancy rate	Total number of inpatient service days for a given period × 100	Total number of inpatient bed count days for the same period
Inpatient bed occupancy rate for adults and children (A&C)	Total number of inpatient service days for A&C for a given period × 100	Total number of inpatient bed count days for A&C for the same period
Newborn (NB) bed occupancy rate	Total number of NB inpatient service days for a given period × 100	Total number of bassinet bed count days for the same period

Source: © AHIMA.

Bed Turnover Rate

The bed turnover rate is a measure of hospital utilization. It includes the number of times each hospital bed changed occupants. The formula for the bed turnover rate is shown in formula 14.7. For example, Community Hospital had 2,120 discharges and deaths for the month of October. Its bed count for October averaged 700. The bed turnover rate is 3.1 (2,120/700). This simply means that on average, each hospital bed had three occupants during October.

Formula 14.7 Calculating the bed turnover rate

$$\text{Bed turnover rate} = \frac{\text{Total number of discharges, including deaths, for a given period}}{\text{Average bed count for the same time period}}$$

Check Your Understanding 14.4

Answer the following questions.

1. On July 1, Community Hospital expanded the number of patient beds from 165 to 200. Use the following information in table 14.6 to determine the inpatient bed occupancy rate for January to June; July to December; and the total for the year (non-leap year).
2. Fill in table 14.5 with the inpatient bed occupancy rate for each of the following patient care units at Community Hospital for the month of September. Calculate to one decimal point.
3. Use the information in table 14.5 to determine the inpatient bed occupancy rate for Community Hospital—all A&C (exclude newborns). Calculate to one decimal point.

Table 14.5 Community Hospital occupancy rate for September

Inpatient unit	Service days	Bed count	Occupancy rate
Medicine	680	38	
Surgery	790	37	
Pediatric	235	20	
Psychiatry	927	40	
Obstetrics	252	12	
Newborn	252	16	

Source: © AHIMA.

Table 14.6 Community Hospital number of service days and bed count

Months	Service days	Bed count
January–June	25,720	165
July–December	27,852	200

Source: © AHIMA.

Length of Stay Data

LOS data is calculated for each patient after he or she is discharged from the hospital. It is the number of calendar days from the day of patient admission to the day of patient discharge. When the patient is admitted and discharged in the same month, the LOS is determined by subtracting the date of admission from the date of discharge. For example, the LOS for a patient admitted on June 12 and discharged on June 17 is five days (17 – 12 = 5).

When the patient is admitted in one month and discharged in another, the calculations must be adjusted. One way to calculate the LOS in this case is to subtract the date of admission from the total number of days in the month the patient was admitted and then add the total number of hospitalized days for the month in which the patient was discharged. For example, the LOS for a patient admitted on June 28 and discharged on July 6 is eight days ([June 30 – June 28 = two days] and [July 1 – July 6 = 6 days]; LOS = 8 days).

When a patient is admitted and discharged on the same day, the LOS is one day. A partial day's stay is never reported as a fraction of a day. The LOS for a patient discharged the day after admission also is one day. Thus, the LOS for a patient who was admitted to the ICU on June 10 at 9:00 a.m. and died at 3:00 p.m. on the same day is one day. Likewise, the LOS for a patient admitted on June 12 and discharged on June 13 is one day.

Table 14.7 Length of stay for five patients discharged June 9

Patient	LOS
1	3
2	7
3	2
4	1
5	19
Total	**32**

Source: © AHIMA.

When the LOS for all patients discharged for a given period of time is summed, the result is the **total length of stay (discharge days)**. As an example, five patients were discharged from the pediatric unit on June 9. The LOS for each patient was as follows in table 14.7.

In the preceding example, the total LOS is 32 days (3 + 7 + 2 + 1 + 19). The total LOS is also referred to as the number of days of care provided to patients who were discharged or died (discharge days) during a given period of time.

The average length of stay (ALOS) is calculated from the total LOS. The total LOS divided by the number of patients discharged is the ALOS. Using the data in the preceding example, the ALOS for the five patients discharged from the pediatric unit on June 9 is 6.4 days (32/5).

The general formula for calculating ALOS is shown in formula 14.8. As with the measures already discussed, the ALOS for adults and children is reported separately from the ALOS for newborns. Table 14.8 reviews the formulas for ALOS. Table 14.9 displays an example of a hospital statistical summary prepared by the HIM department using census and discharge data.

Formula 14.8 Calculating the average length of stay

$$\text{Average length of stay} = \frac{\text{Total length of stay for a given period}}{\text{Total number of discharges, including deaths, for the same period}}$$

Table 14.8 Calculation of LOS statistics

Indicator	Numerator	Denominator
Average LOS	Total length of stay (discharge days) for a given period	Total number of discharges, including deaths, for the same period
Average LOS for adults and children (A&C)	Total length of stay for A&C (discharge days) for a given period	Total number of discharges, including deaths, for A&C for the same period
Average LOS for newborns (NB)	Total length of stay for all NB (discharge days) for a given period	Total number of NB discharges, including deaths, for the same period

Source: © AHIMA.

Table 14.9 Statistical summary, Community Hospital, for the period ending July 20XX

	July 20XX		Year-to-Date 20XX	
Admissions	**Actual**	**Budget**	**Actual**	**Budget**
Medicine	728	769	5,075	5,082
Surgery	578	583	3,964	3,964
OB/GYN	402	440	2,839	3,027
Psychiatry	113	99	818	711
Physical medicine and rehab	48	57	380	384
Other adult	191	178	1,209	1,212
Total adult	2,060	2,126	14,285	14,380
Newborn	294	312	2,143	2,195
Total admissions	**2,354**	**2,438**	**16,428**	**16,575**
	July 20XX		**Year-to-Date 20XX**	
Average length of stay	**Actual**	**Budget**	**Actual**	**Budget**
Medical	6.1	6.4	6.0	6.1
Surgical	7.0	7.2	7.7	7.7
OB/GYN	2.9	3.2	3.5	3.1
Psychiatry	10.8	11.6	10.4	11.6
Physical medicine and rehab	27.5	23.0	28.1	24.3
Other adult	3.6	3.9	4.0	4.1
Total adult	6.3	6.4	6.7	6.5
Newborn	5.6	5.0	5.6	5.0
Total ALOS	**6.2**	**6.3**	**6.5**	**6.3**

continued

Table 14.9 Statistical summary, Community Hospital, for the period ending July 20XX *(continued)*

	July 20XX		Year-to-Date 20XX	
Patient Days	**Actual**	**Budget**	**Actual**	**Budget**
Medical	4,436	4,915	30,654	30,762
Surgical	4,036	4,215	30,381	30,331
OB/GYN	1,170	1,417	10,051	9,442
Psychiatry	1,223	1,144	8,524	8,242
Physical medicine and rehab	1,318	1,310	10,672	9,338
Other adult	688	699	4,858	4,921
Total adult	12,871	13,700	95,140	93,036
Newborn	1,633	1,552	12,015	10,963
Total patient days	**14,504**	**15,252**	**107,155**	**103,999**
	July 20XX		**Year-to-Date 20XX**	
Other key statistics	**Actual**	**Budget**	**Actual**	**Budget**
Average daily census	485	482	498	486
Average beds available	677	660	677	660
Clinic visits	21,621	18,975	144,271	136,513
Emergency visits	3,822	3,688	26,262	25,604
Inpatient surgery patients	657	583	4,546	4,093
Outpatient surgery patients	603	554	4,457	3,987

Source: © AHIMA.

Check Your Understanding 14.5

Use the data provided for patient discharges in table 14.10 to answer the questions that follow. Round to two decimal points.

Table 14.10 Patient discharges

Day	Number of patients discharged	Discharge days
September 1	10	82
September 2	12	75
September 3	17	68
September 4	8	153
September 5	9	43
September 6	11	101
September 7	18	77
September 8	12	93
September 9	13	42
September 10	15	97

Source: © AHIMA.

1. Calculate the number of patients discharged.
2. Calculate the total length of stay.
3. Calculate the average length of stay.
4. Calculate the ALOS for September 10th.
5. Calculate the ALOS for September 1st to (and including) September 5th.

Patient Care and Clinical Statistical Data

The collection of data related to morbidity and mortality is an important aspect of evaluating the quality of hospital services. Morbidity and mortality rates are reported for all patient discharges within a certain time frame. They also may be reported by service or by physician or other variable of interest to identify trends, issues, or opportunities for improvement that may require corrective action. The most frequently collected morbidity and mortality rates are presented in this section.

Hospital Death (Mortality) Rates

The hospital death rate is based on the number of patients discharged, alive and dead, from the hospital. Deaths are considered discharges because they are the end point of a period of hospitalization. In contrast to the rates discussed in the preceding section, newborns are not counted separately from adults and children. The following sections discuss the different statistics for death including gross, net, newborn, fetal, and maternal death rates.

Gross Death Rate

The gross death rate is the proportion of all hospital discharges that ended in death. It is the basic indicator of mortality in a healthcare organization. The gross death rate is calculated by dividing the total number of deaths occurring in a given time period by the total number of discharges, including deaths, for the same time period. The formula for calculating the gross death rate is shown in formula 14.9.

Formula 14.9 Calculating the gross death rate

$$\text{Gross death rate} = \frac{\text{Total number of inpatient deaths, including NBs, for a given period} \times 100}{\text{Total number of discharges, including A\&C and NB deaths, for the same period}}$$

As an example, Community Hospital experienced 15 deaths (A&C and NBs) during the month of June. There were 278 total discharges, including deaths. The gross death rate is 5.4 percent ([15/278] × 100).

Net Death Rate

The net death rate is an adjusted death rate. It is calculated with the assumption that certain deaths should not count against the hospital. The net death rate is an adjusted rate because it does not include patients who die within 48 hours of admission. The reason for excluding these deaths is that historically it has been believed that 48 hours is not enough time to positively affect patient outcome. In other words, the patient was not admitted to the hospital in a manner timely enough for treatment to have an effect on his or her outcome. The formula for calculating the net death rate is shown in formula 14.10.

Formula 14.10 Calculating the net death rate

$$\text{Net death rate} = \frac{\text{Total number of inpatient deaths, including NBs, minus deaths} < 48 \text{ hours for a given period}}{\text{Total number of discharges, including A \& C and NB deaths, minus deaths} < 48 \text{ hours for the same period}} \times 100$$

Continuing with the preceding example of the 15 patients who died at Community Hospital in June, three died within 48 hours of admission. Therefore, the net death rate is 4.4 percent ([{15 – 3}/{278 – 3}] × 100). The fact that the net death rate is less than the gross death rate is favorable to Community Hospital because lower death rates may be an indicator of better care.

Newborn Death Rate

Even though newborn deaths are included in the hospital's gross and net death rates, the newborn death rate is often calculated separately. Newborns include only infants born alive in the hospital. The newborn death rate is the number of newborns who died in comparison to the total number of newborns discharged, alive and dead. To qualify as a newborn death, the newborn must have been delivered alive. A stillborn infant is not included in either the newborn death rate or the gross or net death rate. The formula for calculating the newborn death rate is shown in formula 14.11.

Formula 14.11 Calculating the newborn death rate

$$\text{Newborn death rate} = \frac{\text{Total number of NB deaths for a given period}}{\text{Total number of NB discharges, including deaths, for the same period}} \times 100$$

For example, Community Hospital experienced three newborn deaths during the month of June. There were 47 newborn discharges (including these three deaths). The newborn death rate is 6.4 percent ([3/47] × 100).

Fetal Death Rate

In healthcare terminology, the death of a stillborn infant is called a fetal death. A fetal death is defined as a fetus who is spontaneously expelled from the uterus at any time during the pregnancy. Fetal death more commonly occurs later in pregnancy- usually at 20 weeks of gestation or more. Thus, fetal deaths are neither admitted nor discharged from the hospital. A fetal death occurs when the fetus fails to breathe or show any other evidence of life, such as a heartbeat, a pulsation of the umbilical cord, or a movement of the voluntary muscles.

Fetal deaths also are classified into categories based on length of gestation or weight (see table 14.11). To calculate the fetal death rate, divide the total number of intermediate and late fetal deaths for the period by the total number of live births and intermediate and late fetal deaths for the same period. The formula for calculating the fetal death rate is shown in formula 14.12. For example, during the month of June, Community Hospital experienced 97 live births and 3 intermediate and 2 late fetal deaths. The fetal death rate is 4.9 percent ([{3 + 2}/{97 + 3 + 2}] × 100).

Table 14.11 Classifications of fetal death

Classification	Length of gestation	Weight
Early fetal death	Less than 20 weeks	500 g or less
Intermediate fetal death	20 weeks completed, but less than 28 weeks	501 to 1,000 g
Late fetal death	28 weeks completed	Over 1,000 g

Source: © AHIMA.

Formula 14.12 Calculating the fetal death rate

$$\text{Fetal death rate} = \frac{\text{Total number of intermediate and late fetal deaths for a given period}}{\text{Total number of live births plus total number of intermediate and late fetal deaths for the same period}} \times 100$$

Maternal Death Rate

Hospitals are also interested in calculating maternal death rates (hospital based). A maternal death is the death of any woman from any cause related to, or aggravated by, pregnancy or its management, regardless of the duration or site of the pregnancy. Maternal deaths that result from accidental or incidental causes are not included in the maternal death rate.

Maternal deaths are classified as either direct or indirect. A direct maternal death is the death of a woman resulting from obstetrical (OB) complications of the pregnancy, labor, or puerperium (the period including the six weeks after delivery). Direct maternal deaths are included in the maternal death rate. An indirect maternal death is the death of a woman from a previously existing disease or a disease that developed during pregnancy, labor, or the puerperium that was not due to obstetric causes, although the physiological effects of pregnancy were partially responsible.

The maternal death rate may be an indicator of the availability of prenatal care in a community. The hospital also may use it to help identify conditions that could lead to a maternal death. The formula for calculating the maternal death rate is shown in formula 14.13. For example, during the month of June, Community Hospital experienced 150 maternal discharges. Two of these patients died. The maternal death rate for June is 1.33 percent ([2/150] × 100). Table 14.12 summarizes hospital-based mortality rates.

Formula 14.13 Calculating the maternal death rate

$$\text{Maternal death rate} = \frac{\text{Total number of direct maternal deaths for a given period}}{\text{Total number of maternal (OB) discharges, including deaths, for same period}} \times 100$$

Table 14.12 Calculation of hospital-based mortality rates

Rate	Numerator (*x*)	Denominator (*y*)
Gross death rate	Total number of inpatient deaths, including NBs, for a given period × 100	Total number of discharges, including A&C and NB deaths, for the same period
Net death rate (institutional death rate)	Total number of inpatient deaths, including NBs, minus deaths <48 hours for a given period × 100	Total number of discharges, including A&C and NB deaths, minus deaths <48 hours for the same period
Newborn death rate	Total number of NB deaths for a given period × 100	Total number of NB discharges, including deaths, for the same period
Fetal death rate	Total number of intermediate and late fetal deaths for a given period × 100	Total number of live births plus total number of intermediate and late fetal deaths for the same period
Maternal death rate	Total number of direct maternal deaths for a given period × 100	Total number of maternal (obstetric) discharges, including deaths, for the same period
Infant death rate	Number of deaths under one year of age during a given time period	Number of live births during the same time period

Source: © AHIMA.

Check Your Understanding 14.6

Use the data provided on deaths and discharges at Community Hospital for the past calendar year in table 14.13 to answer the questions that follow. Round to two decimal points.

Table 14.13 Community Hospital death and discharge data

Type of death or discharge	Total
Total discharges, including deaths (A&C)	2,703
Total deaths (A&C)	43
Deaths less than 48 hours after admission (A&C)	2
Fetal deaths (intermediate and late)	5
Live births	175
Newborn deaths	1
Newborn discharges, including deaths	175
Maternal deaths (direct)	1
OB discharges, including deaths	175

Source: © AHIMA.

1. Calculate the gross death rate for adults and children.
2. Calculate the gross death rate for adults and children and newborns combined.
3. Calculate the net death rate for adults and children.
4. Calculate the net death rate for adults and children and newborns combined.
5. Calculate the newborn death rate.
6. Calculate the fetal death rate.
7. Calculate the maternal death rate (direct).

Autopsy Rates

An autopsy is the postmortem (after death) examination of the organs and tissues of a body to determine the cause of death or pathological conditions, also known as a postmortem examination or necropsy examination. An autopsy is a powerful tool for medical or legal purposes. The postmortem examination can establish the cause and manner of death and can determine whether disease or injury was present at the time of death. In addition, the autopsy can alert family members to conditions or diseases for which they may be at risk.

Two categories of hospital autopsies are conducted in acute-care hospitals: hospital inpatient autopsies and hospital autopsies. A **hospital inpatient autopsy** is an examination performed on the body of a patient who died during an inpatient hospitalization by a hospital pathologist or a physician of the medical staff who has been delegated the responsibility.

A **hospital autopsy** is a postmortem examination on the body of a person who at some time in the past was a hospital patient but was not a hospital inpatient at the time of death. A pathologist or some other physician on the medical staff performs this type of autopsy as well. The following sections describe the different types of autopsy rates calculated by acute-care hospitals.

Gross Autopsy Rates

A **gross autopsy rate** is the proportion or percentage of deaths that are followed by the performance of autopsy (see formula 14.14). For example, during the month of June, Community Hospital experienced 19 deaths. Autopsies were performed on three of the patients. The gross autopsy rate is 15.8 percent ([3/19] × 100).

Formula 14.14 Calculating the gross autopsy rate

$$\text{Gross autopsy rate} = \frac{\text{Total inpatient autopsies for a given period}}{\text{Total number of inpatient deaths for the same period}} \times 100$$

Net Autopsy Rates

The bodies of patients who have died are not always available for autopsy. For example, a coroner or medical examiner may claim a body for an autopsy for legal reasons. A **coroner** is the official (elected or appointed, physician or nonphysician) who is responsible for determining the cause, time, and manner of death in unattended, violent, or unexplained deaths, or a case where a law may have been broken. Coroners may also have other duties depending on their state.

In some areas of the country, the coroner has been replaced with a **medical examiner (ME)**. The ME is usually an appointed official who is a physician, commonly holding a specialty in pathology or forensic medicine. Large metropolitan areas usually have a forensic pathologist who acts as the coroner and performs the postmortem examination. In smaller areas, the coroner may be a physician practicing in the community who is not trained as a pathologist. Or a mortician or sheriff may serve as the coroner. A body released to a coroner or ME is not available for autopsy by the hospital pathologist (Horton 2017).

The hospital calculates a **net autopsy rate**. In calculating the net autopsy rate, bodies that have been removed by the coroner or ME are excluded from the denominator because they were not available for an autopsy. The formula for calculating the net autopsy rate is shown in formula 14.15. Continuing with the example in the preceding section, the ME claimed three of the patients for autopsy. The numerator remains the same because three autopsies were performed by the hospital pathologist. However, because three of the deaths were identified as ME's cases and removed from the hospital, 3 is subtracted from 19. The net autopsy rate is 18.8 percent ([3/{19 – 3}] × 100).

Formula 14.15 Calculating the net autopsy rate

$$\text{Net autopsy rate} = \frac{\text{Total inpatient autopsies on inpatient deaths for a given period}}{\text{Total number of inpatient deaths minus unautopsied coroners' or medical examiners' cases for the same period}} \times 100$$

Hospital Autopsy Rates

A third type of autopsy rate is called the **hospital autopsy rate**. This is an adjusted rate that includes autopsies on anyone who may have been a hospital patient. The formula for calculating the hospital autopsy rate is shown in formula 14.16. The hospital autopsy rate includes autopsies performed on any of the following:

- Bodies of inpatients, except those removed by the coroner or ME. When the hospital pathologist or other designated physician acts as an agent in the performance of an autopsy on an inpatient, the death and the autopsy are included in the percentage.
- Bodies of other hospital patients, including ambulatory care patients, hospital home care patients, and former hospital patients who died elsewhere, but whose bodies have been made available for autopsy to be performed by the hospital pathologist or other designated physician. These autopsies and deaths are included in computations of the percentage.

Formula 14.16 Calculating the hospital autopsy rate

$$\text{Hospital autopsy rate} = \frac{\text{Total number of hospital autopsies for the period}}{\text{Total number of deaths of hospital patients with bodies available for hospital autopsy for the period}} \times 100$$

Generally, it is difficult to determine the number of bodies of former hospital patients who may have died in a given time period. In the formula, the phrase *available for hospital autopsy* involves several conditions, including the following:

- The autopsy must be performed by the hospital pathologist or a physician who treated the patient at some time at the hospital.
- The report of the autopsy must be filed in the patient's health record and in the hospital laboratory or pathology department.
- The tissue specimens must be maintained in the hospital laboratory.

Figure 14.5 explains how to calculate the hospital autopsy rate.

Newborn Autopsy Rates

Autopsy rates usually include autopsies performed on newborn infants unless a separate rate is requested. The formula for calculating the **newborn autopsy rate** is shown in formula 14.17.

For example, three newborn deaths occurred at Community Hospital in June, and one of the deaths was autopsied. This represents 33.3 percent ([1/3] × 100).

Formula 14.17 Calculating the newborn autopsy rate

$$\text{Newborn autopsy rate} = \frac{\text{Total number of autopsies on NB deaths for a given period of time}}{\text{Total number of NB deaths for the same period}} \times 100$$

Figure 14.5 Calculation of hospital autopsy rate

In June, 19 inpatient deaths occurred at Community Hospital. Three of these were medical examiner's cases. Two of the bodies were removed from the hospital and so were not available for hospital autopsy. One of the medical examiner's cases was autopsied by the hospital pathologist. Three other autopsies were performed on hospital inpatients that died during the month of June. In addition, autopsies were performed in the hospital on:

- A child with congenital heart disease who died in the emergency department
- A former hospital inpatient who died in an extended care facility and whose body was brought to the hospital for autopsy
- A former hospital inpatient who died at home and whose body was brought to the hospital for autopsy
- A hospital outpatient who died while receiving chemotherapy for cancer
- A hospital home care patient whose body was brought to the hospital for autopsy
- A former hospital inpatient who died in an emergency vehicle on the way to the hospital

Calculation of total hospital autopsies:

1 autopsy on medical examiner's case
+3 autopsies on hospital in patients
+6 autopsies on hospital patients whose bodies were available for autopsy
10 autopsies performed by the hospital pathologist

Calculation of number of deaths of hospital patients whose bodies were available for autopsy:

19 inpatient deaths
−2 medical examiner's cases
+6 deaths of hospital patients
23 bodies available for autopsy

Calculation of hospital autopsy rate:

$$\text{Hospital autopsy rate} = \frac{\text{Total number of hospital autopsies for the period}}{\text{Total number of deaths of hospital patients with bodies available for hospital autopsy for the period}} \times 100$$

(10 × 100)/23 = 43.5%

Source: © AHIMA.

Fetal Autopsy Rates

Oftentimes, fetal autopsy rate will be calculated independently of the overall hospital autopsy rate. This is done to provide data which may be used in determining fetal cause of death. Fetal autopsies are performed on stillborn infants who have been classified as either intermediate or late fetal deaths (see table 14.11). This is the proportion or percentage of autopsies performed on intermediate or late fetal deaths out of the total number of intermediate or late fetal deaths. The formula for calculating the fetal autopsy rate is shown in formula 14.18.

Formula 14.18 Calculating the fetal autopsy rate

$$\text{Fetal autopsy rate} = \frac{\text{Total number of autopsies on intermediate and late fetal deaths for a given period of time}}{\text{Total number of intermediate and late fetal deaths for the same period}} \times 100$$

In a previous example there were five intermediate and late fetal deaths at Community Hospital during a year. Three of the deaths were autopsied. The fetal autopsy rate is 60.0 percent ([3/5] × 100).

Table 14.14 summarizes the different hospital autopsy rates.

Table 14.14 Calculation of hospital autopsy rates

Rate	Numerator	Denominator
Gross autopsy rate	Total number of autopsies on inpatient deaths for a given period × 100	Total number of inpatient deaths for the same period
Net autopsy rate	Total number of autopsies on inpatient deaths for a given period × 100	Total number of inpatient deaths minus unautopsied coroner or medical examiner cases for the same period
Hospital autopsy rate	Total number of hospital autopsies for a given period × 100	Total number of deaths of hospital patients whose bodies are available for hospital autopsy for the same period
Newborn (NB) autopsy rate	Total number of autopsies on NB deaths for a given period × 100	Total number of NB deaths for the same period
Fetal autopsy rate	Total number of autopsies on intermediate and late fetal deaths for a given period × 100	Total number of intermediate and late fetal deaths for the same period

Source: © AHIMA.

Check Your Understanding 14.7

Use the information in the following table to answer the questions that follow. Round to one decimal point.

Community Hospital January through June	Total
Number of inpatient deaths (all deaths)	35
Hospital inpatient autopsies (all autopsies)	9
Coroner's cases	2
Former patient brought to hospital for autopsy	1
Newborn deaths	5
Newborn autopsies	1
Fetal deaths (intermediate and late)	12
Fetal autopsies	1

1. Calculate the hospital autopsy rate.
2. Calculate the gross autopsy rate for this month.
3. Calculate the net autopsy rate for this month.
4. Calculate the newborn autopsy rate.
5. Calculate the fetal autopsy rate.

Healthcare-Associated Infection Rates

The most common morbidity rates calculated for hospitals are related to hospital-acquired infections, called **nosocomial (hospital-acquired) infections**. Morbidity refers to the state of being ill. The hospital must continuously monitor the number of infections that occur in its various patient care units because infection can adversely affect the course of a patient's treatment and possibly result in death. Examples of the different types of infections are respiratory, gastrointestinal, surgical wound, skin, urinary tract, septicemias, and infections related to intravascular catheters. Hospitals strive for a low infection rate which is an indicator of quality patient care.

Healthcare-Associated Infection Rates

Hospital-acquired (nosocomial) infection rates, now referred to as healthcare-associated infections (HAIs) by the CDC, may be calculated for the entire hospital or for a specific unit in the hospital. They also may be calculated for the specific types of infections. Ideally, the hospital should strive for an infection rate of zero. The formula for calculating the hospital-acquired, or nosocomial, infection rate is shown in formula 14.19. For example, Community Hospital discharged 226 patients during the month of June, 13 of whom experienced hospital-acquired infections. The hospital-acquired infection rate is 5.8 percent ([13/226] × 100). If, of those 13 patients who had infections, there were 8 who had a catheter-associated urinary tract infection (CAUTI), the rate would be 61.5 percent ([8/13] × 100). This information would be extremely important to the Infection Control Committee because, if they could control CAUTIs, then more than half of the infections would be eliminated.

Formula 14.19 Calculating the nosocomial infection rate

$$\text{Hospital acquired infection rate} = \frac{\text{Total number of hospital-acquired infections for a given period of time}}{\text{Total number of discharges, including deaths, for the same period}} \times 100$$

Many healthcare organizations report their infection rates to the CDC. The CDC is primarily interested in central line-associated bloodstream infection (CLABSI), catheter-associated urinary tract infection (CAUTI), surgical site infection (SSI), and ventilator-associated pneumonia. These rates are reported as indicators of unsafe practices such as failure to wash hands and other means to reduce infections.

Postoperative Infection Rates

Hospitals often track their **postoperative infection rate**. The postoperative infection rate is the proportion or percentage of infections in clean surgical cases out of the total number of surgical operations performed. A clean surgical case is one in which no infection existed prior to surgery. The postoperative infection rate may be an indicator of a problem in the hospital environment or of some type of surgical contamination.

Two terms must be considered here—*surgical procedure* and *surgical operation*. A **surgical procedure** is any single, separate, systematic process upon or within the body that can be complete in itself. It is normally performed by a physician, dentist, or some other licensed practitioner, with or without instruments, to do the following:

- Restore disunited or deficient parts
- Remove diseased or injured tissues
- Extract foreign matter
- Assist in obstetrical delivery
- Aid in diagnosis

A **surgical operation** involves one or more surgical procedures that are performed at one time for one patient by way of a common approach (means by which the surgery was performed) or for a common purpose. An example of a surgical operation is the resection of a portion of both the intestine and the liver in a cancer patient. This involves two procedures, removal of a portion of the liver and removal of a portion of the colon; but it is considered only one operation because there is only one operative approach or incision. In contrast, an esophagogastroduodenoscopy (EGD) and a colonoscopy performed at the same time are two procedures with two different approaches. In the former, the approach is the upper gastrointestinal tract; in the latter, the approach is the lower gastrointestinal tract. In this case, the two procedures do not have a common approach or purpose.

The formula for calculating the postoperative infection rate is shown in formula 14.20. For example, Community Hospital reported that 258 surgical operations were performed during the month of June. There were two postoperative infections in clean surgical cases. The postoperative infection rate is 0.78 percent ([2/258] x 100).

Formula 14.20 Calculating the postoperative infection rate

$$\text{Postoperative infection rate} = \frac{\text{Number of infections in clean surgical cases for a given period of time}}{\text{Total number of surgical operations for the same period}} \times 100$$

Consultation Rates

A consultation is the response by one healthcare professional to another healthcare professional's request to provide recommendations or opinions regarding the care of a particular patient or resident. The attending physician requests the consultation and explains his or her reason for doing so. The consultant then examines the patient and the patient's health record and makes recommendations in a written report. The formula for calculating the consultation rate is shown in formula 14.21.

During June, Community Hospital had 226 discharges and deaths. Of those, 57 patients received consultations. The consultation rate for June is 25.2 percent ([57/226] × 100).

Formula 14.21 Calculating the consultation rate

$$\text{Consultation rate} = \frac{\text{Total number of patients receiving consultations for a given period of time}}{\text{Total number of discharges and deaths for the same period}} \times 100$$

Check Your Understanding 14.8

Answer the following questions. Round all answers to two decimal point.

1. Use the following information to answer the questions that follow.
   a. Calculate the postoperative infection rate.
   b. Calculate the consultation rate.
2. During the month of September, Community Hospital discharged 278 patients. Of those 278 patients, 12 were seen by a consultant. Six patients had an infection acquired in the hospital.
   a. Calculate the consultation rate.
   b. Calculate the healthcare-associated infection rate.

Case-Mix Statistical Data

Case mix is a description of a patient population based on any number of specific characteristics including age, gender, type of insurance, diagnosis, risk factors, treatment received, and resources used. It is generally used as a distribution of patients into categories reflecting differences in severity of illness or resource consumption. An example of case mix is male patients under the age of 35 who present with right lower quadrant pain and undergo an appendectomy. Medicare severity diagnosis-related groups (MS-DRGs) are often used to determine case mix in hospitals. MS-DRGs are the US government's revision of the DRG system. MS-DRGs were developed to allow the CMS to provide greater reimbursement to hospitals who serve severely ill patients. MS-DRGs are covered in chapter 15, *Revenue Management and Reimbursement*.

When calculating case mix using MS-DRGs, the case-mix index (CMI) is the average relative weight of all cases treated at a given healthcare organization or by a given physician, which reflects the resource intensity or clinical severity of a specific group in relation to the other groups in the classification system. (Chapter 15 also discusses case mix in more detail.)

The CMI is a measure of the resources used in treating the patients in each hospital or group of hospitals. A sample of a case-mix report by payer (table 14.15), by physician (table 14.16), and by top 10 MS-DRGs (table 14.17) is given for Community Hospital. As shown in formula 14.22 the

Table 14.15 Case-mix index by payer, Community Hospital, 20XX

Payer	CMI	*N*
Commercial	1.8830	283
Government managed care	0.9880	470
Managed care	1.4703	2,326
Medicaid	1.3400	962
Medicare	2.0059	1,776
Other	1.3251	148
Self-pay	1.3462	528
Average case mix by payer	**1.4798**	**6,493**

Source: © AHIMA.

Table 14.16 Case mix of physicians, 20XX

Physician	CMI	*N*
A	1.0235	71
B	1.6397	71
C	1.1114	86
Average case mix by physician	**1.2582**	**228**

Source: © AHIMA.

CMI is calculated by multiplying the number of cases for each MS-DRG by the relative weight of the MS-DRG, summing the result (696.205) and dividing by the total number of cases (484). In other words, CMI is calculated by adding the MS-DRG relative weights for all Medicare discharges and dividing by the number of Medicare discharges. By convention, the CMI is calculated to five decimal points and rounded to four.

Formula 14.22

Sum total of MS-DRG relative weights for all Medicare discharges = CMI
Total number of Medicare discharges

696.205 / 484 = 1.4384

The CMI can be used to indicate the average reimbursement for the hospital. From table 14.15, the reimbursement is approximately 1.4798 multiplied by the hospital's base rate. It also is a measure of the severity of illness of Medicare patients.

Table 14.17 Calculation of case-mix index for the top 10 MS-DRGs, Community Hospital, 20XX

MS-DRG	Number (*N*)	MS-DRG weight	*N* X MS-DRG weight
286	84	2.1240	178.4160
293	62	0.6762	41.9244
982	61	2.8150	171.7150
986	51	1.0453	53.3103
434	45	0.6229	28.0305
391	43	1.1976	51.4968
378	41	1.0021	41.0861
287	40	1.1290	45.1600
871	31	1.8072	56.0232
689	26	1.1172	29.0472
Total	**484**		**696.2095**
CMI			**1.4384**

Source: © AHIMA.

In table 14.15, you can see that Medicare patients, as expected, have the highest CMI at 2.0059.

Other data analyzed by MS-DRG include LOS and mortality rates. LOS and mortality data are benchmarked against a particular hospital and national data. The process of benchmarking involves comparing the hospital's performance against an external standard or benchmark. An excellent source of information for benchmarking purposes is the Healthcare Cost Utilization Project database (HCUPnet). HCUPnet is an online query system that provides access to statistics from the Healthcare Cost and Utilization Project (HCUP, pronounced "H-Cup"). HCUP is a family of healthcare databases and related software tools and products developed through a Federal-State-Industry partnership and sponsored by the Agency for Healthcare Research and Quality (AHRQ). HCUP databases bring together the data collection efforts of state data organizations, hospital associations, private data organizations, and the federal government to create a national information resource of encounter-level healthcare data (HCUP 2019). HCUP includes the largest collection of longitudinal hospital care data in the United States, with all payer, encounter-level information beginning in 1988. These databases enable research on a broad range of health policy issues, including cost and quality of health services, medical practice patterns, access to healthcare programs, and outcomes of treatments at the national, state, and local market levels (HCUP 2019).

A comparison of hospital and national data for MS-DRG 293 appears in table 14.18.

Gross analysis of the data indicates that Community Hospital's mortality rate and ALOS are slightly better than the national average. But, at the same time, the hospital's average charges are higher than the national average.

Table 14.18 Benchmark data, Community Hospital versus national average for MS-DRG 293, Heart failure and shock without complication/comorbidity/major complication/comorbidity (CC/MCC)

	ALOS	Mortality rate	Average charges
Community Hospital	2.5	0.9%	$22,375
National average	2.6	1.1%	$18,192

Source: © AHIMA.

Check Your Understanding 14.9

Answer the following questions. Round to four decimal points.

1. A name given to describe an infection acquired in a healthcare organization is ________.
2. Identify the term the CDC uses for hospital-acquired infections.
3. During June, Community Hospital had 127 patients discharged. Of those 127 patients, 57 patients had consultations from specialty physicians. What was the consultation rate for June?
4. Last month, Community Hospital had 68 discharges from its medicine unit. Six patients developed a catheter-associated urinary tract infection (CAUTI) while in the hospital. Calculate the CAUTI rate for the last month.
5. Dr. Green discharged patients from medicine service during the month of August. Table 14.19 presents the number of patients discharged by Dr. Green by MS-DRG. Determine the total number of patients, calculate the total weight for each MS-DRG, and the CMI for Dr. Green.

Table 14.19 Community Hospital number of patients Dr. Green discharged by MS-DRG, August, 20XX

MS-DRG	MS-DRG title	Relative weight	Number of patients	Total weight
179	Respiratory infections and inflammations w/o CC/MCC	0.9693	5	
187	Pleural effusion w/ CC	1.0691	2	
189	Pulmonary edema and respiratory failure	1.2136	3	
194	Simple pneumonia and pleurisy w/ CC	0.9688	1	
208	Respiratory system diagnosis w/ ventilator support < 96 hours	2.2969	1	
280	Acute myocardial infarction, discharged alive w/ MCC	1.7289	3	
299	Peripheral vascular disorders w/ MCC	1.4094	2	
313	Chest pain	0.6138	4	
377	G.I. hemorrhage w/ MCC	1.7775	1	
391	Esophagitis, gastroenteritis, and miscellaneous digestive disorders w/ MCC	1.1976	1	
547	Connective tissue disorders w/o CC/MCC	0.7985	1	
552	Medical back problems w/o MCC	0.8698	1	
684	Renal failure w/o CC/MCC	0.6085	1	
812	Red blood cell disorders w/o MCC	0.8182	2	
872	Septicemia w/o MV 96+ hours w/o MCC	1.0528	1	
918	Poisoning and toxic effects of drugs w/o MCC	0.6412	1	
Total				
Case-mix index =				

Source: © AHIMA.

Ambulatory Care Statistical Data

Ambulatory care includes healthcare services provided to patients who are not hospitalized (that is, who are not considered inpatients or residents and do not stay in the healthcare organization overnight). Such patients are referred to as outpatients. Most ambulatory care services today are provided in freestanding physicians' offices, emergency care centers, and ambulatory surgery centers that are not owned or operated by acute-care organizations. However, hospitals do provide many hospital-based healthcare services to outpatients. Hospital outpatients may receive services in one or more areas within the hospital, including clinics, same-day surgery departments, diagnostic departments, and emergency departments.

Outpatient statistics include health records of the number of patient visits and the types of services provided. Many different terms are used to describe outpatients and ambulatory care services, including the following:

- **Ambulatory care**. Preventive or corrective healthcare services provided on a nonresident basis in a provider's office, clinic setting, or hospital emergency setting
- **Outpatient**. A patient who receives ambulatory care services in a hospital-based clinic or department
- **Emergency patient**. A patient who is admitted to the emergency services department of a hospital for diagnosis and treatment of a condition that requires immediate medical, dental, or allied health services in order to sustain life or to prevent critical consequences
- **Clinic outpatient**. A patient who is admitted to a clinical service of a clinic or hospital for diagnosis or treatment on an ambulatory basis
- **Referred outpatient**. An outpatient who is provided special diagnostic or therapeutic services by a hospital on an ambulatory basis but whose medical care remains the responsibility of the referring physician
- **Outpatient visit**. A patient's visit to one or more units or facilities located in the ambulatory services area (clinic or physician's office) of an acute-care hospital in which an overnight stay does not occur
- **Encounter**. The face-to-face contact between a patient and a provider who has primary responsibility for assessing and treating the condition of the patient at a given contact and exercises independent judgment in the care of the patient
- **Occasion of service**. A specified, identifiable service involved in the care of a patient that is not an encounter (for example, a lab test ordered during an encounter)
- **Ambulatory surgery center or ambulatory surgical center (ASC)**. Under Medicare, an outpatient surgical facility that has its own national identifier; is a separate entity with respect to its licensure, accreditation, governance, professional supervision, administrative functions, clinical services, recordkeeping, and financial and accounting systems; has as its sole purpose the provision of services in connection with surgical procedures that do not require inpatient hospitalization; and meets the conditions and requirements set forth in the Medicare Conditions of Participation. May be referred to as short-stay surgery, one-day surgery, or same-day surgery (White 2020).

Because outpatient care represents a large part of a healthcare organization's activity, statistics are collected and calculated on this group of patients. Many of the statistics covered in this chapter apply to ambulatory care.

Check Your Understanding 14.10

Match the definitions with the terms.

1. __________ Preventive or corrective healthcare services provided on a nonresident basis in a provider's office, clinic setting, or hospital emergency setting
2. __________ A patient who receives ambulatory care services in a hospital-based clinic or department
3. __________ An outpatient who is provided special diagnostic or therapeutic services by a hospital on an ambulatory basis but whose medical care remains the responsibility of the referring physician
4. __________ The face-to-face contact between a patient and a provider who has primary responsibility for assessing and treating the condition of the patient at a given contact and exercises independent judgment in the care of the patient
5. __________ A patient who is admitted to a clinical service of a clinic or hospital for diagnosis or treatment on an ambulatory basis
6. __________ A hospital patient who receives services in one or more of a hospital's facilities when he or she is not currently an inpatient or a home care patient
7. __________ A patient who is admitted to the emergency services department of a hospital for diagnosis and treatment of a condition that requires immediate medical, dental, or allied health services in order to sustain life or to prevent critical consequences
8. __________ An outpatient surgical facility that has its own national identifier; is a separate entity with respect to its licensure, accreditation, governance, professional supervision, administrative functions, clinical services, recordkeeping, and financial and accounting systems; has as its sole purpose the provision of services in connection with surgical procedures that do not require inpatient hospitalization; and meets the conditions and requirements set forth in the Medicare Conditions of Participation
9. __________ An ambulatory surgery center that is owned and operated by a hospital but is a separate entity with respect to its licensure, accreditation, governance, professional supervision, administrative functions, clinical services, recordkeeping, and financial and accounting systems
10. __________ A patient's visit to one or more units or facilities located in the ambulatory services area (clinic or physician's office) of an acute-care hospital in which an overnight stay does not occur
11. __________ A specified, identifiable service involved in the care of a patient that is not an encounter (for example, a lab test ordered during an encounter)

    a. Ambulatory surgery center
    b. Outpatient visit
    c. Encounter
    d. Occasion of service
    e. Referred outpatient
    f. Clinic outpatient
    g. Emergency outpatient
    h. Hospital outpatient
    i. Hospital ambulatory care
    j. Outpatient
    k. Hospital-affiliated ambulatory surgery center

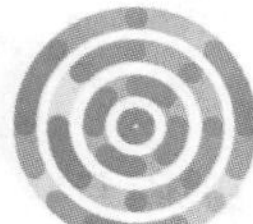

Public Health Statistics and Epidemiological Information

Just as statistics are collected in the healthcare organization, they also are collected on a community, regional, and national basis. Vital statistics are an example of data collected and reported at these levels. The term *vital statistics* refers to the collection and analysis of data related to the crucial events in life: birth, death, marriage, divorce, fetal death, and induced terminations of pregnancy. These statistics are used to identify trends. For example, a higher-than-expected death rate among newborns may be an indication of the lack of prenatal services in a community. A number of deaths in a region due to the same cause may indicate an environmental problem. For example, the World Health Organization (WHO) has found that poor outdoor air quality is a cause of lung cancer deaths.

These types of data are used as part of the effort to preserve and improve the health of a defined population—the public health. The study of factors that influence the health status of a population is called *epidemiology*. The following sections will cover national vital statistics and population-based statistics.

National Vital Statistics System

The National Vital Statistics System (NVSS) is the oldest example of intergovernmental data sharing in the US public health, and the shared relationships, standards, and procedures that form the mechanism by which the National Center for Health Statistics (NCHS) of the Centers for Disease Control and Prevention (CDC) collects and disseminates the nation's official vital statistics. These data are provided through contracts between NCHS and vital registration systems operated in the various jurisdictions and legally responsible for the registration of vital events—births, deaths, marriages, divorces, and fetal deaths.

To facilitate consistent data collection, the NVSS uses standard forms and procedures for the uniform registration of events and recommends that each state use the same forms. The standard certificates represent the minimum basic data set necessary for the collection and publication of comparable national, state, and local vital statistics data. The standard forms are revised about every 10 to 15 years. To effectively implement these new certificates, the NCHS collaborates with its state partners to improve the timeliness, quality, and sustainability of the vital statistics system, along with collection of the revised and new content of the certificates that were originally created in 2003 (CDC 2019a).

The certificate of live birth is used for registration purposes and is composed of two parts. The first part contains the information related to the child and the parents. The second part is used to collect data about the mother's pregnancy. This information is used for the collection of aggregate data only. No identification information appears on this portion of the certificate, nor does it ever appear on the official certificate of birth. Pregnancy-related information includes complications of pregnancy, concurrent illnesses or conditions affecting pregnancy, and abnormal conditions or congenital anomalies of the newborn. Lifestyle factors such as use of alcohol and tobacco also are collected. Thus, the birth certificate is the major source of maternal and natality statistics. A listing of pregnancy-related information appears in figure 14.6.

Data collected from death certificates are used to compile causes of death in the United States. The certificate of death contains decedent information, place of death information, medical certification, and disposition information. The US uses the current edition of the International Classification of Diseases (ICD) for classifying causes of death. Examples of the content of death certificates appear in figure 14.7.

A report of fetal death is completed when a pregnancy results in a stillbirth, regardless of the gestational age. This report contains information on the parents, the history of the pregnancy, and the cause of the fetal death. Information collected on the pregnancy is the same as that recorded on the birth certificate. To assess the effects of environmental exposures on the fetus, the parents' occupational data are collected. A listing of the content of the fetal death certificate appears in figure 14.8.

The report of induced termination of pregnancy records information on the place of the induced termination of pregnancy, type of termination procedure, and patient (see figure 14.9).

A tool for monitoring and exploring the interrelationships between infant death and risk factors at birth is the linked birth and infant death data set. This is a service provided by the NCHS. In this data set, the information from the death certificate (such as age and underlying or

Figure 14.6 Content of US certificate of live birth, 2003

Child's information	**Pregnancy history**
Child's name	Date of first prenatal care visit
Time of birth	Date of last prenatal care visit
Sex	Total number of prenatal visits for this pregnancy
Date of birth	Mother's height
Facility (hospital) name (if not an institution, give street address)	Mother's prepregnancy weight
City, town, or location of birth	Mother's weight at delivery
County of birth	Did mother get Women Infant Child (WIC) food for herself during this pregnancy?
Mother's Information	Number of previous live births
Current legal name	Number now living
Date of birth	Number now dead
Mother's name prior to first marriage	Date of last live birth
Birthplace	Number of other pregnancy outcomes
Residence (state)	Other outcomes
County	Date of last other pregnancy outcomes
City, town, or location	Cigarette smoking before and during pregnancy
Street number	Principal source of payment for this delivery
Apartment number	Date last normal menses began
Zip code	Mother's medical record number
Inside city limits?	Risk factors in this pregnancy
Mother's mailing address	Infections present and treated during this pregnancy
Mother married?	Obstetric procedures
If no, has paternity acknowledgment been signed in the hospital?	Onset of labor
Social Security number (SSN) requested for child?	Characteristics of labor and delivery
Mother's SSN	Method of delivery
Education	Maternal mortality
Hispanic origin?	Newborn Information
Race	Newborn medical record number
Place where birth occurred	Birth weight
Attendant's name, title, and National Provider Identifier	Obstetric estimate of gestation
Mother transferred for maternal, medical, or fetal indications for delivery?	Apgar score (1 and 5 minutes)
Father's Information	Plurality
Current legal name	If not born first (born first, second, third)
Date of birth	Abnormal conditions of newborn
Birthplace	Congenital anomalies of the newborn
Education	Was infant transferred within 24 hours of delivery?
Hispanic origin?	Is infant living at time of report?
Race	Is infant being breastfed at discharge?
Father's SSN	

Source: CDC 2019a.

Figure 14.7 Content of US certificate of death, 2003

Decedent information	**Medical certification**
Name	Date pronounced dead
Sex	Time pronounced dead
Social Security number	Signature of person pronouncing death
Age	Date signed
Under 1 year—month; days	Actual or presumed date of death
Under 1 day—hours; minutes	Actual or presumed time of death
Date of birth	Was medical examiner contacted?
Birthplace	Immediate cause of death
Residence (state)	Due to ______________
County	Due to ______________
City or town	Due to ______________
Street and number	Other significant conditions contributing to death
Apartment number	Was an autopsy performed?
Zip code	Were autopsy findings available to complete the cause of death?
Inside city limits?	Did tobacco use contribute to death?
Ever in US armed forces?	If female, indicate pregnancy status
Marital status at time of death	Manner of death
Surviving spouse's name (if wife, give name prior to first marriage)	For deaths due to injury:
Father's name	Date of injury
Mother's name (prior to first marriage)	Time of injury
Informant's name	Place of injury
Relationship to decedent	Injury at work?
Mailing address	Location of injury
Decedent's education	Describe how injury occurred
Hispanic origin?	If transportation injury, specify if driver or operator, passenger, pedestrian, other
Race	**Certifier information**
Disposition information	Certifier
Method of disposition	Name, address, and zip code of person completing cause of death
Place of disposition (cemetery, crematory, other)	Title of certifier
Location—city, town, and state	License number
Name and complete address of funeral facility	Date certified
Signature of funeral service licensee or other agent	
License number	
Place of death information	
Place of death	
If hospital, indicate inpatient, emergency department or outpatient, dead on arrival	
If somewhere other than hospital, indicate hospice, nursing home or long-term care facility, decedent's home, other	
Facility name	
City or town, state, zip code	
County	

Source: CDC 2019a.

Figure 14.8 Content of US standard report of fetal death, 2003

Mother's information	Number of other pregnancy outcomes
Name of fetus (optional—at the discretion of the parents)	Other outcomes
Time of delivery	Date of last other pregnancy outcomes
Sex	Cigarette smoking before and during pregnancy
Date of delivery	Date last normal menses began
City, town, or location of delivery	Plurality
Zip code of delivery	If not born first (born second, third)
County of delivery	Mother transferred for maternal, medical, or fetal indications for delivery?
Place where delivery occurred	**Medical and health information**
Facility name	Risk factors in this pregnancy
Facility ID	Infections present and treated during this pregnancy
Mother's current legal name	Method of delivery
Date of birth	Maternal mortality
Mother's name prior to first marriage	Congenital anomalies of the newborn
Birthplace	**Father's information**
Residence of mother (state)	Current legal name
County	Date of birth
City, town, or location	Birthplace
Street number	**Disposition**
Apartment number	Method of disposition
Zip code	**Attendant and registrant information**
Inside city limits?	Attendant's name, title, and National Provider Identifier
Education	Name of person completing report
Hispanic origin?	Date report completed
Race	Date received by registrar
Mother married at delivery, conception, or any time between?	**Cause of fetal death**
Date of first prenatal care visit	Initiating cause or condition
Date of last prenatal care visit	Other significant causes or conditions
Total number of prenatal visits for this pregnancy	Weight of fetus
Mother's height	Obstetric estimate of gestation at delivery
Mother's pre-pregnancy weight	Estimated time of fetal death
Mother's weight at delivery	Was an autopsy performed?
Did mother get WIC food for herself during this pregnancy?	Was a histological placental examination performed?
Number of previous live births	Were autopsy or histological placental examination results used in determining the cause of fetal death?
Number now living	
Number now dead	
Date of last live birth	

Source: CDC 2019a.

Figure 14.9 Content of US standard report of induced termination of pregnancy, 1997

Place of induced termination	Hispanic origin?
Facility name	Race
City, town, or location of pregnancy termination	Education
County of pregnancy termination	Elementary/secondary
Patient information	College
Patient identification	Date last normal menses began
Age at last birthday	Clinical estimate of gestation
Marital status	Previous pregnancies
Date or pregnancy termination	Live births
Residence (state)	Other terminations
County	Type of termination procedure
City, town, or location	**Other information**
Inside city limits?	Name of attending physician
Zip code	Name of person completing report

Source: CDC 2019a.

multiple causes of death) is linked to the information in the birth certificate (such as age, race, birth weight, prenatal care, maternal education, and so on) for each infant who dies in the United States, Puerto Rico, the Virgin Islands, and Guam. The purpose of the data set is to use the many additional variables available from the birth certificate to conduct a detailed analysis of infant mortality patterns.

Birth, death, fetal death, and termination of pregnancy certificates provide vital information for use in medical research, epidemiological studies, and other public health programs. In addition, they are the source of data for compiling morbidity, birth, and mortality rates that describe the health of a given population at the local, state, or national level. Because of their many uses, the data on these certificates must be complete and accurate.

Population-Based Statistics

Population-based statistics are based on the mortality and morbidity rates from which the health of a population can be inferred. The entire defined population is used in the collection and reporting of these statistics. The size of the defined population serves as the denominator in the calculation of these rates, which are discussed in the following sections.

Birth Rates and Measures of Infant Mortality

Two community-based rates that are commonly used to describe a community's health are the crude birth rate and measures of infant mortality. WHO's definition of a live birth is "the complete expulsion or extraction from its mother of a product of conception, irrespective of the duration of the pregnancy, which after such separation, breathes or shows other evidence of life such as beating of the heart, pulsation of the umbilical cord, or definite movement of voluntary muscles, whether or not the umbilical cord has been cut or the placenta is attached" (WHO 2019).

Rates that describe infant mortality are based on age. Therefore, the definitions for the various age groups must be strictly followed. Table 14.20 summarizes the calculations for community-based birth and infant mortality rates. These mortalities, or death, rates are broken down as follows.

Crude birth rate is the number of live births divided by the population at risk, meaning the population affected (as shown in table 14.20). Community rates are calculated using the multiplier 1,000, 10,000, or 100,000. The purpose is to bring the rate to a whole number, as discussed earlier in the chapter. The result of the formula is stated as the number of live births per 1,000 population. Formula 14.23 for calculating the crude birth rate is as follows.

Table 14.20 Calculation of community-based birth and infant death (mortality) rates

Measure	Numerator (x)	Denominator (y)	10^n
Crude birth rate	Number of live births for a given community for a specified time period	Estimated population for the same community and the same time period	1,000
Neonatal mortality rate	Number of deaths of infants from birth up to, but not including, 28 days of age during a given time period	Number of live births during the same time period	1,000
Postneonatal mortality rate	Number of deaths of infants from 28 days of age up to, but not including, one year of age during a given time period	Number of live births minus neonatal deaths during the same time period	1,000
Infant mortality rate	Number of deaths of infants under one year of age during a given time period	Number of live births during the same time period	1,000

Source: © AHIIMA.

Formula 14.23 Calculating the crude birth rate

$$\text{Crude birth rate} = \frac{\text{Number of live births for a given community for a specified period of time}}{\text{Estimated population for the same community and the same time period}} \times 1{,}000$$

For example, if there were 5,392 live births in a community of 500,000 in 20XX, the crude birth rate for that year would be 10.8 per 1,000 population ([5,392/500,000] × 1,000).

The neonatal mortality rate can be used as a measure of the quality of prenatal care and the mother's prenatal behavior (for example, alcohol, drug, or tobacco use). The neonatal period is the period of an infant's life from the hour of birth through the first 27 days, 23 hours, and 59 minutes of life. In the formula for calculating the neonatal mortality rate, the numerator is the number of deaths of infants in the neonatal period during a given time period and the denominator is the total number of live births during the same time period. See formula 14.24 to calculate the neonatal mortality rate.

Formula 14.24 Calculating the neonatal mortality rate

$$\text{Neonatal mortality rate} = \frac{\text{Number of deaths of infants from birth up to, but not including, 28 days of age during a given time period}}{\text{Number of live births during the same time period}} \times 1{,}000$$

For example, in your community there were 5,392 live births and 12 infants who died within the neonatal period in 20XX. The neonatal mortality rate is 2.2 per 1,000 live births for the period ([12/5,392] × 1,000).

The postneonatal mortality rate is often used as an indicator of the quality of the home or community environment of infants. The postneonatal period is from 28 days of age up to, but not including, one year of age. In the formula for calculating the postneonatal mortality rate, the numerator is the number of deaths among infants from 28 days of age up to, but not including, one year of age during a given time period and the denominator is the total number of live births minus the number of neonatal deaths during the same time period. The formula for calculating the postneonatal mortality rate is shown in formula 14.25.

Formula 14.25 Calculating the postneonatal mortality rate

$$\text{Postneonatal mortality rate} = \frac{\text{Number of deaths of infants from 28 days of age up to, but not including, one year of age during a given time period}}{\text{Number of live births minus neonatal deaths during the same time period}} \times 1{,}000$$

For example, in your community there were 5,392 live births, 12 neonatal deaths, and 9 postneonatal deaths during 20XX. The postneonatal mortality rate is 1.7 per 1,000 live births minus neonatal deaths for the period ([9/{5,392 – 12}] ×1,000).

The infant mortality rate is the summary of the neonatal and postneonatal mortality rates. In the formula for calculating the infant mortality rate, the numerator is the number of deaths among infants under one year of age (364 days, 23 hours, and 59 minutes from the moment of birth) and the denominator is the number of live births during the same period. The infant mortality rate is the most commonly used measure for comparing health status among nations. All the rates are expressed in terms of the number of deaths per 1,000 live births. The formula for calculating the infant mortality rate is found in formula 14.26.

Formula 14.26 Calculating the infant mortality rate

$$\text{Infant mortality} = \frac{\text{Number of deaths of infants under one year of age during a given period of time}}{\text{Number of live births during the same period}} \times 1{,}000$$

For example, in your community there were 12 neonatal deaths, 9 postneonatal deaths, and 5,392 live births in 20XX. The infant mortality rate is 3.9 per 1,000 live births in that year ([{12 + 9}/5,392] × 1,000).

Other Death (Mortality) Rates

Other measures of mortality with which the HIM professional should be familiar include the following.

Crude death/mortality rate is a measure of the actual or observed mortality in a given population. Crude death rates apply to a population without regard to characteristics such as age, race, and sex. They measure the proportion of the population that has died during a given period of time (usually one year) or the number of deaths in a community per 1,000 for a given period of time. In the formula, the numerator is the total number of deaths in a population for a specified time period and the denominator is the estimated population for the same time period. The formula for calculating the crude death/mortality rate is found in formula 14.27.

Formula 14.27 Calculating the crude death/mortality rate

$$\text{Crude death/mortality rate} = \frac{\text{Total number of deaths for a population during a specified period of time}}{\text{Estimated population for the same time period}} \times 1{,}000$$

For instance, in our previous examples we used a community population of 500,000. There were 1,327 deaths in 20XX. Dividing 1,327 by 500,000 equals 0.002654. Using a multiplier of 1,000 gives a crude death rate of 2.7 deaths per 1,000 population for 20XX ([1,327/500,000] × 1,000).

As its name indicates, the cause-specific mortality rate is the rate of death due to a specified cause. It may be calculated for an entire population or for any age, sex, or race. In the formula, the numerator is the number of deaths due to a specified cause for a given time period and the denominator is the estimated population for the same time period. Table 14.21 displays cause-specific mortality rates for men and women due to influenza and pneumonia for the year 2013. The cause-specific death rates for each age group are consistently higher for men than for women, but the overall rate is higher for women. This information could lead to an investigation of why this occurs. The formula for calculating the cause-specific mortality rate can be found in formula 14.28.

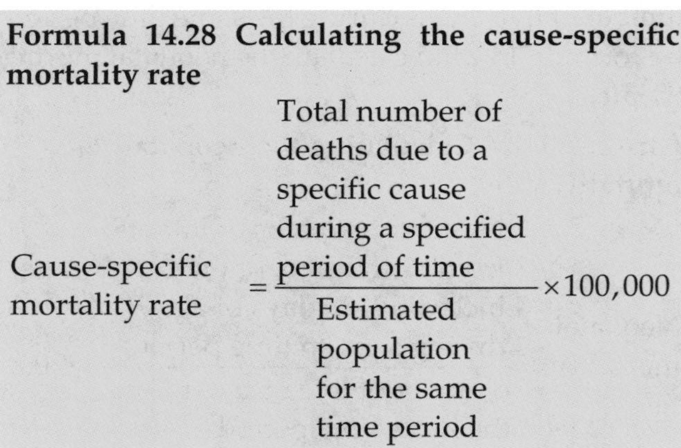

Formula 14.28 Calculating the cause-specific mortality rate

$$\text{Cause-specific mortality rate} = \frac{\text{Total number of deaths due to a specific cause during a specified period of time}}{\text{Estimated population for the same time period}} \times 100{,}000$$

Table 14.21 Cause-specific mortality rates, by sex, due to influenza and pneumonia (ICD-10 codes J09–J18.9), age 45+, in the United States, 2017

	Women			Men		
Age group	**Population**	**Deaths**	**Rate/100,000**	**Population**	**Deaths**	**Rate/100,000**
45–54	21,468,595	937	4.4	20,906,357	1,076	5.1
55–64	21,737,855	2,219	10.2	20,257,803	2,826	14.0
65–74	15,806,306	4,002	25.3	13,877,140	4,782	34.5
75–84	8,298,676	6,746	81.3	6,407,875	7,056	110.1
85+	4,189,013	14,430	344.5	2,279,669	9,846	431.9
Total	71,500,445	28,334	39.62	63,728,844	25,586	40.1

Source: CDC 2019b.

The case fatality rate measures the total number of deaths among the diagnosed cases of a specific disease, most often acute illness. In the formula for calculating the case fatality rate, the numerator is the number of deaths due to a specific disease that occurred during a specific time period and the denominator is the number of diagnosed cases during the same time period. The higher the case fatality rate, the more virulent the infection. The formula for calculating the case fatality rate is found in formula 14.29.

Formula 14.29 Calculating the case fatality rate

$$\text{Case fatality rate} = \frac{\text{Total number of deaths due to a specific disease during a specified period of time}}{\text{Total number of cases due to a specific disease during the same time period}} \times 100$$

For example, in our community there were seven cases of meningitis resulting in two deaths. The case fatality rate of meningitis is 28.6 percent ([2/7] × 100).

The proportionate mortality rate (PMR) is a measure of mortality due to a specific cause for a specific time period. In the formula for calculating the PMR, the numerator is the number of deaths due to a specific disease for a specific time period and the denominator is the number of deaths from all causes for the same time period. Table 14.22 displays the PMRs for influenza and pneumonia in the United States in 2017 by age groups. The formula for calculating the proportionate mortality rate is found in formula 14.30.

Formula 14.30 Calculating the proportionate mortality rate

$$\text{Proportionate mortality rate} = \frac{\text{Total number of deaths due to a specific cause during a specified period of time}}{\text{Total number of deaths from all causes during the same time period}} \times 100$$

The maternal mortality rate (community based) measures the deaths associated with pregnancy for a specific community for a specific period of time. It is calculated only for deaths that are directly related to pregnancy. In the formula for calculating the maternal mortality rate, the numerator is the number of deaths attributed to causes related to pregnancy during a specific time period for a given community and the denominator is the number of live births reported during the same time period for the same community. The maternal mortality rate is expressed as the number of deaths per 100,000 live births. The formula for calculating the maternal mortality rate (community based) is found in formula 14.31.

Formula 14.31 Calculating the maternal mortality rate

$$\text{Maternal mortality rate} = \frac{\text{Total number of deaths due to pregnancy-related conditions during a specified period of time}}{\text{Total number of live births during the same time period}} \times 100{,}000$$

Table 14.22 Proportionate mortality rates for influenza and pneumonia (ICD-10 codes J09–J18.9), all ages, in the United States, 2017

Age group	Influenza and pneumonia deaths	Total deaths	PMR/100
< 1 year	157	22,335	0.70
1–4	104	3,880	2.68
5–14	113	5,571	2.03
15–24	190	32,025	0.59
25–34	405	60,215	0.67
35–44	782	79,796	0.98
45–54	2,013	170,142	1.18
55–64	5,045	372,006	1.36
65–74	8,784	531,610	1.65
75–84	13,802	657,759	2.10
85+	24,276	878,035	2.76

Source: CDC 2019b.

Table 14.23 Calculation of community-based mortality rates

Measure	Numerator (*x*)	Denominator (*y*)	10^n
Crude death/mortality rate	Total number of deaths for a population during a specified time period	Estimated population for the same time period	1,000 or 10,000 or 100,000
Cause-specific mortality rate	Total number of deaths due to a specific cause during a specified time period	Estimated population for the same time period	100,000
Case fatality rate	Total number of deaths due to a specific disease during a specified time period	Total number of cases due to a specific disease during the same time period	100
Proportionate mortality rate	Total number of deaths due to a specific cause during a specified time period	Total number of deaths from all causes during the same time period	N/A
Maternal mortality rate	Total number of deaths due to pregnancy-related conditions during a specified time period	Total number of live births during the same time period	100,000

Source: CDC 2019b.

For example, there were 3,932,181 live births and 1,111 maternal deaths. This is a maternal mortality rate of 29 maternal deaths per 100,000 live births ([1,111/3,932,181] × 100,000). Table 14.23 shows how to calculate community-based mortality rates.

Measures of Morbidity

Two measures are commonly used to describe the presence of disease in a community or specific location (for example, a nursing home)—incidence and prevalence rates. *Disease* is any illness, injury, or disability. Incidence and prevalence measures can be broken down by race, sex, age, or other characteristics of a population.

An incidence rate is used to compare the frequency of new cases of disease in populations. Populations are compared using rates instead of raw numbers because rates adjust for differences in population size. The incidence rate is the probability or risk of illness in a population over a period of time. The denominator represents the population from which the case in the numerator arose, such as a nursing home, school, or organization. For 10^n, a value is selected so that the smallest rate calculated results in a whole number. In a small population such as a nursing home you might select 100, in studying a larger population you might select 1,000. For example, in a local nursing home of 174 patients, 8 new cases of H1N1 (a strain of influenza A virus) occurred during January. Using this formula, the incidence rate is 5.5 percent ([8/147] × 100). The formula for calculating the incidence rate is found in formula 14.32.

Check Your Understanding 14.11

Use the information in table 14.24 to answer the questions that follow. Round to one decimal point.

1. Review the mortality data in table 14.24 to answer the questions that follow.
   a. Calculate the crude death rate per 10,000 for men of all ages.
   b. Calculate the crude death rate per 10,000 for women of all ages.
   c. Calculate the crude death rate per 10,000 for the entire group.
   d. Calculate the crude death rate per 10,000 for men ages 15 to 24.
   e. Calculate the crude death rate per 10,000 for women ages 15 to 24.
2. In a community of 750,000, 4,899 live births were reported. Calculate the crude birth rate.
3. In this same community eight infants died in the neonatal period. Calculate the neonatal mortality rate.
4. In this same community 14 children died in the neonatal period. Calculate the postneonatal mortality rate.

Table 14.24 Mortality Rates, United States, 2017

	Female		Male	
Age group	**Population**	**Deaths**	**Population**	**Deaths**
Less than 1 year	1,924,145	9,867	2,015,150	12,468
1–4 years	7,818,747	1,648	8,180,818	2,232
5–14	20,109,479	2,302	20,973,213	3,269
15–24	21,100,662	8,522	22,149,633	23,503
25–34	22,351,311	18,066	22,991,361	42,149
35–44	20,506,270	29,004	20,369,100	50,792
45–54	21,468,595	66,338	20,906,357	103,804
55–64	21,737,855	146,671	20,257,803	225,335
65–74	15,806,306	227,679	13,877,140	303,931
75–84	8,298,676	321,088	6,407,875	336,671
85+	4,189,013	543,169	2,279,669	334,866
Total				

Source: CDC 2019b.

5. Calculate the infant mortality rate in this community.
6. In this same community there were 4,012 live births. Two mothers died of causes associated with their pregnancies. Calculate the maternal mortality rate.
7. In this same community there were 4,225 deaths. Calculate the crude death rate.
8. In this same community, 125 people died of lung cancer. Calculate the cause-specific mortality rate.
9. In this same community, 37 people reported a *Clostridium difficile (C. diff)* infection; of these, four people died. What is the case fatality rate?
10. What is the proportionate mortality rate for *Clostridium difficile (C. diff)* in this community?

Formula 14.32 Calculating the incidence rate

$$\text{Incidence rate} = \frac{\text{Total number of new cases of a specified disease during a given period of time}}{\text{Total population at risk during the same time period}} \times 10^n$$

The **prevalence rate** is the proportion of persons in a population who have a particular disease at a specific point in time or over a specified period of time. The prevalence rate describes the magnitude of an epidemic and can be an indicator of the medical resources needed in a community for the duration of the epidemic. For example, in a community of 750,000 individuals, 1,875 individuals were identified as having AIDS and an additional 93 cases were identified in 20XX. The prevalence rate is 2.6 cases per 1,000 population ([{1,875 + 93}/750,000] × 1,000). The formula for calculating the prevalence rate is found in formula 14.33.

Formula 14.33 Calculating the prevalence rate

$$\text{Prevalence rate} = \frac{\text{All new and preexisting cases of a specific disease during a given period of time}}{\text{Total population during the same time period}} \times 10^n$$

It is easy to confuse incidence and prevalence rates. The distinction is in the numerators of their formulas. The numerator in the formula for the incidence rate is the number of new cases occurring in a given time period. The numerator in the formula for the prevalence rate is all cases present during a given time period. In addition, the incidence rate includes only patients whose illness began during a specified time period whereas the prevalence rate includes all patients from a specified cause regardless of when the illness began. Moreover, the prevalence rate includes a patient until he or she recovers or passes away.

National Notifiable Diseases Surveillance System

In 1878, the US Congress authorized the US Marine Hospital Service, the precursor to the Public Health Service, to collect morbidity reports on cholera, smallpox, plague, and yellow fever from US consuls overseas. This information was used to implement quarantine measures to prevent the spread of these diseases to the United States. To provide for more uniformity in data collection, Congress enacted a law in 1902 that directed the surgeon general to provide standard forms for the collection, compilation, and publication of reports at the national level. In 1912, the states and US territories recommended that infectious diseases be immediately reported by telegraph. By 1928, all states, the District of Columbia, Hawaii, and Puerto Rico were participating in the national reporting of 29 specified diseases. In 1961, the CDC assumed responsibility for the collection and publication of data concerning nationally notifiable diseases.

A **notifiable disease** is one that must be reported to a government agency so that regular, frequent, and timely information on individual cases can be used to prevent and control future cases of the disease. The list of notifiable diseases varies over time and by state. The Council of State and Territorial Epidemiologists (CSTE) collaborates with the CDC to determine which diseases should be reported. State reporting to the CDC is voluntary. However, all states generally report the internationally quarantinable diseases in accordance with WHO's International Health Regulations. Completeness of reporting varies by state and type of disease and may be influenced by a number of factors; for example, type of illness and resources for reporting.

Information that is reported includes date, county, age, sex, race and ethnicity, and disease-specific epidemiologic information; personal identifiers are not included. A strict CSTE Data Release Policy regulates dissemination of the data. A list of nationally notifiable infectious diseases appears in figure 14.10. The list is updated annually; the list in figure 14.10 is not an exhaustive list.

Selected national morbidity data are reported weekly by the 50 states, New York City, the District of Columbia, and the US territories. Then they are collated and published by the CDC in the Morbidity and Mortality Weekly Report. Public health managers and providers use the reports to rapidly identify disease epidemics and to understand patterns of disease occurrence. Case-specific information is included in the reports. Changes in age, sex, race and ethnicity, and geographic distributions can be monitored and investigated as necessary (CDC 2019c).

Figure 14.10 Nationally notifiable infectious and noninfectious diseases in the United States, 2017

Anthrax	Measles (Rubeola)
Arboviral neuroinvasive and non-neuroinvasive diseases	Meningococcal disease
Babesiosis	Mumps
Botulism, *C.botulinum*	Novel influenza A virus infections
Brucellosis	Pertussis (Whooping cough)
Campylobacteriosis	Pesticide-related illness and injury, acute
Cancer	Plague
Carbon monoxide poisoning	Poliomyelitis, paralytic
Chancroid	Poliovirus infection, nonparalytic
Chlamydia trachomatis, infection	Psittacosis (Ornithosis)
Cholera	Q fever
Coccidioidomycosis/Valley fever	Rabies, animal
Congenital syphilis	Rabies, human
Cryptosporidiosis	Rubella (German measles)
Cyclosporiasis	Rubella, congenital syndrome (CRS)
Dengue virus infections	Salmonellosis
Diphtheria	Severe acute respiratory syndrome–associated coronavirus (SARS) disease
Ehrlichiosis and anaplasmosis	Shiga toxin-producing *Escherichia coli* (STEC)
Food-borne disease outbreak	Shigellosis
Giardiasis	Silicosis
Gonorrhea	Smallpox (Variola)
Haemophilus influenzae, invasive disease	Spotted fever rickettsiosis
Hansen disease and leprosy	Streptococcal toxic-shock syndrome (STSS)
Hantavirus infection, non-Hantavirus pulmonary syndrome	Syphilis
Hantavirus pulmonary syndrome (HPS)	Tetanus, *c. tetani*
Hemolytic uremic syndrome, post-diarrheal (HUS)	Toxic-shock syndrome (other than streptococcal) (TSS)
Hepatitis A, B, and C, acute; Hepatitis B chronic and perinatal infection	Trichinellosis (Trichinosis)
HIV infection (AIDS has been reclassified as HIV stage III) (AIDS/HIV)	Tuberculosis (TB)
Influenza-associated pediatric mortality	Tularemia
Invasive pneumococcal disease (IPD), *Streptococcus pneumoniae*, invasive disease	Typhoid fever
Lead, elevated blood levels	Vancomycin-intermediate *Staphylococcus aureus* and vancomycin-resistant *Staphylococcus aureus* (VISA/VRSA)
Legionellosis (Legionnaire's disease) or Pontiac fever	Varicella (Chickenpox)
Leptospirosis	Varicella deaths
Listeriosis	Vibriosis
Lyme disease	Viral hemorrhagic fevers (VHF)
Malaria	Waterborne disease outbreak
	Yellow fever
	Zika virus

Source: CDC 2019d.

HIM Roles

The health information management (HIM) professional has a vital role in managing information within all healthcare arenas. As managers of data flow, HIM professionals utilize technology to link clinical settings, public health agencies, research institutions, and consumers with health information. HIM professionals serve traditional roles in ensuring quality, collection, storage, organization, interpretation, analysis, security, and sharing of data. Moreover, the role of HIM has extended outside the traditional hospital setting. As technology and the accessibility to health information have increased, the role HIM professionals play in public health research and policy development has expanded.

The HIM professional generates health statistics that provide various healthcare providers with reliable and multidimensional information. Health statistics include data related to health, such as mortality, morbidity, risk factors, health service coverage, and health systems. Health statistics provide information for understanding, monitoring, and planning the use of resources to improve the overall health and well-being of populations.

Health statistics provide data to assist healthcare providers, researchers, health planners, policy makers, legislators, and consumers. Researchers and physicians use data-driven statistics to study the health problems that describe the characteristics of specific populations. By identifying statistical trends, public health officials can monitor local diseases and injuries in comparison to state, national, and international trends. Health planners use data to understand and allocate health resources. Legislators reference health statistics when enacting laws, conducting program oversight, and considering funding. The consumer uses health information and statistics to understand their personal risks, illnesses, and health status compared to the general population.

The HIM professional has the knowledge and skills to assume the lead role in statistical analysis practices in the healthcare environment. Increasingly, roles and responsibilities have resulted in diversified employment opportunities in areas such as data analytics, informatics, and information governance.

Check Your Understanding 14.12

Answer the following questions.

1. What is a notifiable disease?
2. What are the definitions of the terms *incidence rate* and *prevalence rate*?
3. Calculate the incidence rate, per 100,000, for the following hypothetical data: In 20XX, 189,000 new cases of coronary artery disease were reported in the United States. The estimated population for 20XX was 301,623,157.
4. In a community of 50,000, there were four cases of hantavirus pulmonary syndrome during the first half of 20XX. Calculate the incidence rate.
5. In the same community, three more cases of hantavirus pulmonary syndrome were reported for the remaining months of the year. Calculate the prevalence rate.

Real-World Case 14.1

The performance improvement committee of Community Regional Medical Center wanted to study MS-DRG 689 kidney and urinary tract infections with MCC (major complication or comorbidity) because of wide variations in length of stay (LOS) and total charges (refer to chapter 15, *Revenue*

Management and Reimbursement, for more information on MS-DRGs and MCCs). The committee asked the HIM director to prepare a profile of patients discharged from MS-DRG 689. A summary of the patients discharged from MS-DRG 689 at Community Hospital was prepared using information found in the hospital's online database. Further research was performed on the individual patient records to determine if there was a correlation between the LOS and the MCCs for the patients.

Real World Case 14.2

University Hospital is preparing for an upcoming onsite survey with the Joint Commission. With an expanded focus on patient safety, the Joint Commission has identified infection prevention as a focal area in the survey process. Surveyors will specifically target prevention strategies and outcomes during reviews of the hospitals infection control policies and procedures since infections can lead to serious complications, longer patient stays, and death.

A low infection rate can be an indicator of quality care. University Hospital has determined that the infection rate for each physician should be 1 percent or lower.

University Hospital
Physician Profile
January – June 20XX

Physician number	Medical service	Number of discharges	Number of infections	Infection rate
101	Surgery	275	3	3/275 x 100 = 1.09%
111	Surgery	130	4	4/130 x 100 = 3.08%
125	Surgery	366	3	3/366 x 100 = 0.82%
216	Medicine	567	5	5/567 x 100 = 0.88%
302	Medicine	132	2	2/132 x 100 = 1.52%
420	Medicine	154	0	0/154 x 100 = 0%
502	Obstetrics	288	2	2/288 x 100 = 0.69%
517	Gynecology	132	1	1/132 x 100 = 0.76%
815	Newborn	176	2	2/176 x 100 = 1.14%
927	Pediatrics	154	1	1/154 x 100 = 0.65%
TOTAL		2,374	23	23/2,374 x 100 = 0.97%

References

American Health Information Management Association. 2017. *Pocket Glossary of Health Information Management and Technology*, 5th ed. Chicago: AHIMA.

BusinessDictionary.com. 2019. Likert Scale. http://www.businessdictionary.com/definition/Likert-scale.html.

Centers for Disease Control and Prevention. 2019a. "2003 Revisions of the U.S. Standard Certificates of Live Birth and Death and the Fetal Death Report." 1 Jan. 2019.

Centers for Disease Control and Prevention. 2019b. CDC Wonder. http://wonder.cdc.gov.

Centers for Disease Control and Prevention. 2019c. Morbidity and Mortality Weekly Reports.

Centers for Disease Control and Prevention. 2019d. National Notifiable Conditions. https://wonder.cdc.gov/nndss/nndss_annual_tables_menu.asp.

Healthcare Cost and Utilization Project. 2019. https://www.hcup-us.ahrq.gov/overview.jsp.

White, S. 2020. *Calculating and Reporting Healthcare Statistics*, 6th ed. Chicago: AHIMA.

World Health Organization. 2019. Health Statistics and Information Systems. http://www.who.int/healthinfo/statistics/indmaternalmortality/en/.

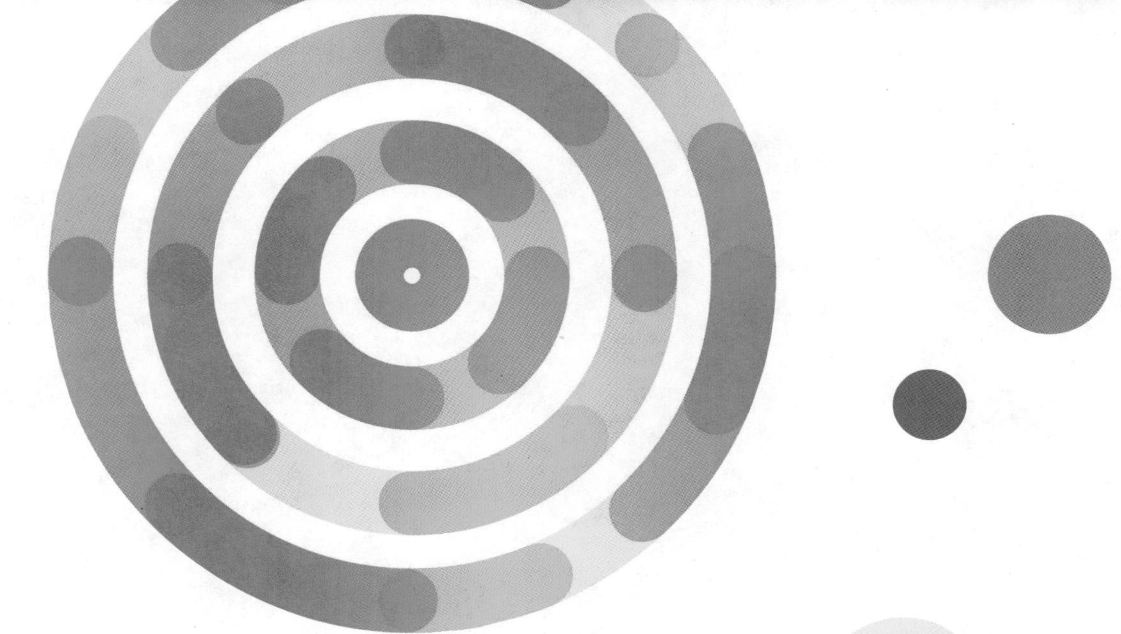

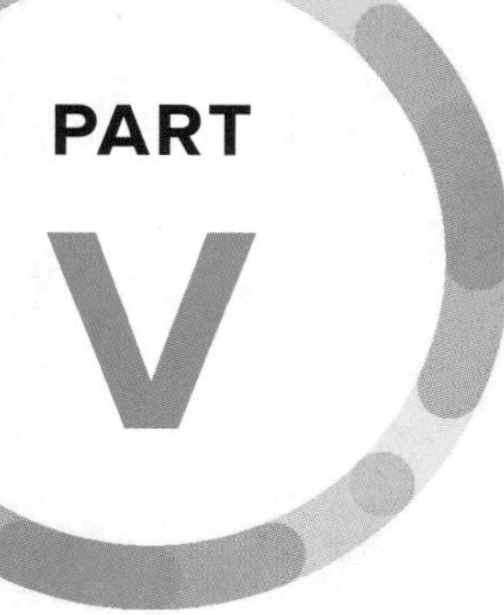

Revenue Cycle Management and Compliance

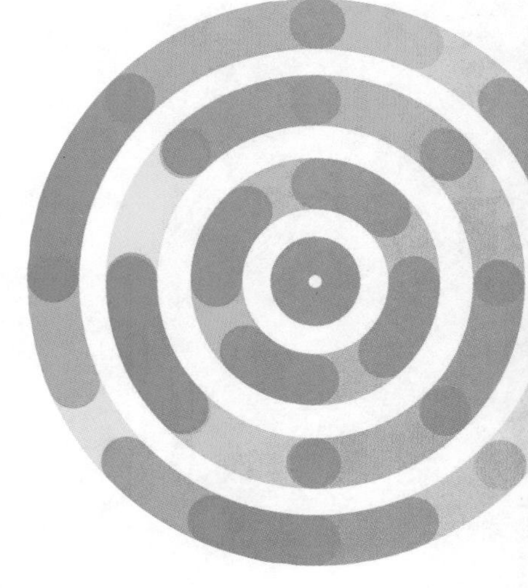

Revenue Management and Reimbursement

Morley L. Gordon, RHIT

Learning Objectives

- Identify health insurance and how it is used in the United States
- Identify revenue cycle management
- Examine new trends in revenue management
- Identify how utilization management is performed in healthcare settings
- Examine how case management is performed in healthcare settings
- Identify healthcare reimbursement methodologies

Key Terms

Accept assignment
Adjudication
Affordable Care Act (ACA)
Ambulatory payment classification (APC)
Ambulatory surgery center (ASC)
Ambulatory surgery center (ASC) payment rate
Balance billing
Beneficiaries
Capitation
Case management
Case-mix index (CMI)
Centers for Medicare and Medicaid Services (CMS)
Charge description master (CDM)
Chargemaster
Children's Health Insurance Program (CHIP)
Civilian Health and Medical Program of the Department of Veterans Affairs (CHAMPVA)
Claims
Clinical data
Coinsurance
Concurrent review
Consumer-directed health plans (CDHP)
Coordination of benefits (COB)
Cost sharing
Copayment
Deductible
Demographic data
Disproportionate share hospital (DSH)
Dual eligible
Eligibility
Episode-of-care (EOC) reimbursement
Exclusive provider organizations (EPO)
Explanation of benefits (EOB)
Federal poverty level (FPL)
Fee-for-service reimbursement
Fee schedule
Global payment
Health insurance marketplace or exchange
Health maintenance organization (HMO)
Healthcare insurance
Home health prospective payment system (HH PPS)
Hospital-acquired condition HAC)
Indian Health Service (IHS)
Inpatient prospective payment system (IPPS)
Managed care
Managed care organization (MCO)
Mandatory eligibility groups
Medicaid
Medical necessity
Medicare

Medicare Access and CHIP Reauthorization Act (MACRA)
Medicare administrative contractors (MAC)
Medicare Advantage (MA) Plan
Medicare Part A
Medicare Part B
Medicare Part D
Medicare severity diagnosis-related groups (MS-DRGs)
National Committee for Quality Assurance (NCQA)
Out of pocket
Outpatient prospective payment system (OPPS)
Patient Assessment Instrument
Point-of-service plans (POS)
Policy
Policyholder
Precertification
Preferred provider organization (PPO)
Premium
Present on admission (POA)
Preventive services
Prior approval
Private healthcare insurance
Professional component
Prospective payment system (PPS)
Prospective review
Quality Payment Program
Reimbursement
Remittance advice (RA)
Resource-based relative value scale (RBRVS)
Retrospective review
Revenue cycle
Skilled nursing facility prospective payment system
Technical component
Third-party administrator (TPA)
Third-party payer
Traditional fee-for-service reimbursement
TRICARE
Usual, customary, and reasonable (UCR) charges
Utilization management (UM)
Value Based Purchasing (VBP)
Veterans Health Administration (VA)
Workers' compensation

Payment for healthcare services, called **reimbursement**, is very complex in the United States. Reimbursement begins before a patient enters a healthcare facility with the collection of **demographic data** which is patient-specific data like date of birth, address, and insurance coverage information. The process ends with the final **adjudication** of all medical charges. *Adjudication* is a term used by the insurance industry that refers to the process of paying, denying, and adjusting claims based on the patient's healthcare insurance coverage benefits. Information about a patient is collected during the course of receiving healthcare services. This includes demographic data, used to identify an individual, and **clinical data**, which is the patient's medical condition or treatment. This information is used to bill for healthcare services. Reimbursement for services is what keeps healthcare providers and organizations in business. Healthcare providers submit **claims**, which represent the services and supplies provided to a patient during his or her encounter with the facility or provider, for reimbursement to insurance companies on behalf of patients. Health information management (HIM) professionals play a vital role in the submission of accurate claims by ensuring the documentation supports the services billed, assigning proper diagnostic and procedure codes, and ensuring accurate information is captured throughout the patient's encounter with the healthcare organization. Accurate information is paramount to the success of healthcare organizations. The balance of care provided, and getting paid for the service delivered, relies on the accuracy of documentation and codes for reimbursement.

This chapter discusses healthcare insurance, revenue cycle management, reimbursement systems (including private and government plans), new trends, managed care, utilization and case management, and healthcare reimbursement methodologies.

Healthcare Insurance

Healthcare is expensive in the United States, and health insurance can be unaffordable for some people. Therefore, millions of Americans go without health insurance. Americans without health insurance must pay for healthcare expenses **out of pocket**, meaning they pay for the services provided with their own funds, or they do not get the services they need (Henry J. Kaiser Family Foundation 2018). **Healthcare insurance** protects a person from paying the full cost of healthcare by prepaying for a healthcare coverage plan. Before the early 1900s, Americans paid for their entire healthcare services out of pocket. There was not an organized way to pay for services and charging patients and paying for services was done through trial and error between the provider of the services and the patient. The cost of healthcare in the early 1900s was not a significant part of an American family's budget and the need for healthcare insurance was not considered by people of that time. During this time hospitals were places for injured soldiers, those who were very sick, the poor, and those who had contagious diseases. Hospitals were known as a last resort—a place where people went to die (Ferenc 2014). By the 1920s, with modern medicine and the discovery of antibiotics, hospitals started marketing themselves as places with positive health outcomes. In return for those positive outcomes, hospitals began to charge more than most people could afford. In 1929, in Dallas, Texas, Baylor Hospital started a prepaid hospital insurance program with a local teachers' union. This program began to pre-pay for future hospital services and became the predecessor to Blue Cross (Griffin 2017).

Health insurance coverage for all Americans began to be a political hot topic as early as 1912. While campaigning for the US presidency, Theodore Roosevelt called for a national healthcare insurance program. He did not win the presidency and, therefore, national healthcare insurance was not implemented at that time (CMS 2015a). Many politicians and presidents throughout the years championed for universal health coverage and almost 100 years after Theodore Roosevelt campaigned for national health coverage, the **Affordable Care Act (ACA)** was signed into law in 2010, providing health coverage for all Americans. The ACA mandated many changes in reimbursement methodologies, which are discussed in this chapter. (Chapter 2, *Healthcare Delivery Systems*, covers ACA in more detail.)

To understand the process of healthcare reimbursement as defined later in this chapter, it is important to understand basic terms used in insurance reimbursement. When a person has healthcare insurance, they receive a **policy**, which is a contract between the insurer and the person, in which they pay a **premium**, which is a set amount per month or per year—to help cover the cost of medical expenses. The **policyholder** is the person covered by the policy. The purchaser of a healthcare insurance policy can be an individual, group, or employer.

Revenue Cycle Management

The **revenue cycle** is the process of patient financial and health information moving into, through, and out of the healthcare organization, culminating with the healthcare organization receiving reimbursement for services provided. HIM professionals are vital to the management of the revenue cycle. The revenue cycle begins with patient registration, known as the front end of the cycle. The documentation of the encounter in the health record, charge capture, coding, and charge entry comprise the middle section of the cycle. The back end of the revenue cycle includes claims transmission and accounts receivable management. The HIM professional provides vital expertise in coding, documentation management, and accounts receivable management and other knowledge of the revenue cycle. Financial viability of the healthcare organization rests with the revenue cycle and every aspect of it having accurate and complete information and data capture. Management of the revenue cycle is the process of supervising the entire claims process, including determining patient eligibility for insurance, collecting money owed on copayments (co-pays) and deductibles, and ensuring correct and timely capture of all charges. Monitoring, or working, the revenue cycle from the patient's first contact with the organization to the final account balance of zero includes numerous steps and professionals (NueMD 2018).

Patient Registration

Patient registration is the first step to ensuring that claims submitted to a payer will receive proper reimbursement. Responsibilities include preregistration, registration, insurance verification, and prior approval (authorization) for some services.

The patient registration department of a hospital is frequently called Patient Access and is responsible for capturing demographic information for each patient. If correct information is not captured on the front end, it will delay the entire process and cause extra work with resubmitting denied claims and cleaning up the errors. Capturing a patient's demographic information begins before the patient encounter with preregistration, which involves collecting the patient's name, date of birth, insurance coverage, and address. If a patient is not covered by an insurance plan, he or she is considered a self-pay patient and is responsible for all charges incurred during his or her encounter. The term third-party payer is used to identify an insurance company that pays for the medical care of covered individuals. The terms *first party*, the patient, and *second party*, the healthcare provider, are not used as frequently.

If a patient is covered by more than one insurance, coordination of benefits (COB)—determining which insurance coverage is the primary, secondary, and tertiary payer—takes place. For example, a patient is covered under the group plan A offered at her place of work and is also covered under the group plan B, offered at her spouse's place of work. Her own insurance A is primary and her spouse's insurance B is billed after her plan A has made its payment. For children covered by both their parents' insurance, the birthday rule is used to determine which coverage is billed first. The parent whose birthday falls first in the calendar year (not who is oldest, or who has insurance for the longest amount of time) is primary; for example, if the mother's birthday is January 21 and the father's birthday is March 14, the mother's insurance plan is primary because her birthday is in January and falls first in a calendar year.

Some medical procedures require prior approval (authorization) for services, which involves obtaining approval from the insurance company before receiving services. The registration staff monitors the healthcare organization's appointments and schedules and is responsible for contacting the health insurance carriers for procedures that require prior approval. For example, a patient with a strong family history of breast cancer may require a breast ultrasound yearly. If this service does not receive prior approval, the insurance company may deny the claim for payment.

Documentation, Coding, and Charge Capture

Healthcare services should be documented in the health record and captured through an electronic system or manually entered into the patient's financial account as they are provided. The charge capture process involves entering codes for all procedures and supplies provided during patient care. The codes include diagnoses, procedure, and supply codes.

A charge description master (CDM), sometimes called chargemaster, is a financial management list that contains information about the organization's charges for healthcare services it provides to patients. As the patient is seen at the healthcare organization, charges are captured for services such as the following:

- Accommodations (room and board)
- Room use (for example, emergency department, recovery room, operating room)
- Supplies used during the course of stay (bandages, splints, venipuncture tray)
- Ancillary services (such as radiology, laboratory, pharmacy)
- Clinical services (such as anesthesia, cardiology, physician rounds)

Hospitals charge facility fees—the technical component of healthcare services, for laboratory and radiology tests. It covers the cost and overhead for providing the service. The portion of work performed by a physician or other healthcare professional is the professional component of the charge capture. More information on the professional and technical components of healthcare charges is found in the global payment section of this chapter. The charge capture process flow for a physician practice is outlined in figure 15.1. When the patient checks in, the front office staff records demographic information in the electronic health record (EHR) or on paper, verifies payment

Figure 15.1 Charge capture process for a physician practice

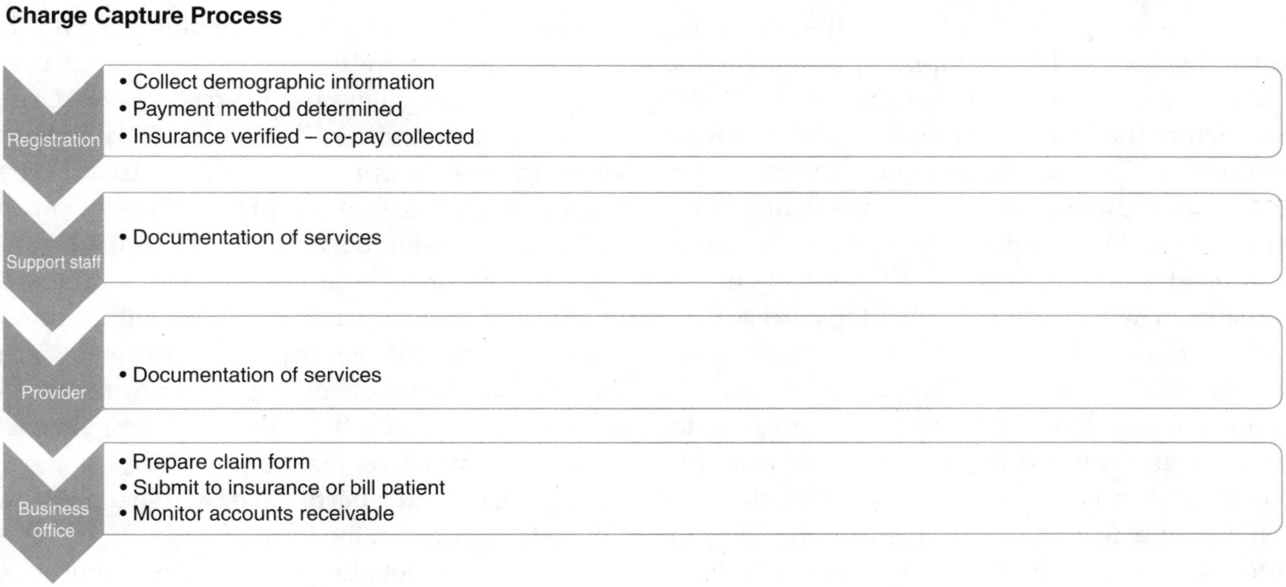

Charge Capture Process

Registration	• Collect demographic information • Payment method determined • Insurance verified – co-pay collected
Support staff	• Documentation of services
Provider	• Documentation of services
Business office	• Prepare claim form • Submit to insurance or bill patient • Monitor accounts receivable

Source: © AHIMA.

method and insurance coverage, and collects the copayment for the visit. The clinical support staff and physicians or providers update the EHR as services are rendered. The front office staff then discharge the patient. Finally, the business office prepares the claim for billing and send it to the insurance company. The business office monitors the claim for payment and follow-up as needed. If the patient does not have insurance coverage, the front office staff collects the payment for services rendered (NueMD 2018).

Healthcare Claims Processing

After all the charges for an episode of care are captured, the healthcare organization creates a claim for reimbursement based on the CDM fees listed for each service. The Health Insurance Portability and Accountability Act (HIPAA) mandated the use of electronic transactions for healthcare claims using the *HIPAA X12 837 Healthcare Claim: Professional* for professional charges and *HIPAA X12 837 Healthcare Claim: Institutional* for facility and technical component claims. Claim forms include *International Classification of Diseases, Tenth Revision, Clinical Modification* (ICD-10-CM) and *International Classification of Diseases, Tenth Revision, Procedure Coding System* (ICD-10-PCS) codes that classify the diagnosis for the inpatient encounter. The ICD-10-CM and ICD-10-PCS codes reflect the reason the patient is being treated. Healthcare Common Procedure Coding System (HCPCS) codes are used to identify healthcare procedures, supplies, and equipment for outpatient encounters and have dollar values associated with them. (Chapter 5, *Clinical Terminologies, Classifications, and Code Systems,* covers ICD-10 CM/PCS, and HCPCS codes in more detail.)

The third-party payer receives the claim for reimbursement and determines the eligibility of the patient for coverage and the medical necessity of the services. **Eligibility** is verification that the patient is covered by the plan on the date of service and the services provided are covered by the plan. **Medical necessity** is the determination that the services provided will benefit the patient and are needed. For example, a patient receiving plastic surgery to improve the look of his or her face may not be covered; however, if the surgery is being done to repair scars from an accident, it may be covered.

The insurance policy determines the amount the patient pays for deductible, coinsurance, and copayment. Deductible is the amount of cost, usually annually, the policyholder must incur before the plan will assume liability for the remaining covered expenses. For example, a person who has a $1,000 deductible must pay that amount each year before the insurance policy will start paying for services. Coinsurance is a pre-established percentage of eligible expenses after the deductible is met (such as 20 percent, though the amount varies by policy). Copayment (co-pay) is a cost-sharing measure in which the policyholder pays a fixed dollar amount (flat fee) per service, such as $15 per physician office visit. Out-of-pocket costs are healthcare costs a patient must pay because the total cost is not covered by insurance. For example, David Sanders is seen in the urgent care clinic for removal of a fishhook from his thumb. The provider was not sure about the placement of the hook and needed to take an x-ray of the hand before removal. After the hook was removed, the wound was cleaned and Mr. Sanders was given a shot of cefitraxone antibiotic. Mr. Sanders is covered by his employer's healthcare plan, ABC HealthCare, which has a $500 yearly family deductible, 20 percent coinsurance, and $15 co-pay for physician visits. Table 15.1 displays how the payer will process the claim.

A provider may choose to accept assignment, meaning payment is based on a fee schedule, a list of services and the amount that the healthcare insurance plan will pay for healthcare claims. The provider will accept the amount paid as payment in full for the service, as opposed to balance billing where the provider charges the patient for the remainder of the costs not paid by the insurance plan. Therefore, there may be different payments of services within a healthcare organization for the same service depending on the contracted price for that service with each third-party payer. Using the previous example with Mr. Sanders, if the provider accepts assignment from ABC HealthCare, the physician agrees to accept $75.00 for the physician visit instead of his normal $100.00 fee.

Healthcare insurance payers have a variety of reimbursement plans and contracts with individual providers and employers for payment such that the same type of service to two different patients may be paid differently depending on each patient's contract or insurance. After a claim is processed, the third-party payer will send notification to the patient in the form of an explanation of benefits (EOB), detailing how the payer processed the claim for payment. The third-party payer will also send a remittance advice (RA) to the healthcare provider explaining the process used for the claim and how much it is paying the healthcare provider.

Working the Accounts Receivable

Billing department employees (billers) are responsible for maintaining and working the organization's accounts receivable (AR). AR is a record of the payments owed to the organization by outside entities such as third-party payers and patients. Billers work the AR by monitoring charges, payments, adjustments, and write-offs. If a claim has not been paid, billers will resubmit the claim to insurance carriers or determine why the claim has

Table 15.1 Example of claim processing

Service	Cost (fee schedule)	Deductible ($500 per year)	Coinsurance (20%)	Copayment ($15 per visit)	Total insurance pays	Patient responsibility
Physician visit	$100.00	$50.00	$10.00	$15.00	$25.00	$75.00
Comment		Patient has already paid $450 this year, he has now met his deductible	20% of cost of visit after the deductible is paid. $100 – $50 = $50 and 20% of $50 = $10	Patient pays $15 out of pocket for each visit		
X-ray	$250.00	$0.00	$50.00	$0.00	$200.00	$50.00
Antibiotic	$50.00	$0.00	$10.00	$0.00	$40.00	$10.00
Total	**$400.00**	**$50.00**	**$70.00**	**$15.00**	**$265.00**	**$135.00**

Source: © AHIMA.

not been paid. When a healthcare organization has a contract with a third-party payer for services, the difference between what the healthcare provider charges and what is paid by the payer is the contractual adjustment (NueMD 2018). The billing department has a detailed list of adjustment codes to monitor all adjustments made to AR.

If the payer accepted a claim, but payment was denied for any reason, it is important for the billers to explore the reason for the denial and correct any errors in the claim or submit additional documentation requirements requested by the payer. This process is called denials management.

Check Your Understanding 15.1

Match the definitions with the terms.

1. Fixed amount paid by policyholder per month
2. Pre-established percentage of eligible expenses after the deductible is met, such as 20 percent
3. Policy or contract in which the purchaser (insured) pays a set amount to help cover the cost of medical expenses
4. Paying for services provided with own funds
5. Amount of cost (usually annually) the policyholder must incur before the plan will assume liability for the remaining covered expenses
6. Process of how patient financial and health information moves into, through, and out of the healthcare facility
7. A list of services and the amount that the healthcare insurance plan will pay for healthcare claims.
8. A financial management list that contains information about the organization's charges for healthcare services it provides to patients

   a. Healthcare insurance
   b. Premium
   c. Fee Schedule
   d. Chargemaster
   e. Out of pocket
   f. Deductible
   g. Coinsurance

Healthcare Insurers

Healthcare insurance types include commercial, managed care, and government-sponsored plans. Each insurer or payer has its own set of reimbursement guidelines, defined by payer contracts with providers, or insurers may follow federal regulations for payment of healthcare claims. This section discusses the different types of healthcare insurers.

Commercial Insurance

Many Americans are covered by commercial insurance plans. The plans may be obtained through their employer, purchased individually, or through a group, such as a professional association. For example, a healthcare organization may pay for its employees to have commercial insurance, or a person may purchase coverage individually from a commercial company. A person who is a member of a national association or group may purchase coverage through that company. Healthcare plans can be private, employer-based self-insurance, not-for-profit, and for-profit.

Private Healthcare Insurance

Individuals, self-employed professionals, and groups of people (such as associations and religious organizations) are able to purchase commercial insurance, called private healthcare insurance, for themselves and their dependents. Typically, these plans have high deductibles (for example $2,500 per year) or limited covered services (for example, a policy may only cover emergency services and not dental and vision services). A premium for coverage is paid each month to the third-party payer and those funds are used to help pay for healthcare services. Private healthcare insurance plans use the premiums collected from policyholders to pay for healthcare incurred by all the members of the plan who are covered during a particular month.

Employer-Based Coverage

Employer-based coverage is obtained when employees and employers share the cost of premium payment—the employer contributes a portion of the premium amount and the employee also contributes, usually with a direct deduction from his or her paycheck. For example, an employer might pay for 80 percent of the cost of coverage and the employee would cover the additional 20 percent of the premium. Employees are usually able to pay an additional premium amount to cover dependents. For example, Sue's Safe Shelter for Women employs 74 people and pays to enroll the employees and their dependents in a Blue Cross Blue Shield plan. Blue Cross Blue Shield offered the first healthcare plans in the United States in 1929 and remains an insurer to this day. Employers with fewer than 50 full-time employees are not required to provide healthcare insurance to their employees.

Employer-Based Self-Insurance Plans

In the 1970s, large companies started to self-insure employees instead of paying into private plans. Companies set aside the cost they would have paid for premiums for health coverage and used those funds to pay the healthcare claims. Employer-based self-insurance is a self-funding arrangement in which an employer funds medical expenses for the covered beneficiaries (individuals who are eligible for benefits from a health plan) and contracts with a third-party administrator (TPA) to provide the administrative oversight to process the medical claims payments for the employer. A third-party administrator is responsible for payment of healthcare claims on behalf of the company. For example, Community Hospital has 4,000 employees and offers healthcare insurance coverage for those employees. Community Hospital is self-insured and contracts with ABC Insurance Provider to administer the insurance plan for the hospital. Community Hospital sets aside the amount of money they would pay for premiums for healthcare coverage. When an employee healthcare claim is sent to ABC Insurance Provider, the claim is paid from the funds Community Hospital has allocated. Many factors affect an employer's decision to self-fund, particularly the ability to assume the risk involved when a claim for high-cost services is experienced. For example, one case of cancer in an employee may cost the employer a large amount of money in a short period of time causing the employer to not be able to assume the risk for future high-cost medical cases.

Not-for-Profit and For-Profit Healthcare Plans

Commercial healthcare insurance plans are either not-for-profit or for-profit plans. Not-for-profit third-party payers do not focus on making money; the premiums collected pay for the administrative costs of running the company and the company receives tax breaks that the for-profit plan does not. As part of the Affordable Care Act (ACA), Consumer Operated and Oriented Plans, or CO-OPs, were created. CO-OPs allow nonprofit, customer-owned health insurance companies to provide insurance coverage to nonprofit organizations through low-interest loans CO-Ops offer insurance to individuals and small businesses (CMS 2015b).

A for-profit plan exists to make money from the premiums collected. The ACA requires healthcare insurance companies to report the amount of premium revenue that is spent on clinical services and quality improvement; this is known as the medical loss ratio (MLR). The MLR requires companies to spend at least 80 percent of premium money on medical care. The ACA also requires the company to issue rebates to enrollees if the percentage falls below these standards (CMS 2018a).

Managed Care

Managed care is a healthcare delivery system, or network, organized to manage cost, utilization, and quality. Managed care plans contract with healthcare providers and medical facilities to provide care for members of the plan at reduced costs. Plans restricting choices usually cost less while a flexible plan will cost more. There are three types of managed care plans addressed. They are the following:

1. Health maintenance organizations (HMO)
2. Preferred provider organizations (PPO)
3. Point of service (POS) (NLM 2019)

A managed care organization (MCO) is a type of healthcare organization that delivers medical care and handles all aspects of the care and payment for care by limiting providers of care, discounting payment to providers of care, or limiting access to care. For example, a provider may agree to see enrollees of an MCO for a set payment per member per month (PMPM), also referred to as capitation, which is discussed in full later in the chapter. Members of an MCO are called enrollees and have access to services including physician, inpatient, preventive, prenatal, emergency, and home healthcare (Casto 2018). The National Committee for Quality Assurance (NCQA) is a private, not-for-profit organization whose mission is to improve healthcare quality by accrediting, assessing, and reporting the quality of managed care plans. Enrollees can find information regarding the quality of care, access, and cost, and compare managed care plans, because the Centers for Medicare and Medicaid Services (CMS) collects data via the Healthcare Effectiveness Data and Information Set (HEDIS) (NCQA 2019). CMS is the Department of Health and Human Services (HHS) agency responsible for Medicare and parts of Medicaid.

Health Maintenance Organizations

A health maintenance organization (HMO) is an entity that combines the provision of healthcare insurance and the delivery of healthcare services. It is characterized by an organized healthcare delivery system to a specific geographic area. The HMO has a set of basic and supplemental health maintenance and treatment services that are provided to voluntarily enrolled members. The members pay a predetermined fixed amount per month or year as prepayments for coverage. HMOs provide for care within their network, where patients are seen by providers and within healthcare organizations the HMO controls and owns. HMOs offer healthcare services such as family health, gynecology, well-child visits, radiology, surgical, obstetrics, inpatient, or therapies. Typically, HMOs offer a broader range of preventative healthcare services than other managed care plans (CMS 2016a).

HMOs started as a way to provide healthcare at reduced cost to the consumer. The Health Maintenance Organization Act of 1973 established federal rules defining the operation of HMOs. The Act made it easier for HMOs to grow and attract clients and required all employers that offered traditional healthcare to their employees to sign up for an HMO if they had more than 25 employees. Under all types of HMOs, every employer pays the same monthly premium for services. Each employee is assigned a primary care physician—a physician who bears the ultimate responsibility for ensuring the employee receives the medical care he or she needs. If an employee has a medical condition, he or she first visits the primary care physician. If the condition is beyond the physician's expertise or scope, the physician refers the employee to another physician within the HMO. If emergency treatment is needed, the employee is referred to hospitals within the HMO; likewise, the employee obtains medication from pharmacies within the HMO network. Most HMOs are extensive enough to offer a wide variety of providers, described as the following:

- *Group model HMOs*. In this model the HMO contracts with more than one physician; for example, a medical group that includes physicians in multiple fields of expertise.

The members of the medical group provide the care to the HMO enrollees on a fee-for-service basis (Casto 2018).

- *Open-panel model or independent practice associations*. This model is created when the HMO contracts with a physician who has his or her own practice and the physician agrees to see the patients who belong to the HMO in addition to their regular patients (Casto 2018).
- *Network model HMOs*. In this model the HMO contracts with a network of providers who provide multispecialty group practices. Reimbursement for healthcare is either on a fee-for-service or capitation basis.
- *Staff model HMOs*. In this model the HMO employs the physicians. Physicians see only members of the HMO and are paid a salary by the HMO. The premiums paid by enrollees to the HMO are used to cover the cost of services and facilities.

Preferred Provider Organizations

A preferred provider organization (PPO) is a managed care contract-coordinated care plan with the following elements:

- Contains a network of providers who have agreed to a contractually specified reimbursement for covered benefits with the organization offering the plan
- Provides for reimbursement for all covered benefits regardless of whether the benefits are provided with the network of providers
- Offered by an organization that is not licensed or organized under state law as an HMO (CMS 2016b)

A PPO is a form of managed care closest to a fee-for-service plan where providers agree to accept lower fees from the insurer for services to be part of the network, with the patient paying a set copayment. If a patient sees a provider outside the network, the patient will pay a higher fee. The PPO can be local or regional. Local PPOs offers plans within a specific area, usually consisting of one or more counties, and this area is approved by CMS. Regional PPOs were introduced to help beneficiaries who live in rural areas. There are specific locations established by CMS (CMS 2016b).

Point-of-Service Plans

A point-of-service (POS) plan allows enrollees to choose between an HMO or PPO each time they are in need of care. For example, a patient is able to choose an in-network primary provider but is also able to seek care outside of the network. Payment for services outside of the network is covered by the plan with the patient paying a percentage of the bill. If the primary care provider refers a patient outside the network of providers, the plan pays all or most of the bill. If the patient sees a provider outside the network and the service is covered by the plan, the patient will have to pay a percentage of the bill as coinsurance, or if the service is not covered by the plan, the patient will pay out of pocket for the entire bill.

Exclusive Provider Organizations

Exclusive provider organizations (EPO) are hybrid MCOs in that they provide benefits to subscribers only when network providers perform healthcare services. Self-insured (self-funded) employers or associations use this model that has characteristics of both HMOs and PPOs.

Government-Sponsored Healthcare Plans

The US government is the largest payer of healthcare insurance. According to CMS, 100 million people are covered through Medicare, Medicaid, the Children's Health Insurance Program (CHIP), and the Health Insurance Marketplace (CMS 2015c). Medicare Part A, Part B, and Part D; the Medicare Advantage Plan; and the Conditions of Participation will be described in the sections that follow, as well as Medicaid eligibility criteria, services, the Medicare–Medicaid relationship, State Children's Health Insurance plans, TRICARE, the Veterans Health Administration, CHAMPVA, Indian Health Services, and workers' compensation.

Medicare

Medicare was enacted as the Title XVIII amendment to the Social Security Act of 1935. Implemented in 1965, Medicare extended health coverage to most Americans age 65 or older or those receiving retirement benefits from Social Security or the Railroad Retirement Board (CMS 2015d). Medicare is financed through payroll taxes paid by workers. CMS is responsible for management of the Medicare program. To be eligible for Medicare coverage, enrollees—called beneficiaries—must fall into one of six benefit categories: be age 65 or older, be a retired federal employee who is enrolled in the civil service retirement system, have end-stage renal disease, be a disabled adult, have become disabled before the age of 18, or be a spouse of an entitled individual. Medicare contracts with Medicare Administrative Contractors (MAC), which are private insurance companies that serve as Medicare's agents in the administration of the Medicare program, including processing and paying claims (CMS 2015e).

The next section will define Medicare Parts A and B, Part C (also known as the Medicare Advantage Plan), and Medicare Part D. The Medicare Conditions of Participation are also discussed.

Medicare Part A Hospital Insurance Medicare Part A hospital insurance assists in covering inpatient care in hospitals, including critical access hospitals and skilled nursing facilities (not custodial or long-term care). It also assists in covering hospice care and some home healthcare. Beneficiaries must meet certain conditions to receive these benefits such as having paid enough Medicare taxes while they were working, being age 65 or older, or being disabled before the age of 65 (CMS 2015f). Most people do not have to pay for Part A coverage because they, or a spouse, paid Medicare and payroll taxes while working which funds their Part A coverage. Individuals may be able to buy coverage if they are not entitled to Medicare, if they did not pay enough Medicare taxes while working. Some states may help people with limited income and resources pay for Part A (CMS 2018b).

Medicare Part B Medical Insurance Under Medicare Part B, medical insurance is an optional and supplemental portion of Medicare for which beneficiaries pay a monthly premium. Part B assists with coverage for physicians' services and outpatient care. It also insures other medical services not covered under Part A, such as some physical and occupational therapists' services, and some home healthcare. Part B pays for these covered services and supplies when they are medically necessary (CMS 2018b). Services covered may include physicians' services, outpatient care, home health, durable medical equipment, ambulance, and preventive services. Preventive services include healthcare services to prevent illness (for example, vaccinations to prevent diseases like polio) or early detection tests and diagnostic tools, when treatment is most likely to be effective (CMS 2018b).

Medicare Advantage Plans Medicare Advantage (MA) Plans were created as part of the Balanced Budget Act (BBA) of 1997. They are sometimes called Part C or MA Plans and are managed care plans offered by private companies approved by Medicare. For example, United Healthcare insurance plan contracts with Medicare to cover beneficiaries who choose this plan. MA Plans cover all Medicare services, but may also offer extra coverage, such as dental, vision, and acupuncture. Beneficiaries who join a MA Plan have Medicare Part A and B coverage through the MA Plan and not from original Medicare Part A (CMS 2018c).

Medicare pays a fixed amount for the beneficiary's care each month to the companies offering MA Plans. Each MA Plan can charge different out-of-pocket costs and have different guidelines for how services are received; for example, requiring a referral before seeing a specialist (CMS 2018c).

Medicare Part D, Prescription Drug Coverage Medicare Part D provides various plan options for beneficiaries to obtain prescription drug coverage. The Medicare Prescription Drug Improvement and Modernization Act (MMA) created Medicare Part D in 2003. Under this Act, Medicare contracts with private insurance companies to provide drug coverage to beneficiaries. Enrollment is voluntary and only available to people who are covered under Parts A and B. Benefits and cost vary by the plan in which the beneficiary is enrolled, and can be as low as $15 per month, with an annual deductible and co-pay required (CMS 2018d).

Out-of-Pocket Expenses and Medigap Insurance Medicare does not pay 100 percent of billed medical claims by healthcare organizations and providers. Medicare beneficiaries pay out of pocket for the deductible, co-pay, and non-covered services portions of healthcare claims. Beneficiaries may purchase supplemental insurance—known as Medigap—to help cover those expenses.

Medicaid

Medicaid helps with medical costs for millions of Americans with low incomes and limited resources including the mandatory eligibility groups of children, pregnant women, elderly adults, people with disabilities, and low-income adults. The US federal government, and state governments, both help fund this program (CMS 2018d). Each state administers its own Medicaid program, and determines the type, amount, duration, and scope of services above and beyond the basic broad federal guidelines. This means that Medicaid programs can vary widely between states. The federal government establishes a set of mandatory benefits and states can choose to provide additional optional benefits beyond the required benefits.

States can apply to CMS for a waiver of federal law to expand health coverage beyond the mandatory eligibility groups. Many states have opted to expand Medicaid coverage, especially for children, above the federal minimums because they feel that the federal minimums do not provide enough coverage. Medicaid eligibility criteria, services, the Medicaid–Medicare relationship, and the state Children's Health Insurance Plan are defined as follows.

Medicaid Eligibility Criteria Medicaid eligibility is based on the annual income of a person or his or her family and is calculated in relation to a percentage of the federal poverty level (FPL), which is the minimum amount of gross income that a family receives in a year. The FPL is determined by HHS and is updated annually on the Medicaid website (CMS 2015c). The ACA set the national Medicaid minimum eligibility level at 133 percent of the FPL for nearly all Americans under the age of 65. This means if the FPL for a family of one is $11,770 per year, the 133 percent FPL would be $15,651 (11,770 × 133% = 15,651).

Non-financial eligibility criteria include proof of federal and state residency, immigration status, and documentation of US citizenship.

Medicaid Services States establish and administer Medicaid programs and determine the type, amount, duration, and scope of services within broad federal guidelines. Common mandatory benefit services include coverage of the following care and services:

- Inpatient hospital
- Outpatient hospital
- Nursing facility
- Physician
- Home healthcare
- Rural health clinic
- Laboratory and x-ray
- Family planning
- Tobacco cessation

Common optional benefits include coverage of the following care and services:

- Prescription drugs
- Physical, occupational, speech, hearing, and language therapy
- Optometry
- Dental
- Chiropractic
- Hospice

The Medicare–Medicaid Relationship

The Federal Coordinated Healthcare Office (Medicare–Medicaid Coordination Office) serves people who are enrolled in both Medicare and Medicaid and are known as dual eligible, meaning they are covered under both Medicare and

Medicaid. The goal is for enrollees who are dual eligible to have full access to seamless, high-quality healthcare and to make the system as cost-effective as possible (CMS 2018e). The Medicare–Medicaid Coordination Office, established by the ACA, works across federal and state agencies to align coordination of benefits (COB) between the programs. COB determines the financial responsibility for payment of medical claims when one or more payers are involved. The goals of the office are to do the following:

- Provide access to people who are covered by both Medicare and Medicaid
- Make the process easier for dual-eligible people
- Provide quality healthcare
- Help with understanding the programs
- Eliminate regulatory conflicts
- Prevent shifting costs from one program to the other
- Improve the transitions of care
- Improve the quality of service and suppliers (CMS 2018e)

State Children's Health Insurance Plan The Children's Health Insurance Program (CHIP) provides healthcare coverage to eligible children through both Medicaid and individual state CHIP programs. Eligibility is based on a percentage of the family's annual income based on the FPL for the current year. Like all Medicaid programs, CHIP is administered by states according to federal requirements and is funded jointly by states and the federal government. States can choose to impose limited enrollment fees, premiums, deductibles, coinsurance, and copayments for children and pregnant women, usually 5 percent of a family's annual income. Cost sharing is prohibited for some services. Cost sharing is the amount that a patient pays for a medical service out of pocket; for example, a healthcare provider who performs a well-baby check must accept the amount Medicaid pays as payment in full.

TRICARE

The US Department of Defense operates TRICARE, which is a major part of the Military Health System and is the healthcare program for uniformed service members (active, Guard or Reserve, and retired) and their families. TRICARE is managed by the Defense Health Agency under leadership of the Assistant Secretary of Defense for Health Affairs and is a regionally managed healthcare program with an expansive provider network that combines the resources of military hospitals and clinics with civilian healthcare networks (DHA 2018). Several healthcare plan options are available for members, depending on their circumstances, and include emergency care, urgent care, preventive services, hospitalization, dental, and pharmacy coverage. Table 15.2 displays some of the plan options.

Veterans Health Administration

The US Department of Veterans Affairs operates the nation's largest integrated healthcare system, the Veterans Health Administration (VA), with more than 1,700 hospitals, clinics, community living centers, domiciliary, readjustment counseling centers, and other facilities. The VA offers a variety of healthcare services from basic primary care to nursing home care for eligible veterans. The number of veterans who can be enrolled in the healthcare program is determined by the amount of money Congress gives the VA each year.

Civilian Health and Medical Program of the Department of Veterans Affairs

The Civilian Health and Medical Program of the Department of Veterans Affairs (CHAMPVA) is a comprehensive healthcare program in which the VA shares the cost of covered healthcare services and supplies with eligible beneficiaries. The Chief Business Office Purchased Care (CBOPC) administers the program. CHAMPVA covers most healthcare services that are medically and psychologically necessary. To be eligible for CHAMPVA, a person cannot be eligible for TRICARE and must be in one of the following categories:

- The spouse or child of an eligible veteran
- The spouse or child of a veteran who died as the result of a service injury

Table 15.2 TRICARE options

Option	Definition	Annual fee	Annual deductible	Co-pay amount
TRICARE Prime and Prime Remote	Managed care option offering the most affordable and comprehensive coverage Prime remote covers remote US stations Overseas options for active duty families living overseas	No annual fee	No deductible	No co-pay
TRICARE Standard and Extra	A fee-for-service plan available to all nonactive duty beneficiaries Most freedom to choose providers	No annual fee	$50/Individual $100/Family	15% of negotiated fee
TRICARE Reserve Select and Retired Reserve	A premium-based healthcare plan that qualified National Guard and Reserve members may purchase	Monthly premiums apply	$50/Individual $100/Family	No co-pay
TRICARE For Life	Offers secondary coverage to people who have Medicare Parts A and B	No annual fee but must have Medicare	No deductible	No co-pay
TRICARE Young Adult Options	A premium-based, worldwide healthcare plan that qualified adult children of eligible sponsors may purchase	Monthly premiums apply	No deductible	$12 per visit outpatient $11 per day inpatient
US Family Health Plan	Available through networks of community-based, not-for-profit healthcare systems in six areas of the United States	Enrollment is required with one year commitment to receive care from the plan	No deductible	No co-pay

Source: Adapted from TRICARE 2015.

- The spouse or child of a veteran who was totally disabled at the time of his or her death
- The spouse or child of a military member who died while serving in the military (VA 2018)

Indian Health Services

The Indian Health Service (IHS) is an HHS agency responsible for providing healthcare to American Indians and Alaska Natives within the United States. The provision of health services to members of federally recognized Native tribes grew out of a special government-to-government relationship between the federal government and Indian tribes. The Indian Self-Determination Act of 1975 turned control of healthcare organizations and programs over to Native and Indian tribes within the United Sates (IHS 2019). Each tribal government is responsible for the healthcare of its tribal members. The IHS is divided into 12 physical areas of the United States, Alaska, Albuquerque, Bemidji, Billings, California, Great Plains, Nashville, Navajo, Oklahoma, Phoenix, Portland, and Tucson. Each area works collaboratively to provide healthcare services to all American Indians and Alaska Natives who live within its areas (IHS 2019). For example, a Native Alaskan living in California can receive care at an IHS facility in California. If an IHS facility is not available for a patient, the tribe may use contract funds to pay for coverage at another healthcare organization. This relationship, established in 1787, is based on Article I, Section 8 of the Constitution. Numerous treaties, laws, Supreme Court decisions, and executive orders are responsible for what the agency is today. The IHS is the principal federal healthcare provider and health advocate for American Indian and Native people, and its goal is to raise their health status to the highest possible level (IHS 2019). Every IHS facility in the United States sets its own standard of coverage and services. For example, in Alaska there are 10 service areas, some with hospitals, clinics, or small rural health centers.

Workers' Compensation

Most employers in the United States are required to carry workers' compensation insurance to cover employees who are injured on the job. Workers' compensation laws are regulated by state and federal government and vary by state. The employee and provider complete a notice of injury report, which details what happened and how the injury occurred, for claim payments to be processed. The healthcare provider adds details to the report indicating the diagnosis and anticipated healthcare services that will be required. When a claim is sent to the workers' compensation insurance carrier the notice of injury report must be submitted with each claim for payment.

Federal Workers' Compensation Funds Federal employees are covered under the Federal Employees' Compensation Act (FECA) of 1916. The Department of Labor's Office of Workers' Compensation Programs (OWCP) administers four major disability compensation programs for federal employees or their dependents if the employee is injured at work. The four programs include the following:

1. Division of Federal Employees' Compensation (DFEC)
2. Division of Energy Employees Occupational Illness Compensation (DEEOIC)
3. Division of Longshore and Harbor Workers' Compensation (DLHWC)
4. Division of Coal Mine Workers' Compensation (DCMWC)

The benefits include disability, wage replacement, medical treatment, and vocational rehabilitation for workers injured on the job (DOL 2015).

State Workers' Compensation Funds Before state workers' compensation laws were introduced, companies were reluctant to provide insurance coverage for employees because of the high costs for workers injured on the job. Most states addressed the concern by introducing state workers' compensation insurance funds as a source of coverage for claims occurring because of workplace injury. State workers' compensation funds are maintained by each state from employer-paid premiums. Benefits may include compensation for burial, life insurance coverage for dependents upon death, compensation for lost income, and health coverage for medical care (Casto 2018).

Check Your Understanding 15.2

Answer the following questions.

1. The number of beneficiaries who can be enrolled in the healthcare program for military members is determined by the amount of money Congress allocates to the _______________ each year.
   a. VA
   b. TRICARE
   c. CHAMPVA
   d. Workers' compensation
2. Mandatory eligibility groups fall under which insurance?
   a. CHAMPVA
   b. Medicare
   c. IHS
   d. Medicaid

3. Identify the insurance that provides coverage to most Americans age 65 or older.
   a. TRICARE
   b. IHS
   c. Medicare
   d. Medicaid
4. What is a healthcare delivery system or network organized to manage cost, utilization, and quality?
   a. HMO
   b. Managed care
   c. Not-for-profit
   d. Employer-Based Self-Insurance
5. Which health insurance typically has a high deductible or limited covered services?
   a. Private Healthcare Insurance
   b. CHAMPVA
   c. Medicare
   d. CHIP
6. An employee for the HIM department is on their way to a forms committee meeting when they trip going up the stairs and twist their knee. Which type of insurance would they be eligible for?
   a. Workers' compensation
   b. Medicaid
   c. IHS
   d. TRICARE
7. Which government health program was introduced out of a special government-to-government relationship?
   a. Medicare
   b. Tricare
   c. IHS
   d. Workers' compensation

New Trends

Revenue management and reimbursement professionals must stay current with changes in laws and regulations that affect the revenue cycle and billing guidelines. New trends in recent years include the healthcare insurance marketplace, consumer-directed healthcare plans, hospital-acquired conditions, ACA, Medicare Access and CHIP Reauthorization Act (MACRA), and present on admission indicator reporting. These trends can affect reimbursement positively or negatively, which means keeping up with these regulations is imperative.

Health Insurance Marketplace or Exchange

The Patient Protection and Affordable Care Act (ACA) was signed into law in 2010. The ACA established a **health insurance marketplace or exchange** where uninsured, eligible Americans are able to purchase federally regulated and subsidized healthcare insurance. People who are not covered by insurance through a job, Medicare, Medicaid, CHIP, or another source are able to purchase insurance through a marketplace exchange. The exchange offers healthcare insurance to members based on their income. Most people who apply qualify for premium tax credits, which lower the cost of coverage. All plans cover essential health benefits, pre-existing conditions, and preventive care (HealthCare 2017).

Consumer-Directed Health Plans

Consumer-directed health plans (CDHP), also known as high-deductible plans (HDPs) because the deductible is at least $1,200 per year, are managed care organizations that influence patients and clients to select cost-efficient healthcare through the provision of information about health benefit packages and through financial incentives. Employers shift payment responsibility to plan members causing employees to opt for the HDP option to save money on premiums. The ACA mandates that HDPs purchased after March 2010 provide free preventive services even if the deductible has not been met.

Hospital-Acquired Conditions and Present on Admission Indicator Reporting

The ACA established the hospital-acquired conditions (HAC) reduction program to encourage hospitals to reduce HACs. An HAC is a reasonably preventable condition that a patient did not have upon admission to a hospital, but that developed during the hospital stay. Examples of HACs include foreign object retained after surgery, blood incompatibility, falls, and infections.

Hospital performance under the HAC reduction program is determined based on a hospital's total HAC score, which can range from 1 to 10. The higher a hospital's total HAC score, the worse the hospital performed under the HAC reduction program. Hospitals are given an opportunity to review their data and request a recalculation of their scores if they believe an error in the score calculation has occurred. The law requires the Secretary of HHS to reduce payments to hospitals that rank in the quartile of hospitals with the highest total HAC scores by one percent (CMS 2015d). Present on admission (POA) indicates that a condition was present at the time the patient was admitted to the hospital. When submitting claims to Medicare for MS-DRG reimbursement the POA indicator includes:

Y: Diagnosis was present at the time of admission

N: Diagnosis was not present

U: Documentation is insufficient to determine if condition was present

W: It is clinically undetermined if the condition was present (CMS 2015e)

Medicare Access and CHIP Reauthorization Act

The Medicare Access and CHIP Reauthorization Act (MACRA) was signed into law in April of 2015. MACRA created the Quality Payment Program, which requires providers to concentrate their healthcare efforts on the value of the care they provide instead of the volume, or number of patients, they see in a day. Providers' performance is measured through data collection reports that measure the following four areas:

1. Quality: Providers measure six areas of performance for their practice, including avoiding harm to patients, providing effective service, providing respectful care, reducing wait times, avoiding waste, and providing quality care that is equitable for all patients.
2. Improvement activities: This performance area measures the activities a provider uses to increase the coordination of care for patients, include the patient in the decision-making process for care, and expand access to care for all patients.
3. Promoting interoperability: This performance area measures the activities a provider uses to proactively share electronic health information with other providers by sharing test results and plans to coordinate healthcare.
4. Cost: This performance area measures the total cost of care for a year or for a hospital inpatient encounter.

MACRA created two ways to participate in the Quality Payment Program. One is a Merit-Based Incentive Payments System (MIPS) that streamlines multiple quality payment programs into one system. It was created to tie healthcare payments to the quality and cost efficiency of care. with the goals of improving healthcare processes and outcomes and reducing costs while increasing providers' use of healthcare information when treating patients (CMS 2018a). The MIPS uses the calendar year for providers to report data to be eligible for an increase in payment or to avoid a reduction for the next year. Providers must report data by March 31 of each year. The other program is the Advanced Alternative Payment Models (APMs) where providers are able to earn a Medicare incentive payment if they participate in an innovative payment model. For example, a medical practice can apply for payment under an APM if they invest in practice innovation and care redesign and enhance the coordination of care for their patients. MACRA also required social security numbers to be removed from Medicare cards by April 2019 to help prevent Medicare fraud (CMS 2018a).

Patient Protection and the Affordable Care Act

The ACA includes a number of provisions designed to encourage improvements in the quality of care and includes comprehensive healthcare insurance reforms. For example, Medicare's hospital readmissions reduction program requires a reduction in payment to a hospital if the hospital has what is considered excessive readmission rates. A readmission includes hospital admission within 30 days of a subsequent hospitalization (CMS 2015d). Another outcome of the ACA is the creation of accountable care organizations (ACOs). The ACO agrees "to be held accountable for improving the health and experience of care for individuals and improving the health of populations while reducing the rate of growth in healthcare spending" (CMS 2015d).

Utilization Management

Utilization management (UM) is the evaluation of the medical necessity, appropriateness, and efficiency of the use of healthcare services, procedures, and facilities under the provisions of the applicable health benefits plan, sometimes called utilization review. Prospective review refers to the review that takes place prior to elective procedures and admissions. This is achieved through a precertification process for elective admissions, certain diagnostic procedures, and outpatient surgeries. Utilization management professionals, who may be clinical nurses, physicians or mid-level providers, use clinical screening processes to apply consistent standards when determining if a service is medically necessary. One tool is preauthorization, which reviews proposed surgeries and other inpatient and outpatient healthcare services before the patient is admitted. Concurrent review involves screening for medical necessity and the appropriateness and timeliness of the delivery of medical care from the time of admission until discharge. Retrospective review includes review and analysis of actual utilization data after the patient has been discharged. The retrospective review may be conducted by a committee of the organization or an outside quality improvement organization (QIO), which is an organization hired by CMS to perform medical peer review of coding information for completeness, adequacy, and quality of care, as well as the appropriateness of payments. An outside review may find errors in daily operations performance that the organization missed. The UM professionals monitor inpatient utilization daily by reviewing a list of all patients, their diagnoses, the requested length of stay versus the actual length of stay, and other information that helps to continually manage inpatient activity to determine medical necessity as well as reimbursement for the inpatient stay.

Case Management

Case management is collaboration between healthcare and service providers to aid in the process of assessment, planning, facilitation, care coordination, evaluation, and advocacy to meet the comprehensive health needs of an individual or family. This is accomplished through communication and coordination of available resources to promote quality and cost-effective outcomes. The primary reason for case management is the facilitation of care across the continuum of care for the patient. For example, a patient newly diagnosed with cancer may require surgery, laboratory services, chemotherapy, radiation, and counseling services. Case management helps navigate all the services and providers for the patient.

The goal of case management is for the individual to reach the optimum level of wellness and functional capability. A case manager is usually a nurse, physician, or social worker who arranges all services that are needed by a patient and his or her family; for example, continued care or social services. They accomplish this by identifying the continued needs of the patient and determining the resources that are available to the patient. Case managers use a multi-disciplinary approach to optimize the outcome. This approach brings together many services from medical, social service, therapies, and such (CMS 2018f).

Healthcare Reimbursement Methodologies

Healthcare services can be reimbursed in a number of ways depending on the type of insurance coverage and the type of service provided. This section discusses fee-for-service reimbursement, episode-of-care reimbursement, capitation, global payment, resource-based relative value scale, skilled nursing payment, and prospective payments.

Fee-for-Service Reimbursement

Fee-for-service reimbursement is a reimbursement method through which providers retrospectively receive payment based on either billed charges for services provided or annually updated fee schedules. A provider submits a claim form to a healthcare plan with all charges itemized. In fee-for-service reimbursement, the itemized charges are individually assessed and paid based on the healthcare insurance coverage the patient holds. For example, if a healthcare provider submits a claim for services for an annual exam and the patient's healthcare coverage includes annual exam coverage, the healthcare insurance plan will pay the claim.

Value-Based Purchasing

Value-based purchasing (VBP) is a type of incentive to improve clinical performance using the EHR and resulting in additional reimbursement or eligibility for grants or other subsidies to support further health information technology efforts. Examples of types of incentives used include better healthcare for patients and populations of people and lower healthcare costs. The goal is to improve the quality, efficiency, and overall value of healthcare. The ACA expands the use of pay for performance in Medicare with the idea that paying providers to achieve better outcomes should improve those outcomes (CMS 2017).

The typical VBP program provides a bonus to healthcare providers if they meet or exceed agreed-upon quality or performance measures; for example, reductions in catheter-associated urinary tract infections. Each year measures are added or deleted to ensure patient safety is the highest priority. The programs may also reward improvement in performance over time, such as year-to-year decreases in the rate of avoidable hospital readmissions (CMS 2017).

Traditional Fee-for-Service Reimbursement

In traditional fee-for-service (FFS) reimbursement systems, third-party payers or patients issue payments to healthcare providers after healthcare services have been received (for example, after the patient has been discharged from the hospital). Payments are based on the specific services delivered.

After services are rendered, an itemized claim for all service charges is submitted to a healthcare plan for payment. Payment is based on the billed charges, taking into account discounted charges, negotiated rates, and usual or customary charges for a geographic area. Usual, customary, and reasonable (UCR) charges is a type of fee-for-service payment method in which the third-party payer remunerates fees that are usual for the provider's practice, customary for the community, and reasonable for the situation. For example, the amount of reimbursement for a mammogram at a rural hospital may be significantly more than for a large urban hospital because the cost of doing business in the rural area is higher and justified for that geographic area.

Many commercial insurance companies use the traditional FFS reimbursement methodology for visits to physician's offices.

Managed Fee-for-Service Reimbursement

Managed FFS reimbursement involves utilization controls for reimbursement under traditional fee-for-service insurance plans, in that managed care plans control costs by handling their members' use of healthcare services. Managed care plans negotiate with providers to develop discounted fee schedules.

Controlling utilization of services includes both prospective and retrospective reviews of planned healthcare services. Precertification is a type of prospective review. For example, a patient with a strong family history of colon cancer needs prior approval to receive a screening colonoscopy before the age approved by a healthcare plan.

The retrospective utilization review process involves evaluation of utilization information after the patient has been discharged or the care has been completed. Utilization review also includes discharge planning—coordinating the activities related to the release of a patient when inpatient hospital care is no longer needed. The managed care plan controls costs by providing a less intensive, and therefore less expensive, care setting as soon as possible.

Episode-of-Care Reimbursement Methodologies

An episode-of-care (EOC) reimbursement is given for a relatively continuous medical treatment provided by the healthcare professional in relation to a particular clinical problem or situation. For example, an obstetrician who charges a patient a flat fee for the entire episode of pregnancy and delivery or a patient receiving follow-up care for the first 60 days after a stroke. In home health services, all services and supplies provided to a patient for a 60-day period are paid by EOC reimbursement.

Capitation

Capitation is a specified amount of money paid to a healthcare plan or physician to cover the cost of a healthcare plan member's services for a certain length of time (CMS 2016c). The healthcare plan negotiates with an employer or agency for a preestablished amount of money to care for the health services of members. The MCO agrees to provide health services for a period of time, usually one year. Capitated premiums are calculated on the projected cost of providing covered services PMPM.

Global Payment

Global payment methodology involves payment that combines the professional and technical components of a procedure and disperses payments as a lump sum to be split between the physician and the healthcare organization. The professional component of a service is considered the part of the service supplied by physicians (for example, the radiologist). The technical component (for example, supplies, equipment, and support services) is supplied by a hospital or freestanding surgical center. For example:

A patient receives a chest x-ray.
Professional component: Services of the radiologist
Technical component: Radiology department use, x-ray equipment
Global payment: The facility received a lump-sum payment for the radiologist reading the x-ray and the facility fees to take the x-ray

Prospective Payment

A prospective payment system (PPS) is a method of reimbursement in which Medicare payment is made based on a predetermined, fixed amount. The payment amount for a particular service is derived based on the classification system of that service. CMS uses separate PPSs for reimbursement of the following:

- Acute inpatient hospitals
- Home health agencies
- Hospice
- Hospital outpatient
- Inpatient psychiatric facilities
- Inpatient rehabilitation facilities
- Long-term care hospitals
- Skilled nursing facilities (CMS 2014b)

Medicare Acute Inpatient Prospective Payment System

The inpatient prospective payment system (IPPS) under Medicare Part A is a payment methodology in which payment is based on the diagnosis of the patient. An inpatient stay is categorized into a Medicare severity diagnosis-related group (MS-DRG). A DRG is a unit of case-mix classification in a PPS where diseases are placed into groups because related diseases and treatments tend to consume similar amounts of healthcare resources and incur similar amounts of cost to the hospital. A patient's hospitalization may fall into one of more than 500 diagnostic classifications in which cases demonstrate similar resource consumption and length of stay patterns. Hospitals are paid a set fee for treating patients in a single DRG category, regardless of the actual cost of care. A hospital may receive an adjustment or an additional reimbursement if it is a disproportionate share hospital (DSH), a hospital that treats a high percentage of low-income patients (CMS 2015e). The IPPS works in conjunction with coding and ICD-10 CM/PCS, where the codes are grouped together. This data is used to look at quality measures, such as readmission rates and HACs. An inpatient rehabilitation hospital or unit within a hospital is a free-standing facility that provides an intensive rehabilitation program for patients. Patients must be able to tolerate three hours of intense rehabilitation services per day. These facilities are paid under the IRF PPS. A patient assessment instrument (PAI) is completed on Medicare patients shortly after admission and upon discharge. Based on the patient's condition, services, diagnosis, and medical condition, a payment level is determined for the inpatient rehabilitation stay. Comprehensive outpatient rehabilitation facilities have separate Medicare guidelines.

Medicare Severity Diagnosis-Related Groups

The DRG system was updated to MS-DRG to better account for severity of illness and resource use for inpatient services. The three levels of severity in the MS-DRG system are the following:

1. Major complication/comorbidity (MCC): The patient has a medical condition that arises during an inpatient stay, like a wound infection (complication) or a medical condition that coexists with the primary reason for admission and affects the patient's treatment or length of stay (comorbidity)
2. Complication/comorbidity (CC): The patient has a medical condition that is not considered major
3. Non-CC: All severity levels are based on the secondary diagnosis; this level of severity indicates the patient does not have a CC (CMS 2016b)

A hospital's case-mix index (CMI) represents the average MS-DRG relative weight for a particular hospital. The CMI is calculated by looking at the Medicare discharges for a defined period of time (month, quarter, year), adding them together, then dividing by the number of total discharges within that period of time. The CMI allows administration to measure the hospital's performance based on MS-DRG cases. CMIs are calculated using both transfer-adjusted cases and unadjusted cases, meaning that a patient who is transferred from facility A to facility B to receive a higher level of care and is only at facility A for one day will not receive the entire DRG payment for the patient's diagnosis because the patient was transferred out of the first facility. The payment rate is based on the type of case and resources required to treat the patient. By analyzing the CMI of a facility a manager is able to compare the CMI against other similar facilities in the area, or the year-to-year changes of the facility in its CMI. This analysis allows coding managers to correct coding errors resulting in improper MS-DRG payments in a timely manner and allows administrators to understand the type of patient in the healthcare organization to allow and plan for future clinical allocations.

Resource-Based Relative Value Scale System

A resource-based relative value scale (RBRVS) system is a payment methodology in which physician payments are determined by the resource costs needed to provide care. The RBRVS contains national uniform relative values for all physicians' services. The relative value of each service must be the sum of relative value units representing the physicians' work, practice expenses net of malpractice insurance expenses, and the cost of professional liability insurance. The calculation for payment is based on the three components listed. There may also be an adjustment based on geographical resource costs (CMS 2017).

Skilled Nursing Facility Prospective Payment System

Skilled nursing facilities (SNFs) are paid based on a case-mix classification system under the skilled nursing facility prospective payment system, the SNF Value-Based Purchasing Program (VBP), and the SNF Quality Reporting Program (QRP). This payment methodology shows a commitment by CMS to shift payment models from volume to value based systems. The case-mix model is called the Patient-Driven Payment Model (PDPM), and the focus is on the condition and care requirements of the patient rather than on the amount of care provided to the patient in order to determine the Medicare payment. The payment system also encourages SNFs to innovate in terms of meaningful quality measure reporting, reducing paperwork and administrative costs. The goal is for SNFs to treat the needs of the whole patient not just the services the patient receives, which requires substantial paperwork to track.

Outpatient Prospective Payment System

As part of the BBA, CMS started using the outpatient prospective payment system (OPPS)—the Medicare prospective payment system used for hospital-based outpatient services and procedures that is predicated on the assignment of ambulatory payment classifications (APC). A single payment is made for all outpatient services that fall within an APC, which is a group consisting of diagnoses and procedures that are similar in terms of resources used, complexity of illness, and conditions represented. A single payment is made for the outpatient services provided. A single visit can result in multiple APC groups. APC groups consist of five types of services: significant procedures, surgical services, medical visits, ancillary services, and partial hospitalization. The OPPS reimburses some hospital outpatient services and certain Medicare Part B services furnished to hospital inpatients when Part A payment cannot be made; for example, implantable devices used in diagnostic testing (CMS 2014a).

Ambulatory Surgery Center Prospective Payment System

For Medicare purposes, an ambulatory surgery center (ASC) is a distinct entity that operates exclusively for the purpose of furnishing surgical services to patients who do not require hospitalization and when the expected duration of services does not exceed 24 hours following admission. This definition applies to the ASC no matter who pays for the ASC's services (CMS 2019c. Medicare makes a single payment to ASCs for covered surgical procedures, including ASC facility services furnished in connection with the covered procedure; this is known as the ambulatory surgery center (ASC) payment rate. Examples of ASC-covered services include nursing, surgical dressing, administrative costs for the facility, and ancillary services (CMS 2019a).

Home Health Prospective Payment System

The home health prospective payment system (HH PPS) was mandated by the BBA. The HH

PPS uses the Patient-Driven Groupings Model (PDGM) for payment, which is based on a 30-day period of time for service. The 30-day periods of time are categorized into 432 case-mix groups and 5 subgroups, which include source of admission, timing, clinical grouping, functional impairment level, and comorbidity adjustments (CMS 2018b; CMS 2019b).

Ambulance Fee Schedule

The BBA mandated the implementation of a national ambulance fee schedule for Medicare Part B. Ambulance transport includes both vehicular and air travel. Medicare will determine the medical necessity for the transportation of a patient by ambulance and if the facility to which the patient is taken is appropriate. For example, a patient living on an island with only a small clinic healthcare facility is in a motor vehicle crash, resulting in a broken femur. The clinic calls an air ambulance service to transport the patient to a larger trauma center on the mainland. Payment for ambulance services includes a base rate payment plus a mileage payment to the nearest healthcare organization. So, if the base rate for air ambulance for the patient with the broken femur is $3,000 and the mileage was 100 miles at $45 per mile, the total payment would be $3,000 (base rate) + $4,500 ($45 per mile) for a total of $7,500. Rates vary based on geographic area across the United States (CMS 2019c).

HIM Roles

During almost every legislative session of Congress, changes are made to healthcare reimbursement methodologies and healthcare coverage options for Medicare and Medicaid patients. Health insurance providers make great efforts to ensure they are paying for services that are medically necessary, reasonable, and covered by their plans. Healthcare reimbursement methodologies are very complex and change based on the type of service, location, type of provider, and so on. HIM professionals know the complexities of reimbursement rules and regulations. They help organizations understand incentive programs that focus on quality and provide the data and information needed for reporting purposes for reimbursement. They provide knowledge on different reimbursement models, which is invaluable to healthcare organizations. Professional coders use their expertise to ensure compliance with regulations for reimbursement; for example, a coder will determine the code needed for POA requirements. HIM auditors are able to review claim denials to determine what documentation is needed to process a claim form for reimbursement.

Check Your Understanding 15.3

Match the terms to the descriptions.

a. Resource-based relative value scale
b. Concurrent review
c. Utilization management
d. Hospital-acquired conditions
e. Ambulatory surgery center

1. Payments for services are determined by the resource costs needed to provide them.
2. The evaluation of the medical necessity, appropriateness, and efficiency of the use of healthcare services, procedures, and facilities under the provisions of the applicable health benefits plan.
3. A group of reasonably preventable conditions that patients do not have upon admission to a hospital, but which develop during the hospital stay.
4. A distinct entity that operates exclusively for the purpose of furnishing surgical services to patients who do not require hospitalization.
5. Screening for medical necessity and the appropriateness and timeliness of the delivery of medical care from the time of admission until discharge.

Real-World Case 15.1

David, a student from an accredited HIM program, was given a professional practice experience project that required him to review reimbursement denials for Medicare patients over the course of the past year. He noticed that the denials were higher when the claim included services from the radiology department. He researched the claims and resubmitted them with additional documentation. Through this process, he discovered that the additional documents required were similar for each claim. Also, because of the settings on the organization's EHR, the required diagnosis codes for the radiological services performed were not being submitted on the claim form, although the procedure code was included on the claim. David communicated his findings to the manager, and they discussed potential next steps.

Real-World Case 15.2

Emily Kelley was taken to Kirklake Community Hospital for pain in her side. She was admitted and taken into surgery, where her appendix was removed. In recovery her temperature spiked, and after looking at Emily's labs it was determined that she had developed an infection from the surgery. This was not the first surgery where an infection subsequently developed, and the current total HAC score for this hospital was 8. As a result of the high HAC score, the reimbursement to the hospital for Emily's surgery was less than it should have been based on APC grouping. The billers noticed a decrease in reimbursement and discussed it with the manager. The HIM manager approached the performance improvement manager to discuss the spike in HACs. She was able to provide the data to support an investigation into why this was happening. It was determined that the infections were occurring when a particular provider was on staff.

References

American Health Information Management Association. 2017. *Pocket Glossary of Health Information Management and Technology*, 5th ed. Chicago: AHIMA.

American Medical Association. 2015. Overview of the RBRVS. http://www.ama-assn.org/ama/pub/physician-resources/solutions-managing-your-practice/coding-billing-insurance/medicare/the-resource-based-relative-value-scale/overview-of-rbrvs.page.

Case Management Society of America. 2015. http://www.cmsa.org/.

Casto, A.B. 2018. *Principles of Healthcare Reimbursement*. 6th ed. Chicago: AHIMA.

Centers for Medicare and Medicaid Services. 2019a. Hospital Outpatient Prospective Payment System. http://www.cms.gov/Outreach-and-Education/Medicare-Learning-Network-MLN/MLNProducts/downloads/HospitalOutpaysysfctsht.pdf.

Centers for Medicare and Medicaid Services. 2019b. Skilled Nursing Facility Prospective Payment System. http://www.cms.gov/Outreach-and-Education/Medicare-Learning-Network-MLN/MLNProducts/downloads/snfprospaymtfctsht.pdf.

Centers for Medicare and Medicaid Services. 2019c. Ambulatory Surgical Center Fee Schedule. https://www.cms.gov/Outreach-and-Education/Medicare-Learning-Network-MLN/MLNProducts/downloads/AmbSurgCtrFeepymtfctsht508-09.pdf.

Centers for Medicare and Medicaid Services. 2094d. Home Health Prospective Payment System. http://www.cms.gov/Outreach-and-Education/Medicare-Learning-Network-MLN/MLNProducts/Downloads/Home-Health-Prospective-Payment-System-Text-Only.pdf.

Centers for Medicare and Medicaid Services. 2019e. Ambulance Fee Schedule. http://www.cms.gov/Medicare/Medicare-Fee-for-Service-Payment/AmbulanceFeeSchedule/.

Centers for Medicare and Medicaid Services. 2018a. MACRA. https://www.cms.gov/Medicare/Quality-Initiatives-Patient-Assessment-Instruments/Value-Based-Programs/MACRA-MIPS-and-APMs/MACRA-MIPS-and-APMs.html.

Centers for Medicare and Medicaid Services. 2018b. Medicare Advantage Organizations, Cost Plans and Prescription Drug Plan Sponsors. https://www.cms.gov/Medicare/Medicare-Advantage/Plan-Payment/Downloads/Release-of-Medical-Loss-Ratio-MLR-Reporting-Tool-for-Contract-Year-2017.pdf.

Centers for Medicare and Medicaid Services. 2018e. Medicare Part A. https://www.cms.gov/Medicare/Medicare-General-Information/MedicareGenInfo/Part-A.html.

Centers for Medicare and Medicaid Services. 2018f. Medicare Part B. https://www.cms.gov/Medicare/Medicare-General-Information/MedicareGenInfo/Part-B.html.

Centers for Medicare and Medicaid Services. 2018g. Health Plans—General Information. https://www.cms.gov/Medicare/Health-Plans/HealthPlansGenInfo/.

Centers for Medicare and Medicaid Services. 2018h. Medicaid and CHIP Eligibility Levels. http://www.medicaid.gov/medicaid-chip-program-information/program-information/medicaid-and-chip-eligibility-levels/medicaid-chip-eligibility-levels.html.

Centers for Medicare and Medicaid Services. 2019i. Federal Policy Guidance. http://www.medicaid.gov/federal-policy-guidance/federal-policy-guidance.html.

Centers for Medicare and Medicaid Services. 2018j. About the Medicare-Medicaid Coordination Office. Advancing Care for People with Medicaid and Medicare. https://www.cms.gov/Medicare-Medicaid-Coordination/Medicare-and-Medicaid-Coordination/Medicare-Medicaid-Coordination-Office.

Centers for Medicare and Medicaid Services. 2017. Hospital Value-Based Purchasing. https://www.cms.gov/Outreach-and-Education/Medicare-Learning-Network-MLN/MLNProducts/downloads/Hospital_VBPurchasing_Fact_Sheet_ICN907664.pdf.

Centers for Medicare and Medicaid Services. 2016a. Capitation. https://www.cms.gov/apps/glossary/search.asp?Term=capitation&Language=English&SubmitTermSrch=Search.

Centers for Medicare and Medicaid Services. 2016b. Medicare Managed Care Manual: Chapter 1—General Provisions. https://www.cms.gov/Regulations-and-Guidance/Guidance/Manuals/downloads/mc86c01.pdf.

Centers for Medicare and Medicaid Services. 2016c. Resource-Based Relative Value Scale. https://www.cms.gov/apps/glossary/search.asp?Term=resource-based+relative+value&Language=English&SubmitTermSrch=Search.

Centers for Medicare and Medicaid Services. 2015a. Tracing the History of CMS Programs: From President Theodore Roosevelt to President George W. Bush. https://www.cms.gov/About-CMS/Agency-Information/History/Downloads/PresidentCMSMilestones.pdf.

Centers for Medicare and Medicaid Services. 2015b. Loan Program Helps Support Customer-Driven Non-Profit Health Insurers. https://www.cms.gov/CCIIO/Resources/Grants/new-loan-program.html.

Centers for Medicare and Medicaid Services. 2015c. Medicare. https://www.cms.gov/Medicare/Medicare.html.

Centers for Medicare and Medicaid Services. 2015d. History: CMS' Program History. https://www.cms.gov/About-CMS/Agency-Information/History/index.html?redirect=/History/.

Centers for Medicare and Medicaid Services. 2019. Fact Sheet: Medicare issues fiscal year 2019 payment & policy changes for skilled nursing facilities. July 31, 2018 https://www.cms.gov/newsroom/fact-sheets/medicare-issues-fiscal-year-2019-payment-policy-changes-skilled-nursing-facilities

Defense Health Agency. 2015. TRICARE. http://www.tricare.mil.

Department of Health and Human Services. 2018. About the Affordable Care Act. https://www.hhs.gov/healthcare/about-the-aca/index.html.

Ferenc, D. 2014. *Understanding Hospital Billing and Coding*, 3rd ed. St. Louis, MO: Elsevier.

Griffin, J. 2017 (March 7)."The History of Healthcare in America." Employee Benefits Consultants - JP Griffin Group. https://www.griffinbenefits.com/employeebenefitsblog/history_of_healthcare.

Indian Health Service. 2019. https://www.ihs.gov/.

The Henry J. Kaiser Family Foundation. 2018 (December 10). "Key Facts about the Uninsured Population." https://www.kff.org/uninsured/fact-sheet/key-facts-about-the-uninsured-population/.

National Committee for Quality Assurance. 2019. About NCQA Overview. http://www.ncqa.org/AboutNCQA.aspx.

National Library of Medicine, MedlinePlus. 2019. Managed Care Summary. https://www.nlm.nih.gov/medlineplus/managedcare.html.

NueMD. 2018 (November 19). Revenue Cycle Management 101. https://www.nuemd.com/revenue-cycle-management/rcm-101.

TRICARE. 2015. Compare Plans. http://www.tricare.mil/Plans/ComparePlans.aspx.

US Department of Labor. 2015. Office of Workers' Compensation Programs (OWCP). http://www.dol.gov/owcp/.

US Department of Veterans Affairs. 2018. CHAMPVA Family Members Insurance. http://www.va.gov/hac/forbeneficiaries/champva/handbook.asp.

Fraud and Abuse Compliance

Darline A. Foltz, RHIA, CHPS, CPC
Karen M. Lankisch, PhD, MHI, RHIA, CHDA, CPC, CPPM

Learning Objectives

- Differentiate among fraud, abuse, and waste
- Identify the elements of a compliance program
- Examine the legal and regulatory requirements related to the management of a compliance program
- Examine the purposes of audits
- Examine the benefits of a coding compliance plan
- Explore the need for the involvement of health information management (HIM) professionals in clinical documentation integrity
- Identify clinical documentation integrity metrics
- Differentiate between the organizations involved in the federal regulations and initiatives

Key Terms

Abuse
Anti-Kickback Statute
Appeal
Audit
Automated review
Balanced Budget Act of 1997
Clinical documentation integrity (CDI)
Clinical validation audit
Coding audit
Coding compliance plan
Compliance
Compliance program
Complex review
Comprehensive Error Rate Testing (CERT)
Computer-assisted coding (CAC)
Denial
Exclusions Program
False Claims Act
Fraud
Health Care Fraud Prevention and Enforcement Action Team (HEAT)
Health Insurance Portability and Accountability Act (HIPAA)
Medical necessity audit
Medicare Fraud Strike Force
Merit-Based Incentive Payment System (MIPS)
Natural language processing (NLP)
Noncovered services
Office of Inspector General (OIG)
Overpayment
Physician Self-Referral Law
Qui tam
Reasonable cause
Reasonable diligence
Recovery audit contractor (RAC)
Risk analysis
Semi-automated reviews
Stark Law
Unbundling
Upcoding
Waste
Whistleblower Protection Act (WPA)
Willful neglect

Payers of healthcare services, including federal and state governments, private insurance companies, and patients trust that physicians and all healthcare professionals render high-quality medical care to their patients and submit accurate claims for payment while upholding the highest ethical standards. While most healthcare professionals strive to meet these expectations, there are some dishonest healthcare professionals who illegally exploit the healthcare system for personal gain. In addition to dishonest healthcare professionals, there are healthcare organizations that have poor billing policies and procedures or improperly trained billing and coding staff resulting in unintentional billing errors. These instances have created the need for laws to combat fraud and abuse to ensure proper reimbursement.

While the terms *fraud* and *abuse* are often used together, there is a distinct difference between them. **Fraud** is "when someone intentionally executes or attempts to execute a scheme to obtain money or property of any healthcare benefit program" (CMS 2017c, 4). The key word in this definition is *intentionally*. Some examples of fraud are the following:

- Billing for services not provided to the patient
- Falsely documenting in health records, such as documenting a higher severity of diagnosis or completely falsifying diagnoses; for example, a diagnosis of malnutrition that does not meet the definition of or have the supporting health record documentation of severe protein calorie malnutrition should not be coded to this level of severity as additional reimbursement may result from this incorrect coding
- Directing others to falsely document or bill
- Paying for or getting paid for referring patients

Abuse occurs "when healthcare providers or suppliers perform actions that directly or indirectly result in unnecessary costs to any healthcare benefit program" (CMS 2017c, 4). In the case of abuse, the healthcare provider is entitled to payment but requests more reimbursement than he or she deserves. Mistakes happen in the course of doing business, so one or two errors will not usually result in accusations of abuse. It is only when a consistent pattern is evident that abuse allegations occur. Some examples of abuse include a pattern of coding errors such as upcoding or unbundling.

Unbundling is the practice of using multiple procedure codes to bill for the various individual steps in a single procedure rather than using a single code that includes all of the steps of the comprehensive procedure code. For example, a code for a complete laboratory blood count should be used rather than individual codes for a red blood count, a white blood count, a hematocrit, and all the other tests that make up a complete blood count. Unbundling can result in the healthcare organization receiving an overpayment and is considered abuse as it violates coding guidelines.

Upcoding is the practice of assigning diagnostic or procedural codes that results in higher payment rates than the codes that actually reflect the services provided to patients; for example, billing with the procedure code for an open procedure when the procedure was actually laparoscopic. This difference in surgical approach would provide the healthcare provider with an **overpayment**—a higher reimbursement than deserved. Overpayments typically occur in the following situations:

- There is insufficient documentation to support the amount billed
- A treatment or service does not meet the definition of medically necessary (*medically necessary* is defined as the likelihood that a healthcare service will have a reasonably beneficial effect for the patient)
- Duplicate payments for the same service are made
- There are administrative or processing errors (CMS 2017a)

Noncovered services are healthcare services that are not reimbursable under a healthcare plan. These services vary by medical plan. Some examples of healthcare services that might be considered noncovered are cosmetic surgery such as liposuction and breast augmentation. Infertility treatments, weight loss programs, mental health services, and dental services are treatments and procedures that are not typically covered by medical insurance.

Another related term is **waste**. Waste is the overutilization or inappropriate utilization of services and the misuse of resources. Waste is typically not a criminal or intentional act. Examples of waste include having too many supplies on hand and being required to destroy them when the expiration date passes or ordering more ancillary tests than may be required to treat the patient (CMS 2018b).

Any inappropriate payment made to a healthcare organization for any reason is considered an improper or inappropriate payment. Improper payments are discussed later in this chapter. Mistakes will occur in the process of billing for healthcare services and may result in an incorrect payment to a healthcare organization. A mistake is considered the most innocent of improper payments since there is no intent to falsely receive an incorrect payment from a healthcare plan. The next level in the spectrum of improper payment is inefficiencies. This is a more serious type of error that occurs when billing insurance companies since ongoing inefficiencies may demonstrate a lack of effort to bill correctly, resulting in improper payments and waste of insurance plan staff and resources. Bending the rules is the next level of improper payments, and meets the definition of abuse, since it demonstrates that a healthcare provider consistently chooses to bill in the provider's favor when billing rules allow for some interpretation. Intentional deception is clearly the most serious and highest level of improper payments since this reflects a healthcare provider's purposeful incorrect billing to result in improper payments, falling under the definition of fraud. This progression is shown in figure 16.1.

The risk for fraud and abuse exists in all organizations so compliance measures must be taken. **Compliance** is the process of establishing an organizational culture that promotes the prevention, detection, and resolution of instances of conduct that do not conform to federal, state, or private payer healthcare program requirements or the healthcare organization's ethical and business policies. In other words, compliance actively prevents fraud and abuse. This chapter will review fraud and abuse regulations and initiatives related to coding and billing fraud and abuse. Programs and tools used by healthcare organizations to ensure accurate coding and billing, such as compliance and clinical documentation integrity programs, will also be discussed.

Figure 16.1 Progression, types, and causes of inappropriate payments

Type of inappropriate payment	Mistake	Inefficiencies	Bending the rules	Intentional deception
Cause of inappropriate payment	Error	Waste	Abuse	Fraud
Example	Accidentally charging the wrong patient for a physician office visit	Failure to run software edits on a claim, which results in the following: the insurance company rejects the claim, the healthcare organization has to rebill, and the insurance company reprocesses the claim—a waste of staff time and resources	Hospital coders that consistently select the higher paying DRG when more than one DRG is acceptable to bill	Purposely selecting the wrong principal diagnosis to upcode claims

Moderate → **Serious**

Source: CMS 2014a.

Federal Regulations and Initiatives

While there is no way to accurately measure how much healthcare fraud exists in the United States, from the audits conducted by the federal government and commercial insurance companies, billions of dollars are involved. With the federal government as the largest payer of healthcare services, federal laws, programs, and enforcement are necessary to protect the monies available to the citizens of the United States. Fraud and abuse of federal funds earmarked for healthcare puts beneficiaries' health and welfare at risk as monies paid for fraudulent claims reduce the amount of funds available for legitimate healthcare services. A discussion of the federal government regulations and initiatives for the control and prevention of healthcare fraud and abuse follows.

Office of the Inspector General

The Office of Inspector General (OIG) works to combat fraud, waste, and abuse and to improve the efficiency of Health and Human Services (HHS) programs (OIG 2019a). The HHS is the principal agency of the US federal government that is responsible for protecting the health of all Americans and providing essential human services. The HHS reports to the OIG. The mission of the OIG is to protect the integrity of the HHS programs as well as the health and welfare of individuals enrolled in federal programs such as Medicare and Medicaid. The OIG is responsible for monitoring Medicare and Medicaid, which provide health insurance to one in three Americans at the cost of hundreds of billions of taxpayer dollars annually. The sheer size of Medicare and Medicaid make these programs vulnerable to criminals. One of the vital roles of the OIG is to keep these programs less prone to waste, fraud, and abuse. The OIG has the federal government's largest team of auditors and is the premier healthcare law enforcement agency. Every year the OIG investigates, prosecutes, and convicts hundreds of individuals who misuse or steal taxpayer dollars. This results in the annual recovery of billions of dollars for the federal government (OIG 2019a).

The majority of the OIG's resources go to the oversight of Medicare and Medicaid, but also extend to programs under other HHS institutions, including the Centers for Disease Control and Prevention (CDC), the, National Institutes of Health (NIH), and the Food and Drug Administration (FDA) (OIG 2019a).

The OIG is organized into five divisions, categorized as follows and illustrated in figure 16.2.

1. *Office of Audit Services*. The Office of Audit Services is responsible for auditing HHS programs to ensure the agencies and their contractors are meeting their responsibilities. Their findings can be used in criminal and other investigations.
2. *Office of Evaluation and Inspections*. This division evaluates HHS programs to make them more effective and to prevent fraud, abuse, or waste within HHS.
3. *Office of Management and Policy*. This division ensures that the OIG has the resources that they need to fulfill their responsibilities.
4. *Office of Investigations*. This is the OIG division responsible for monitoring and enforcing fraud and abuse regulations in HHS programs, operations, and beneficiaries. These efforts include operating the fraud hotline where individuals can call and report fraudulent activities, working with the Department of Justice (DOJ) to coordinate fraud investigations, protecting the Secretary of HHS and participating in public safety and security management activities, and working to enforce and update the fraud and abuse efforts of the OIG to continue to improve programs.
5. *Office of Counsel to the Inspector General*. The Office of Counsel to the Inspector General provides legal advice to the OIG (OIG 2019a).

Figure 16.2 OIG organizational structure

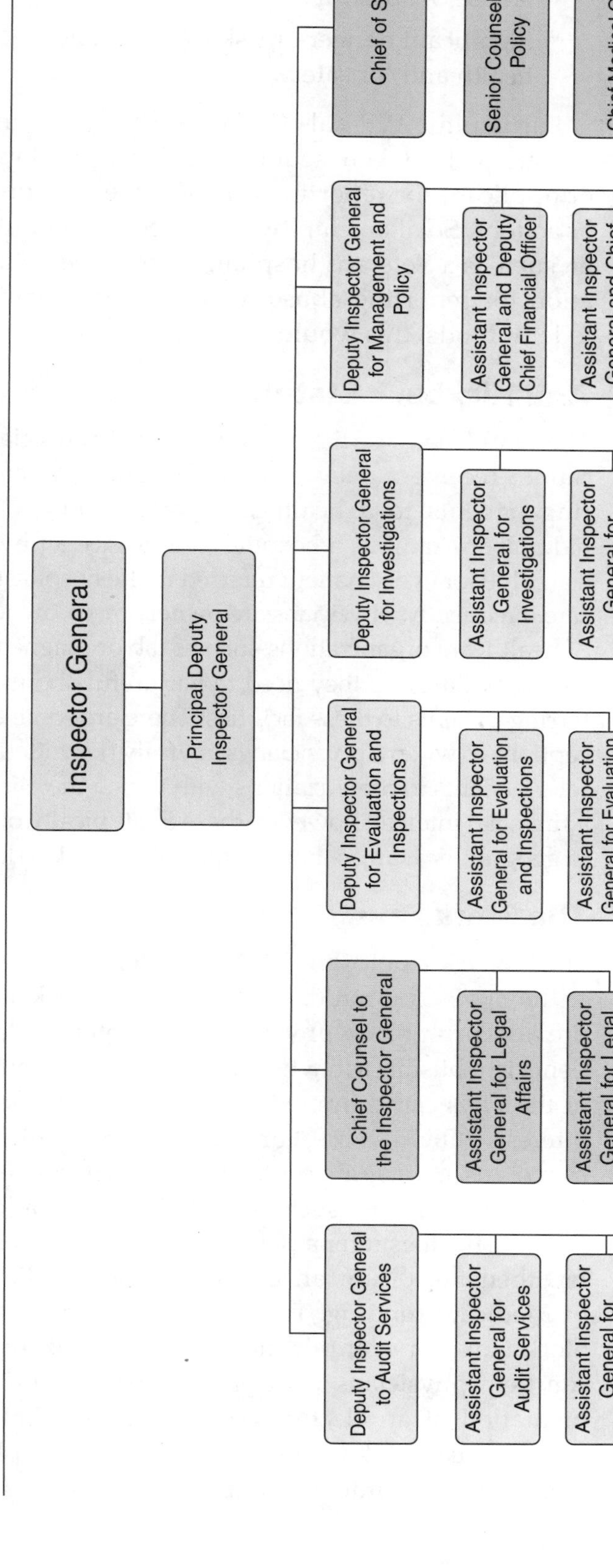

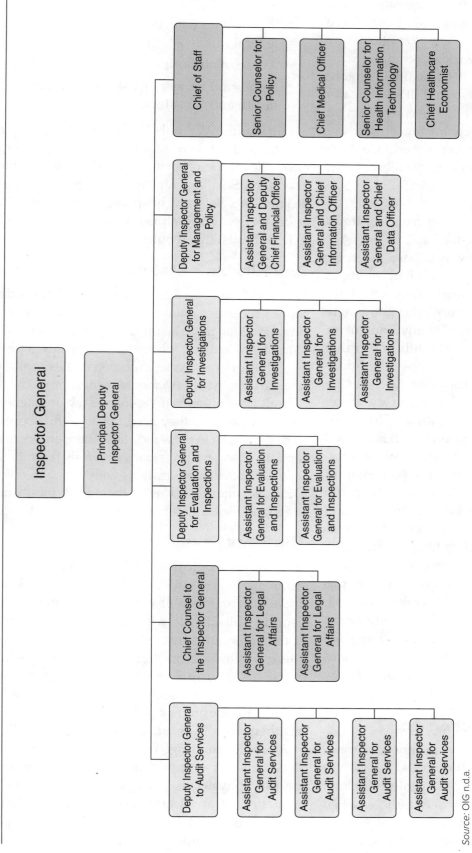

Source: OIG n.d.a.

There are a number of federal regulations and initiatives used to combat fraud and abuse. These include the False Claims Act, Whistleblower Protection Act (WPA), Anti-Kickback Statute, Stark Law, Balanced Budget Act of 1997, Health Insurance Portability and Accountability Act (HIPAA), Health Care Fraud Prevention and Enforcement Action Team, OIG, recovery audit contractor, quality improvement organizations, Recovery Audit Contractor, and Quality Improvement Organizations.

False Claims Act

Individuals have been committing crimes of fraud for hundreds of years. In fact, the False Claims Act, also known as Lincoln's Law, was passed during the Civil War to address the fraudulent billing of Union Army supplies. The False Claims Act allows penalties to be awarded to those who knowingly submit fraudulent claims to the US government for payment. "Knowingly" does not only mean that the individual has actual knowledge of the fraudulent claim but also includes deliberately being ignorant regarding the fraudulent claim and disregard of the fraudulent claims (FindLaw 2019). The law has been the foundation upon which fraud and abuse efforts have been based, with revisions and other legislation added to it over the years. One of the key components of the False Claims Act is qui tam. Qui tam is the whistleblower provisions of the False Claims Act—private persons, known as relators, may enforce the Act by filing a complaint, under seal (meaning kept secret), alleging fraud committed against the government. For example, if a coder is told to assign codes in violation of coding rules, then he or she can anonymously report the healthcare organization for fraud. The individual who submits the allegations can receive as much as 30 percent of the penalties collected by the federal government (DOJ 2018a).

Whistleblower Protection Act

A whistleblower is someone who reports wrongdoing by an organization or individual. The Whistleblower Protection Act (WPA) protects federal employees and applicants for federal jobs when they report situations or actions that they believe qualifies as one of the following situations:

- Violation of law
- Significant mismanagement or waste of federal funds
- Abuse of authority
- Significant danger or risk to the public health and/or safety

Further, the WPA also prevents any personnel actions to be taken against a federal employee or applicant for reporting one of these situations or actions. So, if an employee of a federal employer, such as a Veterans hospital, experiences retaliation for reporting abuse, violation, or waste of federal funds, this would be unlawful.

Anti-Kickback Statute

The Anti-Kickback Statute dictates that physicians cannot receive money or other benefits for referring patients to a healthcare organization (OIG n.d.b). For example, a hospital cannot give a physician $100 for every patient referred to the hospital for care. Frequently, physicians are owners or co-owners of healthcare organizations such as lab or diagnostic testing facilities, so they need to be careful about referring patients to these facilities. There are some exceptions to when a physician is lawfully permitted to refer patients to organizations with which they have a financial interest; however, these are typically only in geographical areas that are sparsely populated.

The Stark Law

The Physician Self-Referral Law, otherwise known as the Stark Law, builds on the Anti-Kickback Statute and prohibits a physician from referring patients to a business in which he or she or a member of the physician's immediate family has financial interests (OIG n.d.b.). For example, if the physician owns an imaging center, he or she cannot refer a patient for images such as x-rays at that location. If he or she does refer a patient to the imaging center, then the physician cannot receive Medicare or Medicaid funding. There are exceptions to the Stark Law; for example, healthcare organizations can help physicians with limited costs of implementation of an electronic health record (EHR), and in areas of low population per geographic area such as a rural area, patient referrals may be made to physician-owned or family-owned businesses if there are no other options available.

Balanced Budget Act of 1997 and the Exclusions Program

The Exclusions Program is a database of individuals and healthcare organizations that are not permitted to participate in or receive payment from any federal healthcare program due to past healthcare-related crimes they committed against the federal government. The Balanced Budget Act of 1997 (BBA) is the law that gives the OIG the authority to exclude individuals and healthcare organizations that are convicted of healthcare-related crimes from receiving payment from any federal healthcare program, including Medicare and Medicaid programs. In addition, the BBA does not allow healthcare providers or healthcare organizations to hire or contract with someone on the excluded database. Healthcare providers and healthcare organizations that hire or contract with an excluded individual or healthcare organization are in violation of law and may be penalized or fined. The terms of an individual's or healthcare organization's exclusion is based on a number of factors such as whether the crime is a felony or misdemeanor, whether this is a first conviction, the scope of the crime, and so forth. However, mandatory terms for a felony begin at five years of exclusion from the Medicare and Medicaid programs and three years for a misdemeanor. Reinstatement of the excluded individual or healthcare organization is not automatic at the end of the time period, rather the individual or organization must apply to the OIG for reinstatement to participate in federal healthcare programs (OIG 2019b).

The BBA also permits Medicare to refuse to allow convicted felons into the Medicare program and educates Medicare beneficiaries on how they can assist in preventing fraud as well as how to report fraud when they identify it. It also gives Medicare beneficiaries the right to receive a copy of their detailed bill from the healthcare provider (BBA 1997).

Health Insurance Portability and Accountability Act

The Health Insurance Portability and Accountability Act (HIPAA) of 1996 addresses many topics such as privacy and security of health information as well as fraud and abuse. HIPAA created a joint venture between the HHS and the DOJ (HHS 2009). HIPAA also increased the civil monetary penalty for fraud and abuse convictions. The penalty was increased from $2,000 per incident to $10,000 per incident plus three times the total amount of the fraudulent claims (OIG 1998). Every year the penalties are increased to account for inflation. Incidents occurring after January 29, 2018, increased to $11,463 per incident (OIG 2019c). For additional information on HIPAA, refer to chapter 9, *Data Privacy and Confidentiality*, and chapter 10, *Data Security*. Figure 16.3 is an example of how civil monetary penalties work. It is clear from this example that committing fraud and abuse can have significant monetary consequences for individuals and healthcare organizations.

Healthcare providers must make a concerted effort to comply with best practices regarding reimbursement and monitoring for fraud and abuse. Best practices include monitoring and auditing (covered later in this chapter). When HHS determines the civil monetary penalties for the instance of fraud or abuse, the level of efforts that a healthcare provider or healthcare organization has put into fraud and abuse prevention is considered. These efforts can be grouped into the three categories that follow.

Figure 16.3 Example of civil monetary penalties

ABC Hospital submitted 150 claims where they unbundled laboratory charges. They were overpaid $100 on each claim. If the OIG considered this to be fraud or abuse, the civil monetary penalty/fine would be three times the overpayment plus $11,463 for each incident.

150 claims x $100 overpayment = $15,000

3 x total amount of overpayment = $15,000 x 3 = $45,000

$11,463 x 150 claims (each claim is considered an incident) = $1,719,450+45000

ABC Hospital would be fined $1,764,450.

Source: Adapted from OIG 2019c and OIG n.d.b.

1. Reasonable cause. It would be unreasonable to expect the healthcare provider to comply with the requirements of HIPAA
2. Reasonable diligence. The healthcare provider has taken reasonable actions to comply with the legislative requirements
3. Willful neglect. Intentionally failing to comply with or being indifferent to the HIPAA provisions (45 CFR 160.401)

Health Care Fraud Prevention and Enforcement Action Team

Since 2009 the Health Care Fraud Prevention and Enforcement Action Team (HEAT) and the Medicare Fraud Strike Force teams, which are a component of HEAT, have worked to fight healthcare fraud. HEAT is one of many programs used to combat Medicare fraud. It combines the efforts of HHS, OIG, and the DOJ (DOJ 2016).

The Medicare Fraud Strike Force teams consist of local, state, and federal law enforcement individuals who combine their resources and data analytics to identify instances of fraud. Strike forces are located in specific areas of the country where instances of fraud are high. Strike forces exist in Miami, Florida; Los Angeles, California; Detroit, Michigan; Houston, Texas; Brooklyn, New York; Baton Rouge and New Orleans, Louisiana; Tampa and Orlando, Florida; Chicago, Illinois; Dallas, Texas; Washington, DC; Newark, New Jersey, Philadelphia, Pennsylvania; and the Appalachian Region. The Appalachian strike force, the most recent strike force to be added, was established in October 2018 to combat illegal opioid prescriptions. HEAT and the strike forces have been successful in their efforts to identify fraud and to recoup monies for the federal government. As of January 2018, strike force statistics were as follows:

- Criminal Actions Identified: 1,938
- Indictments Made: 2,498
- Money Recouped: $3,005,849,223 (OIG 2019d)

Many fraudulent activities involve kickbacks, bribes, and unnecessary opioid prescriptions as well as fraudulent coding and billing. For example, in November 2018, two clinic workers were sentenced for their roles in a $5.9 million case of fraudulent coding and billing of physical therapy services that were not done and for falsely documenting in health records (OIG 2019d).

Recovery Audit Contractor

Recovery Audit Contractor (RAC) is a governmental program whose goal is to identify improper payments made on claims of healthcare services provided to Medicare beneficiaries. Improper payments may be overpayments or underpayments. RACs review claims on a post-payment basis for the purposes of detecting and correcting past improper payments so that Centers for Medicare and Medicaid Services (CMS), fiscal intermediaries, and Medicare Administrative Contractors (MACs) can implement actions that will prevent future improper payments (CMS 2019a).

RAC was established as a demonstration project to test the Medicare program on payments made to healthcare providers. The program was found to be effective by identifying over one billion dollars in overpayments and so it was implemented across the country as per the Tax Relief and Health Care Act of 2006. Medicare contracted with several organizations to conduct the audits required by the program (OIG 2013). The RAC program has significantly impacted the workload of health information management (HIM) departments primarily in the functions of release of information, coding, and auditing. The RAC program requests copies of health records to conduct the post-payment audits so the release of information staff in hospitals and other providers have seen a tremendous increase in workload, some receiving hundreds of requests per year. The increased scrutiny of coding with the RAC audits has providers focused on coding practices and accuracy, resulting in more internal audits and education of coders, adding to their workload.

A request for additional documentation from a healthcare provider to support the submitted claim is an additional documentation request (ADR). ADRs are sent to providers on a 45-day cycle. A baseline annual ADR limit is established for each healthcare provider, such as a hospital. Table 16.1 provides an example of how to calculate ADR.

Most affected are HIM departments that handle the health record requests for an entire healthcare enterprise. *Enterprise* is a term that describes all of the healthcare providers within one company. For example, an enterprise may consist of a hospital, multiple physician offices, ambulatory surgical centers, outpatient therapy sites, a rehabilitation facility, and a long-term care facility, all of which are owned by one company. An HIM department that handles all HIM functions for an enterprise would experience a significant increase in workload since they would be handling health record requests for all of the healthcare providers in the enterprise. HIM departments of healthcare providers that have a higher Medicare payment denial rate also experience a higher number of ADRs, because CMS associates a high payment denial rate with potential coding and billing errors and therefore increases the number of RAC audits for these healthcare organizations to ensure compliance as noted above.

CMS publishes the areas that are the focus of RAC audits and those that are being proposed for future audits. HIM departments should consider conducting coding audits prior to billing claims in the areas that RAC audits are targeting with the goal of avoiding coding and billing errors. Coding audits are good professional practice because they not only potentially improve the accuracy of claims processing but also provide data for health information managers regarding areas of education needed for coders.

RACs utilize three review processes to identify improper payments. These review processes are automated, semi-automated and complex. Data analysis of claims data is conducted during the **automated review** process. **Semi-automated reviews** begin with the automated review process and convert to a semi-automated review when providers opt to submit supporting documentation to substantiate the claim. A **complex review** involves the review of health records by a qualified healthcare coder or clinician as the type of review warrants. If the RAC review identifies an improper payment, overpayment or underpayment, the healthcare provider is sent an informational letter that describes the RAC determination. Letters describing complex review findings are more detailed than those describing automated and semi-automated review determinations and also include information to assist providers in avoiding future billing errors. The letters regarding overpayments include instruction to refund the improper payment (CMS 2016a).

The healthcare organization has the right to appeal the request for the refund and needs to make a decision whether or not to appeal the RAC findings. An **appeal** is a request for reconsideration of a denial of coverage or rejection of claim decision. Table 16.2 provides some potential reasons for appealing or not appealing the RAC findings.

The five levels in the appeal process are displayed in figure 16.4 and described as the following:

1. *Redetermination*. A redetermination is the first level of appeal after the initial determination on a claim. It is a look at the claim by MAC staff not involved in the initial determination.
2. *Reconsideration by a Qualified Independent Contractor (QIC)*. If the redetermination does not rule in their favor, the healthcare organization has the right to appeal to the qualified independent

Table 16.1 Calculation of Additional Documentation Request (ADR)

Rule	Example	Calculation
This baseline ADR number is based on the number of Medicare claims paid to the hospital in a previous 12-month period multiplied by one half of one percent (0.5%).	A hospital that billed and received payment for 22,530 Medicare claims in a previous 12-month period would not receive more than 14 ADRs in a 45-day period.	22,530 claims x 0.005, which is 112.65, the annual ADR limit. 112.65/8 = 14.08 112 is the limit of ADRs for the year, 8 is the number of 45-day cycles in a year. With rounding, the maximum number of ADRs in a 45-day cycle is 14.
	A hospital bills and receives payment for 255,000 Medicare claims in a previous 12-month period.	The ADR limit for a 45-day cycle is 159. (255,000 x 0.005 =1,276; 1,276/8 = 159).

Source: CMS 2018a.

Table 16.2 Appealing RAC findings

Reasons to appeal after review of the RAC findings by the coding manager or physician reviewer	Reasons not to appeal after review of the RAC findings by the coding manager or physician reviewer
The healthcare provider's review of the health record referenced in the demand letter does not match the findings of the RAC audit.	When the healthcare provider's review of the health record referenced in the demand letter matches the findings of the RAC audit; there would not be any point to an appeal and would be a waste of the organization's time and money.
The amount of repayment specified in the demand letter is significant and the staff time involved in an appeal will be time well spent	The amount of repayment specified in the demand letter is such a low amount that it would not be worth the healthcare organization's time and money to file an appeal as appeals can be very labor intensive in terms of staff reviewing the record

Source: ©AHIMA

Figure 16.4 Five levels in the RAC Appeal Process

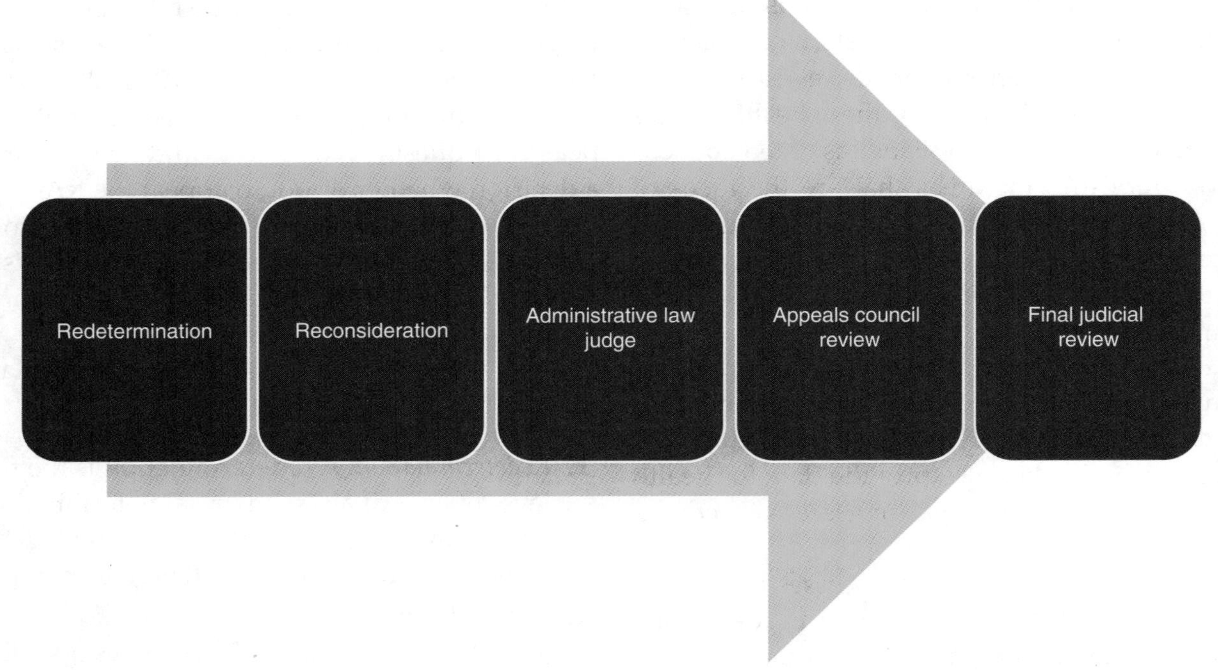

Source: ©AHIMA.

contractor, an outside organization contracted by Medicare to audit the reconsideration.

3. *Administrative Law Judge (ALJ) Hearing or Review by Office of Medicare Hearings and Appeals (OMHA)*. There are two options in the third level of appeal, a hearing by an administrative law judge or a review by the Office of Medicare Hearings and Appeals (OMHA).
4. *Review by the Medicare Appeals Council*. The fourth level of appeal is a Council review, which is conducted by the HHS Departmental Appeals Board (DAB) Medicare Operations Division.
5. *Judicial review in US District Court*. The final level of appeal is to the US District Court (CMS 2017b).

Quality Improvement Organization

A Quality Improvement Organization (QIO) is a group of health quality experts, clinicians, and consumers organized to improve the quality of care delivered to people with Medicare and is one of the largest federal programs that is dedicated to increasing the quality of care for Medicare beneficiaries. QIOs have gone through a number of transitions since their inception in 1972 when they were known as Medicare Professional Standards Review Organizations (MPSRO). In 1982, the MPSROs transitioned to Peer Review Organizations (PROs). In 2002, the PROs became Quality Improvement Organizations (QIOs) (QIO 2019a) and most recently, in 2014, the QIOs went through another restructuring. With each evolution, the quality of care for Medicare beneficiaries has been the focus of the mission. The 2014 restructuring of the QIOs separated them into two types of QIOs: Beneficiary and Family Centered Care (BFCC)-QIOs and Quality Innovation Network (QIN)-QIOs. The (BFCC)-QIOs handle the Medicare beneficiary complaints and quality of care reviews such as, appeals of a healthcare provider's decision to discharge a Medicare beneficiary from a hospital or discontinue other types of services; or review of validity of hospital diagnosis and procedure coding data completeness, adequacy, and quality of care; and appropriateness of prospective payments for outlier cases and nonemergent use of the emergency department. While the RAC audits focus on payments, the QIO audits focus on the quality of patient care.

There are fourteen (14) regions of Quality Innovation Networks (QIN-QIOs). Each QIN-QIO region encompasses between two to six states, depending on population size. The QIN-QIOs are composed of Medicare beneficiaries, healthcare providers, and community representatives whose goals are to identify ways to increase patient safety, make communities healthier, better coordinate post-hospital care, and improve clinical quality by engaging in data-driven initiatives, such as "reducing disparities in access and quality for priority populations, increasing use of health information technology, reducing adverse events related to healthcare-acquired infections, increasing care efficiency by promoting value within the health system, and improving the quality of life for patients nearing the end of life by alleviating pain with palliative care measures" (QIO 2019b).

Because of their role in monitoring coding quality, QIOs are an important part of Medicare's fraud and abuse efforts. QIOs are required to report any evidence of fraud that they identify. Obviously, the QIOs must review health records to be able to carry out the duties listed previously and they request copies of health records from the HIM department. Healthcare organizations should analyze the QIO requests for patterns related to specific diagnosis-related groups, diagnoses, procedures, and physicians to identify opportunities for education and improvement.

Merit-Based Incentive Payment System

Merit-Based Incentive Payment System (MIPS), which includes the program that was originally known as Meaningful Use (MU) is a regulation that was issued by CMS on July 28, 2010, outlining an incentive program for eligible professionals (EPs), hospitals, and critical access hospitals participating in Medicare and Medicaid programs that adopt and successfully demonstrate meaningful use of certified EHR technology (ONC 2019).

MIPS was a three-stage program with specific requirements for the use of certified EHR technology for each stage. Each stage became gradually more sophisticated in the demands of the EHR. EPs were not mandated to implement certified EHR technology but those who chose not to implement certified EHR technology forfeited the incentive payments and realized reduced Medicare payments at the end of the program (ONC 2019).

In 2015, with the introduction of the Medicare Access and CHIP Reauthorization Act (MACRA), MU was renamed the Medicare EHR Incentive Program (later renamed Promoting Interoperability Program), and was transitioned to become one of the three components of the new Merit-Based Incentive Payment System (MIPS), which itself is part of MACRA. MIPS took the existing CMS quality programs, including meaningful use, the Physician Quality Reporting System, and Value-Based Payment Modifiers and consolidated these multiple, quality programs into a single program to improve quality care (ONC 2019). Figure 16.5 illustrates the structure of MIPS. (Quality improvement is discussed in more detail in chapter 18, *Performance Improvement*.)

Timely access to health information is key in monitoring fraud and abuse. With healthcare providers implementing EHRs health data will be more readily available for analysis by the OIG, Medicare Fraud Strike Force, and others involved in fighting fraud and abuse.

Figure 16.5 Merit-Based Incentive Payment System (MIPS)

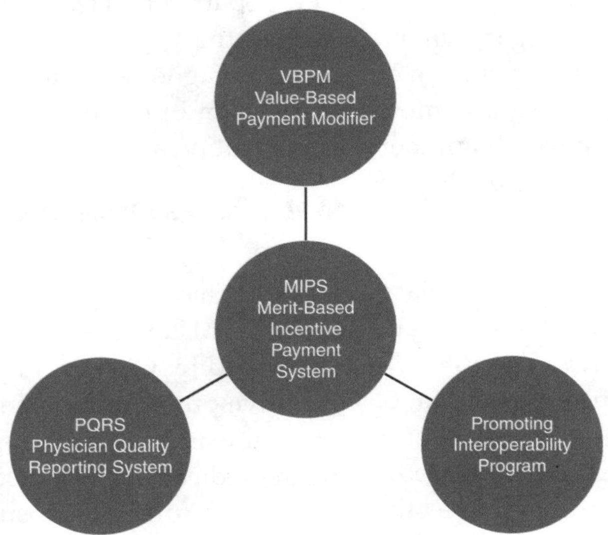

Source: ONC 2019

Check Your Understanding 16.1

Answer the following questions.

1. A hospital's baseline ADR limit is adjusted by which of the following?
   a. A percentage (%) that is set by CMS on a quarterly basis
   b. The hospital's denial rate
   c. The focus topics established by RAC on an annual basis
   d. The number of claims billed by the hospital in a previous 12-month period
2. Identify the organization that is responsible for coordinating the Medicare fraud programs.
   a. Quality improvement organizations
   b. Recovery audit contractor
   c. Office of Inspector General
   d. The Joint Commission
3. Identify which of the federal fraud and abuse laws prohibits a physician's referral of designated health services for Medicare and Medicaid patients if the physician has a financial relationship with the entity.
   a. False Claims Act
   b. Anti-Kickback Statute
   c. Stark Law
   d. HIPAA
4. Identify an example of fraud.
   a. Accidentally overbilling for healthcare services
   b. Charging an inappropriate amount for healthcare services or supplies
   c. Knowingly submitting bills for healthcare services not provided
   d. Unbundling codes
5. Identify an example of abuse.
   a. Billing for healthcare services
   b. Knowingly charging an inappropriate amount for healthcare services or supplies
   c. Unbundling codes
   d. Consistently upcoding to receive higher payments

Compliance Program

Every healthcare organization should have a compliance program. A **compliance program** is a set of internal policies and procedures that a healthcare organization puts into place to comply with applicable state and federal laws. An effective compliance program can enhance a healthcare organization's operations, improve quality of care, reduce overall costs, as well as reduce the organization's liability with regards to fraud and abuse. The compliance program can help the healthcare organization identify problems and correct them before they become systemic and costly.

There are seven basic elements that should be included in an effective compliance program. They are the following:

1. *Policies, procedures, and standards of conduct.* A healthcare organization should put all policies, procedures, and standards of conduct related to their compliance program in writing. These are discussed later in this chapter.
2. *Identifying a compliance officer and committee.* The chief compliance officer and compliance committee are responsible for the overall compliance program for the healthcare organization. Besides the chief compliance officer, the compliance committee should consist of representatives from the healthcare organization's departments that have the most responsibility for monitoring compliance within the healthcare organization. These departments would likely include HIM, revenue cycle management, patient billing, medical staff, and patient accounting. The privacy officer, general counsel, and risk management should also be represented on the committee. A healthcare organization may also want to include members from administration such as the chief executive officer or chief operations officer as the support and involvement of upper management signifies that the healthcare organization has a high level of commitment to compliance. The healthcare organization may consider adding a member of the governing board to the compliance committee since the compliance committee typically reports directly to the governing board. The governing board has ultimate responsibility of compliance for the healthcare organization. The compliance committee will also review the OIG work plan and then determine what items they want to include in their compliance activities and review for the upcoming year. This plan will change from year to year as the OIG focus and the needs of the healthcare organization change.
3. *Educating staff.* It is imperative that all staff be trained in compliance policies, procedures, and standards of conduct as they apply to their position in the healthcare organization. The level of knowledge and competency of understanding of compliance varies depending on the position within the healthcare organization. For example, the compliance officer needs to know everything about compliance in order to educate and answer questions within the Health Information Management Department. A coder needs to understand compliance in regards to coding and reimbursement, whereas an insurance claim specialist needs a more basic knowledge of compliance compared to a coder. This training should occur, at a minimum, in their orientation training and on an annual basis. This is discussed later in this chapter.
4. *Establish communication channels.* There should be methods in place for employees to report fraud and abuse; this can be a confidential hotline or comment box where employees can report fraud and abuse without fear of reprisal.
5. *Perform internal monitoring.* Healthcare organizations must be diligent to ensure compliance with policies and procedures such as through the use of audits and data analysis. Audits are discussed later in this chapter.
6. *Penalties for noncompliance with standards.* There should be appropriate consequences for employees who do not comply with policies and procedures and who participate in fraud and abuse activities. These consequences might include some form of disciplinary

action or termination, depending on the severity of the employee's action.

7. *Taking immediate corrective action when a problem is identified*. Healthcare organizations must take action when fraud and abuse are identified such as completing an internal review to determine where the problem first occurred and implementing specialized training on problem areas; failure to do so could increase their risk of fraud and abuse accusations (OIG n.d.).

These elements of an effective compliance program as they relate to fraud and abuse prevention strategies and audits are discussed in the following sections.

Fraud and Abuse Prevention Strategies

Healthcare providers can use a number of prevention strategies to protect themselves from fraud and abuse allegations. These strategies include the following:

- *Policies and procedures*. Policies and procedures are a critical part of a compliance program and tell "who" and "what" should be done to combat fraud and abuse. Policies should include internal coding procedures, how and when to write physician queries, billing practices, and audits. Healthcare providers that have written policies and procedures in place and are diligent about enforcing these policies and procedures with their staff demonstrate a commitment to compliance. Not only is compliance the right and ethical thing to do but it may also save a provider from higher penalties and fines if abuse is identified.
- *Risk analysis*. Healthcare providers should regularly conduct a risk analysis, which is the process of identifying areas of compliance risk. The risk analysis can then be used to establish work plans and auditing schedules with the goals of eliminating or controlling the risk of fraud and abuse. Individuals should not conduct a risk analysis of their own areas of responsibility; however, they should participate in a review of the findings and creation of audit and work plans. For example, the supervisor of coding should not conduct the risk analysis of the coding department and staff but should be an integral part in establishing work plans and audit schedules for eliminating or controlling the risks of fraud and abuse that are identified in the results of the risk analysis (CMS 2013).
- *Education of employees and medical staff of the healthcare organization*. Laws and regulations change regularly. A healthcare organization's employees and medical staff must be kept up to date on all changes in laws and regulations that impact the work they do. Employees and medical staff members must also understand their role in preventing fraud and abuse and what to do if they are requested to act in a fraudulent manner. Anyone that plays a role in the coding and billing of healthcare services such as billers, coders, physicians, case managers, documentation improvement specialists, and others must stay informed of annual changes in codes and coding guidelines. A component of compliance training is typically a part of a healthcare organization's orientation programs for newly hired employees and newly appointed medical staff members. All employees need basic information about compliance such as what constitutes fraud and abuse, how to report any concerns, annual compliance training for rules and regulations, rights and responsibilities, incident reporting process, and standards. More detailed and complex compliance training should be conducted for employees whose positions in the healthcare organization require a more in-depth knowledge and understanding of the rules and regulations surrounding healthcare compliance. For example, employees involved in the revenue cycle should receive education regarding the False Claims Act and coders should receive frequent education regarding current coding guidelines and results of coding audits.

- *Routine review of coding and billing reports.* There are billing and coding reports that healthcare organizations use on a routine basis to gauge the status of the billing and coding processes. A routine review of these coding and billing reports can be useful in the identification of significant changes in coding and billing practices as they could show changes in the most frequently assigned codes or other significant changes in coding practices. Identified coding changes may or may not be justified. For example, there may have been a change in coding rules that would justify the use of different codes. A consultant may have given the healthcare organization improper information regarding coding, billing, or other reimbursement practices that resulted in changes that should not have occurred. Another example is reviewing coding and billing reports for the frequency of code use may identify codes that are being over- or underused, identifying topics for continuing coder education. The data that can be reviewed are discussed later in this chapter.
- *Clinical documentation strategies.* A strong clinical documentation integrity (CDI) program is important to fighting fraud and abuse through the focus on quality and accuracy. CDI is discussed later in this chapter. An example of a documentation issue is the use of the copy and paste functionality in an EHR. Although this practice saves time by allowing clinicians to duplicate previous documentation and insert it into current notes, it also creates an opportunity for incorrect data to be carried forward and may result in the appearance of fraud or abuse (AHIMA 2016). Refer to chapter 3, *Health Information Functions, Purpose, and Users,* for more information regarding documentation requirements.
- *Documentation of compliance activities.* It is imperative for a healthcare provider to detail documentation of their compliance activities including the risk analyses, work plans, audit plans, meeting minutes, results of audits, completion of planned compliance activities, education of employees, medical staff, contracted organizations, and so forth. In the health information world, the phrase, "if it wasn't documented, it wasn't done" is well-known and applies to compliance activities as well. Providers will want to maintain a thorough, complete record of documentation activities to prove to auditors and surveyors that they are committed to and striving to ensure compliance within their healthcare organization.
- *Share successes.* Healthcare providers may want to internally share their successful compliance efforts by publishing dashboards, scorecards, self-assessment tools, and other mechanisms to demonstrate the healthcare provider's commitment to compliance. This will keep compliance in the minds of all employees. Obviously, senior management and legal counsel should review the data that are shared to ensure confidential information was not inadvertently published (CMS 2013).

Audits

An **audit** is a function that allows retrospective reconstruction of events, including who executed the events in question, why, and what changes were made as a result. An audit is also an independent review of electronic system records and activities in order to test the adequacy and effectiveness of data security and data integrity procedures and to ensure compliance with established policies and procedures. Audits are an important tool in a compliance program as issues can be identified by watching for changes in practices, violations of policies, comparisons between periods (such as year to year), and more.

Types of Audits

Internal audits or reviews are conducted routinely by employees of healthcare organizations whereas external audits are conducted by a third-party payer, hired consultant, accrediting agency, and any other individual or group that is not employed by the healthcare organization. Audits can be a one-time occurrence or may be performed on an ongoing basis such as monthly, annually, or by some other schedule. Audits allow the healthcare organization to confirm that the policies and procedures of the healthcare organization are being met and to identify problems that need to be addressed and corrected. Audits that are fraud and abuse related serve a number of the following purposes:

- Reducing improper reimbursement
- Improving the accuracy of healthcare claims
- Improving patient care
- Showing commitment to complying with laws and regulations

The types of audits that relate to fraud and abuse include coding, medical necessity, clinical validation, and comprehensive error rate testing audits.

Coding audits are conducted to ensure claims are being coded correctly as incorrect coding may result in over- and underpayments. Providers may conduct internal coding audits for new coding staff, for previously identified problematic areas, and for high-risk areas that have been identified by external reviewers such as CMS and OIG. Internal reviews should only be considered as a first step in achieving coding compliance. Providers should also contract with coding consultant(s) to provide expert coding audits. Using only an internal auditing process increases the risk of accepting incorrect coding as correct because that is how claims have always been coded. In addition, if a coding supervisor or lead coder incorrectly interprets one or more coding guidelines, this could lead to a systemic process of incorrect coding. The following questions should be asked when monitoring and auditing the coding process at a healthcare organization:

- Is the diagnosis-related group correct?
- Is there any unbundling?
- Are the codes assigned for the appropriate level of service?
- Are codes changed so that a noncovered service is billed as a covered service?
- Is there a discrepancy between the codes provided by the physician and the hospital (Prophet 1997)?

Medical necessity audits are conducted to determine if healthcare services performed were needed based on the patient's condition and prognosis. Medicare and other payers do not pay for procedures that are not medically necessary. There are obvious procedures that are not medically necessary such as elective cosmetic surgeries but there are many situations that are less obvious because of the patient's physical condition or prognosis for recovery. For example, open heart surgery on a patient that has terminal cancer with a one-month life expectancy would not be considered medical necessary. In fact, an ethical provider would probably consider surgery to be an unnecessary cause of pain. Most unnecessary procedures that are performed are simple diagnostic procedures such as preoperative tests that do not warrant being performed due to the condition of the patient or the type of planned surgery. For example, a patient without a history of heart disease or related conditions would not need a preoperative EKG in preparation for a simple eye surgery such as cataract surgery. The American Board of Internal Medicine (ABIM) created a foundation to advance the core values of medical professionalism as a force to improve the quality of care. This foundation started an initiative in 2010 called Choosing Wisely as a type of collaborative between physicians and patients to reduce the provision of unnecessary procedures. With this initiative physicians and patients are recommended to ask, "Does this patient really need this procedure? Do I really need this procedure?" (ABIM 2019). Medical necessity audits will continue to be an important part of fighting fraud and abuse and will continue to become more sophisticated as more health data and data analysis become available with increased use and complexity of the EHR.

Clinical validation audits are conducted to determine if health records contain the necessary documentation, such as lab results, diagnostic test results, operative reports, and so forth to support the diagnoses made by the physician. Historically, physicians were able to diagnose conditions and diseases without supportive proof; however, those days are in the past. Providers who do not have health record documentation that substantiates their diagnoses based on clinical criteria generally accepted by the medical community will likely experience reductions in payment or denials of payment. Clinical validation audits can be conducted internally or externally. External clinical validation audits are typically conducted on Medicare patients by RACs and, as discussed earlier in this chapter, there are appeal mechanisms in place for providers if they do not agree with a RAC audit. The appeal process can be expensive though when staff time and legal counsel expenses (if used) are factored in so each provider must make a decision on a case by case basis of whether or not to appeal a RAC decision. Knowing that clinical validation audits may be conducted, coders are also responsible for ensuring that the documented diagnoses are substantiated prior to finalizing coding (Butler 2018). Again, long gone are the days of coding directly from a physician-documented list of final diagnoses.

The Improper Payment Elimination and Recovery Improvement Act (IPERIA) of 2012 requires federal agencies to audit programs they administer annually to ensure payments have been made properly and requires the agencies to recover improper payments. Included in the audits, each agency must identify programs that might be susceptible to improper payments, which may indicate patterns of fraud and abuse; to estimate the amount of improper payments; to report this information to the US Congress and the public; and to describe the actions taken by the agency to reduce future improper payments. The **Comprehensive Error Rate Testing (CERT)** program is the program that CMS uses to measure payment compliance with Medicare Fee-For-Service (FFS) program federal rules, regulations, and requirements. The CERT process involves a random sampling of claims followed by requests for health records. Medical professionals, including physicians, nurses, and certified coders, review the claims and health record documentation. The reviewers determine whether the claim was paid properly or denied properly, such as through a RAC audit, according to Medicare coverage, coding, and billing rules and regulations. When the reviewers identify an improper payment, they assign one of the following improper payment categories:

- Insufficient documentation—the health record documentation submitted does not support the claim
- Medical necessity—the health record documentation submitted does not support the medical necessity of the services provided
- Incorrect coding—the health record documentation submitted does not support the code that was billed; or indicates that the service was performed by a provider other than the billing provider; or that the billing service was unbundled; or that an incorrect discharge disposition was coded
- No documentation—the provider did not submit any health record documentation to repeated requests
- Other—there was an improper payment that does not fall into one of the previous categories (CMS 2019b)

Improper payments (both under- and overpayments) are calculated and recouped from the providers and then a calculation of the improper payment rate is calculated and reported to the US Congress and the public. Refer to figure 16.6 for an example of a coding audit tool.

The following section addresses preparing for and conducting internal and external audits.

Preparing for and Conducting Audits

Before an audit can be conducted, the healthcare organization must identify the objective of the audit. For example, an objective of an audit may be to monitor billing practices or coding quality. Once the objective is established, the audit method can be determined. Audit methods include analyzing electronic data, reviewing documents, collecting data,

Figure 16.6 CERT Process

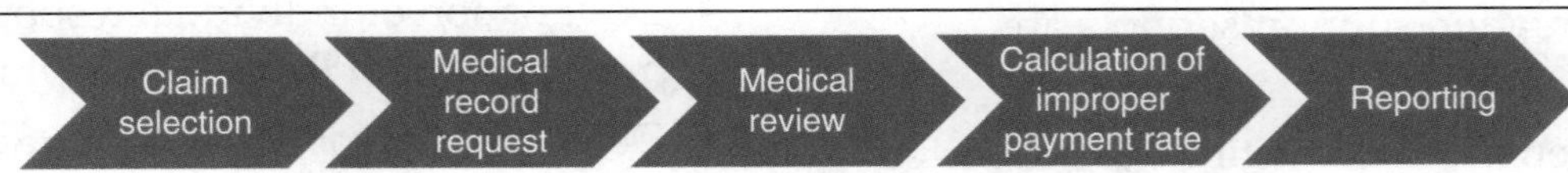

Source: CMS 2019b

adding and inputting it into a database, or assembling data using a manual data collection tool. The method will control the resources needed such as the health record, bills, queries, and so forth. The number of cases needed and how the cases will be identified must be established using statistical methods and are therefore outside the scope of this chapter. For example, the healthcare organization may determine that it needs to review 20 percent of the queries written every month. The following are the statistical methods that can be used to select the specific queries:

- *Simple random sampling*. This model gives every bill, patient, and so forth so that each has the same chance of being chosen.
- *Systematic random sampling*. In this model, a pattern such as selecting every 10th patient admitted is used.
- *Convenience sampling*. In this model, the bills, for example, are chosen based on which ones are available to the auditor.

While audits vary based on what is being audited, there is a basic process—identify areas of risk that need to be monitored, conduct audits on these areas of risk, document the findings of the audit, analyze the data, and correct any problems identified. To conduct the audit, the auditors need access to the resources being audited. The areas of risk can be HHS focus areas, problems that have previously been identified at the healthcare organization, or areas where problems are suspected. There should be a database, spreadsheet, or other tool where the audit is recorded. The data elements collected during the audit vary based on the audit objective. For example, auditing a claim for healthcare services in the emergency department might consider the following areas:

- Procedures are reported at the appropriate level
- Claims are not submitted more than once
- Coding guidelines such as not unbundling are followed
- Documentation support services are reported on the claim
- Copayments and deductibles are collected from the patient (CMS 2015)

The general rule for documentation in the health record is "if it is not documented, it was not done". That is true in compliance as well. The documentation of audits is a significant part of this proof. The documentation should include where the data was obtained, why it was gathered, what was done with the data, what the healthcare organization learned and what the audit tells the organization (CMS 2015).

The HIM professional is the keeper of the health record and, therefore, must control the release of data needed for the audit. In preparation for an audit, the HIM professional must review the audit request documents to validate the auditor's right to review the health record. The HIM professional must also ensure the audit will take place in an atmosphere that maintains the security of protected health information (PHI) during audit activities. The healthcare organization will be best served if the audit processes in place are proactive rather than reactive. A proactive approach enables a healthcare organization to identify areas of concern, opportunities for documentation improvement, and educational needs, and to address and correct these issues prior to any audit request from an external organization such as a RAC.

The HIM professional should plan audit activities, keeping in mind that both internal and external audit requests can arrive at any time. Audit planning should include the following:

- Identification of the audit requestor
- Information requested
- Information needed
- Identification of individuals from the healthcare organization that need to be involved in the audit, keeping in mind that these individuals may be from other departments such as patient accounting, revenue management, charge description master control, clinical services, clinical documentation integrity (CDI), or utilization review (UR)
- Timeline of audit activities
- Designation of individual responsible for the management of the audit activities
- Determination of when audit results will be reviewed and who will review them

The traditional role of the HIM professional in the audit process typically includes providing the health records to be audited or auditing health records. The audit may have particular requirements, specifications, and criteria regarding the health records to be included. Then the HIM professional will apply privacy regulations and organizational policies and procedures to ensure the audit is lawful and that the health record may be used or released.

External Audits

External audits are performed to confirm that a healthcare organization's internal audits are valid; in other words, that the internal audits are identifying all of the compliance issues. External auditors are hired by a healthcare organization to conduct the review. The auditors are impartial and typically have not had a previous relationship with the healthcare organization. An external audit ensures the healthcare organization's policies and procedures are in compliance with laws, regulations, and their own policies and procedures. An example of an external audit is an audit of coders to validate their accuracy. Another example is an external audit to determine the compliance with the Joint Commission standards regarding patient's rights. The goal of an external audit is to determine the healthcare organization's level of compliance.

Denials and Appeals

A **denial** is when a bill has been returned unpaid for any of several reasons (for example, sending the bill to the wrong insurance company, patient not having current coverage, inaccurate coding, lack of medical necessity, and so on). For example, Mary Smith's admission was denied due to lack of medical necessity. The claim had already been paid so the Medicare Administrative Contractor takes back the funds.

When the healthcare organization receives a denial or the insurer either does not submit payment for healthcare services or takes back payment that was previously paid for healthcare services, the healthcare organization must review the denial to determine if it agrees or disagrees. Based on the review of the health record and the denial, the healthcare organization can appeal a denial. An appeal is a request for reconsideration of a denial of coverage or rejection of claim decision. A healthcare organization generally has a limited amount of time to submit the appeal. A common appeals process that a healthcare organization follows includes the following:

- Review the notification of denial from the insurer
- Determine the type of denial (medical necessity, coding change, and so forth)
- Route the denial to the appropriate department or individual (HIM, utilization management, and so forth)
- Determine if the denial is warranted (agree or disagree with the insurer's findings)
- Write an appeal letter if warranted
- Document the decision, including a copy of the appeal letter, as per policy

The individuals or departments that address an appeal depend on the type of appeal. For example, the physician would write a medical necessity appeal letter, and the coding supervisor would write an appeal letter related to a change in coding. Generally, the health record would be reviewed to determine whether or not an appeal is appropriate. For example, the coding supervisor may review the health record and determine that the coder made a mistake and the codes assigned in the denial are appropriate.

An appeal letter would identify the claim being denied including the patient name, dates of service, reason for denial, and other identifying information. The appeal letter would then explain the reason why the healthcare organization deserves the reimbursement that has been denied. For example, with a medical necessity denial, the physician would explain why the patient needed hospitalization. This could be through content from the health record or additional information. For a denial letter that addresses a change in coding, the coding supervisor would quote from the health record the documentation that supported the original code or quote from the coding rules. Supporting evidence from the health record should be attached when appropriate.

The healthcare organization should track the activities related to denials and appeals. This includes the number of denials, number of appeals, types of denials, and whether the denial was upheld or overturned. This can help the healthcare organization identify patterns and take the necessary steps to reduce the number of denials.

Coding and Fraud and Abuse

Codes are used to determine reimbursement; therefore, code assignment is critical since the healthcare organization's revenue is involved. With the ever-increasing focus on proper payments by federal, state, and private healthcare payers, accurate coding is imperative and is constantly scrutinized by these payers, creating additional responsibilities and pressures for coders. With accusations of improper payments, some falling under the definitions of fraud or abuse, it is more important than ever for coders to follow AHIMA's Standards for Ethical Coding (see inside front cover for how to access the Standards on the student website). These 11 standards should be reviewed thoroughly and completely as part of a coder's orientation to a coding position and as a part of routine continuing education. Coding compliance relies on these ethical standards. Refer to the AHIMA Standards of Ethical Coding which is found in the online resources (see inside front cover to register for access).

Coders who follow official coding guideline rules and regulations, follow their employer's policies and procedures, follow AHIMA's Ethical Standards of Coding (see inside front cover for how to access the Standards on the student website), and so forth will still make mistakes. Mistakes are made in all jobs, coding included, but it is how mistakes are handled when they are identified that determines whether the same mistakes will be prevented in the future. Coders and all provider employees are best served, both personally and professionally, by being upfront and honest, which includes reporting incorrect or improper coding practices of their own or others (Bryant 2018).

The following section addresses coding compliance and computer-assisted coding.

Coding Compliance

Healthcare organizations should have a **coding compliance plan** in addition to the healthcare organization's compliance plan. A coding compliance plan focuses on the rules and guidelines specifically related to coding and the responsibility of coders. It should contain the same components as the healthcare organization's compliance plan but with the focus on coding. Benefits of the coding compliance plan include the following:

- Improved documentation in the health record
- Retention of a high standard of coding
- Reduction in denials of healthcare services reimbursement based on coding errors
- Correction of coding-related risks (Schraffenberger and Kuehn 2011)

The coding compliance plan should include expectations for coding quality, such as 98 percent accuracy in code assignment, use of official coding guidelines and official resources such as the American Health Association's Coding Clinic for ICD-10-CM and ICD-10-PCS and CPT Assistant. Coding staff are expected to be almost perfect in their code assignments as there is so much at stake for the healthcare organization based on the codes used for billing, including the accurate reimbursement for healthcare services rendered as well as the external audits conducted by the federal government and commercial insurance payers.

The following are strategies that can be used to combat fraud and abuse in coding:

- Provide ongoing training to all coding staff
- Implement comprehensive policies and procedures
- Examine the quality of coding through the use of audits
- Ensure the coding practices follow official coding guidelines

- Ensure there is a corresponding or supporting diagnosis code for each procedure code
- Support codes with health record documentation
- Support evaluation and management code assignment with the documentation
- Educate physicians on how to improve their documentation
- Use best practices to write a query to clarify documentation
- Disseminate memorandums on changes in regulations and insurers' policies
- Verify the advice of consultants prior to implementation of their recommendations
- Monitor changes in regulations
- Compare organization metrics with national data
- Monitor claims denials and coding changes
- Review data to identify any significant changes in the organization's case-mix index or coding practices
- Ensure the person maintaining the chargemaster is knowledgeable in coding, billing, and documentation
- Report any possible fraud to the healthcare organization's compliance officer or attorney (Prophet 1997)

Other issues that must be addressed in the coding compliance plan include upcoding and unbundling, discussed earlier in this chapter.

Queries

A query is "a communication tool or process used to clarify documentation in the health record" (Bossoondyal et al. 2019). For example, a query should be written if one place in the health record states the fracture is the left arm and in another, it says right arm. When documentation issues are identified, the coder should query the physician. The query should be clearly written and should address the problem with the documentation rather than any impact on reimbursement. The question should include the documentation that needs clarification. The query should never direct the physician what to document. For example, the coder should never tell the physician to add a diagnosis or ask a question that can only be answered yes or no. Another best practice is that the physician should always have access to the health record when asked to make a decision. The query can be written or electronic.

The use of queries should be monitored to ensure it meets the best practices for writing queries. The monitors should include whether queries were only written to increase documentation or not, the appropriateness of the query, and whether or not it meets the other best practices.

The query should become a permanent part of the health record and the physician's response to the query should be documented in the health record by the physician.

Computer-Assisted Coding

Computer-assisted coding (CAC) is the process of extracting and translating dictated and then transcribed free-text data (or dictated and then computer-generated discrete data) into *International Classification of Diseases, Tenth Revision, Clinical Modification* (ICD-10-CM) and Current Procedural Terminology (CPT) codes for billing and coding purposes. CAC assists to reduce issues with fraud and abuse by incorporating coding principles and guidelines (Garvin et al. 2006). CAC does this by incorporating prompts and decision-support tools to assist in the accurate and timely selection of correct codes. CAC facilitates the creation of an audit trail to identify coding errors (Rudman et al. 2009).

CAC uses **natural language processing (NLP)** to review the documentation in the EHR and assign diagnosis and procedure codes. NLP is a technology that converts human language into data that can be translated then manipulated by computer systems and is a branch of artificial intelligence. In 2013, the AHIMA Foundation conducted a research study to determine whether coding timeliness and accuracy are affected by the use of CAC. The study determined that the best scenario for coding accuracy is for a credentialed coder to code in conjunction with the use of a CAC. Study results demonstrated that credentialed coders that used a CAC were able to reduce the amount of time it took to code a health record by 22 percent. A coder that did not use a CAC or the use of a CAC alone without a credentialed coder resulted in lower coding accuracy (AHIMA 2013).

CAC does not eliminate the need for coders, but the role of the coder changes as he or she will validate the codes assigned by the computer rather than assign the code. The CAC can help prevent fraudulent coding and ensure consistent, complete coding due to the NLP. Inaccurate coding results in inaccurate reimbursement and possibly charges of fraud or abuse. Figure 16.7 is an example of how the EHR documentation is used to assign codes via computer-assisted coding.

Check Your Understanding 16.2

Answer the following questions.

1. True or false: Internal monitoring should be part of a compliance program.
2. True or false: In systematic random sampling a pattern such as every 10th patient admitted is used to select patients.
3. True or false: A compliance program is a reconstruction of events that include who executed the events in question, why, and what changes were made as a result.
4. Identify a benefit of a compliance plan.
   a. Reduction in denials
   b. Elimination of denials
   c. Maintenance of the status quo
   d. Documentation audits
5. The coder assigned separate codes for individual tests when a combination code exists. This is an example of:
   a. Upcoding
   b. Complex coding
   c. Query
   d. Unbundling

Figure 16.7 ICD-10-CM CAC example

In this example, the CAC software assigned the code T15.91xA based on documentation in the emergency department record that states the patient had a "foreign body in the right eye." The coder is presented with the decision to accept the code or reject it based on further analysis.

Review of the documentation revealed that the foreign body was located on the edge of the cornea, which changes the fourth character in ICD-10-CM from 9 to 0. The coding professional replaces the T15.91xA with T15.01xA, Foreign body in cornea, right eye.

Emergency Department Record

A patient is brought to the emergency department with a foreign body in the right eye. He was working with metal, and a piece flew in his eye. He reports slight irritation to the right eye but no blurred vision. A slit lamp shows a foreign body approximately 2 to 3 o'clock on the edge of the cornea. The foreign body appears to be metallic. The iris is intact.

Procedure:

Two drops of Alcaine were used in the right eye. Foreign body is removed from the right eye.

Computer-Generated Codes:

T15.91xA, Foreign body, external eye, right

Final Coding Decision:

Coding professional selects the more specific code for foreign body of cornea, T15.01xA

Source: Smith and Bronnert 2010.

Clinical Documentation Integrity

Clinical documentation Integrity (CDI) is the process a healthcare organization undertakes to improve clinical specificity and documentation. The role of a HIM professional in CDI is to educate physicians and other healthcare professionals on best documentation practices. The HIM professional is uniquely qualified because of their clinical understanding and knowledge of documentation, coding, and reimbursement systems. The improved documentation will allow coders to assign more precise diagnosis and procedure codes; for example, ensuring that the organism for pneumonia is documented and coded. The CDI process can be performed either concurrently or retrospectively to the patient encounter. Concurrent CDI is performed while the patient is admitted and still in the hospital and can enhance the quality of care as the improved documentation is available for all care providers. Retrospective CDI is performed after the patient is discharged. The review is frequently performed during the coding process. The CDI review of the health record looks for "conflicting, incomplete, or nonspecific provider documentation" (AHIMA 2015). The improved documentation helps ensure the documentation supports code assignment. For example, the documentation should indicate whether the fractured arm is the left or right one so that the proper code can be chosen. This is important because reimbursement is based on the codes that are assigned according to the documentation. If the documentation is open to interpretation, the healthcare organization could be accused of fraud or abuse. Refer to chapter 6, *Data Management*, for more information on CDI. The following sections address the role of information systems in CDI, metrics used in monitoring CDI, and clinical outcome measures and monitoring.

Information Systems and CDI

Information systems are used throughout the CDI process – from initial documentation to monitoring the CDI program. The EHR and other information systems can assist with documentation through edits, reminders, structured data (chapter 3, *Health Information Functions, Purpose, and Users*), and more. Suggestions for improvement in documentation can be made by these information systems throughout the patient's care. These suggestions can improve the specificity of the documentation in the EHR, indicate conditions that might need to be added, and so forth. Information systems can also be used in the query process to request clarification from physicians. An electronic query can save the physician a trip to the HIM department and therefore may result in a quicker turnaround time. Queries may be retained in an information system and become part of the healthcare organization's legal health record. Information systems can monitor the metrics regarding the CDI program (Arrowood et al. 2016).

Clinical Documentation Integrity Monitoring and Metrics

The CDI program must be monitored to determine how successful it is. A monthly dashboard showing the metrics (something that is measured) for the month should be created. These metrics can be used to compare results from month to month and year to year. The metrics can address volume of reviews, number of queries, physician response to queries, turnaround time, case-mix index, diagnosis-related group proportions, trends, physicians who were queried the most, denials, and more. A threshold should be created as a target for the CDI program to meet. For example, physicians should agree with the CDI specialist 90 percent of the time. Monitoring the metrics in the dashboard will indicate areas of concern to address. For example, if the number of queries suddenly increases, the healthcare organization will need to research the reason for the increase. It could be due to a new physician, a new service, or another reason. The action(s) to be taken will vary based on the findings but could include training, revision of the program, and more (Arrowood et al. 2016).

HIM Roles

HIM professionals are actively involved in fraud and abuse compliance. Two common roles are CDI specialist and coding auditor.

- *CDI Specialist*. A CDI specialist works with physicians on documentation issues, monitors metrics collected, and addresses issues that are identified. The CDI specialist must understand classification systems and the health recommend documentation.
- *Coding Auditor*. A coding auditor monitors the quality of the codes assigned by the coders and addresses any issues identified through training and other communication. The coding auditor may also handle coding denials that are received by the healthcare organization.

Real-World Case 16.1

In June 2018, HHS and OIG along with state and federal law enforcement charged more than 600 individuals with participating in false billings of Medicare and Medicaid totaling about $2 billion in Medicare and Medicaid losses. This is the largest ever healthcare fraud law enforcement action. Of the 600 defendants, 165 were medical professionals including physicians, nurses, and pharmacists. Many of the defendants were charged for their roles in prescribing and distributing opioids and other dangerous narcotics. Other defendants participated in submitting false claims for treatments that were not medically necessary and often never provided. Some patient recruiters, beneficiaries, and others received kickbacks in return for supplying beneficiary information to providers for the purpose of submitting fraudulent claims to Medicare. It is particularly disconcerting to note that almost every healthcare fraud scheme requires a corrupt medical professional to be involved for the fraud to be successful. These medical professionals preyed on vulnerable patients who turned to them for care and treatment (DOJ 2018b).

Real-World Case 16.2

The University of New Mexico Hospitals had a number of unsuccessful efforts to improve the quality of documentation in the health record. These efforts failed due to a lack of physician buy-in and qualified staff. Subsequently they created a CDI program that utilized physician advisors to educate physicians on the importance of clinical documentation in the health record. The focus was on the accuracy of patient's record. Physicians focused on documentation of Severity of Illness (SOI), Risk of Mortality (ROM), and the patient's condition. In the first five months of 2015, the University of New Mexico Hospitals realized an increase in revenue of more than $1.8 million as a result of improved documentation. In the first 16 months of the program, the hospitals' CMI improved by 18.6 percent. The hospitals have also seen improvement in the quality of care they provide based on SOI and ROM measures (Precyse n.d.).

References

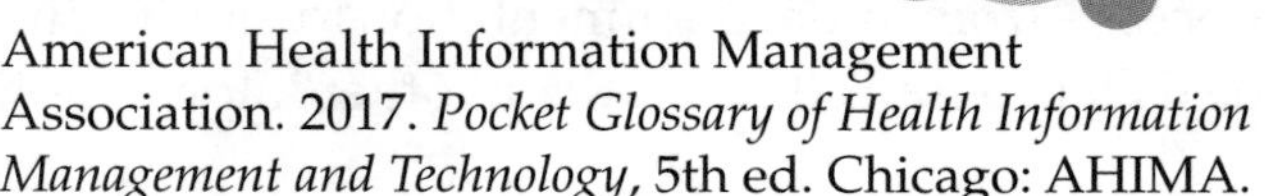

American Board of Internal Medicine. 2019. Choosing Wisely, An Initiative of the ABIM Foundation. http://www.choosingwisely.org/.

American Health Information Management Association. 2017. *Pocket Glossary of Health Information Management and Technology*, 5th ed. Chicago: AHIMA.

American Health Information Management Association. 2016. Standard of Ethical Coding. http://bok.ahima.org/CodingStandards#.XDqGEM17nIU.

American Health Information Management Association. 2015. So What Exactly is Clinical Documentation Improvement? http://bok.ahima.org/doc?oid=300922#.XQrV-3dFyUk.

American Health Information Management Association. 2013. Study Reveals Hard Facts on CAC. http://bok.ahima.org/doc?oid=106668#.Vu9SIebx2b8.

Arrowood, D., L. Bailey-Woods, E. Barnette, T. Combs, M. Endicott, and J. Miller. 2016. Clinical Documentation Improvement Toolkit. http://library.ahima.org/PdfView?oid=301829.

Balanced Budget Act of 1997. Public Law 105-32. https://www.govinfo.gov/content/pkg/BILLS-105hr2015enr/pdf/BILLS-105hr2015enr.pdf.

Bryant, G. 2018. Coding Compliance and Ethics: A Culture and a Process. http://bok.ahima.org/PdfView?oid=302483.

Bossoondyal, S., G. Bryant, T. Combs, K. DeVault, M. Endicott, C. Ericson, O. Ewoterai, K. Good, T. Grier, W. Haik, T. Hicks, F. Jurak, K, Kozlowski, C. Mogbo, B. Murphy, L. Prescott, S. Schmitz, C, Seluke, S. Wallace, M. Wieczorek, and A. Yuen. 2019. http://bok.ahima.org/doc?oid=302673#.XXBWTnspCUk.

Butler, M. 2018. You Got Proof? Payers, Auditors Increase Clinical Validation Checks. *Journal of AHIMA* 89(7):16–19.

Centers for Medicare and Medicaid Services. 2019a. Medicare Fee for Service Recovery Audit Program. https://www.cms.gov/Research-Statistics-Data-and-Systems/Monitoring-Programs/Medicare-FFS-Compliance-Programs/Recovery-Audit-Program/.

Centers for Medicare and Medicaid Services. 2019b. Comprehensive Error Rate Testing Program-Improper Payment Measurement in the Medicare Fee-For-Service (FFS) Program. https://www.cms.gov/Research-Statistics-Data-and-Systems/Monitoring-Programs/Medicare-FFS-Compliance-Programs/CERT/Downloads/IntroductiontoComprehensiveErrorRateTesting.pdf.

Centers for Medicare and Medicaid Services. 2018a. Medicare Fee-for-Service Recovery Audit Program Additional Documentation Limits for Medicare Providers (Except Suppliers and Physicians). https://www.cms.gov/Research-Statistics-Data-and-Systems/Monitoring-Programs/Medicare-FFS-Compliance-Programs/Recovery-Audit-Program/Downloads/ADR-Limits-Institutional-Provider-Facilities-May-2016-revised-12-21-18508ao.pdf.

Centers for Medicare and Medicaid Services. 2018b. Medicare Learning Network: Combating Medicare Parts C and D Fraud, Waste and Abuse. https://www.cms.gov/Outreach-and-Education/Medicare-Learning-Network-MLN/MLNProducts/Downloads/CombMedCandDFWAdownload.pdf.

Centers for Medicare and Medicaid Services. 2017a. Medicare Learning Network Fact Sheet-Medicare Overpayments. https://www.cms.gov/Outreach-and-Education/Medicare-Learning-Network-MLN/MLNProducts/downloads/overpaymentbrochure508-09.pdf.

Centers for Medicare and Medicaid Services. 2017b. Medicare Learning Network Medicare Parts A & B Appeals Process. https://www.cms.gov/Outreach-and-Education/Medicare-Learning-Network-MLN/MLNProducts/downloads/MedicareAppealsprocess.pdf.

Centers for Medicare and Medicaid Services. 2017c. Medical Learning Network Medicare Fraud and Abuse: Prevention, Detection and Reporting. https://www.cms.gov/Outreach-and-Education/Medicare-Learning-Network-MLN/MLNProducts/downloads/fraud_and_abuse.pdf.

Centers for Medicare and Medicaid Services. 2016a. Recovery Auditing in Medicare Fee-For-Service for Fiscal Year 2016. https://www.cms.gov/Research-Statistics-Data-and-Systems/Monitoring-Programs/Medicare-FFS-Compliance-Programs/Recovery-Audit-Program/Downloads/FY-2016-Medicare-FFS-Report-Congress.pdf.

Centers for Medicare and Medicaid Services. 2015. Self-Audit Toolkit. https://www.cms.gov/Medicare-Medicaid-Coordination/Fraud-Prevention/Medicaid-Integrity-Education/documentation-matters.html.

Centers for Medicare and Medicaid Services. 2014a. Medicare Fraud and Abuse. https://www.cms.gov/Outreach-and-Education/Medicare-Learning-Network-MLN/MLNProducts/downloads/fraud_and_abuse.pdf.

Centers for Medicare and Medicaid Services. 2013. Compliance Program Element VI, Monitoring, Auditing and Identification of Compliance Risks. https://www.cms.gov/Medicare/Compliance-and-Audits/Part-C-and-Part-D-Compliance-and-Audits/Downloads/Element-VI-Focused-Training-Power-Point-.pdf.

Department of Health and Human Services. 2009. Testimony. http://www.hhs.gov/asl/testify/2009/10/t20091028a.html.

Department of Justice. 2018a. Justice Department Recovers Over $2.8 Billion from False Claims Act

Cases in Fiscal Year 2018. https://www.justice.gov/opa/pr/justice-department-recovers-over-28-billion-false-claims-act-cases-fiscal-year-2018.

Department of Justice. 2018b. National Health Care Fraud Takedown Results in Charges Against 601 Individuals Responsible for Over $2 Billion in Fraud Losses. https://www.justice.gov/opa/pr/national-health-care-fraud-takedown-results-charges-against-601-individuals-responsible-over.

Department of Justice. 2016. Fact Sheet: The Health Care Fraud and Abuse Control Program Protects Consumers and Taxpayers by Combating Health Care Fraud. https://www.justice.gov/opa/pr/fact-sheet-health-care-fraud-and-abuse-control-program-protects-conusmers-and-taxpayers.

FindLaw. 2019. What is the False Claims Act? https://employment.findlaw.com/whistleblowers/what-is-the-false-claims-act.html.

Office of Inspector General. 2019a. About Us. http://oig.hhs.gov/about-oig/about-us/.

Office of Inspector General. 2019b. Exclusions Program. https://oig.hhs.gov/exclusions/index.asp.

Office of Inspector General. 2019c. Civil Monetary Penalties Inflation Adjustment https://www.federalregister.gov/documents/2019/02/07/2019-00603/civil-monetary-penalty-adjustments-for-inflation.

Office of Inspector General. 2019d. Medicare Fraud Strike Force. https://oig.hhs.gov/fraud/strike-force/.

Office of Inspector General. n.d.a. Organizational Chart. http://oig.hhs.gov/about-oig/organization-chart/index.asp.

Office of Inspector General. n.d.b. A Roadmap for New Physicians: Fraud & Abuse Laws. https://oig.hhs.gov/compliance/physician-education/01laws.asp.

Office of Inspector General. 2013. Medicare Recovery Audit Contractors and CMS's Actions to Address Improper Payments, Referrals of Potential Fraud, and Performance. http://oig.hhs.gov/oei/reports/oei-04-11-00680.pdf.

Office of Inspector General. 1998. 42 CFR Parts 1003, 1005 and 1006. Health care programs: Fraud and abuse; revised OIG civil money penalties resulting from the Health Insurance Portability and Accountability Act of 1996. *Federal Register*. 63(57):14393-14402. http://oig.hhs.gov/authorities/docs/hipaacmp.pdf.

Office of Inspector General. n.d. Health Care Compliance Program Tips. http://oig.hhs.gov/compliance/provider-compliance-training/files/Compliance101tips508.pdf.

Garvin, J.H., V. Watzlaf, and S. Moeini. 2006. Automated Coding Software: Development and Use to Enhance Anti-Fraud Activities. https://www.ncbi.nlm.nih.gov/pmc/articles/PMC1839655/.

Office of the National Coordinator for Health Information Technology. 2019. Meaningful Use. https://www.healthit.gov/topic/meaningful-use-and-macra/meaningful-use.

Office of the National Coordinator for Health Information Technology. n.d. Organizational Chart. https://oig.hhs.gov/about-oig/organization-chart/index.asp.

Quality Improvement Organizations. 2019a. The History of the QIO Program. https://qioprogram.org/qionews/articles/history-qio-program.

Quality Improvement Organizations. 2019b. QIO Program 11th Scope of Work 2014-2019. https://www.cms.gov/Medicare/Quality-Initiatives-Patient-Assessment-Instruments/QualityImprovementOrgs/Current.html.

Precyse. n.d. UNM Hospitals Turns the Tide on Clinical Documentation. https://www.precyse.com/resources/Precyse%20UNMH%20CDI%20Success%20Story%20Web%20Version.pdf.

Prophet, S. 1997. Fraud and abuse implications for the HIM professional. *Journal of AHIMA* 68(4): 52–56.

Rudman, W. J., J. S.Eberhardt, W. Pierce, and S. Hart-Hester. 2009. Healthcare fraud and abuse. *Perspectives in Health Information Management* 6(Fall):1g.

Schraffenberger, L.A. and L. Kuehn. 2011. *Effective Management of Coding Services*, 4th ed. Chicago: AHIMA.

Smith, G. and J. Bronnert. 2010. Transitioning to CAC: The skills and tools required to work with computer-assisted coding. *Journal of AHIMA* 81(7):60–61. http://library.ahima.org/doc?oid=101090#.VxUObfkrLDc.

45 CFR 160.401: Definitions. 2009.

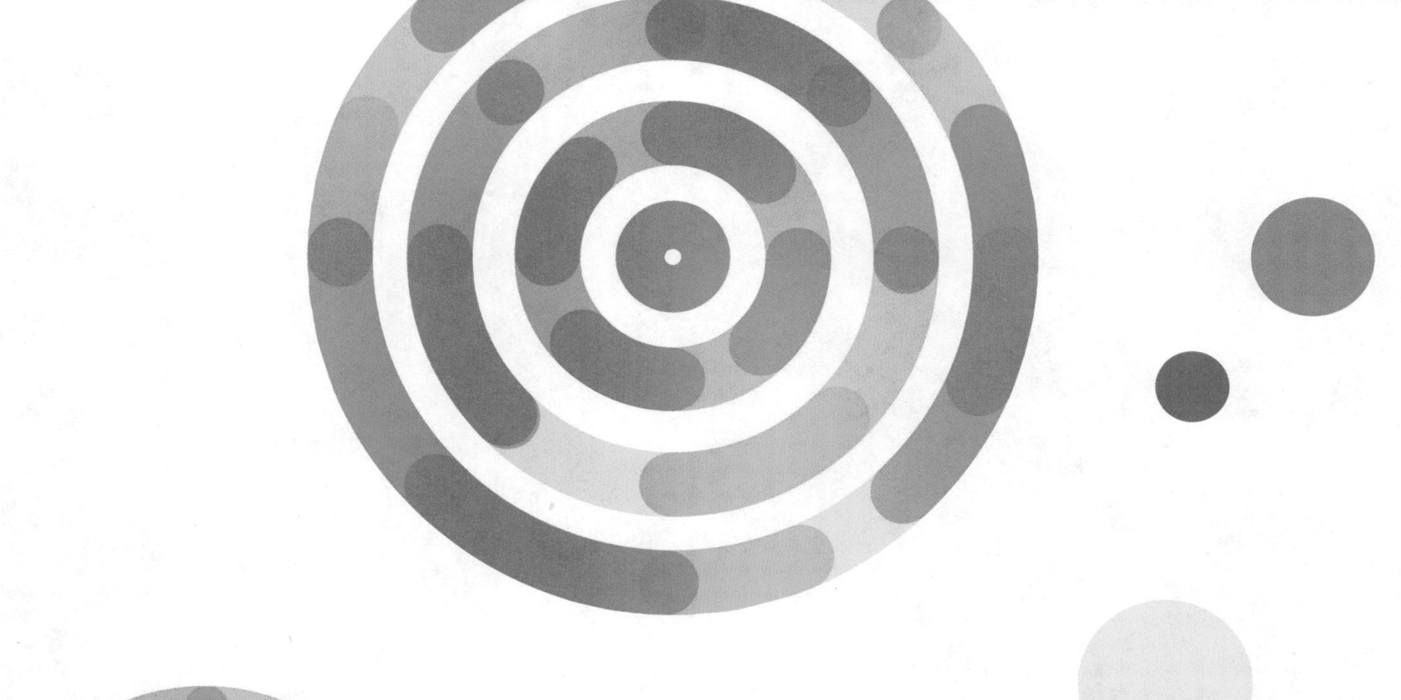

PART VI Leadership

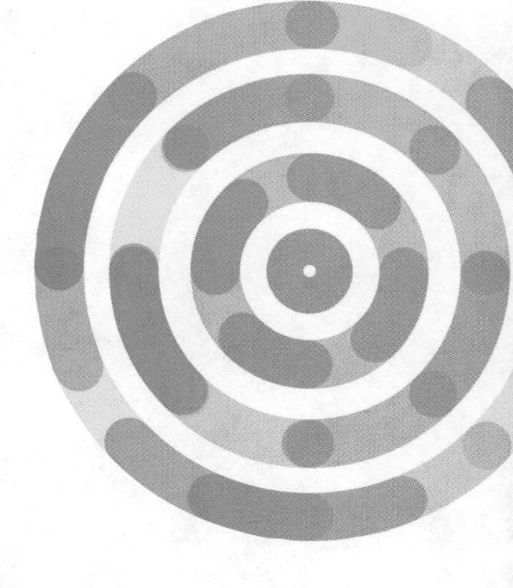

Management

Leslie L. Gordon, MS, RHIA, FAHIMA

Learning Objectives

- Identify the four functions involved in management
- Examine the principles of organizational behavior
- Articulate the organizational structure in a healthcare organization
- Verify the process for strategic and operational planning
- Analyze the basics and tools of project management, including work analysis and change management
- Examine financial management in healthcare
- Analyze the management and allocation of resources used in healthcare
- Examine the management of venders and contracts in healthcare
- Utilize enterprise information management
- Analyze the management of mergers in healthcare
- Examine the management of corporate compliance and patient safety

Key Terms

Accounting
Accrual accounting
Budget
Budget adjustment
Budget management
Budget variance
Cash basis accounting
Change management
Controlling
Corporate compliance
Cultural competence
Enterprise information management (EIM)
Executive management
Expenses
External analysis
Financial management
Gantt chart
Impact analysis
Internal analysis
Job classification
Job description
Job evaluation
Leading
Management
Market assessment
Mergers
Middle management
Operational planning
Organization
Organizational behavior
Organizational chart
Organizational structure
Planning
Policies
Principles of organization
Procedures
Program evaluation and review technique (PERT) chart
Project management
Project management life cycle
Resource allocation
Revenue
Risk management

Staffing
Strategic information systems planning
Strategic plan
Strategic planning
Strategy
Supervisory management
Supply management
SWOT analysis
Variable costs
Work analysis
Workflow

All organizations, from businesses with a small number of employees to large corporations with several thousand employees, use the practice called management. Management is the process of planning, controlling, leading, and organizing the activities of an organization. In healthcare, management is necessary for the entire organization, as well as for the departments making up the organization. Securing effective management practices within an organization or department establishes a positive direction to successfully deliver end results, and to do this, strategic planning is necessary. A strategy is a course of action designed to produce a desired (business) outcome and a strategic plan is the document in which the leadership of a healthcare organization identifies the overall mission, vision, and goals to help define the long-term direction of the organization as a business entity. Strategic planning includes an analysis of how an organization will react to changes in the external environment in the foreseeable future. Successful management practices also encompass work processes, project management and finance, all of which are described throughout this chapter.

Management

The practice of health information management (HIM) ensures the availability, accuracy, and protection of the clinical information needed to deliver healthcare services and to make appropriate healthcare-related decisions. HIM managers, directors, and supervisors use the four functions of management—planning, controlling, leading, and organizing—in the day-to-day and long-term operations of the HIM department to ensure the healthcare organization complies with laws and regulations that mandate the management of HIM functions.

The HIM director uses the planning function of management to develop goals for the department. Planning is the examination of the future and preparation of action strategies to attain goals of the department or healthcare organization; for example, a director in the HIM department may use the planning function to prepare for the future state of the department after the implementation and installation of a new electronic health record (EHR) application. She will determine the impact of the EHR on the policies and procedures, the budget, and other aspects of the department. The director will anticipate the changes in staffing, processes, and procedures to determine what changes will be necessary in preparing, implementing, and managing the new information system. Short-term planning may involve staffing coverage for an employee who is taking leave time.

Controlling is the function in which performance is monitored according to policies and procedures (defined later in the chapter). In HIM, controlling includes monitoring the performance of employees for quality, accuracy, and timeliness of completion of duties. For example, the policy of the department may include a 97 percent accuracy rate for all codes for surgical procedures. The coding supervisor will monitor accuracy for all coders to ensure compliance with this standard. If an employee falls below the stated standard, training will be provided to the employee.

Leading is the function in which people are directed and motivated to achieve the goals of the healthcare organization. In an HIM department, leading involves assigning responsibilities to the tasks the department needs to accomplish. For example, in the case of a disaster where multiple patients are brought to the healthcare organization, the HIM director may ask all personnel to report to the emergency staging area to help with health record management. The day-to-day operations of the department require the director to understand the policies and procedures to determine when a change may be needed.

The HIM director uses the function of organizing on a daily basis, for both long-term and short-term tasks and goals. **Organization** is coordinating all of the tasks and responsibilities of a department to guarantee the work to be accomplished is completed correctly and in a timely manner. A director or supervisor is responsible for the decisions concerning the division of labor for the HIM department, such as coding responsibilities and information disclosure. The billing department may have a priority list of health records to complete first for reimbursement purposes. The supervisor will ensure the employees are responsible for specific health records first.

Organization is the planned coordination of activities of multiple people to achieve a common purpose or goal. For a healthcare organization, organization is vital for structure and allows employees at all levels to understand their job duties, to whom they report, and what is expected of them. Managers at all levels use the following **principles of organization** to manage in an effective manner:

- *Unity of command.* In this management principle, each employee reports to one manager. The employees in the scanning department report to the scanning department supervisor and the supervisor reports to the HIM director.
- *Span of control.* The number of employees a person manages is called the span of control and is influenced by the size of the organization (such as a department with only two employees compared to a department with 100 employees), the skill level of the employees (entry-level employees require more supervisor time), and the responsibilities of the supervisor and employees. Span of control can be high, where there are a lot of employees to manage, or low, with few employees to manage. High span of control may cause the manager to be ineffective because too many people report to him or her, or a manager with low span of control may feel he or she is not being used effectively and is capable of more responsibility.
- *Specialization.* All employees have special qualifications or skills that allow them to perform their job to the best of their ability; managers who employ this principle assign work among their reporting employees according to their specialization, such as assigning the most complex coding cases to the coder who has the highest quality performance on coding reviews. The manager can divide and conquer the work of the department using each employee's strengths, which results in a positive outcome for the healthcare organization.
- *Delegation.* The process by which managers distribute work to the employees of the department along with the authority to make decisions and to act on those decisions.
- *Directing.* The process of assigning the tasks for the day to employees and providing training, instructions, and advice to help with accomplishing the responsibilities.
- *Coordinating.* The process of ensuring activities happen in the order they need to. It is important, for example, for the coding process to be completed before the billing is performed.
- *Controlling.* Performance is monitored in accordance with policies and procedures and changed based on the situation at hand at each moment of the day (McConnell 2019).

This chapter discusses management roles as they relate to healthcare organizations. Organizational behavior and structure, the fundamentals of work planning, change management, project management, financial management, resource and vendor management, enterprise information and management of mergers, corporate compliance, patient safety, and risk management are also addressed.

Organizational Behavior

Humans are social by nature and usually live within groups of their own kind. Organizational behavior is a field of study that explores how people act within organizations and their behavior individually, in a group, and collectively across a department. Understanding management must include the study of organizational behavior and the culture of people. Cultural competence is the ability to accept and understand the beliefs and values of other people and groups and is vital to the overall health of an organization. Cultural competence is discussed in detail in chapter 21, *Ethical Issues in Health Information Management,* and is important for healthcare professionals to understand because they are required to work with different people, both as coworkers and as patients, from diverse backgrounds who have varying beliefs, values, and goals. The organizational behavior of a healthcare organization affects the way its members interact with each other. For example, if an HIM director works in a healthcare organization that does not have clear lines of supervision defined, multiple people may direct him or her, causing confusion and frustration. A data analyst supervisor speaking negatively about the HIM director to the people who report to him demonstrates the organizational behavior of that particular department, meaning the supervisor is creating a behavior of negativity within the department and the supervisor's direct employees may view such speech as an indication that it is acceptable to speak negatively about others in the department and about the people above them. Supervisors and managers should be aware of the culture of their department and control the organizational behavior, as best as they are able, to provide positive human interaction and work environment.

Organizational Structure

Healthcare organizations have an organizational structure—the framework of authority and supervision for the employees within the organization. The organizational structure defines the hierarchy of reporting and responsibility for each level of decision-making authority and the responsibilities within the institution. The structure follows a chain of command, or the hierarchical structure within an organization. This helps employees to know whom they report to and who reports directly to them. A person should never report to more than one person at a time for a given task because it could cause frustration and confusion if they are being told different things. Some people may split their time between departments and could, therefore, report to more than one person but never for a single task. For example, a person who works in the registration department in the morning reports to the registration manager; in the afternoon that employee works in the billing department and reports to the billing manager for those responsibilities. It is difficult for a manager to supervise a lot people, and it could make them less effective. The ideal number of direct reports for a supervisor is a hotly debated topic, with the general consensus being 5 to 11.

Organizational structure is how the organization is arranged in terms of functions or responsibilities. It starts at the top with a board of directors and ends with employees throughout the institution. The board of directors is an elected or appointed group of people who bear ultimate responsibility for the successful operation of the organization. Managers and directors are responsible for different aspects of the business and operations of the organization. It is important to understand management levels and organizational tools, including organizational charts; mission, vision, and values; and policies and procedures and how they direct and govern individual departments and entire organizations. These management levels are discussed in this section. The organizational tools are discussed later in this chapter.

Management Levels

Management generally includes three levels: executive, middle, and supervisory. Executive management is the senior management of a healthcare organization, the people who oversee a broad functional area or group of departments or services. This level of management establishes the organization's future direction and monitors the organization's operations in those areas. The executive manager includes the chief information officer (CIO) who is responsible for HIM and information technology (IT). CIOs are responsible for the strategic direction for the organization in terms of information governance (IG) and the technology related to IG (chapter 6, *Data Management*). Middle management involves the people within the organization who oversee the operation of a broad scope of functions; for example, the HIM manager may oversee coding, transcription, and disclosure of information at the departmental level or they may oversee a defined product or line of service, such as in the case of a radiology department manager. Supervisory management oversees the staff-level employees and monitors the effectiveness of everyday operations and individual performance against pre-established standards. In HIM a coding supervisor is an example of this level of management—this individual may have inpatient and outpatient coders, discharge analysts, and clerks reporting to him or her. The focus of this chapter is management, not leadership. Leadership is covered in chapter 19, *Leadership*.

Organizational Tools

Managers and supervisors rely on tools to help with their functions. These tools include organization charts, policies, procedures, strategic planning, and the organization's mission, vision, and values: Each of these is discussed in further detail.

Organizational Chart

An organizational chart, sometimes called an org chart, is a visual graphic or diagram showing the structure and reporting relationships between positions, departments, and employees of an organization. The org chart shows the relation of one department to another and a department org chart shows the relationships among staff, supervisors, and managers within a single department. Figure 17.1 is an example of an org chart for a healthcare organization and figure 17.2 is an example of an org chart for an HIM department.

Mission, Vision, and Values Statements

Chapter 1, *Health Information Management Profession*, defines mission, vision, and values—which are tools healthcare organizations use to set the direction and define their purpose and philosophies. A mission statement is a written statement that identifies the core purpose and philosophies of a healthcare organization; it defines the healthcare organization's general purpose. The vision statement is a short description of an organization's ideal future state, and the values statement is a short description that communicates an organization's social and cultural belief system. These statements can range from analytical to creative, but they are always a screenshot of what the healthcare organization represents, its goals for

Figure 17.1 Organizational chart for a healthcare organization

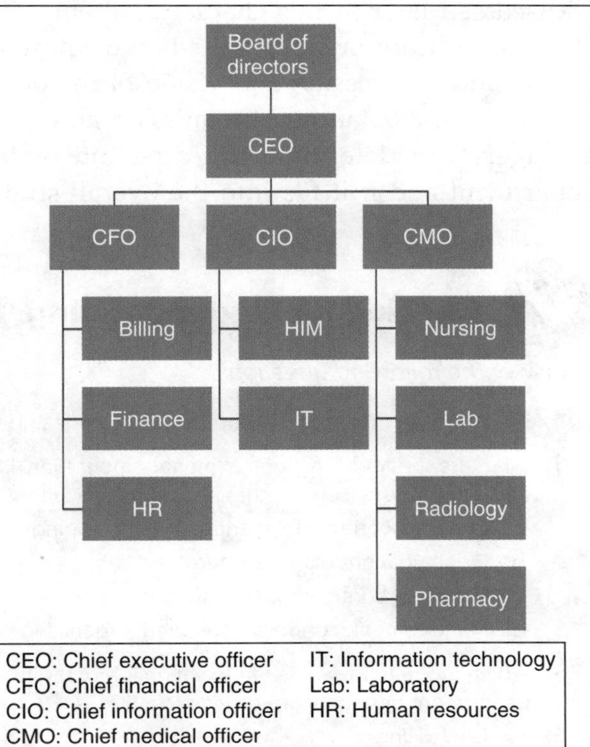

Source: ©AHIMA.

Figure 17.2 Organizational chart for an HIM department

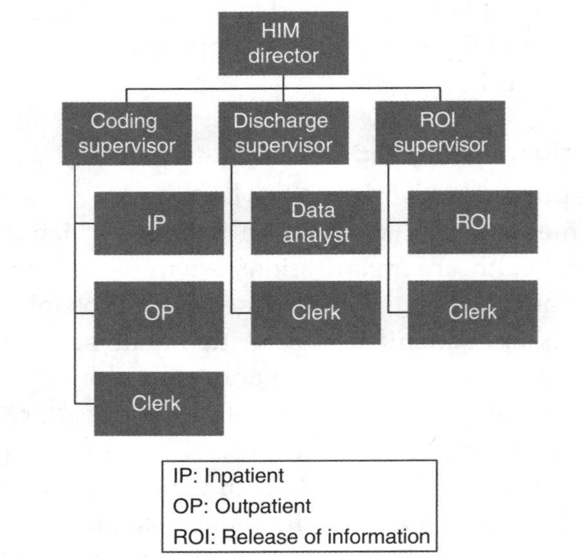

Source: ©AHIMA.

the future, and what the healthcare organization believes (McNamara n.d.).

Healthcare organizations update their mission and vision statements regularly as part of the strategic planning processes (strategic planning is discussed later in this chapter). All employees of the healthcare organization should know and understand the mission and vision of the organization. By understanding the mission and vision, managers can determine the direction of their department and if it fits into the overall strategy of the organization. For example, if the mission of a healthcare organization includes serving only female patients, managers will not look at expanding services to male patients with prostate cancer. Figure 17.3 provides examples of vision and mission statements from various healthcare organizations.

Policies and Procedures

Policies are the principles describing how a department or an organization will handle a specific situation or execute a specific process. They are clear, simple statements of how an HIM department will conduct its services, actions, or business; and a set of guidelines and steps to help with decision-making. For example, the American Health Information Management Association (AHIMA) has a privacy policy on their website stating: "AHIMA is committed to honoring the privacy of its members and general users who access the website" (AHIMA 2015). The policy goes on to state what information is collected and for what purpose.

Once policies are in place, **procedures** define the processes by which the policies are put into action. Procedures are written documents that describe the steps involved in performing a specific function. The procedure could be how to code a health record or how to abstract data. It includes steps taken to adhere to the policy. Figure 17.4 gives an example of a policy and procedure from AHIMA on the external Americans with Disabilities Act (ADA) Accommodations for taking certification examinations.

Check Your Understanding 17.1

Answer the following questions.

1. True or false: Planning is a course of action designed to produce a desired (business) outcome.
2. What are the four functions of management that HIM directors use in the day-to-day and long-term operation of the department to ensure the healthcare organization complies with management of HIM functions?
   a. Strategy, controlling, management, planning
   b. Planning, controlling, strategy, leading
   c. Planning, controlling, leading, organizing
   d. Management, controlling, leading, organizing
3. Which of the following is the examination of the future and preparation of action plans to attain goals of the department or healthcare organization?
   a. Controlling
   b. Leading
   c. Organizing
   d. Planning

4. What is the coordination of all the tasks and responsibilities of a department to ensure the work that needs to be accomplished is completed correctly called?
   a. Organizing
   b. Specialization
   c. Controlling
   d. Strategy
5. What is a written statement that identifies the core purpose and philosophies of a healthcare organization?
   a. Vision
   b. Values
   c. Organization
   d. Mission

Figure 17.3 Sample mission and vision statements

General Hospital Affiliated with a Larger Healthcare System

Lutheran hospital's **mission** is to improve the health of the communities we serve by providing high-quality services in a responsible and caring way.

Our **vision** is to become the leader in promoting healthy lifestyles in an atmosphere of spiritual support, dignity, compassion, and mutual respect for all.

Community General Hospital

Anytown General Hospital's **mission** is to provide quality health services and technology to meet the changing healthcare needs of the people of southwestern Minnesota.

Anytown General Hospital's **vision** is to become the hospital of choice for residents of Polk, Sunny Isle, and Spring counties, a position we strive to strengthen by our long-term commitment to:

- Teamwork
- Service excellence
- Compassionate care
- Cost consciousness
- Continuous improvement

Academic Medical Center

Prairie University Hospital's **mission** is to provide the most up-to-date medical and surgical services available in the three-state area and to train medical students and graduate physicians to meet current and future challenges in healthcare.

Our **vision** is the achievement of healthy communities and progress toward the future of healthcare for Montana, western North Dakota, and northwestern South Dakota.

Specialty Hospital

The **mission** of Women's hospital of Somewhereville is to meet the healthcare needs of our patients and to exceed their service expectations.

Our **vision** is of a hospital:

- Providing services with compassion and kindness
- Striving for performance improvement
- Fostering pride and integrity
- Aiming for increased cost-effectiveness and productivity

Specialty Clinic within an Academic Medical Center

The **mission** of the Midwest Asthma Center is to:

- Provide optimal medical care for persons with asthma and related illnesses
- Develop new knowledge about asthma and its management through medical research programs and materials for our patients, for other healthcare providers, and for the community

The **vision** of the Midwest Asthma Center is to provide the highest quality of integrated comprehensive care for persons with asthma and related illnesses and to be one of the centers of excellence in the world for asthma treatment, research, and education.

Primary Care Physicians' Practice

The **mission** of Coastal Shores Primary Care Associates is to serve the unique needs of individuals and families by providing high-quality, coordinated, primary care medical services through and efficient, accessible, and responsive network of caring providers.

Our **vision** is to be the primary care medical group of choice in the Atlantic County area by delivering high-quality, individualized, and efficient patient care.

Source: Kellogg 2012, 1086–1087.

Figure 17.4 Example policy and procedure for ADA accommodations

AHIMA External ADA Policies and Procedures

HOW TO REQUEST TEST ACCOMMODATIONS FOR THE AHIMA CERTIFICATION EXAMINATIONS

1. The applicant must personally submit a written request.
2. Requests by a third party (such as an evaluator, employer, etc.) will not be considered.
3. If an applicant has a documented disability covered under the Americans with Disabilities Act (ADA) and ADA Amendments Act (ADAAA) and requires test accommodations, s/he must notify AHIMA in writing each time s/he requests accommodations.
4. The request should indicate the nature of the disability and the specific test accommodations needed.
5. A qualified professional must provide documentation verifying the disability and explaining the test accommodations that are needed.
6. Applicants will be notified in writing whether their accommodation request has been approved.
7. **The request (application form and documentation) must accompany the AHIMA examination application, and must be received by the normal application closing date.**

What to Do:

- Read the AHIMA Disability Documentation Guidelines carefully and share them with the qualified professional who will be providing supporting documentation for your request.
- Complete the AHIMA Test Accommodation Request form
- Attach documentation of the disability and your need for accommodation.
- **Compare your documentation with the AHIMA Disability Documentation Guidelines** to ensure a complete submission.
- **Incomplete documentation will delay processing of your request.**

Source: AHIMA 2019.

Strategic and Operational Planning

The strategic plan of a healthcare organization is a map to the future state of the company. The plan outlines the outcomes and goals for the long range. Strategic planning involves how the organization will react to changes in the external environment in the foreseeable future. Usually the time frame is three to five years into the future. In the healthcare environment a strategic plan must take into consideration any federal, state, and local regulations, laws, and accreditation standards that affect the organization currently and in the foreseeable future (Johnson 2017). The steps for creating a strategic plan, which include internal and external analysis of the environment in which the healthcare organization is functioning, will be explored in more detail in this chapter.

By analyzing the environment every few years (three to five), executive management is able to stay abreast of the changes in regulation, technology, culture, and direction of the organization. The strategic plan process helps organizations understand the environment in which they operate and identify the plan they will follow to reach their desired future state (Buchbinder and Shanks 2017).

Operational planning is the specific day-to-day tasks required in operating a healthcare organization or an HIM department. The operational plan is the road map to guide a healthcare organization or department toward the goals of the strategic plan. The operational plan is a shorter and more defined time frame than the strategic plan. Department managers are involved in creating an operational plan for their departments to propose how to staff and accomplish the work tasks for the coming year. Supervisors use operational planning on a daily basis to organize the work of their teams to keep up with department workload.

Healthcare organizations review the inner working of the organization to determine strengths and weaknesses of the business practice and process. This process is an internal analysis. For example, an internal analysis of the coding department may reveal that 10 of the coders are credentialed and have at least 10 years of experience; however, the top 5 coders are all leaving their employment within the next three months. An external analysis involves exploring the factors outside the control of the organization to determine what is happening within the same market. The development of the market assessment determines what opportunities and threats to the future of the organization exist. For example, an external analysis is performed by healthcare organization A within the service area in which it operates. The analysis determines that at healthcare organization B, operating within the same service area, coders are paid 25 percent more than what healthcare organization A is paying. Healthcare organization A concludes that the reason experienced coders are not applying for open coding positions is because they can be paid more at healthcare organization B. Healthcare organization A has the external analysis information needed to understand it must increase the wages of coders to be competitive within its' service area. An assessment of the market would involve determining the number of coding positions on the market and the eligible workforce looking for work (Buchbinder and Shanks 2017).

Developing Strategic and Operational Plans

The process to develop a strategic and operational plan begins with a SWOT (acronym for strengths, weaknesses, opportunities, and threats) analysis. In a SWOT analysis, key leadership personnel determine the strengths of the organization (what the company does well) and the weaknesses (areas for improvement), and establish future opportunities (and evaluate threats to those opportunities). An example SWOT analysis performed by an HIM department found the following:

- **S**trengths. Coders are all credentialed
- **W**eaknesses. Staff is not trained in a new information system that is being implemented within the next three months
- **O**pportunities. The new information system will increase productivity in the department by 45 percent
- **T**hreats. Some members of the staff are opposed to change and there is a time delay with implementing the new information system (Buchbinder and Shanks 2017)

By exploring SWOT in detail an organization's management is able to determine what the future state of the organization could and should be. It gives an honest portrayal of the current and future state of the healthcare organization. The strengths and weakness are usually internal to the organization, with opportunities and threats being external (Buchbinder and Shanks 2017). Healthcare organizations have information management strategic plans to guide the overall enterprise management of information and information systems.

Information Management Strategic Plan

Information is a strategic asset. A high level of oversight is required for information to be used effectively for organizational decision-making, performance improvement, cost management, and to lower risk to the company. A strategic plan for information management is vital for an organization to stay within the guidelines of legal and regulatory laws. Strategic information systems planning is described in the next section.

Strategic Information Systems Planning

Strategic information systems planning is the process of identifying and prioritizing various upgrades and changes that might be made in an organization's information systems. The Office for the National Coordinator (ONC) for Health Information Technology released a Federal Health IT Strategic Plan for the years 2015 through 2020. The four federal health IT goals in this plan are the following:

- **Goal 1:** Advance person-centered and self-management health with the objectives to empower health management engagement and to foster partnerships
- **Goal 2:** Transform healthcare delivery and community health by improving healthcare quality and access, supporting high-value healthcare, and protecting public health
- **Goal 3:** Foster research, scientific knowledge, and innovation by increasing access to information, accelerating the development of innovative technologies, and investing in research on how health IT can improve health and care delivery
- **Goal 4**: Enhance the nation's health IP infrastructure (ONC 2015)

Healthcare organizations should use the ONC strategic plan in the development of their own IT strategic plan to ensure compliance with federal guidelines. The healthcare organization should include representation from all stakeholders who use health IT. For example, a laboratory manager may want to implement a new technology that does not submit data to the EHR to perform lab tests. The HIM manager may want to implement a release of information software system, but it does not keep an audit trail of releases, which is required by law. After the strategic and operational plans are developed and implemented, a healthcare organization will analyze the workflow and process and determine ways for improvement. (The ONC strategic plan for health IT is discussed in chapter 11, *Health Information Systems*.)

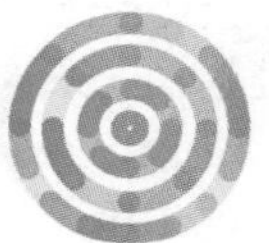

Work Analysis, Change Management, and Project Management

The leaders of healthcare organizations must understand what it takes to accomplish everyday workflow—the process and steps it takes to complete a task. With new technology and advances in healthcare delivery and processes, healthcare managers are required to manage change. Knowledge of the workflow makes needed changes easier to identify. Work analysis is the process of gathering information about what it takes to get a job done. For example, a person tracks everything they do over a period of time, (a week or month), and how long it takes to do each task. Analysis of that information determines what the job responsibilities are. Change management is the formal process of introducing change, adopting the change, and diffusing it throughout the organization. This section will explain work analysis and design, change management, and the impact of change on processes.

Work Analysis and Design

Work analysis involves mapping the steps required to complete a task from start to finish. It is the technique used to study the flow of operations and is sometimes called operations analysis or workflow analysis. Similar to following a complex recipe while cooking a dish, the work analysis for completing a trauma registry for the state would include many steps, including running a report on all trauma codes, analyzing the records that belong on the registry, completing the trauma registry, and sending the report to the state. A work analysis breaks down the workflow into its component parts. The goal is to determine if there are areas that slow the process of the job task under review. Figure 17.5 shows a workflow diagram for completing the trauma registry.

Figure 17.5 Workflow diagram trauma registry

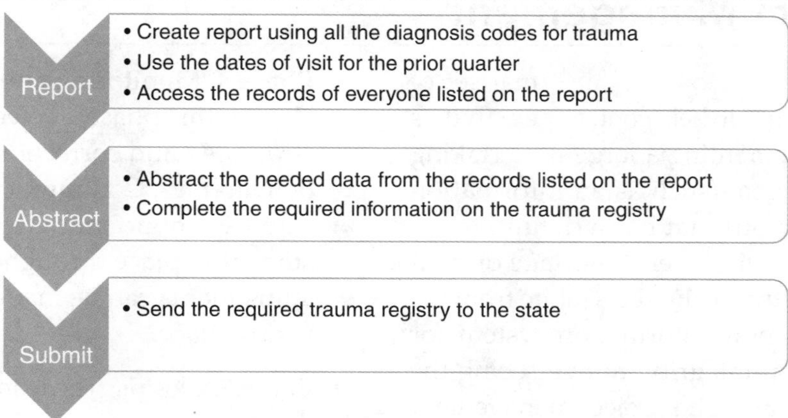

Report
• Create report using all the diagnosis codes for trauma
• Use the dates of visit for the prior quarter
• Access the records of everyone listed on the report
Abstract
• Abstract the needed data from the records listed on the report
• Complete the required information on the trauma registry
Submit
• Send the required trauma registry to the state

Source: ©AHIMA.

After analyzing the workflow, a job description, job classification, and job evaluation are created. A **job description** is a list of duties, reporting relationships, working conditions, and responsibilities for a particular job. **Job classification** is a method of job evaluation that compares a written position description with the written descriptions of various classification grades, which make up the formal salary structure of an organization. **Job evaluation** is the process of applying predefined compensable factors to determine their worth. It allows the company to have guidelines and clear boundaries of the scope of individual jobs; for example, education level and credentials. The company is able to measure the work being done, and place employees in positions that best fit the needs of the company. Advances in technology and information systems happen quickly. Healthcare workers are constantly changing their processes and job tasks due to these advances and need to stay on top of the analysis of their workflow.

Change Management

Managing change is a challenging yet necessary task for healthcare supervisors. Healthcare rules, regulations, and laws are passed with each congressional session in the United States. Changes in payment methodologies, privacy, and security guidelines and other regulations, as well as updates in technology and healthcare delivery directly affect HIM professionals regularly. The US military uses a change management system called VUCA, which is an acronym for volatility, uncertainty, complexity, and ambiguity. *Volatility* means the situation is not stable and it is unknown how long it may last. To combat volatility, one should be prepared. *Uncertainty* is not knowing if change will or will not happen. The approach to uncertainty is investing in information – collecting, interpreting, and sharing it. *Complexity* means the situation may have interconnected variables. Resources can be built to manage complexity. *Ambiguity* is the fact that no precedents exist and it is not known what is not known. The strategy for dealing with ambiguity is to experiment with different situations and find the best solutions. Healthcare organizations and employers can implement these change management strategies to help with the fear and resistance to change. The more information an employee is given the more buy-in they will have in the changes taking place in their jobs (Butler 2019).

The key to having a smooth transition is in the planning. By thoroughly analyzing how change is going to affect the workflow and work procedures, the organization will be able to determine the best course of action. **Impact analysis** is a collective term used to refer to any study that determines the benefit of a proposed project, including cost-benefit analysis, return on investment, benefits realization study, qualitative benefit study, or how change affects workflow.

Project Management

Project management is a formal set of principles and procedures to help control the activities associated with implementing a large undertaking to achieve a specific goal (such as an information system implementation) that has a definitive beginning and end. There is never a shortage of projects to manage in healthcare. Projects range from the implementation of a new information system for clinical documentation integrity to overseeing the meaningful use program. The project management life cycle, methodologies, tools and techniques, and the project management profession are discussed in the following sections.

Project Management Life Cycle

The project management life cycle is the period in which the processes involved in carrying out a project are completed, including the definition, planning and organization, tracking and analysis, revisions, change control, and communication. The following is an example of a project management life cycle as applied to HIM.

The life cycle of project management includes the following five phases. Figure 17.6 shows the life cycle of a project, similar to figure 17.5; however, a project has a closing and is not continuous.

- **Phase 1.** Project initiation: This phase outlines an overview of the project, the high-level scope and project risks, the charter and support from people affected by the project. This phase will have a statement of work, a business plan, and a contract between stakeholders.
- **Phase 2.** Planning: Strategic planning, which is the overall approach of the project, and implementation planning, which is how the project will be executed, take place during this phase. Also, a budget is created.
- **Phase 3.** Execution: This phase involves procuring resources for the project, executing tasks, and ensuring the performance of team members. This is the largest phase, where the action takes place and the project is carried out.
- **Phase 4.** Monitoring and Controlling: During this phase, project deviations are addressed and corrections made based on deliverables. Communication of project status is important in this phase. This vital step takes place throughout the project so adjustments can be made as the project is taking place.
- **Phase 5.** Closing: The team confirms that the project scope and deliverables were met, including lessons learned and customer satisfaction (Eramo 2019). Closure of the project is an important tool to help identify areas that can be improved upon in future endeavors.

Project Management Tools

Project management is made easier by utilizing tools to track and analyze the steps and tasks within the project. Tools needed for project management include a project plan, Gantt charts, and PERT charts.

A detailed project plan identifies the individual steps to complete the project. Gantt and PERT charts are visual tools used to manage the elements or steps of a project. A Gantt chart is a graphic tool used to plot tasks and shows the duration of project tasks (start and stop dates) and overlapping tasks (tasks that can be performed at the same time); in other words, it is used as a method to illustrate the time needed for each task. It also includes who is responsible for the task. A program evaluation and review technique (PERT) chart is a project management tool that diagrams a project's time lines and tasks as well as its interdependencies. Gantt charts focus on the percentage of completion for each task and may show a link between one or more tasks with a critical path that identifies the sequence of activities that must happen before the next one can start. In the example mentioned earlier, the charts will indicate the time it takes to complete the task of converting the filing system for records. Figure 17.7 is a display of a Gantt chart; figure 17.8 is a display of a PERT chart.

Figure 17.6 Project management life cycle

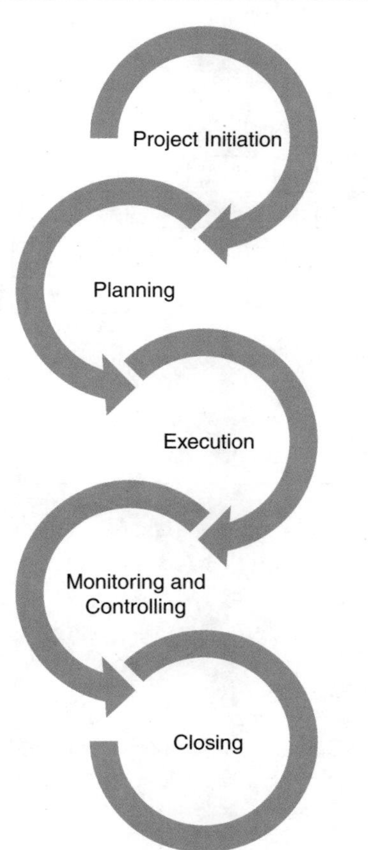

Source: ©AHIMA.

Project Management Professional

A project management professional (PMP) certification is a credential offered by the Project Management Institute (PMI). Individuals with this certification demonstrate competency in the project manager role and lead and direct projects and teams. The certification examination covers the areas of initiating, planning, executing, monitoring, controlling, and closing the project (PMI 2015). The HIM professional needs to understand project management to manage the implementation of new information systems, the EHR, or new processes mandated by laws; for example, the implementation of the Health Insurance Portability and Accountability Act (HIPAA) mandated new privacy and security policies for healthcare organization. The PMP certification is a highly desirable and valued certification that could benefit HIM professionals looking to work as a project manager or wanting the knowledge and background of a PMP.

The PMP credential certifies a person's skills in the five project phases and the tasks associated with each phase. The knowledge, skills, and abilities of a PMP include communication, human resource, finance management, integration, procurement, quality, risk management, project scope, stakeholder management, and time management (Eramo 2019).

Figure 17.7 Gantt chart

Implementation of New Coding Software Hospital Wide

				6/1–6/7	6/8–6/14	6/15–6/21	6/22–6/28	6/29–7/5	7/6–7/12	7/13–7/19	7/20–7/26
	Task	**Start**	**Complete**	1	2	3	4	5	6	7	8
Phase 1	**Design**										
1.1	Identify Requirements	1	1								
1.2	Acquire Software	2	2								
1.3	Test Software	3	3								
Phase 2	**Construct**										
2.1	Develop Training Program	3	4								
2.2	Train Coders	4	4								
2.3	Test Application	4	5								
2.3.1	Unit Testing	5	5								
2.3.2	System Testing	6	7								
Phase 3	**Pilot**										
3.1	Implement Software	7	8								
3.2	Conduct System Training	7	8								
3.3	Support Pilot	8	8								
Ongoing	**Pre / Post Production**										
	Weekly Team Meetings	1	8								
	Engage Stakeholders	2	8								

Source: Najduch 2015a.Used with permission

Figure 17.8 PERT chart

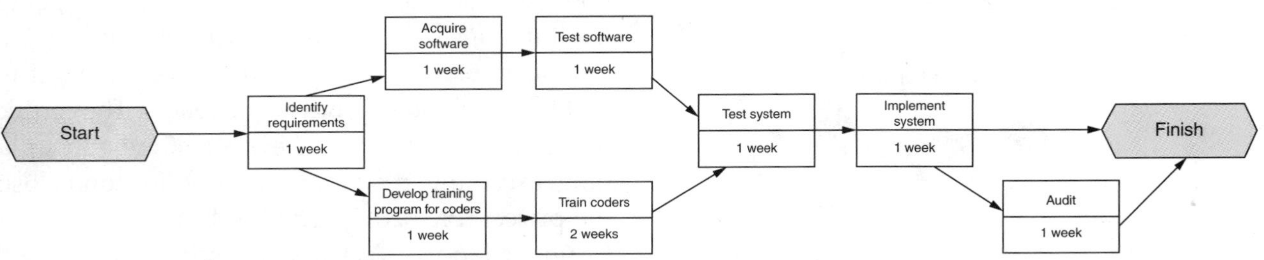

Source: Najduch 2015a. Used with permission

Check Your Understanding 17.2

Answer the following questions.

1. What is a useful general tool for guiding day-to-day decisions?
   a. Operational plan
   b. SWOT
   c. Strategies
   d. Strategic plan
2. What analysis shows the honest portrayal of the current and future state of the healthcare organization?
   a. External analysis
   b. Workflow analysis
   c. Supply management analysis
   d. SWOT analysis
3. True or false: Values are a process by which the policies are put into action.
4. What is the formal process of introducing change, adopting the change, and diffusing it throughout the organization?
   a. SWOT
   b. Change management
   c. Supply management
   d. Workflow
5. Which of the following is the management and control of the supplies used within an organization?
   a. Work analysis
   b. Staffing
   c. Supply management
   d. Strategic plan

Financial Management

Financial management is the mechanism that all businesses use to fully comprehend and communicate their financial activities and status. Top-level executives are usually responsible for financial management with input from department leaders. Knowledge of accounting and budgets is important for those tasked with the financial management of an institution.

Accounting

Accounting is the process of collecting, recording, and reporting an organization's financial data including the assets, expenses (defined later), and liabilities of the company. It is important for the HIM professional to understand accounting methodologies and budgets so they are prepared to manage a department. The viability of a healthcare organization relies on financial management and the revenues that enter the institution rely heavily on the functions of the HIM department (for example, correct coding for reimbursement). Assets include the human, financial, and physical resources of an organization such as the employees, financial holdings, and physical buildings owned by the organization. Expenses are the amount of money charged as a cost to the organization, such as the cost of utilities. Liabilities include the amounts the organization owes to others, like loans.

The financial stability of the healthcare organization depends on the ability to understand the revenue and overall expenses each year. Revenue is the recognition of income earned and the use of appropriated capital from the rendering of services during the current period (CMS 2018), while expenses are the amounts charged as costs by an organization to the current year's activities of operation. Revenue is earned through coding and billing for healthcare services. Management must consider that they will not receive the entire amount billed for services due to adjustments to claims. An HIM manager may choose to hire an independent coding consultant who can audit Medicare claims, which can result in higher revenue for the organization. Expenses are either variable or fixed costs, with variable costs including resources that change like supplies, while fixed costs remain constant like rent, wages, and equipment rental.

There are two ways to record the transactions in the financial books—cash basis accounting and accrual accounting. Cash basis accounting is registering the transaction when it occurs, meaning when money is received for services provided, or paid for expenses incurred. This type of accounting is usually used in small businesses, because it is easier to manage. A small health clinic operating in a remote village in Alaska may use cash basis accounting for healthcare services rendered because they do not bill health insurance and patients pay for services as they are delivered. Accrual accounting involves recording known transactions in the appropriate time period before cash payments (receipts) are expected or due. A company records the revenue when it is earned and records expenses as the transactions happen, not when it receives the cash or makes a payment. For example, a large rehabilitation center will write on their books the exercise classes that they provide, even if they have not been paid for those classes yet. In healthcare, most organizations use accrual accounting where cash or revenue reflects the amount the organization expects to receive for the services provided. The HIM department may use the accrual accounting system for the release of information function, charging for the service of copying records, with revenue reflecting the amount expected from the patient.

Budgets

A budget is a plan that converts the organization's goals and objectives into targets for revenue and spending. A comprehensive organization master budget includes forecasted revenue (amount of money expected for the year) and forecasted expenses (cost of doing business for the year). In reality, the budget of a healthcare organization is several budgets, each addressing a specific need. For example, the budget for an HIM department includes what is needed to staff and manage the required functions of the department. The HIM department manager can use the budget to provide information that allows her to forecast success or difficulty for the department by analyzing the projected staff available to work during the upcoming holiday season when many employees are requesting time off. There are many types of budgets, including the following operating, cash, and capital budgets:

- *Operating budget*. This budget summarizes the anticipated expenses for the day-to-day routine operations
- *Cash budget*. This is the forecast of expenses and revenue for one year; it includes the

expenses predicted, the revenue forecast, cash outflow and inflow, and the ending cash on hand

- *Capital budget*. This budget refers to the long-term plans for facilities and equipment (Buchbinder and Shanks 2017)

Budget management involves the process of maintaining financial viability by ensuring operating revenues for the year are sufficient to cover the operating expenditures (Harrison and Harrison 2013). Managers control their budgets throughout the year by making adjustments or amendments when needed. A budget adjustment is the approval to move funds from one budget to another. For example, an HIM department manager has a coding employee vacancy for a period of time. The amount of money budgeted to pay for that employee is not used, so a budget adjustment could be made to move the unused money into a different fund to cover the cost of something else such as overtime pay for employees who are covering for the unmanned position. A budget variance is a difference in the budgeted revenue or expense amount; for instance, an HIM manager budgeted $10,000 for training coders during the current year and training actually cost the department $11,500. Therefore, the department has a negative budget variance of $1,500. Ideally, a positive variance occurs when the projected revenue is higher or the expenses are lower than projected, meaning the expenditures are within or below the amount that was budgeted. Part of the budgeting process involves supplies and staffing management. The planning includes maintenance of contracts and services, utilities, and employee salary increases.

Supply management

Supply management is the management and control of the supplies used within an organization. It can be physical goods, services, information, or any resources needed to run the organization. Knowing the supplies needed to run the healthcare organization vastly improves and helps in managing a successful organization. In an HIM department it is important for the manager to anticipate and include in the budget the costs that the department incurs with supplies, pens, paper, copy costs, coding books, and regulation documentation requirements.

Staffing

Staffing is the managerial function that involves proper and effective selection, appraisal, and training of personnel. The HIM manager must be aware of (and budget for) the staffing needs of the department and take into consideration employee paid time off, leave, and illness. When it comes to staffing, the manager should keep the following in mind:

- Staff recruitment and selection
- Performance management
- Staff retention
- Employee relations and fair treatment
- Staffing planning and scheduling
- Productivity
- Training and development

For additional information on staffing and the managerial functions of staffing, see chapter 20, *Human Resources Management*.

Management of Resources and Allocation

Healthcare organizations have limited resources. Resources include money, people, tools, and technology. Resource allocation is a process and strategy of deciding where resources should be used to achieve the mission, values, and goals of the organization. For example, the HIM department budget includes an amount of money to be used for information systems and the manager must decide between purchasing a software system to help with clinical documentation integrity or an information system to track information needed for various registries because there is not enough funding for both. The manager must prioritize the needs of the department with legal and regulatory issues that may affect the choice of resources. For example, the coding department must have the current coding guidelines each year and cannot work with outdated codes; thus, the department must purchase updated code books each year.

Management of Vendors and Contracts

A vendor is a company outside the healthcare organization with which an HIM department conducts business; for example, coders may use an encoder that is owned and operated by an external company (vendor). A contractor is an outside company or individual who provides or performs a service for the HIM department; for example, the coding functions could be contracted to a company that specializes in coding. HIM professionals must understand the process for selection, implementation, and managing of outside vendors and contractors. A contract is a legal document that details the relationship between two entities—for instance, between the contracted coders and the HIM department. In this case the vendor is outside the coding department and the HIM department manager is contracting with the vendor for coding services. Choosing a vendor or contractor includes identifying the need, designing the system, submitting a request for information (ROI), analyzing the ROI, submitting a request for proposal (RFP), and establishing a contract for services with the chosen vendor.

Enterprise Information Management

Enterprise information management (EIM) ensures the value of information assets, requiring an organization-wide perspective of information management functions; it calls for explicit structures, policies, processes, technology, and controls. It also includes the infrastructure and processes to ensure the information is trustworthy and actionable. EIM is the set of functions used by organizations to plan and organize, and coordinate people, processes, technology, and content for managing information as a corporate asset that ensures data quality, safety, and ease of use (Johns 2014). With executive-level management decisions relying on the data and information found within the organization's health information systems, the importance of accurate, complete, and quality data becomes clear. Management of information from the entire enterprise perspective is vital to quality patient care and business viability.

Management of Mergers

Mergers are business situations where two or more companies combine—one of them continues to exist as a legal business entity while the other(s) cease to exist legally and their assets and liabilities become part of the continuing company. Mergers commonly occur in healthcare with healthcare providers and organizations attempting to streamline their operations and improve their competitive positions. A merger may entail a consolidation where two entities combine to form one new entity (the surviving entity), or it may be an acquisition where one entity acquires part or all of the assets of the other; or it may be a stock acquisition where one entity acquires the stock of the other entity. All organizations must determine the licensure, regulatory, and accreditation requirements before the operational issues of a merger.

The HIM professional understands the operational issues related to the management of information and the functions of the department and how they will be affected by the merger. Operational issues for the HIM manager include the following:

- Single or multiple locations for HIM functions
- Integration of information systems
- Completion of health records
- Merging of department employees
- How the master patient index (MPI) will be handled (MPI information is found in chapter 3, *Health Information Functions, Purpose, and Users*)
- How release of information will be handled

The function of the HIM department must be reviewed to guarantee compliance with state licensure and regulatory requirements (AHIMA 2012).

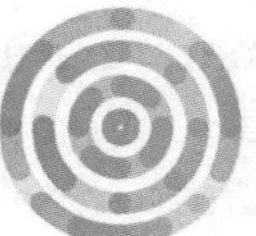

Management of Corporate Compliance and Patient Safety

Corporate compliance is the process of establishing an organizational structure that promotes the prevention, detection, and resolution of instances of conduct that do not conform to federal, state, or private payer healthcare program requirements nor to the healthcare organization's ethical and business policies. In HIM, compliance includes managing a coding or billing department according to the laws, regulations, and guidelines that govern it. A compliance officer is a designated individual who monitors the compliance process at a healthcare organization. (Compliance is discussed in more detail in chapter 16, *Fraud and Abuse Compliance*.) The HIM manager is responsible for knowing and obeying laws that govern the management of HIM functions including coding and billing. A formal compliance program plan is the process that helps a healthcare organization accomplish its goal of providing high-quality healthcare and efficiently operating a business under various laws and regulations. The plan will include internal controls that promote adherence to applicable federal and state guidelines. Improving the quality and safety of healthcare delivery should be a goal of all healthcare organizations; risk management and analysis determine how the healthcare organization is reaching the goal of quality healthcare and safety of patients. Customer satisfaction is critical to the health of an organization—when customers are not happy, the organization will not stay solvent because unhappy customers will not return for services and will tell their friends and family about their experience.

Risk Management and Risk Analysis

Risk management is a comprehensive program of activities intended to minimize the potential for injuries to occur in a healthcare organization and to anticipate and respond to ensuring liabilities for those injuries that occur. Risk management includes the processes that are in place to identify, evaluate, and control risk, defined as the organization's risk of accidental financial liability. A healthcare organization as a whole has a risk management director or department to evaluate and manage the potential for injuries that happen during the course of doing business—for example, patient falls, patient infections occurring while being treated, or surgery on the wrong body part. HIM managers must handle risk in terms of coding and billing fraud and abuse (discussed in chapter 16, *Fraud and Abuse Compliance*). Managers must know the laws and regulations governing HIM functions and educate staff on those items. Risk management programs is discussed in more detail in chapter 10, *Data Security.*

Risk management begins with a risk analysis, which includes identifying weaknesses in an organization's operations and determining how likely it is that any given threat may occur. An HIM manager performs a risk analysis of the HIM functions and procedures (such as coding and billing) to ensure the functions are being performed properly.

Customer Satisfaction

Customer satisfaction is important to the healthcare organization and to the HIM department. Customer satisfaction is a measurement of a customer's expectations, either by falling short, meeting, or exceeding the expectations. Customer satisfaction is usually determined using surveys that measure satisfaction with services provided. In an HIM department, the manager may want to assess customer satisfaction with the process of attaining copies of patient immunization records. Customers can be considered internal or external based on their relationship to the service. An internal customer needing a copy of immunization records could be a surgeon who works for the healthcare organization. An external customer might be a parent who needs their child's health records so the child can play baseball at the local community center. A sample satisfaction survey is displayed in figure 17.9.

Figure 17.9 Customer satisfaction survey

Customer Satisfaction Survey
City Community Hospital
123 Main Street
Your City, ST 00111
800-555-5555

Who received services at City Community Hospital?

- ☐ Me
- ☐ My dependent

Were your important questions answered regarding your condition or treatment by your healthcare providers (physician, nurses)?

- ☐ Yes, always
- ☐ Yes, sometimes
- ☐ No
- ☐ I didn't have any questions

Were the answers you were given presented in a way that you could understand?

- ☐ Yes, always
- ☐ Yes, sometimes
- ☐ No
- ☐ I do not have any questions

How would you rate the skills of our staff in meeting or exceeding your expectations?

- ☐ Excellent
- ☐ Very good
- ☐ Good
- ☐ Fair
- ☐ Poor

How would you rate how well the staff worked together on your behalf?

- ☐ Excellent
- ☐ Very good
- ☐ Good
- ☐ Fair
- ☐ Poor

Overall, how satisfied were you with the treatment and care you received at City Community Hospital?

- ☐ Excellent
- ☐ Very good
- ☐ Good
- ☐ Fair
- ☐ Poor

Overall, how satisfied were you with your provider?

- ☐ Excellent
- ☐ Very good
- ☐ Good
- ☐ Fair
- ☐ Poor

Would you recommend City Community Hospital to your family or friends?

- ☐ Yes, definitely
- ☐ Yes, probably
- ☐ No

If no, why not?

Comments:

Source: ©AHIMA.

HIM Roles

The roles for HIM professionals in terms of management are varied and vast. HIM professionals understand the principles of management as well as the delivery of healthcare across the continuum of care. With the understanding of the technology and systems used in a healthcare setting the HIM professional is uniquely qualified to work in many settings, not only directly in healthcare but in related fields, for example insurance claims management, revenue cycle management, and enterprise information management.

Healthcare organizations are concern about compliance with regulatory agency policies as well as patient safety. The process improvement and patient safety department of healthcare organizations address quality standards for care, for which HIM professionals are able to understand, monitor and correct processes that need to be changed within the work flow of patient care.

Check Your Understanding 17.3

Answer the following questions.

1. What process should an organization use to see if there are resources available to help accomplish the mission, values, and goals of the organization?
   a. Measuring
   b. Process improvement
   c. Resource allocation
   d. PERT chart
2. What is a formal set of principles and procedures that help control the activities associated with implementing a large undertaking?
   a. Resource allocation
   b. Project management
   c. Project improvement
   d. Financial management
3. What project management tool focuses on the percentage completion of a task and may show a link between one or more tasks?
   a. PERT chart
   b. Project management
   c. Planning and design
   d. Gantt
4. Which of the following is the process that all organizations and businesses use to fully comprehend and communicate financial activities and status?
   a. Financial management
   b. Cash basis accounting
   c. Budgets
   d. Resource allocation
5. The process of maintaining financial viability by ensuring operating revenues for the year are sufficient to cover the operating expenditures is called what?
   a. Budge adjustment
   b. Budget management
   c. Budget variance
   d. Accrual accounting

6. Which of the following are amounts charged as costs by an organization to the current year's activities of operation?
   a. Budgets
   b. Accrual accounting
   c. Revenue
   d. Expenses

Real-World Case 17.1

Central Community Hospital hired Susan Davis as the new manager to work in the health information management (HIM) department. One of the first items Susan reviewed was the workflow process for how documents were handled between the intake department and HIM. The intake department is responsible for assuring all documentation needed for a new admission to the hospital is received from the clinic that is admitting the patient. She noticed that the two departments were managing a lot of the same work, which created duplicate documents in the health record. Intake would scan documents and then send them to HIM. HIM would receive the documents and scan them as well. HIM would also copy the documents to send them to the utilization review nurse who is responsible for ensuring that reimbursement authorizations are in place and managed. When Susan asked Intake why they sent the documents to HIM, the answer was "because that's how it has always been done." When thinking about other ways the situation could be handled, Susan came up with the following ideas:

- Have Intake scan the documents into the electronic health record (EHR), and then hand the copy to the utilization review nurse, leaving HIM out of the process; or
- Once Intake is done with the document, instead of scanning it into the EHR, hand it directly to HIM, and continue with the rest of the process.

Real-World Case 17.2

The HIM department of a small critical access hospital in Alaska purchased telehealth technology to allow the hospital to communicate with providers from across the state and the nation. The HIM director indicates that she has the skills needed to manage the new telehealth project from start to finish. Her supervisor asked her to manage the project and discovered within a few weeks that the director didn't have the skills needed to manage the project. The supervisor sent the director to training in project management applications and processes. The director was able to use project management tools and resources and gain the skills needed to complete the project successfully.

References

American Health Information Management Association. 2019. Register Health Information Administrator Candidate Guide. *AHIMA External ADA Policies and Procedures*.

American Health Information Management Association. 2015. Privacy Statements for AHIMA's websites. http://www.ahima.org/privacy.

American Health Information Management Association. 2017. *Pocket Glossary of Health Information Management and Technology*, 5th ed. Chicago: AHIMA.

American Health Information Management Association. 2012. Identifying issues in facility and provider mergers and acquisitions. *Journal of AHIMA* 83(2):50–53.

Butler, M. 2019. Weathering the storm: How to lead through the chaos of change. *Journal of AHIMA* 90(1):12–15.

Buchbinder, S.B. and N.H. Shanks. 2017. *Introduction to Health Care Management*, 3rd ed. Burlington, MA: Jones & Bartlett Learning.

Centers for Medicare and Medicaid Services. 2018. https://www.cms.gov/apps/glossary/.

Eramo, L. 2016. HIM, meet project management, why project management is a skill growing in importance for HIM. *Journal of AHIMA* 87(1):20–23.

Harrison, C and Harrison, W. 2013. Introduction to Health Care Finance and Accounting. Delmar, Cengage Learning. Clifton Park, NY.

Johns, M.L. 2015. *Enterprise Health Information Management and Data Governance*. Chicago: AHIMA.

Johnson, T. 2017. Strategic Planning in the Healthcare Industry. https://www.balancedscorecard.org/BSC-Basics/Blog/ArtMID/2701/ArticleID/1119/Strategic-Planning-in-the-Healthcare-Industry.

Kellogg, D. 2012. Principles of Organization and Work Planning. Chapter 18 in *Health Information Management Technology: An Applied Approach*, 4th ed. Edited by N.B. Sayles. Chicago: AHIMA.

McConnell, C. 2019. *The Effective Health Care Supervisor.* Burlington, MA: Jones & Bartlett Learning.

McNamara, C. n.d. Basics of Developing Mission, Vision, and Values Statements. https://managementhelp.org/strategicplanning/mission-vision-values.htm.

Office of the National Coordinator for Health Information Technology. 2015. Federal Health IT Strategic Plan. https://www.healthit.gov/sites/default/files/9-5-federalhealthitstratplanfinal_0.pdf.

Project Management Institute. 2015. PMI Certifications. http://www.pmi.org/certification.aspx.

Performance Improvement

Darcy Carter, DHSc, MHA, RHIA
Miland N. Palmer, MPH, RHIA

Learning Objectives

- Examine performance measurement principles
- Examine quality improvement principles
- Discuss various performance improvement tools and techniques used to facilitate communication, identify root causes, and collect, analyze, and report data
- Verify the fundamental principles of continuous performance improvement
- Examine formal performance improvement activities
- Verify team-based performance improvement principles
- Explain team-based performance improvement processes
- Examine the concept of quality and its importance in healthcare
- Correlate the importance of patient safety and national patient safety goals
- Apply the elements of a quality assessment program
- Identify major organizations that publish clinical quality standards and guidelines
- Articulate ways in which healthcare organizations manage the prevention and occurrence of adverse events
- Examine the management of quality and performance improvement principles
- Discuss the importance of collecting and analyzing process data for performance improvement
- Verify clinical quality management initiatives in healthcare
- Explain the role of utilization management in regard to performance improvement
- Identify the various process improvement methodologies used in healthcare to improve quality and patient safety

Key Terms

Accountable Care Organization (ACO)
Affinity grouping
Agency for Healthcare Research and Quality (AHRQ)
Benchmark
Brainstorming
Cause-and-effect diagram
Checksheet
Claims management
Clinical practice guidelines
Clinical protocols
Common-cause variation
Customer
Dashboards
Data abstracts
DNV GL Healthcare
External customers
Financial indicators
Fishbone diagram
Flow chart
Force-field analysis
High Reliability Organization (HRO)

Incident or occurrence report
Inputs
Internal customers
ISO 9001 certification
The Joint Commission
Lean
Lean Six Sigma
Medication Reconciliation
Multivoting technique
National patient safety goals (NPSGs)
Nominal group technique
Opportunity for improvement
Outcome indicators
Outcome measures
Outputs
Patient advocacy
Performance improvement (PI)
Performance indicators
Performance measurement
Potentially compensable event
Process indicators
Process measure
Process redesign
Productivity indicators
Quality indicators
Risk
Risk management program
Root-cause analysis
Run chart
Scorecards
Sentinel event
Six Sigma
Special-cause variation
Standard
Statistical process control chart
Statistics-based modeling
Structure indicators
Structured brainstorming
Systems thinking
Time ladders
Unstructured brainstorming method
Utilization management (UM)

Throughout history and continuing today, there are many individuals involved in the provision of healthcare services who are trying to improve the way services are provided, thereby enhancing outcomes or improving performance. Performance improvement (PI) is the continuous study and adaptation of a healthcare organization's functions and processes to increase the likelihood of achieving desired outcomes. To be successful, these improvement activities require the participation of everyone involved at every level of the process. In the US, the healthcare system needs improvement, achievement, and success. A death due to a medical error should never happen and healthcare organizations are always finding ways to improve the way processes occur to prevent errors and tragedies in the future. This can be accomplished through continual growth and progress guided by quality and process improvement both departmentally and system-wide.

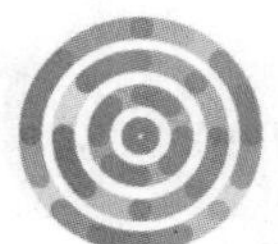

Performance Measurement and Quality Improvement

Performance measurement is the process of comparing the outcomes of an organization, work unit, or employee against pre-established performance plans and standards. Performance measurement is one of the most important concepts in the introductory discussion of quality improvement. Healthcare professionals struggle with where to focus their resources for quality improvement because there are so many areas in need of process improvement. According to the theoretical writings of general industry quality masters, the key to improvement rests in the measurement of the important characteristics of individual organizations.

Performance is "the execution of an activity or pattern of behavior; the application of inherent or learned capabilities to complete a process according to prescribed specifications or standards" (Meisenheimer 1997). Performance is measured using one or more performance indicators—a measure used by healthcare organizations to assess the quality, effectiveness, and efficiency of their services. Examples include financial indicators and productivity indicators. Financial indicators are a set of measures designed to routinely monitor the current financial status of a healthcare organization or one of its constituent parts. An example of a financial indicator would be the average cost per radiology exam compared to the average insurance reimbursement amount received. Productivity indicators are a set of measures designed to routinely monitor the output and quality of products or services provided to an individual, a healthcare organization, or one of its constituent parts; used to help determine the status of a productivity bonus. An example of a productivity indicator would be the number of patients seen per physician per day. It is important to measure the aspects of performance that reflect quality and point conclusively to the aspects of performance that require improvement. The traditional performance improvement process and sentinel events will be discussed in the next sections.

Traditional Performance Improvement Process

Although a number of terms and acronyms represent the PI concept (for example, continuous quality improvement [CQI] and total quality management [TQM]), this chapter uses PI. The key feature of PI as implemented in today's healthcare organizations is that it is a continuous cycle, starting with identification of the measures, performance measurement, analysis and comparison, opportunities for improvement, and ongoing monitoring as displayed in figure 18.1.

A logical starting point is to identify areas to monitor performance including important organization functions, particularly those that are high-risk, high-volume, or problem-prone (such as discharge not final billed [DNFB], coding compliance, or patient safety issues). Outcomes of care, customer feedback, and the requirements of regulatory agencies are additional areas that healthcare organizations consider when prioritizing performance measures. Once the scope and focus of performance monitoring are determined, the data collection requirements for each performance measure are defined (Shaw and Carter 2019).

As shown in step 2 in figure 18.1, measuring performance depends on the identification of performance measures for each service, process, or outcome determined important to track. A performance measure is a quantitative tool (for example, a rate, ratio, index, or percentage) that provides an indication of an organization's performance in relation to a specified process or outcome. A performance indicator is one measure and performance measures include multiple indicators that would be looked at to measure performance. Monitoring selected performance measures can help an organization determine process stability or identify improvement opportunities. Specific criteria define the

Figure 18.1 Organization-wide PI process

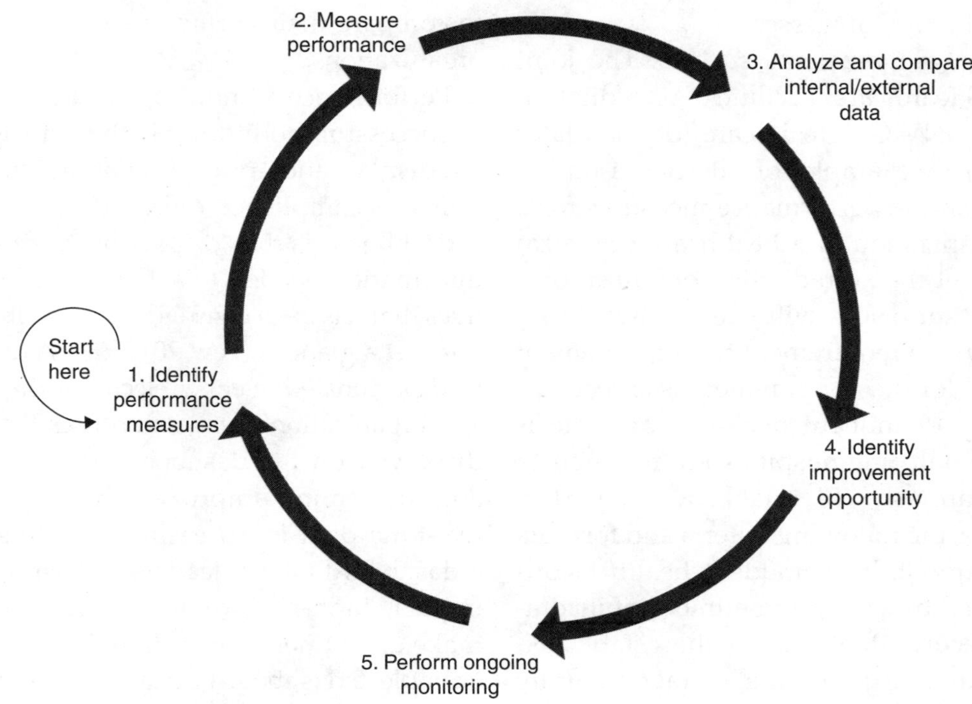

Source: ©AHIMA.

organization's performance measures. Components of an effective performance measure include a documented numerator statement, a denominator statement (such as an error rate in coding with the number of correctly coded health records as the numerator and the total number of health records coded as the denominator), and a description of the population to which the measure is applicable. In addition, the measurement period, baseline goal, data collection method, and frequency of data collection, analysis, and reporting must be identified (Shaw and Carter 2019). An example of this would be managing the DNFB report. A measurement period is set monthly with a baseline goal of the DNFB being under a specific dollar amount (such as $500,000). Data collection would occur weekly and include the value of the charges on the outstanding health records. The health information management (HIM) professional may then analyze (step 3 of figure 18.1) the DNFB weekly and report both weekly and monthly averages to the chief financial officer (CFO). Based on the DNFB data, performance improvement activities may be initiated if a pattern of high DNFB is observed. The sum total of the performance measures applicable to a healthcare organization make up the performance measurement system required in the hospital accreditation processes.

Accreditation organizations such as The Joint Commission, Healthcare Facilities Accreditation Program, and DNV GL Healthcare (defined later in this chapter) are examples of external resources used to establish the performance measures for a healthcare organization. If a healthcare organization fails to meet the accreditation organization's standards, site surveyors will cite the healthcare organization with a requirement for improvement if the threshold for the measurement is exceeded.

The monthly delinquent health record rate is one important outcome hospitals are required to monitor continuously. To establish this performance measure, the following criteria and formula are used. The monthly delinquent health record rate is calculated by taking the number of incomplete health records that exceed the established standard and dividing it by the average monthly discharges.

$$\frac{\textit{Number of incomplete health records that exceed the established standard}}{\textit{Average monthly discharges}}$$

Tracking this outcome allows the hospital to continuously monitor its deficiency rate or percentage of delinquent health records. If the health record delinquency rate exceeds the hospital's established performance standards (an internal comparison) or nationally established performance standards (external comparison), an **opportunity for improvement** has been identified (step 4 of figure 18.1). Corrective action must be taken when a healthcare organization fails to meet a performance indicator.

Step 5 is a culmination of the prior steps. Monitoring performance based on internal and external data is the foundation of all PI activities. Each healthcare organization, using its mission, scope of care, and services it provides, must identify and prioritize which processes and outcomes (in other words, which types of data) are important to monitor. For example, a healthcare organization would monitor its performance on patient satisfaction using both internal data that have been collected from patients regarding their level of satisfaction and external data from other organizations to compare their performance with that of similar organizations.

Performance monitoring is data driven. The key to successful monitoring is the appropriate analysis, display, and application of measurement data. This is accomplished efficiently with **dashboards**. A dashboard is the "display of the most important information needed to achieve one or more objectives that has been consolidated… so it can be monitored at a glance" (Few 2013, 26). A dashboard can be disseminated in either electronic or paper format. The organization's leadership uses the information displayed on the dashboard to guide operations and determine improvement projects. Having real-time data in an easily accessible format like a dashboard allows leaders to keep track of high-impact, high-risk, or high-value processes and make adjustments on a daily basis if needed. For example, a dashboard can show the DNFB at different healthcare facilities within an organization.

Additional information on data presentation is in chapter 13, *Research and Data Analysis*.

Every department in a healthcare organization should continuously monitor its key performance indicators. The following are tips for identifying and monitoring key performance indicators for HIM functions:

- Collect information at the appropriate level of detail needed to monitor performance
- Monitor the overall performance of the department using a number of indicators appropriate for the size and complexity of the department
- Divide the department into the units where specialized work is performed
- Find measures that describe the unit's performance over time, recording on a daily basis and reporting on a weekly basis
- Design a report that can track data over time, including percentage measures to identify problem areas
- Design a dashboard that can be used to monitor key indicators in real time

When all departments in a healthcare organization continuously monitor their performance, they are better able to address situations that may lead to an adverse patient outcome.

Sentinel Events

The Joint Commission requires healthcare organizations to conduct in-depth investigations of occurrences that resulted—or could have resulted—in life-threatening injuries to patients, medical staff, visitors, or employees. The Joint Commission uses the term sentinel event for such occurrences.

A sentinel event, therefore, describes an occurrence with an undesirable outcome usually happening only once. The occurrence, however, points to serious issues involved in care processes that must be resolved so this does not happen again.

Examples of sentinel events include medical errors, explosions and fires, acts of violence, removal of the wrong body part, and obstetric death. When these occur, the healthcare organization is required to prepare a detailed report of its investigation to explain the root cause of the event in order to avoid recurrence of similar events in the future. The Joint Commission issues sentinel event alerts when it detects a pattern of similar events reported by the healthcare facilities it accredits and uses its sentinel events data as a basis for its National Patient Safety Goals.

Quality Dimensions of Performance Improvement

There are three types of quality indicators, or standards against which patient care is measured to identify a level of performance for that standard.

1. Structure indicators measure the attributes of the healthcare setting, such as number and qualifications of the staff, adequacy of equipment and facilities, and adequacy of organizational policies and procedures.
2. Process indicators measure steps in a process and tasks people, or devices do, from conducting appropriate tests, to making a diagnosis, to carrying out a treatment.
3. Outcome indicators measure the actual results of care for patients and populations, including patient and family satisfaction (Donabedian 1988).

Quality has both a technical and an interpersonal dimension. The technical dimension recognizes that caregivers must have the knowledge and judgment to arrive at an appropriate strategy for providing service and the technical skills to execute it. The interpersonal aspect recognizes that caregivers must have the communication skills and social attributes necessary to serve patients appropriately. The interpersonal aspect of quality recognizes the importance of empathy, honesty, respectfulness, tactfulness, and sensitivity to others. It is far easier to measure quality's technical dimension than its interpersonal dimension (Donabedian 1988).

Contemporary Approach to Process Improvement

The contemporary approach to process improvement is much more proactive than the traditional quality management approach. Although process improvement uses several traditional quality management techniques such as quality indicators, most often its primary focus is on continually making small, targeted changes for improvement that over time lead to significant overall improvement. Process improvement is a mindset that, when adopted into organizational culture, can produce significant and continuous improvement. Process improvement is a proactive cycle that ensures key processes, products, and services are performed efficiently and within set quality standards. One key to successful process improvement is proactively measuring, monitoring, and improving indicators before the process or indicator is considered broken or unacceptable. An example would be putting an effective coding compliance plan in place that includes measuring, monitoring, and improving the coding in the facility before a negative outside audit or noncompliance fine is assessed and the in-house auditing process or coding product is determined to be unacceptable. Opportunities for improvement are identified by gathering and analyzing data on an ongoing basis. Process improvement assumes that organizations should continuously and systematically identify and test small, planned changes in processes and systems.

As process improvement practices have evolved, an important focus on the opinions of customers has developed. Many organizations and quality experts define *quality* as meeting or exceeding customer expectations. External customers are those people outside the organization for whom it provides services. For example, the external customers of a hospital would include patients, third-party payers, and the department of health. Organizations also have internal customers such as employees. The employees receive services from other areas in the organization that make it possible for them to do their jobs. For example, a nurse in an intensive care unit would be an internal customer of the hospital pharmacy; the nurse depends on the pharmacy to provide the medications needed to fill the physician's orders for his or her patients. As the importance of the perceptions and requirements of external healthcare customers becomes clear, the need for a standardized comparable way to measure their perceptions and opinions is apparent.

The Centers for Medicare and Medicaid Services (CMS) and the Agency for Healthcare Research and Quality (AHRQ) collaborated to develop the Hospital Consumer Assessment of Healthcare Providers and Systems (HCAHPS) survey. This was the first standardized survey used to compare hospital performance and quality at the national level. Hospitals are required to administer and participate in this survey if they provide services to Medicare patients. The results from this survey are informative to process improvement projects within hospitals as hospitals can use these results to identify areas that need improvement. Consumers may also access the results of the surveys at the US Department of Health and Human Services (HHS) website and use the information to make informed decisions about which providers and hospitals they would like to use. Depending on the indicators used by the hospital and the information needs to measure those indicators, organizations may use supplemental survey tools to gather that information. Often, contractors or consultants design and administer the surveys; only approved contractors can administer the HCAHPS survey.

Another means by which customers can see how a healthcare organization performs is through the publication of scorecards. As discussed earlier, quality has many dimensions. Healthcare leaders cannot just focus on one aspect of quality (such as financial measures) without also considering other aspects (such as patient satisfaction or clinical quality) or they miss the whole picture. Scorecards are tools that present metrics from a variety of quality aspects in one concise report. They may present measures of clinical quality (such as infection rates), financial quality, volume, and patient satisfaction. Several sources, including healthcare organization as well as local and national agencies provide scorecards.

Check Your Understanding 18.1

Answer the following questions.

1. The administration at Community Hospital has received several complaints about food services from patients recently discharged from the hospital. Administration has decided to review the patient responses to the survey they provide to patients upon discharge in order to monitor the performance of food services at the hospital. In this example, which of the following is driving the performance monitoring?
   a. The mission of the organization
   b. The process improvement team
   c. Data
   d. Experts
2. Which of the following provides real-time process measure metrics in a consolidated format?
   a. Structure indicator
   b. Outcome indicator
   c. Dashboard
   d. Time ladder
3. Fifty percent of the HIM staff has a nationally recognized credential. This is an example of which type of indicator?
   a. Outcome
   b. Process
   c. Structure
   d. Internal
4. The focus of PI should be on which of the following?
   a. Interpersonal skills
   b. Customers
   c. Financial stability of the organization
   d. Employees
5. University Hospital tracks the number of patients that are diagnosed with a urinary tract infection that was not present when the patient was admitted to the facility. This is an example of a(n):
   a. Financial indicator
   b. Outcome indicator
   c. Process indicator
   d. Structure indicator

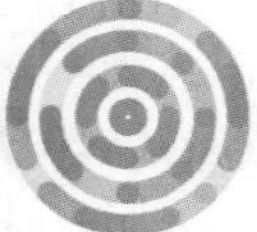

Fundamental Principles of Continuous Performance Improvement

The fundamental principles of performance improvement include the following:

- The problem is usually the system
- Variation is constant
- Data must support PI activities and decisions
- Support must come from the top down
- The organization must have a shared vision
- Staff and management must be involved in the process
- Setting goals is critical
- Effective communication is important
- Success should be celebrated

These principles are discussed in detail in the sections that follow.

The Problem Is Usually the System

Problems in patient care and other areas of the healthcare organization are usually symptoms of shortcomings inherent in a system or a process. A system is a set of related and highly interdependent components that are operating for a particular purpose. Every system has **inputs** or data entered into a hospital information system (for example, in the hospital's Admission Discharge Transfer - Registration (ADT-R) system, the patient's knowledge of his or her condition, the admitting clerk's knowledge of the admission process, and the computer with its admitting template are all inputs). The system processes the inputs and eventually produces **outputs**, or the outcomes of inputs into a system (for example, the output of the admitting process is the patient's admission to the hospital). One system's outputs may then become inputs for another system. Healthcare organizations are large systems; each department in a healthcare organization is a system with numerous subsystems.

The admitting department in a hospital is a system that exemplifies inputs, outputs, and the interrelationship between processes. When a patient enters the hospital, he or she presents to the admitting clerk. The clerk uses a computer to collect data for the ADT-R system. This information system collects data on patients admitted to the healthcare organization. The process begins with the clerk asking for the patient's address, insurance coverage, and reason for admission, as well as the patient's responses. The output of the process is the patient's admission to the hospital and a completed face sheet (which includes patient information, demographics, insurance information, emergency contact) for his or her health record. These outputs are viewed as inputs into the next system which in the hospital is the EHR.

Systems thinking is a vital part of PI and is an objective way of assessing work-related ideas and processes with the goal of allowing people to uncover ineffective patterns of behavior and thinking and then finding ways to make lasting improvement. This requires individuals to think about patterns and interrelationships between work units in the organization.

Variation Is Constant

Every system has some degree of variation built into it. No system produces the exact same output every time. It is desirable to reduce variation within systems as much as possible so that system output can be more predictable, better controlled, and the system can be more reliable (Omachonu 1999). Variation that is inherent within the system is **common-cause variation**. For example, when a nurse takes a patient's blood pressure, she may believe she is performing the procedure in exactly the same way every time, but in practice she will get slightly different readings each time. Although the blood pressure cuff, patient, and nurse are all the same inputs into the system, variations can occur. For example, the cuff may be applied to a different place on the patient's arm. The patient may have a slightly different emotional or physiological status at the time of the measurement. The nurse may have a different level of focus or concentration. Any one of these (or other) factors can affect the values obtained. However, they are potentially present in every single episode of blood pressure measurement in every single patient. It is important to recognize not every variation is a defect. The variation may just be an example of common-cause variation.

Factors outside of the system may cause variations. This type of variation is **special-cause variation**. If the special cause produces a negative effect, identify the special cause and eliminate it, if possible. If the special cause produces a positive effect, reinforce it so this positive effect will continue and perhaps be expanded into the processes of others in the organization. An example of this type of variation occurs when a patient is diagnosed with hypertension and the physician prescribes a blood pressure medication for the patient. After the patient takes the blood pressure medication, there is a substantial drop in the blood pressure measurement. All the factors (diet, exercise, stress, family history) have remained unchanged demonstrating that the medication caused the decrease in blood pressure values, which is considered a special cause. In this situation, the variation is intentional and desired. In other situations, the variation may produce an undesirable and unintentional effect. For example, if a patient is upset about a phone call he received just before the nurse came in to take his vitals, his blood pressure may register exceptionally high. The change in values occurred due to a special cause (phone call) and resulted in a blood pressure reading much higher than expected.

Similar examples of special-cause variation exist in HIM operations. For example, common-cause variation can be observed in the number of health records that can be coded each day. On a day when one of the regular coders is out sick, the number of health records coded might drop significantly because the coder will have no productive work time while home sick leaving the team short staffed. This would be an example of special-cause variation. Ideally, the goal is to remove special causes if they create an undesirable effect. When trying to control and reduce variation in a process it is important to remember there are staff with differing levels of expertise and patients with diverse levels of severity.

Data Must Support Performance Improvement Activities and Decisions

PI activities should be guided and driven by data in order to ensure an informed process. PI activities conducted without the use of reliable data are just a guess. In the burgeoning era of big data, organizations and teams must be careful not to become overloaded with data. Data, transformed into information through proper analysis, are a key tool to the success of PI activities. Collection and analysis of appropriate data will provide a solid foundation for PI activities and improve the chances of success (Strome 2013). Before PI was a generally accepted practice, healthcare organizations relied on unsupported assumptions about which processes were functioning well and which ones were not. However, objective and accurate assessment cannot occur without concrete data. Collecting and analyzing data provides information about the current processes, their effectiveness, and their potential areas for improvement efforts as well as the success of changes already implemented.

PI activities must identify the best method for obtaining timely, accurate, and relevant data. Examples of data collection methods and instruments include retrospective health record review with specific quality criteria, surveys, direct observation, and individual or focus group interviews. Electronic health records (EHRs) have allowed healthcare organizations to implement and automate data collection. Data collection alone is not enough. Careful data analysis is required to build knowledge and inform process improvement efforts.

Support Must Come from the Top Down

PI must become a part of the healthcare organization's culture. It is vital that the executive leaders of the organization believe in its value for it to permeate the entire organization. Leaders must also ensure their management teams are well versed in the principles and techniques of continuous PI. More information on organizational culture is in chapter 21, *Ethical Issues in Health Information Management*.

The Organization Must Have a Shared Vision

The organization's executive leaders and board of directors are responsible for developing and communicating a clear vision of the organization's future. The organization's vision, mission, and values set its direction and support the norms it considers important. These statements guide employees as they make their own contributions to the organization in fulfilling their professional responsibilities. See chapter 1, *Health Information Management Profession*, for more information on mission and vision.

Staff and Management Must Be Involved in the Process

PI depends on everyone in the organization actively seeking to meet the spoken or anticipated needs of internal and external customers. This is particularly important for employees who have direct contact with external customers as they may be in the best position to recognize when customer needs are met. Often employees offer helpful ideas for improvement. Staff should be empowered to make a difference for their fellow employees and the patients they serve.

Setting Goals Is Critical

All PI programs must have established goals or targets the organization strives to achieve in a given PI program year. Each goal should be specific and define measurable end results. For end results to be measurable there must be data collection and evaluation of that data. An example of an organizational goal might be: To provide high-quality patient care that is cost-effective.

After establishing goals, specific, measurable objectives that can be completed within a certain time frame should be identified. An objective associated with the previously mentioned goal might be: By the end of the year, a high-quality, cost-effective care program will be designed for the management of diabetes patients.

Effective Communication Is Important

Effective communication is essential for the PI process to work. Communication must exist at all levels of the organization and in all directions.

Openly identifying and discussing problems is not always comfortable or easy. However, an organization that is committed to serving its customers must view problems as opportunities for improvement. Two-way communication is effective and requires clear, articulate, and tactful speaking. More importantly, it requires careful, attentive listening and understanding. Organizations need to listen to their customers—both internal and external—so they can hear information about which services need improvement.

Success Should Be Celebrated

Although PI demands healthcare organizations focus on identifying and addressing problems, it also must celebrate the organization's successes. A celebration of success communicates to everyone the participants' efforts are applauded, success can result from such efforts, and others should be encouraged to participate in PI initiatives. The people involved in improving the process are recognized and appreciated.

Formal Performance Improvement Activities

Managers should feel empowered to monitor all processes within their supervision and responsibility, making small adjustments where necessary, and identifying when a more in-depth, formal approach is appropriate. Daily monitoring and minor process adjustments performed by a single manager are informal and more of a maintenance activity. Once a manager identifies an issue through the monitoring process, it requires a structured, formal PI intervention. The scope of the process, complexity of the problem, and involvement of other systems or departments should influence how formal the process should be and who should be involved.

Data collection and analysis is a vital part of PI; and benchmarking is an important PI data analysis tool. When an organization compares its current performance to its own internal historical data, or uses data from similar external organizations, it helps establish an organizational benchmark. A benchmark is a systematic comparison of one healthcare organization's measured characteristics with those of another similar organization or with internal, regional, or national standards. For example, an HIM department will track their health record deficiencies on a monthly basis and compare their deficiency rate to that of similar sized facilities. Often, further study or more focused data collection on a performance measure is warranted when data collection results fall outside the established benchmark. This is the "monitoring and improving customer satisfaction" process (Shaw and Carter 2019, 114). Opportunities for improvement are often discovered when unintended events and patterns are observed during continuous monitoring. This technique is best represented as the "team-based performance improvement process" (Shaw and Carter 2019, 28–30). The interdependency and interrelation of these processes is important and will be discussed later in this chapter.

PI initiatives use a number of tools and techniques. Some of the tools facilitate communication among employees while others help people determine the root causes of performance problems. Some tools indicate areas of agreement or consensus among team members. Others permit the display of data for easy analysis.

Checksheets

A checksheet is a data collection tool that records and compiles observations or occurrences. The checksheet consists of a simple list of categories, issues, or observations on the left side of the health record and a place on the right to record incidences by placing a checkmark (see figure 18.2). When the data collection is finished, the checkmarks are counted to reveal any patterns or trends. A checksheet is a simple way to obtain a clear picture of the basic facts. After data are collected, other tools may be used to display the data and help analyze them more easily.

Data Abstracts

Data abstracts are a defined and standardized set of data points or elements common to a patient population that can be regularly identified in the health records of the population and coded for use and analysis in a database management system. The data abstracts are used in clinical process monitoring where data is collected on each patient from the health record and recorded in the specified fields of an abstract on paper or electronically.

Time Ladders

Time ladders support the collection of data that must be oriented by time; they specify intervals of time necessary to address the problem under consideration listed down the right side of one, two, or three columns. Then, as the data collector observes, he or she records events next to the time of occurrence. For example, a receptionist could record on a time ladder when a patient arrives at his or her workstation and then record again on the same time ladder when the patient goes to an exam room. To visualize how the receptionist's other duties have an impact on his or her interactions with patients, he or she could also be asked to record timing of phone calls, provider requests for assistance, and other competing tasks. Collecting time ladder data over an appropriate period develops a detailed, clear picture of the workflow or process. Another example is a time ladder created from computer-based data. For example, the EHR could be used to generate a report documenting the time of arrival for patients without appointments. Using this data from a substantial period of a month or more, clinic management could anticipate the need to keep a specific number of appointment slots available for walk-ins. Figure 18.3 shows an example of a time ladder.

Figure 18.2 Checksheet

	Coders		
Issue Observed	1	2	**Total**
Missing documentation	卌	||||	9
Missing authentication	|||	||	5
Physician query required	|||	卌	8

Source: ©AHIMA.

Figure 18.3 Time ladder

Patient #1 arrived	9:00	3 calls from patients Request to make call from clinician
Patient #2 arrived Patient #3 arrived	9:15	4 calls from patients Print forms for patient #1
Patient #1 to exam room	9:30	3 calls from patients Print forms for patient #2 Request for specialist consult patient #1
Patient #4 arrived Patient #2 to exam room Patient #5 arrived	9:45	5 calls from patients Print forms for patient #3 Print forms for patient #4
Patient #3 to exam room Patient #4 to exam room	10:00	1 call from patient Print forms for patient #5
Patient #5 to exam room	10:15	Schedule appointment for patient #2

Source: ©AHIMA.

Statistics-Based Modeling Techniques

With increased implementation of EHRs, the amount of data collected by and available to healthcare facilities is growing exponentially. The best way to use and apply this data is through statistics-based modeling. Statistics-based modeling is the use of analytical and graphical techniques to assist in the display and interpretation of raw data. Two common statistical-based modeling techniques are run charts and process control charts. A run chart displays data points for a specific time frame to provide information about performance (see figure 18.4). In a run chart, the measured points of a process are plotted on a graph at regular time intervals to help team members identify whether there are substantial changes in the numbers over time. For example, suppose an HIM professional wished to reduce the number of incomplete health records in the HIM department. He or she might first plot the number of incomplete health records each month for the past six months. Based on an analysis of the health records process, he or she then might enact a change designed to improve the process. The data collection should continue after the change is made to determine its effect on the process. If the run chart then indicated that the number of incomplete charts had decreased post-change, the HIM professional could attribute the decrease to the improvement effort. A run chart is an excellent tool for providing visual verification of how a process is performing and whether an improvement effort has worked.

A statistical process control chart looks like a run chart except that it has reference lines indicating the upper control limit (UCL) and lower control limit (LCL) drawn horizontally at the top and bottom of the chart. The upper line represents the UCL, and the lower line represents the LCL. In figure 18.5, the middle line represents the mean and the line above represents two standard deviations above the mean. The line below the mean represents two standard deviations below the mean. Remember, two standard deviations from the mean statistically include 95 percent of the observations of a process and three standard deviations include 99 percent (see chapter 13, Research and Data Analysis, for more information on calculating statistics). Like the run chart, the statistical process control chart plots points to show how a process is performing over time. However, the two control limit lines permit the evaluator to use the rules of probability to interpret whether the process is stable (in other words, predictable and within the bounds of probability) or out of control (many points of data outside the second or third standard deviations).

The statistical process control chart makes it possible to see whether the variation within a process is the result of a common cause or a special cause. It lets the PI team know whether the team needs to try to reduce the ordinary variation

Figure 18.4 Run chart

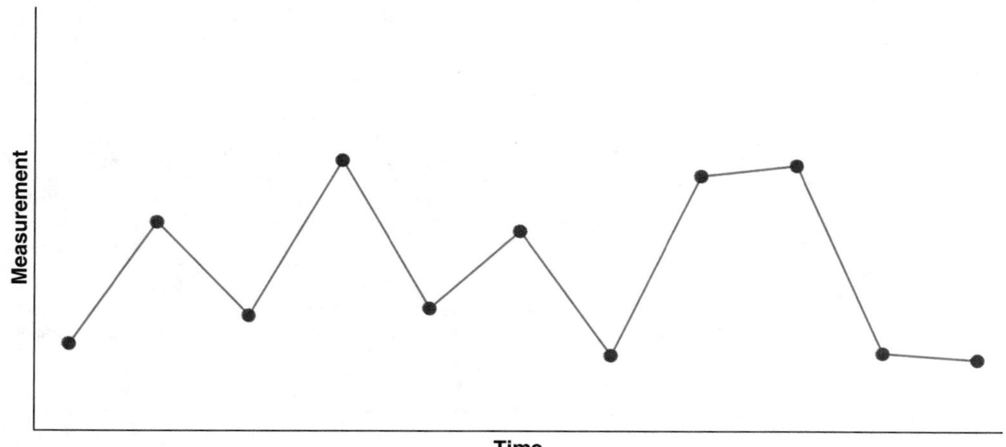

Source: ©AHIMA.

Figure 18.5 Statistical process control chart

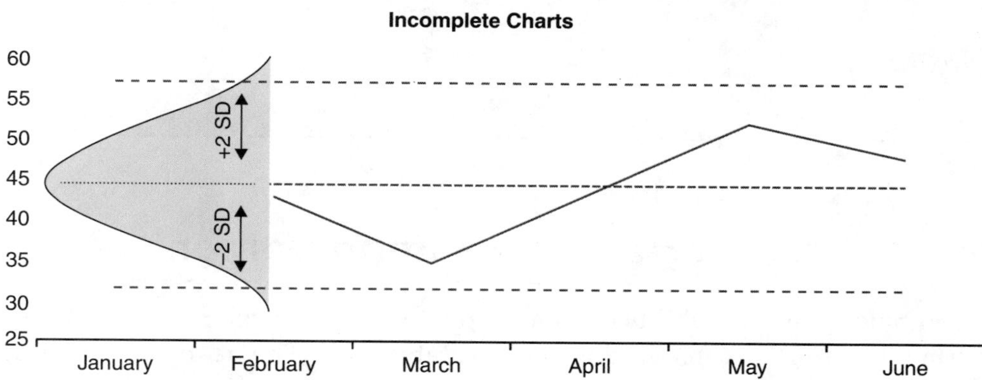

Source: ©AHIMA.

occurring through common cause or to seek out a special cause of the variation and try to eliminate it. Removing the variation will bring the upper and lower control limit lines closer together. Common-cause variation would produce patterns that would stay within the two or three standard deviations of the mean, whereas a special-cause variation is more likely to produce patterns that will exceed the limits of chance of the two or three standard deviations.

Check Your Understanding 18.2

Answer the following questions.

1. The type of variation caused by factors outside a system is a(n):
   a. Input or output
   b. Processes
   c. Common-cause variation
   d. Special-cause variation
2. Which tool displays performance data over time?
   a. Benchmark
   b. Run chart
   c. Checksheet
   d. Time ladder
3. Community Hospital has reviewed their nosocomial infection rate for the past quarter and found that it is 0.2 percent. Community Hospital then compares their rate with that of a similar hospital across town and finds that the other hospital has a rate of 0.3 percent. This is an example of which of the following?
   a. Checksheet
   b. Data abstract
   c. Run chart
   d. Benchmark
4. Lisa is a coding auditor at a local hospital. As part of her coding review process she is tallying each instance that a coder incorrectly assigns the discharge disposition for a patient. Which of the following data collection tools is Lisa using?
   a. Checksheet
   b. Flow chart
   c. Time ladder
   d. Fishbone diagram

5. A set of related and highly interdependent components that are operating for a particular purpose is called a:
   a. System
   b. Benchmark
   c. Statistics-based model
   d. Run chart

Team-Based Performance Improvement

The combined cognitive ability of teams can be an important tool in PI because of the complex issues faced in healthcare. Team-based PI begins with the assembly of the team. Staff with knowledge and background in the process under examination should be included. In addition, staff members accept change and transition easier when they have been part of the decision-making process.

The team's success depends on the following nine elements:

1. Establishing ground rules for the team (described in chapter 19, *Leadership*)
2. Stating the team's purpose or mission (described in chapter 19)
3. Identifying customers and their requirements
4. Documenting current processes and identifying barriers
5. Benchmarking
6. Collecting current process data
7. Analyzing process data
8. Process redesign
9. Recommendations for process change

Except where noted, these team-based performance elements are discussed in detail in the sections that follow.

Identifying Customers and Their Requirements

The PI team must identify the customers associated with the processes under discussion. Keep in mind customers are both internal (for example, the healthcare organization's business office) and external (for example, third-party payers). Once customer groups are identified, their needs related to the process need to be explored and established. The team can then work toward modifying the process to meet the customers' requirements.

Documenting Current Processes and Identifying Barriers

The process improvement team members work together to discuss and document current processes and identify barriers to establishing successful processes. For this step, the team's knowledge is vital because members must answer the following questions:

- What is the current process?
- Where are the start and end points of the process?
- What are the inputs, outputs, and interdependencies?
- What is the potential for error in the process?
- What are the barriers to the process?
- What are the gaps to meeting the customer's needs?

Benchmarking

Benchmarking compares an organization's performance against that of external standards. Healthcare organizations routinely use benchmarking as a way to measure their performance. When benchmarking for PI, a healthcare organization compares its performance data with that of a similar healthcare facility and uses the findings to determine areas that need improvement. Benchmarking also increases motivation to improve processes and outcomes through comparison to potential competitors and similar departments.

Collecting Current Process Data

Once performance monitoring identifies an improvement opportunity, the first task of the PI process team is to research and define performance expectations for the process targeted. For example, performance monitoring of coding productivity identifies that coding staff is consistently not meeting previously set productivity standards.

PI teams have a variety of tools they employ, such as flow charts, brainstorming, diagramming, and force-field analysis (described in the following sections) that make it easier to gather and analyze information; and they help team members remain focused on PI activities and move the process along efficiently. The PI team should also use any information from routinely monitored processes as relevant to the targeted process.

Flow Chart Current Process

A **flow chart** is a graphic tool that uses standard symbols to visually display detailed information, including time and distance of the sequential flow of work of an individual or a product as it progresses through a process. A flow chart should be created to illustrate the current process used because the team must first examine and understand the current process before making improvements. Each team member has a unique perspective on and significant insight into how a portion of the process works. Flow charts help all the team members understand the process in the same way (see figure 18.6).

Figure 18.6 Flow chart

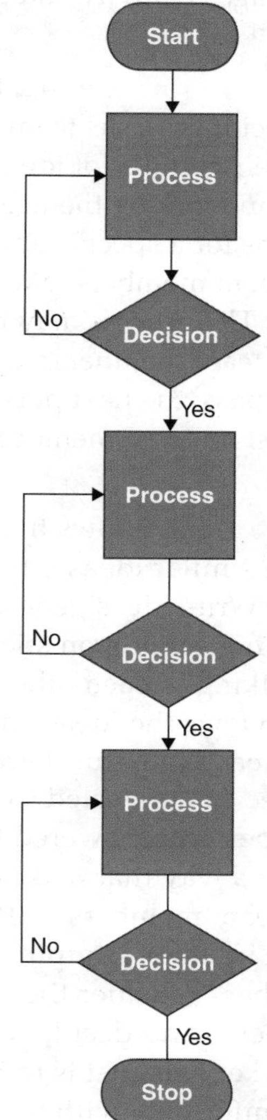

Source: ©AHIMA.

The work involved in developing the flow chart allows the team to understand every step in the process as well as the sequence of steps. The flow chart provides a visual picture of each decision point and event in the process. It exposes places where there are redundancies and complex and problematic areas.

Brainstorm Problem Areas

Brainstorming is a technique used to generate a large number of creative ideas from a group. It encourages PI team members to think outside the box and offer original ideas to address problems in the process. Brainstorming is highly effective for identifying a number of potential process steps that may benefit from improvement efforts and for generating solutions to specific problems. It helps people to begin thinking in new ways and involves them in the process. It is an excellent method for facilitating open communication. There are a number of approaches to brainstorming, including the following:

- The **unstructured brainstorming method** results in a free flow of ideas. The team leader or facilitator writes the ideas on a chart or board when presented. This allows everyone to see the list as it forms. There should be no discussion or evaluation of the ideas at this point. The goal of brainstorming is to encourage creativity and generate many ideas.

- In structured brainstorming, the team leader or facilitator asks team members to create their own list of ideas. Team members can work by themselves or in small groups for a specific amount of time. Then, the team members take turns offering a new idea. The process may take several rounds. As team members run out of new ideas, they pass; the next person then offers an idea until no team member can produce a fresh idea.
- Affinity grouping allows the team to organize similar ideas into logical groupings. Write ideas generated in a brainstorming session on sticky notes. Without talking to each other, each team member reviews the ideas on the notes and places each in natural groupings that seem related or connected to each other. Each member is empowered to move the ideas in a way that makes the most sense. As team members shift the ideas or place them in other groupings, the other team members consider the merits of the placements and decide what further action to take. The goal is to have the team become comfortable with the arrangement. Finally, label the natural groupings that emerge. An example of an affinity diagram is in figure 18.7.
- Nominal group technique is a process used to reach consensus about an issue or an idea that the team considers most important. Each team member ranks each idea according to importance. For example, if there were six ideas, the most important idea is ranked with the number six (giving it six points); the second most important idea is ranked the number five, and so on. After each individual team member has had a chance to rank the list of ideas, the scores for each idea are totaled. The nominal group technique demonstrates where the team's priorities lie.
- The multivoting technique is a variation of the nominal group technique and serves the same purpose. Instead of ranking each issue or idea, team members rate issues by marking them with a distribution of points. In weighted multivoting, a team member distributes his or her allotment of points among as few or as many issues as he or she wants. For example, the team member might give 13 out of 25 points to one issue of importance, 3 points each to four other issues, and no points to the remaining issues. After the voting, the sum of the numbers

Figure 18.7 Affinity diagram

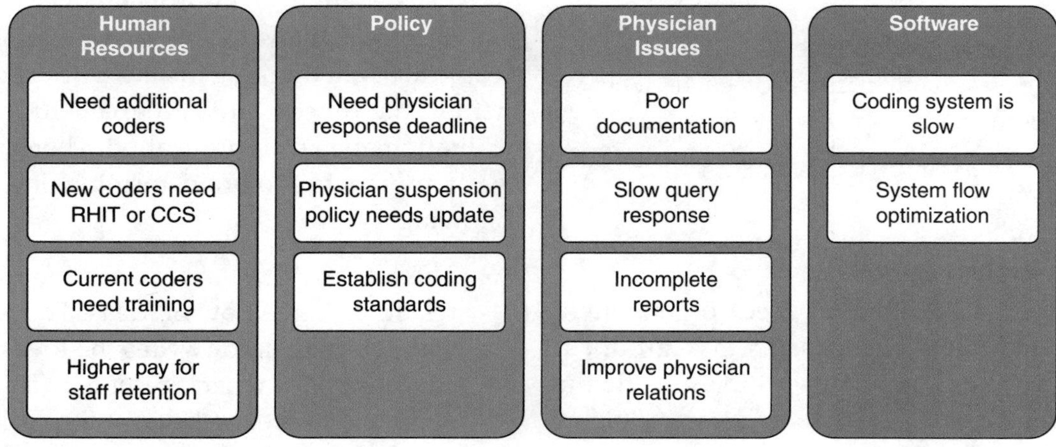

Source: ©AHIMA.

given to each issue determines the issue with the highest priority. Thus, the team will be able to see which issue emerged as particularly important to the entire team.

Cause-and-Effect Diagram

One of the common quality improvement tools used for risk management purposes is the cause-and-effect diagram. A cause-and-effect diagram, also known as fishbone diagram because of its characteristic fish shape (see figure 18.8), is an investigational technique that facilitates the identification of the various factors that contribute to a problem. It facilitates root-cause analysis, or the analysis of an event from all aspects (human, procedural, machinery, material), to identify how each contributed to the occurrence of the event and to develop new systems that will prevent recurrence. The problem or reason for the quality improvement exercise is written clearly in a box on the right side of the diagram. A horizontal line is drawn and diagonal lines resembling ribs connect the boxes above and below the main horizontal line (or backbone). Each box contains a different category of information.

The categories may represent broad classifications of problem areas. For example, possible categories include people, methods, equipment, materials, policies, procedures, environment, or measurement. The team determines how many categories it needs to classify all the possible sources of the problem.

After constructing the diagram, the team brainstorms the possible root causes of the problem. Brainstorming continues until all the team's ideas about causes are exhausted. The purpose of this tool is to permit the team to explore, identify, and graphically display all of the root causes of a problem.

Force-Field Analysis

Force-field analysis is another tool used to display data generated through brainstorming. Force-field analysis identifies specific drivers of and barriers to an organizational change, so that positive factors can be reinforced and negative factors reduced (figure 18.9). Team members brainstorm the

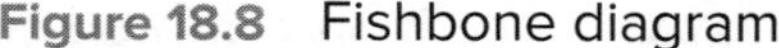

Figure 18.8 Fishbone diagram

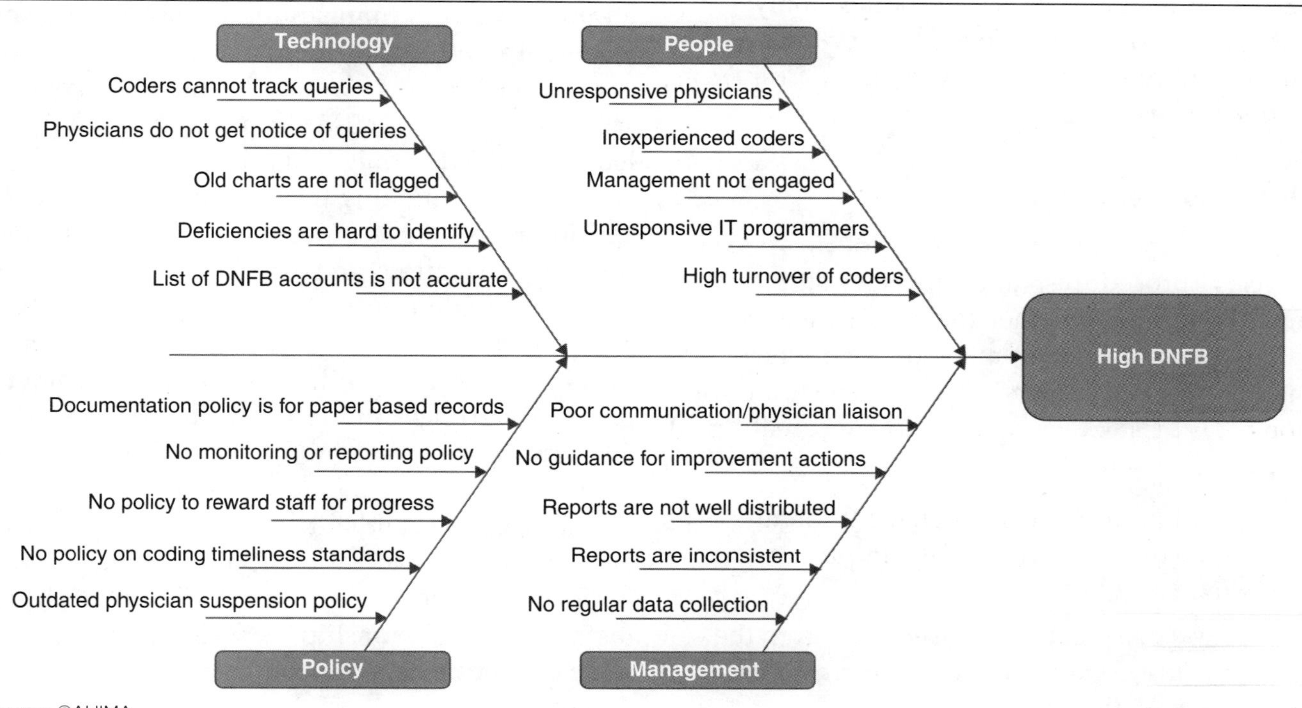

Source: ©AHIMA.

Figure 18.9 Force-field analysis

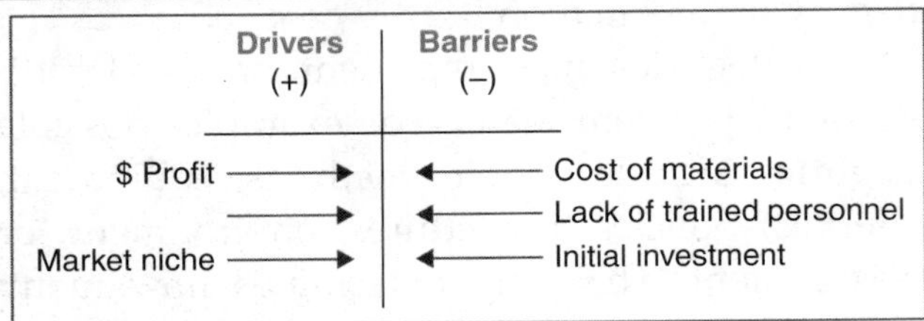

Source: ©AHIMA.

reasons or factors that would encourage a change for improvement and those that might create barriers. The team leader places the factors in the appropriate column on the chart.

Force-field analysis enables team members to identify factors that support or work against a proposed solution. Often the next step after force-field analysis is to develop ways that would eliminate barriers or reinforce drivers.

Analyzing Process Data

Following the collection of data, it is important for the team to consider the data in a meaningful way. Again, PI tools and techniques can assist the team by providing meaningful documents from which conclusions can be drawn. Teams can use bar graphs, histograms, scatter diagrams, and Pareto charts to better analyze the data. For additional information on these tools and techniques, refer to chapter 13, *Research and Data Analysis.*

Process Redesign

Following in-depth examination of all the data, policies, procedures, and interviews, the team must determine whether the process will receive minor adjustments or a major restructuring to make it meet customers' expectations. If the solution is process redesign, the following are the next steps.

- Incorporate findings or changes identified in the research phase of the improvement process
- If necessary, collect focused data from the prioritized problem areas to further clarify process failure or variation
- Create a flow chart of the redesigned process.
- Develop policies and procedures that support the redesigned process.
- Educate involved staff about the new process including justifications for the change.

Recommendations for Process Change

The process improvement team is responsible for putting the outcome of its work in a report format, along with recommendations for improving the process. Determine the recommendations after receiving and analyzing all data. The data include findings from the appropriate tools and techniques discussed previously. The recommendations should consider anything that might have an impact on the organization, including the following:

- Utilization of staff
- Effect on the budget
- Change in productivity
- Effects on customer requirements

Recommendations are viewed by the appropriate manager or administrator, considered by the leadership group and top management for an organization-wide problem, or by the management group heading the HIM department if the problem is confined to only that unit.

After implementing the new process, the team continues to measure performance against customers' expectations and established performance standards to determine if there is a need for further improvement (refer to figure 18.1). When measurement data indicates the improvement is effective (for example, error rate dropped by 50 percent), ongoing monitoring of the process resumes.

The team disbands at this point in the cycle, and routine organizational monitoring of the performance measures resumes. Figure 18.10 illustrates the relationship between organization-wide performance monitoring and team-based PI processes.

Figure 18.10 Organization-wide and team-based PI model

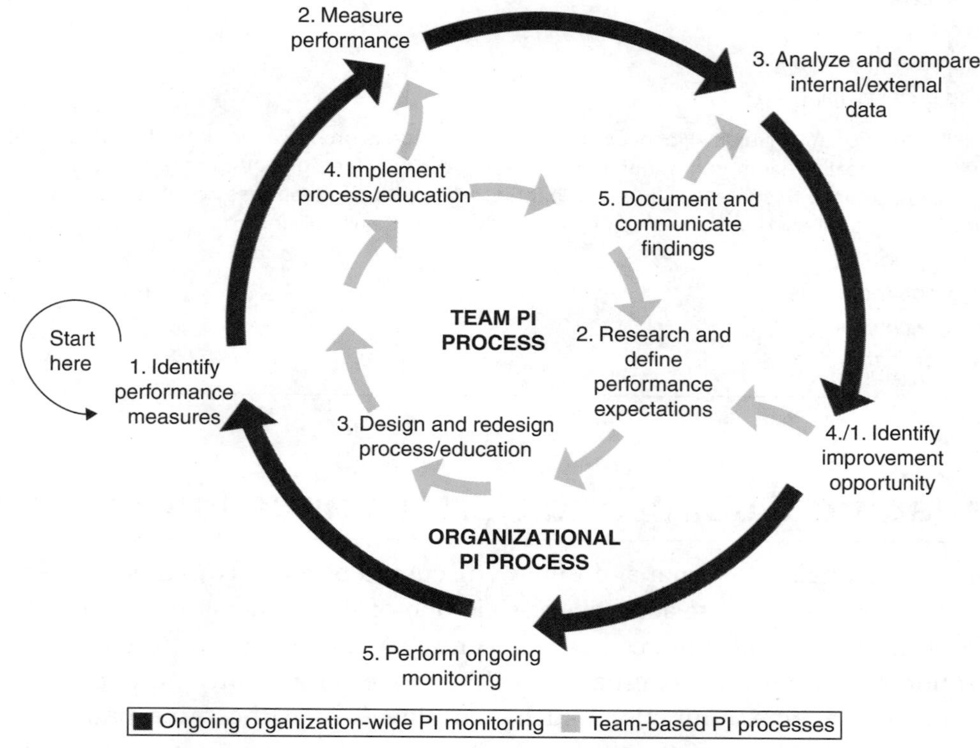

Source: Shaw and Carter 2019.

Check Your Understanding 18.3

Answer the following questions.

1. A PI team has been tasked with improving the patient admitting process because the hospital has received patient complaints. Before creating a new process, the team has diagrammed the current process. Which of the following tools would the team have used to when they diagrammed the current process?
   a. Flow chart
   b. Force-field analysis
   c. Unstructured brainstorming
   d. Structured brainstorming
2. Which of the following is used to compare an organization's performance against that of external standards?
   a. Affinity grouping
   b. Benchmarking
   c. Scorecards
   d. Brainstorming
3. Which of the following is an investigational technique that facilitates the identification of the various factors that contribute to a problem?
   a. Affinity grouping
   b. Cause-and-effect diagram
   c. Force-field analysis
   d. Nominal group technique

4. In what technique do team members rate issues by distribution of points?
   a. Affinity grouping
   b. Nominal group technique
   c. Multivoting technique
   d. Structured brainstorming

5. Kevin is the HIM Director at University Hospital. He is looking for ideas on how to improve the process for requesting employee vacation time. In their monthly staff meeting, Kevin asks each employee to create a list of ideas. Each team member has an opportunity to share their ideas with the group. When the team has no more ideas to share, this process ends. What team-based performance improvement tool is Kevin utilizing?
   a. Affinity grouping
   b. Nominal group technique
   c. Multivoting technique
   d. Structured brainstorming

Managing Quality and Performance Improvement

HIM professionals must manage quality and the PI process to ensure these activities accomplish the important and vital changes needed by the organization's internal and external customers. Traditional management functions such as planning, organizing, leading, and controlling should be applied to PI initiatives. See chapter 19, *Leadership,* for information on management functions. External entities should be considered during a healthcare organization's quality deliberations, discussions, and decision-making. External entities include agencies that offer voluntary accreditation services, are involved in the reimbursement cycle, administer licensure services, and offer national quality policy and direction. In order to meet a healthcare organization's goals and mission, all relevant agencies must be factored into their approach to achieving superior quality. Components of PI activities include organizational factors, standards of organizational quality, utilization management, and risk management.

Organizational Components of PI

To be successful in implementing PI programs, healthcare organizations may have to restructure and create a new culture to accommodate the vast changes and competition that exist in today's healthcare environment. PI is most successful in organizations that have an interdisciplinary and participative management approach. As discussed previously in this chapter, shared vision is one of the cornerstones of a successful PI program. A shared vision puts everyone—including the governing board, upper management, and employees—on the same path to organizational success. Changing to a shared leadership environment can create a new organizational culture of shared vision, responsibility, and accountability. Because every employee is a vital part of this shared leadership, this type of environment helps to increase employee motivation and empowerment. For more information on change management, please refer to chapter 17, *Management.*

In addition to an enterprise-wide vision, a shared leadership framework is essential for implementing PI. Shared leadership essentially means that organizations ensure all their employees participate in an integrated, continuous PI program. When various organizational frameworks or structures are developed, it encourages shared leadership by encouraging employee participation and instilling ownership.

Large healthcare organizations are complex both in size and in geographical location requiring focused effort to standardize and facilitate necessary changes. The organizational structures and processes that constitute a PI program need to be accomplished across the entire healthcare organization, meaning that every location and department within the organization takes part in the PI program. To be effective, the organizational unit responsible for PI must be able to communicate with all areas of the healthcare organization and foster interdisciplinary cooperation. Many healthcare organizations have created a PI department to help the organization pursue its quality efforts. Many PI departments assume leadership in the assessing and tracking of organizational compliance with accreditation standards, focus areas, and patient safety goals.

The following are the basic responsibilities of the PI department:

- Helping departments or groups of departments with similar issues to identify potential quality problems
- Assisting determination of the best methods for studying potential problems (for example, survey, chart review, interview with staff, or data mining)
- Participating in regular meetings across the organization as appropriate, and training organization members on quality and PI methodology, tools, and techniques

A permanent multidisciplinary committee should coordinate the program and ensure the uniformity of clinical quality assessment (QA) processes throughout the organization. The committee should include representatives of the medical staff, nursing staff, and infection control team. Consult representatives from other areas as needed.

Standards of Organizational Quality in Healthcare

A number of private and government entities develop and maintain standards of organizational quality for healthcare. These entities include agencies and departments of the federal government, accreditation organizations, private for-profit organizations, and not-for-profit organizations such as medical societies and organizations dedicated to research on a specific disease or condition. Standards of quality include descriptive statements known as standards of care, quality of care standards, performance standards, accreditation standards, and practice standards.

A **standard** is a written description of the expected features, characteristics, or outcomes of a healthcare-related service. Standards provide a minimum level of performance. Four types of standards relevant within the context of clinical quality assessment are addressed in the following sections:

- Clinical practice guidelines and clinical protocols
- Accreditation standards
- Government regulations
- Licensure requirements

The sections that follow will discuss each of these standards in detail.

Clinical Practice Guidelines and Protocols

Standards of clinical quality include both clinical practice guidelines and clinical protocols. **Clinical protocols** are detailed, step-by-step instructions used by healthcare practitioners to make knowledge-based clinical decisions directly related to patient care. The **Agency for Healthcare Research and Quality (AHRQ)** is an agency within HHS. AHRQ's mission is to improve the quality, safety, efficiency, and effectiveness of healthcare for all Americans. **Clinical practice guidelines** are developed to standardize clinical decision-making. As the word *guideline* suggests, clinical practice guidelines are not meant to be inflexible and do not apply in every case.

In contrast to clinical practice guidelines, clinical protocols are treatment recommendations based on guidelines. They are specific instructions for performing clinical procedures established by authoritative bodies, such as medical staff committees, and intended to be applied literally and universally. One example of a clinical protocol is the step-by-step description of the accepted procedure for preparing intravenous solutions at a specific acute-care hospital.

Accreditation Standards

In the US, many different organizations monitor the quality of healthcare services and offer accreditation programs for healthcare organizations. These programs base accreditation on a data collection and submission process followed by a comprehensive survey process. Participation in accreditation programs is voluntary. (See chapter 3, *Health Information Functions, Purpose, and Users,* for a discussion of accreditation.) The Joint Commission, DNV GL, and other voluntary accreditation organizations are addressed in the following sections.

Joint Commission The Joint Commission (discussed in chapter 8, *Health Law*) emphasizes PI in their accreditation standards. All hospitals and long-term care facilities are required to report outcome measures. Outcome measures document the results of care for individual patients as well as for specific types of patients grouped by diagnostic category. For example, an acute-care hospital's overall rate of postsurgical infection is an outcome measure. Process measures focus on a process that leads to a certain outcome, meaning that a scientific basis exists for believing that the process, when executed well, will increase the probability of achieving a desired outcome. An example is the percent of stroke patients receiving appropriate medication (Tissue Plasminogen Activator [TPA]) within the appropriate time frame. Outcome and process measures have evolved into quality measures now called accountability measures. Accountability measures focus on four main components: research, proximity, accuracy, and adverse effects. These measures are the key to improving patient care and quality, thus improving patient outcomes. The Joint Commission scores healthcare organizations on compliance with specific National Patient Safety Goals (NPSGs). The NPSGs outline the areas of organizational practice that most commonly lead to patient injury or other negative outcomes that can be prevented if standardized procedures are used. For example, an NPSG requires the healthcare provider to eliminate wrong-site, wrong-patient, and wrong-procedure surgery. To accomplish this, healthcare organizations must create and use a preoperative verification process, such as a checklist, to confirm the patient's identity and that appropriate documents (for example, health records, imaging studies) are available. They also must implement a process to mark the surgical site and involve the patient in the marking process.

The data collected are used to help focus the accreditation survey on patient safety and high-quality patient care and to select specific patients to "trace" during the on-site survey. This approach, known as tracer methodology, consists of following (tracing) a few patients through their entire stay at the hospital to identify quality and patient safety issues that might indicate quality problems or patterns of less than optimum care. A trace of a surgical patient, for example, might reveal a missing updated history and physical (H&P) on the patient's health record within 24 hours before surgery. Following this lead, the surveyor might discover that the healthcare organization is having an ongoing problem with H&Ps in general; a problem with obtaining the required updated H&P within 24 hours before surgery, or perhaps a problem with just one particular physician.

DNV GL and Other Voluntary Accreditation Organizations DNV GL Healthcare is a voluntary accreditation organization that has operated in the US since the late 1800s but is relatively new to healthcare. The organization is recognized by CMS to have *deemed status,* which means healthcare organizations accredited by DNV GL are recognized as meeting the Medicare Conditions of Participation, which are the administrative and operational guidelines and regulations under which healthcare organizations can take part in the Medicare and Medicaid programs. Medicare and Medicaid are discussed in chapter 15, *Revenue Management and Reimbursement.*

Other voluntary accreditation organizations include: Healthcare Facilities Accreditation Program (HFAP), which focuses accreditation activities on general acute-care specialty hospitals and long-term acute-care hospitals; The National Committee on Quality Assurance (NCQA), which focuses on health plans and outpatient provider organizations; and The Commission on the Accreditation of Rehabilitation Facilities (CARF), which focuses on long-term and mental health rehabilitation facilities.

Government Regulations and Licensure Requirements

Various agencies and departments of the federal, state, and local governments also review the quality of services provided in healthcare organizations. However, government regulations and licensure requirements are compulsory rather than voluntary.

Medicare Conditions of Participation. To participate in the Medicare program, healthcare providers must comply with federal regulations known as the Conditions of Participation. The CMS develops the Conditions of Participation.

Quality improvement organizations. Quality improvement organizations (QIOs) are responsible for monitoring the quality of care provided to Medicare patients. CMS and the QIOs collaborate with practitioners, beneficiaries, providers, plans, and other purchasers of healthcare services to achieve the following key functions:

- Improve quality of care for Medicare beneficiaries
- Protect the integrity of the Medicare Trust Fund by ensuring Medicare only pays for services that are reasonable, necessary, and appropriate
- Protect beneficiaries by addressing complaints

QIOs use medical peer review, data analysis, and other tools to identify patterns of care and outcomes that need improvement. They then work cooperatively with facilities and individual physicians to improve care. CMS established a comprehensive program in which QIOs use a data-driven approach to monitoring care and outcomes and a shared approach to working with the healthcare community to improve care.

State and local licensure requirements. To maintain its licensed status, each healthcare organization must adhere to the state regulations that govern it such as quality of care. For additional information, refer to chapter 8, Health Law.

Check Your Understanding 18.4

Answer the following questions.

1. Which of the following is a written description of the expected features, characteristics, or outcomes of a healthcare-related service?
   a. Flow chart
   b. Standard
   c. Pareto chart
   d. Ground rules
2. Midtown Hospital is currently under construction in an urban area. The administration is planning to treat Medicare patients at this new facility. In order to participate in the Medicare program and treat these patients the facility must comply with which federal regulation?
   a. Conditions of Participation
   b. National Patient Safety Goals
   c. Clinical Practice Guidelines
   d. Utilization Management Review
3. QIOs use peer review, data analysis, and other tools to:
   a. Evaluate whether or not a healthcare facility is meeting standards for accreditation and licensing
   b. Calculate reimbursement
   c. Penalize healthcare organizations
   d. Identify areas that need improvement

4. The NPSG scores organizations on areas that:
   a. Commonly lead to financial stability of the organization
   b. Affect customers
   c. Affect compliance with state law
   d. Commonly lead to patient injury
5. Which of the following is a voluntary accreditation organization that is relatively new to healthcare?
   a. DNV GL
   b. AHRQ
   c. The Joint Commission
   d. ACO

Utilization Management

Utilization management (UM) is composed of a set of processes used to determine the appropriateness of medical services provided during specific episodes of care. In most hospitals, UM programs perform three important functions—utilization review, case management, and discharge planning. Utilization management is an important part of quality patient care as it helps to ensure necessary and appropriate care, effectiveness of the services provided to the patient, and timely and safe discharge of patients. See chapter 15 for a complete discussion on utilization management.

Risk Management

In healthcare, risk is any occurrence or circumstance that might result in a loss. Loss includes any damage to an entity's person, property, or rights, including physical injury, cognitive injury, emotional injury, wrongful death, and financial loss. In this chapter, the focus is on how risk management relates to quality. For additional information about risk, refer to chapter 10, *Data Security.*

The purpose of the risk management program is to link risk management functions to the related processes of quality assessment and PI. The aims of the program are to (1) help provide high-quality patient care while also enhancing a safe environment for patients, employees, and visitors, and (2) minimize financial loss by reducing risk through prevention and evaluation.

The basic functions of healthcare risk management programs are similar for most organizations and including the following:

- Risk identification and analysis
- Loss prevention and reduction
- Claims management

The sections that follow will discuss each of these healthcare risk management programs in detail.

Risk Identification and Analysis

The role of the risk manager is to collect and analyze information on actual losses and potential risks and to design systems that mitigate potential losses in the future. Risk managers use information from a variety of sources to identify areas of risk exposure within the organization. The following are some sources for risk management information:

- Incident reports (sometimes called occurrence reports or occurrence screens)
- Current and past liability claims against the organization
- Performance improvement reports
- Internal inspections of the organization's physical plant and medical equipment
- Reviews conducted by the organization's insurance carriers
- Survey reports from state and local licensing agencies
- Survey reports from accreditation organizations
- Reports of complaints from patients, visitors, medical staff, and employees

An incident (or occurrence) report is a structured tool used to collect data and information about any event *not* consistent with routine operational procedures, such as a wrong-side surgery or foreign body left in following surgery. In the language of risk management, the documentation of these events is used to identify potentially compensable events. A potentially compensable event is an occurrence, such as an accident or medical error that may result in personal injury or loss of property to patients, staff, visitors, or the healthcare organization.

Incident reports are prepared to help healthcare organizations identify and correct problem areas and prepare for legal defense. An incident report documents the event for operational purposes and is not used for patient care, so it is considered an extremely confidential document that is never filed in the health record and should not be photocopied or prepared in duplicate. The healthcare provider should never document that an incident report was completed. Incident reports are not part of the legal health record and are not discoverable in event of legal action (Farenholz 2017). See figure 18.11 for an example of an incident report.

Loss Prevention and Reduction

The risk manager is responsible for developing systems to prevent injuries and other losses within the organization. Performance improvement actions are often initiated in response to suggestions offered by the risk manager. Education also is an invaluable tool in risk management and sometimes is the only activity required to prevent potential safety problems.

Risk managers in many healthcare organizations are responsible for developing policies and procedures aimed at preventing accidents and injuries and reducing the organization's risk exposure.

Claims Management

Claims management is the process of managing the legal and administrative aspects of the healthcare organization's response to injury claims (injuries occurring on the healthcare organization's property). Claims management may be handled differently depending on the size and type of organization. Accordingly, the role of the risk manager in managing claims varies. Many organizations place the entire process in the hands of their liability insurance vendors. In such cases, the risk manager may act as the healthcare organization's liaison with the insurance company. However, some healthcare organizations are self-insured, meaning that they establish a dedicated fund for financing future liability settlements. Organizations manage claims and risk by incorporating patient advocacy, incorporating regulatory and accreditation requirements, and having an organizational incident response mechanism in place.

Patient Advocacy

Many large healthcare organizations such as acute-care hospitals have instituted patient advocacy programs. In such programs, a patient representative (sometimes called an ombudsperson) responds personally to complaints from patients and their families. Often, patients and their families are looking for nothing more than an explanation of an adverse occurrence or an apology for a mistake or misunderstanding. Patient representatives can handle minor complaints and seek remedies on behalf of patients. They can also recognize serious problems that need to be forwarded to performance improvement or risk management personnel.

Accreditation Requirements for Risk Management in Acute-Care Hospitals

Anything that undermines patient safety is a risk issue. According to accreditation standards, all hospital activities must be evaluated as to the potential risk to the patient or the organization. Leadership is responsible for ensuring adequate resources for patient safety.

Incident Response Patient safety should be of utmost importance to healthcare organizations and all employees within the organization. Healthcare organizations need to create a culture of safety within their facilities in order to focus on error elimination. Steps must be taken to ensure patient safety and adequate response to an adverse event occurring within the organization. Healthcare organizations must be equipped to recognize an adverse event and then have a plan and protocols in place to care for the affected patient and to mitigate the situation in order to prevent further adverse events. Once the situation has been appropriately resolved, the organization should initiate a PI process to identify what improvements and changes to the systems and processes are needed to prevent future adverse events.

Figure 18.11 Partial example of incident or occurrence report (including the necessary data elements for this incident)

Med Rec #: 00-05-45
Name: Jackson, Julia
Date of Birth: 06-22-23
Street: 6401 Fremont Ave
City: Western City, CA

Risk Management use only: __________

Patient ID/Name of individual involved.
Use addressograph for patient.

INSTRUCTIONS: (1) Fill out the first page of the Incident Report Form. (2) Select the type of incident from the bottom of page 2. (3) Fill out all appropriate sections as directed. The report must be dated and filled out by the end of the shift in which the incident occurred or was discovered. **DO NOT COPY THIS FORM.** Please print; this report must be legible. **Please fill out all applicable parts of this form.** Upon completion of this form, route it to your Nurse Manager or Supervisor. Do not leave this form in the patient's chart.

Date of incident: 05/29/XX Time (2400 Clock): 1645 Hospital Unit: Med/Surg

What day of the week did it occur?

Sun	[√]	Thurs	[ ]
Mon	[ ]	Fri	[ ]
Tues	[ ]	Sat	[ ]
Wed	[ ]		

Did the incident occur during:

Day 0701–1500	[ ]
Evening 1501–2300	[√]
Night 2301–0700	[ ]

Employee involved worked a(n):

8 Hour shift	[√]
10 Hour shift	[ ]
12 Hour shift	[ ]
Double shift	[ ]
Other ________	

Where did the incident occur? patient room

Description of incident. Include follow-up care given (i.e., vital signs, x-ray, laboratory tests, etc.).
Pt. developed a macular rash over trunk and extremities after 10 mg dose of Compazine given for postop nausea. Compazine stopped and Benadryl given IM.

IMMEDIATE EFFECT OF THE INCIDENT: Severe macular rash over trunk

Involved Person Data

Date of Admission: 05/29/XX
What sex is the person?
Male [ ]
Female [√]

What is the person's age? ______

Inpatient	[√]
Outpatient	[ ]
Student	[ ]
Employee	[ ]
Visitor	[ ]
Volunteer	[ ]
Other: ________	

Current Diagnosis/Reason for visit: Bowel Obstruction

Is the involved person aware of the incident? Yes [√] No [ ]
Is the family aware of incident? Yes [ ] No [√]

continued

Figure 18.11 Partial example of incident or occurrence report (including the necessary data elements for this incident) *(continued)*

DO NOT COPY

****** PLEASE PRINT ******

Person preparing report (Signature): Gwen Nelson, R.N. Print: Gwen Nelson, R.N.

Name of individual witnessing incident (Print): Bob Patterson, R.N.

Dept/Address: Med/Surg Team Leader

Name of employee involved in incident: Gwen Nelson, R.N. Dept/Address: Med/Surg

Name of employee discovering incident: Gwen Nelson, R.N. Dept/Address: Med/Surg

****** STAFF TO NOTIFY ATTENDING PHYSICIAN AND/OR DESIGNATED RESIDENT/NURSE PRACTITIONER OF INCIDENT ******

I notified Dr./NP: Jeff Cook at: 1650 (time).

M.D./NP responded ☐ in person ☑ by phone at: 1705 (time).

Was the attending physician notified?

Yes [✓] Date: 05/ 29/ XX Time: 1650

No [ ] Why not? ____________________

Examining Physician/Nurse Practitioner statement regarding condition/outcome of person involved:

Pt. was examined by me at 1700 hours. Trunk and extremities show a macular rash on them. One dose of Benadryl given IM to pt. and rash began to subside. Compazine stopped.

Examining MD/NP signature: Tom Lander, M.D. House Staff

Examining MD/NP name (print): Tom Lander, M.D.

Date: 05 / 29 / XX Time: 1700 Clinical Service: Medicine

CHOOSE THE TYPE OF INCIDENT YOU ARE REPORTING. Use the index below to locate the type of incident you are reporting, go to that section and mark the appropriate box(es). THERE MAY BE MORE THAN ONE ITEM APPLICABLE IN A SECTION. CHECK BOX(ES) IN APPROPRIATE SECTIONS.

Medication/IV Incident	Page 3, Section 1	Patient Behavioral Incident	Page 5, Section 6
Blood/Blood incident	Page 3, Section 2	Safety Incident	Page 5, Section 9
Burn	Page 5, Section 7	Security Incident	Page 5, Section 8
Equipment Incident	Page 5, Section 10	Surgery Incident	Page 5, Section 4
Fall	Page 4, Section 3	Treatment/Procedure Incident	Page 5, Section 5
Fire Incident	Page 5, Section 11		

CONFIDENTIAL: This material is prepared pursuant to Code Annotated, §26-25-1, et seq., and 58-12-43(7, 8, and 9), for the purpose of evaluating healthcare rendered by hospitals or physicians and is NOT PART of the medical record.

continued

Figure 18.11 Partial example of incident or occurrence report (including the necessary data elements for this incident) *(concluded)*

DO NOT COPY

SECTION 1 MEDICATION/IV INCIDENT

1A. TYPE OF MEDICATION

Fill in specific medication/solution on the adjacent line.

Analgesic ____________
Anesthetic agent ____________
Antibiotic ____________
Anticoagulant ____________
Anticonvulsant ____________
Antidepressant ____________
Antiemetic Compazine
Antihistamine ____________
Antineoplastic ____________
Bronchodilator ____________
Cardiovascular ____________
Contrast media ____________
Diuretic ____________
Immunizations ____________
Immunosuppressive ____________
Insulin ____________
Intralipids ____________
Investigational drug ____________
IV solution ____________
Laxative ____________
Narcotic ____________
Oxytocics ____________
Psychotherapeutic ____________
Radionuclides ____________
Sedative/tranquilizer ____________
TPN ____________
Vasodilator ____________
Vasopressor ____________
Vitamin ____________
Other ____________

1B. TYPE OF MEDICATION OR IV INCIDENT

Adverse reaction . . . . . [ ] 1B01
Allergic/contraindication . . . . . [ ] 1B02
Delayed stat order . . . . . [ ] 1B03
Improper order (MD/NP) . . . . . [ ] 1B04
Incompatible additive . . . . . [ ] 1B05
Incorrect additive . . . . . [ ] 1B06
Incorrect dosage . . . . . [ ] 1B07
Incorrect drug . . . . . [ ] 1B08
Incorrect narcotic count . . . . . [ ] 1B09
Incorrect patient . . . . . [ ] 1B10
Incorrect rate of flow . . . . . [ ] 1B11
Incorrect route . . . . . [ ] 1B12
Incorrect schedule . . . . . [ ] 1B13
Incorrect solution/type . . . . . [ ] 1B14
Incorrect time . . . . . [ ] 1B15
Incorrect volume . . . . . [ ] 1B16
Infiltration . . . . . [ ] 1B17
Given before culture taken . . . . . [ ] 1B18
Medication given before lab results returned . . . . . [ ] 1B19
Medication missing from cart . . . . . [ ] 1B20
Not documented . . . . . [ ] 1B21
Not prescribed . . . . . [ ] 1B22
Omitted . . . . . [ ] 1B23
Outdated . . . . . [ ] 1B24
Out-of-sequence . . . . . [ ] 1B25
Patient took unprescribed medication . . . . . [ ] 1B26
Repeat administration . . . . . [ ] 1B27
Transcription error . . . . . [ ] 1B28
Other ____________ 1B29

1C. ROUTE OF MEDICATION ORDERED:

IM . . . . . [ ] 1C01
IV . . . . . [ ] 1C02
PO . . . . . [ ] 1C03
Other Suppository 1C04

1D. MEDICATION DISPENSING INCIDENT

Meds not sent/delayed from pharmacy . . . . . [ ] 1D01
Incorrectly labeled . . . . . [ ] 1D02
Incorrect dose . . . . . [ ] 1D03
Incorrect drug sent . . . . . [ ] 1D04
Incorrect IV additive . . . . . [ ] 1D05
Incorrect IV fluid . . . . . [ ] 1D06
Incorrect route (IV, PO, IM, PR) . . . . . [ ] 1D07
Mislabeled . . . . . [ ] 1D08
Other ____________ 1D09

SECTION 2
BLOOD/BLOOD COMPONENT INCIDENT

2A. BLOOD/BLOOD COMPONENT TYPE

Albumin . . . . . [ ] 2A01
Cryoprecipitate . . . . . [ ] 2A02
Factor VIII (AHF) . . . . . [ ] 2A03
Factor IX (Konyne) . . . . . [ ] 2A04
Fresh frozen plasma . . . . . [ ] 2A05
Packed red blood cells (PRBC) . . . . . [ ] 2A06
Plasmanate® . . . . . [ ] 2A07
Platelets . . . . . [ ] 2A08
RhoGAM® . . . . . [ ] 2A09
Washed red blood cells (WRBC) . . . . . [ ] 2A10
Whole blood . . . . . [ ] 2A11
Other ____________ 2A12

2B. TYPE OF BLOOD/BLOOD COMPONENT INCIDENT

Crossmatch problem . . . . . [ ] 2B01
Improper unit verification . . . . . [ ] 2B02
Inappropriate IV fluids administered with blood components . . . . . [ ] 2B03
Inappropriate documentation . . . . . [ ] 2B04
Inappropriate storage . . . . . [ ] 2B05
Incomplete patient ID . . . . . [ ] 2B06
Incorrect patient . . . . . [ ] 2B07
Incorrect rate . . . . . [ ] 2B08
Incorrect type . . . . . [ ] 2B09
Incorrect volume . . . . . [ ] 2B10
Patient refused . . . . . [ ] 2B11
Other ____________ 2B12

CONFIDENTIAL: This material is prepared pursuant to Code Annotated, §26-25-1, et seq., and 58-12-43(7, 8, and 9), for the purpose of evaluating healthcare rendered by hospitals or physicians and is NOT PART of the medical record.

Source: Shaw and Carter 2019.

Clinical Quality Management Initiatives

Initiatives and processes seeking to ensure high-quality care and patient safety became a focus in healthcare as the 21st century commenced. Stemming from the Institute of Medicine (IOM) 1999 and 2001 reports on the quality of healthcare in America, a consensus developed around the need to use information technology as both a methodology and a pathway for managing and improving healthcare quality.

The beginning of the 21st century witnessed an increased link between clinical quality and reimbursement for health services. Pay-for-performance initiatives by the federal government, Joint Commission, and private payers began rewarding organizations for quality outcomes. These incentives, such as Meaningful Use, encouraged healthcare providers to invest in technology that will improve patient care and safety. For additional information on these topics, refer to chapter 15.

In recent years, CMS has become an advocate for pay for performance within the Medicare program. One of its efforts requires hospitals participating in the Medicare program to collect and report on proven clinical hospital quality measures. To qualify for full inpatient prospective payment the hospital must report on all measures required by CMS. Those that do not report data on these measures face a payment reduction per case. Medicare expects hospitals to compare their own data to national and regional averages in order to identify areas for quality improvement.

The early part of the 21st century witnessed new and creative efforts to encourage medical error reporting. The Patient Safety and Quality Improvement Act of 2005 allows for the voluntary reporting of medical errors, serious adverse events, and their underlying causes (HHS 2017). Subsequent emphasis by The Joint Commission on patient safety issues has resulted in voluminous research and new programs sponsored by The Joint Commission to assist its accreditation customers in improving this important area of healthcare organization functioning.

Accountable care organizations, PI methodologies, ISO-9001 certification, and medication reconciliation are key components of clinical quality management.

Accountable Care Organizations

Accountable Care Organizations (ACOs) are a part of the Affordable Care Act (2010). ACOs are a network of physicians, hospitals, and other healthcare providers and suppliers working together to coordinate and improve care for patients with Medicare. This coordination of care includes sharing patient information among providers to eliminate duplication of tests and prevent medical errors. Participation in an ACO is voluntary. ACOs focus on improving the quality of care of patients and decreasing healthcare spending. As ACOs meet the requirements of the model, they share in the savings. Patients who receive care from an ACO maintain all of their rights as a Medicare beneficiary (CMS 2018). For more information on the Affordable Care Act and ACOs, refer to chapter 2, *Healthcare Delivery Systems*.

Robust Process Improvement Methodologies

As discussed earlier, benchmarking is an important quality tool in healthcare quality programs. However, some healthcare organizations have begun to benchmark against other industries (for example, a hospital's handoff from surgery to intensive care compared against the race-car industry's handoff during a pit stop) and are selecting models that may be adapted to the healthcare industry. These methodologies can be used in healthcare as part of the PI process. Some of these are Lean, Six Sigma, Lean Six Sigma, and high reliability.

Lean

Lean is a process improvement methodology focused on eliminating waste and improving the flow of work processes. Healthcare organizations have found ways to apply the Lean methodology, such as eliminating waste in processes by streamlining workflow and tasks to remove time-consuming and unnecessary steps. Healthcare has a growing burden to improve the quality of patient care while also decreasing and controlling costs. In many ways, Lean is a good fit for healthcare organizations and many of the principles of Lean are transferrable from its origins in the automotive industry to other industries, including healthcare (Meyer 2010). Because of the complex nature of healthcare, there are abundant opportunities to incorporate Lean methodology to reduce waste and improve efficiency.

Six Sigma

Six Sigma uses statistics for measuring variation in a process with the intent of producing error-free results. Sigma refers to the standard deviation used in descriptive statistics to determine how much an event or observation varies from the estimated average of the population sample. Six Sigma was chosen as a target statistic because even two or three standard deviations would not be acceptable in certain scenarios. A 2.5 percent error rate for making correct change at a movie theater may be acceptable, but that error rate in healthcare can be catastrophic. Even one preventable adverse event or death should not occur. Therefore, it is important to keep this PI approach in proper perspective when applying it to healthcare. The Six Sigma measure indicates no more than 3.4 errors per 1 million encounters (Pyzdek and Keller 2018). Consider the challenge of achieving no more than 3.4 errors per 1 million prescriptions, surgeries, or diagnoses. In certain areas, this standard may seem unattainable; and in others, it may not be rigorous enough.

Deploying Six Sigma in healthcare requires the identification of elements of a product line that are critical to quality, or CTQs. The healthcare organization should conduct focus groups or interviews of customers to elicit the CTQs. Typically, in healthcare the customers will be the patients and the providers or physicians. All others involved—the corporations, payers, accreditors or licensers—are identified as stakeholders, entities with an important interest in the product that do not have consumer relationships to it. Supporting the CTQs are elements critical to process (CTPs). Techniques such as focus groups or interviews help to determine the CTPs.

Lean Six Sigma

Combining Lean and Six Sigma is a way to combine elements from both techniques into an integrated program to improve process flow and quality (Sperl and Ptacek 2013). This Lean Six Sigma methodology utilizes elements of elimination of waste from Lean and critical process quality characteristics from Six Sigma. Using these tools in a combined format allows for quality improvement and overall efficiencies within healthcare organizations—improving both product and process.

High Reliability Organizations

High reliability organizations (HROs) are organizations that focus on creating an environment that eliminates or minimizes error. HRO methodology comes from the airline, wildland firefighting, and nuclear power industries and is now being used in healthcare. HROs are concerned with noticing weak signals in order to prevent a potential negative outcome, and these weak signals receive a substantial response within this model. In healthcare, as with other types of industries, there are often small signals that are ignored. Healthcare organizations can become HROs by paying attention to these small signals. For example, a housekeeper may notice a problem with a patient. Within an HRO organization, that housekeeper would be empowered and motivated to report this concern to a clinician. An important part of this model and one way that HROs notice weak signals is mindfulness—a keen awareness and a necessary characteristic for all employees of an HRO. When employees are mindful and focused on their duties, there is less room for error. For example, a distracted physician may be more prone to error. Organizational reliability is improved, and errors are reduced when sources of distraction are eliminated and mindfulness is emphasized within a healthcare organization. HROs are preoccupied with failure and use these failures as learning experiences to improve processes and quality in order to eliminate error (Weick and Sutcliffe 2015).

ISO 9001 Certification

If healthcare organizations expand into global entities, they are required to deal with the same issues other industries face when doing business outside the US. ISO 9001 certification is part of a PI system required to conduct business in certain foreign countries. The International Organization for Standardization in Geneva, Switzerland, first published ISO 9001 standards in 1987. ISO 9001 sets specification standards for quality management with regard to process management and product control. In the healthcare setting, product control is quality control of patient care activities. Companies that document and demonstrate compliance with ISO 9001 standards can receive certification by independent ISO auditors (Rakhmawati et al. 2014).

Medication Reconciliation

Medication adjustments and changes often occur during patient encounters with health services, as patients are admitted, discharged, or transferred to another hospital unit or to another healthcare organization. Healthcare providers may not have access to a listing of current medications the patient was taking prior to admission or encounter with health services. As the patient transfers within the healthcare organization or to an outside healthcare organization, there is potential for missing medication dosages, omitted medications, or information on drug interactions and allergies. All of these factors put patients at risk for adverse drug events. **Medication reconciliation**, such as ensuring that the patient is receiving the right dose of medication, is the process that monitors and confirms that the patient receives consistent dosing across all healthcare facility transfers, such as on admission, from nursing unit to surgery, and from surgery to the intensive care unit. Healthcare organizations use the medication reconciliation process to eliminate medication error and improve care for the patient. Medication reconciliation is also part of the Joint Commission's NPSGs.

HIM Roles

Healthcare organizations use measures to determine their level of performance on quality and safety. These measures focus on outcomes, the structure of the healthcare organization, patient surveys, and organizational systems; and are used by healthcare organizations, private payers, and accrediting organizations to ensure they provide exceptional care. Organizations use internal measures as quality standards for their organization. External measures are used by accrediting organizations and private payers for payment based on performance as well as value-based purchasing initiatives. Payment for healthcare services is linked to quality measures. As more and more information is collected and analyzed in relation to quality, the information must maintain integrity. Consumers rely on information regarding quality, such as Hospital Compare data, to make healthcare decisions. This information is an asset and should be governed with accountability (Kloss 2015).

Health information management professionals are uniquely qualified to practice in the field of performance improvement. They understand the practice of collecting, analyzing, and interpreting performance data for healthcare organizations. HIM professionals understand where and how data is collected throughout a patient's encounter with a healthcare organization, which allows them to help organizations achieve quality clinical outcomes. HIM professionals also understand data quality, data analysis, and other aspects of data management.

Check Your Understanding 18.5

Answer the following questions.

1. Which of the following is a basic function of a healthcare risk management program?
   a. Claims management
   b. Discharge plan
   c. Time ladders
   d. Workflow analysis

2. Which of the following is a group of processes that determine the appropriateness of medical services?
   a. Utilization management
   b. Incident management
   c. Case management
   d. Risk management
3. John is currently a patient at Community Hospital. He is dissatisfied with the care he is being provided. He addressed this concern with his nurse; however, the care did not improve. Who should the patient contact at the hospital to discuss his concerns about his care?
   a. Utilization review coordinator
   b. Risk manager
   c. Patient representative or advocate
   d. Discharge planner
4. A woman dies in labor and delivery. The Joint Commission would call this type of outcome a(n):
   a. Sentinel event
   b. Clinical protocol
   c. Screening criteria
   d. Occurrence screen
5. Fred is a patient at Community Hospital. He fell out of bed during his second day at the facility. Which of the following steps should now occur?
   a. Review conditions of participation
   b. Conduct a continued stay utilization review
   c. Perform claims management functions
   d. Complete an incident report

Real-World Case 18.1

Memorial Hospital has been undergoing significant growth over the past few years. After the hospital implemented their new electronic health record (EHR) system, the HIM department scanned the paper health records that were being stored in the filing room and the filing room was no longer needed to store health records. Because of the growth within the healthcare facility, the filing room was recently transformed into a space for the clinical documentation integrity (CDI) team. This space is directly adjacent to the coding area. The proximity of the CDI team to the coding team has facilitated significantly increased interaction between the two groups. The CDI team often approaches members of the coding team regarding cases they are working on. Gina is the coding manager at Memorial Hospital, and she has been reviewing the last two quarterly coding audits of her team. She finds that the coding quality has dropped over the past six months. Performance indicators on productivity have also dropped during this period. Using benchmarking, Gina compares her coding team's productivity and quality metrics with similar-sized hospitals within her organization. As she anticipated, her facility's coding quality and productivity are below that of other healthcare facilities in her organization. Gina conducts a root-cause analysis to help identify the cause of the decline in both the productivity and quality of the coding being performed by her team.

Real-World Case 18.2

A large acute-care hospital located in the US was plagued with a poor reputation, high readmission rate, and weak profitability. As a last resort, the hospital board of directors fired the CEO and conducted a national search for a replacement. The new CEO selected by the board had been running a very successful hospital in a different part of the country. This new recruit was skilled and knowledgeable in PI. She had first-hand experience with methods like Lean Six Sigma and HROs. She came on board and immediately initiated training and much-needed culture changes. Hospital-wide PI teams were assembled to assess and prioritize the improvement needs of the hospital. Taking each of the highest priority issues, following the process of identifying measures, measuring performance, analyzing data, identifying the improvement opportunity, and continually monitoring performance they were able to make drastic changes in every department. Through this transition process and over the course of a year the new CEO realized sizeable cost savings. Through the PI process, priorities for new equipment and infrastructure were set. One high priority item was a new surgical suite with updated technology. The board approved the construction of the new suite and purchase of the new equipment. Because of the implemented PI processes and monitoring, one month after the surgical suite opened the hospital epidemiologist noticed a spike in postsurgical infections. A PI team was assembled with representatives from the surgery service, housekeeping, nursing, infection control, and HIM. The team meticulously evaluated and improved each of the procedures related to the new surgical suite. Continued monitoring only demonstrated minor improvements in postoperative surgeries. Having exhausted the expertise and ideas of the internal PI team, the CEO contacted external experts and assembled a team to come and consult with the internal PI team. Both teams were put into a small conference room and given five hours to review the collected data and the changes that had been made with little to no results. The external view of the outside experts, along with a detailed decomposition of the processes related to the suite, pointed to the construction process. Pulling the specifications and reports from the construction process, the team had questions for the construction contractors about the grade of materials used in the room. Specifically, they were concerned that the walls and flooring were too porous to be properly sterilized. The contractor confirmed the suspicion and came up with a solution to recover the walls and floor with appropriate materials. Monitoring infection rates closely, the suite reopened for use. Weekly dashboard reports were given to all stakeholders and showed no postoperative infections. At a review meeting at one month, the postoperative infection rate had dropped to a level lower than before the new surgical suite was opened.

References

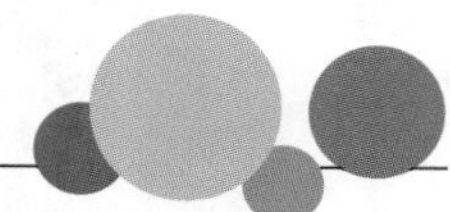

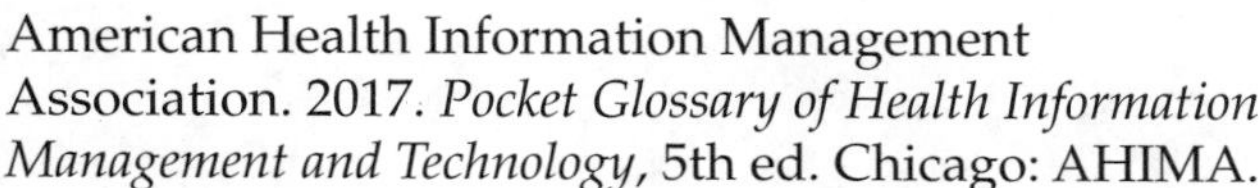

American Health Information Management Association. 2017. *Pocket Glossary of Health Information Management and Technology*, 5th ed. Chicago: AHIMA.

Centers for Medicare and Medicaid Services. 2018. Accountable Care Organizations. http://www.cms.gov/Medicare/Medicare-Fee-for-Service-Payment/ACO/.

Department of Health and Human Services. 2017. The Patient Safety and Quality Improvement Act of 2005. https://www.hhs.gov/hipaa/for-professionals/patient-safety/statute-and-rule/index.html.

Donabedian, A. 1988. The quality of care: How can it be assessed? *Journal of the American Medical Association* 260(12):1743–1748.

Farenholz, C. 2017. *Documentation for Health Records*, 2nd ed. Chicago: AHIMA.

Few, S. 2013. *Information Dashboard Design: Displaying Data for At-a-Glance Monitoring*, 2nd ed. Burlingame, CA: Analytics Press.

Institute of Medicine. 2001. *Crossing the Quality Chasm: A New Health System for the 21st Century*.

Washington, DC: National Academies Press.

Institute of Medicine. 1999. *To Err Is Human: Building a Safer Health System*. Washington, DC: National Academies Press.

Kloss, L. 2015. *Implementing Health Information Governance: Lessons from the Field*. Chicago: AHIMA.

Meisenheimer, C. 1997. *Improving Quality: A Guide to Effective Programs,* 2nd ed. Burlington, MA: Jones & Bartlett Learning.

Meyer, H. 2010. Life in the "lean" lane: Performance improvement at Denver Health. *Health Affairs* 29(11):2054–2060.

Omachonu, V. K. 1999. *Healthcare Performance Improvement*. Norcross, GA: Engineering and Management Press.

Pyzdek, T. and D. Keller. 2018. *The Six Sigma Handbook,* 5th ed. New York, NY: McGraw-Hill.

Rakhmawati, T., S. Sumaedi, and N. Astrini. 2014. ISO 9001 in health service sector: A review and future research proposal. *International Journal of Quality and Service Sciences* 6(1):17–29. http://doi.org/10.1108/IJQSS-12-2012-0025.

Shaw, P. and D. Carter. 2019. *Quality and Performance Improvement in Healthcare: A Tool for Programmed Learning,* 7th ed. Chicago: AHIMA.

Sperl, T. and R. Ptacek. 2013. *The Practical Lean Six Sigma Pocket Guide for Healthcare.* Chelsea, MI: MCS Media.

Strome, T. 2013. *Healthcare Analytics for Quality and Performance Improvement*. Hoboken, NJ: John Wiley & Sons.

Weick, K. and K. Sutcliffe. 2015. *Managing the Unexpected: Sustained Performance in a Complex World.* Hoboken, New Jersey: John Wiley & Sons, Inc.

Leadership

Leslie L. Gordon, MS, RHIA, FAHIMA

Learning Objectives

- Compare different leadership theories
- Differentiate among leadership styles
- Identify the impact of change management on processes, people, and systems
- Examine critical thinking skills
- Examine the difference between leadership and management
- Examine the fundamentals of team leadership
- Examine the process to execute and facilitate team meetings
- Examine business-related partnerships
- Identify leadership roles
- Summarize health information-related leadership roles

Key Terms

Active listening
Authoritarian leadership
Behavior theory
Benevolent autocracy
Bureaucracy
Business-related partnerships
Change management
Chief executive officer (CEO)
Chief financial officer (CFO)
Chief information officer (CIO)
Coercive power
Conflict management
Consensus building
Consensus-oriented decision-making model (CODM)
Consultative leadership
Contingency theory
Critical thinking
Democratic leadership
Distal attributes
Emotional intelligence (EI)
Empathy
Expert power
Exploitive autocracy
Great Person theory
Laissez-faire leadership
Leader–member relations
Leadership
Leadership criteria
Leadership grid
Leading
Leading by example
Legitimate power
Managing
Motivation
Participative leadership
Power and influence theory
Proximal attributes
Referent power
Reward power
Self-awareness
Self-regulation
Situational leadership
Social skill
Team building
Team charter
Team leader
Team member
Team norms
Theory X and Y
Timekeeper
Trait theory
Transactional leadership
Transformational leadership
Transitional model

Leadership is a process whereby an individual influences a group of individuals to achieve a common goal (Northouse 2019). Leading is one of the four functions of management (others are planning, organizing, and controlling) in which people are directed and inspired toward achieving specific goals. Leaders should not be confused with managers, because managers have people who work for them, whereas leaders have people who follow them. This concept will be explored throughout this chapter. Yet, while leaders provide direction, they must also use the skills of a manager to guide their followers to successful results in an effective and efficient way. By inspiring others, creating a vision, and mapping out what needs to be done, a leader can ensure that everyone in the group or team is successful.

Former President Dwight D. Eisenhower once said that "leadership is the art of getting someone else to do something you want done because he wants to do it." How a person perceives himself or herself as a leader may be different than an employee's view of that person as a leader. There are numerous definitions for leadership with multiple approaches to identify and explain the multifaceted factors that shape leadership and how it is accomplished. These theories evaluate the relationship of the leader to others and examine styles of leadership, adding to the general knowledge of leader behavior and effectiveness.

Though created over 50 years ago, Robert Blake and Jan Mouton's leadership grid is still one of the most used tools to determine leadership style and presents five different personal leadership styles that depend on a person's concern for people (plotted on the y-axis) versus their concern for production (plotted on the x-axis) (see figure 19.1).

Figure 19.1 Blake and Mouton's leadership grid

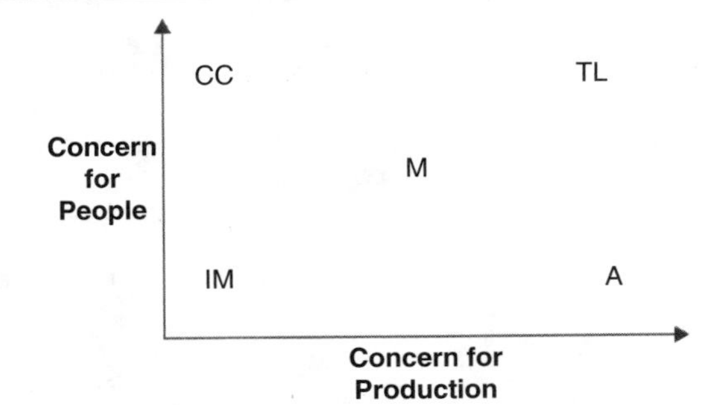

Source: ©AHIMA.

The first style is *impoverished management* (IM) where a leader has a low concern for people and a low concern for production (near the zero point on a graph). The *country club* (CC) style shows that a leader has a high concern for people and yet still has a low concern for production. The *authoritarian* (A) leadership style reflects a very low concern for people and a very high concern for production. The *team leader* (TL) style has a very high concern for people and also a very high concern for production. Finally, the *middle of the road* (MR) leadership style produces medium results with a medium concern for both people and production (Blake and Mouton 1964).

This chapter will discuss the various leadership theories, styles, patterns of leadership, and transformational leadership, as well as characteristics of leaders who create, motivate a group of people, and deliver an inspiring vision of the future. Also discussed are change management, critical thinking, and identifying the executive level of management. The chapter concludes with discussions of teams including team leadership and business-related partnership and holding meetings.

Leadership Theories

There are four major theories on leadership. Each theory defines a different way in which a person is perceived as a leader. Each theory is discussed in the following sections.

1. *Trait theory*. Originally called Great Man theory, the belief is that leadership is an inherited set of traits and not learned. A leader is born a leader and is not created by education or training.
2. *Behavior theory*. Leadership can be learned.
3. *Contingency theory*. Leadership is based on the situation and context.

4. *Power and influence theory*. Leadership can be based on position and title.

Each of the four theories is discussed in the following sections.

Trait Theory

Trait theory is one of the earliest leadership theories, sometimes referred to as the "Great Person Theory," which states that some people have innate leadership skills that are not due to training and exercises but, rather, to their natural ability. Leadership is considered a unique property of extraordinary people that cannot be learned (Galton 1869).

Traits can be divided into three divisions: distal attributes, proximal attributes, and leadership criteria. Distal attributes—such as personality, cognitive abilities, motives, and values—are traits that surround the leader as a person. Proximal attributes—such as problem-solving skills, social appraisal skills, and expertise and tacit knowledge—are derived from the distal attributes and are part of a leader's operating environment. From these proximal attributes, a leader possesses leadership criteria—leader emergence, meaning they are developing into a leader, leader effectiveness, meaning they are a successful leader, as well as advancement and promotion. Criticisms of the trait theory are that it is too simplistic –perceptions of leaders by their followers does not necessarily reflect the effectiveness of the leader, the context of the leader's position is not considered, and it focuses too much on personality traits and not on social skills and problem-solving ability.

Behavior Theory

A group of researchers, in response to the trait theory advocates, proposed the behavior-based theory to better define what makes a leader. Whereas the proponents of the trait theory believe leaders are born with these characteristics, the behaviorists determined leaders can be made and that successful leadership is based on definable, learnable behavior.

The behavior theory opened the door to leadership development rather than looking for those individuals who were born into a leadership role. The difference between great leaders and good ones isn't their intelligence or technical abilities it is their *emotional intelligence* (EI). There are five skills that allow leaders to capitalize their performance and their employees' performance. They are the following:

1. Self-awareness. The ability to know oneself in terms of strengths, weaknesses, desires, values, and impact on other people.
2. Self-regulation. The ability to change and control moods and impulses in oneself.
3. Motivation. The general willingness to achieve what one desires to do or be.
4. Empathy. The ability to understand other people.
5. Social skill. The ability to build relationships and rapport with people.

Contingency Theory

Contingency theory states leadership exists between persons in social situations, and persons who are leaders in one situation may not necessarily be leaders in other situations (Stogdill 1948). The first contingency approach, in terms of team performance, to leadership stated that leadership effectiveness depends on the relationship between the leader's task motivations and certain aspects of the situation. Task motivation is a leader who set goals and structures responsibilities to be measurable outcomes. This model postulates that the leader's task motivations are dependent on whether he or she can control and predict the team's outcomes. Whether those outcomes are in alignment with the situation (context) depends on three calculations: (1) whether the leader perceives supportive relations with team members (leader–member relations); (2) whether the task is highly structured with standardized procedures and measures of performance (task structure); and (3) whether the leader's position of authority is harsh or satisfying to the team members (position power) (Fielder 1964).

Many contingency theories have defined leadership effectiveness in terms of team performance or satisfaction. However, a decision model created by Victor Vroom and Arthur Jago emphasized that situational factors are more important than leadership behaviors (Vroom and Jago 1995). The model relies on decision-making to determine leadership style. Five different decision-making strategies range on a continuum from directive to participative decision-making. These strategies include two types of autocratic styles, in which one person has complete control and decision-making authority (type A1: the leader decides alone, and type A2: leader collects information from followers and then decides alone), two types of consultative styles (type C1: leader consults followers individually and then decides alone, and type C2: leader consults followers as a group and then decides alone), and a group decision-making option (group consensus). Figure 19.2 illustrates the relationships between the leader and followers.

Power and Influence Theory

The power and influence theory of leadership takes a different approach in that there are various ways leaders use authority, control, and their influence on others to get things done. Perhaps the best-known of these theories is the model that social psychologists John R. P. French Jr. and Bertram Raven proposed listing five forms of power (French and Raven 1960). Positional power is the authority a person has because of their position in the organization's structure. Personal power is the influence a person has over others based on their skill and ability to influence others.

Positional power is divided into legitimate power, reward power, and coercive power. Legitimate power is afforded by a person's position or status within the organization such as the department director. The team leader expects the team members to follow their orders and their status allows the leader to act as a liaison between the team and upper management. Use caution when relying too much on legitimate power as it is only effective in situations in which the team believes the team leader has the right or power to influence them.

Reward power is based on the leader's ability to give rewards to team members for outstanding work such as letters of recommendation, additional training or responsibilities, and additional compensation for working on the team. Reward power and legitimate power go hand in hand as the leader can only provide rewards if they are in a position of power.

Finally, coercive power, considered the opposite of reward power, occurs when the team leader uses threats and punishments to get their way. For example, the team member may be threatened with termination. Extensive use of coercive power should be avoided as many leaders abuse this power and use it inappropriately (French and Raven 1960).

Personal power is divided into referent power and expert power. Referent power (also known

Figure 19.2 Vroom and Jago's decision-making strategies

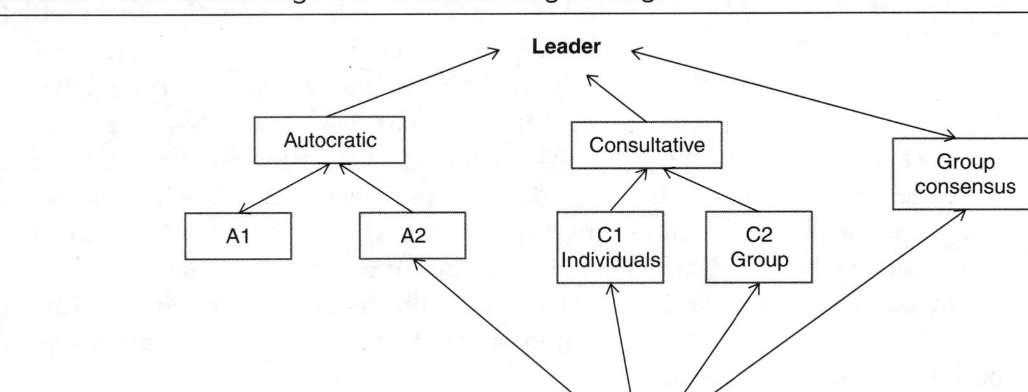

Adapted from: Vroom and Jago 1995.

as charismatic power) is the ability of the team members to identify with leaders who have desirable resources or personal traits. This may come from the leader's energy, endurance, empathy, toughness, humor, or charm. **Expert power** refers to leaders who are experts in their field or have knowledge or skills that are in short supply. Team members tend to listen to those who demonstrate expertise. A person does not have to be in a position of power to have expert power. A team leader can take maximum advantage of expert power by using their knowledge to offer guidance and support to the team to motivate them. A leader should not be a know-it-all and must listen to the concerns of the team members to create credibility and respect. The team leader does not have to have all the knowledge and expertise in the group and should acknowledge the expertise of other team members (French and Raven 1960).

Two additional power and influence theories are transactional leadership and leading by example. **Transactional leadership** assumes that the team members will accept and complete their responsibilities for no other reason than to receive rewards. Therefore, leaders need to design a task and reward system to ensure the team's work progresses at a satisfactory pace. **Leading by example** places the leader in a role model position, which allows a person to display, through their actions, how they would expect others to act. If the team members see the leader assume responsibilities and complete them on time, then the team members are likely to do the same (French and Raven 1960).

Leadership Styles

After all leadership styles are evaluated, they can be divided into three basic groups: authoritarian, democratic, and laissez-faire. **Authoritarian leadership** is a domineering style of leadership in which decisions are made at a distance from the workers they affect. Rulemaking, task assignments, and problem-solving are done solely by the leader and enforced through punishment, threats, demands, orders, and regulations (Lewin et al. 1939). A result to this type of leadership is that the decisions are made by one person and usually not allowed to be questioned. A disadvantage is the team members are often afraid of the leader and the consequences of making of mistake and being punished.

The **democratic leadership** style is participative and supports collective decision-making by offering others in the group choices and then empowering group members by facilitating group deliberations and encouraging and rewarding active member involvement. The leader gains authority by taking personal responsibility for the group's outcomes and accepts accountability for the results. The pluses for this type of leadership style are that it builds consensus of the group members, encourages creativity, builds commitment, and creates a shared vision. The negative aspects of the democratic style is that it is not particularly effective when decisions have to be made quickly and the group feels the leader is not leading but, rather, depending too heavily on the group. This style is difficult to use when there is little communication and the group is comprised of inexperienced people. A type of leadership style included in the democratic method is value-based leadership—an approach that emphasizes values, ethics, and stewardship as central to effective leadership (Lewin et al. 1939).

The third leadership style is **laissez-faire leadership** (also known as delegative leadership). This style reflects a leader who holds a title and responsibility but is strictly hands-off and has everyone else perform the work. This style is commonly associated with negative outcomes though it can be highly effective if the group members are already highly accomplished and motivated. Some of the negatives associated with laissez-faire leadership include some group members may need direction and guidance, some group members may be inexperienced and struggle with the task at hand, and the leader may appear to be uninterested. A type of leadership style associated with laissez-faire is path–goal leadership, which emphasizes the role of the leader in removing barriers to goal achievement but otherwise having a hands-off attitude after the group is established (Lewin et al. 1939).

Patterns of Leadership

Leadership can be defined as a continuum of six distinct styles (see figure 19.3). On one side of the continuum is exploitive autocracy—the harshest form of leadership, as the leader wields absolute power and uses the team to serve their own personal interests. This is followed by benevolent autocracy where the leader also wields absolute power but is generally kind and sincere in the use of the team for the good of the organization. Subsequently, in a bureaucracy the leader relies primarily on rules and regulations but sometimes those rules and regulations become more important than the team's purpose. Next is consultative leadership where the leader remains open to input from members of the team but still retains full decision-making authority. Situational leadership involves the leader who changes the approach based on the needs of the team and situation. At the most lenient end of the continuum is participative leadership where plans and decisions are made by the team and the leader is there to provide advice and assistance (McConnell 2018).

Leader–member relations—the acceptance of and confidence in the leader by the team members, as well as the loyalty and commitment they show toward the leader—is vital for any leadership style because the lack of acceptance and confidence in a leader by the team will cause the leader to fail.

Douglas McGregor investigated the theory that leadership styles may be related to a leader's philosophy about the members in a group or team, and his research resulted in Theory X and Y. Theory X is pure authoritative leadership, in which the team leader believes team members perform best under supervision that involves close control, centralized authority, authoritarian practice, and minimal participation of the group members in the decision-making process. The leader feels that the team is lazy, has no motivation, and will do nothing productive if not overseen closely. In theory X, leaders are pessimistic about the team members and the quality of their work, and assume the average person dislikes work and must be forced to accomplish the group's goals. This theory may be self-fulfilling because if the leader believes the team members are lazy, they may, indeed, become lazy (McGregor 1960).

Theory Y relates to participative leadership where the team leader believes team members are eager to do well, have the motivation to perform their best, and are capable of doing so. In theory Y, leaders are optimistic about the team members and expect great results from their work. The Theory Y leader assumes that work is not avoided, self-motivation and inherent satisfaction will work toward the benefit of the group, and each group member seeks responsibility. Leaders will delegate tasks and responsibilities as much as possible and open communication is encouraged (McGregor 1960).

While the reality is that neither of these theories is used exclusively by leaders, there are elements of each that reflect how people anticipate working with others. As an example of Theory X, some people may dread being placed on a particular team feeling they will have to do all the work because other members of the team will not carry their weight. However, there are some groups for which people volunteer either because they know other people in the group or believe the work is worthwhile. In this theory Y example, leaders rarely have to threaten, punish, or look over the shoulders of the team members because the members enjoy being a part of that group.

Figure 19.3 The continuum of leadership styles

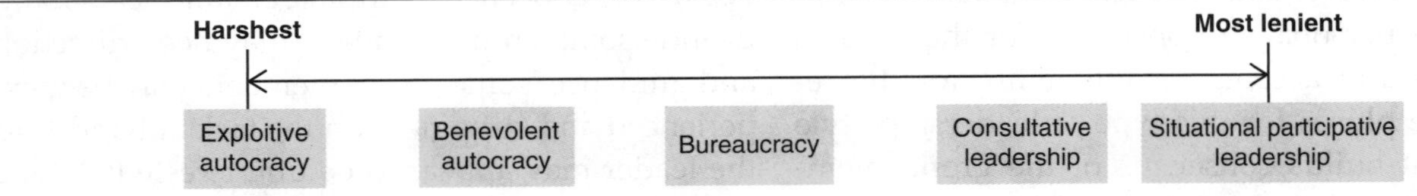

Source: ©AHIMA.

Transformational and Transactional Leadership

Leaders who inspire and motivate a group of people, and create a vision of the future exemplify transformational leadership. The leader becomes a role model who coaches and builds a team of committed members. The leader identifies a needed change, creates the vision of how to accomplish this change, and aligns the group members with tasks that will not only achieve the goals and objectives of the vision but also enhance the performances of group members.

There are four common components of transformational leaders. First, leaders serve as a role model to the group, referred to as idealized influence (II). Second, leaders have the ability to inspire and motivate their followers, also known as inspirational motivation (IM). Third, leaders demonstrate individualized consideration (IC), or a genuine concern for the needs and feelings of their followers. Finally, leaders challenge their followers to be innovative and creative, referred to as intellectual stimulation (IS).

Transformational leaders recognize many of today's problems cannot be solved with the same solutions of the past. New problems require new answers. Therefore, transformational leaders need to think outside of the box for new and innovative solutions and inspire their group members to do the same.

The theory of transactional leadership assumes people are motivated by reward and punishment, such as monetary rewards or disciplinary actions as punishment. The understanding of the worker is that they are there to do a job and be told what to do, with a clear chain of command. The transactional leader operates as if performance to a certain standard is expected and clear from the beginning. There is no need to praise or correct unless expectations exceed or fall below the standards for the job.

Check Your Understanding 19.1

Answer the following questions.

1. In which of the following theories would a leader feel that they can trust group members and do not have to micromanage?
   a. Theory X
   b. Theory Y
   c. Transformational leadership theory
   d. Participative leadership theory
2. The belief that a person may be a leader in one situation but not in another is the basis of what leadership theory?
   a. Trait
   b. Behavioral
   c. Contingency
   d. Power and Influence
3. True or false: Leading is one of the four management functions in addition to planning, consolidating, and controlling
4. According to Vroom and Jago's decision-making strategies, the "c" stands for which of the following?
   a. Chief
   b. Clinical
   c. Consultative
   d. Coordination
5. What is the type of power given to leaders who are authorities in their fields or have knowledge or skills that are in short supply?
   a. Expert
   b. Referent
   c. Legitimate
   d. Influence

Change Management

Managing change in a healthcare setting is a constant responsibility for leaders and is often impacted by internal and external forces outside of their control. Within an organization, change generally occurs when there is a need for a process or procedural improvement. It is the role of the leader to influence and guide others through the change so the group feels the change was worthwhile and they are not threatened by the final result—whether by loss of employment, change in work responsibilities, or reduced income.

Methods of Change Management

Change management is a controlled method to ensure change can be managed smoothly. The underlying tenet is all human beings prefer doing things that have the most meaning for themselves. When people believe change is going to be harmful to themselves or their careers, they are resistant to change. To overcome this resistance, leaders need to patiently sell the idea of change by educating and training their team and carefully disseminating information. The following sections explain various methods of change management: Kotter's eight-step method to leading change, Lewin's change management model, and Bridge's transitional model of change.

Kotter's Eight-Step Method to Leading Change

While a professor at Harvard's Business School, John Kotter developed an eight-step method of leading change within an organization. The eight steps to creating a climate of change within an organization include the following. A climate of change starts with establishing a sense of urgency, building a team to guide change, and developing an informed vision and strategy to deal with the change. To engage and enable change in the entire organization or within a department includes generating short-term wins, empowering broad-based action, and communicating the change vision to all employees. To implement and sustain change includes consolidating gains and anchoring the new approaches within the culture of the organization (see table 19.1) (Kotter 1995). An example of this method of change management in health information management (HIM) is the implementation of a new electronic system in the radiology department for physician orders. A new system may change the way the HIM department processes physician orders for radiology tests. The manager of the HIM department could follow Kotter's eight-step method to alleviate the anxiety caused by the required change.

Table 19.1 Kotter's eight-step method of leading change

Create a climate of change	Engage and enable change in the whole organization	Implement and sustain change
1. Establish a sense of urgency	4. Generate short-term wins	7. Consolidate gains
2. Build a team to guide change	5. Empower a broad-based action	8. Anchor changes in organizational culture
3. Develop vision and strategy	6. Communicate vision to all employees	

Source: Kotter 1995.

Lewin's Change Management Model

Kurt Lewin, one of the first researchers in social psychology, proposed an alternative model of change management by advocating that organizations must first *unfreeze*, or disrupt, current processes, meaning the organization's existing mindset is interrupted. Often organizations continue using the same work processes believing the "if it ain't broke, don't fix it" adage. However, the organization's recognition that change must occur is the unfreezing of current work processes. This stage can lead to employees and management having feelings of denial and anxiety that must be overcome before the organization can move on to the second stage.

The second stage—*create the change*—occurs when people resolve their uncertainty and look for new ways to do things. This is typically a period of confusion and even anger and fear as they realize change must occur. There is usually resistance as the change is not clearly defined yet; however, the organization is beginning to move in a positive direction.

The final stage is *refreezing* the environment, so the change is integrated into the processes and procedures within the organization. The change now becomes the status quo and produces a positive impact in the organization (Lewin 1947). An example of using Lewin's model within an HIM department is the implementation of a new reimbursement methodology in the US. Unfreezing would involve preparing for the implementation date. Transition and refreezing would involve getting all staff and teams comfortable with the change and then getting productivity back up to where it was prior to unfreezing.

It is not the change itself that leads to misunderstanding, it is the manner in which a change is introduced. Leaders should introduce and conduct training for the change well in advance of the change's implementation so employees can adapt to and learn the idea, consider the implications, and ask questions for more clarification. Involving employees in change management will reduce their uncertainty and potentially increase their acceptance rather than them feeling the change was thrust upon them without their input.

When providing the information and directives of how the change will occur, a leader must consider the types of employees impacted by the change, the work situation where the change will occur, and how supervisors will work with their staff—including their attitudes toward their staff members. Care must be given to how the directive for change is presented to the staff. For example, directives should be reasonable, intelligible, worded appropriately, compatible with the desired end result of the change, and indicate that the change can occur within a reasonable time frame.

Presenting the directive for change takes a great deal of forethought on the part of a leader and is not to be rushed into without considering how the staff will react. Employees will be better able to acknowledge the directive if they understand the purpose behind the change. A better-informed employee is more likely to accept the change. However, do not provide too much information as this may result in the leader spending excessive time clarifying the minute details rather than focusing employees on the bigger picture.

Bridge's Transitional Model of Change

William Bridges, a management consultant, focused his research on transitional process rather than change implementation. He created a **transitional model** that defines three stages: (1) ending, losing, and letting go; (2) the neutral zone; and (3) new beginnings. Each stage identifies changing emotions employees experience as their daily work is either changed or replaced. The emotions associated with stage 1 are fear, denial, anger, sadness, disorientation, frustration, uncertainty, and a sense of loss. In stage 2 people may experience resentment toward the change initiative; low morale and productivity; anxiety about their role, status, or identity; and skepticism about the change initiative. Finally, in stage 3 employees may experience high energy, openness to learning, and renewed commitment to the group or their role in the organization (table 19.2). Understanding what a member of a group is feeling during the change process will help a leader anticipate potential issues and allow the leader to better guide the employees to a successful resolution (Bridges 2016).

Table 19.2 Bridges' list of feelings for a transitional model

Stage 1	Stage 2	Stage 3
Fear	Resentment	High energy
Denial	Low morale and productivity	Openness to learning
Anger	Anxiety about role, status, or identity	Renewed commitment
Sadness	Skepticism	
Disorientation		
Frustration		
Uncertainty		
Sense of loss		

Source: Bridges 2016.

Mergers

Mergers involve the joining of two or more companies into one; this is a major source of change management as hospitals and other healthcare organizations are combined. During and after the merging of two healthcare organization, employees will wonder if there will be duplication or replacement of positions. Will the new entity need two HIM directors or can one position handle both departments? Perhaps the healthcare organization will create a corporate HIM position and only have supervisors at each location. The employee might wonder if their pathway to advancement has been lost as a result of a change in the organizational culture. One entity may have an organizational culture that encourages promotion from within while another entity may see the benefit of bringing in professionals from outside the healthcare organization. Which entity will dominate and thus offer an advantage to that company's employees? Will one entity's staff be given preference over the other? Mergers can create unsettling times but by being prepared for a leadership role an individual can provide extra security as either an asset in the new entity or by moving to another healthcare organization that can better appreciate their leadership abilities.

Electronic Record Systems

Another major source of change is the development and implementation of the electronic health record (EHR) in a healthcare organization. Traditionally, HIM has been very labor intensive with people whose sole job is to move paper; from patient care sites, to analysis and assembly, to incomplete files, to coding, and then to permanent files—not to mention moving paper for disclosure of information and off-site storage. However, with the creation of the EHR most document movement is handled electronically, thus reducing staffing levels previously necessary in HIM departments (see chapter 3, *Health Information Functions, Purpose, and Users,* for more information about change within the EHR environment. This change is significant and affects all employees as the physical size of the department may be reduced since there is less paper to be stored and used for patient care. It is a leader's duty to explain the benefits of the change to staff and set a vision of where the department needs to transform; and clarify that while some jobs may be eliminated (file clerks) new jobs may be created (scanning). A leader must feel comfortable with their role and convey that sense of job security to the other employees in the department.

Leadership

The difference between leading and managing is sometimes hard to distinguish and the terms are often used interchangeably. It is important to understand the difference, especially in terms of leading an organization, department, or team of employees. Managing is the process of planning, controlling, leading, and organizing activities. Managing is a process and it includes leading. Leading refers to a person's ability to understand and influence situations, and motivate and encourage others, while intervening when necessary, toward success or to a desired end goal. More information on managing can be found in chapter 17, *Management*. To better understand how to become an effective leader it is important to explore leadership competencies, emotional intelligence, and leading others.

Leadership Competencies

The main competencies for effective leaders include being emotionally stable, having the ability to get the job done, being a good communicator, being unafraid, being credible, having the ability to develop committed followers, and exhibiting charisma. The first competency of being emotionally stable can be learned and developed by understanding emotional intelligence, discussed next. The ability to get the job done includes providing direction, expectations, and standards of what is expected. Communication is key to providing clear instructions and making sure that everyone who needs to know the directions understands them. The ability to be unafraid means leaders take responsibility, take risks, and keep fears to themselves. Credibility means being truthful and keeping commitments. The ability to develop committed followers happens with leaders who are willing and able to help out wherever they are needed and who care about those who are following them. Charisma, which is the charm that inspires others, can be learned, especially by making a point of recognizing people doing the right things for the project (McConnell 2018).

Emotional Intelligence

Emotional intelligence (EI) includes five skills good leaders try to master to maximize their performance and the performance of their team. These skills are: self-awareness, self-regulation, motivation, empathy, and social skill. **Self-awareness** is the ability to know one's self, to understand one's strengths and weakness and personal values and the effect that has on others. For example, a leader knows that she gets very angry when a team member is late for a meeting; knowing this she is able to control that anger. She can develop the skills to prevent herself from getting angry or change the start time of the meeting to combat her own anger. **Self-regulation** is the ability to control or direct impulses and moods. Expanding on the same example, the leader may consider the possible reasons the team member is always late and may explore solutions with them. **Motivation** is a person's desire to do something, the thing that compels a person. For example, a leader should consider what motivates them as a person as well as what motivates their team members. People are motivated by different things including money, success, mentoring, learning something new, a job well done, or being a part of a team. **Empathy** is the ability to understand another person's emotions. For example, a coworker recently lost his father and is therefore distracted from the project at hand. Empathy is the ability to imagine how that may feel and what can be done to help this team member through this difficult time. Finally, **social skill** is the ability to build and maintain rapport with others to motivate them in a desired direction. Humans communicate in many different ways using both verbal language and body language. Some cultures have different acceptable social interactions, for example eye contact or body proximity. Leaders need to understand the culture of the people they are working with to ensure their behaviors are socially acceptable in a particular culture. Developing and practicing those skills are important for a leader (Bradberry and Greaves 2009).

Leading Others

The ability to be a leader and to lead others can be learned and developed through education and practice of leadership skills. Leading is the ability to analyze and understand the situation, project, or department and what needs to be accomplished; for example, leading a department through the change needed for implementation of a new computer system. The leader is responsible for energizing and engaging others and intervening where needed to get the best out of followers and team members (Kansas Leadership Center 2016).

Critical-Thinking Skills

HIM leaders are continuously confronted with a changing profession, whether it is in reimbursement, technology, or disclosure of protected health information. One of the most useful tools an HIM leader can possess is to think critically. **Critical thinking** is a disciplined process of actively and skillfully conceptualizing, analyzing, synthesizing, applying, and evaluating information. The information can be gathered from or generated by observation, experience, reflection, reasoning, or communication, and used as a guide to belief and action (The Foundation for Critical Thinking 2018). Through analysis and evaluation of an issue one is able to create an understanding of the issue. Critical thinking involves the examination of the purpose, problem, or question; any assumptions, concepts, reasoning leading to conclusions, implications and consequences, or objections from alternative viewpoints, and a frame of reference. Critical thinking has two components—belief generating and processing skills, or the habit of using those skills to guide behavior (The Foundation for Critical Thinking 2018).

Critical thinking varies according to the individual's underlying motivation. When used for selfish purposes, it is often revealed as the skillful handling of ideas for the personal interest of an individual or group. When used in good faith, it is seen as ethical and perhaps idealistic, especially by those with other agendas. Critical thinking of any kind is never universal—everyone is subject to episodes of undisciplined or irrational thought. The quality of critical thinking is a matter of degree and dependent on, among other things, the quality and depth of experience in a given domain of thinking or with respect to a particular class of questions. The development of critical-thinking skills is a lifelong endeavor as no one thinks critically in all situations (The Foundation for Critical Thinking 2018).

The list of core critical-thinking skills includes observation, interpretation, analysis, inference, evaluation, explanation, and metacognition (The Foundation for Critical Thinking 2018). There are tools that can be used to help with critical thinking in a group. These include brainstorming, nominal group technique, and Ishikawa diagrams. Brainstorming is the aggregation of ideas from a group, where no response is considered bad and the goal is to generate quantity, not necessarily quality. Using the nominal group technique, the group writes down their suggestions anonymously and then votes on which ideas are the most appropriate for the context of the discussion. This technique focuses on finding a communally acceptable solution. An Ishikawa diagram (also referred to as a root-cause diagram) is used to determine the root causes of a problem by constantly asking, Why?

C-Suite

The HIM department reports to administrators in the C-suite (also referred to as the C-level). The C-suite is a slang term for the uppermost management level in an organization and refers to the executive titles that start with the letter C, referring to the word *chief* as in chief executive officer (CEO), chief information officer (CIO), and chief financial officer (CFO). It is important to note these executives report to the board of directors and the decisions they make affect the subordinate levels in an organization. More information about hospital structure and the board of directors can be found in chapter 2, *Healthcare Delivery Systems*. At this level of management, technical and functional expertise matters less than leadership skills and a strong grasp of business fundamentals. The leadership skills discussed earlier in this chapter are vital for an effective CEO.

Chief Executive Officer

The chief executive officer (CEO) is generally accountable solely to the board of directors (see chapter 2 for more information about the board of directors). The major responsibilities of the CEO are to develop and implement high-level strategies; set a vision; make major organizational decisions; manage the overall operations and resources of a company; build culture; set the budget to be presented to the board of directors for approval; and act as the main point of communication between the board of directors, the corporate operations, and the public (SHRM 2018). The CEO position requires strong communication and collaboration skills, approachability, transparency, and the ability to transform an organization (Hanke 2018).

Chief Information Officer

The chief information officer (CIO) is responsible for leading, planning, budgeting, resourcing, and training the information technology (IT) staff. The CIO needs to know how to create business models and make rigorous decisions based on the analysis of the return on investment for addition of purchasing technology for the organization. Healthcare organizations are continually purchasing technology to improve the way they conduct business. In addition to a deep understanding of technology and the interoperability of electronic records, the CIO needs a good understanding of change management.

Chief Financial Officer

The chief financial officer (CFO) typically reports to the CEO or board of directors and is the chief financial spokesperson for the organization. Most CFOs have a master's in business administration (MBA) or are a certified public accountant (CPA). Along with leadership skills a CFO must possess a strong understanding of corporate finance methodologies, cash management, and accounting principles. A healthcare organization's CFO has the added responsibility of understanding healthcare reimbursement methodologies and the organization's cost reports. A cost report contains information on the costs and charges of an organization.

Check Your Understanding 19.2

Match the emotional intelligence terms with the definitions.

1. Self-awareness
2. Self-regulation
3. Motivation
4. Empathy
5. Social skill

   a. Controlling or redirecting
   b. Managing relationships
   c. Knowing one's self
   d. Being driven
   e. Considering others

Team Leadership

HIM professionals often work with other healthcare professionals (such as nurses, information technologists, informaticists, therapists) throughout the organization. As such, they should be a part of any team within an organization where their expertise is needed. By assembling a diverse group of people with technology knowledge as well as users and stakeholders, teams provide a valuable asset to the future of any healthcare organization. It should be noted that teams and committees are not the same; teams have a relatively short life span, whereas committees are part of the formal organizational structure. The **team leader** is someone who provides leadership, instruction, and direction to a team for the purpose of achieving a set goal or objective. It is the team leader who is responsible for the team's outcomes and ensuring everyone on the team contributes in a meaningful way. A good team leader possesses the qualities of compassion and integrity, which can be developed through training (Scott 2018).

A team leader must project certain leadership traits and qualities to the team members to ensure the team's objectives are met. These include the following:

- *Communication*. This is an essential function to ensure all the members of the team are aware of and understand their role and responsibilities.
- *Organization*. This skill allows the team to perform at the optimal level by maintaining order to meet goals and objectives.
- *Confidence*. Through their actions, the team leader must show the team that they are confident not only in their abilities, but also in the abilities of the team members.

- *Respectful*. All members of the team have to be shown respect for their input and who they represent on the team.
- *Fair*. All members of the team must be treated equitably and no favoritism shown because of title or relationship to the team leader.
- *Integrity*. The team's leader must not appear to change or waiver when difficulties occur but rather keep a constant viewpoint and direction.
- *Influential*. The team leader must be able to bring the team to a consensus when differences of opinion occur to achieve a common outcome.
- *Delegation*. The team leader cannot do it all; therefore, various tasks and objectives should be delegated to different team members.
- *Facilitator*. When disagreements occur among the team members, it is the team leader's responsibility to keep everyone on task and focused on the projected outcomes.
- *Negotiator*. When a stalemate occurs on the team's decision regarding the final deliverable, it is the team leader's responsibility to work toward a common agreement (Scott 2018).

Factors that contribute to the success of a team include a team leader and team members who have effective and excellent communication skills and all roles and responsibilities of members being clearly defined. When there is disagreement among members, it needs to be productive disagreement instead of accusations; and when decisions are made, all parties must agree to support those decisions. Next, the team needs to have strong external relationships with not only executive management but the other stakeholders who have an interest in the team's goals and objectives. Finally, the team needs to perform a routine self-assessment to determine what worked and what were the bottlenecks to finding the end result.

Teams that fail often have unclear goals or changing objectives so the team is constantly trying to achieve a moving target. Leadership is ineffective when there is no clear decision maker in the group and the lack of leadership results in conflicts between team members as they struggle to understand and take ownership of the process.

As with all new initiatives, support from the upper levels of management is essential for a team to accomplish its targeted goals. The support is often in the form of a team charter, providing a team purpose, help with team member selection, and creation of team norms. Without executive support, the team loses its champion to defend the team before the other top executives and the board. Executive support also ensures the team will have the resources (time, personnel, and money) needed to complete the team's objectives successfully.

Team Charter

The team charter, provided by upper management, is the document that explains the issues the team was created to address, describes the team's goal /or vision, and lists the initial members of the team and their respective departments. A team must understand their purpose and direction to be successful. A clear charter helps define the purpose for the members (Heathfield 2018).

Team Purpose

The main purpose for creating teams is to provide a formal framework so its members can participate in planning, problem-solving, and decision-making to better serve the organization. Therefore, the team purpose needs to be well defined by the team charter. When everyone knows the team's objectives then the team will not waste time with unnecessary or unproductive communication.

Team Selection

Once management determines a team should be formed to accomplish a set of specific goals and objectives and a person has been delegated as the team leader, it is time to appoint the team members. Every team should have the input and expertise of people from different parts of the organization who have direct relationships to the outcomes associated with the goals and objectives of the team. Membership should include people with technical expertise, knowledge of the process under consideration, employees who work with the process after the changes have been integrated, as well as other people who may affect or be affected by the outcomes of the team. Effective teams have good interpersonal communication skills and understand the roles of each member of the team.

The size of the team depends on the scope of the outcomes required. For example, in a large organization strategic planning may have as many as 100 members who are then placed on teams and subcommittees to work on specific objectives. On the other hand, deciding what documents need to be scanned in an HIM department may only need five or six members to accomplish the task.

Team and Member Participation

Comprising a team of diverse members is a risky venture that can prolong the desired outcomes of the team. This is especially true if the team members do not know each other, each member's area of expertise, or the task ahead. It can also occur when multiple managers are placed on one team as each might try to take control from the team leader. Ideally, the team leader should be clearly known to team members and should start by leading the team in team building exercises at the beginning of the process so the members can learn to work as a group rather than individually. An example of a team building exercise is dividing the team into groups of three to five members and having them use toothpicks and 3 x 5 cards to design a boat that will float for one minute without falling over or sinking.

Diversity of team members is vital to ensure the members are examining all the facts and remain objective. Diversity allows members to understand their own biases, perspectives, and decision-making processes (Rock and Grant 2016). Diversity includes not only team members from different departments but also cultural differences. More information on cultural competence can be found in chapter 21, *Ethical Issues in Health Information Management*.

Each team goes through group dynamics that often take the form proposed by Bruce Tuckman (a professor at The Ohio State University). Referred to as Tuckman's model of forming-storming-norming-performing, this four-stage model is a simple way to determine where a team dynamic is at any given point. *Forming* is the process of putting the team together. This is the first exposure of the team members to each other and making first impressions that are either on target or off base from reality. These first impressions will color a person's viewpoint of other team members throughout most of the team's existence. *Storming* is the phase when personalities clash as team members are trying to find their role on the team and attempting to establish their position in the team dynamics. During this time the leader may have to institute conflict management, which focuses on working with individuals to find a mutually acceptable solution (Tuckman 1965). For more information on managing diversity and conflict management, see chapter 20, *Human Resources Management*. *Norming* is the phase where conflicts are reduced, everyone knows their positions and responsibilities, and actual work to achieve the goals and objectives can begin. Finally, *performing* is the phase where actual results are obtained as the team is productive and reaches its final outcomes and deliverables.

Each of these phases can exist for different times depending on the composition of the team and people's personalities. For example, if a team is comprised of members who have worked before on other teams, then the storming phase can be shortened. However, if the team is comprised of members that have never met or are representing different departments that have not traditionally worked well together, than the storming phase can take up a lot of time that could otherwise have been productive (Tuckman 1965).

Eventually team members must work together to reach the common goals and objectives of the team. Each member must take the responsibility to communicate not only with the team leader but with each other, not blame others but support group members' ideas, leave the egos at the door and not brag, use active listening (a communication method that requires the listener to provide feedback to the speaker), and get involved by being a participant, not a bystander. The four rules for active listening are: (1) seek to understand before you seek to be understood; (2) be nonjudgmental; (3) give your undivided attention to the speaker; and (4) use silence effectively (Department of State 2018).

Team Norms

Team norms help determine acceptable and unacceptable behavior for a team. Team norms may be *explicit* as in rules and regulations or *unwritten behavior* that is formed over time or through peer pressure. Most newly created teams start out with a preliminary set of norms that will be reviewed and modified frequently as conflicts or disagreements among team members occur. Some teams review norms at the beginning or end of each meeting and discuss which are working effectively and which need to be retooled. The establishment of and adherence to team norms helps build team discipline and trust among team members, and supports a safe environment.

Some norms that are common to most teams include the following:

- Meetings will start on time.
- Members will listen and not interrupt.
- Everyone will be able to speak.
- The team leader will moderate the discussion.
- Members will avoid cultural humor.
- Members will speak respectfully.
- All members' concerns will be addressed to come to consensus (Berea College, Brushy Fork Institute 2018)

Team Meetings

Once the team has been formed, a leader has been selected, team members have established their roles on the team, and a charter has been presented by upper management, it is then the team leader's responsibility to set an agenda, schedule meetings, conduct the meeting, build consensus, and handle any follow-up tasks required to ensure the next meeting runs smoothly. The frequency of meetings is determined by the time constraints given in the team charter. Some teams may meet once a month while others need to meet weekly or more often to reach a goal within the time frame given. For example, moving the HIM department to an off-site location may require teams meeting more infrequently when compared to implementing computer-assisted coding.

Scheduling of Meetings

One of the most difficult parts of organizing and running a team is the scheduling of meetings. The greater the number of team members, the more difficult it is to arrange a meeting. Ensure team members are informed in advance of the meeting to reduce scheduling conflicts.

Conducting Effective Meetings

Everyone on the team must be ready to participate and be an active member on the team. This means members coming prepared for the meeting by reading any material issued beforehand, being ready to discuss the material, and understanding what will be covered in the meeting. Often team members represent a division or unit within the organization, so the team member should collaborate with other people in their department and bring their collective views to the meeting. This will provide a richer discussion as a single person might not have considered all of the nuances that someone else from the department might have observed and shared with the team member representing the unit.

Prior to the meeting, the team leader should send requests to team members for input on meeting agenda items. This is not to say everything suggested will be included, but it is a starting point and indicative of what members feel are important issues that need discussion. The team leader controls the amount of information and discussion presented in the meeting to a reasonable amount so the meeting does not exceed its allotted time. The agenda and any other materials to be read should be sent to the members well in advance (four to five days) of the meeting so they have enough time to review and prepare for the meeting.

The team leader must start the meeting on time to be cognizant and respectful of the members' schedules. The meeting should begin with a review of the agenda and ask for any additional comments before continuing. A team member delegated to be secretary will take notes (minutes) during the meeting. It is also helpful to have a member be a **timekeeper** to ensure the meeting stays on track without too many digressions. When confronted with numerous tasks to complete in a limited amount of time, the team leader must delegate several tasks and responsibilities to the team members, which allows everyone to share in the decision-making process.

At the end of the meeting, the leader should conduct a review of what was discussed and remind everyone who is responsible for individual tasks for future meetings. Be sure to end the meeting on time or even a little early; the team members will appreciate the thoughtfulness behind an efficient meeting. Finally, once the secretary has completed their notes, they should be distributed to the team members for review and clarification, if needed.

Consensus Building

When a group of people converge from diverse backgrounds to search for a solution to a problem, conflicts and differences of opinion often occur. It is the responsibility of the team leader to use **consensus building**—a decision-making method that seeks consent of all participants to resolve those differences so an acceptable result can be found. Note that a successful result does not mean it is favored by all, but only that it is acceptable to the members of the team.

The **consensus-oriented decision-making model (CODM)** presents a six-step progression that allows groups the flexibility to come to a consensus by approaching important topics with open discussion rather than presenting a preformulated proposal; gathering a list of all the needs and concerns expressed by the group to form a list of conditions for possible proposals to address; taking turns in a unified attempt to shape each idea into the best possible proposal before choosing among them; and using empathy in the closure stage to address any unresolved feelings from the process.

The six CODM steps include the following:

1. Discussion
2. Identify the emerging proposal
3. Identify unsatisfied concerns
4. Collaboratively modify the proposal
5. Assess the degree of support
6. Finalize the decision or circle back to the first steps (Hartnett 2018)

Consensus building is needed so the team is inclusive and not limited in their perspective. The team members represent diverse backgrounds, and everyone should be encouraged to participate and all voices should be heard. Team members need to collaborate for further development of ideas into final results. Consensus building seeks to have everyone reach a common agreement so that implementation of the team's deliverables will be acceptable to all parts of the organization. It also results in more informed, collaborative decisions and outcomes as everyone on the team has ownership of the results and can relay them to their counterparts in their respective organizational units (Hartnett 2018).

Communication

Communication is vital for a leader to be effective. Direct communication with team members is important so they understand everything that concerns their work on the team. Communication can take different forms, whether through the use of meetings, minutes, reports (a summary of the data collection, conclusions, and recommendations of the team at a specific period of time), and storytelling (which is used to summarize an entire project using words, pictures, or graphs in a fashion that permits listeners to grasp the team's accomplishments and to understand its specific application).

Figure 19.4 Stages of communication

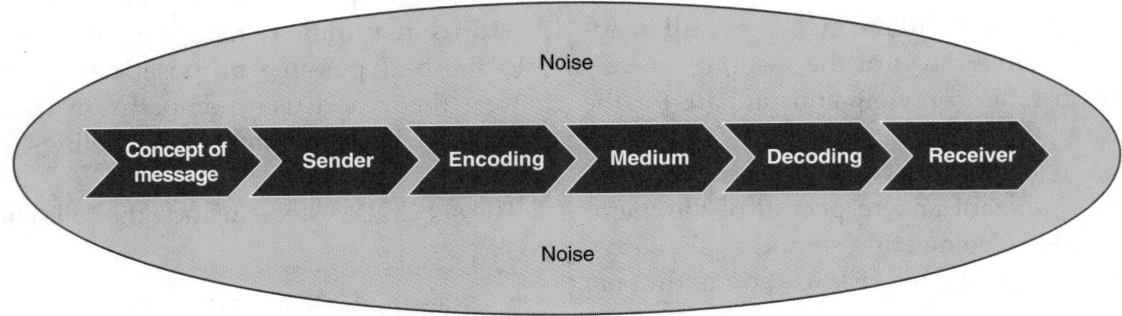

Source: ©AHIMA.

Most forms of communication use the same process shown in figure 19.4. They follow the six stages below

Stage 1: Determine the concept of the message (ideation). This is the most difficult part of the process as the message must be clearly and concisely formulated prior to sending the message to the receiver.

Stage 2: Designate the sender. It is usually the team leader who communicates to people outside of the team and ensures the message is sent to each team member.

Stage 3: Encoding. The message is put into a format that is clear and understandable to everyone. For example, when communicating with a person who is not an HIM professional, it would be important not to use jargon (specialized language for a group) and acronyms that HIM professionals use such as Master Patient Index, ROI, or DRG.

Stage 4: Select the medium by which the message should be sent—via email, letter, text, telephone or face-to-face conversation, or posting on the organization's intranet. Each type of medium has a specific intimacy for the receiver that may not be appropriate depending on the circumstances.

Stage 5: Decoding. The receiver acquires the message and must internalize the message accurately, so the meaning is not lost.

Stage 6: The communication process is understood by the receiver. This impacts not only the concept of the message but also the encoding, medium, and decoding. Surrounding the entire message is the background noise, those things that are distracting to the receiver when interpreting the message being received; for example, the tone of voice and mannerisms of the person attempting to communicate.

It is also important to know that while much of the communication a team leader oversees is verbal, there is a great amount of nonverbal communication that adds to the message. Nonverbal communication is both written (text and graphs) and visual (behavior, body language, clothing, and intentional and unintentional signals). Team leaders who are successful communicators adapt to the intended receivers' learning styles. Those learning styles include sensory (people who learn by doing), personality (some people prefer to work at night and sleep during the day), information processing (reading and writing out notes), social interaction (forming study groups), and instructional and environmental preference (some people prefer to learn in a classroom rather than online).

Last, there are barriers to effective communication. The first is *selective perception*, which means an individual will tune out information if it does not meet their preconceived ideas or conclusions. The next is *information overload*. Healthcare professionals are constantly being presented with an excess of information and data, often much more than they need to accomplish their jobs. Having too much information slows down the communication process by making it difficult to distinguish what is of value and what is not. *Emotions* often interfere with the coding and decoding of a message. *Attitude* will determine if the receiver is receptive to a message presented by the team leader. In the US today, *language* can be a barrier to effective communication. Many hospitals in western states are now looking for bilingual employees to speak with employees and patients whose primary language is Spanish. *Silence* can be used effectively as a communication tool (namely, waiting until someone responds to a message) or as a barrier (indicating the receiver is either ignoring or in disagreement with the message). Some people have *communication apprehension* and do not like to speak in front of a group or present ideas that conflict with the group's opinion. Sometimes *differences in gender* can result in a single message having multiple interpretations based on the gender of the receiver. Another barrier to communication is *political correctness* where the intent of the message may be skewed so as to not offend the receiver. In this case, the message may be completely different than the original intent, and the true intent of the message may not be received. Finally, the actual *presentation of the information* may create a barrier. Many times, a clearer message can be received better visually rather than through a narrative format. For example, this paragraph is over 300 words long. Many people would grasp this information better in the form of bullets, as the following:

- Selective perception
- Information overload
- Emotions
- Attitudes
- Language
- Silence
- Communication apprehension
- Differences in gender
- Political correctness
- Presentation of information

Check Your Understanding 19.3

Match the terms with the descriptions

1. _____ Team building
2. _____ Team charter
3. _____ Team leader
4. _____ Team member
5. _____ Team norms

a. The rules, both explicit and implied, that determine both acceptable and unacceptable behavior for the group
b. The process of organizing and acquainting a team and creating skills for dealing with team processes
c. Responsible for championing the activities of the team
d. Explains the issues the team was initiated to address, and describes goals and vision
e. Responsible for participating in the team

Business-Related Partnerships

Often it is beneficial for people in leadership positions to make **business-related partnerships**. A business-related partnership, which can be internal or external to the healthcare organization, is an agreement between two parties to cooperate for the advancement of their mutual interests and the entity's strategic goals. To create a successful partnership, each party must agree on a shared vision and mission and ensure each partner's needs and expectations will be met. It is important to identify the strengths and weaknesses of each partner so the tasks and accountability can be assigned to each partner appropriately.

Internal Business Partnerships

Within a healthcare organization, business partnerships can exist between individual managers or across entire departments. This is necessitated by the need to share resources, whether it is project funding, capital equipment, knowledge, expertise, or personnel. The main advantage of developing a partnership within an organization is that two heads are often better than one—sometimes great ideas can be generated with input from and the perspective of two people. Also, high-caliber employees can be made partners to compensate for a leader's areas of weakness. However, when two or more people are brought together the potential risk of disagreement and its resolution may be problematic. Common business partners for the HIM department are the billing office, compliance, and information services. Internal relationships in HIM are discussed in chapter 3, *Health Information Functions, Purpose, and Users.*

External Business Partnerships

External business-related partnerships often occur with the various vendors providing services to HIM professionals, whether they are HIM consultants, EHR providers, or off-site storage companies. With external business partnerships, areas of responsibility as well as how success is evaluated and measured for both parties must be determined beforehand. It is imperative that the HIM professional assume a leadership role so the vendor will provide what the organization needs, not what is easiest for the vendor to provide, or what is the bare minimum from the vendor. Often projects fail because vendors want to install what they have already developed rather than meet the deliverables required by the healthcare organization. It is important that HIM professionals exert their leadership capabilities for the betterment of the organization as well as their own professional development.

Leadership Roles

While leaders may be managers, not all managers are leaders. A leader can be anyone in a department or organization who may or may not have an organizational title. For example, Ben works in a large HIM department where he rarely sees the HIM director, who is often in meetings in another part of the medical center. The department is transitioning to computer-assisted coding software and Ben is running into an issue with the software accurately assigning the right codes when the physician does not articulate the proper documentation required by ICD-10-CM/PCS (*International Classification of Diseases, 10th revision, Clinical Modification/Procedure Coding System*). Rather than go to the department director (who has the title) he instead turns to Emily, the coder who sits next to him, who has experienced the same problems in the past and has experience in correcting the errors.

While titles do not necessarily guarantee a leader, it does give a person a platform to develop and exhibit leadership qualities. The titles available to HIM professionals listed in the following section are taken from the interactive Career Map published by the American Health Information Management Association (AHIMA). The Career Map lists the different job titles at various levels of mastery of the HIM profession and divides the jobs into different career paths; for example, coding and revenue cycle, informatics, data analytics, and information governance. The following jobs listed are at the advanced and master level—those that best show leadership potential (AHIMA 2018).

HIM Roles

There are many opportunities for developing leadership skills in the HIM profession. Health information management professionals are instrumental in compliance and risk management, education and communication, informatics and data analysis, information technology and infrastructure, health information administration, and revenue cycle management. These roles are the following:

- *Compliance and risk management*. HIM professionals already hold the positions of compliance auditor, compliance officer, and chief compliance officer. Other positions include chief privacy officer and business analyst. These positions are becoming increasingly important as payers are connecting reimbursement to successful outcomes.
- *HIM education and communication*. Professionals with advanced degrees can teach the next generation of HIM professionals what they need to start a career in addition to the skills needed five years in the future. These positions include the different ranks of professor, program director, or department chairperson. In addition, healthcare organizations are seeking knowledgeable people to train their employees in coding as well as compliance, the EHR, and privacy and security.
- *Informatics and data analysis*. HIM professionals with additional training and knowledge in project management, data analytics, and mapping between nomenclatures are highly valued. These are leaders who can forecast future needs and see a job through to a successful conclusion.
- *IT and infrastructure*. Data quality managers are needed to ensure the data collected throughout the healthcare organization (not just diagnosis and procedure codes) conform to the Data Quality Management Model of AHIMA where 10 characteristics of data quality were identified—accuracy, accessibility, comprehensiveness, consistency, currency, definition, granularity, precision, relevance, and timeliness (AHIMA Task Force on Data Quality Management 1998).
- *Health information administration*. To run an efficient department, managers must also lead. Traditional leadership roles are the director and assistant director, manager and supervisor, and regional director of HIM who oversees multiple healthcare organizations. In addition, HIM professionals with special skills in certain areas have taken the lead by becoming consultants who aid organizations with their expertise; for example, an HIM professional skilled in auditing may offer consultative services in auditing.
- *Revenue cycle management*. HIM professionals have a unique position within any healthcare organization as the claim for services cannot be sent to an insurer until the HIM medical coder has analyzed the patient chart and assigned both diagnosis and procedure codes prior to submission to the billing department. As such, HIM professionals have an opportunity to demonstrate leadership in positions like director of coding, coding manager, revenue cycle manager, and reimbursement and insurance manager.

All these positions offer HIM professionals an opportunity to demonstrate leadership to their organization by understanding the organizational strategic plan and ensuring their staff will provide support. However, a title does not guarantee leadership, so HIM professionals must constantly seek out opportunities by volunteering for assignments that will provide additional leadership skills and build a network of professionals both internal and external to the organization.

- *Chief learning officer*. This position is dedicated to the training of employees so their learning is in alignment with the organization's mission, goals, and objectives. Another responsibility of this position is identifying what manpower the organization will need in the near future and ensuring that organizational resources are used strategically and applied to achieve maximum results.
- *E-MPI manager*. This position is dedicated to resolving issues with the master patient indices (MPIs) when an enterprise decides to combine the MPIs from various healthcare organizations into an electronic format. The e-MPI manager works with registration to reduce duplicates and changes, and contributes to the design of the e-MPI to ensure coordination with local healthcare organization leadership through the use of improved practices. It is highly recommended that this person has extensive information system programming skills as well as HIM departmental experience.
- *Information governance officer*. This position is dedicated to developing an organization-wide framework for managing information throughout the information's life cycle and ensuring the information collected supports the organization's strategic plan and initiatives. This position requires knowledge of all of the health information systems as well as data analytics.
- *Meaningful Use specialist*. This position is focused on end-user issues, workflow processes, and issues with the EHR, and requires an overall understanding of the issues related to the implementation of the EHR and the federal government's Meaningful Use initiative. Not only must this individual understand the information technology aspects of the EHR but also the regulatory and healthcare reform issues that are focused on payment based on performance.
- *Practitioner consultant*. This position works closely with clinicians and IT specialists to develop and provide solutions that have both a clinical and financial impact. The practitioner consultant needs to be well versed in medical terminology and nomenclature, disease processes, and the billing and revenue cycle.
- *Research and development scientists*. This position helps support the development of solutions for health IT as well as being part of the educational system to help train future IT professionals. This position normally requires a PhD (doctorate).
- *Vice president of coding*. This position is responsible for managing the different coding divisions in facilities , establishing performance guidelines, forecasting the needs of the organization and its employees, and participating in process improvement opportunities. Since the organization is dependent on well-trained and knowledgeable medical coders, this position is vital for the financial health of the organization.
- *Vice president of security*. This position provides a workforce focused on the protection of information security focused not only on the EHR but also on the patient-centered health record as typified in patient portal access.

Real-World Case 19.1

Changes in healthcare are impacting all healthcare organizations. The HIM professional is desired for their expertise in reimbursement, HIPAA (Health Insurance Portability and Accountability Act), and the integration of the health record from a paper to an electronic format. Because of an increased demand on the HIM professional's time, leaders need to delegate to staff within the department.

Jonathan is the director of the HIM department and is also a member (or leader) of additional committees within his medical center. His workday is now 9 to 10 hours long due to his day-to-day duties and the additional committee work. Therefore, Jonathan has decided to delegate his oversight of the release of information unit to Mary, a credentialed member of the HIM department workforce. Jonathan needs to feel confident that Mary is responsible and can successfully complete this assignment. He also needs to be aware that even though he is focusing his time on other issues and meetings, he is also ultimately responsible for any task that he delegates to someone else. While Jonathan may be delegating a task to Mary to relieve some of his work pressure, this is also a great opportunity for him to test Mary for future assignment of duties and, potentially, promotion.

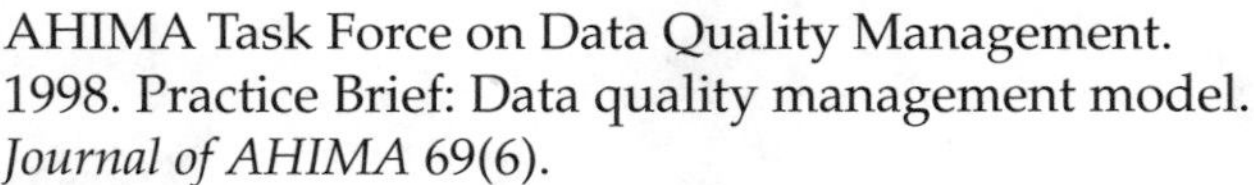

Real-World Case 19.2

Kaleb has been working at Valley Hospital for four years as a clinical informaticist and wants to further his career by developing his skills and eventually taking on more responsibilities for leadership opportunities within the hospital. He begins by exploring his emotional intelligence and leadership competencies to better understand himself and what skills he needs to improve to become a leader. He continually volunteers within his department and the hospital to serve on teams and committees. After a year of self-exploration, teamwork, and training, Kaleb was promoted to department manager and continues to explore ways to hone his skills and abilities to continue to be a great leader.

References

AHIMA Task Force on Data Quality Management. 1998. Practice Brief: Data quality management model. *Journal of AHIMA* 69(6).

American Health Information Management Association. 2018. Career Map. https://my.ahima.org/careermap.

American Health Information Management Association. 2017. *Pocket Glossary of Health Information Management and Technology*, 5th ed. Chicago: AHIMA.

Berea College, Brushy Fork Institute. 2018. Establishing Group Norms. https://www.berea.edu/brushy-fork-institute/establishing-group-norms/.

Blake, R.R. and J.S. Mouton. 1964. *Managerial Grid: The Key to Leadership Excellence.* Houston: Gulf Publishing Company.

Bradberry, T. and J. Greaves. 2009. *Emotional Intelligence 2.0*, San Diego: TalentSmart.

Bridges, W.B. 2016. *Managing Transitions, Making the Most of Change*, 4th ed. Philadelphia: Da Cappo Press.

Department of State. 2018. Active Listening. https://www.state.gov/m/a/os/65759.htm.

Fielder, F.E. 1964. A Theory of Leadership Effectiveness. In *Advances in Experimental Social Psychology.* Edited by L. Berkowitz. New York: Academic Press.

French, J. P. R. Jr. and B. Raven. 1960. The Bases of Social Power. Chapter 20 in *Group Dynamics*. Edited by D. Cartwright and A. Zander. New York: Harper and Row.

Galton, F. 1869. *Hereditary Genius*. New York: Appleton.

Hanke, S. 2018 (May 30). Five top skills for CEOs to maintain influence. *Forbes*. https://www.forbes.com/sites/forbescoachescouncil/2018/05/30/five-top-skills-for-ceos-to-maintain-influence/#12cbf755b48e.

Hartnett, T. 2018. The Basics of Consensus Decision-Making. https://www.consensusdecisionmaking.org/.

Heathfield, S. 2018 (Nov 4). How to Build a Successful Work Team. https://www.thebalancecareers.com/how-to-build-a-successful-work-team-1918515.

Kansas Leadership Center. 2016. *Redefine Leadership*. www.kansasleadershipcenter.org.

Kotter, J. 1995. *Leading Change*. Boston: Harvard Business Review.

Lewin, K. 1947. Frontiers of group dynamics. *Human Relations* 1:5–41.

Lewin, K., R. Lippitt, and R.K. White. 1939. Patterns of aggressive behavior in experimentally created social climates. *Journal of Social Psychology* 10:271–301.

McConnell, C.R. 2018. *Umiker's Management Skills for the New Health Care Supervisor*, 7th ed. Burlington, MA: Jones & Bartlett Learning.

McGregor, D. 1960. *The Human Side of Enterprise.* New York: McGraw Hill.

Northouse, P. 2019. *Leadership: Theory and Practice*. London: SAGE Publications.

Rock, D. and H. Grant. 2016 (Nov 4). Why diverse teams are smarter. *Harvard Business Review*. https://hbr.org/2016/11/why-diverse-teams-are-smarter.

Scott, S. 2018 (June 28). The 10 effective qualities of a team leader. *Small Business Chronicle*. https://smallbusiness.chron.com/10-effective-qualities-team-leader-23281.html.

Society for Human Resource Management (SHRM). 2018. http://www.shrm.org/templatestools/samples/jobdescriptions/pages/cms_001618.aspx.

Stogdill, R.M. 1948. Personal factors associated with leadership: A survey of the literature. *Journal of Psychology* 25:35–71.

The Foundation for Critical Thinking. 2018 (Feb 16). Defining Critical Thinking. https://www.criticalthinking.org/pages/defining-critical-thinking/766.

Thye, L.K. 2010. Leadership Traits and Behavioral Theories. http://www.slideshare.net/robertsonlee/leadership-traits-and-behavioral-theories.

Tuckman, B. 1965. Developmental sequence in small groups. *Psychological Bulletin* 63:384–399.

Vroom, V.H. and A.G. Jago. 1995. Situation effects and levels of analysis in the study of leader participation. *Leadership Quarterly* 6:169–181.

Human Resources Management

Valerie S. Prater, MBA, RHIT, FAHIMA

Learning Objectives

- Identify human resources management roles and responsibilities
- Identify major provisions of employment laws
- Apply ethical principles to human resources management responsibilities
- Examine workforce planning
- Analyze the role of job analysis in the employee recruitment and selection process
- Examine management practices used to organize and schedule work
- Analyze performance of employee productivity and performance standards
- Identify management actions that promote positive communication and fair handling of workplace disputes
- Apply labor law to supervision in a union environment
- Recommend training methods for workplace scenarios
- Create an employee career development plan

Key Terms

Adverse impact
Age Discrimination in Employment Act of 1967
Americans with Disabilities Act (ADA) of 1990
ADDIE model
Authorization cards
Autonomy
Bargaining unit
Behaviorally anchored rating scale (BARS)
Benchmarking
Bias
Bona fide occupational qualification (BFOQ)
Career development
Civil Rights Act of 1991 (CRA 1991)
Classroom-based learning
Coaching
Collective bargaining
Comparison system
Competencies
Compressed workweek
Contingent or contract work
Critical incident method
Development
Disciplinary action
Discrimination
Dismissal
Disparate treatment
Distributional errors
Downsizing
Dysfunctional conflict
Employee engagement
Employee relations
Equal Employment Opportunity Commission (EEOC)
Equal employment opportunity law
Equal Pay Act of 1963
Exempt employees
Exit interview
Fair Labor Standards Act (FLSA) of 1938
Family and Medical Leave Act (FMLA) of 1993

Flextime
Forced distribution
Full-time equivalent (FTE)
Genetic Nondiscrimination Act (GINA) of 2008
Graphic rating scale
Grievance process
Halo-horns effect
Harassment
Hostile work environment
Human capital
Human resources management (HRM)
Job analysis
Job description
Job interview
Job sharing
Job specifications
Justice
Layoff
Line authority
Mentoring
National Labor Relations Act (NLRA)
National Labor Relations Board (NLRB)
Negligent hiring
New employee orientation
Nonexempt employees
Occupational Safety and Health Act
Occupational Safety and Health Administration (OSHA)
Offshoring
Onboarding
Online learning
On-the-job training
Outsourcing
Parallel work division
Part-time employee
Performance appraisal
Performance management
Performance measurement
Pregnancy Discrimination Act
Process
Progressive penalties
Protected class
Quid pro quo
Reasonable accommodation
Recruitment
Reliability
Right-to-work laws
Selection
Selection test
Serial work division
Sexual harassment
Simulation
Staffing
Strike
Taft-Hartley Act
Telecommuting
Termination
Termination at will
Title VII of the Civil Rights Act of 1964
Training
Turnover
Union
Validity
Variance
Work measurement
Worker Adjustment and Retraining Notification (WARN) Act
Workflow analysis
Work distribution analysis
Workforce planning
Wrongful discharge

The healthcare industry is the largest employer in most states in the United States—a dramatic change from 1990, when manufacturing was dominant, and from 2003 when retail was the largest employer (BLS 2014). The Bureau of Labor projects 19% overall growth in healthcare sector employment through 2024, with the Medical Records and Health Information Technicians occupation category expected to grow by 13% through 2026; drivers of growth include aging of the US population (AHIMA House of Delegates 2017).

With employment growth and opportunity come workforce challenges. The healthcare industry is complex and continues to experience rapid change, including advances in technology. Healthcare organizations must deal with pressures to reduce costs, demonstrate evidence of quality and safety improvement, manage a growing volume of data, and meet the needs of a variety of internal and external customers, all while facing competition.

This chapter begins with an introduction to human resources management, a foundation in employment law and ethical principles. Next, human resources management functions and the importance to healthcare organizations and to the health information management (HIM) profession are presented. These include workforce planning and job analysis, recruitment and selection, staffing and performance management, retention and employee relations, and training and development. Principles of fairness and respect are applied across topics. Focus is on the roles and responsibilities of HIM supervisors and managers. Intended as an overview, the chapter is not a comprehensive review of all aspects of human resources management.

Human Resources Management

Human resources management (HRM) is defined as "the process of acquiring, training, appraising, and compensating employees, and of attending to their labor relations, health, safety, and fairness concerns" (Dessler 2016, 2). The need to fill positions with qualified candidates and effectively manage human resources has never been more important in healthcare than it is today. Despite increased emphasis on technology, healthcare remains a service industry with people as the most important and valuable asset. In financial accounting terms, discussed in chapter 17, *Management*, an asset is something of value to an organization that appears on the positive side of the financial statement. The human assets of an organization are often referred to as **human capital**, the sum of the knowledge, skills, creativity, and problem-solving abilities of the workforce (Momand 2018). While employee salaries are shown on the financial statement as costs to an organization, it is noted that organizations have a greater chance of success when people are managed as assets to be grown and developed versus as costs, or liabilities (Momand 2018). Human resources management is crucial as healthcare organizations seek to improve financial and quality performance.

Roles and Responsibilities

Health information management leaders can contribute directly to effective and efficient management of an organization's human resources. They support the organization's mission and financial health by helping to make the organization a place where people want to work and can grow professionally. It is said that that all managers are human resources managers, and therefore the HRM concepts are relevant to all managers (Fried and Fottler 2018). Managers who have **line authority** in an organization are those who supervise one or more employees, can give orders, and are responsible for getting work done by directing the work of others (Dessler 2016).

There are many HIM manager roles with line authority across all types and sizes of healthcare organizations; examples of titles include HIM Director, Disclosure of Information Manager, and Coding Supervisor. The HRM functions performed by these managers can vary, but typically include direct, day-to-day involvement in one or all of the areas addressed in this chapter—from recruitment and staff selection to performance management and training. With more work today done in teams and dependent upon collaboration, all employees, regardless of management title, can benefit from having HRM knowledge and skills (Fried and Fottler 2018).

Healthcare organizations, unless very small, have a human resources department with a human resources manager. The human resources department serves line managers in an advisory role, supporting performance of HRM functions. In a large healthcare system, the human resources department typically includes employees who specialize in recruiting, compensation, training, or other areas; these staff assist both individual employees and line managers. The human resources department is responsible for organization-wide functions such as human resource strategic planning, payroll, and benefits administration, and for compliance with personnel policies and procedures consistent with the organization's mission. In a smaller healthcare business, a single human resources manager may handle all human resources responsibilities. A cooperative relationship among the organization's human resources manager, departments, and line managers is essential for effective overall HRM in an organization. Key roles and responsibilities for HIM line managers are explored across the chapter.

Employment Law and Ethics

As a basis for HRM responsibilities, major federal laws addressing the employer-employee relationship in the US are reviewed in this section. Addressed are **equal employment opportunity law**, efforts to ensure equal access to employment and fairness in employment without regard to certain characteristics such as race if unrelated to a job, and labor law outlining rules for the employer-employee-labor union relationship. While state law is not reviewed here, managers should be aware that most states have laws in one or more of the areas noted. A basic understanding of employment law is important for supervisory and middle-level managers for the following major reasons:

- Compliance is ethically the right thing to do
- People want to work where they are treated fairly, consistent with law
- Managers have responsibility to communicate organizational policies based on law to staff
- Violations of law can result in significant legal and financial liability for the organization

Ethical principles are introduced in this section and referenced throughout the chapter as related to HRM. Chapter 21, *Ethical Issues in Health Information Management*, discusses ethical principles in more detail

Ethical Principles

Ethics refers to the formal, intentional process used to make clear and consistent decisions involving personal and professional values (Harman 2006). Ethical principles, combined with employment law, provide guidance to support managers in making fair and respectful decisions when supervising employees. The two ethical principles that stand out as particularly applicable to human resources management in the healthcare field are the following:

1. The principle of justice recognizes the importance of treating people fairly and applying rules consistently.
2. The principle of autonomy, or respect for an individual's voluntary choice, recognizes that employees need a voice in what happens to them in the workplace (Beauchamp and Childress 2013).

The American Health Information Management Association (AHIMA) Code of Ethics obligates HIM professionals to demonstrate actions that reflect ethical principles, including to "respect the inherent dignity and worth of every person" (AHIMA 2019). Showing respect for employees without favoritism or discrimination is consistent with the AHIMA Code of Ethics, the intent of equal opportunity laws, and is essential to ethical human resources management. Discrimination refers to treating a person differently based on individual characteristics, such as race, or group membership, such as religious affiliation; if in violation of a law, it is illegal. To support legal concepts and ethical principles, managers should "…avoid making employment decisions on the basis of personal attributes, characteristics, or behaviors unless they can be shown to be directly related to job performance" (Filerman et al. 2014, 192). Discrimination and its relationship to job performance are discussed below from a legal perspective in presenting Title VII of the Civil Rights Act of 1964 and the Age Discrimination in Employment Act of 1967.

In each section of this chapter, consider specific ways a manager can uphold the ethical principles of justice and autonomy, and avoid illegal discrimination, in effectively carrying out HRM responsibilities.

Fair Labor Standards Act of 1938

Amended several times since its passage, the Fair Labor Standards Act (FLSA) of 1938 sets the minimum wage requirements for overtime pay, and child labor standards; it is administered and enforced by the Wage and Hour Division of the US Department of Labor (DOL) and applies to most US work settings (DOL 2014).

Employees are classified as nonexempt or exempt based on job title, duties, and salary level; nonexempt employees are covered by FLSA minimum wage and overtime provisions, exempt employees are not covered (Dessler 2016). Examples: top executive salaried positions are exempt, clerical jobs paid hourly are nonexempt; managers who are expected to work hours as needed to keep operations running are typically exempt. Administrative, professional, and technical positions must be carefully analyzed in consultation with the human resources department to determine if FLSA minimum wage and overtime pay rules apply. Current definitions of exemption are published online by the DOL.

Equal Pay Act of 1963

The Equal Pay Act requires that men and women in the same workplace receive equal pay for performing equivalent work. Comparison of job content, rather than job title, is used to determine whether one job is substantially equivalent to another (EEOC n.d.a.). The Equal Pay Act covers essentially all employers and all forms of pay including salary, overtime, bonuses, vacation and holiday pay, benefits, and reimbursement for business travel expenses (EEOC n.d.a).

Title VII of the Civil Rights Act of 1964

Title VII of the Civil Rights Act of 1964 and its amendments represent perhaps the most important and sweeping of the federal antidiscrimination laws. Commonly referred to simply as Title VII, this act applies to employers with 15 or more employees and prohibits employment decisions, including those involving hiring, compensation, dismissal, or working conditions, based on an individual's race, color, religion, sex, or national origin (Gomez-Mejia et al. 2016). Unlawful employment practices as defined in this law are shown in figure 20.1.

Title VII established the Equal Employment Opportunity Commission (EEOC) as the federal agency with responsibility to administer and enforce equal opportunity employment laws, investigate complaints, and file discrimination charges in court.

The following definitions are important to human resources management developed from Title VII court cases:

- Protected class. Identified groups of people, with characteristics as described in figure 20.1, who are protected by law based on past history of employment discrimination affecting these groups
- Disparate treatment. Illegal employment discrimination based on intentional unequal treatment of an individual who is a member of a protected class
- Adverse impact. Unequal discriminatory effect of an employment practice (for example, requiring a passing score on a test that does not cover job-related knowledge or skills) on members of a protected class (Gomez-Mejia et al. 2016)

Hiring managers and supervisors should be aware that employment discrimination based on a characteristic associated with a protected class, such as a racial or ethnic group, is illegal unless the characteristic can be shown to directly interfere with job performance; for example, where cultural dress impacts ability to meet a job safety standard (EEOC n.d.c). In very narrowly interpreted situations, employers may be able to defend as a bona fide occupational qualification (BFOQ) the use of an otherwise discriminatory characteristic in making an employment decision if the characteristic is directly related to business necessity; for example, preference for a particular religious affiliation for teaching at a religious-affiliated school (Dessler 2016). Job analysis, discussed later in the chapter, must be used to justify job-related qualifications for a position. Amendments to Title VII that address issues surrounding harassment and

Figure 20.1 Title VII of the Civil Rights Act of 1964: unlawful employment practices

From the text of Title VII of the Civil Rights Act of 1964 (Pub. L. 88-352) (Title VII)
Unlawful employment practices SEC. 2000e-2. *[Section 703]*

(a) Employer practices

It shall be an unlawful employment practice for an employer—

(1) to fail or refuse to hire or to discharge any individual, or otherwise to discriminate against any individual with respect to his compensation, terms, conditions, or privileges of employment, because of such individual's race, color, religion, sex, or national origin; or

(2) to limit, segregate, or classify his employees or applicants for employment in any way which would deprive or tend to deprive any individual of employment opportunities or otherwise adversely affect his status as an employee, because of such individual's race, color, religion, sex, or national origin.

Source: EEOC n.d.b.

pregnancy discrimination in the workplace are described in the sections that follow.

Harassment

Harassment, including sexual harassment, is covered as a form of illegal discrimination under Title VII. Harassment involves unwelcome workplace conduct based on an individual's race, color, religion, gender, national origin, age, disability, or genetic information (EEOC n.d.d). To be considered illegal, enduring the offensive conduct becomes a condition of the individual's continued employment, or is severe enough to create a hostile work environment (EEOC n.d.d). A hostile work environment is a setting in which intimidating and abusive workplace conduct that interferes with an employee's job performance takes place; the unwanted conduct goes beyond a minor or occasional annoyance. Examples of such unwanted conduct by a supervisor, coworker, or nonemployee include telling offensive jokes, name calling, and acts involving physical threat or insult (EEOC n.d.d).

A type of harassment based on sex is sexual harassment; this may include verbal comments, unwanted physical contact, sexual advances, or requests for sexual favors (EEOC n.d.d). Sexual harassment complaints can arise based on a hostile work environment where repeated and unwelcome sexually oriented conduct makes a workplace uncomfortable or may be based on direct ***quid pro quo*** advances where sexual favors are requested in exchange for a job benefit or continued employment (McWay 2016). Sexual harassment can apply to workers regardless of gender and can be committed by supervisors, coworkers, or nonemployees. In a real-world example, a hospital employer paid a court-ordered financial settlement in a case brought by a group of women who alleged sexual harassment by a physician during employment-related medical examinations; the hospital had received complaints, but had failed to take action (McNair et al. 2007).

The best management strategies to address workplace harassment focus on prevention, featuring clear policies, open communication, and antiharassment training. Supervisors should inform employees of the organization's complaint procedure, take all complaints seriously, and document prompt follow-up action.

Pregnancy Discrimination Act of 1978

Title VII was amended with the Pregnancy Discrimination Act of 1978 to protect women from sex discrimination based on pregnancy, and conditions related to pregnancy or childbirth (EEOC n.d.e). This act further specifies that women should be treated the same as other employees with respect to eligibility for health plan benefits and with regard to their ability to work.

Supervisors and managers who are responsible for staff selection, scheduling, or performance appraisal (addressed later in the chapter) should be familiar with the major provisions of this legislation, and with all other equal opportunity employment laws.

Age Discrimination in Employment Act of 1967

The Age Discrimination in Employment Act of 1967 prohibits age discrimination against job applicants or workers age 40 and older, making hiring, compensation, and other employment decisions based on age illegal (EEOC n.d.f). Age presents an area of legal risk for managers and supervisors particularly in the candidate selection process or when a staff layoff is necessary. To avoid violation of this law, hiring and continuing employment decisions should focus on job requirements and performance standards. Retaining qualified experienced older workers can help maintain stability within an organization's workforce.

In narrowly defined situations, employers may be able to defend age as a BFOQ if they can show that age is directly related to job performance based on job analysis. An example based on job safety is the age 65 requirement for mandatory retirement of airline pilots (FAA 2012).

Occupational Safety and Health Act of 1970

The Occupational Safety and Health Act of 1970, as amended in 2004, states as its purpose the following:

> To assure safe and healthful working conditions for working men and women; by authorizing enforcement of the standards developed under the Act; by assisting and

> encouraging the States in their efforts to assure safe and healthful working conditions; by providing for research, information, education, and training in the field of occupational safety and health (OSHA 2004).

This legislation created the Occupational Safety and Health Administration (OSHA) agency within the DOL to administer and enforce the law and provide education on workplace safety. Employers are expected to provide a physically safe work environment and to report all job-related illnesses, injuries, and fatalities. Supervisors and managers should be mindful of potential workplace safety hazards, knowledgeable of OSHA injury and illness reporting requirements, and work with the organization's human resources department and safety officer to ensure that employees receive required safety orientation and training.

Americans with Disabilities Act of 1990

The Americans with Disabilities Act (ADA) prohibits discrimination in employment against people with disabilities, applies to employers with 15 or more workers, and is enforced by the EEOC (DOL 2015).

The ADA applies to qualified job applicants and to current employees; its scope continues to evolve as courts rule on complaints. In a complaint, a disabled individual alleges that an employer failed to provide a reasonable accommodation, or workplace adjustment that does not present an undue (significant) hardship to the organization, and that this failure interfered with the qualified individual being hired or with his or her ability to perform a job. In order to comply with this law and demonstrate fair employment practices, managers should have an appreciation of the key ADA terms and concepts explained with examples in figure 20.2 and work closely with the organization's human resources department.

Civil Rights Act of 1991

The Civil Rights Act of 1991 (CRA 1991) amended Title VII of the Civil Rights Act of 1964 and the Americans with Disabilities Act. CRA made it easier for the plaintiff (complaining party, such as a former employee or job applicant in a protected class) to sue for damages claiming adverse impact or disparate treatment. The CRA made clear it is the employer's responsibility to prove that illegal hiring and workplace discrimination did not occur.

Family and Medical Leave Act of 1993

The Family and Medical Leave Act (FMLA) of 1993 covers public agencies and private employers

Figure 20.2 Americans with Disabilities Act of 1990: key terms for compliance

Disability: Refers to a physical or mental impairment that substantially limits one or more major life activities, such as the ability to see, hear, stand, walk, or learn.

Essential job functions: Duties required to be performed by every person in a job in order to meet job performance standards. During an interview, an employer can legally ask a disabled (or any) job applicant about their ability to perform these job functions. A thorough job analysis and clearly written job description define the essential functions of a job. Example for a coder: Accurately assign diagnostic codes using *International Classification of Diseases, Tenth Revision, Clinical Modification* (ICD-10-CM)

Reasonable accommodation: Action taken by an employer to allow a disable applicant or employee access to a work opportunity. A disable person is typically expected to request the accommodation. Examples of reasonable accommodations include actions such as altering the work schedule and modifying office equipment or software. A coder with a vision impairment, for example, may need additional workspace lighting or a larger computer monitor with adjustment to screen magnification.

Undue hardship: An accommodation that would present a significant cost, cause extreme difficulty, or have a negative impact on organizational operations. The employer is ultimately responsible for evaluating a request for accommodation and determining what is reasonable and appropriate in a given job situation. Example of accommodation for a coder that may represent undue hardship: Alteration in workflow projected to negatively affect the organization's revenue cycle.

Source: Adapted from Gomez-Mejia et al. 2016; McWay 2016.

with 50 or more employees working in 20 or more workweeks in a calendar year (DOL 2012). Administration and enforcement of the FMLA is by the DOL's Wage and Hour Division for non-federal employers and by the US Office of Personnel Management (OPM) for federal employers (DOL 2012). Provisions of the law include the following:

- Employees who have worked at least 12 months are eligible to take unpaid, job-protected leave of up to 12 workweeks for specified family and medical reasons including the birth or adoption of a child, care of a seriously ill family member or the employee's own serious health condition, or for an emergent issue related to a family member's active military status
- Employees are required to comply with an employer's existing policies regarding request for leave, advance notice, or for use of accrued sick leave and vacation time (DOL 2012)

Genetic Nondiscrimination Act of 2008

The ability to conduct genetic tests and generate sensitive genetic information resulted from the Human Genome Project. This major public research project identified and mapped a complete set of DNAs, the chemical compound with genetic code that provides building blocks for the human body (NIH 2018). Concern that highly personal information, such as the potential to develop a particular disease, could be used by insurers to deny health coverage or by employers in making employment decisions led to passage of the Genetic Nondiscrimination Act (GINA) of 2008. GINA prohibits employers' use of genetic information in making decisions regarding hiring, promotion, benefits, pay, and termination, and restricts disclosure of genetic information about applicants, employees, and their families (Brodnik and Sharp 2017).

Major Labor Laws

In 1935, Congress passed the Wagner Act, also known as the National Labor Relations Act (NLRA); this gives employees the right to form labor unions and bargain collectively, regulates union-employer relations, and formed the National Labor Relations Board (NLRB) as the federal agency to enforce the law (Brodnik and Sharp 2017). Major provisions of this act include that it is unlawful for employers to do the following:

- Threaten employees with loss of jobs based on union vote or activity
- Question employees about their union views
- Promise special benefits to employees to discourage union support
- Punish employees for engaging in legal union activity, as by firing or by transferring to a more difficult job (NLRB 2018a)

Labor organizations are prohibited under the NLRA from such actions as using threats or coercive tactics in an effort to gain employees' support for the union, or striking over issues not related to employment terms or conditions (NLRB 2018a).

The NLRA excludes managerial and supervisory staff from protections of the law and from participation in a bargaining unit and differentiates employees from supervisors. A supervisor is defined in the NLRA as one who has authority and uses independent judgment "in the interest of the employer, to hire, transfer, suspend, lay off, recall, promote, discharge, assign, reward, or discipline other employees, or responsibly to direct them, or to adjust their grievances, or effectively to recommend such action" (29 USC 152(11)).

The definition of who is a supervisor or manager in a healthcare organization, and therefore who can be a member of a collective bargaining unit, has also been addressed by the courts. Summarized as follows, the ruling in a landmark case provides an example where certain nurses were considered managers based on job responsibility, and not part of the bargaining unit:

> The facility had classified six nurses as supervisors, excluding them from the union bargaining unit. The NLRB disagreed, indicating that these nurses' exercise of professional judgment did not place them in a supervisory role; the employer was cited for unfair labor practice. The US

> Supreme Court disagreed with the NLRB's ruling, saying it contradicted the wording of the NLRA statute describing use of independent judgment by supervisors; the nurses could in fact be classified as managers. (*NLRB v. Kentucky River Community Care, Inc.* 2001, 1)

The Taft-Hartley Act of 1947 made changes to the employer-employee labor relationship by doing the following:

- Giving employers freedom to express their views to employees regarding unionization
- Allowing the US president to issue a temporary ban on strikes that might impact national health and safety
- Giving states permission to enact right-to-work laws prohibiting forced union membership as a condition of employment (Dessler 2016)

Since the Taft-Hartley Act, right-to-work laws have been enacted in many states. The 1974 Healthcare Amendments to the Taft-Hartley Act clarified that employees of private, not-for-profit hospitals are covered under federal labor law and that healthcare unions must provide 10-day advance notice of strike (Fried and Fottler 2011). More on unions and supervising in a union environment is presented later in the chapter.

The Worker Adjustment and Retraining Notification (WARN) Act of 1988 requires organizations of more than 100 employees to provide at least 60-days advance notice of a workforce layoff or downsizing (Maurer 2017). Supervisory roles in the event of layoff or downsizing are addressed later in the chapter.

Check Your Understanding 20.1

Answer the following questions.

1. Managers with _____authority in an organization supervise one or more employees, direct the work of others, and have HRM responsibilities.
   a. Line
   b. Staff
   c. Legal
   d. Personal
2. By law________ are excluded from an employee union bargaining unit.
   a. Clerical staff
   b. Supervisors
   c. Non-managers
   d. Clinical professionals
3. Which of the following refers to the sum of the knowledge, skills, creativity, and problem-solving abilities of an organization's workforce?
   a. Labor
   b. Management
   c. Human capital
   d. Human resources management
4. Which ethical principle recognizes the importance of treating people fairly and applying rules consistently?
   a. Autonomy
   b. Justice
   c. Respect
   d. Morality

5. Which of the following laws established the EEOC as the federal agency to administer and enforce equal opportunity employment laws?
   a. Equal Pay Act of 1963
   b. Title VII of the Civil Rights Act of 1964
   c. Age Discrimination Act of 1967
   d. Civil Rights Act of 1991
6. Title VII of the Civil Rights Act of 1964 prohibits discrimination in employment that impacts members of a protected class. Which of the following does NOT describe a protected class under this act?
   a. Race or ethnic group
   b. Religious affiliation
   c. Women
   d. Disabled persons
7. Which of the following statements is TRUE of the federal Age Discrimination in Employment Act?
   a. Employment discrimination against aged individuals with disabilities is prohibited.
   b. The Act sets standards to protect benefit and retirement plans of older workers.
   c. Discrimination against workers age 40 and older is illegal.
   d. The practice of mandatory retirement based on age can never be defended.
8. The HIM department's receptionist is paid an hourly rate and is eligible for overtime pay, consistent with the Fair Labor Standards Act. According to this law, her position is classified as which of the following?
   a. Exempt
   b. Nonexempt
   c. Full-time
   d. Professional
9. An employer should offer reasonable accommodation, such as by modifying office equipment, to a qualified applicant or employee based on physical or mental impairment. This is a provision of the:
   a. Genetic Nondiscrimination Act of 2008
   b. Occupational Safety and Health Act of 1970
   c. Civil Rights Act of 1991
   d. Americans with Disabilities Act of 1990
10. This Act formed the National Labor Relations Board as the federal agency to enforce labor law.
   a. National Labor Relations
   b. Taft-Hartley
   c. Equal Opportunity Employment
   d. Fair Labor Standards

Workforce Planning and Job Analysis

An effective (and cost-effective) staff recruitment and selection process begins with an understanding of the positions to be filled. This understanding involves workforce planning, job analysis, and job description, which are presented in this section. In some cases, new positions are created, or positions are redesigned, as a result of changes in HIM or in the health care environment. For example, clerks that used to assemble paper health records may now prepare and scan documents into an electronic health record and perform quality control. Whether existing or new, thorough understanding of a job and the qualifications for the position are essential as a foundation for the recruitment and selection process, presented in a later section of the chapter.

Workforce Planning

Reviewing national demographic, social, and economic data and trends, and relating these to an organization's workforce needs, is central to workforce planning. While workforce planning (deciding what positions are needed) is a top management responsibility, HIM managers contribute by staying abreast of data and trends relevant to the HIM profession that may impact recruitment, staffing, and other HRM needs.

External sources of HIM workforce data include government reports provided by the DOL and the Health Resources and Services Administration's Bureau of Health Professions, as well as AHIMA reports. For example, the AHIMA House of Delegates 2018 Environmental Scan Report noted the following trends expected to impact the HIM workforce through 2026:

- An aging workforce, with more workers age 55+
- Continued growth in healthcare employment outside of hospital settings
- Projected overall increase in employment of health information technicians and health services managers, with the exception being in coding
- Continued automation and outsourcing of HIM jobs
- Projected need for higher levels of education across the HIM workforce (AHIMA House of Delegates 2017)

This report also shows that employment of coding professionals has declined somewhat in the past 10 years due to efficiencies in management and use of technology (AHIMA House of Delegates 2017).

Staying current on external workforce data can assist managers and the organization in doing the following:

- Forecasting and planning for the right number and types of workers needed to staff HIM positions;
- Describing HIM jobs and the qualifications required to perform these jobs as workforce needs change
- Planning recruitment efforts to find qualified employees

The next section of the chapter will present the HRM functions of job analysis, job description, and job specifications.

Job Analysis

Job analysis involves collecting and analyzing information about a job in order to better understand the significant duties of the job, and to identify the skills and characteristics required of an employee who can successfully perform the job. The completed job analysis provides information to create, revise, or redesign a job description and job specifications required for employee recruitment and selection. Job analysis also supports other HRM functions addressed later in the chapter such as performance appraisal, staffing, and training.

The three major steps in conducting a job analysis are to do the following:

1. *Clarify the purpose of the analysis.* Identify the job to be analyzed. If the current job is being redesigned or the unit or department is undergoing restructure, more than one job may be involved. Consider relationships among jobs in determining which jobs to analyze. To do this, a workflow analysis may be needed, if this has not already been conducted. Workflow analysis is a detailed step-by-step assessment of how work moves from one task to the next and from one employee to the next within a work process. A chart or workflow diagram may be used to show the beginning-to-end process. Workflow analysis is also discussed in chapter 17 Management.
2. *Collect information about the job.* Sources of information for an existing job include documents such as organization charts, job descriptions, and job procedures (covered in chapter 17). An interview with an employee who currently holds the position can be valuable due to that individual's

detailed knowledge of the job. A list of specific questions for the employee interview should be developed (Examples: What are your primary job duties? What equipment do you use? What education, skill, or certification is required to perform your job? How is your work evaluated?) Other data collection methods include observing the job being performed, conducting a survey, or having employees keep a log of job activity over a period of time. External sources of information for job analysis, such as the DOL's O*NET, can also be useful (DOL 2019). Use of a variety of data sources and collection methods is recommended; see examples in figure 20.3.

3. *Identify the job's primary duties and the competencies required to perform them.* Based on data collected, what essential work is done? Are some duties more important than others? If so, indicate priority such as by showing rank order, a scaled value, or amount of time spent on each duty. What is required to competently perform these primary job duties? Competencies are clear action-oriented statements identifying measurable knowledge, skills, abilities, or other characteristics required of an individual to successfully perform the work duty (OPM 2018). An example of a competency for a disclosure specialist might read like this: Able to apply policies and procedures to process requests for disclosure of health information with 99 percent accuracy. Ability to comprehend policies and procedures and attention to detail would be among characteristics required of the job.

Job Description and Job Specifications

A job description, also called a position description, is a written explanation of a job and the duties it entails and is based on information provided by the job analysis. A job description helps the human resources department, the hiring manager, the employee's direct supervisor, and the employee understand the job duties and expectations. While formats may vary across organizations, most job descriptions contain section headings similar to the following heads:

- Job title or identification
- Job summary
- Reporting relationships (reports to, supervises as applicable)
- Duties (responsibilities)
- Standards of performance
- Working condition

The most useful job descriptions are very clear and detailed yet concise. The relationships section can include internal reporting and supervisory relations, as well as significant contacts outside of the unit (for example, medical staff committee chairs, or vendors). Priority in job duties can be

Figure 20.3 Data collection for job analysis

Sources of data

- Organizational chart (discussed in chapter 19, Leadership)
- Job description
- Job procedures
- Workflow analysis (discussed in chapter 19)
- Employee
- Supervisor

Methods of data collection

- Interviews (employee, supervisor)
- Direct observation of work (best for jobs involving physical tasks)
- Survey questionnaire (to employee, delivered in person or online)
- Diary or log (by employee)
- External sources:
  - Online databases for job analysis
  - Professional association websites (research and practice briefs, sample job descriptions, sample survey, and interview questions for job analysis)
  - Proprietary websites (sample descriptions)
  - Consultants

Sources: Adapted from Fried and Fottler 2011; Dessler 2016.

indicated in various ways, such as by showing percentage of time typically spent on a duty or by ranking responsibilities in order of importance. Standards of performance indicate an expectation, such as volume or quality of work (for example, code an average of X inpatient health records per week with Y or fewer errors). Statements on working conditions address health or safety issues.

In the rapidly changing field of HIM, job descriptions should be updated often, at least annually and always when changes to the job are made or when a new policy, procedure, technology, or regulation is introduced.

Most job description formats include a section on job specifications, titled such as "required knowledge, skills, and experience," or these may be provided as a separate document. **Job specifications** describe the individual qualifications required to perform the job outlined in the job description. Based on job analysis, specifications list the education level, experience, skills, personal characteristics, physical strength requirements, licensure, or credential needed to do the job (for example, associate's degree required, RHIT [registered health information technician] preferred).

Specifications must be job related and justified by job analysis data. This is necessary to support fair hiring decisions, consistent with the principle of justice and with equal employment opportunity law as discussed earlier in the chapter. For example, job specifications for a Clinical Documentation Integrity Specialist position might show an associate's degree and three years of experience in clinical documentation Integrity as the required minimum based on job analysis, with a bachelor's degree and the Clinical Documentation Improvement Professional (CDIP) credential as preferred or desired (AHIMA 2013a).

Figure 20.4 provides an example of a job description with job specifications.

Figure 20.4 Disclosure specialist job description

Disclosure specialist job description

Job title: Disclosure specialist
Department: Health Information Management
Department supervisor's title: Disclosure manager

General summary

Purpose: To provide coverage for disclosure of health information functions, including written and verbal requests for health information. Duties include: managing incoming requests, verification of proper authorization for requests, using master patient index to obtain health record numbers, using chart location system to locate paper charts, using EHR system to locate electronic health information, copying health information, billing for copies of health information when applicable, entering all releases into correspondence tracking system, answering telephone calls related to the disclosure function, and numerous other associated duties.

Decision-making authority: Routine decisions include verification of appropriate authorization, prioritizing requests, problem-solving record locations, problem-solving in customer service for internal and external departmental personnel.

Supervisory responsibility: No formal supervisory responsibility.

Essential duties:

Duty A	**Processes incoming requests for the disclosure area with 98% accuracy.**	**Time %: 15%**	**Relative Impor tance = 5 (1–5 scale)**

Task #1: Opens and date stamps 100% of all requests received each day.
Task #2: Screens each request for disclosure requirements and verifies proper authorization.
Task #3: Utilizes facility computer system to obtain health record numbers and dates of service.
Task #4: Enters health record number, name, requestor, requestor type, date received, and other data items into correspondence tracking system.

Duty B	**Identifies locations of and retrieves health records needed to complete disclosure request with 98% accuracy.**	**Time %: 20%**	**Relative Importance = 5**

Task #1: Locates patient charts, utilizing the chart tracking system.
Task #2: Locates older charts on microfilm using the microfilm system.
Task #3: Locates and obtains records from other departments not housed in the health records or HIM department.

continued

Figure 20.4 Disclosure specialist job description *(concluded)*

Duty C	**Tracks health records during disclosure request processing with 98% accuracy.**	**Time %: 5%**	**Relative Importance = 4**

Task #1: Transfers location of chart in the chart location system.
Task #2: Returns all health records to correct location.

Duty D	**Processes authorizations and subpoenas with 98% accuracy.**	**Time %: 25%**	**Relative Importance = 5**

Task #1: Determines information requested on authorization.
Task #2: Communicates with requestor regarding possible charges.
Task #3: Photocopies requested information.
Task #4: Calculates invoice and determines whether prepayment is required.
Task #5: Determines disposition and mails out copies (pick-up, mail, overnight).
Task #6: Completes request in correspondence tracking system, entering date processed, documents sent, and such.

Duty E	**Processes STAT (needed immediately) and walk-in requests same day with 98% accuracy.**	**Time %: 10%**	**Relative Importance = 4**

Task #1: STAT requests are completed according to the need of the patient for patient care purposes.
Task #2: Assist walk-in requestors in filling out authorization for release of confidential medical information form.

Duty F	**Processes problem requests.**	**Time %: 5%**	**Relative Importance = 4**

Task #1: Researches request.
Task #2: Returns request with letters stating reason for return.
Task #3: Sends final notices on requests pending more than two months.
Task #4: Cancels unpaid prepayment requests after three to four months.

Duty G	**Answers phone calls related to disclosure.**	**Time %: 20%**	**Relative Importance = 4**

Task #1: Assists requestors with verbal continuity of care requests.
Task #2: Assists callers concerning status of requests.

Required knowledge and skills (job specifications):

Component	*Description*
Knowledge	Working knowledge of health records functions to include chart order and assembly, terminal digit order filing, and record flow of department. Required for completely satisfactory performance in this job is knowledge of health record format, computerized registration inquiry process and back-up manual registration system, as well as admissions process. Working knowledge of computerized access systems. Knowledge of policies and procedure surrounding disclosure of protected health information preferred.
Skills	Required for completely satisfactory performance in this job is the ability to communicate effectively, provide good customer service, problem solve routine health record issues, prioritize tasks, be punctual and dependable regarding work tasks, work independently, and pay attention to detail. Must utilize well-organized work habits along with good written and verbal communication skills, utilize electronic messaging, and perform accurate data entry, verification, and updating. Able to learn and apply detailed policies and procedures. Computer skills proficiency.
Formal education and experience	The formal education normally associated with completely satisfactory performance in this job is a high school diploma or the equivalent. A minimum of two years of experience in health record department or equivalent is required. Experience processing disclosure requests preferred.

Working conditions: Conditions that differ from the normal work environment include stress when communicating with parents, patients, physicians, attorneys, telephones constantly ringing, meeting deadlines, and frequent distractions.

These statements are intended to describe the essential responsibilities being performed by people assigned to this job. They are not intended to be an exhaustive list of the responsibilities assigned to these people.

APPROVED BY
NAME:
TITLE:

Source: AHIMA 2013b.

Recruitment and Selection

Recruitment and selection of employees is costly to an organization, so making the most of this investment of time and dollars is important. A cost-effective staff recruitment and selection process begins with an understanding of the positions to be filled, as discussed in the previous section. Whether existing or new, a thorough understanding of the job and qualifications for a position is essential. With a job analyzed and clearly described, recruitment for an open position can begin. Selection tools are then applied in an effort to find the best person for the job. This section of the chapter presents detail on the HRM functions of employee recruiting and selection, linking these to the functions of job analysis and job description. See overview in table 20.1.

Recruitment

Recruitment is the way an organization attracts a pool of qualified job applicants. The best way to recruit talent is to build an environment where people want to work; factors supporting this include treating employees with respect and offering opportunities for growth (AHIMA 2013a).

An HIM manager typically works in cooperation with the human resources department to recruit employees to fill jobs. Sources of qualified job candidates can be broadly classified as internal and external. Internal sources of candidates include promotion or transfer of employees from within the organization. Internal candidates have the advantages of being known by the organization and will need less orientation than external candidates. Promotion from within can be a motivator for employees. A disadvantage is that the healthcare organization is not bringing in new talent when hiring from within, and may in turn create another open position to fill. Also, a rejected internal applicant may harbor negative feelings that impact individual or team performance. A summary of the pros and cons of internal vs. external recruiting is presented in figure 20.5.

Table 20.1 HRM functions: Workforce planning, recruitment, and selection

Opportunity or challenge	HRM functions
Understand position to fill	Conduct, review, and revise job analysis
	Prepare, review, and revise job description
Know job requirements such as skills and education required	Prepare, review, and revise job specifications
Develop a pool of qualified candidates	Attract and recruit candidates, both internally and externally
Select the right candidate	Check, test, interview, select, and hire the best candidate
Comply with legal and regulatory requirements	Stay informed on applicable laws and consult human resources department as needed

Source: @AHIMA

Methods to identify qualified candidates include internal job posting, employee referral, online (the healthcare organization's web page, job boards, social media sites), and print advertising (local newspaper, professional journals). College recruiting efforts such as job fairs can be valuable to fill entry-level positions but are time-consuming. Employment agencies are another option, including those run by government agencies. Use of private agencies involves payment of a fee, an option typically reserved for top executive or hard-to-recruit technical positions.

Use of online recruiting methods has become prevalent across many organizations, with advantages and disadvantages. Online recruiting typically generates more responses faster and at a lower cost than other methods. However, many of the applicants may not be qualified, and fewer minority applicants may respond. Therefore, use of more than one recruiting method is recommended, using clear information on the job duties and job specifications.

Selection

Selection is the process of choosing the individual to hire who best fits the job and the organization from among the pool of qualified prospects generated by recruiting, making the best investment in human capital (Mondy and Martocchio 2016). Hiring the right person for a job can positively impact

Figure 20.5 Internal versus external job candidate: advantages and disadvantages

Internal candidate	External candidate
Advantages • Known individual (strengths, weaknesses) • Morale boost with new opportunity, promotion • Needs less orientation • Knows organization and the culture • Faster, less costly hiring process	**Advantages** • Represents a larger, more diverse pool of applicants • Brings fresh ideas from outside • May already have specialized training (saving time and money) • Not involved in organizational politics
Disadvantages • Strong candidates may not be available or have not been developed • Morale problem may develop among applicants not selected • Can lead to stagnation, lack of new ideas • May need specialized training • Another vacancy to fill	**Disadvantages** • Reliance on references for information about candidate • Working relationships with internal applicants not selected may be strained • Requires orientation • Needs time for socialization into organization (may not fit culture) • More complex, costly hiring process

Source: ©AHIMA

overall staff morale and productivity, and the ability of the organization to reach its goals (Mondy and Martocchio 2016).

Careful selection is also necessary to avoid the negative impact of placing the wrong person in a job. For example, an underqualified or overqualified individual may perform poorly, or may not fit with the organizational culture, leading to the need for replacement after a short time. Ruling out candidates with a history of problematic behavior can help to avoid disciplinary issues, as well as turnover (employees leaving the organization, discussed later in the chapter). Courts have held employers liable for **negligent hiring**, hiring individuals with criminal backgrounds or other problems without applying proper safeguards to protect customers' information or property (Dessler 2016, 149). The importance of verifying candidate work history and of conducting reference and background checks to avoid negligent hiring cannot be underestimated, especially in a field where employees have access to protected health information. Hiring managers should work closely with human resource managers on the background checking aspects of selection. Additional techniques common to a successful employee selection process are testing and interviewing, discussed as follows.

Testing

When used as one component of the candidate selection process, a well-constructed **selection test** can assess job skills and abilities or identify job-related attitudes that may not surface in an interview. Disadvantages of tests include inability to measure motivation to work, as well as risk of discrimination. According to the federal *Uniform Guidelines on Employee Selection Procedures*, regulatory standards to assist employers in avoiding discriminatory practices, selection tests used must be necessary to appropriately evaluate the knowledge, skills, and abilities identified in job analysis as needed to perform the job (SHRM 2018a).

To be fair, legal, and effective, selection tests should be designed to meet standards for validity and reliability. **Validity** of a selection test refers to the test's ability to accurately measure the job skill, knowledge, or behavior it was meant to measure. The type of test and test questions should be consistent with the knowledge, skills, and abilities required of the job, as supported by job analysis and job description (Mondy and Martocchio 2016). For example, a selection test for a coder might include performance on an encoder application exercise or on a pencil-and-paper coding test. Other types of selection tests include cognitive (mental) ability, physical ability, and personality tests.

Reliability refers to the degree to which a selection test produces consistent scores on test and retest. Using the coder example above, if a candidate scored 150 on a coding test, then on retake of the same test the following day scored 70, test reliability could be questioned; validity (accuracy) of this test would also be in question (Mondy and Martocchio 2016). Hiring managers are advised to work closely with the human resources department in evaluating the cost of testing and in determining valid, reliable testing tools and techniques for a particular job.

Interviewing

A job interview is a conversation in which a hiring manager and a job applicant exchange information. It is goal oriented and designed to support the selection process based on the candidate's oral responses. Job interviews can be classified by type as structured (planned in advance; each candidate is asked the same questions) or unstructured (open-ended; interviewer asks each candidate questions that come to mind). Within a job interview, different types of questions can be asked. Structured-type questions include the following:

- Situational, where candidates are asked how they would handle a given job-related scenario;
- Behavioral, where candidates are asked to relate a behavior used in the past to handle a job situation; and
- Knowledge, where candidates are asked direct questions about job knowledge or skill.

Open-ended type questions, such as, "What is your greatest strength?" encourage a job candidate to talk and allow the interviewer to probe for more information.

Structured interviews using structured, job-related questions have the advantages of being consistent across candidates, objective, and legally defensible. Interview types, examples of common types of questions, and major advantages and disadvantages of each are summarized in table 20.2.

Methods of interviewing include the familiar one-on-one, face-to-face candidate meeting with an interviewer, arranged as a single event or as a sequence of individual interviews. Use of phone and video has become common, especially for initial screening interviews. Phone interviews are a fast, low-cost method to determine a candidate's eligibility for a position, to assess oral communication skills, and to decide on further investment in a face-to-face meeting (SHRM 2018b). Group interviews, where several candidates meet with one or more interviewers, and panel interviews where one candidate is interviewed by several interviewers at the same time, are also common with use of face-to-face and video methods.

While used for nearly all positions, interviews unfortunately are not always a reliable predictor of candidate success. Factors contributing to this

Table 20.2 Types of job interviews and questions

Interview types	Interview question types	Advantages and disadvantages
Unstructured: Interviewer asks questions that come to mind	Open-ended, probing: For example, "What is your greatest professional strength, and how have you used it to advance your career?"	• Flexible; may uncover information missed in structured interview • Not standardized; different information obtained across job candidates cannot be rated or scored • Candidate encouraged to talk, may volunteer information not related to job • Potentially discriminatory • Time consuming
Structured: Each candidate for a job is asked the same questions planned in advance	*Situational:* Ask how candidate would handle a given scenario (for example, "What would you do if a physician became angry when you queried her about documentation in a record?") *Behavioral:* Ask candidate to relate behavior from the past to a job situation (for example, "Describe a situation where you had to deal with a subordinate's chronic tardiness, and explain how you handled it.") *Knowledge:* Straightforward job knowledge questions (for example, "What encoder software have you used?")	• Standardized • Answers can be rated or scored • Questions are job related, based on job analysis • More objective and consistent than unstructured interview • Legally defensible • Time efficient • Not flexible

Source: Adapted from Fried and Fottler 2011; Dessler 2016.

include use of general questions unrelated to job skills. Hiring managers can improve effectiveness of job interviews by doing the following:

- Use well-written situational or behavioral questions based on the job description (see examples of these question types in table 20.2)
- Use structured interviews, asking all interviewees the same questions
- Participate in interviewer training (or by providing training for hiring managers)

Combined with other techniques, such as selection testing, interviewing is useful in screening job qualified candidates, further evaluating candidates' communication skills, attitude, professionalism, and motivation, and in learning more about an individual's fit for the position (SHRM 2018b). Planning and preparation are required to support effective interviewing and an overall effective candidate selection process.

Check Your Understanding 20.2

Answer the following questions.

1. Reviewing workforce data and trends and deciding what positions are needed in an organization is consistent with responsibility for conducting:
   a. Workforce planning
   b. Workflow analysis
   c. Job description
   d. Job analysis
2. Collecting and analyzing information about a job in order to better understand the significant duties of the job, and to identify the skills and characteristics required, is consistent with:
   a. Workforce planning
   b. Workflow analysis
   c. Job description
   d. Job analysis
3. Job analysis is needed to support several HRM functions performed by managers. Name two of these HRM functions.
4. True or false: Advantages of internal recruiting include both less orientation for the candidate selected and a positive impact on applicants who are not selected.
5. Information in ______ is used as the basis for development of a job description.
   a. A job interview
   b. An employee performance appraisal
   c. Job specifications
   d. A job analysis
6. Listing of duties and responsibilities required of a job would be found in which of the following?
   a. Job summary
   b. Job description
   c. Job specifications
   d. Job interview
7. Where would the following information be found? Qualifications required: Bachelor's degree and two or more years of healthcare management experience.
   a. Job summary
   b. Job description
   c. Job specifications
   d. Job interview

8. Which of the following refers to the ability of a selection test to measure the job skill, knowledge, or behavior the test was intended to measure?
   a. Reliability
   b. Impact
   c. Performance
   d. Validity
9. "Describe a situation in the past where there was team conflict and how you handled it" is an example of which type of interview question?
   a. Open-ended
   b. Behavioral
   c. Situational
   d. Knowledge

Staffing

Staffing, as an HRM function, involves management decisions about the types of employees needed, how many employees are needed, how work will be organized, and how employees are scheduled in a work unit. Addressing the types and number of employees needed and filling those needs starts with workforce planning and job analysis, followed by recruitment and selection, as presented in the previous chapter section. Managers must also decide how to organize the work of the unit and how best to schedule the employees, as discussed in this section.

Organizing Work

Much of the work in HIM involves processes, such as activities in data management, the revenue cycle, disclosure of health information, or in conducting a job analysis. Process refers to systematic steps or actions taken in order to accomplish a goal, or to create a product or service (Johns 2016).

The following are the two major ways that process-type work is organized in HIM:

1. Serial work division are tasks or steps in a process are handled separately in sequence by individual workers, as with an assembly line, to complete a process.
2. Parallel work division are the same tasks are handled simultaneously by several workers; each completes all steps in the process from beginning to end, working independently of the other employees (Oachs 2016).

As an example, the triggering event in the disclosure process would be receipt of a request for disclosure. In serial work division, a clerk might open the mail and log a request in a disclosure of information tracking system. A disclosure specialist would then complete the remaining steps to validate and process the request, unless a paper health record must be retrieved in which case that step would be completed by a request to a file clerk. With parallel work division, several disclosure specialists are each responsible for receiving, logging, tracking, validating, and processing requests including retrieving the necessary health records. The specialists' work may be divided in various ways, such as by type of request (for example, attorneys, insurers, medical providers, patients). Volume of work and skill level of employees should be considered in determining which pattern of work division is the best fit.

To view the efficiency of work in a process, managers can conduct a workflow analysis, (discussed earlier in the chapter and in chapter 19, *Leadership*) identifying each step in a process sequence and how steps relate to each other. Results can help identify redundancies or roadblocks in the process.

A work distribution analysis can also be conducted. This is a process of data collection to determine the type and appropriateness of a unit's work assignments, the time allowed for the tasks, and the employees doing the work. This analysis can be accomplished by having employees log time spent on key tasks or functions (as outlined in job descriptions) during a given period of time. Results of work distribution analysis can be used to create a chart or spreadsheet to help a manager identify the following:

- Enough time is being spent on priority job functions versus minor tasks
- Some employees are working over capacity, and others are underutilized
- There is duplication of work (Oachs 2016)

Based on workflow analysis and work distribution analysis, revision in job descriptions, procedures, physical space plans, work division, or staff schedules may be made to improve work quality and productivity.

Scheduling Work

When the type, amount, steps, and distribution of work have been determined, a plan for scheduling staff can be developed that provides effective coverage of services and that is fair to employees.

Understanding the organizational definition of the workday and workweek is important in the development of standard scheduling. General rules are as follows: one **full-time equivalent (FTE)** employee is expected to work 8 hours per day, 5 days per week, 40 hours per week, 52 weeks per year, 2,080 hours in a year. There are variations, such as the alternative scheduling arrangements discussed later in this chapter. Typically, a **part-time employee** is one who consistently works less than 30 hours per week; employers define part-time and full-time employee status internally based on state and federal law (SHRM 2019).

The workweek typically begins on Sunday or Monday, with nonexempt employees paid at a higher rate for working on weekends and holidays. HIM services often cover daytime business hours, Monday through Friday. Evening and weekend hours may also be needed, or even 24-hour, seven-day-per-week coverage for specific functions or in larger organizations. The organization's hours of operation and the types and volume of services provided drive decisions regarding the number of FTEs needed to cover required HIM job functions and hours.

An equitable system of staff rotation where evening, weekend, and holiday coverage is required is important to establish so that staff feel the burden is fairly shared. Some healthcare organizations hire staff to work solely on the weekend. It is necessary for managers to be familiar with vacation policy and to plan staff vacation schedules in advance. Options for work coverage during staff vacations, or for other absences such as illness, include reassigning employees who have been cross-trained to perform several jobs, hiring temporary workers to fill in, or distributing work across other staff during the absence (Oachs 2016). Anticipating work disruptions when new systems are introduced is also important; it may be necessary to make scheduling adjustments or hire supplemental temporary workers while full-time staff attends training.

Beyond standard schedules, alternative work scheduling arrangements can allow employees more control over their schedules, offer a response to employee and family needs, may result in a morale boost and improved productivity, and can provide a recruitment feature. Adjustment to orientation and training offerings may be needed where employees are not on a standard schedule or at a single location. Alternatives described by various sources include the following:

- **Flextime**, or flexible work hours. An employee is able to choose his or her start and departure times, accommodating personal needs while completing a set number of hours each day required for a shift (typically 7 to 8) and cover the department's core busy time period (for example, 10 a.m. to 3 p.m.) (Oachs 2016).
- **Compressed workweek**. An employee works longer days to complete 40 hours of work in less than five days, perhaps on a 10-hour, four-day schedule. While presenting an advantage to some workers, downsides to this strategy include that

long days may lead to fatigue and lower productivity.

- **Job sharing**. Two or more employees split one full-time job over a day, a week, or a month. Employees in the arrangement must be compatible. A significant scheduling challenge can arise if one employee leaves the organization and a match to the sharing arrangement is not available (Oachs 2016).
- **Contingent or contract work**. In these arrangements, temporary workers supplement full-time employees for a given period of time, often as part-time workers without benefits. This offers flexibility to both parties, can be useful in transitional situations such as for special projects or in cases of a staffing vacancy. Clear contract terms are essential (Oachs 2016).
- **Telecommuting**. Also called remote or virtual work, the employee uses technology to perform work and link with the organization from home or another out-of-office location. The organization usually provides a computer and the required software. Coding, editing transcribed documents, and disclosure are HIM examples of where telecommuting can work. Advantages for the employee include reduced expense of commuting and increased productivity as there will often be fewer distractions. However, separating work from personal time and social isolation can present employee challenges. Lack of frequent communication with the employee and security concerns are challenges for the employer. An approach is to have the employee sign a telecommuting agreement with the supervisor that outlines mutual expectations such as for location, hours, communication frequency, security, and confidentiality (LeBlanc 2016).

Where shortages of qualified staff or cost considerations are concerns, some organizations have turned to **outsourcing** HIM work. With outsourcing, the organization contracts with an outside vendor firm having expertise in an area to provide staff and assume responsibility for a function such as transcription, disclosures, coding, or billing. The hired firm provides the services on-site or via telecommuting. The HIM manager's job then becomes vendor contract and relationship management (LeBlanc 2016). Advantages include not having to recruit qualified staff or to directly supervise individual employees, reducing overall cost. Disadvantages for the manager include less hands-on control over quality of work and the need to monitor vendor performance.

Offshoring, a type of outsourcing, is where employees of the vendor firm are based outside of the US. Wages are often lower than those in the US, offering a cost benefit; quality control, cultural and language differences, privacy, and security represent areas of concern (Hickman and Karban 2014). Before considering offshoring, an HIM department should have a solid technology infrastructure and strong privacy and security policies in place; vendors should be verified and contract terms carefully managed to reduce the potential for risk (Hickman and Karban 2014).

Creative approaches to staff scheduling have become more commonly used to meet a variety of human resources and business needs. Given the availability of technology to support work, pressure to reduce costs in healthcare, and the changing needs of the workforce, the use of alternative approaches to staff scheduling is expected to continue.

Measuring and Improving Performance

Performance management provides the big picture context for the relationships among important HRM functions presented in the chapter, from job analysis to recruitment, to performance appraisal to training, as represented visually in figure 20.6. Performance management, performance measurement, and performance appraisal are presented in this section of the chapter.

Figure 20.6 Relationship of HRM functions to performance management

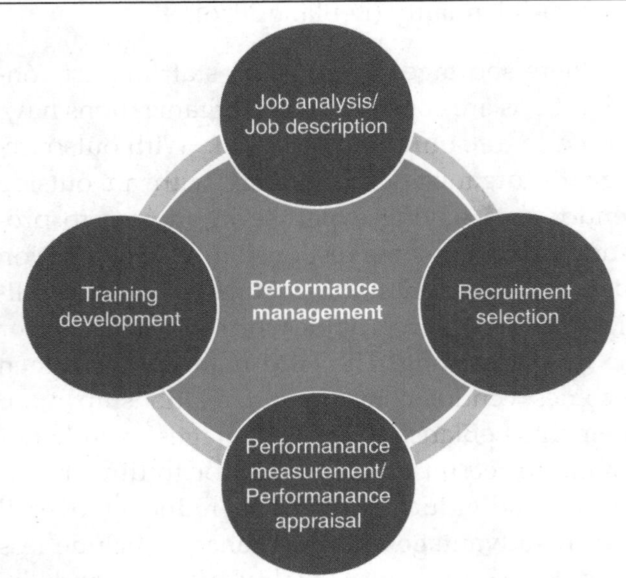

Source: Adapted from Fried and Fottler 2011, 2018; Oachs 2016.

Performance Management

The term performance management includes the full range of activities involved in measuring, reviewing, and improving employee performance, including defining job expectations, setting goals, monitoring performance, providing feedback, and designing strategies to improve performance (Fried and Fottler 2018). Performance management is not a single, scheduled review; it is an ongoing process continually fed by, and related to, other important HRM functions. For example, job analysis, previously discussed, supports the development of performance standards used for measuring performance and for performance appraisal. Information from performance appraisal can help management assess not only individual and group performance, but the effectiveness of employee recruitment and selection activities. Both job analysis and performance appraisal help to identify employee needs for training, discussed later in this chapter. Measurement of performance and development of performance standards are presented next.

Performance Measurement

Employees need to know what is expected of them, and how they are doing relative to expectations. Managers need to be able to report on the volume (amount), efficiency, and quality of work being done in a unit. Setting performance standards and measuring performance can address the needs of both. Performance measurement compares work outcomes to the established performance standards; results are typically expressed in quantifiable terms, such as rates (Oachs 2016). Examples of performance measures expressed as rates include the incomplete record delinquency rate (volume), coding productivity rate (volume), and coding accuracy rate (quality). Data on actual practice in identified performance areas are collected and reviewed.

Analysis of employee performance data based on standards can support the following:

- Employee performance appraisals
- Staffing decisions
- Job analysis and job description redesign
- Productivity and quality improvement initiatives

Developing Standards

Two methods for developing performance standards commonly used in HIM are benchmarking and work measurement. Benchmarking is based on comparison of external performance data on similar functions performed in similar organizations, collected through research. Sources of data for benchmarking include reports and articles published by national, state, and local professional associations, or through contact with peer institutions. To initiate benchmarking, a manager should first identify the work function to be benchmarked (such as coding or disclosure), the type of performance measure (such as number of health records coded or requests for information processed) and a time period (per hour or day) (Oachs 2016). The external search for relevant performance standards can then be conducted. As an example, a study of *International Classification of Diseases, Tenth Revision, Clinical Modification* (ICD-10-CM) coding productivity at a large urban teaching hospital revealed an average of 1.6 inpatient health records coded per hour in 20XX (Alakrawi et al. 2017). Any external standard should be assessed as a match to the unit's job function, organization size, patient type and volume, classification system, and health record system, and adjusted as appropriate. Internal performance data collected on the same measure can be compared to the external data to support validity of the standard.

Work measurement to develop standards is based on assessment of internal data collected on actual work performed within the organization and calculation of time it takes to do the work. The method starts by identifying the work function(s) to be measured. The following are several techniques that can be used to gather this information:

- *Analyze historical performance data*. Total hours worked on a job can be obtained from payroll records. Tracking reports in HIM information systems typically provide data by employee and job task.
- *Supervisor performs the work, logging time spent*. This gives management an understanding of the work, but the time-on-task will likely be slower than that of a skilled employee who performs the work daily, and this may not be the best use of management time.
- *Employees self-report data*. Ask employees to log what they do, time spent on tasks, units of work received and processed each day. Do this for a defined period of time, such as over two weeks excluding holidays. A log or tracking form should be provided to each participating employee for consistency of data capture. For example, a daily log entry for ICD-10-CM coding might contain: number of hours worked, number of health records received, and number coded. A basic unit/time productivity statistic can then be calculated, dividing the number of coded health records produced by time worked. For example, 24 health records coded divided by 8 hours equals a 3 record-per-hour coding productivity rate. Where multiple employees perform the same job, average data across employees to determine a productivity standard for the job.
- *Observe a sample of job functions*. Identify the job functions to be observed and define the time period (number of days or weeks) of the study. Physical functions or those that can easily be visually observed fit best with this technique. Identify and train observers on what information is to be gathered, when, and how it should be collected including observation schedule and forms. Inform the employees to be observed of the purpose of the study and how the information will be used and shared (Oachs 2016).

Determining which work measurement technique to use involves consideration of time, budget, and personnel available and willing to participate. Once developed, performance standards should be approved by upper management.

Measuring Performance

Once standards have been developed and approved, the manager can then establish a plan for ongoing measuring and monitoring of performance. Not every task needs to be monitored (that is, tracked and analyzed). The manager and the healthcare organization decide on outcomes to monitor, such as volume, turnaround time, or accuracy of key services. Data on actual practice in the identified performance areas are then collected and reviewed.

Routine methods of accurate performance data collection and review should be established. Suggestions for managers include the following:

- Require employees to complete a weekly or monthly productivity report; use an electronic format such as a spreadsheet for efficiency. See figure 20.7 for a sample employee productivity report.
- Review work volume reports available from organizational information systems, such as payroll, or from applications used by HIM employees (for example, encoders) to supplement or to validate employees' individual productivity reports.
- Include quality measures such as accuracy rate in addition to work volume statistics.

- Meet with each supervised employee (and with teams) regularly (weekly, monthly, as needed) to review data collected and discuss issues related to standards not met.

Reported performance data should be regularly analyzed for variance—where actual performance does not meet or is significantly different from the standard. Questions the manager should first consider in analyzing variances include: Does the figure represent a trend? Is there an obvious explanation: a new employee, a temporary staffing shortage due to a holiday, or a spike in work volume? Is more information or additional monitoring needed to fully assess the variance? After further review, consider if action is needed; for example, change in procedure, staffing adjustment, additional training, or counseling of an individual employee. Does the standard need review? Review table 20.3 showing a sample productivity report; consider how a manager might interpret and use this report.

Performance Appraisal

Performance appraisal refers to the formal system of review and evaluation to assess, and ultimately to improve, employee or team performance (Mondy and Martocchio 2016). Performance appraisal supports critical data collection and communication roles in performance management. Organizations need legally defensible performance data to support employee decisions such as those on pay rate, promotion, dismissal, or training and career development plans, as well as to help forecast recruitment needs. Most employees want to know where they stand and can handle constructive feedback. In a survey, 92 percent of employees responded positively to the statement, "Negative feedback, if delivered appropriately, is effective at improving performance" (Folkman 2014).

Planning and implementation of an effective and fair appraisal system involves attention to the following factors:

- Job-related criteria for employee assessment, determined through job analysis
- Clear performance expectations, agreed on in advance between manager and subordinate
- Standardization of methods, instruments, and time periods for data collection and appraisal interview with formal documentation for legal protection

Figure 20.7 Sample manual productivity report for disclosure specialist

Name: Best Employee	Mon	Tue	Wed	Thur	Fri	Sat	Sun	Weekly total	Comments
Date									
Total hours worked									
Total requests received (#)									
Requests logged into tracking system by type (#)									
Authorization verified (#)									
Processed; records sent (#)									
Media used to deliver information (**M** = mail; **E** = electronic; **F** = fax; **P** = in person; **O** = other									
Invoice sent (#)									
Unable to process and letter sent (#)									
Other work (not disclosure)									
Meetings (hours)									
Training (hours)									
Additional activity (hours); explain at Comments									

Source: Adapted from Tooley 2007; AHIMA 2012.

Table 20.3 Sample inpatient health information management productivity report

Indicator: Standard	January 2015	February 2015	March 2015
Discharges (actual volume)	5,000	5,400	5,360
Incomplete record delinquency rate: < 50%	35%	45%	50%
Days in accounts receivable due to uncoded records: < 5 days	3	5	5
Charts coded per day: ≥ 24	26	22	23
Coding accuracy: 99%	99%	95%	98%
Turnaround transcribed history and physical (H&P): < 24 hours	12	16	24
Disclosure routine requests received (actual)	200	245	300
Disclosure routine request turnaround: < 4 days	3*	3	6
Budgeted FTEs: 50 (actual)	50	50	48
Resignations: < 1%	0	0	4% (2)
Training hours (required)	4	16	8

*Background: This figure shows the average number of days it took to respond to routine disclosure requests in January based on these data: 100 requests responded to within 2 days; 100 responded to within 4 days; 200 total routine requests. Calculate turnaround: [(100 x 2 days) + (200 x 4 days)]/200 = 3 days average response rate. Average response met the standard of less than 4 days.

Source: Adapted from Oachs 2016.

- Training of appraisers in areas such as how to provide unbiased ratings, how to conduct appraisal interviews, and how to give effective feedback
- Continuous communication and feedback before and after the appraisal interview to support performance improvement and avoid surprises
- Formal grievance (complaint) procedure should the need for appeal of appraisal results arise (Mondy and Martocchio 2016)

An employee's immediate supervisor is traditionally the primary evaluator (appraiser) of performance. The supervisor has authority over and is ultimately responsible for performance of a unit, and typically is in a good position to observe an individual employee's performance. Ideally, performance data have been regularly collected, analyzed, and reviewed with employees (as discussed in the previous section). Additional sources of performance appraisal data include subordinates, peers or team members, multiple raters, and self-appraisal. Gathering performance appraisal data from additional sources allows the supervisor to consider input from others in close contact with the employee, and helps the supervisor avoid bias, also referred to as favoritism or partiality. The supervisor typically remains involved, even when additional sources are included. Pros and cons of sources of performance appraisal data are outlined in table 20.4.

Performance Appraisal Methods

Methods used in performance appraisal must meet criteria for validity and reliability concepts described previously for selection testing. Management decisions on pay, promotion, or dismissal based on a performance appraisal are subject to defense in discrimination lawsuits. The human resources department provides guidance as to an organization's accepted standard performance appraisal method(s). Some common methods are briefly described as follows:

- Graphic rating scale. A checklist is used to numerically rate employees on general traits, like job knowledge or attendance. While simple and easy to use, because this method often lacks job-related specifics, its validity and reliability may be limited in determining future job performance (Schermerhorn and Bachrach 2018).
- Comparison system. Appraiser ranks an employee compared to all others in a group or unit based on overall performance or a list of traits; employees are ranked highest to

Table 20.4 Sources of performance appraisal data: pros and cons

Appraiser	Pros	Cons
Immediate supervisor	• Often in best position to know and observe employee's work • Responsible for unit performance to which employee is a contributor • Appraisal data supports unit's employee training and development plan	• May not be familiar with all aspects of employee's job or projects (may lack technical expertise; employee may work in a different geographic location, or with multiple teams or units) • Potential for bias (positive or negative) if supervisor is the only appraiser
Subordinates	• Offers insight into manager's strengths and weaknesses • Feedback can be useful for career development	• May be perceived as "popularity" rating of limited value • If not anonymous (as in small unit or organization), subordinates may fear reprisal and not offer honest input
Peers or team members	• Provides close-up view of employee performance • Multiple opinions reduce bias • Peer pressure of evaluation can motivate team members to be more productive	• Reluctance to criticize teammates or peers • May focus on one specific problem or conflict that occurred providing an unbalanced overall assessment
Multiple sources (also called multi-rater, 360-degree rating)	• Bias is reduced by including multiple perspectives from inside and outside the organization (that is, managers, subordinates, peers, customers) • Development-focused • Emphasizes team and customer relationships	• If not anonymous (as in small unit or organization), raters may not offer honest input • Can be expensive to include multiple parties; use of an online rating system recommended • Training of appraisers and employee on purpose and procedures is required • Less useful for promotion, compensation decisions
Self	• Encourages employee involvement in appraisal process • Employees in ideal position to evaluate own performance, and identify their development goals • Provides opportunity for employee to keep supervisor informed of accomplishments, issues	• Can be manipulated to overstate good performance or minimize negatives • Not recommended for compensation decisions

lowest. This system tends to be subjective, can be difficult to apply where several employees have performed at a similar level, or where factors outside of an employee's control such as illness have impacted performance data (Mondy and Martocchio 2016).

- **Forced distribution**. Managers are required to place appraised employees into predetermined performance categories; for example, 15 percent rated as top performers, 75 percent rated average, 10 percent at the bottom. While this system can help to avoid distributional errors in ratings (see below), the rigidity can be unforgiving. Unless managers are allowed some flexibility to adjust the percentages, results can negatively impact morale among productive employees (Dessler 2016).
- **Critical incident method**. Employee and supervisor identify critical job behaviors, both positive and negative; the supervisor then observes the employee and keeps an ongoing evaluation record during the appraisal period. The need for close observation and detailed documentation represent both the strengths and weaknesses of this system (Mondy and Martocchio 2016).
- **Behaviorally anchored rating scale (BARS)**. This system links specific examples of measurable job-related behaviors, both positive and negative, to a scaled rating. For example, team leadership might be rated from 1 to 5 (Never to Always): Employee consistently volunteers to lead project teams. Objectivity, validity, and reliability are improved; rating format is typically lengthy, must be updated to reflect job changes (Mondy and Martocchio 2016).

Ensuring performance appraisal fairness can be challenging for managers and supervisors. One problem area, as noted earlier, is bias. Bias is clearly illegal when a manager allows race, color, religion, age, gender, or disability to influence performance ratings. More subtle forms of bias include a manager's tendency to rate an employee higher or lower based on a trait, such as personal appearance or punctuality, regardless of the trait's actual effect on performance. Another risk area is placing more weight on a behavior observed immediately preceding the appraisal meeting and not considering the entire review period. A ratings fairness trap for managers, the **halo-horns effect**, occurs when an employee is strong (halo) or weak (horn) in one rated area and the supervisor unfairly generalizes that performance to rate the employee high or low across all other areas on the performance appraisal (SHRM 2018c). For example, an employee gets along very well in teams and is good with conflict management; the halo effect of these strengths leads to a high overall appraisal rating despite the employee not having consistently met standards for work accuracy. **Distributional errors** in ratings are also seen: these are errors of inequity like central tendency, where a manager rates all employees satisfactory regardless of performance in order to avoid conflict, or leniency or strictness where some managers are overly generous or strict compared to other raters (Fried and Fottler 2018). Manager training is the best strategy to address these appraisal rating issues.

In the appraisal interview, supervisor and employee meet to review the performance appraisal. The following steps help the appraising supervisor plan and implement a meaningful interview:

1. *Preparation*. Review the employee's job description, performance standards, and prior appraisals. Provide the employee with advance notice (at least one week) and set a mutually agreed-upon time to meet. Identify a private place for the interview; avoid interruptions. Set aside enough time (at least an hour).
2. *Make the appraisal objective and defensible*. Base the appraisal on job-related criteria, performance standards, and data. Offer clear, specific examples to help managers and the employee interpret the appraisal consistently. Managers should avoid getting personal on the appraisal but rather compare the employee's performance to the established standards.
3. *Encourage the employee to speak, share ideas, and offer solutions*. Ask open-ended questions, such as, What do you think is causing X?
4. *Agree on an action plan going forward*. Identify what is going well and areas for improvement; specify expectations and timelines (Dessler 2016).

Check Your Understanding 20.3

Answer the following questions.

1. The HRM function that involves decisions about scheduling employees to cover a workday and workweek is known as:
   a. Work measurement
   b. Staffing
   c. Benchmarking
   d. Outsourcing
2. Which of the following refers to the range of activities involved in measuring, reviewing, and improving employee performance?
   a. Performance management
   b. Staffing
   c. Performance appraisal
   d. Workflow analysis

3. One disclosure specialist handles requests from insurance and managed care companies; another handles requests from attorneys and courts. Each completes all steps in the process from beginning to end. This is an example of which of the following?
   a. Serial work division
   b. Job sharing
   c. Job rotation
   d. Parallel work division
4. Mary can start work at her office anytime between 8 a.m. and 10 a.m. and work an 8-hour day, Monday through Friday. This is an example of what type of alternative staffing?
   a. Compressed workweek
   b. Flextime
   c. Telecommuting
   d. Contract
5. Coding is done by a vendor whose employees are in China. This is an example of which of the following?
   a. Contingent work
   b. Job sharing
   c. Outsourcing
   d. Offshoring
6. To develop performance standards for disclosure turnaround time, the manager conducted a literature search and contacted peer institutions. Which method did she use?
   a. Workflow analysis
   b. Benchmarking
   c. Work measurement
   d. Productivity analysis
7. Results of which of the following can help a manager assess prioritization of work, duplication of work, or underutilization of employees?
   a. Work distribution analysis
   b. Work measurement
   c. Benchmarking
   d. Workflow analysis
8. When reviewing the monthly performance report, a manager noticed the coding accuracy rate was below standard. She considered whether this difference might be related to a recent change in systems or to another factor. This manager is performing which of the following?
   a. Performance measurement
   b. Workforce planning
   c. Work observation study
   d. Variance analysis
9. The performance appraisal method that links specific job-related performance to each rating level is the:
   a. Graphic rating scale
   b. Critical incident technique
   c. Behaviorally anchored rating scale
   d. Forced distribution method
10. Which of the following is a positive aspect of using employee self-appraisal as a source of data for performance appraisal?
   a. Employees are in the best position to provide objective reviews without overstatement.
   b. The supervisor is kept informed of the employee's accomplishments.
   c. Appraiser and employee training on the purpose and procedures of this process is required.
   d. Peer pressure of evaluation can motivate team members to be more productive.

Employee Engagement and Retention

Given investment in job analysis, employee recruitment, selection, staffing, and performance management, the retention of employees is important to an organization. Turnover reflects the rate at which employees leave a firm and must be replaced. This rate includes voluntary employee exits and dismissals (involuntary termination of employment, discussed in the next section of the chapter). The high cost of turnover includes the costs of recruitment, the interview and testing processes in selection, pay during a new employee's orientation period when productivity may be low, and the cost of management time needed for orientation and on-the-job training.

This section explores areas where line managers, particularly immediate supervisors, can impact retention by helping to influence employee engagement within the organization and reduce costly voluntary employee turnover.

Employee Engagement

Employee engagement refers to the level of commitment employees demonstrate, their willingness to continue working for the organization and to go above and beyond the minimum expectations (SHRM 2017). Disengaged employees are described as those who have mentally quit, but remain on the job working at a low productivity level. Engagement is especially important in healthcare, an industry where cost-containment, quality of care and service, and competition are major forces. High levels of employee engagement have been linked to an organization's favorable productivity and profitability (SHRM 2017).

Factors shown to positively impact employee engagement include opportunities for improved work-life balance, such as flexibility in scheduling and work location; and job stability, where the organization is seen as growing and including the employee's role in the its growth (AHIMA House of Delegates 2017). While the employee shares responsibility for remaining engaged, managers do make a difference. Research has shown that employee engagement increases significantly when an employee's relationship with their direct supervisor is positive and includes the following:

- Clear job expectations and feedback
- Necessary equipment to do the job
- Authority to accomplish job tasks
- Freedom to make decisions about assigned work (SHRM 2017)

Reducing Turnover

Employees leave an organization voluntarily for a variety of personal reasons, including for a career change, retirement, or due to family circumstances. Managers can, however, employ the following strategies, working with the human resources department, to help retain strong performers and reduce voluntary turnover:

- *Investigate the issue*. Identify, review, and track the unit's turnover rate; analyze exit interviews (addressed later in this chapter) for issues or trends. Are new hires leaving quickly? Are top performers leaving? Why?
- *Improve selection*. Improve effectiveness of candidate testing and interviewing (presented earlier in the chapter) to help choose an individual who is the best fit with the job and the organization. Provide a realistic picture of a job to applicants, including negative aspects.
- *Provide clear expectations and feedback.* Provide clear job descriptions and effective performance appraisals, as previously discussed, supported by ongoing employee communication and feedback.
- *Provide professional growth opportunities.* Training and career development programs, addressed later in this chapter, demonstrate management's investment in an employee's long-term success.
- *Improve compensation and recognition.* Advocate for appropriate pay rates

for employees using job analysis data. Create non-pay opportunities, such as awards, to recognize employees' good work.

- *Recognize the need for work-life balance*: Consider alternative work scheduling options (addressed earlier in this chapter), where feasible (Dessler 2016, 264).

Employee Relations and Fair Treatment

Employee relations is a broad term referencing management activity focused on establishing and maintaining positive employer-employee relationships that contribute to job satisfaction, productivity, and fair discipline (Dessler 2016). Communication, respect, and fair handling of work-related disputes are themes of positive employer-employee relationships.

Communication Strategies

Without a communication system in place, managers may be unaware of problems or suggestions for improvement until a crisis has brewed. Employees like to be informed about what goes on in the organization, feel they are involved, and have a means to voice their ideas and complaints. Line managers often need training on ways to gather employee feedback, and to listen openly and respectfully to voiced complaints. The following are practical suggestions of ways to foster communication:

- Keep an open-door policy to show that a manager is accessible; this can include a physically open door, or use of a website, email, or other communication tools
- Walk around to informally connect with staff, ask open-ended questions about how things are going
- Conduct staff meetings and focus groups to encourage two-way communication
- Promote organizational options such as hotlines, suggestion boxes, or surveys for employees to voice ideas and concerns

Reviewing results of employee surveys and exit interviews conducted by the human resources department can help managers better understand employee attitudes and concerns. Exit interview refers to the final meeting an employee has with his or her employer; the meeting provides an opportunity to collect feedback on issues or problem areas, including what may have caused the employee to leave (LeBlanc 2016).

Most employees want to make suggestions. An active approach to increase employee involvement in problem-solving is appointment of a temporary suggestion team focused on a specific work-related issue (Dessler 2016). This team is given a specific charge, such as to improve workflow in an area, provided meeting space or a website, and asked to propose ideas to management by a target date.

Conflict Management

Despite efforts at employee communication, some conflict is to be expected where people work together, especially in teams. The type and intensity of conflict are of concern to managers. Some level of healthy disagreement is necessary to encourage new ideas and creativity in an organization, but too much conflict becomes distracting and harmful. Dysfunctional conflict is a destructive type of struggle that becomes emotionally draining and harms productivity.

There are many sources of conflict, from individual personalities and beliefs to organizational issues such as role confusion, scarce resources, and tasks that are interdependent across employees or departments. Healthcare organizations have become more culturally, racially, and gender diverse, increasing the potential for greater creativity and problem-solving along with the potential for employee conflict. Organizations that have been successful in managing diversity and minimizing conflict have in common a commitment to valuing diversity and inclusion, to treating employees as individuals rather than as members of a group, and to accommodation of family needs (Gomez-Mejia et al. 2016).

When dysfunctional conflict does occur, avoidance of the disruption may be a natural management response, and in some situations may be the appropriate approach. But avoidance does not resolve the issue. True conflict resolution requires collaboration; this approach takes time and requires the willingness of all parties to participate (Schermerhorn and Bachrach 2018). Determining the best approach to conflict management involves consideration of time, budget, the importance and complexity of the issues at play, and the potential for long-term damage if conflict is not resolved. Table 20.5 identifies common conflict management strategies and suggests when each should be used.

Disciplinary Action

When an employee fails to follow rules, policies, or procedures, or fails to meet performance standards, organizations have processes in place for applying disciplinary action in the form of performance counseling or penalty. Efforts to ensure fairness of disciplinary action and to show respect for employees are critical in supporting positive employee relations. Supervisors do this by investigating facts before taking disciplinary action, by not acting when angry, by remaining objective, avoiding bias, and clearly explaining discipline policy and right of appeal to an employee (Dessler 2016). Failure to follow and apply disciplinary policy consistently across all employees may lead to EEOC charges of discrimination and even to lawsuits from employees in a protected class.

Fair discipline in most organizations includes a system of progressive penalties that calls for applying the minimum action necessary based on the severity of the offense. The goal is to formally communicate the issue to an employee and allow for a change in behavior. Progressive disciplinary actions typically follow a sequence starting with a documented verbal warning for first offense of minor severity, such as for dress code violation, with a written warning for the second instance. For serious rule violations, such as bringing a weapon to work, immediate dismissal may be the appropriate initial penalty (Mondy and Martocchio 2016).

As with conflict management, avoidance does not address discipline problems and can compound the disciplinary process. For example, an overly lenient annual performance appraisal rating of an employee with poor productivity provides weak background documentation when a manager ultimately faces discipline of that employee. The employee may complain, perhaps justly, that no feedback was provided.

Handling Grievances

Issues related to promotion, transfer, and layoff top the list of sources of employee complaints, followed by performance appraisal, work assignment, and scheduling (Dessler 2016). A grievance process is a formal procedure for management review of employee complaints designed to ensure fair treatment (Dessler 2016). Facing an employee grievance can be challenging for a manager, but most large (and all unionized) organizations have

Table 20.5 Approaches to conflict management

Method	When to apply
Avoidance: Ignore the issue; withdraw or back off	Where focus on a higher priority issue is urgent, or where parties involved need time to "cool off"
Accommodation: Downplay differences, focus on similarities and areas of agreement; conflict remains, peaceful co-existence is achieved	An issue is minor and more important to an employee than to the manager or organization; when seeking team harmony and moving on is the goal
Compromise: Bargaining, trade-offs; each side gives up something, gains something; risk is that conflict may reoccur	For complex issues where a temporary or rapid resolution is needed where time is limited
Collaboration: Problem-solving; addresses the issues, differences, and underlying conflict to arrive at a mutually beneficial resolution; all parties invest in the process	Ideal for long-term problem-solving and true conflict resolution, but takes time (costly); depends on willingness of all parties to participate openly in process
Command: Authority figure issues a directive to resolve the issue	When quick action is needed, as in a crisis, or when a law, policy, or an unpopular decision must be enforced

Source: Adapted from Schermerhorn and Bachrach 2018, 278.

policy and a multistep procedure in place for handling grievances to make the process clear for both employee and employer. Supervisors should be familiar with the organization's grievance process.

Guidelines for handling grievances start with efforts to recognize and correct sources of dissatisfaction before formal grievances occur, such as by developing open communication with employees and with fair approaches to performance appraisal and discipline, as noted earlier. For example, the opportunity for employees to voice their views, such as on performance ratings, may be handled using informal communication channels like the open-door policy previously described.

Points to address when handling a formal grievance process include the following:

- Inform the next level of management of the grievance
- Be familiar with the organization's formal grievance policy and procedure, including required forms
- Work with the union representative, as applicable
- Investigate the situation thoroughly;
- Review the employee's personnel file and any prior grievance reports
- Meet with the employee in private to discuss the grievance; listen
- Stay focused on facts
- Respond within time limits specified by organizational policy or labor union contract (Dessler 2016)

Managers should be prepared to work through any next steps in the grievance process, which may include working on a solution with the employee (and union representative where applicable), a hearing, or appeal of the grievance decision. Ineffective handling of grievances can put a healthcare organization at risk of costly liability should an employee take legal action to dispute the grievance decision.

Dismissal

Termination of employment is a broad term encompassing both voluntary separation by the employee, as well as dismissal of the employee by the employer. **Dismissal** is the involuntary termination of employment.

The legal concept of **termination at will** generally recognizes that the employer or the employee can terminate employment for any reason unless prohibited by law (SHRM 2018d). However, employees do have protections against wrongful discharge based on statutes (for example, Title VII), contracts, and court decisions. **Wrongful discharge** is unfair dismissal due to failure of the employer to comply with law, organizational policy, or a contract. For example, an employee who is a member of a protected class is dismissed based on performance; annual performance appraisals show that performance standards had been met. Wrongful discharge based on discrimination under Title VII would a concern in this scenario. A wrongfully discharged employee may take their case to court.

Appropriate reasons for dismissal of an employee fall into the following four general groups:

1. *Performance*. Consistent failure to perform assigned job duties, or to meet specified performance standards, as documented
2. *Conduct*. Intentional violation of the organization's policies or rules
3. *Qualifications*. Inability to perform skills or to meet other specified qualifications of the assigned job; training and job transfer have been explored
4. *Elimination*. Elimination of work, the job, or change in job requirements (Dessler 2016)

Dismissal is obviously a very serious HRM action. This step should be taken when needed, but only after careful planning and consultation with the human resources department to ensure that all documentation is in order and that law, policy, and (where applicable) union contract are followed. The employee should not be surprised by the decision if clear feedback and support have been given via performance appraisal and in the progressive disciplinary process. Yet, involuntary loss of employment can be traumatic even for the well-informed employee who may feel fear, failure, disappointment, or anger; dismissal is also difficult on the manager making the decision (Mondy and Martocchio 2016).

Best practices include scheduling a dismissal interview early in the week to allow the dismissed employee to begin an immediate job search. Avoid dates of special significance to the employee, such as birthday or religious holiday, to show respect. The employee's direct supervisor should conduct the meeting; a human resources representative should be asked to attend to confirm what occurred during the dismissal meeting (SHRM 2018d).

These following additional guidelines are recommended for the dismissal interview:

- Conduct the well-planned meeting in person, scheduled for about 10 minutes
- Use a conference room or other neutral location (not manager's office). Have phone numbers for security available in case medical attention is needed or a threatening situation develops
- Get to the point. Briefly describe the situation in a few clear sentences using facts; state the decision
- Listen to the employee but leave no options.
- Provide severance information and final paycheck (arranged in advance with the human resources department)
- Close the interview; tell the employee where they should go next (Dessler 2016)
- Ensure that keys and other organization property are collected and the employee's access to computer systems has been blocked (SHRM 2018d)

Solid hiring decisions, as discussed earlier in this chapter, are the best strategy for reducing the need for disciplinary-based dismissals.

For economic reasons, an employer may initiate nondisciplinary dismissal of one or more employees in the form of a layoff or downsizing. **Layoff** is a temporary dismissal where employees are told there is no work available now, but that they may be recalled if work becomes available; in **downsizing**, the number of employees is permanently reduced (Dessler 2016).

Senior management makes the strategic layoff or downsizing decision and is responsible for compliance with applicable law, such as the WARN Act described earlier in the chapter. Supervisors may have roles in determining which employees stay on the job and of informing staff of the outcome; handling the situation with fairness and respect is important. This involves keeping all employees informed and basing fair decisions as to who stays on job descriptions, performance appraisals, or on seniority. Layoff and downsizing decisions can have a negative effect on morale for those remaining at work. It is important to acknowledge the feelings of remaining employees and to communicate concern for those who have been dismissed, sharing facts regarding provision of any severance packages or services provided (Maurer 2017).

Labor Relations

While unions are not present in all work settings, it is worthwhile to examine what a union is and to consider the management relationship in a unionized environment. A **union** is an organization formed by employees for the purpose of acting as a group when dealing with management regarding work issues (Fried and Fottler 2018). Research from a variety of sources indicates that pay and benefits, along with employee concerns regarding employer fairness, job security, and lack of recognition are among the factors that drive interest in labor unions (Carrell and Heavrin 2013).

The right of workers to unionize is recognized from an ethical perspective as a human right consistent with the principle of autonomy, presented earlier in the chapter. In the US, workers' right to unionize and to bargain collectively with management is protected by labor law, also presented earlier in the chapter. Union membership in the US was 10.5 percent of the total workforce in 2018, essentially unchanged from 2017, but down significantly from 20.1 percent in 1983; union membership is highest among public sector workers (BLS 2019). In 2018, SEIU Healthcare, part of the Service

Employees International Union (SEIU), was the largest healthcare union in North America at more than 1.1 million members (SEIU 2018). A brief overview of the union-organizing process and key concepts for supervisors in union settings are presented in this section.

Union Organization

In the initial phase of union development within a workplace, labor union officials attempt to gauge the level of employee interest in joining a union. Union representatives provide employees information (outside of scheduled work hours) about unionization and solicit signing of authorization cards. An authorization card is a document that indicates an employee's interest in having a union represent him or her. The next step is for the union to petition the NLRB for an election to become the employees' representative. The NLRB verifies the signed authorization cards and recognizes a group of employees within the organization to be the bargaining unit, those who will be represented by the union. By law, supervisors and managers are excluded from the employee bargaining unit.

Once a bargaining unit is certified, an election is scheduled to decide whether the union will represent the employee group (bargaining unit). Prior to the vote, a campaign takes place where both management and the union can make appeals to employees, consistent with law. A simple majority of votes cast by workers in the bargaining unit is typically required to win the election. If the union does win the right to represent employees, collective bargaining begins. The NLRB describes collective bargaining as a mutual obligation of the employer and union "to meet at reasonable times to bargain in good faith about wages, hours, vacation time, insurance, safety practices and other mandatory subjects" and negotiate agreement (NLRB 2018a). Labor law defines the types of items required in collective bargaining (for example, wages) versus those that are voluntary (such as budget for continuing education). The concept of good-faith bargaining assumes that both sides are participating and willing to negotiate an agreement.

Ultimately, if there is failure to agree after repeated attempts, unionized employees may initiate a strike, a temporary work stoppage called in an effort to express an employment contract negotiation demand. A strike obviously represents a low point in labor union–management relations, and is distressing for all parties. Managers in unionized healthcare organizations should work with the human resources department to understand the rules for communication with employees and the plans for worker replacement to support essential functions in case a strike scenario develops.

Supervising in a Union Environment

Organizations may see labor unions as interference with management. Top management may take an opposing view during a union-organizing effort, actively presenting its "side" to employees using a variety of communication methods. Once a union officially represents employees, the collective bargaining process may become contentious.

Demonstrating respect for employees' right to join unions, along with knowledge of the laws in place, provides a foundation for front-line managers in a union environment to best work with their employees. Managers and supervisors facing union-organizing campaigns are advised to be truthful in providing information to employees and to avoid interfering with legal unionizing activity. Managers should be aware of and consistently enforce rules in a nondiscriminatory manner, such as those regarding union solicitation and distribution of union literature. As offered by the NLRB on this topic:

> Working time is for work, so your employer may maintain and enforce nondiscriminatory rules limiting solicitation and distribution, except that your employer cannot prohibit you from talking about or soliciting for a union during non-work time, such as before or after work or during break times… (NLRB 2018b).

Two easy-to-recall acronyms, TIPS and FORE, offer terms and concepts to help managers remember what to do or to avoid in a union environment, consistent with respect for employees' right to unionize, the ethical principle of justice, and labor law compliance. See table 20.6.

Table 20.6 TIPS and FORE: Useful acronyms for supervisors during a union-organizing drive

Term	Example
Threaten	Do not threaten loss of job, reduce hours, or discipline because of employees' union election or other union activity. Intimidating behavior risks long-term damage to the employer–employee relationship.
Interrogate	Do not ask an employee, "How are you going to vote?" or "Have you signed a union authorization card?" Do not schedule mandatory one-on-one meetings with employees to discuss union representation.
Promise	Do not promise a salary increase, promotion, or favor in exchange for a union vote.
Spy	Do not go to union meetings or try to listen in on conversations about the union during employee breaks.
Facts	Do state facts, such as that signing an authorization card makes the union an employee's legal representative. Review current human resource policies related to solicitation. Do this in a way that is informative, avoids distortion, and is not intimidating.
Opinion	Do voice your professional opinion on the value of a union, when asked by an employee, without telling the employee(s) what to do. Be honest.
Rules	Do accurately review what the law permits, such as regarding worker replacement in the event of a strike. Again, be informative as opposed to threatening. Consistently enforce rules on solicitation and distribution of any non-work-related information during work hours, not just during a union drive.
Experience	Do share your personal experience, positive or negative, in working with or as a member of a labor union. Be honest and factual.

Source: Adapted from Carrell and Heavrin 2013.

Check Your Understanding 20.4

Answer the following questions.

1. The rate at which employees leave an organization and must be replaced is known as:
   a. Dismissal
   b. Turnover
   c. Engagement
   d. Retention

2. An employee's positive relationship with a direct supervisor who offers clear job expectations and feedback has been shown to increase:
   a. Dismissal
   b. Turnover
   c. Engagement
   d. Communication

3. Strategies to reduce voluntary turnover include all of the following *except:*
   a. Improve candidate testing and interviewing
   b. Provide professional growth opportunities for employees
   c. Investigate turnover issues
   d. Use a system of progressive penalties

4. Fair approaches to performance appraisal and disciplinary processes can help to prevent:
   a. Strike
   b. Turnover
   c. Grievances
   d. Wrongful discharge

5. An employee's dismissal interview should be conducted by:
   a. The Director of Human Resources
   b. The employee's immediate supervisor
   c. The Director of Security
   d. A manager familiar with the employee's work
6. An employee indicates interest in having a union represent him by:
   a. Participating in a strike
   b. Speaking with management
   c. Signing an authorization card
   d. Participating in collective bargaining
7. Communication strategies a manager can use to help build positive employer-employee relations include all the following *except:*
   a. Conducting staff meetings and focus groups
   b. Walking around to observe and critique performance
   c. Having an open-door policy
   d. Promoting use of suggestion boxes and hotlines
8. A conflict occurred within a workgroup. The issue was minor, but had become a distraction. The team leader felt it was important to get the group back on track and move on. Which of the following conflict management approaches would be best in this situation?
   a. Avoidance
   b. Accommodation
   c. Compromise
   d. Command
9. Juan arrived late to work; when asked, he explained his commuter train had been delayed. This was his first tardy incident. His supervisor reminded Juan of the policy for notification should this happen again. Juan was issued a verbal warning, consistent with:
   a. Employment at will
   b. The disciplinary process
   c. A system of progressive penalties
   d. Accommodation
10. Respecting employees' free choice to join a labor union, a manager can legally do which of the following during a union-organizing drive?
   a. Threaten reduced hours or loss of job based on an employee's union vote.
   b. Interrogate employees regarding union activity.
   c. Promise a party, pay raise, or other favor based on union vote.
   d. State facts, such as the organization's policy prohibiting solicitation during work time.

Training and Development

As HIM roles continue to evolve and become more complex, higher skill levels are needed to support success. Greater use of technology, production of more data, and pressure to improve healthcare efficiency are among drivers of need for more HIM employees with analytical, critical-thinking, and leadership skills (AHIMA House of Delegates 2017). Changes in jobs and roles impact essentially all HRM functions from job analysis to staff recruitment and selection to training and development. Strategies to address skill gaps include hiring new workers, retraining existing workers for new roles, bringing back and retraining retirees, and shifting workers into different roles within the unit or the organization (Fried and Fottler 2018). In healthcare, the training function is typically decentralized. This means that departments or units are responsible for their specific training needs; the human resources department manages education programs required for employees organization-wide (for example, OSHA compliance) and for management training (for example, equal employment opportunity law compliance). Accrediting agencies such as the Joint Commission require documentation of staff training; this may be managed centrally to ensure compliance. The process of connecting employees to the organization and initiating training begins with new employee orientation, discussed in the next section.

New Employee Orientation

New employee orientation includes a group of activities that welcome new employees and introduce them to the healthcare organization; to the assigned department, unit, or workgroup; and to the specific job to be performed. It is the first step in helping the employee to feel knowledgeable, competent, and satisfied (Patena 2016). Formats vary, though large healthcare facilities typically have a formal process for new employee orientation. Some activities may be conducted one-on-one, others in a group of new employees, and some activities may be computerized. An aspect of successful orientation is onboarding, time spent upfront to welcome, socialize, and integrate a new employee into the values and culture of an organization, benefitting both employee and employer (Harden 2017). An example of a best practice that demonstrates this approach is shown in figure 20.8.

Because there is so much for the new employee to absorb, orientation typically takes places over several days or even weeks. While orientation responsibility is typically shared between the human resources department staff and the line manager, peers can also play a role. Some organizations assign a buddy or mentor (current senior employee) to each new employee to help them get adjusted. Each healthcare facility and job has unique orientation content, but some topics are commonly addressed with respect to the employee, the organization, and the job; see table 20.7.

Regardless of the specific schedule or content of orientation, obtaining evaluation feedback from new employees is essential to support improvement going forward. Orientation sets the stage for further employee training and development, discussed next.

Employee Training and Development

Training, a term mentioned throughout this chapter, refers to providing new or current employees with knowledge, skills, and abilities related to the competencies needed to perform their present jobs. Training can also fulfill legal requirements or support essential organizational goals, such as

Figure 20.8 New employee onboarding best practice: example

New employee onboarding at The Mayo Clinic, Rochester, Minnesota

Goals of the strategic onboarding process:

- Engage the new employee
- Affirm the employment decision
- Introduce the organization's culture
- Prepare the new employee to be a successful contributor

On the first day: New employee is met at the door by an assigned mentor, a senior employee who has already been in contact and who becomes an onboarding mentor. The mentor escorts the newcomer to human resources to finalize paperwork, most of which has been taken care of in advance. The mentor next guides the new employee to the assigned office area, introduces her to individuals with whom she will be working directly, and then takes her to a welcome reception with colleagues were food is served.

The focus is on introducing the organization's people and culture, providing a positive first impression, and setting the stage to keep momentum going on the job.

Source: Adapted from Harden 2017.

Table 20.7 Common types of content covered during new employee orientation

Employee-centered • Compensation (pay, holidays) and benefits (insurance, retirement) • Career development opportunities, career planning resources
Organization-centered • Organization overview: history, mission, structure, services, customs, culture • Health and safety information and procedures • Privacy and security policies and procedures; related system access and training • Employment policies and procedures (sick leave, vacation, discipline and grievance processes) • How to file a discrimination or harassment complaint • Information on employee activities and events • Tour of facility • Networking/socialization activity • Evaluation of orientation
Job- or department-centered • Job description, job duties, schedule, performance standards • Department policies and procedures • Introduction to workspace and equipment • Department tour • Socialization activity with coworkers • Meeting with supervisor; question and answer session, feedback on orientation
Unique considerations for outsourced workers • Contractual expectations for quality control, such as performance measures • Training to address cultural, language, legal differences (for offshore workers)

Source: Adapted from Fried and Fottler 2011; Patena 2016.

valuing diversity. Diversity awareness training educates employees, including managers, on specific cultural and gender differences and how to respond to these in the workplace (Gomez-Mejia et al. 2016). **Development** has a longer-term focus designed to increase or enhance employee skills, knowledge, or abilities needed for the employee's career advancement and by the organization in the future (Gomez-Mejia et al. 2016). Both training and development are learning strategies that support employee recruitment, productivity, performance improvement, and engagement, serving organizations well in a competitive environment. Investment in employee training and development is necessary but comes at a cost to the organization. Therefore, careful planning and implementation are required to support effectiveness. Training is discussed first in the chapter, followed by career development.

Planning and Implementation

Numerous experts in the HRM and instructional design fields have recommended the **ADDIE model** as a general guide to planning and implementing employee training programs. The following are the ADDIE model steps:

1. *Analyze*. Assess and document a learning need for the training. Sources of information for this step include job analyses, performance reports, performance appraisals, external requirements of law or accreditation, trends noted in literature, employee surveys, focus groups, and exit interviews.
2. *Design*. Establish objectives for the training, and to use as criteria for evaluating the training when complete. Identify the target employee audience for the training and the delivery method(s). Develop a realistic budget; obtain any required approvals.
3. *Develop*. Create the training program content and lesson plans; identify instructor(s), equipment, and supplies needed. (Alternately, purchase from a vendor a packaged training program that meets the identified need, objectives, and budget, and that fits the target audience.) Consider a pilot or test run of the training program before full implementation, if possible.
4. *Implement*. Schedule, publicize, and provide the training to the identified employee audience.

5. *Evaluate*. Conduct evaluation of the training. Evaluation criteria may include employee reactions (Did employees find the training valuable?) or measurement of job performance improvement after training. Analyze evaluation results. If additional training needs are identified, restart the planning process at step 1.

The nature of the audience—adult learners—is important to consider in planning effective employee training. Most adults are challenged to some degree with balancing work, home, and personal demands; time is valuable. Concepts to consider in supporting adult learners that can also contribute to successful training, include the following:

- *Motivation*. Adults are more likely to remember material that is relevant to their life and work and that has practical value to them. Positive training participation and outcomes are more likely when employees see a direct connection between the training and an interesting work goal or to an opportunity for growth.
- *Knowledge of results*. Adults appreciate feedback, ideally immediately, on their performance.
- *Reinforcement*. Motivators to participate in training include incentive pay or rewards, a convenient training schedule that saves time, and immediate feedback on performance (Patena 2016).

Additional considerations regarding training include attention to learning styles and special needs of the target audience. Some workers and groups respond more enthusiastically than others to social interaction; plan accordingly. A mix of methods can be used to address different sensory needs of learners: use of sound for the auditory learner, reading material for the visual learner, and simulated practice for the hands-on learner (Patena 2016). As required by the ADA, employers must make reasonable accommodations for access to training by employees with disabilities. For example, to accommodate trainees with hearing impairment, include captioning in videos.

Delivery Methods

Multiple delivery options are available for training. The one(s) selected should be based on training objectives, audience, content, and budget. Major training delivery methods are described in this section.

Classroom-based learning refers to instructor-led, face-to-face training; lectures, workshops, and seminars are common formats. Small group discussion can be added to encourage learner interaction, as appropriate to the topic. This method is commonly used by managers because it is familiar and is efficient for offering facts to a large group in the same location at the same time. Scheduling face-to-face classroom-based training can present challenges for employer and employees; training should be conducted during the employee's regular working hours. Classroom sessions can be videotaped for playback to those unable to attend the live meeting. Where face-to-face interaction is needed, such as for team-building or conflict resolution training, live classroom delivery that includes small group work would be an effective choice. Cost of classroom training is a disadvantage where charges for room rental, food, and travel for employees not in the same location are included. Where employees enter training at varying skill levels, self-paced online learning is often a better delivery option (Patena 2016).

Online learning is a broad term referring to the use of electronic media to deliver training instead of face-to-face, classroom-based learning. Typically, online learning is self-paced, with instructor leadership; students and instructor communicate, though often not in real-time. Approaches include use of videoconferencing, webinars, learning management systems, web-based portals, and mobile devices such as smartphones and tablets. Advantages of the online learning method include cost savings, convenience, flexibility of scheduling for employees and trainers not in the same location, and the ability to customize content to workers' needs. Disadvantages include some interpersonal skills, such as team building, are not easily taught outside of the face-to-face classroom (Patena 2016). Webinars to help employees stay current on regulatory or coding changes are examples where online learning can be effective. The self-paced online certification exam preparation courses offered by AHIMA are other examples of this delivery method (AHIMA 2018a).

Simulation training uses physical devices, computer-based scenarios, and video gaming to provide hands-on practice. The learner interacts with a fictional experience as if it were real, chooses actions, and answers questions. The feedback provided in simulation training may enhance motivation to learn. AHIMA's Virtual Lab is an example of an online environment that provides simulations and actual practice using HIM applications (AHIMA 2018b).

On-the-job training refers to an employee learning his or her job by actually doing it as part of a structured training plan. On-the-job training can apply to new employees, as well as to current employees learning a new job or system. Trainers can be the supervisor or an experienced peer employee. A team of experienced employees can be assigned to support a new employee learning an operation; phone or other media can be used to field questions, helpful where employees work remotely (Dessler 2016). The basic steps outlined in figure 20.9 can be used by the trainer(s) to help structure on-the-job training and support the employee receiving training.

Other approaches to on-the-job training include use of job rotation, where an employee moves from one job to the next, learning aspects of each job; this is applicable to supervisors needing to learn various functions within a department or organization. Shadowing, which provides a quick review of a job, is used to show one employee what tasks another employee handles on a daily basis. Cross-training refers to an employee learning to competently perform several jobs within a unit or department. Cross-training provides scheduling flexibility helpful to management and offers high-performing employees an opportunity to develop new skills.

Figure 20.9 Steps for on-the-job training

Step 1	**Prepare the employee** Put the employee at ease Explain the job and find out what the individual already knows about it Get the employee interested in learning the job (motivate to learn) Explain why the job is important (motivate to learn) Clarify standards of performance If using equipment, assure the employee is in the correct position for use Familiarize the employee with equipment and materials needed
Step 2	**Present the operation** Explain and show one important step at a time Stress each key point slowly Instruct clearly, completely, and patiently, but no more than the employee can master Have the employee explain what has been demonstrated
Step 3	**Try out performance** Have the employee do the job and correct any errors Have the employee explain each key point as he or she does the job again Make sure the employee understands the steps; answer any questions Continue until the employee demonstrates confidence Put the employee on his or her own
Step 4	**Follow-up** Designate to whom the employee is to go for help Check frequently and encourage questions Compliment good work; offer constructive feedback Taper off close supervision but continue monitoring work against standards Check back periodically

Source: Adapted from Juran 1995; Dessler 2016.

Career Development

Given the changing healthcare landscape—consolidations, mergers, new technology and regulations—workers may find the need to develop, or redevelop, themselves to fit in. This is true for HIM. Coders' auditing skills have increased in importance with the use of computer-assisted coding. Skills in data analysis are needed as healthcare organizations collect and store more health data. A workforce study showed that in the future HIM professionals anticipated spending less work time on coding tasks; skills in leadership, training, data analytics, and informatics were identified as important, as was the need for advanced education (Marc el al. 2017).

Career development is the process by which employees assess their existing skills, knowledge, experience, and interests, establish career objectives, and develop a course of action; the outcome is an employee career development plan (SHRM 2018e). The greater the overlap between the employee's career interests and objectives and those of the employer, the greater the opportunity for mutual benefit (SHRM 2018e). Career development may include training components, but the purpose is to address the longer-term needs of an individual employee; benefits to the organization are building workforce talent and supporting retention (Elsdon 2012).

Figure 20.10 Sample employee career development plan

Employee career development plan

Employee:
Job title:
Date:

Department or unit:
Supervisor:
Target date for next plan review:

Long-term career goal (desired in 5+ years):

____

____

Short-term objectives (achieve in next 1-5 years) (skills, jobs, education, etc.):

____

____

____

Employee's major strengths: ______________________________

____

____

Career development/training needs to support goal and objectives:

____

____

Action steps (to support short-term objectives)

Description	Target date
Complete self-paced training modules on X	*By x date*
Attend continuing education seminar on X	*As scheduled*
Complete special project	*As assigned by supervisor*
Gather information on three schools offering bachelor's degree completion programs; review with mentor and supervisor	*By end of next quarter*

Signed:

Source: Adapted from Elsdon 2010; SHRM 2018f.

The next sections of this chapter will cover the roles of the employer and employee in addressing employee career development.

Employer Role

Managers can use the performance appraisal process as a career development practice, connecting an employee's job performance, training needs, and career interests. Use of the existing appraisal process is efficient (versus creating a new process) and serves to link the organization's needs to employee career development and career planning. The performance appraisal interview provides a time to discuss the employee's strengths, training and development needs, and career plans, and then to agree on action steps. This can work especially well if employee self-appraisal is a component of the performance appraisal process, is completed in advance of the appraisal interview, and includes questions on the employee's career development needs and objectives. Documenting the manager–employee agreed-upon career development plan with a timeline for tracking progress is important. See figure 20.10 for an example of a format that can be used to document and track an employee career development plan.

Other career development practices are coaching and mentoring, applicable to both new and experienced employees. Coaching, the process of educating and training subordinates, is a managerial skill (Dessler 2016). In addition to offering specific job-related training, an effective coach provides an employee with feedback and support, serving as a professional role model and as a sounding board for career advice. HIM department managers and supervisors who demonstrate interest in their employees' career development, and who are willing to invest the time to provide thoughtful advising, can be effective career coaches. Mentoring involves career advising and counseling of an employee, and can be performed by a manager, but more often is a role for a senior employee. Mentors may be assigned to an employee as part of a formal mentoring program, or chosen informally by the employee. A mentor can assist a fellow employee in making professional connections within the organization and in professional associations and may be able to point the employee toward opportunities that assist in skill-building.

Referral of employees to internal and external resources can support a career development plan. Large organizations may have a career center, career planning workshops, or a budget to support an employee's access to outside continuing education. Best practice for managers is to have a list of internal, as well as external government and professional association, resources available when providing career development advice to employees.

Employers need to be aware of healthcare industry and HIM professional employment trends and share these during employee career development advising. HIM managers can obtain access to online professional resources, such as the most recently published AHIMA workforce study and the Bureau of Labor Statistics' *Occupational Outlook Handbook for Medical Records and Health Information Technicians* published by the DOL (BLS 2018).

Employee Role

While employer guidance is important, employees today need to take personal responsibility for career decisions and be active in their own career planning. Managers can challenge employees to take charge of their career development by suggesting that employees regularly ask themselves (and answer) the following questions:

- Who am I?
- What can I do?
- Where do I want to go? By when?
- How do I get there? (Schermerhorn and Bachrach 2018, 187)

Managers can encourage and support employees' career development by pointing out available career assessment and planning tools and by making time to answer employees' follow-up questions. As examples, the Department of Labor's O*Net offers a free online occupational and career assessment system that helps an employee sort interests, skills, and career options (DOL 2019). AHIMA's Career and Student Center offers online career mapping and other information for HIM professionals

(AHIMA 2018c). Assigning visits to these sites, or asking an employee to write a short essay on his or her dream job, can serve as career planning exercises in advance of a scheduled performance appraisal interview or career development discussion. Employees should be expected to follow through on agreed-upon timelines as part of a documented career development plan, and to proactively seek advice when barriers to accomplishing action steps are encountered.

Return on Investment: Training and Development

Given the cost of employee training and career development (time and dollars), and pressure within the healthcare industry to reduce cost, is it worth the investment. Consider a brief summary of the following points offered across this chapter that support an investment in training and development of an organization's workforce:

- Successful (productive) organizations manage people as assets to be developed
- Managers trained in understanding of employment law can help ensure compliance and avoid legal and financial liability for the organization
- Turnover is costly; top reasons why high-performing employees leave organizations include the lack of career development opportunity

After investing in recruitment, selection, and orientation of employees, designing equitable staffing plans, measuring performance, and conducting performance appraisal, it seems only logical that an organization should invest in training and development to help retain its best employees. Hiring new employees is costly and involves risk. Keeping and developing proven staff, and retraining staff as workforce needs change, are cost-effective HRM strategies.

Check Your Understanding 20.5

Answer the following questions.

1. Educational programs with a longer-term focus, designed to stimulate professional growth by enhancing an employee's skills, knowledge, or abilities needed for career advancement are referred to broadly as:
   a. Training
   b. Development
   c. Coaching
   d. Simulation learning
2. The socialization of new employees into the values and culture of an organization is referred to as:
   a. Training
   b. Development
   c. Onboarding
   d. Orientation
3. Identify which of the following statements is NOT true when providing training to adult learners.
   a. Adult learners appreciate immediate feedback on performance.
   b. A convenient training schedule that saves time provides motivation for adult employees to participate.
   c. Positive training outcomes are more likely when adult employees see a direct connection between the training and an opportunity for growth.
   d. Adults are unlikely to remember practical training material that is relevant to their life or work.
4. The role in career development of counseling and advising an employee that is most often performed by a senior employee is known as:
   a. Training
   b. Coaching
   c. Mentoring
   d. Career planning

5. Using the ADDIE model for training planning and implementation, setting objectives and preparing a budget for training occur during:
   a. Step 1
   b. Step 2
   c. Step 4
   d. Step 5
6. A work unit has identified the need for conflict management training for managers and supervisors. Which of the following would be the best training delivery method?
   a. Classroom-style learning with lecture
   b. Videoconference or webinar
   c. Classroom-style learning with small group exercises
   d. Online learning with discussion boards
7. Using a structured on-the-job-training process, "Check frequently and encourage questions" would occur during which of the following steps?
   a. Step 1: Prepare the employee
   b. Step 2: Present the operation
   c. Step 3: Try out performance
   d. Step 4: Follow up
8. An example of an action an employee might take for himself or herself in the career development and career planning process would be to:
   a. Complete the Department of Labor's O*Net online occupational and career assessment
   b. Provide coaching and mentoring
   c. Connect job performance, training needs, and expressed career interests during the annual performance appraisal advising
   d. Refer to organizational career planning services and external resources

HIM Roles

Throughout the chapter, HRM roles and responsibilities of HIM managers with authority for supervision of HIM employees have been described. In summary, examples where HIM managers may be directly involved in human resources management functions include one or all of the following areas:

- Compliance with employment law and ethical principles
- Workforce planning
- Job analysis and development of job descriptions
- Recruitment and selection of staff
- Organizing and scheduling work
- Performance measurement
- Performance appraisal
- Employee engagement
- Conflict management
- Handling of grievances, discipline, and labor relations
- Training and career development

Health information management managers work with the support and advice of the human resources manager or department of an organization. Completion of an HIM associate degree program provides foundational knowledge and skills needed for participation in day-to-day HRM supervisory roles within an HIM unit as described in this chapter.

The HIM professionals seeking transition to a career focused exclusively on management of human resources will likely need to pursue advanced education in the field. Most jobs with HRM titles, such as Recruiting Specialist or Training and Development Specialist, require a minimum of a bachelor's degree (HumanResourcesEDU 2019). Senior-level positions, such as Human Resources Director and Labor Relations Manager, typically require a master's degree; for example, Master of Science in Human Resources Management or a Master of Business Administration (HumanResourcesEDU 2019). Several recognized human resources professional organizations offer certification, including the Society of Human Resource Management (SHRM); certification is often a preferred job specification for HRM positions (HumanResourcesEDU 2019). Those seeking an HRM-focused career in academia will need a master's or doctoral degree.

Real-World Case 20.1

A busy HIM supervisor with a limited understanding of the duties of a disclosure process was asked to make a hiring decision for a disclosure specialist position at his hospital. An external candidate, a bright African American woman, interviewed well; her references checked out, and she was hired. The new employee participated in general hospital orientation. In a rush to get the employee started, she was given a brief introduction to the job. The normal high-volume of incoming requests continued over the new employee's first three months on the job; however, the disclosure processing rate slowed dramatically. Complaints came to the HIM supervisor's manager. During her 90-day probationary interview, the new employee was given a written warning to speed up. She complained that she had not received the same training on disclosure processing procedures or systems as was provided to other staff. She threatened to file a grievance, then abruptly quit. A job opening notice is once again posted.

Real-World Case 20.2

Sunrise System is a large, multi-specialty provider of health services. Employees in some areas of the organization, including several in HIM, work remotely; coding work is outsourced to a vendor firm. Based on review of quality indicators, Sunrise executive management has announced a strategic initiative to assess and improve teamwork across the organization. In the current performance appraisal system, immediate supervisors rate individual employees annually using a graphic rating scale; items such as attitude, quality of work, productivity, attention to detail, job knowledge, and attendance are scored. You are part of an appointed task force of unit managers and supervisors charged with providing recommendations for redesign of the current employee performance appraisal system in order to better assess teamwork across the workforce.

References

AHIMA House of Delegates. 2017. 2018 Environmental Scan Report. http://bok.ahima.org/PdfView?oid=302420.

Alakrawi, Z., V. Watzlaf, S. Nemchik, and P.T. Sheridan. 2017. New study illuminates the ongoing road to ICD-10 productivity and optimization. *Journal of AHIMA* 88(3):40-45.

American Health Information Management Association. 2019. American Health Information Management Association Code of Ethics. http://bok.ahima.org/doc?oid=105098#.XNMu_o5KhPY.

American Health Information Management Association. 2018a. Certification Exam Prep. http://www.ahima.org/education/onlineed/Programs/examprep.

American Health Information Management Association. 2018b. VLab Overview. http://www.ahima.org/education/vlab?tabid=overview.

American Health Information Management Association. 2018c. Career and Student Center. http://www.ahima.org/careers.

American Health Information Management Association. 2017. *Pocket Glossary of Health Information Management and Technology*, 5th ed. Chicago: AHIMA.

American Health Information Management Association. 2013a. Recruitment, selection, and orientation for CDI specialists. *Journal of AHIMA* 84(7):58–62 [expanded web version]. http://library.ahima.org/doc?oid=106800#.Vxk06PkrK9I.

American Health Information Management Association. 2013b. Release of Information Toolkit. Appendix I Release of Information Specialist Job Description, 56–58. http://library.ahima.org/doc?oid=106371#.Vxk00vkrK9I.

American Health Information Management Association. 2012. Management practices for the release of information (2012 update). *Journal of AHIMA* 83(2). http://bok.ahima.org/doc?oid=105883#.W8Tdw_ZFw2w.

Beauchamp, T.L. and J.F. Childress. 2013. *Principles of Biomedical Ethics,* 7th ed. New York: Oxford University Press.

Brodnik, M.S. and M. Sharp. 2017. Workplace Law Chapter 20 in *Fundamentals of Law for Health Informatics and Information Management,* 3rd ed. Edited by M.S. Brodnik, L.A. Rinehart-Thompson, and R.B. Reynolds. Chicago: AHIMA.

Bureau of Labor Statistics. 2019 (January 18). Union Membership (Annual) News Release. http://www.bls.gov/news.release/union2.htm.

Bureau of Labor Statistics. 2018. Occupational Outlook Handbook, Medical Records and Health Information Technicians. http://www.bls.gov/ooh/healthcare/medical-records-and-health-information-technicians.htm.

Bureau of Labor Statistics. 2014. The Economics Daily. Largest industries by state, 1990–2013. http://www.bls.gov/opub/ted/2014/ted_20140728.htm.

Carrell, M. and C. Heavrin. 2013. Chapter 4 in *Labor Relations and Collective Bargaining: Private and Public Sectors*, 10th ed. Upper Saddle River, NJ: Pearson.

Department of Labor. 2019 (February 5). Employment and Training Administration. O*NET OnLine. http://www.onetonline.org.

Department of Labor. 2015. Disability Resources, Laws, and Regulations. http://www.dol.gov/dol/topic/disability/laws.htm.

Department of Labor, Wage and Hour Division. 2014. Handy Reference Guide to the Fair Labor Standards Act. http://www.dol.gov/whd/regs/compliance/hrg.htm.

Department of Labor, Wage and Hour Division. 2012. Fact Sheet #28: The Family Medical Leave Act. http://www.dol.gov/whd/regs/compliance/whdfs28.pdf.

Dessler, G. 2016. *Fundamentals of Human Resource Management,* 4th ed. Upper Saddle River, NJ: Pearson.

Elsdon, R. 2012 (July 12). Building Workforce Strength. Career Convergence Web Magazine. https://www.ncda.org/aws/NCDA/pt/sd/news_article/31875/_PARENT/CC_layout_details/false.

Elsdon, R. 2010. Building Workforce Strength: Creating Value through Workforce and Career Development. Santa Barbara, CA, USA: ABC-CLIO. ProQuest ebrary.

Equal Employment Opportunity Commission. n.d.a. Equal Pay/Compensation Discrimination. Accessed October 8, 2018. http://www.eeoc.gov/laws/types/equalcompensation.cfm.

Equal Employment Opportunity Commission. n.d.b. Title VII of the Civil Rights Act of 1964. Accessed October 8, 2018. http://www.eeoc.gov/laws/statutes/titlevii.cfm.

Equal Employment Opportunity Commission. n.d.c. Facts About Race/Color Discrimination. Accessed October 8, 2018. http://www.eeoc.gov/eeoc/publications/fs-race.cfm.

Equal Employment Opportunity Commission. n.d.d. Harassment. Accessed October 8, 2018. http://www.eeoc.gov/laws/types/harassment.cfm.

Equal Employment Opportunity Commission. n.d.e. The Pregnancy Discrimination Act of 1978. Accessed October 8, 2018. http://www.eeoc.gov/laws/statutes/pregnancy.cfm.

Equal Employment Opportunity Commission. n.d.f. The Age Discrimination in Employment Act of 1967. Accessed October 8, 2018. http://www.eeoc.gov/laws/statutes/adea.cfm.

Federal Aviation Administration. 2012 (September 20). Information for Operators. https://www.faa.gov/other_visit/aviation_industry/airline_operators/airline_safety/info/all_infos/media/2012/info12017.pdf.

Filerman, G.L., A.E. Mills, and P.M. Schyve, eds. 2014. *Managerial Ethics in Healthcare: A New Perspective*. Chicago: Health Administration Press.

Folkman, J. 2014. (February 19). "Should I Tell You The Good News First?" The Feedback Employees Most Want To Hear. http://www.forbes.com/sites/joefolkman/2014/02/19/should-i-tell-you-the-good-news-first-the-feedback-employees-most-want-to-hear/.

Fried, B.J. and M.D. Fottler, eds. 2018. *Fundamentals of Human Resources in Healthcare,* 2nd ed. Chicago: Health Administration Press.

Fried, B.J. and M.D. Fottler, eds. 2011. *Fundamentals of Human Resources in Healthcare*. Chicago: Health Administration Press.

Gomez-Mejia, L.R., D. Balkin, and R. Cardy. 2016. *Managing Human Resources,* 8th ed. Upper Saddle River, NJ: Pearson.

Harden, J. 2017. (March 9). Orientation and Onboarding: Best Practices. Mayo Clinic Laboratories. Mayo Foundation For Medical Education And Research. https://news.mayocliniclabs.com/2017/03/09/orientation-and-onboarding-best-practices/.

Harman, L.B. 2006. *Ethical Challenges in the Management of Health Information,* 2nd ed. Burlington, MA: Jones & Bartlett Learning.

Hickman, G. T and K. M. Karban. 2014.Trust but verify: Safeguards in contracting for outsourced coding services. *Journal of AHIMA* 85(6):40-44.

HumanResourcesEDU. 2019. HR Degree and Education Options. https://www.humanresourcesedu.org/degrees/.

Johns, M. 2016. Data Governance and Stewardship Chapter 3 in *Health Information Management: Concepts Principles and Practice,* 5th ed. Edited by P.K. Oachs and A.L. Watters. Chicago: AHIMA.

Juran, J. M. 1995. *Managerial Breakthrough: The Classic Book On Improving Management Performance*. Universals for Breakthrough and Control. New York: McGraw-Hill.

LeBlanc, M.M. 2016. Human Resources Management Chapter 23 in *Health Information Management: Concepts Principles and Practice,* 5th ed. Edited by P.K. Oachs and A.L. Watters. Chicago: AHIMA.

Marc, D., J. Robertson, L. Gordon, Z. Green-Lawson, D. Gibbs, K. Dover, and. M. Dougherty. 2017. What the data say about HIM professional trends. *Journal of AHIMA* 88(5):24-31.

Maurer, R. 2017 (April 18). Layoffs Require Communication, Compassion and Compliance. https://www.shrm.org/resourcesandtools/hr-topics/talent-acquisition/pages/layoffs-communication-compassion-compliance.aspx.

McNair, J.H., W. Anglade, and R. Smith. 2007 (March 23). Litigating non-economic compensatory damages: How do you piece together lives shattered by workplace discrimination? Compensatory damages—Maybe, maybe not. *ABA National Conference on EEO Law.* http://www.americanbar.org/content/dam/aba/administrative/labor_law/meetings/2007/2007_eeo_mcnair.authcheckdam.pdf.

McWay, D. 2016. Law and Ethics in the Workplace Chapter 15 in *Legal and Ethical Aspects of Health Information Management,* 4th ed. Clifton Park, NY: Cengage Learning.

Momand, M. Q. 2018. Human as a RESOURCE or CAPITAL. https://www.shrm.org/resourcesandtools/tools-and-samples/member2member/pages/human-as-a-resource-or-capital.aspx.

Mondy, R.W. D. and J. Martocchio. 2016. *Human Resource Management,* 14th ed. Upper Saddle River, NJ: Pearson.

National Institutes of Health. 2018. Human Genome Project. http://report.nih.gov/nihfactsheets/ViewFactSheet.aspx?csid=45.

National Labor Relations Board. 2018a. Employer/Union Rights and Obligations. http://www.nlrb.gov/rights-we-protect/employerunion-rights-and-obligations.

National Labor Relations Board. 2018b. Your Rights During Union Organizing. http://www.nlrb.gov/rights-we-protect/whats-law/employees/i-am-not-represented-union/your-rights-during-union-organizing.

National Labor Relations Board v. Kentucky River Community Care, Inc., 532 U.S. 706; 121 S. Ct. 1861; 149 L. Ed. 2d 939 (2001).

Oachs, P.K. 2016. Work Design and Process Improvement Chapter 25 in *Health Information Management: Concepts Principles and Practice,* 5th ed. Edited by P.K. Oachs and A.L. Watters. Chicago: AHIMA.

Occupational Safety and Health Administration. 2004. Occupational Health and Safety Act of 1970. https://www.osha.gov/pls/oshaweb/owadisp.show_document?p_table=OSHACT&p_id=2743.

Office of Personnel Management. 2018. Assessment and Selection, Job Analysis. Six Steps to Conducting a Job Analysis. http://www.opm.gov/policy-data-oversight/assessment-and-selection/job-analysis/.

Patena, K.R. 2016. Employee Training and Development Chapter 24 in *Health Information Management: Concepts Principles and Practice,* 5th ed. Edited by P.K. Oachs and A.L. Watters. Chicago: AHIMA.

Schermerhorn, J.R., Jr. and D. G. Bachrach. 2018. *Exploring Management,* 6th ed. Hoboken, NJ: John Wiley & Sons.

Service Employees International Union. 2018. What type of work do SEIU members do? Healthcare. https://www.seiu.org/cards/these-fast-facts-will-tell-you-how-were-organized/.

Society for Human Resource Management. 2019. When should a part-time employee be reclassified as full-time? https://www.shrm.org/resourcesandtools/tools-and-samples/hr-qa/pages/legalregulatoryissueswhenshouldapart-timeemployeebereclassifiedasfull-time.aspx.

Society for Human Resource Management. 2018a (September 10). Screening by Means of Pre-Employment Testing. https://www.shrm.org/resourcesandtools/tools-and-samples/toolkits/pages/screeningbymeansofpreemploymenttesting.aspx.

Society for Human Resource Management. 2018b (March 2). Screening and Evaluating Candidates. https://www.shrm.org/resourcesandtools/tools-and-samples/toolkits/pages/screeningandevaluatingcandidates.aspx.

Society for Human Resource Management. 2018c (September 6). Managing Employee Performance. Toolkits. https://www.shrm.org/ResourcesAndTools/tools-and-samples/toolkits/Pages/managingemployeeperformance.aspx.

Society for Human Resource Management. 2018d (August 24). Involuntary Termination of Employment in the United States. https://www.shrm.org/resourcesandtools/tools-and-samples/toolkits/pages/involuntaryterminationof.aspx.

Society for Human Resource Management. 2018e (November 19). Introduction to the Human Resources Discipline of Organizational and Employee Development. https://www.shrm.org/resourcesandtools/tools-and-samples/toolkits/pages/introorganizationalandemployeedevelopment.aspx.

Society for Human Resource Management. 2018f (November 14). Employee Career Development Plan. https://www.shrm.org/resourcesandtools/tools-and-samples/hr-forms/pages/cms_011324.aspx.

Society for Human Resource Management. 2017 (March 17). Developing and Sustaining Employee Engagement. https://www.shrm.org/resourcesandtools/tools-and-samples/toolkits/pages/sustainingemployeeengagement.aspx.

Tooley, P. 2007. Release of information: Strategies to maximize customer service, productivity, and revenue with release of information activity tracking form. *Proceedings of AHIMA's 79th National Convention and Exhibit*. Philadelphia, PA.

29 USC 152(11): National Labor Relations Act (NLRA), Definitions. 1947.

Ethical Issues in Health Information Management

Misty Hamilton, MBA, RHIT

Learning Objectives

- Examine moral values and ethical principles
- Interpret the concepts of morality code of conduct, and moral judgment
- Identify how cultural issues affect health and healthcare quality, cost, and health information management
- Identify cultural competence for healthcare professionals
- Examine the ethical foundations of health information management
- Examine the American Health Information Management Association's (AHIMA) Code of Ethics
- Examine ethical issues related to medical identity theft
- Evaluate the process of ethical decision-making
- Demonstrate methods used to resolve a breach of healthcare ethics
- Identify the important health information ethical problems in healthcare

Key Terms

Autonomy
Beneficence
Bias
Blanket authorization
Breach
Code of ethics
Confidentiality
Culture
Cultural audit
Cultural competence
Cultural diversity
Cultural competence
Double billing
Ethical principles
Ethics
Ethics committee
Excellence
Integrity
Leadership
Managed care
Medical identity theft
Morals
Moral distress
Moral values
Need-to-know principle
Nonmaleficence
Prejudice
Privacy
Respect
Retrospective documentation
Security
Stereotyping
Unbundling
Upcoding
Values

The phrase "first do no harm" is well known in the healthcare industry as a long-standing code of conduct for medical professionals. First and foremost, the goal of a healthcare professional is to not cause harm to those being treated; the legal term for this concept is nonmaleficence. Health information management (HIM) professionals are guided by a similar code of conduct and adhere to a professional code of ethics, a set of principles regarding business practices and professional behavior. HIM professionals do not provide direct patient care, but they do interact with patients in terms of coding, disclosure of information, reimbursement for healthcare services, data quality, and so forth. Ethics is a field of study dealing with moral principles, theories, and values. In healthcare, ethics involves formal decision-making needed to deal with competing perspectives and obligations of the people who have interest in a common problem. For example, a grandmother requests the health records of her grandson. The disclosure of health information specialist states she is not authorized to receive the health records because she is not the child's parent. The grandmother then states she suspects her grandson is being abused, and that is why she is requesting the health records. The disclosure of health information specialist still does not release the health records to the grandmother; however, she does inform her of the steps necessary to report the suspected abuse.

An individual has the right to determine what does or does not happen to them in terms of healthcare delivery and services. Autonomy is a core ethical principle centered on this fact, meaning a patient has the right to choose his or her course of treatment. A clinical application of this concept is a cancer patient's right to refuse chemotherapy, radiation, or surgical treatment. Beneficence is a legal term that means promoting good for others or providing services that benefit others, such as a patient care coordinator clarifying an explanation of medical benefits (EOB) for a patient (see chapter 15, *Revenue Management and Reimbursement,* for more detail about EOBs).

People are guided by their own set of values and ethical principles according to their personal beliefs and cultural upbringings. It is important for HIM professionals to understand cultural competency and diversity to help guide their interactions in the workplace as well as when associating with patients. Understanding a person's background, culture, beliefs, and values makes it possible to comprehend why they may act in a certain way, and can help guide professional interactions. This chapter explores the individual moral values and ethical principles of people and defines cultural competence in the healthcare environment. The ethical foundations of HIM include ethical issues related to medical identify theft, ethical decision-making, and breach of healthcare ethics. Important HIM-specific ethical issues are addressed. Ethical issues related to labor and employment laws can be found in chapter 20, *Human Resources Management*.

Moral Values and Ethical Principles

The concept of morals relates to what is right or wrong in human behavior (Brodnik 2017, 15). Moral values are developed through the "influence of family, culture, religion and society and is a system of principles by which an individual guides their life" (Brodnik 2017, 14). In healthcare, employees need to be mindful of the moral values of the people with whom they work, including fellow employees and patients. The moral values people hold can be deeply set in who they are as a person, which can cause conflict with others who hold opposing values. As an HIM professional it is also important to understand ethical principles, a foundation of principles used to help with decision-making and understand why others may make the decisions they do. The following principles explain the ways in which ethical decisions are made:

- *Altruism*. The belief that other people are more important than an individual person, wherein a personal sacrifice takes place.

An example would be donating a kidney to a stranger (Allen 2013).

- *Autonomy*. An individual's right to make his or her own decisions, or self-determination. The ability to allow a patient to control what happens to his or her body. For example, a person can refuse all medical care after a diagnosis of cancer (Brodnik 2017, 17).
- *Beneficence*. Doing good, promoting the health and welfare of others, demonstrating kindness, showing compassion, and helping others. For example, organizations providing food to the homeless population of a community.
- *Consequentialism*. Considers the consequences before making a decision and is based on the end result; for example, when coding a patient's health record the coder understands that certain medical codes receive higher reimbursement, but the consequence of miscoding could result in legal charges against the provider.
- *Deontology*. The duty or responsibility guiding the decision based on action and not the end result; for example, the HIM department is short staffed and tomorrow the organization's onsite accreditation begins. It is against department policy to work overtime; however, there are still a few tasks that need to be completed for tomorrow's accreditation visit. The HIM staff member clocks out but stays and finishes the tasks for tomorrow's visit. She feels it is her duty to make sure everything is ready for the site visit even if it requires her to clock out to do so.
- *Egoism*. Instead of taking others into consideration, egoism involves only considering oneself in the decision-making process; for example, an information technology manager accepts a gift from an electronic health record (EHR) vendor, even though it is against hospital policy, because she really likes the gift.
- *Least harm*. Occurs with situations where two choices may be less than ideal. One should choose the situation that will do the least amount of harm to the fewest number of people; for example, a physician choosing to treat the patient in the emergency department with the greatest chance for survival instead of the patient with more severe or life-threatening injuries.
- *Utilitarianism*. Deals with situations that provide the greatest advantage or benefit to the most people; for example, your local health department decides to give out free flu shots because the Centers for Disease Control reports that this flu season may be deadly.

Ethical decision-making involves consideration of what is right and what is wrong based on a code of conduct or behavior. An ethical dilemma occurs when one is faced with a choice between two or more situations—for example, should life support be discontinued or continued, or the decision regarding which patient will receive an available kidney. An HIM professional who has strong beliefs against assisted suicide may not be comfortable working in a state where it is legal or at an organization where it is practiced.

Many ethical decisions are based on an individual's **culture**, which includes the values, beliefs, attitudes, languages, symbols, rituals, behaviors, and customs unique to a particular group of people (Simmers et al. 2017). **Values** include the social and cultural belief system of a person or a healthcare organization. Culture is learned, shared, social in nature, dynamic, and changing, meaning people generally have similar beliefs and values based on their upbringing—what they were taught by parents, peers, and surroundings. An individual's values can change over time based on varying environments and social networks. For example, a student who leaves home for the first time to go to college will be exposed to new and different experiences, and as a result the values developed at home may shift and reflect those from his or her college environment.

Health information management professionals have responsibilities to patients, the HIM profession, and to themselves. Patients have the right to decide their course of treatment, deny treatment, and the right to privacy. While normally the patient's rights are of the utmost importance, there are times when the public's rights outweigh the rights of an individual (Allen 2013). Issues related to individual rights in regard to privacy and confidentiality are covered in chapter 9, *Data Privacy and Confidentiality*.

Cultural Competence in the Healthcare Environment

Cultural competence is the ability to accept and understand the beliefs and values of other people and groups and is vital to the overall state of an organization. Cultural diversity is the perceived or actual difference among people. Respecting alternative cultural beliefs is imperative, but respect does not require agreement with alternative beliefs (Ortiz and Casey 2017). Healthcare professionals work with, and care for, many different people each day and cannot let differences in values and beliefs impact the work; therefore, everyone must respect the differences of each person encountered during the day. For example, cultural competence is expressed by referring to a transgender person with the pronoun (he or she) by which the individual identifies. Accepting diversity and the inclusion of all people is important to cultural competence and acceptance. Culture includes the following:

- Ethnicity (classification of people based on national origin or culture)
- Socioeconomic status (classification of people based on economic or social welfare status)
- Religion
- Gender or gender identity
- Sexual orientation
- Age
- Education
- Occupation

Attitudes that affect one's cultural competence include prejudice, stereotyping, and bias. Prejudice is a strong feeling or belief about a person or subject formed without reviewing facts or information (Simmers et al. 2017). Prejudice occurs when a person is judged solely based on one of the cultural factors listed previously; for example, an elderly patient who feels a young physician is not qualified to care for him or her. Stereotyping is an assumption that everyone within a certain group is the same. Stereotypes "labels" individuals and disregards each person's unique characteristics; for example, believing that psychiatrists are not "real" physicians. A bias prevents a person from having an impartial judgment; for example, a physician assuming that low-income patients are less likely to adhere to medical advice. Unconscious bias includes stereotypes about people outside of one's awareness.

Healthcare professionals should be mindful of the differences in culture, beliefs, and values of other people particularly coworkers and patients, and avoid prejudice, stereotyping, and bias. This can be done by appreciating the differences in people, exploring various cultures, values, and beliefs; trying to understand why people believe and act the way they do; and being sensitive to other cultures (Simmers et al. 2017). The following sections will introduce HIM professionals to cultural issues and the effects on health, healthcare quality, and cost. To begin to understand cultural competence, it should first be explored with the process of helping people identify and become self-aware of their own culture perception. The following sections explore training programs related to expanding culture in the workplace, and regulations in regard to cultural competence.

Cultural Disparities in US Healthcare

Many factors influence health and healthcare including a person's health status, disease risk factors, and their access to healthcare. These factors are influenced by the culture in which people live such as lack of affordable transportation and reduced access to employment. The World Health Organization (WHO) defines the social determinants of health as the conditions into which persons are born, grow, live, work, and age (WHO 2018). Health disparities exist disproportionately in certain populations. Data shows that residents in mostly minority communities have lower socioeconomic status, greater barriers to healthcare access, and greater risks for disease compared with the general population (Meyer et al. 2013).

Increased healthcare costs can also be a result of disparities in quality and access to healthcare. Patients who do not have access to quality healthcare are less likely to get the preventive care they need to stay healthy and as a result are more likely to suffer from serious illnesses. The US Department of Health and Human Services Office of Minority Health established national standards for culturally and linguistically appropriate services (CLAS) in health and healthcare with the intention to advance health quality, improve quality of care, and help eliminate healthcare disparities in the United States. The principal standard is to provide effective, equitable, understandable, and respectful quality care while being responsive to diverse cultural beliefs and practices, preferred languages, health literacy, and other communication needs (HHS n.d.).

Healthcare Professionals and Cultural Competence

Healthcare professionals nationally struggle to respond to the needs of people from diverse groups and to incorporate cultural competence in healthcare settings; however, there are many benefits to patients in doing so (Goode and Dunne 2003). The following are some of the reasons to incorporate cultural competence into organizational policies and procedures:

- To reflect the current and projected demographic changes in the US as the American population continues to change as a result of immigration patterns and significant increases among racially, ethnically, culturally, and linguistically diverse populations (Goode and Dunne 2003)
- To eliminate long-standing disparities in the health status of people of diverse racial, ethnic, and cultural backgrounds; the disparities in the incidence of illness and death among people of certain ethnicities is related to the bias, stereotyping, and prejudice of healthcare providers; and incorporation of cultural competence can help improve the disparities (Goode and Dunne 2003)
- To improve the quality of health services and outcomes; healthcare providers who are culturally competent provide a higher level of patient satisfaction, health outcomes, and preventative care (Goode and Dunne 2003)
- To meet legislative, regulatory, and accreditation mandates; for example, the Joint Commission supports standards that require cultural and linguistic competence in healthcare
- To gain a competitive edge in the marketplace; primary care organizations must allow their providers to acquire cultural knowledge and develop skill sets that will enable them to work effectively with diverse patient populations; implementing culturally competent service delivery systems positively impacts provider recruitment and retention as well as patient access to and satisfaction with care (Goode and Dunne 2003)
- To decrease the likelihood of liability or malpractice claims; the ability to communicate well with patients has been shown to reduce the likelihood of malpractice claims; organizations have faced potential claims that their failure to understand beliefs breaches professional standards of care (Goode and Dunne 2003)

Cultural competence means providing quality healthcare to every patient. For an entire healthcare organization, it means the institution and its employees have the capacity to do the following:

- Value diversity
- Conduct self-assessments to determine

the attitudes, practices, and policies of the organization, meaning both the organization as a whole conducts a self-assessment and employees individually assess themselves to align with the culture and attitude of the organization
- Manage the dynamics of difference
- Acquire and institutionalize cultural knowledge
- Adapt to the diversity and cultural context of the communities served (NCCC 2018a)

Assessing the cultural awareness and competence of a healthcare organization's employees involves training to help employees understand their own attitudes and practices toward cultural awareness, as well as understanding and practicing the policies of the organization. Healthcare organizations conduct ongoing assessments of their progress toward reaching the goals of CLAS-related activities with the purpose of assessing performance, monitoring progress, obtaining information about the organization and customers, and assessing the value of activities that fulfill governance, leadership, and workforce responsibilities (HHS n.d.).

One of the assessments an organization measures is the accessibility of interpreters for people who speak a language other than English, including American sign language. Many healthcare organizations maintain lists of interpreters who can be called to help communicate with patients. The assessment is part of an organization's continuous quality improvement activities. Table 21.1 is a sample of measures in performance improvement and outcomes assessments.

Healthcare Organization Cultural Competence Awareness

Cultural competence is a process that evolves over time. Both healthcare organizations and individuals will have various levels of awareness, knowledge, and skills. Addressing how one views language, communication style, belief systems, customs, attitudes, perceptions, and values in others is a way to assess personal cultural competence. Each employee of the healthcare organization should honestly determine if he or she has prejudices or biases and assess whether those affect their actions and views toward fellow employees, patients, healthcare providers, and vendors. This self-assessment should be ongoing and not a one-time process, in order to truly address ongoing or new personal viewpoints.

Healthcare professionals should also assess their department's strengths and weaknesses in the area of accepting diversity. Assessing attitudes, practices, structures, and policies of programs and their personnel is a necessary, effective, and systematic way to plan for and incorporate cultural competency within organizations (NCCC 2018b). It is important for healthcare organizations to educate and train employees in the areas of diversity and cultural competence. For example, the manager of an HIM department could have employees take a cultural competence self-assessment to identify strengths and further areas of development. Once completed the employees could work on their areas of improvement. Employees can do this by exploring a specific culture or ethnicity and helping to understand why people may act the way they do (for instance, in some cultures a person will not make eye contact with a member of the opposite

Table 21.1 Assessment of cultural and linguistic competency

Continuous quality improvement program assessment of cultural and linguistic competency			
Monitor and assess the organization's performance for the prior year in the areas listed	**Outcome**	**Assessment**	**Plan**
Accessibility of interpreter services	Interpreter needed 100 times	Sign language interpreter was not available five times	Hire sign language interpreter
Effectiveness of culture and linguistic competency training for providers	Training provided twice per year	Five healthcare providers did not attend training	Follow up with all providers once per year to confirm training is completed

Source: Adapted from HHS n.d.

sex unless it is a close family member). The following are examples of how an organization can encourage employees and everyone who does business with the organization to improve the cultural acceptance of all who are in contact with the organization:

- Challenge colleagues when they make racial, ethnic, or sexually offensive comments or jokes; for example, if a fellow employee is overheard telling a racially toned joke, other coworkers should let the employee know the behavior is unacceptable.
- Humans by nature are social beings and strive to be with others, and people tend to socialize with those similar to them. Actively seek to connect with people who are different and include diversity in social circles. For example, many people are comfortable with the same group of coworkers and friends while having lunch. Inviting new people to the group increases the cultural competence of the group, which positively affects the organization.
- Do not make assumptions about a person before the facts are verified. For example, if a new person is hired in the HIM department and speaks broken English, a coworker without cultural awareness may assume the new person is not able to perform the job functions because of the language barrier, when in fact he or she may be able to perform the job well.

An understanding and sensitivity to the beliefs and cultures of others can help alleviate misunderstanding and offenses that may happen because someone has not been trained to be sensitive. For example, a cultural miscommunication may occur when a supervisor accentuates the positive attributes of an employee and minimizes the negatives, which leads the employee who is accustomed to direct and honest (even when negative) feedback to think he or she is doing a comprehensively great job. Figure 21.1 shows a four-part model of continuous cultural competence awareness.

Figure 21.1 Cultural competence model

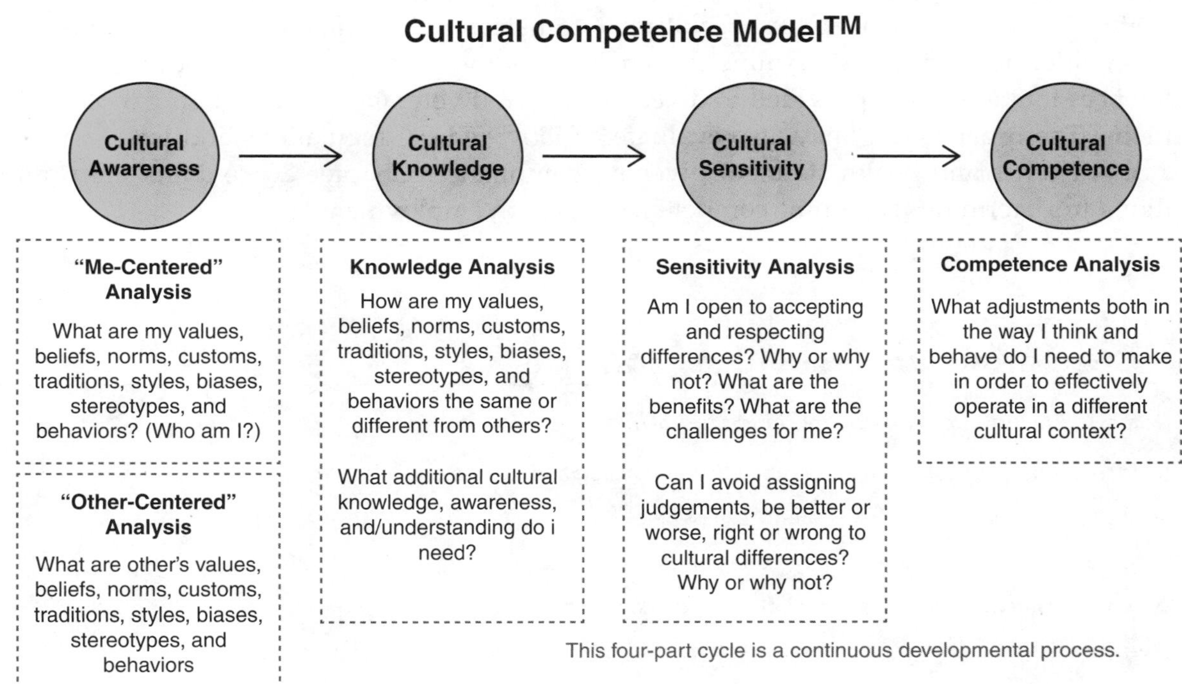

Source: © The Winters Group, Inc. Used with permission.

Training Programs

Cultural awareness training for all employees is an important component of a healthcare organization's overall cultural competence. By providing training, healthcare professionals gain the knowledge, skills, and abilities to understand peoples' beliefs and culture. A cultural audit is a strategy to define a facility's values, symbols, and routines, and identify areas for improvement. Key considerations include the following:

- Conduct a needs and capacity assessment to identify cultural commonalities and differences to be addressed, and the ability of your healthcare organization and staff to address them
- Involve individuals representing the diversity of your community around the planning of your healthcare organization and encourage cross-cultural dialogues between people
- Facilitate both formal and informal opportunities for cross-cultural interactions among staff (HHS 2018)

To perform a cultural audit, an organization may assess the availability of interpreter services and the effectiveness and availability of cultural training provided to staff and determine if there are differences in the services provided to diverse populations. The organization may also evaluate the health outcomes and health status of diverse populations to determine if cultural competency training and awareness helps change the outcomes for patients over time. This list is not comprehensive, and organizations may use other methods to perform a cultural audit.

Healthcare organizations have established continuous quality improvement programs to measure the quality of a service or product through systems or process evaluation and implementation of revised processes that result in better healthcare outcomes. (Quality improvement is discussed in greater detail in chapter 18, *Performance Improvement*.) Organizations incorporate CLAS measures into their ongoing quality improvement activities to determine how well they assess cultural competence.

Regulations for Cultural Awareness

Legal responsibilities of healthcare organizations, as determined by federal law, prohibit discrimination based on ethnicity, religious faith, physical disability, or age. By incorporating cultural awareness training and monitoring across the spectrum of business, a healthcare organization abides by the laws prohibiting discrimination of employees, patients, vendors, or anyone who may have contact with the organization. The Equal Employment Opportunity Commission (EEOC) was established to help provide equal employment opportunities for minority groups, women, people with disabilities, and veterans. Healthcare organizations must follow federal regulations and laws to remain in compliance. Chapter 20 contains more information on employment law.

Check Your Understanding 21.1

Answer the following questions by matching the term with the definition.

1. Duty or responsibility guiding the decision based on action and not the end result
2. The socioeconomic or religious differences in people
3. The individual's right to determine what does or does not happen to him or her in terms of healthcare
4. Only considering oneself instead of taking others into consideration
5. System of principles that guide an someone's life, usually with regards to right and wrong
6. Field of study dealing with moral principles, theories, and values

7. To not cause harm
8. Promoting good for others or providing services that benefit others
9. Strong feeling about a person without reviewing facts
10. Assuming everyone within a certain group is the same

a. Egoism
b. Moral value
c. Nonmaleficence
d. Prejudice
e. Deontology
f. Beneficence
g. Autonomy
h. Ethics
i. Cultural diversity
j. Stereotyping

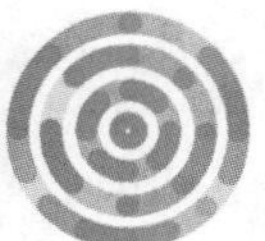

Ethical Foundations of Health Information Management

Ethical principles and values have been important to the HIM profession since its inception in 1928. The first ethical pledge was presented in 1934 by Grace Whiting Myers, a visionary leader who recognized the importance of protecting information in medical records. The HIM profession was launched with recognition of the importance of privacy and the requirement of an authorization for the release of health information:

> I pledge myself to give out no information from any clinical record placed in my charge, or from any other source to any person whatsoever, except upon order from the chief executive officer of the institution which I may be serving (Huffman 1972, 135).

Today, it is the patient who authorizes the disclosure of his or her health information and not the chief executive officer (CEO) of the healthcare organization, as stated in the original pledge. The most important values embedded in this pledge are to protect patient privacy and confidential information and to recognize the importance of the HIM professional as a moral agent in protecting patient information. The HIM professional has a clear ethical and professional obligation not to give any information to anyone unless the release has been authorized (Gordon and Gordon 2016). Disclosure of information is discussed in detail in chapter 3, *Health Information Functions, Purpose, and Users*.

The HIM professionals are responsible for the protection of patient privacy and confidentiality, and for maintaining the security and control of health records. It is important to understand these terms, as they are sometimes used interchangeably (Gordon and Gordon 2016).

- **Privacy** is the right of a patient to control the disclosure of protected health information (PHI) and includes the freedom from unauthorized intrusion in healthcare. For example, a patient has the right to authorize his/her health information be shared with a family member.
- **Confidentiality** is a legal and ethical concept that requires healthcare providers to protect health records and other personal and private information from unauthorized use or disclosure. For example, any information a patient shares with a physician will be kept private between the patient and physician.

- **Security** is privacy and confidentiality that pertains to the physical and electronic protection of information (Brodnik 2017). For example, a healthcare organization having a policy on the creation, safeguarding, and maintenance of employee passwords.

Professionals working in the HIM field are guided by the ethical foundations of privacy, confidentiality, and security that are detailed in a professional code of ethics that outlines values and obligations for HIM professionals. Ethical issues related to medical identity theft, ethical decision-making questions, and specific ethical problems encountered by HIM professionals are explored in detail in the following sections.

Professional Code of Ethics for the Health Information Management Professional

A professional code of ethics is adopted by an organization to guide the members in determining right and wrong conduct when performing the duties of their job. The American Health Information Management Association (AHIMA) Code of Ethics applies to all AHIMA members and is based on the core values of the association. The preamble to the AHIMA Code of Ethics states the following:

> The ethical obligations of the HIM professional include the safeguarding of privacy and security of health information; disclosure of health information; development, use, and maintenance of health information systems and health information; and ensuring the accessibility and integrity of health information.
>
> Healthcare consumers are increasingly concerned about security and the potential loss of privacy and the inability to control how their personal health information is used and disclosed. Core health information issues include what information should be collected; how the information should be handled, who should have access to the information, under what conditions the information should be disclosed, how the information is retained and when it is no longer needed, and how it is disposed of in a confidential manner. All the core health information issues are performed in compliance with state and federal regulations, and employer policies and procedures. Ethical obligations are central to the professional's responsibility, regardless of the employment site or the method of collection, storage, and security of health information. In addition, sensitive information (for example, genetic, adoption, drug, alcohol, sexual, health, and behavioral information) requires special attention to prevent misuse. In the world of business and interactions with consumers, expertise in the protection of the information is required (AHIMA 2019).

HIM professionals may encounter ethical dilemmas while working, including clinical code selection and use, privacy and confidentiality, and fraud and abuse. The code of ethics can be used to help HIM professionals make sound decisions when ethical problems emerge by creating expectations for conduct. HIM professionals have access to sensitive information contained within the health record. Patients trust the information they share with their healthcare provider will be protected. When a celebrity or well-known person receives care, his or her protected health information has a value to the media and may be sold by people without ethical values.

The HIM professional is obligated to demonstrate actions that reflect values, ethical principles, and the ethical guidelines regardless of employment site (for example, acute-care hospital, physician's office, government agency, vendor, and so forth). The seven purposes listed in table 21.2 are descriptions of the values and principles used to guide the conduct of HIM professionals. The code includes enforceable core principles and guidelines. Alleged violation of ethical principles is taken very seriously by AHIMA and reviewed by a team dedicated to that purpose.

Professional Values and Obligations

Health information management professionals are ethically responsible for preserving, protecting, and

Table 21.2 AHIMA Code of Ethics

The Code of Ethics serves seven purposes	
1. Promote high standards of HIM practice	
2. Identify core values on which the HIM mission is based	
3. Summarize broad ethical principles that reflect the profession's core values	
4. Establish a set of ethical principles to be used to guide decision-making and actions	
5. Establish a framework for professional behavior and responsibilities when professional obligations conflict or ethical uncertainties arise	
6. Provide ethical principles by which the general public can hold the HIM professional accountable	
7. Mentor practitioners new to the field to HIM's mission, values, and ethical principles	
Principles and guidelines form the foundation of the Code of Ethics	
Principle	**Example**
1. Advocate, uphold, and defend the individual's right to privacy and the doctrine of confidentiality in the use and disclosure of information.	Safeguard all confidential patient information to include, but not limited to, personal, health, financial, genetic, and outcome information
2. Put service and the health and welfare of persons before self-interest and conduct oneself in the practice of the profession so as to bring honor to oneself, peers, and to the health information management profession.	Act with integrity, behave in a trustworthy manner, elevate service to others above self-interest, and promote high standards of practice in every setting
3. Preserve, protect, and secure personal health information in any form or medium and hold in the highest regard health information and other information of a confidential nature obtained in an official capacity, taking into account the applicable statutes and regulations.	Take precautions to ensure and maintain the confidentiality of information transmitted to other parties through the use of any media, transferred, or disposed of in the event of termination, incapacitation, or death of a healthcare provider
4. Refuse to participate in or conceal unethical practices or procedures and report such practices.	Act in a professional and ethical manner at all times
5. Advance health information management knowledge and practice through continuing education, research, publications, and presentations.	Continually develop and enhance professional expertise, knowledge, and skills (including appropriate education, research, training, consultation, and supervision); contribute to the knowledge base of health information management and share one's knowledge related to practice, research, and ethics
6. Recruit and mentor students, staff, peers, and colleagues to develop and strengthen professional workforce.	Provide directed practice opportunities for students
7. Represent the profession to the public in a positive manner.	Be an advocate for the profession in all settings and participate in activities that promote and explain the mission, values, and principles of the profession to the public
8. Perform honorably health information management association responsibilities, either appointed or elected, and preserve the confidentiality of any privileged information made known in any official capacity.	Perform responsibly all duties as assigned by the professional association operating within bylaws and policies and procedures of the association and any pertinent laws
9. State truthfully and accurately one's credentials, professional education, and experiences.	Claim only those relevant professional credentials actually possessed and correct any inaccuracies occurring regarding credentials
10. Facilitate interdisciplinary collaboration in situations supporting health information practice.	Foster trust among group members and adjust behavior in order to establish relationships with teams
11. Respect the inherent dignity and worth of every person.	Treat each person in a respectful fashion, being mindful of individual differences and cultural and ethnic diversity

Source: Adapted from AHIMA 2019.

securing health information in all mediums. The professional values AHIMA identifies as important are excellence, integrity, respect, and leadership and are demonstrated by the following values:

- **Excellence**. The quality of excelling, being better or the best at something
- **Integrity**. Openness in decision-making, honesty in communication, activity, and

ethical practices that command trust and support collaboration

- **Respect**. Appreciation of the value of differing perspectives, enjoyable experiences, courteous interaction, and celebration of achievements that advance our common cause
- **Leadership**. Visionary thinking, decisions responsive to membership and mission, and accountability for actions and outcomes

An HIM professional's ethical obligations, as outlined by the AHIMA standards, include duty to the patient and the healthcare team to protect health information, provide service to those who seek access to their information, preserve and secure health information, promote the quality and advancement of healthcare, and function within the scope of responsibility and restrain from passing clinical judgment (AHIMA 2019). Obligations also include those to the employer such as reliability; protection of committee deliberations (for example, a committee may make decisions related to who will receive an organ donation from a donation list, and those deliberations are protected much like patient information); compliance with all laws, regulations, and policies that govern the health information system; recognizing the authority and power of the job responsibilities; and to accept compensation only in relationship to work responsibilities. Ethical obligations to the public include advocating for change when patterns or system problems are not in the best interest of the patients, reporting violations of practice standards to the proper authorities, and promoting interdisciplinary cooperation and collaboration. Finally, ethical obligations to self, peers, and professional associations include being honest about degrees, credentials, and work experiences; bringing honor to oneself by committing to lifelong learning; strengthening HIM membership in AHIMA and state associations; representing the HIM profession to the public; and promoting and participating in HIM research (Gordon and Gordon 2016).

There may be times when your professional ethics and personal ethics conflict. Professional responsibilities often require an individual to move beyond personal values and could require a more comprehensive set of values than what someone needs to be an ethical agent in his or her personal life (AHIMA 2019). For example, you may have been taught to always respect your elders; when an 80-year-old female comes into the HIM department and requests her husband's health records without proper authorization, you may struggle with the fact that you cannot release the information to her. However, you can supply her with the proper steps to obtain the information correctly.

HIM professionals are ethically obligated to give back to the HIM community by providing practice opportunities for students, such as being involved in student professional practice experience opportunities. HIM professionals also have a responsibility to pass on knowledge to and mentor new health information management professionals and students.

Ethical Issues Related to Medical Identity Theft

Identity theft is illegally obtaining another person's personal information and using it to commit theft or fraud, usually for the purpose of financial transactions. **Medical identify theft** is the fraudulent use of an individual's identifying information in a healthcare setting. Contamination of the health record with erroneous information (for example, incorrect blood type or drug allergies) is one of the most serious risks because it can pose problems with patient safety, such as misdiagnoses, mistreatment, delayed treatment, or adverse reactions (Eramo 2016). The two primary ways medical identity theft happens is (1) consensual, or knowingly sharing information, and (2) nonconsensual, when someone unknown to the victim, or without the victim's permission, uses his or her information. A thief may use another person's insurance information, including Social Security number, to see a doctor, obtain prescription drugs, or fraudulently bill for healthcare services. Medical identity theft can be difficult to detect because people do not always pay close attention to their medical bills and insurance claims. If healthcare professionals do not recognize this impact on health records and do not fix the error, the theft can remain on the health record of the patient, potentially causing misdiagnosis or incorrect treatment (McNabb and Rhodes 2014). For example, consider a thief using a patient's insurance card to obtain prescription drugs from multiple providers and pharmacies. The patient is unaware of this use; months later the patient returns to his provider and needs medication, but his health record has been flagged as "drug seeking" and his provider will not prescribe the medication he needs. It can take some time for the patient to identify where and when his information was stolen and to clear his health record. The patient and the HIM professional each have a unique perspective on medical identity theft and are each responsible for identifying, reporting, and combating the crime. HIM professionals serve patients well by educating them about what to look for in terms of medical identity theft. For example, HIM professionals should work with patients and explain to them what they should look for if they receive a bill for medical services that they do not recognize, and instruct that they should check for fraudulent behavior in their name on their medical bills and credit reports. Patients can detect medical identity theft by reviewing their credit reports annually. A credit report will indicate accounts opened in the patient's name by healthcare organizations; if the patient does not recognize the organization, he or she can begin the steps to rectify the situation and identify the fraud.

It is important for HIM professionals to help find and correct fraudulent information within a health record. The California Attorney General's Office created an informational web page for consumers—First Aid for Medical Identify Theft: Tips for Consumers (OAG, CA DOJ 2019). This web page describes the following five signs of possible medical identify theft and provides tips on what to do in response to each.

1. If a patient receives a Receipt of a Breach Notice from a healthcare organization, it indicates that the patient's protected health information was involved in a data breach. Depending on the type of information involved in the breach, a security freeze on the patient's credit records may be required. Breach notifications will be discussed in more detail later in this chapter.
2. If a patient notices an unknown item in the Explanation of Benefits he or she receives from an insurance company and does not recognize the service being paid for, the patient must contact the insurer and the provider who billed for the services to correct the information.
3. If a patient receives a notification from the insurance provider that he or she is close to, or has reached the benefit limit for a service (for example, a patient is notified that the limit to the number of refills for a certain medication has been reached), the patient may need to obtain a complete list of all benefits paid on his or her behalf to determine erroneous charges.
4. A call from a debt collector for medical services not received indicates the patient should contact the service provider and obtain a copy of all bills and related documentation of care to determine where the fraud came from and determine if the health record needs to be changed.
5. Patients should listen carefully to the questions asked of them when they are registering for a healthcare visit, meaning they should always verify their own demographic information when being seen by a provider and should always address and correct erroneous information (OAG, CA DOJ 2019).

The HIM professionals assist patients with the process of finding out what happened in cases of medical identity theft and help guide patients to fixing errors that may be in their health record and should help build awareness of medical identity theft in their work setting. HIM professionals should provide consumer education on how to guard against theft, like protecting insurance card information and monitoring statements from one's insurance company and healthcare providers (McNabb and Rhodes 2014).

Ethical Decision Making

When a healthcare professional is faced with ethical decisions and dilemmas, several factors are included in the decision-making process, including but not limited to: cost, technological feasibility, federal and state laws, medical staff bylaws, accreditation and licensing stands, and employer policies, rules, and regulations (Gordon and Gordon 2016).

An example of an ethical decision-making process for a healthcare organization is an elderly patient who is not able to make his own healthcare decisions and has a limited chance of long-time survival. The patient has a daughter who wants the healthcare organization to do everything possible to keep her father alive and her brother wants to remove all care and let the patient pass. The ethics committee considers the cost to the healthcare organization, the technological feasibility to care for the patient, and the bylaws of the organization to make the decision.

Health information management professionals should be guided by the AHIMA Code of Ethics in making ethical decisions because they relate directly to the HIM profession. Most professional organizations are guided by a code of ethical standards of practice for the profession; the American Medical Association (AMA) subscribes to a body of ethical statements for a physician to recognize responsibility to the patient first, as well as to society, other health professionals, and to self (AMA 2018). There may not be one right answer to an ethical dilemma; rather, there may be a range of morally acceptable options, with some options being better or worse than others. The most difficult aspect of ethics is deciding on the best course of action and providing good reasons to support the choice (Harman and Cornelius 2017). For example, a coder encounters a conflict between a coding guideline and a payer requirement. She can contact the compliance department, survey colleagues, or contact the payer for advice to resolve the conflict. The best option is to contact the payer for advice. Figure 21.2 shows seven considerations that should be deliberated by HIM professionals faced with an ethical decision.

Figure 21.2 Ethical decision-making process

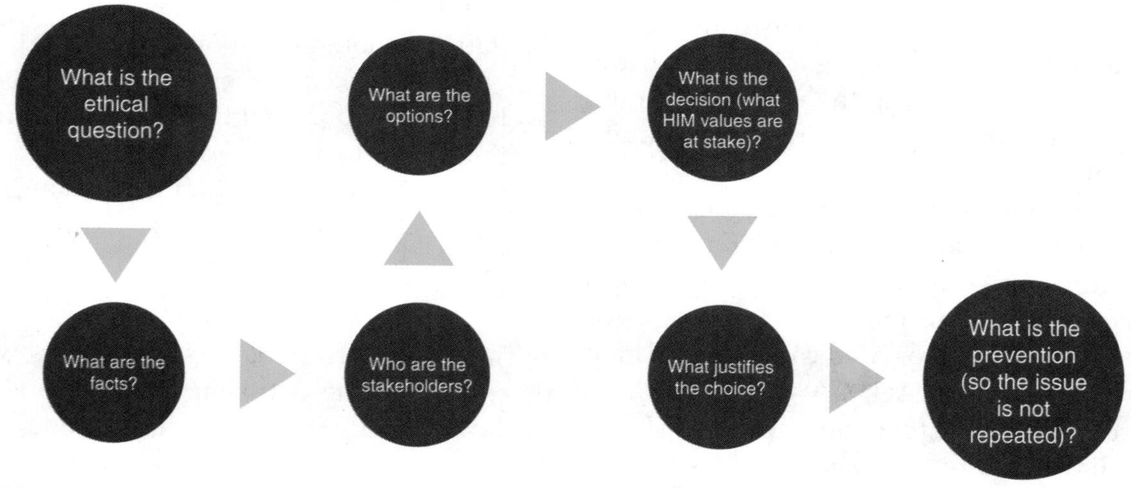

Source: ©AHIMA.

Sarah, who is a new graduate of a health information technology program, sits for the registered health information technician (RHIT) examination and fails. She does not want her employer to know she failed and tells all her coworkers she passed the examination. Sarah then starts using the RHIT credential after her name in work correspondence. A coworker, Nancy, discovers that Sarah is using the RHIT credential fraudulently and notifies the supervisor, Joan. It is the responsibility of both Nancy and Joan as HIM professionals to prevent this activity from happening. Joan should contact AHIMA and report the abuse. Sarah's ethical dilemma is outlined in figure 21.3.

There may be times when the ethical issue is not only between what is the right thing to do, but also how to do it. This is known as **moral distress**. When confronted with an ethical dilemma HIM professionals have the following options:

- Talk with a trusted colleague and get advice
- Approach the problem through the proper channels and document his or her efforts.
- Frame issues for the institution in terms of shared values and the AHIMA Code of Ethics
- Appeal to professional sources as necessary
- Address the issues in some way rather than letting them go unaddressed (Harman and Cornelius 2017)

Breach of Healthcare Ethics

Not all actions are clear code of ethics violations and some breaches simply result from a lack of an employee's code awareness or negligence. A **breach** of healthcare ethics is a situation in which ethics are either intentionally or accidentally violated. For example, a health information specialist releases an entire health record instead of only releasing the documentation of a work-related injury. The most complicated situations often involve colleagues who witness what is, or appears to be, unethical behavior and are unsure how to respond, especially if job security is on the line (Crawford 2017). As discussed in detail in chapter 9, healthcare organizations must disclose when a breach of PHI occurs; as part of the healthcare organization's ongoing monitoring of disclosures

Figure 21.3 Sarah's ethical dilemma outline

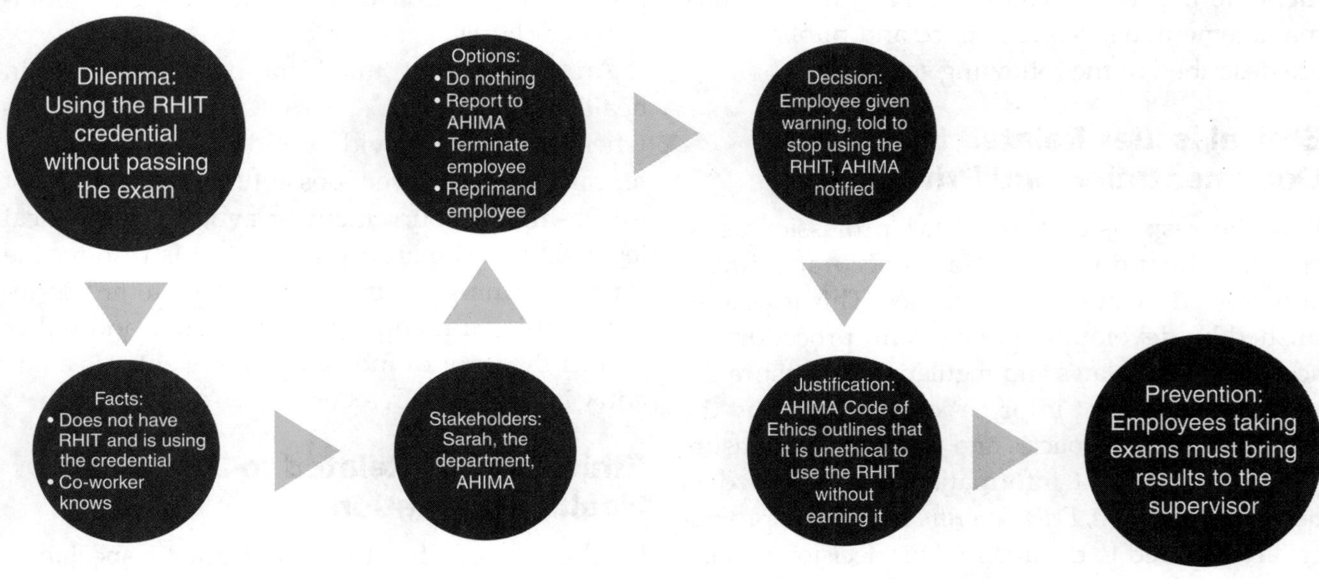

Source: ©AHIMA.

it also tracks ethical violations. For example, a security breach of PHI would occur if a patient asks for a copy of a payment made by her insurance company for a surgery she had last month, and the business office copies the remittance advice (RA) notice the healthcare facility received but fails to delete or remove the PHI for 10 other patients listed on the same RA. An example of a code of ethics breach is a coding supervisor instructing her coders to assign codes that are not supported by health record documentation. A healthcare ethics breach is a physician choosing to perform a clinical procedure that has not been tested or approved for the purpose of interest or study.

Healthcare organizations may establish an ethics committee, a committee tasked with reviewing clinical ethics violations to determine the course of action required to remedy the violations. Most ethics committees involve people from varied backgrounds and have three major functions: (1) providing clinical ethics consultation, (2) developing policies pertaining to clinical ethics, and (3) facilitating education on topical issues in clinical ethics (Pearlman 2016). The goals of the ethics committee include identifying and ensuring the rights of patients, establishing processes to ensure shared decision-making between patients and clinicians, and ensuring the processes do not interfere with the ethical practices of the healthcare organization (Pearlman 2016).

Breaches of healthcare ethics not related to clinical situations are the responsibility of the supervisor or manager where the breach occurred. The business office manager would address the breach of PHI. The coding supervisor's immediate director would address the breach of ethics by the coding supervisor. There is a process to file a complaint with AHIMA Profession Governance if an AHIMA member has violated the Code of Ethics. All suspected violations of the code of ethics are handled through a peer review process which includes the submission of a formal complaint to the staff liaison of the AHIMA Profession Governance – Professional Ethics Committee. A code of ethics cannot guarantee ethical behavior, it offers ethical guidelines an HIM professional can follow and by which actions can be judged. Ethical behaviors result from a personal commitment to engage in ethical practice (AHIMA 2019).

Important Health Information Ethical Problems

Some areas in health information management have specific ethical problems. Documentation, privacy, coding, disclosures, quality management, decision support, and public health are described in the following sections.

Ethical Issues Related to Documentation and Privacy

It is the responsibility of HIM professionals to ensure patient documentation is accurate, timely, and created by authorized parties. This is accomplished by developing policies and procedures in accordance with laws and regulations to ensure the integrity of patient information is upheld by the organization. The policies and procedures to ensure integrity of patient information are described in detail in chapter 10, *Data Security*. Healthcare providers are required to document their decision-making processes; educational sessions are important to provide training on documentation, which can help protect against unethical behaviors and protect the healthcare organization from malpractice claims.

An example of unethical documentation in healthcare is retrospective documentation—when healthcare providers add documentation after care has been given, possibly for the purpose of increasing reimbursement or avoiding a medical legal action. The HIM professional is responsible for maintaining accurate and complete health records and can identify the occurrence and either correct the error or indicate that the entry is a late entry into the health record.

Ethical Issues Related to Disclosure of Health Information

Disclosure of health information specialists should embody the value of integrity. The HIM professional must "release information only with valid authorization from a patient or a person legally authorized to consent on behalf of a patient" (AHIMA 2019). There are two primary ethical issues that arise from disclosures: the need-to-know-principle and blanket authorizations. The need-to-know principle is based on the minimum necessary standard. For example, in responding to a request to verify an admission for lap-band surgery, if the disclosure specialist gives out the history and physical, labs, discharge summary, and operative report to an insurance company, the documentation could reveal more information than requested—which in turn results in a violation of the patient's privacy. The health information specialist must only disclose the need-to-know or the least amount of information necessary, in this case only the admission information.

The other ethical concern for disclosures is misuse of the blanket authorization, which is when the patient signs an authorization allowing the disclosure specialist to release any and all information from that point forward. This is an issue because under a blanket authorization the patient is giving authorization for future diagnoses and treatments, one of which he or she may not want authorized. For example, if the patient signs the blanket authorization today to release annual examination results to his or her employer and in five years the patient is diagnosed with cancer, the employer could find out about the cancer because the information was automatically released to the employer (and the patient may not remember signing the blanket authorization five years prior). Most authorizations will state a set amount of time and for a specific reason, diagnosis, date range, provider, and such. This can be prevented by a blanket authorization having an end date, usually after one year, and will need to be signed again the next year.

Ethical Issues Related to Coding

Codes are associated with reimbursement rates and, therefore, there are inherent incentives to code so the healthcare organization will receive the highest reimbursement dollar amount possible. Coding professionals need to be guided by ethical coding practices because they may be asked by a provider to fraudulently code to receive higher payment for services rendered. It is important for a coder to only assign codes where data is clearly stated in the health record. If more information is needed, or the information needs to be clarified, a query to the physician should be used. The process for a physician query is discussed in chapter 16, *Fraud and Abuse Compliance*.

The standards of ethical coding, based on AHIMA's Code of Ethics, are guidelines outlining the following 11 standards for ethical coding:

1. Apply accurate, complete, and consistent coding practices to produce high-quality healthcare data
2. Report all healthcare data elements required for external reporting purposes completely and accurately, in accordance with regulatory and documentation standards and requirements and applicable official coding conventions, rules, and guidelines
3. Assign and report only the codes and data that are clearly and consistently supported by health record documentation in accordance with applicable code set and abstraction conventions, rules, and guidelines
4. Query provider for clarification and additional documentation prior to code assignment when there is conflicting, incomplete, or ambiguous information in the health record regarding a significant reportable condition or procedure or other reportable data element dependent on health record documentation
5. Refuse to change reported codes or the narratives of codes so that meanings are misrepresented
6. Refuse to participate in or support coding or documentation practices intended to inappropriately increase payment, quality for insurance policy coverage, or skew data by means that do not comply with federal and state statutes, regulations, and official rules and guidelines
7. Facilitate interdisciplinary collaboration in situations supporting proper coding practices

8. Advance coding knowledge and practice through continuing education
9. Refuse to participate in or conceal unethical coding or abstraction practices or procedures
10. Protect the confidentiality of the health record at all times and refuse to access protected health information not required for coding-related activities
11. Demonstrate behavior that reflects integrity and shows a commitment to ethical and legal coding

Upcoding, unbundling, and double billing are coding ethical dilemmas. Upcoding is the practice of assigning diagnostic or procedural codes that represent higher payment rates than the codes that truly reflect the services provided to patients via the documentation. For example, a physician examines a patient briefly for the flu, but the bill submitted for the visit includes an hour-long, complex exam that did not occur. Unbundling is the practice of using multiple codes to bill for the various individual steps in a single procedure rather than using a single code that includes all the steps. For example, a patient goes in for a new cast on a broken leg and instead of billing for one bundled visit (all the services related to treating the fracture are billed as one service), the bill lists codes for each step as individual procedures resulting in a larger reimbursement. Double billing is when two providers bill for one service provided to one patient. An example of this is a surgeon who was an assistant for an operation bills Medicare as if she were the primary surgeon, with the primary surgeon also billing Medicare for the same surgery on the same patient.

Ethical Issues Related to Quality Management, Decision Support, and Public Health

Healthcare costs are increasing, and organizations are trying to find ways to keep costs down while still providing quality services, which can be a difficult task. Some examples of quality outcome problems due to this trend include the following:

- Healthcare organizations falsifying their performance information to the public
- Negative patient outcomes, such as inattentive patient care
- Failure to ensure a physician's license is valid
- Health records being hidden or not available to the surveyors when accreditation or licensure surveys occur
- Repetition of unsuitable healthcare (Gordan and Gordan 2016)

The HIM professional is put in an advocate position so the interest of both the public and the individual patient can be served. An example of this is a global infection or bioterrorism, where it is pertinent to keep the balance between protecting the privacy of those injured or affected and delivering information to the government and healthcare professionals so the medical crisis can be resolved.

Ethical Issues Related to Managed Care

Managed care helps control the cost of healthcare by providing services at a fixed cost. It does this by minimizing variation in clinical practice; for example, all patients seen for hypertension receive the exact same standard of care and service, with little variation for individual patients. Ethical issues that arise with this type of care involve physicians missing a clinical indication a patient needs more than what the standard care provides. In some managed care settings, the goal is to increase productivity while keeping costs the same, where physicians have less time with patients, creating an opportunity for the physician to miss some key information.

Managed care incentives may affect provider behavior or have a negative effect on patient care. Incentives include providing rewards to physicians who provide the lowest cost care or withholding bonuses for physicians who have too many costly diagnostic procedures. A physician may be worried about having too many costly procedures so the physician may not order a needed procedure to save money. These incentives can have a negative effect on patient care because if a physician is worried about having too many costly procedures, patient care can be compromised (Jecker and Braddock 2008).

Ethical Issues Related to Sensitive Health Information

All health information must be protected; however, there is some information that requires special attention because it is considered sensitive health information such as genetic, adoption, drug, alcohol, sexual health, and behavioral information. This type of information not only has strict rules and regulations, but also provides an ethical gray area when it comes to releasing and providing records. For example, Benjamin is being treated for mental health and behavioral problems and upon turning age 18 chooses to receive a copy of all his medical information. Benjamin has the right to receive a copy of his medical information, but it may not be in his best interest to read the medical notes from his teenage years. The mental health clinic where he was treated has a policy that states before the clinic gives a copy of the health record to a patient, the clinic psychiatrist must review the health record with the patient to explain it to him or her.

When developing policies and procedures for disclosure that contain substance abuse, sexually transmitted disease, and mental health information, extra caution is required on the HIM professional's part because there may be competing interests between public safety and patient privacy. Federal and state legislation provides some guidance, but often legal counsel may be needed.

Ethical Issues Related to Research

Research is important for the growth and advancement of the healthcare profession. The Institutional Review Board for the Protection of Human Subjects (IRB) oversees the clinical research that is conducted for healthcare and oversees that appropriate steps are taken to protect the rights and welfare of humans participating as subjects in the research (FDA 2019). Without research, common medications or cures would not exist. However, with research comes an ethical obligation to provide patient safety and protection. This obligation is cited in the Belmont Report, which provides the foundation for ethical research. The Belmont Report protects "the autonomy, safety, privacy, and welfare of human research subjects" (Adams and Callahan 2014). The Belmont Report provides the following three primary ethical principles:

1. *Autonomy*. Autonomy includes the informed consent process for human research subjects and starts with a full disclosure of the nature of the study; the risks and benefits; and gives the participant the opportunity to back out of the study. The idea behind this is that the potential participant has full knowledge of what he or she is doing, and can confidently say yes or no.
2. *Beneficence*. Beneficence occurs when a researcher determines what the maximum potential is for society, compared to the minimum risk of harm done to the participants in the research. An example would be a researcher looking at a trial for finding the cure for the common cold. The risk to the research participants would be low and the maximum potential for the trial is high because the common cold affects a large number of people each year.
3. *Justice*. This principle involves impartial selection of participants in a research study, as it is important to avoid unfairly coercing participants; for example, prisoners have historically been coerced into taking part in medical research against their will (Adams and Callahan 2014).

The HIM department is involved in the IRB process by making the health records of patients enrolled in a research study available to external monitors and auditors. Agreements between the HIM department and researchers assure patient consent and policies and procedures are followed. In the case of electronic health information there are agreements outlining the exact information to be released to researchers. The HIM department offers training to researchers and HIM staff for the procedures in place for the consent process and maintenance of the health records. Research is often provided at large teaching hospitals but is sometimes case specific; for instance, a rare disease is being researched and a small healthcare facility is seeing one patient for follow-up treatment. In this case the HIM professionals of that healthcare facility may not have the policies and procedures for research established and would need to create the process and training.

Ethical Issues Related to Electronic Health Record Systems

The access of electronic health record (EHR) systems is a complex challenge regarding record integrity, information security, linkage of information for continuum of care within different e-health systems, and the development of software for HIM purposes. HIM professionals need to be part of the implementation team for new electronic systems because they provide a unique understanding of the federal rules and regulations regarding privacy and security of health records. The HIM professionals help facilitate a successful implementation of new information systems. See chapter 11, *Health Information Systems,* for more information on EHR implementation.

Healthcare professionals are trained in the ethical issues related to the EHR because staff may have access to more information than what is needed to do their jobs. Employees accessing the EHR should not explore information out of curiosity, as this would be unethical. When a patient's health information is shared or linked within an EHR without his or her knowledge, the patient's autonomy is breached. Providers sometimes may use the copy and paste option to copy information from one patient record to another and may inadvertently add incorrect information into a record. Understanding ethical issues in documentation and HIM processes helps the HIM professional to prevent unethical behaviors and train others in the code of ethics in HIM. HIM professionals must follow the AHIMA Code of Ethics in their work as well as strive for cultural competence in their dealings with others.

Check Your Understanding 21.2

Answer the following questions.

1. Mary signed an authorization allowing her son's schools to receive his annual physicals from now until he graduates from high school. What kind of authorization did Mary sign?
   a. Disclosure authorization
   b. Blanket authorization
   c. Need-to-know authorization
   d. Consent authorization
2. Releasing health information to help a patient receive further healthcare falls under what ethical principle?
   a. Beneficence
   b. Justice
   c. Autonomy
   d. Vulnerable population
3. What is the practice of assigning diagnostic or procedural codes that represent higher payment rates?
   a. Upcoding
   b. Unbundling
   c. Utilization
   d. Managed care

4. Which of the following types of information include areas like genetics, adoption, and drug use that require special attention?
   a. Special information
   b. Scientific information
   c. Sensitive information
   d. Super information
5. The participant in a research group has been given full disclosure on what the study entails and the choice to opt out of the study. This falls under what ethical principle?
   a. Justice
   b. Autonomy
   c. Vulnerable population
   d. Beneficence
6. What is the practice of using multiple codes to bill for various individual steps in a single procedure, rather than using a single code that includes all the steps of the comprehensive procedure?
   a. Utilization
   b. Upcoding
   c. Need-to-know
   d. Unbundling
7. Which of the following has created ethical issues based on security, interoperability, and record integrity?
   a. HIPAA
   b. Advocate
   c. Sensitive data
   d. Electronic health record
8. The minimization of variation in a clinical practice is used in what setting?
   a. Need-to-know
   b. Utilization
   c. Managed care
   d. Quality assurance

HIM Roles

HIM professionals use the AHIMA Code of Ethics in their everyday lives and jobs. It is important for them to understand the proper boundaries in terms of what is the right and wrong way to complete the duties of the profession. HIM professionals work in a variety of settings including third party payers to determine proper reimbursement to the healthcare organization or provider. They research payments made for healthcare services to determine if billing is the result of fraud or abuse.

Real-World Case 21.1

Kelly was a new coder who had never held an HIM job before. She had just graduated from college and passed her RHIT when she was hired by a local clinic and she was excited to start working. A few weeks later, her manager asked to meet with her. The manager closed the door and told Kelly that she wanted her to code the health record for a particular procedure using two codes instead of one so the reimbursement would be higher. The manager then proceeded to divulge information that the clinic was struggling financially so anything extra would help. Kelly got the impression that if she did not comply, they would let her go. She really needed the job and since it was her boss asking, she felt obligated to do as she was told.

Real-World Case 21.2

Monica's best friend Shanna lives out of state and her mom just had a breast biopsy. Shanna calls Monica upset because they have not received the results of the biopsy. Shanna wants to fly home to be with her mom if the results show a malignancy; however, she does not want to purchase her plane ticket until she gets the results due to financial resources. Monica, trying to be helpful, looks up the biopsy results and lets Shanna know that the tumor is benign. Monica feels she did the right thing since the results were benign and she saved Shanna from purchasing an unneeded plane ticket.

References

Adams, L. and T. Callahan. 2014. Research Ethics. Ethics in Medicine, University of Washington School of Medicine. https://depts.washington.edu/bioethx/topics/resrch.html.

Allen, J. 2013. *Health Law & Medical Ethics for Healthcare Professionals*. Upper Saddle River, NJ: Prentice Hall.

American Health Information Management Association. 2019. Code of Ethics. http://library.ahima.org/doc?oid=105098#.Vxk2qPkrK9I .

American Health Information Management Association. 2017. *Pocket Glossary of Health Information Management and Technology*, 5th ed. Chicago: AHIMA.

American Medical Association. 2018. Principles of Medical Ethics. https://www.ama-assn.org/about/publications-newsletters/ama-principles-medical-ethics.

Brodnik, M. S., L. A. Rinehart-Thompson, R. B. Reynolds. 2017. *Fundamentals of Law for Health Informatics and Information Management*, 3rd ed. Chicago: AHIMA.

Crawford, M. 2017. Everyday ethics: AHIMA code of ethics guides daily work, complex situations. *Journal of AHIMA* 82(4):30–33.

Department of Health and Human Services, Office of Adolescent Health. 2018. Cultural Competence. https://www.hhs.gov/ash/oah/resources-and-training/tpp-and-paf-resources/cultural-competence/index.html.

Department of Health and Human Services, Office of Minority Health. n.d. National Standards for Culturally and Linguistically Appropriate Services. https://www.thinkculturalhealth.hhs.gov/pdfs/EnhancedNationalCLASStandards.pdf.

Eramo, L.A. 2016. Stopping thieves in their tracks: What HIM professionals can do to mitigate medical identity theft. *Journal of AHIMA* 87(8):40–43.

Goode, T.D. and C. Dunne. 2003. Policy Brief 1: Rationale for Cultural Competence in Primary Care (revision). Washington, DC: National Center for Cultural Competence, Georgetown University Center for Child and Human Development. http://nccc.georgetown.edu/documents/Policy_Brief_1_2003.pdf.

Gordan, L.L. and M.L. Gordan. 2016. Ethical Issues in Health Information Management. Chapter 21 in *Health Information Management Technology: An Applied Approach*, 5th ed. Edited by N.B. Sayles and L.L. Gordan. Chicago: AHIMA.

Harman, B. H. and Cornelius, F. H. 2017. *Ethical Health Informatics Challenges and Opportunities*, 3rd ed. Burlington, MA: Jones & Bartlett Learning.

Huffman, E.K. 1972. *Manual for Medical Record Librarians*, 6th ed. Chicago: Physicians' Record Company.

Jecker, N.S. and C.H. Braddock III. 2008. Managed Care. Ethics in Medicine, University of Washington School of Medicine. https://depts.washington.edu/bioethx/topics/manag.html.

McNabb, J. and H.B. Rhodes. 2014. Combating the privacy crime that can kill. *Journal of AHIMA* 85(4): 26–29.

Meyer, P., P. Yoon, and R. Kaufmann. 2013. Introduction: CDC Health Disparities and Inequalities Report. http://www.cdc.gov/mmwr/preview/mmwrhtml/su6203a2.htm?s_cid=su6203a2_w.

National Center for Cultural Competence. 2018a. Georgetown University. "Rationale for Self-Assessment." https://nccc.georgetown.edu/assessments/rationale.php.

National Center for Cultural Competence. 2018b. Georgetown University. "Tools and Processes for Self-Assessment." https://nccc.georgetown.edu/foundations/assessment.php.

Office of the Attorney General, California Department of Justice. 2019. First Aid For Medical Identity Theft: Tips for Consumers. https://oag.ca.gov/privacy/facts/medical-privacy/med-id-theft.

Ortiz J. and D. Casey. 2017. Ethics, law, and policy. Dead wrong! the ethics of culturally competent care. *MEDSURG Nursing* 26(4):279–282.

Pearlman, R. 2016. Ethics Committees, Programs and Consultation. Ethics in Medicine, University of Washington School of Medicine. https://depts.washington.edu/bioethx/topics/ethics.html.

Simmers, L., K. Simmers-Nartker, and S. Simmers-Kobelak. 2017. *Simmers DHO Health Science*, Updated 8th ed. Boston, MA: Cengage Learning.

U.S. Food & Drug Administration. 2019. Institutional Review Boards Frequently Asked Questions. https://www.fda.gov/regulatory-information/search-fda-guidance-documents/institutional-review-boards-frequently-asked-questions.

World Health Organization. 2018. Social Determinants of Health. http://www.who.int/social_determinants/sdh_definition/en/.

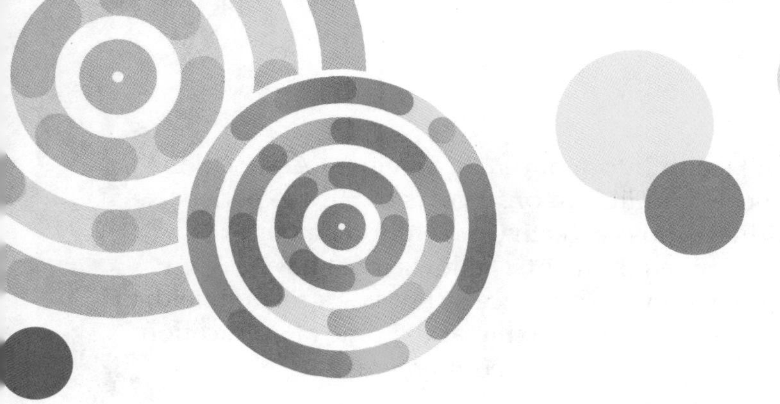

Appendix

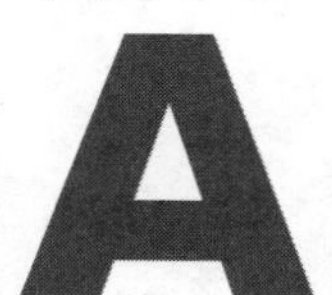

Check Your Understanding Answer Key

Check Your Understanding 1.1

1. **b** The American College of Surgeons recognized the need for improved health records and started the hospital standardization movement.
2. **b** Data analytics is the science of examining raw data with the purpose of drawing conclusions about that information.
3. **a** The health information management (HIM) profession is changing due to factors such as new laws, the electronic health record (EHR), and new technology.
4. **a** Today's HIM profession is focused on the information available in the EHR and other information systems.
5. **b** A credential which is received via a certification process is a formal agreement granting an individual permission to practice in a profession, usually conferred by a national professional organization dedicated to a specific area of healthcare practice; or the accordance of permission by a healthcare organization to a licensed, independent practitioner to practice in a specific area of specialty within that organization.
6. **b** The Commission on Accreditation for Health Informatics and Information Management Education (CAHIIM) is the accreditation organization for health information management educational programs.

Check Your Understanding 1.2

1. **b** Candidacy is the initial accreditation stage when a program is working towards CAHIIM accreditation.
2. **a** Engage is a virtual network that allows health information management (HIM) professionals to consult with each other, share resources, and more.
3. **b** The House of Delegates controls the HIM profession.

4. b I am not eligible for an American Health Information Management Association (AHIMA) Fellowship because I need a minimum of 10 years of HIM experience. Fellowship is open to any individual who is an active or senior member of AHIMA and who meets the eligibility requirements. Fellows must have a minimum of 10 years full-time professional experience in HIM or a related field, a minimum of 10 years continuous AHIMA membership at the time of application, excluding years as a student member, among other requirements.

5. b The Commission on Certification for Health Informatics and Information Management (CCHIIM) credential designed specifically for graduates of an accredited associate degree program is the Registered Health Information Technician (RHIT).

Check Your Understanding 2.1

1. a A hospitalist is a physician who cares for patients primarily when they are in the hospital. After a patient is discharged from the hospital, they return to the care of their primary physician.

2. d Physician assistants are licensed to practice medicine with physician supervision.

3. c Respiratory therapy services are provided by a qualified professional for the assessment, treatment, and monitoring of patients with deficiencies or abnormalities of pulmonary function.

4. d A radiologic technologist uses ultrasound, CT, and MRI equipment.

5. d Orthopedics is a specialty that is surgical in nature.

6. b Registered nurses are required to have a license in the state in which they practice. Every state in the US requires nurses to be licensed within that state.

7. a A clinical laboratory scientist performs tests on body fluids, tissues, and cells.

8. T Health information management professionals are trained in the management of health data and information flow throughout the healthcare organization and are responsible for ensuring the availability, accuracy, and protection of clinical information.

9. T Audiologists do provide comprehensive diagnostic and treatment and rehabilitative services for auditory, vestibular, and related impairments.

10. F The rehabilitation team includes many members of the medical, nursing, and allied health professions.

Check Your Understanding 2.2

1. b The continuum of care refers to the range of healthcare services provided to patients, from routine ambulatory care to intensive acute care, with the emphasis on treating patients at the level of care required by their course of treatment.

2. a The board of directors has the ultimate responsibility for the direction of the hospital.

3. a The Veteran's Administration serves the US military.

4. a A safety net hospital is a medical center that by legal obligation provides healthcare to individuals regardless of their ability to pay.

5. a Permissions for providers to perform procedures is called clinical privileges.

6. **T** Acute-care hospitals provide short-term care to diagnose or treat an illness.
7. **T** Case management is the ongoing, concurrent review to ensure the necessity and effectiveness of clinical services provided to patients.
8. **T** Pharmaceutical services are considered part of the clinical support services.
9. **F** Long-term acute-care hospitals specialize in the treatment of patients with serious medical conditions that require care on an ongoing basis.

Check Your Understanding 2.3

1. **d** Voluntary agencies provide healthcare and healthcare planning services, usually at the local level and to low-income patients.
2. **d** Freestanding ambulatory care centers provide emergency medical services and urgent care for walk-in patients. Urgent care centers provide diagnostic and therapeutic care for patients with minor illnesses and injuries.
3. **b** In general, long-term care is the healthcare rendered in a non-acute-care facility to patients who require inpatient nursing and related services for more than 30 consecutive days.
4. **a** Hospice care is not focused on cure. It is palliative, focusing on pain relief, comfort, and enhanced quality of life for the terminally ill.
5. **a** Artificial intelligence is the ability of a computer program or machine to think and learn.
6. **e** Managed care manages cost, quality, and access to services.
7. **b** Freestanding ambulatory care centers provide emergency medical services and urgent care for walk-in patients.
8. **a** The Human Genome Project was a 13-year-long international effort with three principal goals: (1) to determine the sequence of the three billion DNA subunits, (2) to identify all human genes, and (3) to enable genes to be used in further biological study.
9. **c** Subacute care offers patients access to constant nursing care while recovering at home.
10. **d** Continuum of care is care provided by different caregivers at several different levels of the healthcare system.

Check Your Understanding 2.4

1. **d** *To Error is Human* reported that as many as 98,000 people die each year from preventable medical errors.
2. **b** Healthy People 2020 sets out a plan to improve the nation's health.
3. **c** The National Academy of Medicine was established in 1970 as a nongovernmental agency to provide unbiased advice to decision makers and the public.
4. **a** The Centers for Disease Control and Prevention (CDC) is the leading federal agency charged with protecting the public health and safety through the control and prevention of disease, injury, and disability.

5. **b** *Leadership by Example* addressed the duplication and contrasting approaches to performance measures by the six major governmental healthcare programs that serve nearly 100 million Americans.
6. **T** PCORI is the largest single research funder that has comparative effectiveness research as its main focus.
7. **F** Healthcare policy is established at all levels – national, state, and local.
8. **T** Hospitals and care systems need to redesign how care is delivered to eliminate inefficiencies within the system, leading to better, integrated care, and lowering the total cost of care.
9. **T** The CDC collects, analyzes, and creates national statistical databases and publishes papers on important health issues.
10. **T** Social determinants of health (SDOH) are conditions in the environments and age that impact a wide range of health, functioning, and quality-of-life outcomes and risks.

Check Your Understanding 2.5

1. **b** The HITECH Act is part of the American Recovery and Reinvestment Act.
2. **c** Until World War II, most healthcare was provided in the home.
3. **c** The Tax Equity and Fiscal Responsibility Act of 1982 created the first prospective payment system for Medicare and mandated the creation of others in the future.
4. **c** The American Recovery and Reinvestment Act (ARRA) created the Office of National Coordinator for Health Information Technology.
5. **b** Medicaid is a federal healthcare program that provides healthcare services to low-income people.
6. **e** The Tax Equity and Fiscal Responsibility Act of 1982 required the gradual implementation of a prospective payment system (PPS) for Medicare reimbursement.
7. **d** The Social Security Act of 1935 gave states funds on a matching basis for maternal and infant care, rehabilitation of crippled children, general public health work, and aid for dependent children under 16 years of age.
8. **b** The Public Law 92–603 of 1972 required concurrent review of Medicare and Medicaid patients.
9. **c** The Patient Protection and Affordable Care Act of 2010 provided an individual mandate to have minimum acceptable coverage or pay a tax penalty.
10. **a** The Utilization Review Act of 1977 required hospitals to conduct continued-stay reviews for Medicare and Medicaid patients.

Check Your Understanding 3.1

1. **d** The primary purpose of the health record is patient care.
2. **b** Policy-making users utilize the health record to make changes to reimbursement systems as well as healthcare programs.
3. **c** The electronic health record is a digital record of an individual's health-related information that conforms to nationally recognized interoperability standards and can be created, managed, and consulted by authorized clinicians and staff across more than one healthcare organization.

4. **c** Individual users include patient care providers, patient care managers and support staff, coding and billing staff, patients, employers, lawyers, law enforcement officials, and healthcare researchers and clinical investigators.

5. **b** Deidentified data do not have any identifying data such as name, so public health and research frequently use deidentified data to monitor trends, determine efficacy of drugs, and for other purposes.

Check Your Understanding 3.2

1. **a** Information about multiple admissions can be stored on multiple rolls of microfilm, making it difficult to retrieve.

2. **d** Terminal-digit filing distributes health records evenly throughout the filing units.

3. **a** Rules-based algorithm assigns weights to specific data elements and uses those weights to compare one record to another.

4. **d** There are a number of standards including the assignment of a unique identifier for each form. Minimal color is acceptable but should be limited to highlighting key data.

5. **a** Qualitative analysis is monitoring the quality of the documentation. Quantitative analysis is a review of the health record to determine if there are any missing reports, forms, or signatures.

6. **a** Every healthcare facility should have a clinical forms committee to establish standards for design and approve new and revised forms. The committee should also have oversight of computer screens and other data capture tools.

7. **b** Assembly is organizing the documents in a health record in a specific order.

8. **c** Abstracting can be either the process of extracting information from a document to create a brief summary of a patient's illness, treatment, and outcome, or the process of extracting elements of data from a source document or database and entering them into an automated system.

9. **b** An overlay is when two patients are assigned the same health record number.

10. **b** When a health record is not completed according to the time frame established by the medical staff rules and regulations, the records are delinquent.

Check Your Understanding 3.3

1. **c** Personal health records are electronic or paper health records maintained and updated by an individual for himself or herself; a tool that individuals can use to collect, track, and share past and current information about their health or the health of someone in their care.

2. **d** An amendment is a clarification to the health record documentation. It must be dated, timed, and signed.

3. **b** All versions of a document in the health record must be retained. There must be policies that address which version is displayed.

4. **c** Copying and pasting can save time but there is a risk that outdated or inaccurate information can be copied and pasted.

5. **b** A mask is used to display data. It prevents dashes or other characters from being stored in the database.

Check Your Understanding 4.1

1. **b** The history and physical (H&P) can be documented for every patient no more than 30 days before or 24 hours after admission to the hospital.
2. **d** The goal of documentation standards is to ensure what is documented in the health record is complete and accurately reflects the treatment provided to the patient.
3. **b** The Medicare Conditions of Participation are the standards that a healthcare organization must meet to receive Medicare funding.
4. **a** Deemed status is an official designation indicating that a healthcare organization complies with the Medicare Conditions of Participation.
5. **d** Medical staff privilege is the process of ensuring the physician or other healthcare professional has the education and qualifications required to perform services and procedures in a healthcare organization.

Check Your Understanding 4.2

1. **T** Only individuals authorized by the healthcare organization's policies should be allowed to enter documentation in the health record.
2. **F** Auto-authentication does not meet standards for appropriate timing, dating, and signing-off of documentation by healthcare providers and therefore should not be used.
3. **b** The time and date of each entry (orders, reports, notes) must be accurately documented.
4. **F** Errors must never be obliterated. The original entry should remain legible, and the corrections should be entered in chronological order.
5. **T** Health record entries should be documented at the time the services described are rendered.

Check Your Understanding 4.3

1. **F** The care provided in the home setting as well as the skill level of the healthcare professional providing the care is individualized based upon the needs of the patient.
2. **b** The discharge summary is a concise account of the patient's illness, course of treatment, response to treatment, and condition at the time of patient discharge (official release) from the hospital.
3. **c** Administrative data is coded information contained in secondary records (such as billing records) describing patient identification and insurance. Patient registration and account information would be considered administrative data.
4. **a** Behavioral health records contain a treatment plan that often includes family and caregiver input and information as well as assessments geared toward the transition to outpatient, nonacute treatment.
5. **c** Standing Orders are orders the medical staff or an individual physician established as routine care for a specific diagnosis or procedure.
6. **T** Many services such as surgery, infusions, and other diagnostic procedures that once required a patient to stay overnight in the hospital can be performed on an outpatient basis.

7. d A patient assessment instrument (PAI) is completed on Medicare patients shortly after admission and upon discharge. Based on the patient's condition, services, diagnosis, and medical condition, a payment level is determined for the inpatient rehabilitation stay.

8. b Behavioral health records contain much of the same information as other types of health records such as progress notes, history and physical and more

9. c Ambulatory surgery centers have nurses who call the patient 24 to 48 hours after surgery. This call is documented in the health record.

10. b Fetal monitoring strips. Labor and delivery documentation includes fetal monitoring strips, a record of medications given and stopped, as well as nursing progress notes.

11. a Many of these documents would be found in multiple types of health records. The PAI is the key document that indicates this is a rehabilitation health record.

12. d Informed consent is the process by which the healthcare provider informs or makes the patient knowledgeable about the risks and benefits of the proposed treatment or procedure.

13. a The consultation documents the clinical opinion of a physician other than the primary or attending physician. The consultation is usually requested by the primary or attending physician, but occasionally may be the request of the patient or the patient's family.

Check Your Understanding 4.4

1. d The source-orientated health record format is where the documentation contained within the health record is organized by source or originating department.

2. b The "S" stands for the word subjective.

3. c Pay-for-performance is a reimbursement model where the healthcare provider is paid incentives for providing quality care.

4. b Document imaging is the process by which paper-based documentation is captured, digitized, stored, and made available for retrieval by the end user.

5. T Pay-for-performance is a reimbursement model where the healthcare provider is paid incentives for providing quality care.

Check Your Understanding 4.5

1. d Documentation should be done at the time the service is provided, which makes the documentation timely.

2. T Documentation in the health record is important to health information management (HIM) professionals for coding, claim generation, data quality monitoring, disclosure of health information, and such.

3. T The HIM professional is viewed as the expert to develop workflows and infrastructure around the electronic health record.

4. b Nursing documentation should only be objective in nature.

5. F The HIM professional does not document in the health record.

Check Your Understanding 5.1

1. **T** Category I CPT does include E/M, anesthesia, surgery, radiology, pathology and laboratory, and medicine.
2. **F** The three main core components of SNOMED CT are: concepts, descriptions, and relationships.
3. **F** The preferred term is the description or name assigned to a concept that is used most commonly in a clinical record or in literature for a specific language or dialect.
4. **F** Nursing terminologies are used to represent clinical information generated and used by nursing staff.
5. **T** If data granularity is the goal of collecting the data, clinical terminologies is the best choice.

Check Your Understanding 5.2

1. **a**
2. **c**
3. **b**
4. **e**
5. **d**

Refer to the terms and definitions in the glossary at the back of this textbook.

Check Your Understanding 5.3

1. **LOINC** Logical Observation Identifiers, Names and Codes is used for clinical lab observations.
2. **c** The semantic clinical drug term type includes ingredients plus strength plus dose.
3. **T** HCPCS Level II is standard for supplies under HIPAA.
4. **F** RxNorm is the standard for drugs under the promoting interoperability program.
5. **a** Dental procedures are not published by the Centers for Medicare and Medicaid Services.

Check Your Understanding 5.4

1. **T** Data elements specified in OASIS-D are collected on long-term care patients.
2. **F** The UHDDS was incorporated into the inpatient prospective payment system.
3. **d** Code systems are found in the UMLS Metathesaurus. LOINC is a code system.
4. **c** SNOMED CT is made up of three main components: concepts, descriptions, and relationships.
5. **b** The preferred term is the description assigned to a concept that is used most commonly in a clinical record or in literature for a particular language or dialect.

Check Your Understanding 6.1

1. **T** A data element can be a single or individual fact that represents the smallest unique subset of a larger database sometimes referred to as the raw facts and figures.
2. **b** Data sets are a recommended list of data elements that have defined and uniform definitions that are relevant for a particular use or are specific to a type of healthcare industry.
3. **b** Defining a data dictionary is a fundamental step to understanding data elements, their meaning, and usage. It also supports the creation of well-structured and defined data sets by creating standardized definitions of data elements to help ensure consistency of collection and use of the data.
4. **c** Relational and object-oriented databases are the two most commonly used databases in healthcare.
5. **F** The data dictionary creates a definition for each data element in a database.
6. **F** There are multiple sources of data in a healthcare organization including the electronic health record, indices, and more.

Check Your Understanding 6.2

1. **a** Information governance is the process of managing information within a healthcare organization.
2. **b** The IGAM helps healthcare organizations evaluate the current state of an IG initiative, including identification of best practices, gaps, and areas of opportunity based on risk, strategy, and operations of a healthcare organization.
3. **b** Integrity is creating methods that enable the data generated and maintained by a healthcare organization to be authentic and reliable.
4. **F** To build a successful IG initiative, a healthcare organization must have support from the healthcare organization's executive leadership.

Check Your Understanding 6.3

1. **F** Information and data governance are two different concepts. Information governance focuses on information and how it is used. Data governance focuses on data collection and other aspects of data.
2. **d** The principles of information governance are accountability, transparency, integrity, protection, compliance, availability, retention, and disposition.
3. **T** Data stewardship is principles and practices established to ensure the knowledgeable and appropriate use of data derived from individuals' personal health information.
4. **T** Data sharing is needed regardless of the information system used.
5. **d** Information assets refer to the information collected during day-to-day operations of a healthcare organization that has value within the healthcare organization.

Check Your Understanding 6.4

1. **F** Healthcare organizations must evaluate the data they collect to ensure it is quality data and that it meets the needs of the healthcare organization.
2. **a** The four data quality domains are application, collection, warehousing, and analysis.
3. **c** Data comprehensiveness certifies all required data elements that should be collected throughout the health record are documented.
4. **T** Data granularity is collecting data at the appropriate level of detail.
5. **d** Data integrity ensures the data entered into an information system or maintained on paper are only accessed and amended by individuals given that authority.

Check Your Understanding 6.5

1. **b** Queries can be performed using paper or electronic means.
2. **F** The healthcare organization must establish policies on how to handle queries, including the possibility of including them in the health record.
3. **c** One of the goals of queries is to identify and clarify missing, conflicting, or nonspecific provider documentation related to diagnoses and procedures.

Check Your Understanding 6.6

1. **T** The medical staff bylaws mandate expectations in documentation and data quality.
2. **T** Healthcare organizations must hold healthcare providers accountable for the documentation that they enter in the health record.
3. **b** Accreditation organizations establish standards for documentation that the healthcare organization must meet as part of the accreditation process.
4. **F** Healthcare organizations should hold providers responsible for compliance with contractual requirements. The contract should have disciplinary actions that are taken when requirements are not met.

Check Your Understanding 7.1

1. **a** Data is patient-identifiable if the identity of the patient is given even if it takes several data elements to identify the patient.
2. **d** Data derived from the primary health record, such as an index or a database, are considered secondary data sources.
3. **a** Secondary data are used for quality performance and patient safety, research, population health, and administrative purposes.
4. **F** The patient health record is a primary data source.
5. **F** The patient health record contains patient-specific data. Aggregate data are found in registries.
6. **T** Managers of health information management and other departments use secondary data to make decisions.
7. **T** Secondary data are used for quality performance and patient safety, research, population health, and administrative purposes.

Check Your Understanding 7.2

1. **c** Operation index allows the user to look up the patients according to the procedure, such as a C-section) code.
2. **a** The American College of Surgeon's Commission on Cancer has an approval process for cancer programs that includes the cancer registry.
3. **b** All the data in the cancer registry is tied to the accession number so it is the first step in abstracting the patient into the cancer registry.
4. **d** Data that allow healthcare providers and others to identify the patient are known as identification data.
5. **c** The trauma registry maintains a database on patients injured by an external physical force such as a motor vehicle crash, a gunshot wound, a stabbing, or a fall
6. **b** While the Medicare Provider Analysis and Review (MEDPAR) database is a valuable tool, it is limited in what research can be conducted since it contains only Medicare patients.
7. **a** The Health Care Quality Improvement Act of 1996 established the National Practitioner Data Bank.
8. **a** The protocol is the rules that will be used during the research study.
9. **c** The Healthcare Cost and Utilization Project (HCUP) is a valuable database especially since it contains data on all payer types.

Check Your Understanding 8.1

1. **b** Law is classified as public or private.
2. **c** Administrative law is a type of public law.
3. **b** Arbitration occurs outside the court system to lighten the court dockets and provide less costly and time-consuming alternatives for parties to settle their differences
4. **a** Medical malpractice is a broad term that encompasses negligence, intentional torts, and contract actions. The other options are too narrow.
5. **d** A complaint is how a lawsuit is initiated. The other options do not describe a complaint.
6. **c** Default judgment is rendered against a defendant who fails to answer (participate) in a lawsuit. In this question, the defendant failed to answer a complaint.
7. **a** A tort is a wrongful act that results in injury to another. Torts can be purposeful but can also be unintentional.
8. **b** For a negligence lawsuit to be successful, the plaintiff must prove the following four elements: duty, breach, causation, and injury (harm)
9. **b** Private law is limited to private (nongovernmental) parties.
10. **b** Sources of law are statutory law, constitutional law, administrative law, and common (judicial) law.
11. **d** Only legislative bodies create statutes.

12. **d** Advance directives include the living will, durable power of attorney for healthcare decisions (DPOA-HCD) and do-not-resuscitate order.

13. **a** The physician-patient relationship is established by contract, whether express (articulated, either in writing or verbally) or implied (evidenced by one's actions).

14. **a** Consent is an individual's agreement to receive medical treatment. It is not limited to invasive procedures, only a written agreement, or requires an element of negligence.

15. **c** A cross-claim, or counterclaim, is a lawsuit filed by a defendant against a plaintiff.

Check Your Understanding 8.2

1. **b** Although a patient has an interest in the information in his or her health record, the organization that created and maintains it is the owner of the physical record. Staff members and payers also have an interest in the health record, but they do not own it.

2. **c** Either a court order or subpoena is used to obtain health information for a court that has *jurisdiction* (legal authority to make decisions) over the pending litigation.

3. **b** Authentication is the process by which a health records custodian confirms the legitimacy of a health record, including verifying both the subject patient and that the information in it is valid.

4. **c** The legal health record is the record disclosed upon request.

5. **c** Health organizations must follow their relevant accrediting body standards regarding the content of the health record.

6. **c** Patient care, which documentation of patient treatment and provider communication support, is always the primary purpose of the health record.

7. **c** The National Practitioner Data Bank was created to identify problematic physicians. It is not a reimbursement mechanism, nor is it a type of certification. It has not been repealed.

8. **c** The American Health Information Management Association (AHIMA) recommends 10 years.

9. **b** It is true that retention periods can differ among healthcare organizations. Accreditation requirements are not the only factor. Operational needs should be considered. Retention periods for health information about minors are often longer than for adults.

10. **a** All applicable laws must be considered. It may be in the best interest of an organization not to retain records indefinitely. Thus, it may be best practice to destroy them at a predetermined time. Health records involved in litigation should not be destroyed.

11. **c** Credentialing is the ultimate responsibility of the board of directors and relates to physicians rather than nurses. There are also various levels of privileges.

12. **b** Credentialing is not a reward system for number of patients treated. It is separate from licensure, which is handled by a state's medical board. Medical malpractice premiums are established by professional malpractice insurance carriers in conjunction with state insurance regulations, and not by the organization credentialing physicians.

13. d Clinical privileges are the defined set of services a qualified physician is permitted to perform in an organization. Accreditation refers to the recognition by an external entity, and licensure refers to a designation by a governmental agency or board. Credentialing refers to medical staff appointments in a general sense, but not to the specific set of services or functions that an individual may engage in.

14. a Only licensure describes the designation that allows an individual to practice within a certain professional area; its absence prohibits an individual from practicing.

15. b Degaussing is the method of neutralizing the magnetic field to erase data

Check Your Understanding 9.1

1. b The right of privacy, which does apply to health information, has been granted by court decisions that interpret the US Constitution.

2. c If state laws provide a lesser degree of protection to health information than HIPAA provides, then state law may be preempted. However, state laws that protect health information to a greater extent than HIPAA may supersede HIPAA.

3. a HIPAA does not specify a length of time that protected health information (PHI) must be maintained; however, the right of access exists for as long as the PHI exists.

4. c Where state statute protects PHI to a lesser degree (is less strict) than HIPAA, that state statute will be preempted by HIPAA. This must be analyzed on a case-by-case basis, so preemption is not automatically granted or denied when HIPAA is analyzed relative to a state statute.

5. d The Privacy Rule applies to healthcare providers that conduct transactions electronically, health plans, and healthcare clearinghouses. Together, these constitute covered entities. The Privacy Rule also applies to covered entities' business associates.

6. b The Privacy Rules extends to protected health information in any form or medium, including paper and oral forms

7. d Per the right to request confidential communications, both healthcare providers and health plans may refuse to accommodate the request if the individual does not provide information as to how payment will be handled.

8. a A reasonable cost-based fee is permitted, but it must be based on actual costs incurred for that request. If state statute permits an individual to be charged more than the HIPAA-permitted reasonable cost-based fee then the state statute is preempted by HIPAA.

9. b Organizations outside the covered entity's workforce that use PHI to perform functions on behalf of the covered entity includes the definition of a business associate.

10. b The minimum necessary standard requires that uses, disclosures, and requests be limited to only the amount needed to accomplish an intended purpose.

11. d Business associates must respond to accounting requests that are made directly to them.

12. a Deidentified information does not identify an individual or provide a reasonable basis to believe the individual could be identified. To be deidentified, information has been removed such that it cannot be constituted later or combined to reidentify an individual. Deidentified information is not subject to the HIPAA Privacy Rule.

Check Your Understanding 9.2

1. **b** The HIPAA Privacy Rule requires the Notice of Privacy Practices be available at the site where the individual is treated and posted in a prominent place where patients can reasonably be expected to read them.
2. **c** Privacy Rule gives individuals the right to request restrictions and amendments. It does not give an automatic right for those requests to be granted. Individuals are to receive this PHI at a reasonable cost-based price; it does not allow them to receive it at no cost.
3. **b** Refusal by an individual to sign a HIPAA consent enables the provider to refuse to provide treatment. The HIPAA consent is optional and does not have to be presented or signed at all if the covered entity chooses not to provide it.
4. **d** A covered entity does not have to use it for PHI to be used or disclosed for TPO. The Notice of Privacy Practices informs the individual of TPO uses and disclosures; permission (consent) is not required.
5. **c** Written authorization is not required for inclusion in the facility directory. Inclusion in the facility directory is not automatic upon a patient's admission to a hospital. Facility directory listings cannot include all PHI in a designated record set.
6. **b** The opportunity to agree or object pertains to a patient's verbal agreement (or objection) to being included in the facility directory or to communications with family or friends involved in the patient's care.
7. **a** This disclosure of information is a public interest and benefit exception (regarding decedents). As such, written authorization is not required, and it is not a violation of the Privacy Rule. HIPAA consent is optional by nature, so this disclosure is not subject to the HIPAA consent.
8. **c** Release of vital statistic information is a public interest and benefit exception to the written authorization requirement, so neither consent nor authorization is required. Consent is optional under the Privacy Rule.
9. **d** Research is a public interest and benefit exception to the written authorization requirement. This does not mean that research always results in an exception to authorization. It does mean that an IRB or privacy board, which monitors the ethics of research studies and the human rights of research subjects, has reviewed the study and deemed the standard authorization requirement not necessary.
10. **a** Calling a patient by name is subject to the minimum necessary requirement, but it is a permissible incidental disclosure, necessary for the office to conduct its business. It is a disclosure for operational purposes, not payment purposes.

Check Your Understanding 9.3

1. **a** Medical identity theft is a fraudulent act committed to obtain medical services or goods or to obtain money, and it damages the integrity of an individual's health information.

2. **a** Red flag categories reflect suspicious characteristics. Merely referring to an account held by an elderly person, is not on its face a suspicious characteristic.
3. **a** The covered entity is responsible to train all members of its workforce, not only employees. The retention period for HIPAA-related records is six years.
4. **d** Unless exceptions (such as emancipation) exist, a minor is deemed legally incompetent. Individuals with developmental disabilities must be assessed for legal competence. As such, an adult with a developmental disability may be legally incompetent. An individual assigned to serve as a minor's personal representative, to make healthcare decisions on the minor's behalf, is the most likely of the options to be deemed legally competent without additional facts to indicate otherwise.
5. **c** Individuals must be informed in advance in the Notice of Privacy Practices. Opt-out instructions are required. Prior authorization is required if individuals are targeted for fundraising based on their diagnosis. There are exceptions to the authorization requirement for fundraising.
6. **b** Face-to-face communications do not require written authorization. Not all activities identified as marketing require written authorization. Use of an individual's PHI for the introduction of products or services of nominal value specifically does not require authorization.
7. **a** The HIPAA Privacy Rule does not require the identity of the culprit in a breach be disclosed. All other information must be included when informing an individual about a breach of their PHI.
8. **d** While highly recommended, it is a security measure that does not fall within the usual scope of duties for a privacy officer.
9. **c** Breach notification applies even if only one individual's PHI was breached.
10. **b** Written authorizations do not have to be notarized.

Check Your Understanding 10.1

1. **c** External security threats come from hackers, natural disasters (including tornadoes), and other sources.
2. **a** Data availability ensures the organization can depend on the information system to perform as expected and to provide information when and where it is needed. Preventing loss of data is a key component to ensure the data is available.
3. **b** Access systems for spite or profit. Employees who use patient information for identity theft or other means of fraud or theft fall under the access systems for spite or profit category of threat.
4. **c** Integrity, or data integrity, means data are complete, accurate, consistent, and up to date so the data are reliable.
5. **c** Internal security threats occur within the healthcare organization.
6. **a** A computer worm is a program that copies itself and spreads throughout a network.
7. **d** Baiting involves hackers leaving an infected USB or flash drive in a public area with the hopes that someone will come by, pick it up, and use it out of curiosity.
8. **a** Server redundancy is duplicate information on one or more servers.

9. **d** Patient, employee, and organizational information. A healthcare organization must be concerned with the privacy of not only patient information but employee and organizational information too.
10. **c** Employees are the biggest security risks because they have legitimate access to patient and other information.
11. **b** Phishing is accomplished using email. Hackers send the target individual what appears to be a legitimate email correspondence from a legitimate company or organization requesting the target to click a link within the email. The target is typically asked to provide, log-in and password credentials to an information system or application. It is a type of social engineering.

Check Your Understanding 10.2

1. **d** Access controls ensure individuals are given authorization to access only the data they need to perform their respective jobs.
2. **b** Encryption is a method of encoding data, converting data into unreadable scrambled characters and symbols as they are transmitted through a telecommunication network so the data are not understood by persons who do not have a key to transform the data into their original form.
3. **a** Risk analysis is assessing security threats and vulnerabilities.
4. **b** People are threats to data security through intentional sabotage, unintentional mistakes, and more.
5. **a** A covered entity should have policies on the use of passwords. These policies should include mandatory scheduled password changes.
6. **b** Automatic log-outs, which are simply timed log-outs that reduce the chances a person's account will be used by someone else, can be used to prevent access by unauthorized individuals. It is one of the HIPAA administrative requirements.
7. **b** A firewall is a part of an information system or network that is designed to block unauthorized access while permitting authorized communications. It is a software program or device that filters information and serves as a buffer between two networks.
8. **d** The CIA Trial includes confidentiality, integrity, and availability.

Check Your Understanding 10.3

1. **b** Potential business associate liability was increased under HIPAA. With the implementation of the American Recovery and Reinvestment Act revisions (ARRA), potential business associate liability increased. Business associates are now held directly responsible for not complying with, the administrative, physical, and technical safeguards of the HIPAA Security Rule, as well as the policies and procedures and documentation requirements.
2. **a** Documentation must be retained for six years from the date of its creation or the date when it was last in effect, whichever is later.
3. **d** Data integrity means that data are complete, accurate, consistent, and up to date, so the data are reliable. Reliability is a measure of consistency of data items based on their reproducibility and an estimation of their error of measurement.

4. **d** The technical safeguards are the technology and policies and procedures regarding the use and operation of the technology. They include integrity, audit controls, and access controls, which also includes password management.
5. **a** The designated individual responsible for data security must be identified by every covered entity (CE). HIPAA requires each CE must designate a security official to assume the leadership role.
6. **d** All CEs need a coordinated security program with someone in charge of the program, policies, audits, and other mechanisms in place.
7. **a** A trigger is an event such as an employee not involved in patient care accessing the health record of a celebrity, requiring investigation for potential security violation.
8. **a** The employee and patient have the same last name.
9. **b** An addressable specification is one that a CE can evaluate to determine if implementation is feasible. If not, the CE must document why and how they will address the intent of the standard.

Check Your Understanding 11.1

1. **b** Laboratory information systems are source systems because they originally created the information.
2. **a** A core electronic health record (EHR) component includes computerized provider order entry (CPOE).
3. **a** Clinical decision support allows a provider to check drug and allergy interactions.
4. **a** CDS is the process in which individual data elements are represented in the computer by a special code to be used in making comparison, trending results, and supplying clinical reminders and alerts.
5. **c** E-prescribing is used to send prescriptions to retail pharmacies.
6. **a** The bar-coding system ensures the right drug, dose, route, time, and patient
7. **b** All the healthcare systems must have interconnectivity for the reconciliation to work.
8. **b** During implementation the functionality is added one system at a time.
9. **b** Templates provide data entry support and are created based on the type of patient being treated.
10. **c** The EHR provides data and support for data collection about one patient at a time the other characteristics are the future state of EHRs

Check Your Understanding 11.2

1. **b** Interface is the zone between different computer systems across which users want to pass information.
2. **a** Telehealth is the services given to a patient through an interactive telecommunications system by a practitioner at a distant site (CMS 2017).
3. **b** The Consolidated Clinical Document Architecture (C-CDA) is a collection of healthcare document templates in XML format.
4. **b** An Health information organization (HIO) provides identity management to assure appropriate security services.

5. **T** Cloud computing is a process where data (and software) are housed on remote servers accessible through the internet.
6. **T** The HL7 FHIR standard brings interoperability into the world of web-based connectivity.
7. **F** Direct exchange uses an initiative called the direct project for securely *pushing* patient health information to a known, trusted receiver using secure email technology.
8. **T** A patient is not required to use a patient portal.
9. **F** eHealth Exchange must be purchased by healthcare providers.

Check Your Understanding 11.3

1. **b** The systems development life cycle ensures all the components needed for a system to achieve its desired results are addressed.
2. **b** The systems development life cycle includes feedback and monitoring for continuous quality improvement.
3. **c** Goals should be specific, measurable, attainable, relevant, time-based.
4. **a** Physicians must be included in the organization's technology plans.
5. **d** Due diligence confirms the facts about a product.
6. **c** Negotiations include coming to terms on all the issues before they are agreed on by both parties.
7. **a** Data conversion is moving of data from an old system to a new one.
8. **b** Managing change helps people adapt to new technology.
9. **a** Best of breed happens when multiple vendors throughout a healthcare organization are used.
10. **d** Workflow and process analysis and design is the most often missed step.

Check Your Understanding 12.1

1. **a** A scorecard reports outcome measures.
2. **d** Data mining is extraction and analysis of data.
3. **b** A dashboard reports process measures.
4. **e** Data capture is the process of recording data.
5. **c** Speech recognition is the conversion of speech to text.

Check Your Understanding 12.2

1. **T** The two main types of electronic personal health records (PHR) are standalone or tethered (also known as connected).
2. **F** There is no required functionality for a patient portal. They are all different. Scheduling appointments is just one of the commonly seen functions.
3. **T** Health information such as exercise and diet plans, health goals, and home monitoring system results such as blood pressure levels may be a part of the PHR.

4. **T** There are many different smartphone apps, which are all a part of consumer health IT.
5. **F** The PHR is often sponsored by a healthcare provider and test results and other information are often posted in the PHR.
6. **F** Patient portals are used to provide direct email communication between patients and physicians.
7. **T** Health literacy includes the ability to read and complete health-related forms.
8. **F** There is a wide range of functions seen in the PHR as there is not a data standard.
9. **F** The patient portal is a way to provide patients with information on common diseases.
10. **T** While some data is generated by the healthcare organization, patients can and do generate health data for the PHR.

Check Your Understanding 12.3

1. **c** Consumer-mediated exchange is a type of health information exchange (HIE) that allows patients to control their health information.
2. **a** Patients should always provide a driver's license or other proof of identity to ensure the correct health record is accessed.
3. **c** The entire purpose of HIE is sharing information electronically.
4. **a** Digital Imaging and Communications in Medicine (DICOM) is the standard used to share MRIs, CT scans, and other radiological images.
5. **a** There are several benefits to HIE including a basic level of interoperability.
6. **b** There are a number of capabilities seen in HIEs. Two of them are sharing patient information and e-prescribing.
7. **c** Health insurance exchanges (HIX) give patients the ability to choose their healthcare plan from the health insurance market.
8. **c** The data standard used to share lab tests is LOINC.
9. **T** The purpose of HIE is sharing data. To get the benefit of this shared information, data integrity is key.
10. **F** The HIE model used to share data with the health department is directed exchange.

Check Your Understanding 13.1

1. **a** A Pareto chart can help analyze data about the frequency or causes of problems in a process. In this scenario, the healthcare organization can use the Pareto chart to graphically display why patients are being admitted to hospital. This data can then be used to reduce the number of readmissions.
2. **F** Two-variable bar charts can also display an important summary of healthcare data.
3. **a** A histogram is a graph that represents the frequency distribution of numerical data. A frequency polygon is a graphical means to display a frequency distribution using continuous data in a line form.
4. **c** A bubble chart is like a scatter chart except that it compares three data variables.

5. **a** Value labels assign a value to a specific variable and appear in the output for easy interpretation.
6. **F** A pie chart displays percentage of the whole.
7. **d** A scatter chart, scatter plot, scatter diagram, or scatter graph is used to demonstrate a relationship between two variables.
8. **T** The graphical presentation of data by a box-and-whisker plot provides a visual summarization of several main factors: median, range, and outliers.
9. **a** A Pareto chart is the best graphical form to be use when examining a problem and a process, which makes it a valuable tool in performance improvement.
10. **b** Ratio variables are the most common quantitative variables used in healthcare. These include numbers that can be compared meaningfully with one another.

Check Your Understanding 13.2

1. **c** Descriptive statistics are used to give information on data and for organization and summarization. Generally, descriptive statistics do not provide information on data relationship (such as between groups of data results) or any results focused on cause and effect found by the research. This question asks for frequency, not a relationship.
2. **d** The mean, mode, and percentile are all measures of central tendency, which leaves the Z-score.
3. **a** The mean, median, and mode are all measures of central tendency. They look at how the data are centered around the middle value.
4. **c** The range is simple to calculate by taking the difference between the highest and lowest value.
5. **a** Percentiles show the value below which a percentage of scores fall. For example, 85 percent of the students taking the test scored lower than X score.

Check Your Understanding 13.3

1. **F** When presenting data graphically, if the data follow a symmetrical or bell curve, then the data are termed a normal distribution. In a normal distribution, the mean, median, and mode are equal.
2. **T** The total area under the curve equals 1, so the area of one half of the curve is equal to 0.50 and the area of the other half is equal to 0.50.
3. **F** Z-scores represent the number of standard deviations above or below the mean, so a Z-score of –1.5 represents a score that is 1.5 standard deviations below the mean.
4. **c** Determining if data follow a normal distribution is important because certain statistics can be computed on data that are distributed normally. One way to do this is by computing a Z-score. A Z-score is a standardized unit that provides the relative position of any observation in the distribution and is also the number of standard deviations that the observed value lies away from the mean.
5. **b** One standard deviation from the mean = 68.26 percent of the area, two standard deviations = 95.45 percent of the area, and three standard deviations = 99.74 percent of the area under the curve.

6. **b** When the tail is pulled toward the right side, it is called a positively skewed distribution; when the tail is pulled toward the left side of the curve, it is called a negatively skewed distribution.

7. **a** The formula for calculating the Z-score is:

$$Z-\text{score}=\frac{\text{Observation or x } - \text{Mean } (\mu)}{\text{Standard Deviation } (\sigma)}$$

Z-scores represent the number of standard deviations above or below the mean, so a Z-score of 5.5 represents a score that is 5.5 standard deviations below the mean. The score of 82 percent is 3 standard deviations above the mean.

8. **F** An analysis of variance (ANOVA) is a test used to find and examine the differences in the determined averages (means) within and between data groups. The research must be designed to gather data from two groups of participants.

9. **T** Regression equations are used to determine if there is a relationship between variables and to identify what type of relationship is present.

10. **F** The null hypothesis is centered on the prediction that there will be no difference found between the groups of the research study. The alternative hypothesis is just that, a different or opposite statement of the null hypothesis. It is related to t-tests, not ANOVA.

Check Your Understanding 13.4

1. **d** The first step is determining the object of the information and what you are trying to say with it.

2. **c** Individual data can be used to provide direct care to patients and in quality improvement studies.

3. **a** Data that is evaluated against standards or benchmarks (like hospitals across the state) are known as comparative data.

4. **c** Aggregate data are individual, comparative, or other multiple sources of data that are compiled and analyzed to draw conclusions about a specific topic or area.

5. **b** Descriptive statistics are used to give information on data and for organization and summarization. Inferential statistics is the process of making deductions for a larger population based on the statistical results taken from a sample.

Check Your Understanding 13.5

1. **e** Mixed methods uses a variety of research methods including qualitative and quantitative.

2. **i** A descriptive study is used to learn more about a topic (exploratory) and creates new hypotheses.

3. **j** A correlation study is used to determine if there is a relationship between two variables, such as smoking and cancer.

4. **c** A case control study is also known as a retrospective study. It is one in which the researcher is looking into the past for data; the data is historical and not currently obtained.

5. **d** The Framingham Heart Study is a prospective study. A prospective study is defined as research that is designed to follow the study participants into the future to see if there is a relationship that develops for the study variables.

6. **g** The experimental study design is the most powerful when trying to establish cause and effect. In healthcare, experimental research studies can entail exposing participants to different interventions to compare the results of the interventions with the outcome.
7. **b** The quasi-experimental study is similar to the experimental study except, randomization of participants is not included in a quasi-experimental study, the independent variable may not be manipulated by the researcher, and there may be no control or comparison group.
8. **f** Ethnography is a methodology where the researcher delves into a particular culture or organization in great detail to learn everything there is to know about them and to develop new hypotheses.
9. **h** Grounded theory is a research method that enables the researcher to develop a theory that is substantiated or confirmed by the data. It is a systematic method that can use multiple methods (both quantitative and qualitative findings) and pull it all together to develop a theory.
10. **a** Qualitative research is used to provide robust data on a new topic or provide background for larger studies on the same topic.

Check Your Understanding 13.6

1. **b** The Institutional Review Board (IRB) protects human subjects involved in research activities.
2. **a** HIM researchers are typically involved in IRB exempt research rather than expedited or full board approval.
3. **b** Expedited research includes those studies that pose only minimal risk to human subjects, including those studies that collect information on human subjects that is identifiable and may include sensitive information such as identifiable health information on subjects who are positive for the human immunodeficiency virus (HIV).
4. **c** The Centers for Disease Control and Prevention (CDC) is a US government agency whose mission is to collaborate with the public to create the expertise, information, and tools people and communities need to protect their health, through health promotion, prevention of disease, injury, and disability, and preparedness for new health threats.
5. **c** The Patient-Centered Outcomes Research Institute (PCORI) provides funding to researchers to perform research that is patient-centered and patient-engaged. Every research study funded by PCORI must include patients within all aspects of the research methodology process.
6. **b** The Agency for Healthcare Research and Quality (AHRQ) is a federal agency within the US Department of Health and Human Services (HHS) whose mission is to make healthcare safer, higher in quality, and more accessible, equitable, and affordable.
7. **b** The World Health Organization (WHO) works to direct and coordinate authority on international health through the United Nations.
8. **a** Every research study funded by PCORI must include patients within all aspects of the research methodology process, including the design.

Check Your Understanding 14.1

1. **d**
2. **c**
3. **d**
4. **c**
5. **d**
6. **c**
7. **d**
8. **d**
9. **c**
10. **d**
11. **c**
12. **d**
13. **d**
14. **c**
15. **d**

Discrete data represent separate and distinct values or observations and continuous data are those that represent measurable quantities but are not restricted to certain specified values.

Check Your Understanding 14.2

1. **Ratio**
2. **Proportion**
3. **Ratio**
4. **Proportion**
5. **Proportion**

Ratio compares two quantities and a proportion is a particular type of ratio in which x is a portion of the whole.

Check Your Understanding 14.3

1a. **12** [(10 + 5) –3]
1b. **13** [10 + (5 – 3) + 1]
2a. **14** [12 + 1) + (1 + 1 – 1)]
2b. **15** [(12 + 1) + (1 + 1 – 1) + 1]
3a. **165** [(160 + 20) – 15]
3b. **167** [160 + (20 – 15) + 2]
3c. **167** [160 + (20 – 15) + 2]

Check Your Understanding 14.4

1. **86.1%** Jan-June 31+28+31+30+31+30 = 181; 181 x 165 = 29,865; 25,720/29,865 x 100

   75.7% July-Dec 31+31+30+31+30+31 = 184; 184 x 200 = 36,800; 27,852/36,800 x 100

   80.4% Total for the year
2. **Medicine 59.6%** [680/(38 x 30) x 100]
   Surgery 71.2% [790/(37 x 30) x 100]
   Pediatric 39.2% [(235/20 x 30) x 100]
   Psychiatry 77.3% [927/(40 x 30) x 100]
   Obstetrics 70.0% [252/(12 x 30) x 100]
   Newborn 22.1% [252/(16 x 30) x 100]
3. **65.4%** [2,884/(147 x 30) x 100]

Check Your Understanding 14.5

1. **125** (10 + 12 + 17 + 8 + 9 + 11 + 18 + 12 + 13 + 15)
2. **831** (82 + 75 + 68 + 153 + 43 + 101 + 77 + 93 + 42 + 97)
3. **6.65 days** (831/125)
4. **6.47 days** (97/15)
5. **7.52 days** [(82 + 75 + 68 + 153 + 43)/(10 + 12 + 17 + 8 + 9)]

Check Your Understanding 14.6

1. **1.59%** [(43/2,703) x 100] = 4,300/2,703
2. **1.53%** [(43 + 1)/(2,703 + 175) x 100] = 4,400/2,878
3. **1.52%** [(43 – 2)/(2,703 – 2) x 100] = 4,100/2,701
4. **1.46%** {[(43 + 1) – 2]/(2,703 + 175) – 2] x 100} = 4,200/2,876
5. **0.57%** [(1/175) x 100]
6. **2.78%** [(5/(175 + 5) x 100]
7. **0.57%** [(1/175) x 100]

Check Your Understanding 14.7

1. **30.2%** [(9 + 2 + 1 + 1)/(35 + 2 + 1 + 5) x 100]
2. **25.7%** (9/35 x 100)
3. **27.3%** [9/(35 – 2) x 100]
4. **20.0%** (1/5 x 100)
5. **8.3%** (1/12 x 100)

Check Your Understanding 14.8

1a. **.7.32%** (15/205 x 100)

1b. **1.48%** (3/203 x 100)

2a. **4.32%** (12/278 x 100)

2b. **2.16%** (6/278 x 100)

Check Your Understanding 14.9

1. **Hospital-acquired**
2. **Healthcare-associated infections**
3. **44.9%** [(57/127) x 100]
4. **8.8%** [(6/68) x 100]
5.

MS-DRG	MS-DRG title	Relative weight	Number of patients	Total weight
179	Respiratory infections and inflammations w/o CC/MCC	0.9693	**5**	**4.8465 (0.9693 x 5)**
187	Pleural effusion w/CC	1.0691	**2**	**2.1382 (1.0691 x 2)**
189	Pulmonary edema and respiratory failure	1.2136	**3**	**3.6408 (1.2136 x 3)**
194	Simple pneumonia and pleurisy w/ CC	0.9688	**1**	**0.9688 (0.9688 x 1)**
208	Respiratory system diagnosis w/ ventilator support < 96 hours	2.2969	**1**	**2.2969 (2.2969 x 1)**
280	Acute myocardial infarction, discharged alive w/MCC	1.7289	**3**	**5.1867 (1.7289 x 3)**
299	Peripheral vascular disorders w/ MCC	1.4094	**2**	**2.8188 (1.4094 x 2)**
313	Chest pain	0.6138	**4**	**2.4552 (0.6138 x 4)**
377	GI hemorrhage w/MCC	1.7775	**1**	**1.7775 (1.7775 x 1)**
391	Esophagitis, gastroenteritis. and miscellaneous digestive disorders w/MCC	1.1976	**1**	**1.1976 (1.1976 x 1)**
547	Connective tissue disorders w/o CC/MCC	0.7985	**1**	**0.7985 (0.7985 x 1)**
552	Medical back problems w/o MCC	0.8698	**1**	**0.8698 (0.8698 x 1)**
684	Renal failure w/o CC/MCC	0.6085	**1**	**0.6085 (0.6085 x 1)**
812	Red blood cell disorders w/o MCC	0.8182	**2**	**1.6364 (0.8182 x 2)**
872	Septicemia w/o MV 96+ hours w/o MCC	1.0528	**1**	**1.0528 (1.0528 x 1)**
918	Poisoning and toxic effects of drugs w/o MCC	0.6412	**1**	**0.6412 (0.6412 x 1)**
Total			**30**	**32.9342**
Case-mix index = **1.0978 (32.9342/30)**				

Check Your Understanding 14.10

1. **i**
2. **j**
3. **e**
4. **c**
5. **f**
6. **h**
7. **g**
8. **a**
9. **k**
10. **b**
11. **d**

Refer to the terms and definitions in the glossary at the back of this textbook.

Check Your Understanding **14.11**

1a. **83.9%** (1,305,939/155,651,602 x 10,000)

1b. **80.4%** (1,290,922/160,477,237 x 10,000)

1c. **82%** ([(1,305,939 + 1,290,922)/(155,651,602 + 160,477,237)] x 10,000)

1d. **9.3%** [(20,864/22,525,155) x 10,000]

1e. **3.6%** (7,622/21,429,247 x 10,000)

2. **6.5 births per 1,000 population** (4,899/750,000 x 1,000)
3. **1.6 deaths per 1,000 live births** (8/4,899 x 100)
4. **2.9 deaths per 1,000 live births minus the neonatal deaths** (14/4,899 – 8 x 1,000)
5. **4.5 infant deaths per 1,000 live births** [(8 + 14) / 4,899 x 1,000]
6. **49.9 maternal deaths per 100,000 population** 2/4,012 x 100,000
7. **5.6 deaths per 1,000 population** (4,225/750,000 x 1,000)
8. **16.7 deaths of lung cancer per 100,000 population** (125/750,000 x 100,000)
9. **10.8% deaths due to Clostridium Difficile** 4/37 x 100
10. **0.09% proportionate death rate** 4/4,225 x 100

Check Your Understanding **14.12**

1. **A disease that must be reported to a government agency so regular, frequent, and timely information on individual cases can be used to prevent and control future cases of the disease.**
2. **Incidence rate is a computation that compares the number of new cases of a specific disease for a given time period to the population at risk for the disease during the same time period. Prevalence rate is the proportion of people in a population who have a particular disease at a specific point in time or over a specified period of time.**
3. **62.7 new cases of coronary artery disease per 100,000 population** (189,000/301,623,157) x 100,000
4. **0.8 cases per 10,000 population** (4/50,000) x 10,000
5. **1.4 cases per 10,000 population** (4+3)/50,000 x 10,000

Check Your Understanding **15.1**

1. **c**
2. **h**
3. **a**
4. **f**
5. **g**
6. **b**
7. **d**
8. **e**

Refer to the terms and definitions in the glossary at the back of this textbook.

Check Your Understanding 15.2

1. **a** Congress allocates dollars each year to the Veterans Administration and that determines the number of veterans who can be enrolled in the healthcare program.
2. **d** Medicaid determines a list of mandatory eligibility groups including children, pregnant women, elderly adults, people with disabilities, and low-income adults.
3. **c** Medicare is a federally funded program to assist with the medical costs of Americans 65 years of age and older.
4. **b** Managed care is a healthcare delivery system or network organized to manage costs, utilization, and quality.
5. **a** Private healthcare insurance typically has a high deductible or limited covered services
6. **a** Workers' compensation is insurance coverage for employees who are injured on the job and it is required for employers to carry the coverage.
7. **c** The Indian Health Services was introduced out of a special government-to-government relationship.

Check Your Understanding 15.3

1. **a**
2. **c**
3. **d**
4. **e**
5. **b**

Refer to the terms and definitions in the glossary at the back of this textbook.

Check Your Understanding 16.1

1. **b** The health information management departments of healthcare providers that have a higher Medicare payment denial rate also experience a higher number of additional documentation request (ADRs) as CMS associates a high payment denial rate with potential coding and billing errors.
2. **c** The Office of Inspector General (OIG) is an office in the federal government working to combat fraud, waste, and abuse and to improve the efficiency of Health and Human Services (HHS) programs.
3. **c** The Stark Law prohibits a physician from referring patients to a business in which he or she or a member of the physician's immediate family has financial interests.
4. **c** Fraud is a scheme to obtain funding that is not deserved. This includes knowingly submitting bills for healthcare services that are not provided.
5. **c** Abuse is increasing the costs to an insurer. Unbundling codes is an example of abuse.

Check Your Understanding 16.2

1. **T** There are seven components to a compliance program. One of these is the need for internal monitoring.
2. **T** Systematic random sampling is a pattern used to select patients, such as every 10th patient admitted.
3. **F** A compliance program is a set of internal policies and procedures that a healthcare organization puts into place to comply with applicable state and federal laws.
4. **a** There are a number of benefits of a compliance plan, including a reduction in denials.
5. **d** Unbundling is the practice of using multiple procedure codes to bill for the various individual steps in a single procedure rather than using a single code that includes all the steps of the comprehensive procedure code.

Check Your Understanding 17.1

1. **F** Planning is the examination of the future and preparation of action plans to attain goals. A strategy is a course of action designed to produce a desired outcome.
2. **c** The four functions of management are planning, controlling, leading, and organizing.
3. **d** Planning is the examination of the future and preparation of action plans to attain goals of the department or healthcare organization.
4. **a** Organizing is the coordination of all of the tasks and responsibilities of a department to attain goals of the department or healthcare organization.
5. **d** A mission is a written statement that identifies the core purpose and philosophies of a healthcare organization.

Check Your Understanding 17.2

1. **a** An operational plan guides the day-to-day decisions of an organization.
2. **d** Strengths, weaknesses, opportunities, and threats (SWOT)) guides the day-to-day decisions of an organization.
3. **F** Procedures are the processes by which policies are put into action.
4. **b** Change management is the formal process of introducing change, adopting the change, and diffusing it throughout the organization.
5. **c** Supply management is the management and control of the supplies used within an organization.

Check Your Understanding 18.1

1. **c** Performance monitoring is data driven. The key to successful monitoring is the appropriate analysis, display, and application of measurement data.
2. **c** A dashboard is the display of the most important information needed to achieve one or more objectives that has been consolidated so it can be monitored at a glance.
3. **a** Outcome indicators measure the actual results of care for patients and populations, including patient and family satisfaction.

4. b The performance improvement (PI) team must identify the customers associated with the processes under discussion. Customers are both internal and external. Once customer groups are identified, their needs related to the process need to be explored and established.

5. b Outcome indicators measure the actual results of care for patients and populations, including patient and family satisfaction.

Check Your Understanding 18.2

1. d This type of variation is special-cause variation. If the special cause produces a negative effect, identify the special cause and eliminate it, if possible. If the special cause produces a positive effect, reinforce it so this positive effect will continue and perhaps impact the processes of others in the organization.

2. b A run chart displays data points for a specific time frame. The measured points of a process are plotted on a graph at regular time intervals to help team members identify whether there are substantial changes in the numbers over time.

3. d A benchmark is a systematic comparison of one healthcare organization's measured characteristics with those of another similar organization or with internal, regional, or national standards.

4. a A checksheet is a data collection tool for recording and compiling observations or occurrences. The checksheet consists of a simple list of categories, issues, or observations on the left side of the health record and a place on the right to record incidences by placing a checkmark.

5. a Problems in patient care and other areas of the healthcare facility are usually symptoms of shortcomings inherent in a system or a process. A system is a set of related and highly interdependent components that are operating for a particular purpose.

Check Your Understanding 18.3

1. a A flow chart is a graphic tool that uses standard symbols to visually display detailed information, including time and distance of the sequential flow of work of an individual or a product as it progresses. The flow chart provides a visual image of each decision point and event in the process.

2. b Benchmarking is a systematic comparison of one healthcare organization's measured characteristics with those of another similar organization or with internal, regional, or national standards.

3. b A cause-and-effect diagram is an investigational technique that facilitates the identification of the various factors that contribute to a problem. It facilitates root-cause analysis, or the analysis of an event from all aspects (human, procedural, machinery, material) to identify how each contributed to the occurrence of the event and to develop new systems that will prevent recurrence.

4. c The multivoting technique is a variation of the nominal group technique and serves the same purpose. Instead of ranking each issue or idea, team members rate issues by marking them with a distribution of points.

5. **d** Structured brainstorming is a team-based performance improvement tool. A team leader or facilitator asks team members to create a list of ideas. Team members can work alone or in small groups. Team members take turns offering new ideas. As team members run out of new ideas, they pass; the next person then offers an idea until no team member can produce a fresh idea.

Check Your Understanding 18.4

1. **b** A standard is a written description of the expected features, characteristics, or outcomes of a healthcare-related service. Standards provide a minimum level of performance.
2. **a** To participate in the Medicare program, healthcare providers must comply with federal regulations known as the Conditions of Participation. The CMS develops the Conditions of Participation.
3. **d** Quality improvement organizations (QIO) use medical peer review, data analysis, and other tools to identify patterns of care and outcomes that need improvement. They work cooperatively with facilities and individual physicians to improve care.
4. **d** The Joint Commission scores healthcare organizations on compliance with specific National Patient Safety Goals (NPSGs). The NPSGs outline the areas of organizational practice that most commonly lead to patient injury or other negative outcomes that can be prevented if standardized procedures are used.
5. **a** DNV GL Healthcare is a voluntary accreditation organization that has been in the US since the late 1800s but is relatively new to healthcare. The organization is recognized by CMS to have *deemed status,* which means healthcare organizations accredited by DNV GL are recognized as meeting the Medicare Conditions of Participation, the administrative and operational guidelines and regulations under which healthcare organizations can take part in the Medicare and Medicaid programs.

Check Your Understanding 18.5

1. **a** Claims management is the process of managing the legal and administrative aspects of the healthcare facility's response to injury claims (injuries occurring on the healthcare facility's property).
2. **a** Utilization management (UM) is composed of a set of processes used to determine the appropriateness of medical services provided during specific episodes of care. Utilization management is an important part of quality patient care as it helps to ensure necessary and appropriate care, effectiveness of the services provided to the patient, and timely and safe discharge of patients.
3. **c** Many large healthcare facilities such as acute-care hospitals have instituted patient advocacy programs. A patient representative responds personally to complaints from patients and their families. Patient representatives can handle minor complaints and to seek remedies on behalf of patients. They also can recognize serious complaints that need to be forwarded to performance improvement or risk management personnel.
4. **a** A sentinel event describes an occurrence with an undesirable outcome usually happening only once. The occurrence, however, points to serious issues involved in care processes that must be resolved to avoid a recurrence of the event.

5. **d** An incident (or occurrence) report is a structured tool used to collect data and information about any event *not* consistent with routine operational procedures, such as a wrong-side surgery or foreign body left in following surgery. Incident reports are prepared to help healthcare facilities identify and correct problem areas and prepare for legal defense

Check Your Understanding 19.1

1. **d** Participative leadership theory: a leader feels he or she can trust group members and does not have to micromanage employees.
2. **c** Contingency leadership theory: a person may be a leader in one situation but not in another situation.
3. **b** The four management functions are leading, planning, organizing, and controlling.
4. **c** The "c" is for consultative in Vroom and Jago's decision-making strategies.
5. **a** Expert power is the type of power given to leaders who are authorities in their fields or have knowledge or skills that are in short supply.

Check Your Understanding 19.2

1. **c**
2. **a**
3. **d**
4. **e**
5. **b**

Refer to the terms and definitions in the glossary at the back of this textbook.

Check Your Understanding 19.3

1 **b**
2. **d**
3. **c**
4. **e**
5. **a**

Refer to the terms and definitions in the glossary at the back of this textbook.

Check Your Understanding 20.1

1. **a** Managers who have line authority in an organization are those who supervise one or more employees, can give orders, and are responsible for getting work done by directing the work of others.
2. **b** Per the National Labor Relations Act, supervisors and managers are excluded from an employee union bargaining unit
3. **c** The human assets of an organization are often referred to as human capital, the sum of the knowledge, skills, creativity, and problem-solving abilities of the workforce.

4. b The ethical principle of justice recognizes the importance of treating people fairly and applying rules consistently.

5. b Title VII established the Equal Employment Opportunity Commission (EEOC) as the federal agency with responsibility to administer and enforce equal opportunity employment laws, investigate complaints, and file discrimination charges in court.

6. d Title VII protects individuals from employment discrimination based upon race, color, religion, sex, or national origin. Disability is not mentioned in this Act; also see figure 20.1.

7. c The Age Discrimination in Employment Act of 1967 prohibits age discrimination against job applicants or workers age 40 and older (EEOC n.d.f). This act does not address discrimination based on worker disability or standards for benefit and retirement plans.

8. b The receptionist's position as described in this example is consistent with the nonexempt classification under the Fair Labor Standards Act (hourly paid, eligible for overtime, not a manager).

9. d Per the Americans with Disabilities Act, modification of office equipment would represent a reasonable action for the organization (not an undue financial hardship) to accommodate a qualified job applicant or employee.

10. a The National Labor Relations Act called for formation of the National Labor Relations Board.

Check Your Understanding 20.2

1. a Workforce planning involves review of data and trends and relating these to an organization's workforce needs.

2. d Job analysis involves collecting and analyzing information about a job to better understand job duties and skills required.

3. Human Resource Management (HRM) includes the following functions: employee (staff) recruitment and selection, performance appraisal, staffing, training. Staff recruitment and selection begins with an understanding of the positions to be filled; this understanding involves job analysis. Job analysis also supports the HRM functions of performance appraisal, staffing, and training.

4. F Internal candidates do need less orientation. However, morale problems may develop among internal applicants who are not selected for a position (not a positive impact), making this statement as a whole false.

5. d A job description, a written explanation of a job and the duties it entails, is based on information provided by the job analysis.

6. b A job description is a written explanation of a job and the duties (responsibilities) it entails.

7. c Job specifications describe the individual qualifications required to perform the job outlined in a job description, such as education level, experience, skills.

8. d Validity refers to the ability of a selection test to accurately measure the job skill, knowledge, or behavior it was meant to measure.

9. b Behavioral interview questions is a technique whereby the interviewee is asked to describe past behavior. The candidate is given a situation and asked to describe how he/she handeled it in the past. Behavioral question types are structured.

Check Your Understanding 20.3

1. b Staffing as an HRM function includes management decisions about how employees are scheduled in a work unit.

2. a Performance management includes the full range of activities involved in measuring, reviewing, and improving employee performance; performance appraisal is a part of this.

3. d In parallel work division, the same tasks are handled simultaneously by several workers; each completes all steps in the process from beginning to end, working independently of the other employees, as in the example here.

4. b With flextime, an employee is able to choose his or her start and departure times, accommodating personal needs while meeting scheduling requirements each day.

5. d Offshoring is a type of outsourcing where employees of the vendor firm are based outside of the US, as in this example.

6. b Benchmarking is based on comparison of external performance data on similar functions performed in similar organizations, collected through research. External sources of data for benchmarking include articles and contact with peer institutions, as mentioned here.

7. a Work distribution analysis is a process of data collection to determine the type and appropriateness of a unit's work assignments, the time allowed for tasks, and the employees doing the work. Results can be used to help managers assess work prioritization or duplication, or underutilization of employees.

8. d Reported performance data are analyzed for variance to see where actual performance does not meet or is significantly different from the standard. A manager considers factors that might explain the variance.

9. c The behaviorally anchored rating scale (BARS) system used in performance appraisal links specific examples of measurable job-related behaviors to a scaled rating (a level).

10. b A supervisor being kept informed of the employee's accomplishments is most consistent with the pro aspects of self-appraisal data presented in table 20.4.

Check Your Understanding 20.4

1. b Turnover reflects the rate at which employees leave an organization and must be replaced; this rate includes voluntary employee exits and involuntary termination of employment (dismissals).

2. c Engagement increases when an employee's relationship with a direct supervisor is positive and includes clear job expectations and feedback.

3. d Use of progressive penalties is part of the disciplinary process.

4. c Guidelines for handling grievances start with prevention, efforts to recognize and correct sources of dissatisfaction before formal grievances occur such as with fair approaches to performance appraisal and discipline.

5. b Best practice is for the employee's direct (immediate) supervisor to conduct the dismissal meeting; a human resources representative should be asked to attend to confirm what occurred.

6. c An authorization card is a document that indicates an employee's interest in having a union represent him or her. Signed authorization cards recognize a group of employees within the organization who wish to be represented by a union.

7. b Walking around to observe and critique performance refers to actions consistent with performance management. The other responses represent communication strategies a manager can use to help build positive employee relations.

8. b Accommodation is the approach to apply when an issue is minor; also see table 20.5

9. c A system of progressive penalties was applied in this scenario, with a verbal warning (level of penalty) issued consistent with employee's first tardy incident.

10. d Stating facts such as solicitation policy is legally appropriate for a manager during a union-organizing drive. Threats, interrogation, and promises of pay or benefits are not.

Check Your Understanding 20.5

1. b Development has a longer-term focus designed to increase or enhance employee skills, knowledge, or abilities needed for the employee's career advancement and by the organization in the future.

2. c Onboarding, an aspect of orientation, is time spent upfront to welcome, socialize, and integrate a new employee into the values and culture of an organization, benefitting both employee and employer.

3. d Adult learners are more likely to remember material that is relevant to their life and work, has practical value to them. The other responses are true of training of adult learners.

4. c Mentoring involves career advising and counseling of an employee, and can be performed by a manager, but more often is a role for a senior employee.

5. b In the analyze-design-develop-implement-evaluate (ADDIE) model, setting objectives and preparing a budget for training occur at step 2, Design.

6. c For conflict resolution training, face-to-face classroom delivery that includes small group work would be the most effective choice of method.

7. d "Check frequently and encourage questions" is step 4 of the steps for on-the-job training; also see figure 20.9.

8. a An employee could complete the O*Net assessment on his/her own, with or without encouragement of a manager. The other statements represent actions that could be taken by a manager or mentor.

Check Your Understanding 21.1

1. **e** Deontology – A duty or responsibility guiding the decision based on action and not the result.
2. **i** Cultural diversity – The perceived or actual differences among people.
3. **g** Autonomy – An individual's right to make his or her own decision.
4. **a** Egoism – Only considering oneself in the decision-making process.
5. **b** Moral values is a system of principles that guide an individual's life, usually regarding right and wrong.
6. **h** Ethics – A field of study dealing with moral principles, theories, and values.
7. **c** Nonmaleficence – Not to cause harm.
8. **f** Beneficence – Promoting good for others or providing services that benefit others.
9. **d** Prejudice - Strong feeling about a person without reviewing facts.
10. **j** Stereotyping - Assuming everyone within a certain group is the same.

Check Your Understanding 21.2

1. **b** A blanket authorization is when the patient signs an authorization allowing the disclosure specialist to release any and all information from that point forward.
2. **a** Beneficence is doing good, promoting the health and welfare of others, demonstrating kindness, showing compassion, and helping others.
3. **a** Upcoding is the practice of assigning diagnostic or procedural codes that represent higher payment rates than the codes that truly reflect the services provided to patients via the documentation.
4. **c** Genetic, adoption, drug, alcohol, sexual health, and behavioral information is considered sensitive information and requires special attention.
5. **b** Autonomy, or self-determination, is an individual's right to make his or her own decision; it includes the informed consent process for human research subjects and starts with a full disclosure of the nature of the study, and the risks and benefits, and gives the participant the opportunity to not participate in the study.
6. **d** Unbundling is the practice of using multiple codes to bill for the various individual steps in a single procedure rather than using a single code that includes all the steps.
7. **d** Gaining ccess to electronic health record systems is a complex challenge in regard to record integrity, information security, linkage of information for continuum of care within different e-health systems, and the development of software for health information management purposes.
8. **c** Managed care helps control the cost of healthcare by providing services at a fixed cost. It does this by minimizing variation in clinical practice.

Appendix B Glossary

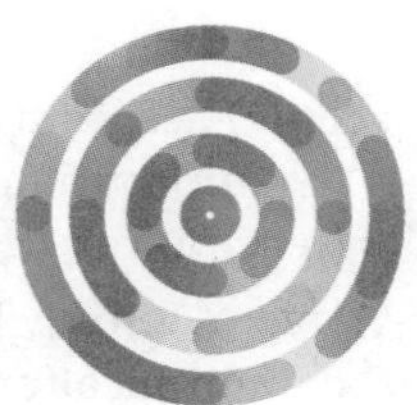

A

Abbreviated Injury Scale (AIS) An anatomically based, consensus-derived global severity scoring system that classifies each injury by region according to its relative importance on a 6-point ordinal scale (1 = minor and 6 = maximal). AIS is the basis for the Injury Severity Score (ISS) calculation of the multiply injured patient

Abstracting 1. The process of extracting information from a document to create a brief summary of a patient's illness, treatment, and outcome 2. The process of extracting elements of data from a source document or database and entering them into an automated system

Abuse Describes practices that, either directly or indirectly, result in unnecessary costs to the Medicare Program. Abuse includes any practice that is not consistent with the goals of providing patients with services that are medically necessary, meet professionally recognized standards, and are fairly priced

Accept assignment A term used to refer to a provider's or a supplier's acceptance of the allowed charges (from a fee schedule) as payment in full for services or materials provided

Access control 1. A computer software program designed to prevent unauthorized use of an information resource 2. As amended by HITECH, a technical safeguard that requires a covered entity must in accordance with 164.306(a)(1) implement technical policies and procedures for electronic information systems that maintain electronic protected health information to allow access only to those persons or software programs that have been granted access rights as specified in 164.308(a)(4) (45 CFR 164.312 2003)

Access safeguards Identification of which employees should have access to what data; the general practice is that employees should have access only to data they need to do their jobs

Accession number A number assigned to each case as it is entered in a cancer registry

Accession registry A list of cases in a cancer registry in the order in which they were entered

Accommodation An employer providing a reasonable adjustment for an employee

Accountable care organization (ACO) A legal entity that is recognized and authorized under applicable state, federal, or tribal law, is identified by a Taxpayer Identification Number (TIN), and is formed by one or more ACO participant(s) that is (are) defined at 425.102(a) and may also include any other ACO participants described at 425.102(b) (42 CFR 425.20 2011)

Accounting 1. The process of collecting, recording, and reporting an organization's financial data 2. A list of all disclosures made of a patient's health information

Accreditation 1. A voluntary process of institutional or organizational review in which a quasi-independent body created for this purpose periodically evaluates the quality of the entity's work against preestablished written criteria 2. A determination by an accrediting body that an eligible organization, network, program, group, or individual complies with applicable standards 3. The act of granting approval to a healthcare organization based on whether the organization has met a set of voluntary standards developed by an accreditation agency

Accreditation Association for Ambulatory Healthcare (AAAHC) An accreditation organization that specializes in ambulatory care

Accreditation organizations A professional organization that establishes the standards against which healthcare organizations are measured and conducts periodic assessments of the performance of individual healthcare organizations

Accredited Standards Committee X12 (ASC X12) A committee accredited by ANSI that is responsible for the development and maintenance of EDI standards for many industries. The ASC "X12N" is the subcommittee of ASC X12 responsible for the EDI health insurance administrative transactions such as 837 Institutional Health Care Claim and 835 Professional Health Care Claim forms

Accrual accounting Recording known transactions in the appropriate time period before cash payment (receipts) are expected or due

Active listening The application of effective verbal communication skills as evidenced by the listener's restatement of what the speaker said

Active membership Individuals interested in the AHIMA purpose and willing to abide by the Code of Ethics are eligible for active membership. Active members in good standing shall be entitled to all membership privileges including the right to vote

Addendum A late entry added to a health record to provide additional information in conjunction with a previous entry. The late entry should be timely and bear the current date and reason for the additional information being added to the health record

ADDIE model Recommended by numerous experts in the HRM and instructional design fields as a general guide to planning and implementation of employee training programs; the steps in this model are analyze-design-develop-implement-evaluate

Adjudication Refers to the process of paying, denying, and adjusting claims based on the patient's health insurance coverage benefits

Administrative data Coded information contained in secondary records, such as billing records, describing patient identification, diagnoses, procedures, and insurance

Administrative law A body of rules and regulations developed by various administrative entities empowered by Congress; falls under the umbrella of public law

Administrative safeguards Under HIPAA, are administrative actions and policies and procedures, to manage the selection, development, implementation, and maintenance of security measures to protect electronic protected health information and to manage the conduct of the covered entity's or business associate's workforce in relation to the protection of that information (45 CFR 164.304 2013)

Administrative simplification As amended by HITECH, authorizes HHS to: (1) adopt standards for transactions and code sets that are used to exchange health data; (2) adopt standard identifiers for health plans, health care providers, employers, and individuals for use on standard transactions; and (3) adopt standards to protect the security and privacy of personally identifiable health information (45 CFR Parts 160, 162, and 164 2013)

Admissibility The condition of being admitted into evidence in a court of law

Adoption Reflects the fact that the organization has implemented all of the major components of technology, although there may be some available technology that is more specialized, costly, or time-consuming to implement that has not yet been implemented

Adverse impact Unequal discriminatory effect of an employment practice (for example, requiring a passing score on a test that does not cover job-related knowledge or skills) on members of a protected class

Affinity grouping A technique for organizing similar ideas together in natural groupings

Affordable Care Act (ACA) A federal statute that was signed into law on March 23, 2010. Along with the Health Care and Education Reconciliation Act of 2010 (signed into law on March 30, 2010), the act is the product of the healthcare reform agenda of the Democratic 111th Congress and the Obama administration

Age Discrimination in Employment Act of 1967 The federal act that states it is unlawful for an employer to discriminate against an individual in any aspect of employment because that individual is 40 years old or older, unless one of the statutory exceptions applies. Favoring an older individual over a younger individual because of age is not unlawful discrimination under the ADEA, even if the younger individual is at least 40 years old. However, the ADEA does not require employers to prefer older individuals and does not affect applicable state, municipal, or local laws that prohibit such preferences (72 FR 36875 2007)

Agency for Healthcare Research and Quality (AHRQ) The branch of the US Public Health Service that supports general health research and distributes research findings and treatment guidelines with the goal of improving the quality, appropriateness, and effectiveness of healthcare services

Aggregate data Data extracted from individual health records and combined to form de-identified information about groups of patients that can be compared and analyzed

AHIMA Foundation An organization that supports AHIMA and the HIM profession through leadership in research, workforce development, scholarships and more

Alert fatigue When an excessive number of alerts are used in an information system, users get tired of looking at the alerts and may ignore them

Allied health professional A credentialed healthcare worker who is not a physician, nurse, psychologist, or pharmacist (for example, a physical therapist, dietitian, social worker, or occupational therapist)

Alphabetic filing system A system of health record identification and storage that uses the patient's last name as the first component of identification and his or her first name and middle name or initial for further definition

Alphanumeric filing system Both alphabetic and numeric characters are used to sort health records in this system

Alternative dispute resolution Methods of resolving legal disputes outside of the court system such as arbitration or mediation

Alternative payment model (APM) New methods of reimbursement used by the federal government

Ambulatory care Preventive or corrective healthcare services provided on a nonresident basis in a provider's office, clinic setting, or hospital emergency setting

Ambulatory payment classification (APC) Hospital outpatient prospective payment system (OPPS). The classification is a resource-based reimbursement system

Ambulatory surgery center/ambulatory surgical center (ASC) Under Medicare, an outpatient surgical facility that has its own national identifier; is a separate entity with respect to its licensure, accreditation, governance, professional supervision, administrative functions, clinical services, recordkeeping, and financial and accounting systems; has as its sole purpose the provision of services in connection with surgical procedures that do not require inpatient hospitalization; and meets the conditions and requirements set forth in the Medicare Conditions of Participation

Ambulatory surgery center (ASC) payment rate The Medicare ASC reimbursement methodology system referred to as the ambulatory surgery center (ASC) payment system. The ASC payment system is based on the ambulatory payment classifications (APCs) utilized under the hospital OPPS

Amendment A clarification made to healthcare documentation after the original document has been signed; it should be dated, timed, and signed

American Academy of Professional Coders (AAPC) The American Academy of Professional Coders provides certified credentials to medical coders in physician offices, hospital outpatient facilities, ambulatory surgical centers, and in payer organizations

American Association of Medical Record Librarians (AAMRL) The name adopted by the Association of Record Librarians of North America in 1944; precursor of the American Health Information Management Association

American College of Surgeons (ACS) The scientific and educational association of surgeons formed to improve the quality of surgical care by setting high standards for surgical education and practice

American College of Surgeons (ACS) Commission on Cancer Established by the American College of Surgeons (ACS) in 1922, the multidisciplinary Commission on Cancer (CoC) establishes standards to ensure quality multidisciplinary and comprehensive cancer care delivery in healthcare settings

American Health Information Management Association (AHIMA) The professional membership organization for managers of health record services and healthcare information systems as well as coding services; provides accreditation, advocacy, certification, and educational services

American Medical Record Association (AMRA) The name adopted by the American Association of Medical Record Librarians in 1970; precursor of the American Health Information Management Association

American Recovery and Reinvestment Act (ARRA) The purposes of this act include the following: (1) To preserve and create jobs and promote economic recovery. (2) To assist those most impacted by the recession. (3) To provide investments needed to increase economic efficiency by spurring technological advances in science and health. (4) To invest in transportation, environmental protection, and other infrastructure that will provide long-term economic benefits. (5) To stabilize state and local government budgets, in order to minimize and avoid reductions in essential services and counterproductive state and local tax increases

Americans with Disabilities Act (ADA) Federal legislation which ensures equal opportunity for and elimination of discrimination against persons with disabilities (Public Law 110-325 2008)

Analysis Review of health record for proper documentation and adherence to regulatory and accreditation standards

Analytics Refers to statistical processing of data to reveal new information

Ancillary services 1. Tests and procedures ordered by a physician to provide information for use in patient diagnosis or treatment 2. Professional healthcare services such as radiology, laboratory, or physical therapy

Ancillary systems Systems that serve primarily to manage the department in which they exist, while at the same time providing key clinical data for the EHR

Anesthesia report The report that notes any preoperative medication and response to it, the anesthesia administered with dose and method of administration, the duration of administration, the patient's vital signs while under anesthesia, and any additional products given the patient during a procedure

Anti-Kickback Statute A statute that establishes criminal penalties for individuals and entities that knowingly and willfully offer, pay, solicit, or receive remuneration in order to induce business for which payment may be made under any federal healthcare program

Appeal 1. A request for reconsideration of a denial of coverage or rejection of claim decision 2. The next stage in the litigation process after a court has rendered a verdict; must be based on alleged errors or disputes of law rather than errors of fact

Appellate courts Courts that hear appeals on final judgments of the state trial courts or federal trial courts

Application controls Security strategies, such as password management, included in application software and computer programs

Application program interface (API) Technology that provides a set of tools for building software applications

Application safeguards Controls contained in application software or computer programs to protect the security and integrity of information

Application service provider (ASP) A third-party service company that delivers, manages, and remotely hosts standardized applications software via a network through an outsourcing contract based on fixed, monthly usage, or transaction-based pricing

Arbitration A proceeding in which disputes are submitted to a third party or a panel of experts outside the judicial trial system

Artificial intelligence (AI) The application of algorithms that analyze data and make applicable recommendations that can be used in decision-making

Assembly The process of ensuring that each page in the health record is organized in a standardized order

Association for Healthcare Documentation Integrity (AHDI) Formerly the American Association for Medical Transcription (AAMT), the AHDI has a model curriculum for formal educational programs that includes the study of medical terminology, anatomy and physiology, medical science, operative procedures, instruments, supplies, laboratory values, reference use and research techniques, and English grammar

Association of Record Librarians of North America (ARLNA) Organization formed 10 years after the beginning of the hospital standardization movement whose original objective was to elevate the standards of clinical recordkeeping in hospitals, dispensaries, and other healthcare facilities; precursor of the American Health Information Management Association

Audit 1. A function that allows retrospective reconstruction of events, including who executed the events in question, why, and what changes were made as a result 2. To conduct an independent review of electronic system records and activities in order to test the adequacy and effectiveness of data security and data integrity procedures and to ensure compliance with established policies and procedures

Audit controls The mechanisms that record and examine activity in information systems

Audit trail 1. A chronological set of computerized records that provides evidence of information system activity (log-ins and log-outs, file accesses) used to determine security violations 2. A record that shows who has accessed a computer system, when it was accessed, and what operations were performed

Authentication 1. The process of identifying the source of health record entries by attaching a handwritten signature, the author's initials, or an electronic signature 2. Proof of authorship that ensures, as much as possible, that log-ins and messages from a user originate from an authorized source 3. As amended by HITECH, means the corroboration that a person is the one claimed. 4. Affirms a health record's legitimacy through testimony or written validation that it is indeed the record of the subject individual and the information in it is valid"

Authoritarian leadership Domineering leadership style where decisions are made at a distance from those affected

Authorization 1. As amended by HITECH, except as otherwise specified, a covered entity may not use or disclose protected health information without an authorization that is valid under section 164.508 2. When a covered entity obtains or receives a valid authorization for its use or disclosure of protected health information, such use or disclosure must be consistent with the authorization (45 CFR 164.508 2013). 3. A right or permission given to an individual to use a computer resource, such as a computer, or to use specific applications and access specific data. It is also a set of actions that gives permission to an individual to perform specific functions such as read, write, or execute tasks

Authorization card A document that indicates an employee's interest in having a union represent him or her

Auto-authentication 1. A procedure that allows dictated reports to be considered automatically signed unless the health information management department is notified of needed revisions within a certain time limit 2. A process by which the failure of an author to review and affirmatively either approve or disapprove an entry within a specified time period results in authentication

Auto-analyzer Device that analyzes the specimen

Automated drug dispensing machine System that makes drugs available for patient care

Automated reviews Reviews performed electronically rather than by humans

Automatic logout Timed logouts of information systems that reduce the chances that one's account will be used by someone else, can be used to prevent access by unauthorized individuals

Autonomy A core ethical principle centered on the individual's right to self-determination that includes respect for the individual; in clinical applications, the patient's right to determine what does or does not happen to him or her in terms of healthcare

Autopsy report Written documentation of the findings from a postmortem pathological examination

Average daily census The mean number of hospital inpatients present in the hospital each day for a given period of time

Average length of stay (ALOS) The mean length of stay for hospital inpatients discharged during a given period of time

Avoidance In business, a situation where two parties in conflict ignore that conflict

Axioms A concept in SNOMED that are true statements, that serve as a starting point for further reasoning and arguments

B

Backdoor program A backdoor program is a computer program that bypasses normal authentication processes and allows access to computer resources, such as programs, computer networks, or entire computer systems

Baiting Hackers leave an infected USB or flash drive in a public area in the hope that someone will come by, pick it up, and use it out of curiosity

Balance billing A reimbursement method that allows providers to bill patients for charges in excess of the amount paid by the patients' health plan or other third-party payer (not allowed under Medicare or Medicaid)

Balanced Budget Act of 1997 Public Law 105-33 enacted by Congress on August 5, 1997, that mandated a number of additions, deletions, and revisions to the original Medicare and Medicaid legislation; the legislation that added penalties for healthcare fraud and abuse to the Medicare and Medicaid programs and also affected the hospital outpatient prospective payment system (HOPPS) and programs of all-inclusive care for elderly (PACE) (Public Law 105-33 1997)

Bar chart A graphic technique used to display frequency distributions of nominal or ordinal data that fall into categories

Bar code medication administration record (BC-MAR) System that uses bar-coding technology for positive patient identification and drug information

Bargaining unit Those individuals who will be represented by the union

Bed count The number of inpatient beds set up and staffed for use on a given day

Bed count day One inpatient bed, set up and staffed for use in a 24-hour time period

Bed turnover rate The average number of times a bed changes occupants during a given period of time

Behavior theory Theory in which proponents believe that leaders can be made and that successful leadership is based on definable, learnable behavior

Behaviorally anchored rating scale Rating system that links specific examples of job-related performance to each rating

Bench trial A trial in which a judge reviews the evidence and makes a determination, without a sitting jury

Benchmark The systematic comparison of the products, services, and outcomes of one organization with those of a similar organization; or the systematic comparison of one organization's outcomes with regional or national standards

Benchmarking The systematic comparison of the products, services, and outcomes of one organization with those of a similar organization; or the systematic comparison of one organization's outcomes with regional or national standards

Beneficence A legal term that means promoting good for others or providing services that benefit others, such as releasing health information that will help a patient receive care or will ensure payment for services received

Beneficiary An individual who is eligible for benefits from a health plan

Benevolent autocracy The leader wields absolute power but is generally kind and sincere in the use of the team for the good of the organization

Best of breed A vendor strategy used when purchasing an EHR that refers to system applications that are considered the best in their class

Best of fit A vendor strategy used when purchasing an EHR in which all the systems required by the healthcare facility are available from one vendor

Bias Favoritism, partiality, or prejudice

Big data Very large volume of data that offers greater reliability and validity

Billing system Information system that generates a bill for healthcare services performed

Biometrics The physical characteristics of users (such as fingerprints, voiceprints, retinal scans, iris traits) that systems store and use to authenticate identity before allowing the user access to a system

Blanket authorization The patient signs an authorization allowing the release of information specialist to release any and all information from that point forward

Board of directors The elected or appointed group of officials who bear ultimate responsibility for the successful operation of a healthcare organization

Bona fide occupational qualification A factor (for example, age) is shown to be directly related to job performance based on documented job analysis

Box-and-whisker plot A visual display that summarizes the median, range, and outliers

Brainstorming A group problem-solving technique that involves the spontaneous contribution of ideas from all members of the group

Breach Under HITECH, the acquisition, access, use, or disclosure of protected health information in a manner not permitted under subpart E of this part that compromises the security or privacy of the protected health information (45 CFR 164.402 2013)

Breach notification As amended by HITECH, a covered entity shall, following the discovery of a breach of unsecured protected health information, notify each individual whose unsecured protected health information has been, or is reasonably believed by the covered entity to have been, accessed, acquired, used, or disclosed as a result of such breach (45 CFR 164.404 2013)

Breach of contract Failure to perform any term of a contract by any party involved in the contract

Bubble chart A type of scatter plot with circular symbols used to compare three variables; the area of the circle indicates the value of a third variable

Budget A plan that converts the organization's goals and objectives into targets for revenue and spending

Budget adjustment The approval to move funds from one budget to another

Budget management The process of maintaining financial viability by ensuring operating revenues for the year are sufficient to cover the operating expenditures

Budget variance A difference in the budgeted revenue or expense amount

Bureaucracy A formal organizational structure based on a rigid hierarchy of decision-making and inflexible rules and procedures

Business associate (BA) 1. A person or organization other than a member of a covered entity's workforce that performs functions or activities on behalf of or affecting a covered entity that involve the use or disclosure of individually identifiable health information 2. As amended by HITECH, with respect to a covered entity, a person who creates, receives, maintains, or transmits protected health information for a function or activity regulated by HIPAA, including claims processing or administration, data analysis, processing or administration, utilization review, quality assurance, patient safety activities, billing, benefit management, practice management, and repricing or provides legal, actuarial, accounting, consulting, data aggregation, management, administrative, accreditation, or financial services (45 CFR 160.103 2013)

Business associate agreement (BAA) As amended by HITECH, a contract between the covered entity and a business associate must establish the permitted and required uses and disclosures of protected health information by the business associate and provide specific content requirements of the agreement. The contract may not authorize the business associate to use or further disclose the information in a manner that would violate the requirements of HIPAA, and requires termination of the contract if the covered entity or business associate are aware of noncompliant activities of the other (45 CFR 164.504 2013)

Business continuity plan A program that incorporates policies and procedures for continuing business operations during a computer system shutdown

Business intelligence (BI) The end product or goal of knowledge management

Business process A set of related policies and procedures that are performed step by step to accomplish a business-related function

Business records exception A rule under which a record is determined not to be hearsay if it was made at or near the time by, or from information transmitted by, a person with knowledge; it was kept in the course of a regularly conducted business activity; and it was the regular practice of that business activity to make the record

Business-related partnerships An agreement between two parties to cooperate for the advancement of their mutual interests and the entity's strategic goals

Bylaws Operating documents that describe the rules and regulations under which a healthcare organization operates

C

Capitation A specified amount of money paid to a healthcare plan or doctor, used to cover the cost of a healthcare plan member's services for a certain length of time

Care area assessments (CAAs) The patient is assessed and reassessed at defined intervals as well as whenever there is a significant change in his or her condition

Care plan The specific goals in the treatment of an individual patient, amended as the patient's condition requires, and the assessment of the outcomes of care; serves as the primary source for ongoing documentation of the resident's care, condition, and needs

Career development The process by which individuals assess their existing skills, knowledge, and experience, explore and establish current and future career objectives, and develop an appropriate course of action

Case definition A method of determining criteria for cases that should be included in a registry

Case fatality rate Rate that measures the total number of deaths among the diagnosed cases of a specific disease, most often acute illness

Case finding A method of identifying patients who have been seen or treated in a healthcare facility for the particular disease or condition of interest to the registry

Case management 1. A process used by a doctor, nurse, or other health professional to manage a patient's healthcare (CMS 2013) 2. The ongoing, concurrent review performed by clinical professionals to ensure the necessity and effectiveness of the clinical services being provided to a patient

Case mix 1. A description of a patient population based on any number of specific characteristics, including age, gender, type of insurance, diagnosis, risk factors, treatment received, and resources used 2. The distribution of patients into categories reflecting differences in severity of illness or resource consumption

Case-mix index (CMI) The average relative weight of all cases treated at a given facility or by a given physician, which reflects the resource intensity or clinical severity of a specific group in relation to the other groups in the classification system; calculated by dividing the sum of the weights of diagnosis-related groups for patients discharged during a given period by the total number of patients discharged

Cash basis accounting Registering the transaction when it occurs, meaning when money is actually received for services provided, or paid for expenses incurred

Causation In law, a relationship between the defendant's conduct and the harm that was suffered

Cause-and-effect diagram An investigational technique that facilitates the identification of the various factors that contribute to a problem

Cause-specific mortality rate The rate of death due to a specified cause

Cause of action Theories under which lawsuits are brought that are related to professional liability such as breach of contract, intentional tort, and negligence

Census The number of inpatients present in a healthcare facility at any given time

Centers for Disease Control and Prevention (CDC) A federal agency dedicated to protecting health and promoting quality of life through the prevention and control of disease, injury, and disability. Committed to programs that reduce the health and economic consequences of the leading causes of death and disability, thereby ensuring a long, productive, healthy life for all people

Centers for Medicare and Medicaid Services (CMS) The Department of Health and Human Services agency responsible for Medicare and parts of Medicaid. Historically, CMS has maintained the UB-92 institutional EMC format specifications, the professional EMC NSF specifications, and specifications for various certifications and authorizations used by the Medicare and Medicaid programs. CMS is responsible for the oversight of HIPAA administrative simplification transaction and code sets, health identifiers, and security standards. CMS also maintains the HCPCS medical code set and the Medicare Remittance Advice Remark Codes administrative code set

Centralized unit filing system All of the patient's encounters are filed together in a single location

Certificate authority An organization that verifies a person's credentials and can revoke the certificate if the credentials are revoked

Certification 1. The process by which a duly authorized body evaluates and recognizes an individual, institution, or educational program as meeting predetermined requirements 2. An evaluation performed to establish the extent to which a particular computer system, network design, or application implementation meets a prespecified set of requirements

Certified tumor registrar (CTR) Credential for a cancer registrar achieved by passing an examination provided by the National Board for Certification of Registrars (NBCR); eligibility requirements for the certification examination include a combination of experience and education

Change control program Assures that there is documented approval for the change to be made and evidence that all elements of implementation, testing, rollout, training, and such are performed

Change management The formal process of introducing change, getting it adopted, and diffusing it throughout the organization

Charge description master (CDM) A financial management form that contains information about the organization's charges for the healthcare services it provides to patients; also called chargemaster

Chargemaster A financial management form that contains information about the organization's charges for the healthcare services it provides to patients; also called charge description master (CDM)

Chart 1. (noun) The health record of a patient 2. (verb) To document information about a patient in a health record. 3. A method of display to present data

Chart conversion An EHR implementation activity in which data from the paper chart are converted into electronic form

Chart tracking A process that identifies the current location of a paper record or information

Checksheet A data collection tool that records and compiles observations or occurrences

Chi-square test Type of inferential statistical testing done to determine and present information on data frequency

Chief executive officer (CEO) The senior manager appointed by a governing board to direct an organization's overall long-term strategic management

Chief financial officer (CFO) The senior manager responsible for the fiscal management of an organization

Chief information officer (CIO) The senior manager responsible for the overall management of information resources in an organization

Chief medical informatics officer (CMIO) A salaried physician (most often part time so that he or she retains credibility with other practicing physicians) who is heavily involved in policy development, workflow and process improvement, and ongoing maintenance of CDS and other systems requiring significant physician input

Chief nursing officer (CNO) The senior manager (usually a registered nurse with advanced education and extensive experience) responsible for administering patient care services

Chief operating officer (COO) An executive-level role responsible at a high level for day-to-day operations of an organization

Chief security officer (CSO) The individual who is responsible for the security program of a healthcare organization

Children's Health Insurance Program (CHIP) Provides health coverage to eligible children through both Medicaid and individual state CHIP programs; like all Medicaid programs, CHIP is administered by states according to federal requirements and is funded jointly by states and the federal government

Circuit court The federal court that hears appeals

Civil law A type of public law that addresses non-criminal laws

Civil Rights Act of 1991 (CRA 1991) The federal legislation that focuses on establishing an employer's responsibility for justifying hiring practices that seem to adversely affect people because of race, color, religion, sex, or national origin (Public Law 102-166 1991)

Civilian Health and Medical Program of the Department of Veterans Affairs (CHAMPVA) The federal healthcare benefits program for dependents (spouse or widow[er] and children) of veterans rated by the Veterans Administration (VA) as having a total and permanent disability, for survivors of veterans who died from VA-rated service-connected conditions or who were rated permanently and totally disabled at the time of death from a VA-rated service-connected condition, and for survivors of persons who died in the line of duty

Claim A request for payment for services, benefits, or costs by a hospital, physician, or other provider that is submitted for reimbursement to the healthcare insurance plan by either the insured party or by the provider

Claims data Information that is required to be reported on a healthcare claim for service reimbursement

Claims management The process of managing the legal and administrative aspects of the healthcare organization's response to injury claims (injuries occurring on the facility's property)

Classifications A clinical vocabulary, terminology, or nomenclature that lists words or phrases with their meanings, provides for the proper use of clinical words as names or symbols, and facilitates mapping standardized terms to broader classifications for administrative, regulatory, oversight, and fiscal requirements

Classroom-based learning Instructor-led, face-to-face training including traditional lectures, workshops, and seminars

Clearinghouse A vendor that processes healthcare claims for a healthcare organization

Client/server system System in which the healthcare organization has commercial software installed on servers housed and maintained within the organization itself, housed within the organization and managed by an outsourced company, or housed and maintained by a contractor for the healthcare organization

Clinic outpatient A patient who is admitted to a clinical service of a clinic or hospital for diagnosis or treatment on an ambulatory basis

Clinical coding Assigning codes to represent diagnoses and procedures

Clinical data The information that reflects the treatment and services provided to the patient as well as how the patient responded to such treatment and services

Clinical data analytics The process by which health information is captured, reviewed, and used to measure quality

Clinical data repository (CDR) A central database that focuses on clinical information

Clinical data warehouse (CDW) A database that makes it possible to access data from multiple databases and combine the results into a single query and reporting interface

Clinical decision support (CDS) The process in which individual data elements are represented in the computer by a special code to be used in making comparisons, trending results, and supplying clinical reminders and alerts

Clinical decision support system (CDSS) CDS that requires the combination of data from more than one source and the ability to deliver the alert back to the appropriate system or systems

Clinical Document Architecture (CDA) An HL7 XML-based document markup standard for the electronic exchange model for clinical documents (such as discharge summaries and progress notes). The implementation guide contains a library of CDA templates, incorporating and harmonizing previous efforts from HL7, Integrating the Healthcare Enterprise (IHE), and Health Information Technology Standards Panel (HITSP). It includes all required CDA templates for Stage I Meaningful Use, and HITECH final rule. It is commonly referred to as Consolidated CDA or C-CDA

Clinical documentation Any manual or electronic notation (or recording) made by a physician or other healthcare clinician related to a patient's medical condition or treatment

Clinical documentation improvement (CDI) The process an organization undertakes that will improve clinical specificity and documentation, which will allow coders to assign more concise disease classification codes

Clinical Laboratory Improvement Amendments (CLIA) of 1988 Established quality standards for all laboratory testing to ensure the accuracy, reliability, and timeliness of patient test results regardless of where the test is (Public Law 90-174 1967)

Clinical observations The observations of physicians, nurses, and other caregivers in order to create a chronological report of the patient's condition and response to treatment during his or her hospital stay

Clinical practice guidelines A detailed, step-by-step guide used by healthcare practitioners to make knowledge-based decisions related to patient care and issued by an authoritative organization such as a medical society or government agency

Clinical privileges The authorization granted by a healthcare organization's governing board to a member of the medical staff that enables the physician to provide patient services in the organization within specific practice limits

Clinical protocols Specific instructions for performing clinical procedures established by authoritative bodies, such as medical staff committees, and intended to be applied literally and universally

Clinical terminology A set of standardized terms and their synonyms that record patient findings, circumstances, events, and interventions with sufficient detail to support clinical care, decision support, outcomes research, and quality improvement

Clinical transformation A fundamental change in how medicine is practiced using health IT systems to aid in diagnosis and treatment

Clinical trial 1. The final stages of a long and careful research process that tests new types of medical care to see if they are safe (CMS 2013) 2. Experimental study in which an intervention or treatment is given to one group in a clinical setting and the outcomes compared with a control group that did not have the intervention or treatment or that had a different intervention or treatment

Clinical validation audit A type of audit conducted to determine if health records contain the necessary documentation

Closed-loop medication management Information systems used to provide patient safety when ordering and administering medications

Cloud computing A practice that uses a vendor to archive data, and in some cases also provide application software, including an EHR, on multiple, disparate servers

Coaching 1. A training method in which an experienced person gives advice to a less-experienced worker on a formal or informal basis 2. A disciplinary method used as the first step for employees who are not meeting performance expectations

Code of ethics A statement of ethical principles regarding business practices and professional behavior

Code systems An accumulation of numeric or alphanumeric representations or codes for exchanging or storing information

Coding The process of assigning numeric or alphanumeric representations to clinical documentation

Coding audit A type of audit conducted to ensure that claims are being coded correctly

Coding compliance plan A component of an HIM compliance plan or a corporate compliance plan modeling the OIG Program Guidance for Hospitals and the OIG Supplemental Compliance Program Guidance for Hospitals that focuses on the unique regulations and guidelines with which coding professionals must comply

Coercive power Power in which a team leader uses threats and punishments to get his or her way

Coinsurance Cost sharing in which the policy or certificate holder pays a pre-established percentage of eligible expenses after the deductible has been met; the percentage may vary by type or site of service

Collaborative Stage Data Set A new standardized neoplasm-staging system developed by the American Joint Commission on Cancer

Collective bargaining A process through which a contract is negotiated that sets forth the relationship between the employees and the healthcare organization

Commission on Accreditation of Rehabilitation Facilities (CARF) An international, independent, nonprofit accreditor of health and human services that develops customer-focused standards for areas such as behavioral healthcare, aging services, child and youth services, and medical rehabilitation programs and accredits such programs on the basis of its standards

Commission on Accreditation for Health Informatics and Information Management Education (CAHIIM) An independent accrediting organization whose mission is to serve the public interest by establishing and enforcing quality accreditation standards for health informatics and health information management educational programs

Commission on Certification for Health Informatics and Information Management (CCHIIM) An independent body within AHIMA that establishes and enforces standards for the certification and certification maintenance of health informatics and information management professionals

Common-cause variation The source of variation in a process that is inherent within the process

Common Clinical Data Set (CCDS) A common set of data types and elements and associated standards for use across several certification criteria

Comparative data Individual data that is organized numerically and collated to make some comparisons against standards or benchmarks

Competencies Demonstrated skills that a worker should perform at a high level

Complaint In litigation, a written legal statement from a plaintiff that initiates a civil lawsuit

Complex review In a revenue audit contractor (RAC) review, this type of review results in an overpayment or underpayment determination based on a review of the health record associated with the claim in question

Compliance 1. The process of establishing an organizational culture that promotes the prevention, detection, and resolution of instances of conduct that do not conform to federal, state, or private payer healthcare program requirements or the healthcare organization's ethical and business policies 2. The act of adhering to official requirements 3. Managing a coding or billing department according to the laws, regulations, and guidelines that govern it

Compliance program A process that helps an organization, such as a hospital, accomplish its goal of providing high-quality medical care and efficiently operating a business under various laws and regulations

Component state associations (CSAs) Component state associations are part of the volunteer structure of AHIMA and are organized in every state, the District of Columbia, and the Commonwealth of Puerto Rico. The purpose of each Component State Association shall be to promote the mission and purpose of AHIMA in its state

Comprehensive Error Rate Testing (CERT) A program used by CMS to measure payment compliance with Medicare Fee-For-Service (FFS) program federal rules, regulations, and requirements

Compressed workweek A work schedule that permits a full-time job to be completed in less than the standard five days of eight-hour shifts

Computer virus A program that reproduces itself and attaches itself to legitimate programs on a computer that can change or corrupt data

Computer worm A type of malware that copies itself and spreads throughout a network. Unlike a computer virus, a computer worm does not need to attach itself to a legitimate program. It can execute and run itself

Computer-assisted coding (CAC) The process of extracting and translating dictated and then transcribed free-text data (or dictated and then computer-generated discrete data) into ICD-10-CM and CPT evaluation and management codes for billing and coding purposes

Computerized provider order entry (CPOE) Electronic prescribing systems that allow physicians to write prescriptions and transmit them electronically. These systems usually contain error prevention software that provides the user with prompts that warn against the possibility of drug interaction, allergy, or overdose and other relevant information

Concept A unique unit of knowledge or thought created by a unique combination of characteristics

Concurrent review Screening for medical necessity and the appropriateness and timeliness of the delivery of medical care from the time of admission until discharge

Conditions for Coverage (CfC) Standards applied to facilities that choose to participate in federal government reimbursement programs such as Medicare and Medicaid

Conditions of Participation (CoP) The administrative and operational guidelines and regulations under which facilities are allowed to take part in the Medicare and Medicaid programs; published by the Centers for Medicare and Medicaid Services, a federal agency under the Department of Health and Human Services

Confidentiality 1. A legal and ethical concept that establishes the healthcare provider's responsibility for protecting health records and other personal and private information from unauthorized use or disclosure 2. As amended by HITECH, the practice that data or information is not made available or disclosed to unauthorized persons or processes (45 CFR 164.304 2013)

Conflict management A problem-solving technique that focuses on working with individuals to find a mutually acceptable solution

Confounding factors Characteristics other than the characteristic of interest (of research) that may also be related to the disease under study

CONNECT Open-source software that implements health exchange specifications; it enables discovery of where there may be information as well as directly retrieving it from the source

Consensus building A decision-making method that seeks consent of all participants to resolve differences so an acceptable result can be found

Consensus-oriented decision-making model (CODM) A seven-step progression that allows groups to be flexible enough to come to a consensus by starting important topics with open discussion rather than by presenting a preformulated proposal; gathering a list of all the needs and concerns expressed by the group to form a list of conditions for possible proposals to address; taking turns in a unified attempt to build each proposal idea into the best possible proposal before choosing among them; and using empathy in the closure stage to address any unresolved feelings from the process. The seven CODM steps are: (1) framing the topic, (2) open discussion, (3) identifying underlying concerns, (4) collaborative proposal building, (5) choosing a direction, (6) synthesizing a final proposal, and (7) closure

Consent 1. A patient's acknowledgment that he or she understands a proposed intervention, including that intervention's risks, benefits, and alternatives 2. The document signed by the patient that indicates agreement that protected health information (PHI) can be disclosed

Consent directive A process by which patients may opt in or opt out of having their data exchanged in the HIE

Consent management systems Systems that help maintain patient preferences about who may have access to their health information

Consolidated Clinical Document Architecture (C-CDA) HL7-created document templates

Constitutional law The body of law that deals with the amount and types of power and authority that governments are given

Consultation rate The total number of hospital inpatients receiving consultations for a given period divided by the total number of discharges and deaths for the same period

Consultation report Documentation of the clinical opinion of a physician other than the primary or attending physician

Consultative leadership The leader remains open to input from members of the team but still retains full decision-making authority

Consumer-directed health plans Managed care organizations that influence patients and clients to select cost-efficient healthcare through the provision of information about health benefit packages and through financial incentives

Context-based access control (CBAC) An access control system that limits users to accessing information not only in accordance with their identity and role, but to the location and time in which they are accessing the information

Contingency plan 1. Documentation of the process for responding to a system emergency, including the performance of backups, the line-up of critical alternative facilities to facilitate continuity of operations, and the process of recovering from a disaster 2. A recovery plan in the event of a power failure, disaster, or other emergency that limits or eliminates access to facilities and electronic protected personal health information (ePHI)

Contingency theory Theory that states leadership exists between persons in social situations, and persons who are leaders in one situation may not necessarily be leaders in other situations

Contingent or contract work Temporary workers supplement full-time employees, often as part-time workers

Continuing education units (CEUs) Training that enables employees to remain current with advancing knowledge in their profession; activities that qualify for CEUs include such things as attending workshops and seminars, taking college courses, participating in independent study activities, and engaging in self-assessment activities

Continuity of care document (CCD) The result of ASTM's Continuity of Care Record standard content being represented and mapped into the HL7 Clinical Document Architecture specifications to enable transmission of referral information between providers; also frequently adopted for personal health records

Continuous data Data that represent measurable quantities but are not restricted to certain specified values

Continuous variables Discrete variables measured with sufficient precision

Continuum of care A system that guides and tracks patients over time through a comprehensive array of health services spanning all levels and intensity of care

Contraindication Medication should not be prescribed due to another medication or condition

Controlling The management function in which performance is monitored according to policies and procedures

Coordination of benefits (COB) Process for determining the respective responsibilities of two or more health plans that have some financial responsibility for a medical claim

Copayment Cost-sharing measure in which the policy or certificate holder pays a fixed dollar amount (flat fee) per service, supply, or procedure that is owed to the healthcare facility by the patient. The fixed amount that the policyholder pays may vary by type of service, such as $20.00 per prescription or $15.00 per physician office visit

Core measures Standardized performance measures developed to improve the safety and quality of healthcare

Coroner The official (elected or appointed, physician or nonphysician) who is responsible for determining the cause, time, and manner of death in unattended, violent, or unexplained deaths, or a case where a law may have been broken

Corporate compliance 1. A facility-wide program that comprises a system of policies, procedures, and guidelines that are used to ensure ethical business practices, identify potential fraudulence, and improve overall organizational performance 2. A program that became common after the Federal Sentencing Guidelines reduced fines and penalties to organizations found guilty of fraud if the organization has a prevention and detection program in place

Correction Edit made to the health record by drawing a single line through the erroneous information and writing the word "error" above the mistake; the practitioner should sign, date, and time the correction

Correlational studies A design of research that determines the existence and degree of relationships among factors

Cost sharing The cost for medical care that patients pay for themselves, like a copayment, coinsurance, or deductible

Council for Excellence in Education (CEE) A group HIM stakeholders including industry representatives, to address issues related to the future of the profession and HIM education

Counterclaim In a court of law, a countersuit

Court of Appeal A branch of the federal court system that has the power to hear appeals on the final judgments of district courts

Court order An official direction issued by a court judge and requiring or forbidding specific parties to perform specific actions

Covered entity (CE) As amended by HITECH, (1) a health plan, (2) a health care clearinghouse, (3) a health care provider who transmits any health information in electronic form in connection with a transaction covered by this subchapter (45 CFR 160.103 2013)

Credential A formal agreement granting an individual permission to practice in a profession, usually conferred by a national professional organization dedicated to a specific area of healthcare practice; or the accordance of permission by a healthcare organization to a licensed, independent practitioner (physician, nurse practitioner, or other professional) to practice in a specific area of specialty within that organization. Usually requires an applicant to pass an examination to obtain the credential initially and then to participate in continuing education activities to maintain the credential thereafter

Credentialing The process of reviewing and validating the qualifications (degrees, licenses, and other credentials) of physicians and other licensed independent practitioners, for granting medical staff membership to provide patient care services

Criminal law A type of public law where the government is a party against an accused who is charged with violating a criminal statute

Critical access hospitals 1. Hospitals that are excluded from the outpatient prospective payment system because they are paid under a reasonable cost-based system as required under section 1834(g) of the Social Security Act 2. Under HITECH incentives, a facility that has been certified as a critical access hospital under section 1820(e) of the Act and for which Medicare payment is made under section 1814(l) of the Act for inpatient services and under section 1834(g) of the Act for outpatient services (42 CFR 495.4 2012)

Critical incident method An ongoing written log of examples of an employee's job-related behavior during the appraisal period

Critical thinking Refers to the process of analyzing, assessing, and reconstructing a situation to provide enhanced solutions and outcomes to a problem

Cross-claim 1. In law, a complaint filed against a codefendant 2. A claim by one party against another party who is on the same side of the main litigation

Crude birth rate The number of live births divided by the population at risk

Crude death/mortality rate The total number of deaths in a given population for a given period of time divided by the estimated population for the same period of time

Cryptography 1. The art of keeping data secret through the use of mathematical or logical functions that transform intelligible data into seemingly unintelligible data and back again 2. In information security, the study of encryption and decryption techniques

Culture The values, beliefs, attitudes, languages, symbols, rituals, behaviors, and customs unique to a particular group of people

Cultural audit A strategy to define an organization's values, symbols, and routines and identify areas for improvement

Cultural competence Skilled in awareness, understanding, and acceptance of beliefs and values of the people of groups other than one's own

Cultural diversity The perceived or actual difference among people

Customer An internal or external recipient of services, products, or information

Customer relationship management (CRM) A database of service providers that may assist patients. These service providers could include transportation companies, home health agencies, meals-on-wheels and others

D

Daily inpatient census The number of inpatients present at census-taking time each day, plus any inpatients who were both admitted and discharged after the census-taking time the previous day

Dashboards Reports of process measures to help leaders follow progress to assist with strategic planning

Data The dates, numbers, images, symbols, letters, and words that represent basic facts and observations about people, processes, measurements, and conditions

Data abstraction The identification of data elements by an individual through health record review

Data abstracts A defined and standardized set of data points or elements common to a patient population that can be regularly identified in the health records of the population and coded for use and analysis in a database management system

Data analytics The science of examining raw data with the purpose of drawing conclusions about that information. It includes data mining, machine language, development of models, and statistical measurements. Analytics can be descriptive, predictive, or prescriptive

Data availability The extent to which healthcare data are accessible whenever and wherever they are needed

Data capture The process of recording healthcare-related data in a health record system or clinical database

Data collection tool A paper or electronic form that contains all of the data elements to be collected in the audit

Data consistency The extent to which the healthcare data are reliable and the same across applications

Data conversion The task of moving data from one data structure to another, usually at the time of a new information system installation

Data definition The specific meaning of a healthcare-related data element

Data dictionary A descriptive list of the names, definitions, and attributes of data elements to be collected in an information system or database whose purpose is to standardize definitions and ensure consistent use

Data element 1. An individual fact or measurement that is the smallest unique subset of a database 2. Under HIPAA, the smallest named unit of information in a transaction

Data governance The overall management of the availability, usability, integrity, and security of the data employed in an organization or enterprise

Data governance framework (DGF) The logical structure for managing all of the healthcare organization's data

Data integrity 1. The extent to which healthcare data are complete, accurate, consistent, and timely 2. A security principle that keeps information from being modified or otherwise corrupted either maliciously or accidentally

Data interchange standards Standards developed to support and create structure with data exchanges to support interoperability; the goal of the data interchange standard is to facilitate consistent, accurate, and reproducible capture of clinical data

Data loss prevention Strategies that are used to limit sensitive data being moved or transferred outside of the healthcare organization

Data management 1. The combined practices of HIM, IT, and HI that affect how data and documentation combine to create a single business record for an organization 2. The definition and structure of data elements and the creation, storage, and transmission of data elements

Data mapping 1. Data mapping allows for connections between two systems. This connection allows for data initially captured for one purpose to be translated and used for another purpose. One system in a map is identified as the source while the other is the target. 2. Process by which two distinct data models are created and a link between these models is defined. 3. A process used in data warehousing by which different data models are linked to each other using a defined set of methods to characterize the data in a specific definition. This definition can be any atomic unit, such as a unit of metadata or any other semantic. This data linking follows a set of standards, which depends on the domain value of the data model used. Data mapping serves as the initial step in data integration

Data mining The process of extracting and analyzing large volumes of data from a database for the purpose of identifying hidden and sometimes subtle relationships or patterns and using those relationships to predict behaviors

Data model 1. A picture or abstraction of real conditions used to describe the definitions of fields and records and their relationships in a database 2. A conceptual model of the information needed to support a business function or process

Data quality The reliability and effectiveness of data for its intended uses in operations, decision-making, and planning

Data quality management The processes used to ensure data integrity

Data quality management model A model, created by AHIMA, that defines the four domains of data quality – application, collection, warehousing and analysis

Data security The process of keeping data, both in transit and at rest, safe from unauthorized access, alteration, or destruction

Data set A list of recommended data elements with uniform definitions that are relevant for a particular use or are specific to a type of healthcare industry

Data standards Agreed-upon specifications for the values acceptable for specific data fields

Data steward The HIM role that is responsible for managing the data in a healthcare organization

Data stewardship The responsibilities and accountabilities associated with managing, collecting, viewing, storing, sharing, disclosing, or otherwise making use of personal health information

Data use Managing data through the use of technology

Data Use and Reciprocal Support Agreement (DURSA) A trust agreement entered into when exchanging information with other organizations using an agreed upon set of national standards, services, and policies developed in coordination with the Office of the National Coordinator for Health Information Technology

Data visualization The use of graphs, charts and other methods to display data

Data warehouse A database that makes it possible to access data from multiple databases and combine the results into a single query and reporting interface

Data warehousing The acquisition of all the business data and information from potentially multiple, cross-platform sources, such as legacy databases, departmental databases, and online transaction-based databases, and then the warehouse storage of all the data in one consistent format used to analyze data for decision-making purposes

Database An organized collection of data, text, references, or pictures in a standardized format, typically stored in a computer system for multiple applications

Database life cycle A system consisting of several phases that represent the useful life of a database, including initial study, design, implementation, testing and evaluation, operation, and maintenance and evaluation

Decision support system (DSS) A computer-based system that gathers data from a variety of sources and assists in providing structure to the data by using various analytical models and visual tools to facilitate and improve the ultimate outcome in decision-making tasks associated with nonroutine and nonrepetitive problems

Decryption Data decoded and restored back to original readable form

Deductible 1. The amount of cost, usually annual, that the policyholder must incur (and pay) before the insurance plan will assume liability for remaining covered expenses 2. Under Medicare, the amount a beneficiary must pay for healthcare before Medicare begins to pay, either for each benefit period for Part A, or each year for Part B, these amounts can change every year

Deemed status An official designation indicating that a healthcare facility is in compliance with the Medicare Conditions of Participation

Default 1. The status to which a computer application reverts in the absence of alternative instructions 2. Pertains to an attribute, value, or option that is assumed when none is explicitly specified

Defendant In civil cases, an individual or entity against whom a civil complaint has been filed; in criminal cases, an individual who has been accused of a crime

Deficiency slip Notification when a document or signature is missing that identifies the pertinent document and what needs to be done (dictated, completed, and signed)

Deidentified information Information from which personal characteristics have been stripped in such a way that it cannot be later constituted or combined to reidentify an individual; it is commonly used in research

Delinquent record An incomplete record not finished or made complete within the time frame determined by the medical staff of the facility

Democratic leadership Participative leadership style that supports collective decision-making by offering choices to the group members and facilitating discussion and member involvement

Demographic data Information used to identify an individual, such as name, address, gender, age, and other information linked to a specific person

Demographics Information used to identify an individual, such as name, address, gender, age, and other information linked to a specific person; also known as demographic data

Denial The decision made by an insurer that the claim will not be paid

Department of Health and Human Services (HHS) The cabinet-level federal agency, and principal agency for protecting the health of all Americans and providing essential human services, especially for those who are at least able to help themselves

Deposition A method of gathering information to be used in a litigation process

Derived classification Classification based on a reference classification such as ICD or ICF by adopting the reference classification structure and categories and providing additional detail or through rearrangement or aggregation of items from one or more reference classification

Descriptive statistics A set of statistical techniques used to describe data such as means, frequency distributions, and standard deviations; statistical information that describes the characteristics of a specific group or a population

Descriptive studies Research that is exploratory in nature and generates new hypotheses from the data that is collected

Designated record set (DRS) As amended by HITECH (1) A group of records maintained by or for a covered entity that is: (i) The medical records and billing records about individuals maintained by or for a covered health care provider; (ii) The enrollment, payment, claims adjudication, and case or medical management record systems maintained by or for a health plan; or (iii) Used, in whole or in part, by or for the covered entity to make decisions about individuals (2) For purposes of this paragraph, the term means any item, collection, or grouping of information that includes protected health information and is maintained, collected, used, or disseminated by or for a covered entity (45 CFR 164.501 2013)

Destruction of records Using a method, such as burning, pulverizing, degaussing, to make health records unreadable

Deterministic algorithm Algorithm that requires exact matches in data elements such as the patient name, date of birth, and social security number

Development Refers to educational programs with a longer-term focus, designed to stimulate an individual's professional growth by increasing or enhancing his or her skills, knowledge, or abilities

Diagnostic studies All diagnostic services of any type, including history, physical examination, laboratory, x-ray or radiography, and others that are performed or ordered pertinent to the patient's reasons for the encounter

Digital certificate An electronic document that establishes a person's online identity

Digital Imaging and Communications in Medicine (DICOM) An ISO standard that promotes a digital image communications format and picture archive and communications systems for use with digital images

Digital signature An electronic signature that binds a message to a particular individual and can be used by the receiver to authenticate the identity of the sender

Direct Project Launched in March 2010 to offer a simpler, standards-based way for participants to send authenticated, encrypted health information directly to known recipients over the internet

Disability A physical or mental condition that either temporarily or permanently renders a person unable to do the work for which he or she is qualified and educated

Disaster recovery plan The document that defines the resources, actions, tasks, and data required to manage the businesses recovery process in the event of a business interruption

Discharge summary A summary of the patient's stay at a healthcare organization that is used along with the postdischarge plan of care to provide continuity of care upon discharge from the facility

Disciplinary action Action taken to improve unsatisfactory work performance or behavior on the job

Disclosure As amended by HITECH, the release, transfer, provision of access to, or divulging in any manner of information outside the entity holding the information (45 CFR 160.103 2013)

Disclosure of health information Providing health information to users outside of the healthcare organization

Discovery The pretrial stage in the litigation process during which both parties to a suit use various strategies to identify information about the case, the primary focus of which is to determine the strength of the opposing party's case

Discrete data Data that represent separate and distinct values or observations; that is, data that contain only finite numbers and have only specified values

Discrete reportable transcription (DRT) Transcription system that combines speech dictation with natural language processing

Discrete variable A dichotomous or nominal variable whose values are placed into categories

Discrimination Treating a person differently based upon individual characteristics or group membership

Disease index A listing in diagnosis code number order of patients discharged from the facility during a particular time period

Disease registry A centralized collection of data used to improve the quality of care and measure the effectiveness of a particular aspect of healthcare delivery

Dismissal Involuntary termination of employment

Disparate treatment Employment discrimination based on intentional unequal treatment of an individual who is a member of a protected class

Disproportionate share hospital (DSH) Healthcare organization that meets governmental criteria for percentage of indigent patients. Hospital with an unequally (disproportionately) large share of low-income patients. Federal payments to these hospitals are increased to adjust for the financial burden

Distal attributes Division of leadership traits that includes personality, cognitive abilities, motives, and values that surround the leader as a person

Distributional errors Errors of inequity like central tendency, where all employees are rated satisfactory regardless of performance in order to avoid conflict, or leniency or strictness where some managers are overly generous or strict compared to other raters

District court The lowest tier in the federal court system, which hears cases involving felonies and misdemeanors that fall under federal statute and suits in which a citizen of one state sues a citizen of another state

DNV GL Healthcare An international certification body and classification society with main expertise in technical assessment, advisory, and risk management created in 2013 with the merger of Det Norske Veritas (Norway) and Germanischer Lloyd (Germany)

Documentation The recording of pertinent healthcare findings, interventions, and responses to treatment as a business record and form of communication among caregivers

Documentation standards Within the context of healthcare, describes those principles, codes, beliefs, guidelines, and regulations that guide health record documentation

Document management system (DMS) System commonly used when transitioning from paper-based to electronic health record that scans the paper record and stores it digitally

Document imaging 1. The practice of electronically scanning written or printed paper documents into an optical or electronic system for later retrieval of the document or parts of the document if parts have been indexed 2. The process by which paper-based documentation is captured, digitized, stored, and made available for retrieval by the end user

Do-not-resuscitate (DNR) order An order written by the treating physician stating that in the event the patient suffers cardiac or pulmonary arrest, cardiopulmonary resuscitation should not be attempted

Double billing Occurs when two providers bill for one service provided to one patient

Downsizing A reengineering strategy to reduce the cost of labor and streamline the organization by laying off portions of the workforce. These layoffs are permanent

Drug knowledge database A subscription service that provides current information about drugs and is accessible to users and the CDS

Dual eligible An individual covered by both Medicare and Medicaid

Due diligence The actions associated with making a good decision, including investigation of legal, technical, human, and financial predictions and ramifications of proposed endeavors with another party

Duplicate health record Occurs when the patient has two or more health record numbers issued; the patient's medical information becomes fragmented with some information under the first number and the remainder under the second

Durable power of attorney for healthcare decisions (DPOA-HCD) A legal instrument through which a principal appoints an agent to make healthcare decisions on the principal's behalf in the event the principal becomes incapacitated

Duty The obligation established by a relationship such as a physician caring for a patient

Dysfunctional conflict A destructive type of struggle that becomes emotionally draining and harms productivity

E

E-discovery Refers to Amendments to Federal Rules of Civil Procedure and Uniform Rules Relating to Discovery of Electronically Stored Information; wherein audit trails, the source code of the program, metadata, and any other electronic information that is not typically considered the legal health record is subject to motion for compulsory discovery

Edit check Helps to ensure data integrity by allowing only reasonable and predetermined values to be entered into the computer

eHealth Exchange A group of federal agencies and non-federal organizations that came together under a common mission and purpose to improve patient care, streamline disability benefit claims, and improve public health reporting through secure, trusted, and interoperable health information exchange. Participating organizations mutually agree to support a common set of standards and specifications that enable the establishment of a secure, trusted, and interoperable connection among all participating exchange organizations for the standardized flow of information

Electronic health record (EHR) An electronic record of health-related information on an individual that conforms to nationally recognized interoperability standards and that can be created, managed, and consulted by authorized clinicians and staff across more than one healthcare organization

Electronic protected health information (ePHI) Health information that is stored digitally and is subject to HIPAA

Eligibility Verification that the patient is covered by the plan on the date of service and the services being provided are covered by the plan

Emergency mode of operations A plan that defines the processes and controls that will be followed until the operations are fully restored

Emergency patient A patient who is admitted to the emergency services department of a hospital for the diagnosis and treatment of a condition that requires immediate medical, dental, or allied health services in order to sustain life or to prevent critical consequences

Emeritus membership AHIMA membership category for members who are 65 years old or older

Emotional intelligence (EI) The five skills that allow leaders to capitalize their performance and that of their employees include Self-awareness, Self-regulation, Motivation, Empathy, and Social skills

Empathy The ability to understand another person's emotions

Employee engagement Refers to the level of commitment employees demonstrate, their willingness to continue working for the organization, and to go above and beyond the minimum expectations

Employee relations Broad term referencing the general management and planning of activities related to developing and improving employee relationships through communication and fair handling of disputes

Encoder Specialty software used to facilitate the assignment of diagnostic and procedural codes according to the rules of the coding system

Encounter The face-to-face contact between a patient and a provider who has primary responsibility for assessing and treating the condition of the patient at a given contact and exercises independent judgment in the care of the patient

Encryption The process of transforming text into an unintelligible string of characters that can be transmitted via communications media with a high degree of security and then decrypted when it reaches a secure destination

End user Persons who will use the system for their daily processes

Engage A virtual network of AHIMA members who communicate via a web-based program managed by AHIMA

Enterprise architecture (EA) The plan used keep up with the technology used by a healthcare organization and how these technologies work together

Enterprise information management (EIM) The set of functions created by an organization to plan, organize, and coordinate the people, processes, technology, and content needed to manage information for the purposes of data quality, patient safety, and ease of use

Enterprise master patient index (EMPI) An index that provides access to multiple repositories of information from overlapping patient populations that are maintained in separate systems and databases

Episode-of-care (EOC) reimbursement Reimbursement methods that include a period of continuous medical care performed by healthcare professionals in relation to a particular clinical problem or situation, and one or more healthcare services given by a provider during a specific period of relatively continuous care in relation to a particular health or medical problem or situation

e-prescribing (e-Rx) When a prescription is written from the personal digital assistant and an electronic fax or an actual electronic data interchange transaction is generated that transmits the prescription directly to the retail pharmacy's information system

e-prescribing for controlled substances (EPCS) The submission of a prescription electronically for narcotics and other controlled substances

Equal Employment Opportunity Commission (EEOC) Title VII established the (EEOC) as the federal agency with responsibility to administer and enforce equal opportunity employment laws, investigate complaints, and file discrimination charges in court

Equal employment opportunity law Government efforts to ensure equal access to and fairness in employment without regard to race, religion, age, disability, gender, or other characteristics not related to a job

Equal Pay Act The federal legislation that requires equal pay for men and women who perform substantially the same work (Public Law 88-38 1963)

Ethical principles Concepts such as altruism, beneficence, consequentialism, deontology, egoism, least harm, and utilitarianism, upon which ethical decisions are made

Ethics A field of study that deals with moral principles, theories, and values; in healthcare, a formal decision-making process for dealing with the competing perspectives and obligations of the people who have an interest in a common problem

Ethics committee A committee tasked with reviewing clinical ethics violations to determine the course of action required to remedy the violations

Ethnography A method of observational research that investigates culture in naturalistic settings using both qualitative and quantitative approaches

Evidence-based medicine (EBM) Healthcare services based on clinical methods that have been thoroughly tested through controlled, peer-reviewed biomedical studies

e-visits Non-face-to-face interaction between patient and provider

Exclusions Program A database of individuals and healthcare organizations that are not permitted to participate in or receive payment from any federal healthcare program due to past healthcare-related crimes they committed against the federal government

Exclusive provider organizations (EPO) Hybrid managed care organization that provides benefits to subscribers only when healthcare services are performed by network providers; sponsored by self-insured (self-funded) employers or associations and exhibits characteristics of both health maintenance organizations and preferred provider organizations

Executive information system (EIS) A system that facilitates and supports senior managerial decisions

Executive management The senior management of a healthcare organization, the people who oversee a broad functional area or group of departments or services; this level of management sets the organization's future direction and monitors the organization's operations in those areas

Exempt employees Specific groups of employees who are identified as not being covered by some or all of the provisions of the Fair Labor Standards Act

Exit interview refers to the final meeting an employee has with his or her employer; the meeting provides an opportunity to collect feedback on issues or problem areas, including what may have caused the employee to leave

Expenses Amounts that are charged as costs by an organization to the current year's activities of operation

Experimental study Study that strives to establish cause and effect; it entails exposing participants to different interventions in order to compare the results of these interventions with the outcome

Expert power Refers to leaders who are experts in their field or have knowledge or skills that are in short supply

Explanation of benefits (EOB) A statement issued to the insured and the healthcare provider by an insurer to explain the services provided, amounts billed, and payments made by a health plan

Exploitive autocracy The leader wields absolute power and uses the team to serve his or her personal interests

Express contract Agreement between physician and patient that is specifically articulated

Expressed consent The spoken or written permission granted by a patient to a healthcare provider that allows the provider to perform medical or surgical services

Extended care facility A healthcare facility licensed by applicable state or local law to offer room and board, skilled nursing by a full-time registered nurse, intermediate care, or a combination of levels on a 24-hour basis over a long period of time

Extension codes Used in ICD-11-MMS, the extension code provides additional information

External analysis Development of the market assessment to determine opportunities and threats to the future of the organization

External customers Individuals from outside the organization who receive products or services from within the organization

External threats Threats that originate outside an organization

F

Facility-based registry A registry that includes only cases from a particular type of healthcare facility, such as a hospital or clinic

Facility directory A directory of patients being treated in a healthcare facility

Fair and Accurate Credit Transactions Act Law passed in 2003 that contains provisions and requirements to reduce identity theft (Public Law 108-159 2003)

Fair Labor Standards Act (FLSA) The federal legislation that sets the minimum wage and overtime payment regulations (52 Stat. 1060 1938)

False Claims Act Legislation passed during the Civil War, amended in 1986, that prohibits contractors from making a false claim to a governmental program; used to reinforce the prevention of healthcare fraud and abuse (Public Law 99-562 1986)

Family and Medical Leave Act (FMLA) The federal legislation that allows full-time employees time off from work (up to 12 weeks) to care for themselves or their family members with the assurance of an equivalent position upon return to work (Public Law 103-3 1993)

Fast Healthcare Interoperability Resource (FHIR) A set of resources that address common use cases in exchanging health information

Federal Health IT Strategic Plan 2015-2020 Issued by the Office of the National Coordinator for Health Information Technology (ONC), this plan describes a vision of high-quality care, lower costs, healthy population, and engaged people and mission to improve the health and well-being of individuals and communities through the use of technology and health information that is accessible when and where it matters most

Federal poverty level (FPL) The income qualification threshold established by the federal government for certain government entitlement programs

Federal Rules of Civil Procedure (FRCP) Rules established by the US Supreme Court setting the "rules of the road" and procedures for federal court cases. FRCP include electronic records and continue to be very important as benchmarks in how these records can be used in courts, not only federal, but state and other courts as well (Public Law 97-462 1983)

Federal Rules of Evidence (FRE) Rules established by the US Supreme Court guiding the introduction and use of evidence in federal court proceedings that are an important benchmark for state and other courts. FRE governs what and how electronic records may be used, and the roles of record custodianship

Federal Trade Commission (FTC) An independent federal agency tasked with dealing with two areas of economics in the United States: consumer protection and issues having to do with competition in business

Fee-for-service reimbursement A method of reimbursement through which providers retrospectively receive payment based on either billed charges for services provided or on annually updated fee schedules

Fee schedule A complete listing of fees used by health plans to pay doctors or other providers

Fellowship program Program of earned recognition for AHIMA members who have made significant and sustained contributions to the HIM profession through meritorious service, excellence in professional practice, education, and advancement of the profession through innovation and knowledge sharing

Fetal autopsy rate The number of autopsies performed on intermediate and late fetal deaths for a given time period divided by the total number of intermediate and late fetal deaths for the same time period

Fetal death (stillborn) The death of a product of human conception before its complete expulsion or extraction from the mother regardless of the duration of the pregnancy

Fetal death rate A proportion that compares the number of intermediate or late fetal deaths to the total number of live births and intermediate or late fetal deaths during the same period of time

Financial indicators A set of measures designed to routinely monitor the current financial status of a healthcare organization or of one of its constituent parts

Financial management The mechanism that all organizations and businesses use to fully comprehend and communicate their financial activities and status

Firewall A computer system or a combination of systems that provides a security barrier or supports an access control policy between two networks or between a network and any other traffic outside the network

Fishbone diagram A performance improvement tool used to identify or classify the root causes of a problem or condition and to display the root causes graphically

Flextime A work schedule that gives employees some choice in the pattern of their work hours, usually around a core of midday hours

Flow chart A graphic tool that uses standard symbols to visually display detailed information, including time and distance, of the sequential flow of work of an individual or a product as it progresses through a process

Force-field analysis A performance improvement tool used to identify specific drivers of, and barriers to, an organizational change so that positive factors can be reinforced and negative factors reduced

Forced distribution Ranking method similar to grading on a curve, where managers place subordinates into predetermined performance categories

Forensics The process of identifying, analyzing, recovering, and preserving data within an electronic environment

Fraud The intentional deception or misrepresentation that an individual knows (or should know) to be false, or does not believe to be true, and makes, knowing the deception could result in some unauthorized benefit to himself or some other person(s)

Free-text data Data that are narrative in nature

Frequency The number of times something occurs in a particular population or sample over a specific period of time

Frequency polygon A type of line graph that represents a frequency distribution

Full-time equivalent (FTE) A statistic representing the number of full-time employees as calculated by the reported number of hours worked by all employees, including part-time and temporary, during a specific time period

Fully specified name (FSN) In SNOMED CT, the unique text assigned to a concept that completely describes that concept

Functioning In International Classification of Functioning, Disability and Health, the umbrella term for body functions, body structures, activities, and participation

Fundraising In these activities that benefit the covered entity, the covered entity may use or disclose to a BA or an institutionally related foundation, without authorization, demographic information and dates of healthcare provided to an individual

G

Gantt chart A graphic tool used to plot tasks in project management that shows the duration of project tasks and overlapping tasks

General consent Explicit consent for routine treatment given to by the patient to the healthcare provider or organization

General jurisdiction Type of court that hear more serious criminal cases or civil cases involving larger sums of money

Genetic Nondiscrimination Act (GINA) Legislation that prohibits genetic discrimination by health insurers and employers

Global membership Type of AHIMA membership for international individuals

Global payment A form of reimbursement used for radiological and other procedures that combines the professional and technical components of the procedures and disperses payments as lump sums to be distributed between the physician and the healthcare facility

Go-live First use of the system in actual practice

Granular level Data consisting of small components or details at the lowest level

Graph A graphic tool used to show numerical data in a pictorial representation

Graphic rating scale A checklist is used to numerically rate employees on general traits related to job performance, like teamwork

Great Person Theory The belief that some people have natural (innate) leadership skills

Grievance process A formal procedure for management review of employee complaints designed to ensure fair treatment

Gross autopsy rate The number of inpatient autopsies conducted during a given time period divided by the total number of inpatient deaths for the same time period

Gross death rate The number of inpatient deaths that occurred during a given time period divided by the total number of inpatient discharges, including deaths, for the same time period

Grounded theory A theory about what is actually going on instead of what should go on

Group membership Allows multiple individuals from an organization to join AHIMA at one time; student and business groups are eligible for this membership type

Grouper 1. Computer program that uses specific data elements to assign patients, clients, or residents to groups, categories, or classes 2. A computer software program that automatically assigns prospective payment groups on the basis of clinical codes

Guidelines In forms control, provides general direction about the design of the form

H

Halo-horns effect Occurs when an employee is strong or weak in one rated area and the supervisor unfairly generalizes that performance to rate the employee high or low across all other areas on the performance appraisal

Harassment The act of bothering or annoying someone repeatedly

Health Care Fraud Prevention and Enforcement Action Team (HEAT) Created by HHS and the Department of Justice, this team's mission is to: prevent waste, fraud, and abuse; identify those who participate in fraud and abuse; reduce healthcare costs; improve the quality of care provided to Medicare and Medicaid patients; provide best practices in combating fraud and abuse; and expand partnership between HHS and the Department of Justice

Health Care Quality Improvement Act of 1986 A 1986 act that requires facilities to report professional review actions on physicians, dentists, and other facility-based practitioners to the National Practitioner Data Bank (NPDB) (Public Law 99-660 1986)

Health informatics The field of information science concerned with the management of all aspects of health data and information through the application of computers and computer technologies

Health information exchange (HIE) The exchange of health information electronically between providers and others with the same level of interoperability, such as labs and pharmacies

Health information management (HIM) An allied health profession that is responsible for ensuring the availability, accuracy, and protection of the clinical information that is needed to deliver healthcare services and to make appropriate healthcare-related decisions

Health information organization (HIO) An organization that supports, oversees, or governs the exchange of health-related information among organizations according to nationally recognized standards

Health information system The term used to describe the full scope of adopting health information technology

Health Information Technology for Economic and Clinical Health (HITECH) Act Legislation created to promote the adoption and meaningful use of health information technology in the United States. Subtitle D of the Act provides for additional privacy and security requirements that will develop and support electronic health information, facilitate information exchange, and strengthen monetary penalties. Signed into law on February 17, 2009, as part of ARRA (Public Law 111-5 2009)

Health insurance marketplace or exchange Offers the purchase of federally regulated and subsidized health insurance to uninsured, eligible Americans based on their income

Health Insurance Portability and Accountability Act (HIPAA) The federal legislation enacted to provide continuity of health coverage, control fraud and abuse in healthcare, reduce healthcare costs, and guarantee the security and privacy of health information; limits exclusion for pre-existing medical conditions, prohibits discrimination against employees and dependents based on health status, guarantees availability of health insurance to small employers, and guarantees renewability of insurance to all employees regardless of size; requires covered entities (most healthcare providers and organizations) to transmit healthcare claims in a specific format and to develop, implement, and comply with the standards of the Privacy Rule and the Security Rule; and mandates that covered entities apply for and utilize national identifiers in HIPAA transactions (Public Law 104-191 1996)

Health IT Under HITECH, hardware, software, integrated technologies or related licenses, intellectual property, upgrades, or packaged solutions sold as services that are designed for or support the use by health care entities or patients for the electronic creation, maintenance, access, or exchange of health information (Public Law 111-5 2009)

Health Level Seven (HL7) Founded in 1987, Health Level Seven International (HL7) is a not-for-profit, ANSI-accredited standards-developing organization dedicated to providing a comprehensive framework and related standards for the exchange, integration, sharing, and retrieval of electronic health information that supports clinical practice and the management, delivery, and evaluation of health services

Health literacy The ability of patients to read and understand health information

Health maintenance organization Entity that combines the provision of healthcare insurance and the delivery of healthcare services, characterized by: (1) an organized healthcare delivery system to a geographic area, (2) a set of basic and supplemental health maintenance and treatment services, (3) voluntarily enrolled members, and (4) predetermined fixed, periodic prepayments for members' coverage

Health plans Another name for health insurer

Health record 1. Information relating to the physical or mental health or condition of an individual, as made by or on behalf of a health professional in connection with the care ascribed that individual 2. A medical record, health record, or medical chart that is a systematic documentation of a patient's medical history and care

Health Services Research Research conducted on the subject of healthcare delivery that examines organizational structures and systems as well as the effectiveness and efficiency of healthcare services

Healthcare clearinghouse An organization that prepares healthcare claims for submission to the healthcare insurer

Healthcare Cost and Utilization Project (HCUP) A family of databases and related software tools and products developed through a Federal-State-Industry partnership and sponsored by AHRQ. HCUP databases are derived from administrative data and contain encounter-level, clinical, and nonclinical information including all listed diagnoses and procedures, discharge status, patient demographics, and charges for all patients, regardless of payer (such as Medicare, Medicaid, private insurance, uninsured), beginning in 1988

Healthcare data analytics The practice of using data to make business decisions in healthcare

Healthcare Facilities Accreditation Program (HFAP) An accreditation organization that establishes standards and conducts surveys. Healthcare providers who are successful in meeting the standards are awarded accreditation

Healthcare Information Management Systems Society (HIMSS) A cause-based, not-for-profit organization exclusively focused on providing global leadership for the optimal use of IT and management systems for the betterment of healthcare

Healthcare insurance Protection from having to pay the full cost of healthcare by prepaying for a plan for healthcare coverage

Healthcare provider A generic term to encompass physicians, healthcare organizations, nurses, physical therapist and others

Healthcare research organizations Organizations that conduct, promote, or support research across healthcare organizations

Hearsay A written or oral statement made outside of court that is offered in court as evidence

High Reliability Organization (HRO) Organizations that focus on creating an environment that eliminates or minimizes error

HIPAA consent A document, required by HIPAA, whereby the patient provides the covered entity permission to release protected health information

HIPAA Security Rule The federal regulations created to implement the security requirements of HIPAA

Histogram A graphic technique used to display the frequency distribution of continuous data (interval or ratio data) as either numbers or percentages in a series of bars

History and physical (H&P) The pertinent information about the patient, including chief complaint, past and present illnesses, family history, social history, and review of body systems

Home health prospective payment system (HH PPS) The case-mix reimbursement system developed by the Centers for Medicare and Medicaid Services in 2008 to cover home health services, including therapy visits and different resource costs provided to Medicare beneficiaries

Home healthcare Limited part-time or intermittent skilled nursing care and home health aide services, physical therapy, occupational therapy, speech-language therapy, medical social services, durable medical equipment (such as wheelchairs, hospital beds, oxygen, and walkers), medical supplies, and other services

Hospice An interdisciplinary program of palliative care and supportive services that addresses the physical, spiritual, social, and economic needs of terminally ill patients and their families

Hospital A healthcare entity that has an organized medical staff and permanent facilities that include inpatient beds and continuous medical or nursing services and that provides diagnostic and therapeutic services for patients as well as overnight accommodations and nutritional services

Hospital-acquired condition (HAC) CMS identified eight hospital-acquired conditions (not present on admission) as "reasonably preventable," and hospitals will not receive additional payment for cases in which one of the eight selected conditions was not present on admission; the eight originally selected conditions include: foreign object retained after surgery, air embolism, blood incompatibility, stage III and IV pressure ulcers, falls and trauma, catheter-associated urinary tract infection, vascular catheter-associated infection, and surgical site infection—mediastinitis after coronary artery bypass graft; additional conditions were added in 2010 and remain in effect: surgical site infections following certain orthopedic procedures and bariatric surgery, manifestations of poor glycemic control, and deep vein thrombosis (DVT)/ pulmonary embolism (PE) following certain orthopedic procedures

Hospital-acquired (nosocomial) infection rate The number of hospital-acquired infections for a given time period divided by the total number of inpatient discharges for the same time period

Hospital autopsy A postmortem (after death) examination performed on the body of a person who has at some time been a hospital patient by a hospital pathologist or a physician of the medical staff who has been delegated the responsibility

Hospital autopsy rate The total number of autopsies performed by a hospital pathologist for a given time period divided by the number of deaths of hospital patients (inpatients and outpatients) whose bodies were available for autopsy for the same time period

Hospital bylaws Written document that govern the staff members, both medical providers and non-physician providers, who create data within the health record for additional support of patient care and reimbursement

Hospital death rate The number of inpatient deaths for a given period of time divided by the total number of live discharges and deaths for the same time period

Hospital in the home New connectivity mechanisms that help monitor patients at home

Hospital inpatient A patient who is provided with room, board, and continuous general nursing services in an area of an acute-care facility where patients generally stay at least overnight

Hospital inpatient autopsy A postmortem (after death) examination performed on the body of a patient who died during an inpatient hospitalization by a hospital pathologist or a physician of the medical staff who has been delegated the responsibility

Hospital newborn inpatient A patient born in the hospital at the beginning of the current inpatient hospitalization

Hospital outpatient A hospital patient who receives services in one or more of a hospital's facilities when he or she is not currently an inpatient or a home care patient

Hospital Standardization Program An early 20th-century survey mechanism instituted by the American College of Surgeons and aimed at identifying quality-of-care problems and improving patient care; precursor to the survey program offered by the Joint Commission

Hospitalist A physician specialty in inpatient care

Hostile work environment A setting in which intimidating and abusive conduct takes place that interferes with an employee's job performance

House of Delegates An important component of the volunteer structure of the American Health Information Management Association that conducts the official business of the organization and functions as its legislative body

Human capital The sum of the knowledge, skills, and abilities of an organization's workforce

Human computer interface (HCI) Any form of input device used by humans, including monitors, keyboards, printers, scanners, and many other devices that enable human interaction with computing technology

Human resources management (HRM) The process of acquiring, training, appraising, and compensating employees, and of attending to their labor relations, health and safety, and fairness concerns

Hybrid health record A combination of paper and electronic records; a health record that includes both paper and electronic elements; also known as hybrid record

I

Identity management (IdM) Provides security functionality, including determining who (or what information system) is authorized to access information, authentication services, audit logging, encryption, and transmission controls

Identity matching algorithm Rules established in an information system that predicts the probability that two or more patients in the database are the same patient

Identity proofing Authentication credentials used to electronically sign prescriptions

Image-based storage Information system used when a document is scanned and storing it digitally on hard drives, CD, or another storage media

Impact analysis 1. A collective term used to refer to any study that determines the benefit of a proposed project, including cost-benefit analysis, return on investment, benefits realization study, or qualitative benefit study 2. An estimate of the impact of threats on information assets

Implementation Refers to technology having been installed, configured to meet the basic requirements of the healthcare organization, and demonstrated to users

Implementation specifications As amended by HITECH, specific requirements or instructions for implementing a privacy or security standard

Implied contract Type of agreement between physician and patient that is created by actions

Incidence rate A computation that compares the number of new cases of a specific disease for a given time period to the population at risk for the disease during the same time period

Incident An occurrence in a medical facility that is inconsistent with accepted standards of care

Incident detection Methods used to identify both accidental and malicious events; detection programs monitor the information systems for abnormalities or a series of events that might indicate that a security breach is occurring or has occurred

Incident or occurrence report A quality or performance management tool used to collect data and information about potentially compensable events (events that may result in death or serious injury)

Independent variable The factors in experimental research that researchers manipulate directly

Index An organized (usually alphabetic) list of specific data that serves to guide, indicate, or otherwise facilitate reference to the data

Indian Health Service The federal agency within the Department of Health and Human Services that is responsible for providing federal healthcare services to American Indians and Alaska natives

Individual The person who is the subject of the protected health information

Individual data Healthcare data that is housed within the electronic health record, or data collected from a case study, a focus group of individuals, or during an interview or survey

Individually identifiable health information As amended by HITECH, information that is a subset of health information, including demographic information collected from an individual, and: (1) is created or received by a health care provider, health plan, employer, or health care clearinghouse; and (2) relates to the past, present, or future physical or mental health or condition of an individual; the provision of health care to an individual; or the past, present, or future payment for the provision of health care to an individual; and (i) that identifies the individual; or (ii) with respect to which there is a reasonable basis to believe the information can be used to identify the individual (45 CFR 160.103 2013)

Infant mortality rate The number of deaths of individuals under one year of age during a given time period divided by the number of live births reported for the same time period

Inference engine A special type of server that supplies the rules that govern clinical decision support

Inferential statistics 1. Statistics that are used to make inferences from a smaller group of data to a large one 2. A set of statistical techniques that allows researchers to make generalizations about a population's characteristics (parameters) on the basis of a sample's characteristics

Informatics A field of study that focuses on the use of technology to improve access to, and utilization of, information

Information Data processed into usable form

Information assets Information that has value for an organization

Information governance The accountability framework and decision rights to achieve enterprise information management (EIM). IG is the responsibility of executive leadership for developing and driving the IG strategy throughout the organization. IG encompasses both data governance (DG) and information technology governance (ITG)

Information Governance Principles of Healthcare Set of principles established by AHIMA which creates the foundation of the IG model

Information technology Computer technology (hardware and software) combined with telecommunications technology (data, image, and voice networks)

Information Technology Asset Disposition (ITAD) Policy that identifies how all data storage devices are destroyed and purged of data prior to repurposing or disposal

Informed consent 1. A legal term referring to a patient's right to make his or her own treatment decisions based on the knowledge of the treatment to be administered or the procedure to be performed 2. An individual's voluntary agreement to participate in research or to undergo a diagnostic, therapeutic, or preventive medical procedure

Injury (harm) In a negligence lawsuit, one of four elements, which may be economic (hospital expenses and loss of wages) and noneconomic (pain and suffering), that must be proved to be successful

Injury Severity Score (ISS) An overall severity measurement maintained in the trauma registry and calculated from the abbreviated injury scores for the three most severe injuries of each patient

Inpatient admission An acute-care facility's formal acceptance of a patient who is to be provided with room, board, and continuous nursing service in an area of the facility where patients generally stay at least overnight

Inpatient bed occupancy rate (percentage of occupancy) The total number of inpatient service days for a given time period divided by the total number of inpatient bed count days for the same time period

Inpatient discharge The termination of hospitalization through the formal release of an inpatient from a hospital

Inpatient prospective payment system (IPPS) A system of payment for the operating costs of acute-care hospital inpatient stays under Medicare Part A

Inpatient service day (IPSD) A unit of measure that reflects the services received by one inpatient during a 24-hour period

Input mask The format in which the data will be displayed in an information system

Inputs Data entered into a hospital system (for example, the patient's knowledge of his or her condition, the admitting clerk's knowledge of the admission process, and the computer with its admitting template are all inputs for the hospital's admitting system)

Institutional Review Board (IRB) An administrative body that provides review, oversight, guidance, and approval for research projects carried out by employees serving as researchers, regardless of the location of the research (such as a university or private research agency); responsible for protecting the rights and welfare of the human subjects involved in the research. IRB oversight is mandatory for federally funded research projects

Integrated delivery network (IDN) A group of hospitals, physicians, other providers, insurers, or community agencies that work together to deliver health services

Integrated delivery system (IDS) A system that combines the financial and clinical aspects of healthcare and uses a group of healthcare providers, selected on the basis of quality and cost management criteria, to furnish comprehensive health services across the continuum of care

Integrated health record A system of health record organization in which all the paper forms are arranged in strict chronological order and mixed with forms created by different departments

Integrity 1. The state of being whole or unimpaired 2. The ability of data to maintain its structure and attributes, including protection against modification or corruption during transmission, storage, or at rest. Maintenance of data integrity is a key aspect of data quality management and security 3. Openness in decision-making, honesty in communication, activity, and ethical practices that command trust and support collaboration

Intentional tort A circumstance where a healthcare provider purposely commits a wrongful act that results in injury

Interface The zone between different computer systems across which users want to pass information (for example, a computer program written to exchange information between systems or the graphic display of an application program designed to make the program easier to use)

Interface engine Technology that manages all of the interfaces for a given entity

Internal analysis Reviewing the inner working of the healthcare organization to determine strengths and weaknesses of the business practice and process

Internal customers Customers within an organization, such as employees

Internal threats Threats that originate within an organization

International Classification of Diseases, 11th Revision, for Mortality and Morbidity Statistics (ICD-11-MMS) Classification system that is a linearization of the ICD-11 foundation component

International Classification of Functioning, Disability, and Health (ICF) Classification of health and health-related domains that describes body functions and structures, activities, and participation

Interoperability The capability of different information systems and software applications to communicate and exchange data

Interrogatories Discovery devices consisting of a set of written questions given to a party, witness, or other person who has information needed in a legal case

Interval-level data Data with a defined unit of measure, no true zero point, and equal intervals between successive values

Interval variables Variables that have equal units with an arbitrary zero point

Intrusion detection The process of identifying attempts or actions to penetrate a system and gain unauthorized access

Intrusion detection system (IDS) A system that performs automated intrusion detection; procedures should be outlined in the organization's data security plan to determine what actions should be taken in response to a probable intrusion

ISO 9000 certification The ISO 9000 family addresses various aspects of quality management and contains some of ISO's best-known standards. The standards provide guidance and tools for companies and organizations that want to ensure that their products and services consistently meet customers' requirements, and that quality is consistently improved

Issues management Any issues that arise during the implementation are documented, brought to the attention of the vendor, and hopefully resolved, or escalated so that resolution is accomplished

J

Job analysis Collecting and analyzing information about a job in order to better understand the significant component duties of the job, and to identify the skills and characteristics required of an employee who can successfully perform the job

Job classification 1. A method of job evaluation that compares a written position description with the written descriptions of various classification grades 2. A method used by the federal government to grade jobs

Job description A detailed list of a job's duties, reporting relationships, working conditions, and responsibilities

Job evaluation The process of applying predefined compensable factors to jobs to determine their relative worth

Job interview A conversation in which a hiring manager and a job applicant exchange information

Job sharing A work schedule in which two or more individuals share the tasks of one full-time or one full-time-equivalent position

Job specifications A list of a job's required education, skills, knowledge, abilities, personal qualifications, and physical requirements

Joinder A complaint against a third party

Joint Commission An independent, not-for-profit organization, the Joint Commission accredits and certifies more than 20,000 healthcare organizations and programs in the United States. Joint Commission accreditation and certification is recognized nationwide as a symbol of quality that reflects an organization's commitment to meeting certain performance standards

Judicial law The body of law created as a result of court (judicial) decisions

Jurisdiction The power and authority of a court to hear, interpret, and apply the law to and decide specific types of cases

Justice Principle that recognizes the importance of treating people fairly, of applying rules consistently, and of fairly distributing cost and risk

K

Key indicator A quantifiable measure used over time to determine whether some structure, process, or outcome in the provision of care to a patient supports high-quality performance measured against best practice criteria

Kiosk Special form of input device geared more to people less familiar with computers

Knowledge The information, understanding, and experience that give individuals the power to make informed decisions

Knowledge source Resources that provide information about the properties of drugs, the latest research about new surgical procedures, and other information needed to support clinical decision-making

L

Laboratory information system (LIS) Health information system that includes hardware; software; communications and network technologies; operational and cultural adaptations that people must make to use the technologies in performing diagnostic studies on various specimens collected from patients and to apply professional judgment in evaluating the quality of the data representing the results; policies and standards from the local organization in which the system is housed as well as accrediting and licensing bodies that must be followed for design of the technology and its use; and workflow and process designs that assure the most efficient and effective use of the technology

Laissez-faire leadership Delegative leadership style that reflects a leader who holds a title and responsibility, but has everyone else perform the work

Layoff A temporary dismissal where employees are told there is no work available now, but that they may be recalled; there is no guarantee of being recalled

Leader–member relations Group atmosphere much like social orientation; includes the subordinates' acceptance of, and confidence in, the leader as well as the loyalty and commitment they show toward the leader

Leadership Visionary thinking, decisions responsive to membership and mission, and accountability for actions and outcomes

Leadership criteria Division of leadership traits that includes leader emergence, leader effectiveness, and leader advancement and promotion

Leadership grid Blake and Mouton's grid that marked off degrees of emphasis toward orientation using a nine-point scale and finally separated the grid into five styles of management based on the combined people and production emphasis

Leading One of the four management functions in which people are directed and motivated to achieve goals

Leading by example The leader is in a role model position and team members follow or emulate the leader's behavior

Lean A process improvement methodology focused on eliminating waste and improving the flow of work processes

Lean Six Sigma Methodology that utilizes elements of elimination of waste from Lean and critical process quality characteristics from Six Sigma

Legal health record Documents and data elements that a healthcare provider may include in response to legally permissible requests for patient information

Legal hold A communication issued because of current or anticipated litigation, audit, government investigation, or other such matters that suspends the normal disposition or processing of records. Legal holds can encompass business procedures affecting active data, including, but not limited to, backup tape recycling. The specific communication to business or IT organizations may also be called a "hold," "preservation order," "suspension order," "freeze notice," "hold order," or "hold notice"

Legitimate power Power derived from your position or status within the organization

Length of stay (LOS) The total number of patient days for an inpatient episode, calculated by subtracting the date of admission from the date of discharge

Licensure The legal authority or formal permission from authorities to carry on certain activities that by law or regulation require such permission (applicable to institutions as well as individuals)

Likelihood determination An estimate of the probability of threats occurring

Limited jurisdiction A type of court that hears cases pertaining to a particular subject (for example, landlord and tenant or juvenile) or involve crimes of lesser severity or civil matters of lower dollar amounts

Line authority The authority to manage subordinates and to have them report back, based on relationships illustrated in an organizational chart

Line graph A graphic technique used to illustrate the relationship between continuous measurements; consists of a line drawn to connect a series of points on an arithmetic scale; often used to display time trends

Linearization a subset of the foundation component in the *International Classification of Diseases 11th Revision* (ICD-11); once created the subset becomes the Tabular list

Litigation A civil lawsuit or contest in court

Living will A legal document, also known as a medical directive, that states a patient's wishes regarding life support in certain circumstances, usually when death is imminent

Logical Observations, Identifiers, Names, and Codes (LOINC) A database protocol developed by the Regenstrief Institute for Health Care aimed at standardizing laboratory and clinical codes for use in clinical care, outcomes management, and research that enable exchange and aggregation of electronic health data from many independent systems

Loose material Documentation that needs to be filed in the health record

M

Machine learning AI applications adjust the algorithms supplied in the software based on additional data, potentially providing evermore sophisticated clinical decision support (Garbade 2018)

Malfeasance A wrong or improper act

Malware Software applications that can take over partial or full control of a computer and can compromise data security and corrupt both data and hard drives

Managed care 1. Payment method in which the third-party payer has implemented some provisions to control the costs of healthcare while maintaining quality care 2. Systematic merger of clinical, financial, and administrative processes to manage access, cost, and quality of healthcare

Managed care organization (MCO) A type of healthcare organization that delivers medical care and manages all aspects of the care or the payment for care by limiting providers of care, discounting payment to providers of care, or limiting access to care

Management The process of planning, organizing, leading, and controlling organizational activities

Managing The process of planning, controlling, leading, and organizing activities

Mandatory eligibility groups Children, pregnant women, elderly adults, people with disabilities, and low-income adults that qualify for Medicaid

Market assessment Determining the number of positions on the market and the eligible workforce looking for work

Marketing As amended by HITECH, means to make a communication about a product or service that encourages recipients of the communication to purchase or use the product or service, or where the covered entity receives financial remuneration in exchange for making communication (45 CFR 164.501 2013)

Master patient index (MPI) A patient-identifying directory referencing all patients related to an organization, which also serves as a link to the patient record or information, facilitates patient identification, and assists in maintaining a longitudinal patient record from birth to death

Maternal death rate (hospital based) For a hospital, the total number of maternal deaths directly related to pregnancy for a given time period divided by the total number of obstetrical discharges for the same time period; for a community, the total number of deaths attributed to maternal conditions during a given time period in a specific geographic area divided by the total number of live births for the same time period in the same area

Maternal mortality rate (community based) A rate that measures the deaths associated with pregnancy for a specific community for a specific period of time

Mean A measure of central tendency that is determined by calculating the arithmetic average of the observations in a frequency distribution

Meaningful Use (MU) A regulation that was issued by CMS on July 28, 2010, outlining an incentive program for professionals (EPs), eligible hospitals, and CAHs participating in Medicare and Medicaid programs that adopt and successfully demonstrate meaningful use of certified EHR technology

Meaningful use program Incentive program to assist qualified healthcare providers to implement the EHR. The name has changed to promoting interoperability

Measurement The systematic process of data collection, repeated over time or at a single point in time

Measures of central tendency The typical or average numbers that are descriptive of the entire collection of data for a specific population

Measures of variability Examination of the spread of different values around the measures of central tendency; these include the range, variance, and standard deviation

Median A measure of central tendency that shows the midpoint of a frequency distribution when the observations have been arranged in order from lowest to highest

Mediation In law, when a dispute is submitted to a third party to facilitate agreement between the disputing parties

Medicaid A joint federal and state program that helps with medical costs for some people with low incomes and limited resources. Medicaid programs vary from state to state, but most healthcare costs are covered if a patient qualifies for both Medicare and Medicaid

Medicaid Fraud Control Units (MFCU) Groups that investigate and prosecute Medicaid fraud as well as patient abuse and neglect in healthcare facilities

Medical device integration Connecting medical devices to the EHR

Medical examiner (ME) Usually an appointed official who is a physician, commonly holding a specialty in pathology or forensic medicine with duties similar to coroner

Medical history Portion of clinical data that addresses the patient's current complaints and symptoms and lists his or her past medical, personal, and family history

Medical home Model of primary care physician practices that is patient-centered, comprehensive, team-based, coordinated, accessible, and focused on quality and safety

Medical identity theft A type of healthcare fraud that includes both financial fraud and identity theft, it involves either (a) the inappropriate or unauthorized misrepresentation of one's identity (for example, the use of one's name and Social Security number) to obtain medical services or goods, or (b) the falsifying of claims for medical services in an attempt to obtain money

Medical Literature, Analysis, and Retrieval System Online (MEDLINE) Medline is the US National Library of Medicine's (NLM) premier bibliographic database that contains over 19 million references to journal articles in life sciences with a concentration on biomedicine

Medical malpractice A type of action in which the plaintiff must demonstrate that a healthcare provider–patient relationship existed at the time of the alleged wrongful act

Medical necessity 1. The likelihood that a proposed healthcare service will have a reasonable beneficial effect on the patient's physical condition and quality of life at a specific point in his or her illness or lifetime 2. As amended by HITECH, a covered entity or business associate may not use or disclose protected health information, except as permitted or required (45 CFR 164.502 2013) 3. The concept that procedures are only eligible for reimbursement as a covered benefit when they are performed for a specific diagnosis or specified frequency (42 CFR 405.500 1995)

Medical necessity audit Type of audit that determines if healthcare services performed were needed based on the patient's condition and prognosis

Medical staff The staff members of a healthcare organization who are governed by medical staff bylaws; may or may not be employed by the healthcare organization

Medical staff bylaws Standards governing the practice of medical staff members; typically voted upon by the organized medical staff and the medical staff executive committee and approved by the facility's board; governs the business conduct, rights, and responsibilities of the medical staff; medical staff members must abide by these bylaws in order to continue practice in the healthcare facility

Medical staff classification Refers to the organization of physicians according to clinical assignment

Medical staff privileges Categories of clinical practice privileges assigned to individual practitioners on the basis of their qualifications

Medicare A federally funded health program established in 1965 to assist with the medical care costs of Americans 65 years of age and older as well as other individuals entitled to Social Security benefits owing to their disabilities

Medicare Access and CHIP Reauthorization Act (MACRA) Law that created the Quality Payment program

Medicare administrative contractors (MACs) Required by section 911 of the Medicare Prescription Drug, Improvement and Modernization Act of 2003, CMS is completing the process of awarding Medicare claims processing contracts through competitive procedures resulting in replacing its current claims payment contractors, fiscal intermediaries and carriers, with new contract entities called MACs. Initially 19 MACs were expected through three procurement cycles. Currently there are 15 A/B MAC jurisdictions that have served as the foundation for CMS's initial series of A/B MAC procurements. CMS will continue to consolidate to 10 A/B MAC jurisdictions

Medicare Advantage (MA) Plan A type of Medicare health insurance plan offered by a private company that contracts with Medicare to provide the beneficiary with all Part A and Part B benefits. These plans include Health Maintenance Organizations, Preferred Provider Organizations, Private Fee-for-Service Plans, Special Needs Plans, and Medicare Medical Savings Account Plans. Enrollees in Medicare Advantage Plans have their services covered through the plan; the services are not paid for under original Medicare

Medicare Conditions of Participation (CoP) Standards that a healthcare organization must meet to receive Medicare funding

Medicare Fraud Strike Force The result of the Health Care Fraud Prevention and Enforcement Action Team, this group uses data analytics to look for evidence of fraud and abuse

Medicare Part A Insurance that assists in covering inpatient care in hospitals, including critical access hospitals, and skilled nursing facilities (not custodial or long-term care). It also assists in covering hospice care and some home healthcare. Beneficiaries must meet certain conditions to get these benefits

Medicare Part B An optional and supplemental portion of Medicare that beneficiaries pay a monthly premium for. Part B assists coverage with doctors' services and outpatient care. It also covers some other medical services that Part A does not cover, such as some of the services of physical and occupational therapists, and some home healthcare. Part B pays for these covered services and supplies when they are medically necessary

Medicare Part D Medicare drug benefit created by the Medicare Modernization Act of 2003 (MMA) that offers outpatient drug coverage to beneficiaries for an additional premium. Starting January 1, 2006, new Medicare prescription drug coverage became available to everyone with Medicare. This coverage assists in lowering prescription drug costs and protects against higher costs in the future

Medicare Provider Analysis and Review (MEDPAR) File A database containing information submitted by fiscal intermediaries that is used by the Office of the Inspector General to identity suspicious billing and charge practices

Medicare severity diagnosis-related groups (MS-DRGs) The US government's 2007 revision of the MS-DRG system better accounts for severity of illness and resource consumption

Medication five rights The right drug, in the right dose, through the right route, at the right time, and to the right patient

Medication reconciliation Process that monitors and confirms that the patient receives consistent dosing across all facility transfers, such as on admission, from nursing unit to surgery, and from surgery to ICU

Mentoring A type of coaching and training in which an individual is matched with a more experienced individual who serves as an advisor or counselor

Merger A business situation where two or more companies combine, but one of them continues to exist as a legal business entity while the other(s) cease to exist legally and their assets and liabilities become part of the continuing company

Merit-Based Incentive Payment System (MIPS) Method under the Quality Payment program that allows multiple quality payment programs into one system

Message format standards Protocols that help ensure that data transmitted from one system to another remain comparable

Metadata Descriptive data that characterize other data to create a clearer understanding of their meaning and to achieve greater reliability and quality of information. Metadata consist of both indexing terms and attributes. Data about data: for example, creation date, date sent, date received, last access date, last modification date

Microfilm Photographic process that reduces an original paper document into a small static image on film

Middle management The management level in an organization that is concerned primarily with facilitating the work performed by supervisory- and staff-level personnel as well as by executive leaders

Minimum Data Set (MDS) for Long-Term Care A federally mandated standard assessment form that Medicare- and Medicaid-certified nursing facilities must use to collect demographic and clinical data on nursing home residents; includes screening, clinical, and functional status elements

Minimum necessary standard Requires that uses, disclosures, and requests must be limited to only the amount needed to accomplish an intended purpose

Misfeasance Relating to negligence or improper performance during an otherwise correct act

Mixed-methodology Research study approach that includes using both quantitative and qualitative data

Mode A measure of central tendency that consists of the most frequent observation in a frequency distribution

Moral distress Situations and times when the ethical issue is not only between what is the right thing to do, but also how to do it

Morals The concept of morals relates to what is right or wrong in human behavior

Moral values A system of principles by which one guides one's life, usually with regard to right or wrong

Morbidity The state of being diseased (including illness, injury, or deviation from normal health); the number of sick persons or cases of disease in relation to a specific population

Motivation A person's desire to do something, the thing that compels a person

Multivoting technique A decision-making method for determining group consensus on the prioritization of issues or solutions

N

National Cancer Registrars Association (NCRA) A not-for-profit association representing cancer registry professionals and certified tumor registrars (CTR). The primary focus is education and certification with the goal to ensure all cancer registry professionals have the required knowledge to be superior in their field

National Center for Health Statistics (NCHS) The federal agency responsible for collecting and disseminating information on health services utilization and the health status of the population in the United States; developed the clinical modification to the International Classification of Diseases, Tenth Revision (ICD-10) and is responsible for updating the diagnosis portion of the ICD-10-CM

National Council for Prescription Drug Programs (NCPDP) A not-for-profit ANSI-accredited standards development organization founded in 1977 that develops standards for exchanging prescription and payment information

National Committee for Quality Assurance (NCQA) A private not-for-profit organization dedicated to improving healthcare quality. Since its founding in 1990, NCQA has been a central figure in driving improvement throughout the healthcare system, helping to elevate the issue of healthcare quality to the top of the national agenda

National Drug Codes (NDC) Codes that serve as product identifiers for human drugs, currently limited to prescription drugs and a few select over-the-counter products

National Labor Relations Act (NLRA) Federal pro-union legislation that provides, among other things, procedures for union representation and prohibits unfair labor practices by unions, such as coercing nonstriking employees, and by employers, such as interference with the union selection process and discrimination against employees who support a union

National Labor Relations Board (NLRB) US government agency that holds elections for labor union representation and that reviews and looks into unfair labor practices

National Library of Medicine The world's largest medical library and a branch of the National Institutes of Health

National Patient Safety Goals (NPSGs) Goals issued by the Joint Commission to improve patient safety in healthcare organizations nationwide

National Practitioner Data Bank (NPDB) A confidential information clearinghouse created by Congress with the primary goals of improving healthcare quality, protecting the public, and reducing healthcare fraud and abuse in the United States. The NPDB is primarily an alert or flagging system intended to facilitate comprehensive review of the professional credentials of healthcare practitioners, healthcare entities, providers, and supplies

National Vital Statistics System (NVSS) The oldest and most successful example of intergovernmental data sharing in public health, and the shared relationships, standards, and procedures that form the mechanism by which the National Center for Health Statistics (NCHS) collects and disseminates the nation's official vital statistics. These data are provided through contracts between NCHS and vital registration systems operated in the various jurisdictions and legally responsible for the registration of vital events—births, deaths, marriages, divorces, and fetal deaths

Natural language processing (NLP) A technology that converts human language (structured or unstructured) into data that can be translated then manipulated by computer systems; branch of artificial intelligence

Need-to-know principle The release-of-information principle based on the minimum necessary standard

Negligence A legal term that refers to the result of an action by an individual who does not act the way a reasonably prudent person would act under the same circumstances

Negligent hiring Occurs when employees with prior criminal records were not subjected to thorough pre-employment screening

Neonatal mortality rate The number of deaths of infants under 28 days of age during a given time period divided by the total number of births for the same time period

Net autopsy rate The ratio of inpatient autopsies compared to inpatient deaths calculated by dividing the total number of inpatient autopsies performed by the hospital pathologist for a given time period by the total number of inpatient deaths minus unautopsied coroners' or medical examiners' cases for the same time period

Net death rate The total number of inpatient deaths minus the number of deaths that occurred less than 48 hours after admission for a given time period divided by the total number of inpatient discharges minus the number of deaths that occurred less than 48 hours after admission for the same time period

Network control A method of protecting data from unauthorized change and corruption at rest and during transmission among information systems

New employee orientation A group of activities that welcome new employees and introduce them to the organization, to the assigned department, unit, or workgroup and to the specific job to be performed

New graduate membership AHIMA membership level for student members who are recent graduates of accredited associate, bachelor's, and master's degree programs as well as AHIMA-approved coding programs

New to AHIMA membership AHIMA membership type all gives a discounted rate to new members for two years

Newborn (NB) An inpatient who was born in a hospital at the beginning of the current inpatient hospitalization

Newborn autopsy rate The number of autopsies performed on newborns who died during a given time period divided by the total number of newborns who died during the same time period

Newborn death rate The number of newborns who died divided by the total number of newborns, both alive and dead

Nomenclature A recognized system of terms that follows pre-established naming conventions; a disease nomenclature is a listing of the proper name for each disease entity with its specific code number

Nominal group technique A group process technique that involves the steps of silent listing, recording each participant's list, discussing, and rank ordering the priority or importance of items; allows groups to narrow the focus of discussion or to make decisions without becoming involved in extended, circular discussions

Nominal-level data Data that fall into groups or categories that are mutually exclusive and with no specific order (for example, patient demographics such as third-party payer, race, and sex)

Nominal variables Variables in which a number is assigned to a specific category; for example, 1 = male and 2 = female

Noncovered services Services not reimbursable under a managed care plan

Nonexempt employees All groups of employees covered by the provisions of the Fair Labor Standards Act

Nonfeasance A type of negligence meaning failure to act

Nonmaleficence A legal principle that means "first do no harm"

Normal distribution A theoretical family of continuous frequency distributions characterized by a symmetric bell-shaped curve, with an equal mean, median, and mode; any standard deviation; and with half of the observations above the mean and half below it

North American Association of Central Cancer Registries (NAACCR) Organization that has a certification program for state population-based registries; certification is based on the quality of data collected and reported by the state registry; NAACCR has developed standards for data quality and format and works with other cancer organizations to align their various standards

Nosocomial (hospital-acquired) infection An infection acquired by a patient while receiving care or services in a healthcare organization

Notice of privacy practices As amended by HITECH, a statement (mandated by the HIPAA Privacy Rule) issued by a healthcare organization that informs individuals of the uses and disclosures of patient-identifiable health information that may be made by the organization, as well as the individual's rights and the organization's legal duties with respect to that information (45 CFR 164.520 2013)

Notifiable disease A disease that must be reported to a government agency so that regular, frequent, and timely information on individual cases can be used to prevent and control future cases of the disease

Numeric filing system A system of health record identification and storage in which records are arranged consecutively in ascending numerical order according to the health record number

Nursing information system System that manages the nursing department, including staffing, credentialing, training, budgeting, and other managerial functions

O

Object-oriented database (OODB) 1. A type of database that uses commands that act as small, self-contained instructional units (objects) that may be combined in various ways 2. An object-oriented database (OODB) is designed to store different types of data including images, audio files, documents, videos, and data elements. OODBs are useful for storing fetal monitoring strips, electrocardiograms, PACs, and more. The OODB is dynamic because it provides the data as well as the object (image and document)

Occasion of service A specified identifiable service involved in the care of a patient that is not an encounter (for example, a lab test ordered during an encounter)

Occupational Safety and Health Act The federal legislation that established comprehensive safety and health guidelines for employers (Public Law 91-596 1970)

Occupational Safety and Health Administration (OSHA) The agency within the DOL to administer and enforce the law and provide education on workplace safety. Employers are expected to provide a physically safe work environment and to report all job-related illnesses, injuries, and fatalities

Office for Civil Rights (OCR) The federal agency within HHS that is responsible for enforcing the Privacy Rule

Office of Inspector General (OIG) Mandated by Public Law 95-452 (as amended) to protect the integrity of HHS programs, as well as the health and welfare of the beneficiaries of those programs. The OIG has a responsibility to report both to the Secretary and to the Congress program and management problems and recommendations to correct them. The OIG's duties are carried out through a nationwide network of audits, investigations, inspections, and other mission-related functions performed by OIG components

Office of the National Coordinator for Health Information Technology (ONC) The principal federal entity charged with coordination of nationwide efforts to implement and use the most advanced health information technology and the electronic exchange of health information. The position of National Coordinator was created in 2004, through an Executive Order, and legislatively mandated in the HITECH Act of 2009

Offshoring Outsourcing jobs to countries overseas, wherein local employees abroad perform jobs that domestic employees previously performed

Onboarding Socialization into the values and culture of an organization

Online analytical processing (OLAP) A data access architecture that allows the user to retrieve specific information from a large volume of data

Online learning Broad term referring to the use of electronic media instead of classroom-based learning to deliver training

Online transaction processing (OLTP) The real-time processing of day-to-day business transactions from a database

On-the-job training A method of training in which an employee learns necessary skills and processes by performing the functions of his or her position

Operating rules Rules that further explain the business requirements so their use is consistent across health plans

Operation index A list of the operations and surgical procedures performed in a healthcare facility, which is sequenced according to the code numbers of the classification system in use

Operational planning The specific day-to-day tasks that are required in operating a healthcare organization or an HIM department

Operative report A formal document that describes the events surrounding a surgical procedure or operation and identifies the principal participants in the surgery

Opportunity for improvement A healthcare structure, product, service, process, or outcome that does not meet its customers' expectations and, therefore, could be improved

Opt in/opt out A type of HIE model that sets the default for health information of patients to be included automatically, but the patient can opt out completely

Optimization Reflects not only good adoption for all routine operations, but also an understanding and appropriate use of the technology's features

Ordinal-level data Data where the order of the numbers is meaningful, not the number itself

Ordinal variables Ranked variables in which a number is assigned to rank a category in an ordered series, but the number does not indicate the magnitude of the difference between any two data points

Organization The planned coordination of the activities of multiple people to achieve a common purpose or goal

Organizational behavior A field of study that explores how people act within organizations and their behavior individually, in a group, and collectively across a department

Organizational chart A visual graphic or diagram showing the structure and reporting relationships between positions, departments, and employees of an organization

Organizational structure The framework of authority and supervision for the employees within the healthcare organization

Out of pocket Paying for the services provided with one's own funds

Outcome indicators An indicator that assesses what happens or does not happen to a patient following a process; agreed upon desired patient characteristics to be achieved; undesired patient conditions to be avoided

Outcome measures 1. The process of systematically tracking a patient's clinical treatment and responses to that treatment, including measures of morbidity and functional status, for the purpose of improving care 2. A measure that indicates the result of the performance (or nonperformance) of a function or process

Outguide A device used in paper-based health record systems to track the location of records removed from the file storage area

Outpatient A patient who receives ambulatory care services in a hospital-based clinic or department

Outpatient prospective payment system (OPPS) The Medicare prospective payment system used for hospital-based outpatient services and procedures that is predicated on the assignment of ambulatory payment classifications

Outpatient visit A patient's visit to one or more units located in the ambulatory services area (clinic or physician's office) of an acute-care hospital in which an overnight stay does not occur

Outputs The outcomes of inputs into a system (for example, the output of the admitting process is the patient's admission to the hospital)

Outsourcing The hiring of an individual or a company external to an organization to perform a function either on-site or off-site

Overlap Situation in which a patient is issued more than one medical record number from an organization with multiple facilities

Overlay Situation in which a patient is issued a medical record number that has been previously issued to a different patient

Overpayment A higher reimbursement than deserved

P

Paper health record Health record that is completely available in paper media

Parallel work division A type of concurrent work design in which one employee does several tasks and takes the job from beginning to end

Pareto chart A bar graph that includes bars arranged in order of descending size to show decisions on the prioritization of issues, problems, or solutions

Part-time employee An employee who works less than the full-time standard of 40 hours per week, 80 hours per two-week period, or 8 hours per day

Participative leadership The team makes plans and decisions and the leader is there to provide advice and assistance

Password A series of characters that must be entered to authenticate user identity and gain access to a computer or specified portions of a database

Pathology report A type of health record or documentation that describes the results of a microscopic and macroscopic evaluation of a specimen removed or expelled during a surgical procedure

Patient account number A number assigned by a healthcare facility for billing purposes that is unique to a particular episode of care; a new account number is assigned each time the patient receives care or services at the facility

Patient acuity staffing The number of nurses and other care providers is based on how sick the patient is

Patient advocacy A healthcare organization program where an employee speaks on a patient's behalf and helps get any information or services needed

Patient assessment instrument (PAI) A standardized tool used to evaluate the patient's condition after admission to, and at discharge from, the healthcare facility

Patient financial system (PFS) Information system that manages patient accounts

Patient-identifiable data Personal information that can be linked to a specific patient, such as age, gender, date of birth, and address

Patient portal Information system that allows patient to log in to obtain information, register, and perform other functions

Patient Protection and Affordable Care Act (ACA) Major healthcare reform law that included, among other provisions, requirement for most individuals to have health insurance

Patient safety Preventing harm to patients, learning from errors, and building a culture of safety

Peer review organization (PRO) Until 2002, a medical organization that performed a professional review of medical necessity, quality, and appropriateness of healthcare services provided to Medicare beneficiaries

Percentile A measure used in descriptive statistics that shows the value below which a given percentage of scores in a given group of scores falls

Performance appraisal Refers to the formal system of review and evaluation methods used to assess employee and team performance

Performance improvement (PI) The continuous study and adaptation of a healthcare organization's functions and processes to increase the likelihood of achieving desired outcomes

Performance indicators A measure used by healthcare facilities to assess the quality, effectiveness, and efficiency of their services

Performance management An ongoing, goal-oriented process focused on productivity and continuous improvement of employees and teams

Performance measurement The process of comparing the outcomes of an organization, work unit, or employee against pre-established performance plans and standards; results are typically expressed in quantifiable terms

Personal health record (PHR) An electronic or paper health record maintained and updated by an individual for himself or herself; a tool that individuals can use to collect, track, and share past and current information about their health or the health of someone in their care

Personal representative Person with legal authority to act on a patient's behalf

Personalized medicine Type of medical care that is designed specifically for an individual

Pharmacy information system This system receives an order for a drug in a hospital, aids the hospital's pharmacist in checking for contraindications, directs staff in compounding any drugs requiring special preparation, aids in dispensing the drug in the appropriate dose and for the appropriate route of administration, maintains inventory (documenting medications in stock using the National Drug Code, the terminology maintained by the Food and Drug Administration [FDA] for use in identifying FDA-approved drugs), supports staffing and budgeting, and performs other departmental operations

Phishing Type of social engineering that uses e-mail to try and obtain passwords and other personal information from individuals

Physical examination The physician's assessment of the patient's current health status after evaluating the patient's physical condition

Physical safeguards As amended by HITECH, security rule measures such as locking doors to safeguard data and various media from unauthorized access and exposures; includes facility access controls, workstation use, workstation security, and device and media controls

Physician champion An individual who assists in communicating and educating medical staff in areas such as documentation procedures for accurate billing and appropriate EHR processes

Physician index A list of patients and their physicians usually arranged according to the physician code numbers assigned by the healthcare facility

Physician orders A physician's written or verbal instructions to the other caregivers involved in a patient's care

Picture archiving and communications system (PACS) An integrated computer system that obtains, stores, retrieves, and displays digital images (in healthcare, radiological images)

Pie chart A graphic technique in which the proportions of a category are displayed as portions of a circle (like pieces of a pie); used to show the relationship of individual parts to the whole

Plaintiff The group or person who initiates a civil lawsuit

Planning 1. Governing principles that describe how a department or an organization is supposed to handle a specific situation or execute a specific process 2. Binding contracts issued by a healthcare insurance company to an individual or group in which the company promises to pay for healthcare to treat illness or injury; such contracts may also be referred to as health plan agreements and evidence of coverage

Point-of-care (POC) charting A system whereby information is entered into the health record at the time and location of service

Point of service (POS) plans A type of managed care plan in which enrollees are encouraged to select healthcare providers from a network of providers under contract with the plan but are also allowed to select providers outside the network and pay a larger share of the cost

Policies 1. Governing principles that describe how a department or an organization is supposed to handle a specific situation or execute a specific process 2. Binding contracts issued by a healthcare insurance company to an individual or group in which the company promises to pay for healthcare to treat illness or injury; such contracts may also be referred to as health plan agreements and evidence of coverage

Policyholder An individual or entity that purchases healthcare insurance coverage

Population-based registry A type of registry that includes information from more than one facility in a specific geopolitical area, such as a state or region

Population-based statistics Statistics based on a defined population rather than on a sample drawn from the same population

Population health Monitoring and preventing disease in a population which can be at a city, county, state or national level

Population health management (PHM) The aggregation of data across multiple health information system resources and the analysis of that data into actions providers can use to improve both clinical and financial outcomes (Phillips 2018)

Portals Windows into information systems

Postneonatal mortality rate The number of deaths of persons aged 28 days up to, but not including, one year during a given time period divided by the number of live births for the same time period

Postoperative infection rate The number of infections that occur in clean surgical cases for a given time period divided by the total number of operations within the same time period

Potentially compensable event An event (for example, an injury, accident, or medical error) that may result in financial liability for a healthcare organization

Power and influence theory Leadership theory noting there are various ways that leaders use authority, control, and their impact to get things done

Power user Users who are able to use technology to significantly improve their productivity

Precertification Process of obtaining approval from a healthcare insurance company before receiving healthcare services

Preemption In law, the principle that a statute at one level supersedes or is applied over the same or similar statute at a lower level (for example, the federal HIPAA privacy provisions trump the same or similar state law except when state law is more stringent)

Preferred provider organization A managed care contract coordinated care plan that: (a) has a network of providers that have agreed to a contractually specified reimbursement for covered benefits with the organization offering the plan; (b) provides for reimbursement for all covered benefits regardless of whether the benefits are provided with the network of providers; and (c) is offered by an organization that is not licensed or organized under state law as an HMO

Preferred term (PT) In SNOMED CT, the description or name assigned to a concept that is used most commonly; in the UMNDS classification system, a representation of the generic product category, which is a list of preferred concepts that name devices

Pregnancy Discrimination Act The federal legislation that prohibits discrimination against women affected by pregnancy, childbirth, or related medical conditions by requiring that affected women be treated the same as all other employees for employment-related purposes, including benefits (Public Law 95-555)

Prejudice Occurs when a person is judged solely based on cultural factors such as ethnicity, religion, age, gender, sexual orientation, or such

Premier membership Level of AHIMA membership that provides additional benefits not available to the other membership levels

Premium Amount of money that a policyholder or certificate holder must periodically pay an insurer in return for healthcare coverage

Presentation software Software used to build slides when presenting a specific topic, idea, research data, or any type of information

Present on admission (POA) A condition present at the time of inpatient admission

Prevalence rate The proportion of people in a population who have a particular disease at a specific point in time or over a specified period of time

Preventive services Healthcare services to prevent illness or early detection tests and diagnostic tools, when treatment is most likely to be effective

Primary care physician (PCP) 1. Physician who provides, supervises, and coordinates the healthcare of a member and who manages referrals to other healthcare providers and utilization of healthcare services both inside and outside a managed care plan. Family and general practitioners, internists, pediatricians, and obstetricians and gynecologists are primary care physicians 2. The physician who makes the initial diagnosis of a patient's medical condition

Primary data source The health record is this type of source because it contains information about a patient that has been documented by the professionals who provided care or services to that patient

Primary purpose The main reason for the health record is for patient care and the day to day business of the healthcare organization

Principles of organization Principles that include specialization, functional definition, span of control, hierarchical chain, and unity of command used by managers at all levels

Prior approval (authorization) Process of obtaining approval from a healthcare insurance company before receiving healthcare services

Privacy The quality or state of being hidden from, or undisturbed by, the observation or activities of other persons, or freedom from unauthorized intrusion; in healthcare-related contexts, the right of a patient to control disclosure of protected health information

Privacy officer A position mandated under the HIPAA Privacy Rule—covered entities must designate an individual to be responsible for developing and implementing privacy policies and procedures

Privacy Rule The federal regulations created to implement the privacy requirements of the simplification subtitle of the Health Insurance Portability and Accountability Act of 1996; effective in 2002; afforded patients certain rights to and about their protected health information

Private healthcare insurance Commercial insurance purchased by individuals, self-employed business people, and groups of people (such as associations and religious organizations), for themselves and for their dependents; typically these plans have high deductibles or limited covered services; a premium for coverage is paid each month to the third-party payer and those funds are used to help pay for the healthcare services

Private key infrastructure Two or more computers share the same secret key and that key is used to both encrypt and decrypt a message; however, the key must be kept secret and if it is compromised in any way, the security of the data is likely to be eliminated; *see also* single-key encryption

Private law The collective rules and principles that define the rights and duties of people and private businesses

Privileged communication The protection afforded to the recipients of professional services that prohibits medical practitioners, lawyers, and other professionals from disclosing the confidential information that they learn in their capacity as professional service providers

Probabilistic algorithm Algorithm that uses mathematical probabilities to determine the possibility that two patients are the same

Problem-oriented health record A patient record in which clinical problems are defined and documented individually

Procedure 1. A document that describes the steps involved in performing a specific function 2. An action of a medical professional for treatment or diagnosis of a medical condition 3. The steps taken to implement a policy

Process Systematic steps or actions taken in order to accomplish a goal, or to create a product or service

Process indicators Specific measures that enable the assessment of the steps taken in rendering a service

Process interoperability The use of workflows and procedures that best support use of technology

Process measures Method of monitoring that focuses on a process that leads to a certain outcome, meaning that a scientific basis exists for believing that the process, when executed well, will increase the probability of achieving a desired outcome

Process redesign The steps in which focused data are collected and analyzed, the process is changed to incorporate the knowledge gained from the data collected, the new process is implemented, and the staff is educated about the new process

Productivity indicators A set of measures designed to routinely monitor the output and quality of products or services provided by an individual, an organization, or one of its constituent parts; used to help determine the status of a productivity bonus

Professional component 1. The portion of a healthcare procedure performed by a physician or other healthcare professional 2. A term generally used in reference to the elements of radiological procedures performed by a physician

Program evaluation and review technique (PERT) chart A project management tool that diagrams a project's time lines and tasks as well as their interdependencies

Progress notes The documentation of a patient's care, treatment, and therapeutic response, which is entered into the health record by each of the clinical professionals involved in a patient's care, including nurses, physicians, therapists, and social workers

Progressive penalties Ensures that the minimum penalty appropriate to the level of offense is applied

Project management A formal set of principles and procedures that help control the activities associated with implementing a usually large undertaking to achieve a specific goal, such as an information system project

Project management life cycle The period in which the processes involved in carrying out a project are completed, including project definition, project planning and organization, project tracking and analysis, project revisions, change control, and communication

Project management office (PMO) PMO departments are found in a larger healthcare organization. In this office, the project manager aids in compiling a project's budget, allocating resources, maintaining a task list, identifying dependencies among tasks, establishing timelines, and managing a schedule

Proportion The relation of one part to another or to the whole with respect to magnitude, quantity, or degree

Proportionate mortality rate (PMR) The total number of deaths due to a specific cause during a given time period divided by the total number of deaths due to all causes

Prospective payment system (PPS) A type of reimbursement system that is based on preset payment levels rather than actual charges billed after the service has been provided; specifically, one of several Medicare reimbursement systems based on predetermined payment rates or periods and linked to the anticipated intensity of services delivered as well as the beneficiary's condition

Prospective review A review of a patient's health records before admission to determine the necessity of admission to an acute-care facility and to determine or satisfy benefit coverage requirements

Prospective study A study designed to observe outcomes or events that occur after the identification of a group of subjects to be studied

Protected class Identified groups, such as racial minorities and women, that are protected by law based on past employment discrimination

Protected health information (PHI) As amended by HITECH, individually identifiable health information: (1) Except as provided in paragraph (2) of this definition, that is: (i) transmitted by electronic media; (ii) maintained in electronic media; or (iii) transmitted or maintained in any other form or medium. (2) Protected health information excludes individually identifiable health information: (i) in education records covered by the Family Educational Rights and Privacy Act, as amended, 20 USC 1232g; (ii) in records described at 20 USC 1232g(a)(4)(B)(iv); (iii) in employment records held by a covered entity in its role as employer; and (iv) regarding a person who has been deceased for more than 50 years (45 CFR 160.103 2013)

Protocol In healthcare, a detailed plan of care for a specific medical condition based on investigative studies; in medical research, a rule or procedure to be followed in a clinical trial; in a computer network, a rule or procedure used to address and ensure delivery of data

Provider Physician, clinic, hospital, nursing home, or other healthcare entity (second party) that delivers healthcare services

Proximal attributes Division of leadership traits that includes problem-solving skills, social appraisal skills, and expertise and tacit knowledge that are derived from the distal attributes and are part of a leader's operating environment

Psychotherapy notes Behavioral health notes that document a mental health professional's impressions from private counseling sessions; information compiled in reasonable anticipation of a civil, criminal, or administrative action or proceeding; or PHI subject to the Clinical Laboratory Improvements Act (CLIA) are all exceptions to the right of access

Public health An area of healthcare that deals with the health of populations in geopolitical areas, such as states and counties

Public key infrastructure (PKI) In cryptography, an asymmetric algorithm made publicly available to unlock a coded message

Public law A type of legislation that involves the government and its relations with individuals and business organizations

Q

Qualitative analysis A review of the health record to ensure that standards are met and to determine the adequacy of entries documenting the quality of care

Qualitative research Research design that collects types of data that includes a participant's perceptions, attitudes, or feelings about a certain subject; methods used to collect qualitative data can include observations, focus groups, case studies, informal conversational interviews, and in-depth interviews

Qualitative variables Categorical variables; all are discrete and include both nominal and ordinal variables

Quality improvement organization (QIO) An organization that performs medical peer review of Medicare and Medicaid claims, including review of validity of hospital diagnosis and procedure coding information; completeness, adequacy, and quality of care; and appropriateness of prospective payments for outlier cases and nonemergent use of the emergency room. Until 2002, called peer review organization

Quality indicator A standard against which actual care may be measured to identify a level of performance for that standard

Quality payment program Program established by MACRA that created Merit-Based Incentive Payments System and the Alternative Payment Models

Quantitative analysis A review of the health record to determine its completeness and accuracy

Quantitative study Data collected for research studies that are collated numerically with descriptive, inferential, or predictive statistics

Quantitative variables Numerical variables; can be broken down into interval and ratio variables

Quasi-experimental study Similar to the experimental study except that randomization of participants is not included in a quasi-experimental study, the independent variable may not be manipulated by the researcher, and there may be no control or comparison group; these studies can be performed over time and may not include individual participants but whole healthcare systems

Query Communication tool for CDI staff to communicate with providers to obtain clinical clarification, provide a documentation alert, get documentation clarification, or ask additional questions regarding documentation

Qui tam The "whistleblower" provisions of the False Claims Act, which provides that private persons, known as relators, may enforce the Act by filing a complaint, under seal, alleging fraud committed against the government

Quid pro quo A favor or advantage given for something expected in return; often in sexual harassment instances, sexual favors are requested in exchange for a job benefit or continued employment

R

Radio-frequency identification (RFID) An automatic recognition technology that uses a device attached to an object to transmit data to a receiver and does not require direct contact

Radiology information system (RIS) Performs functions similar to LIS, receiving an order for a procedure, scheduling it, notifying hospital personnel or the patient if performed as an outpatient, tracking the performance of the procedure and its output, tracking preparation of the report, performing quality control, maintaining an inventory of equipment and supplies, and managing departmental staffing and budget

Randomization The assignment of subjects to experimental or control groups based on chance

Range A measure of variability between the smallest and largest observations in a frequency distribution

Ranking method Appraiser ranks all employees in a group or unit from highest to lowest based on overall performance

Rate A measure used to compare an event over time; a comparison of the number of times an event did happen (numerator) with the number of times an event could have happened (denominator)

Ratio 1. A calculation found by dividing one quantity by another 2. A general term that can include a number of specific measures such as proportion, percentage, and rate

Ratio-level data Data where there is a defined unit of measure, a real zero point, and the intervals between successive values are equal

Ratio variables The most common quantitative variables used in healthcare; these variables include numbers that can be compared meaningfully with one another; zero is truly zero on the ratio scale

Reasonable accommodation workplace adjustment that does not present an undue (significant) hardship to the organization, and that this failure interfered with the qualified individual being hired or with his or her ability to perform a job. In order to comply with this law and demonstrate fair employment practices

Reasonable cause As amended by HITECH, an act or omission in which a covered entity or business associate knew, or by exercising reasonable diligence would have known, that the act or omission violated an administrative simplification provision, but in which the covered entity or business associated did not act with willful neglect (45 CFR 160.401 2013)

Reasonable diligence As amended by HITECH, means the business care and prudence expected from a person seeking to satisfy a legal requirement under similar circumstances (45 CFR 160.401 2013)

Record locator service (RLS) A process that seeks information about where a patient, once identified, may have a health record available to the HIO

Record reconciliation The process of assuring that all the records of discharged patients have been received by the HIM department for processing

Recovery audit contractor (RAC) A governmental program whose goal is to identify improper payments made on claims of healthcare services provided to Medicare beneficiaries. Improper payments may be overpayments or underpayments

Recovery room report A type of health record documentation used by nurses to document the patient's reaction to anesthesia and condition after surgery

Recruitment The process of finding, soliciting, and attracting employees

Red Flags Rule Consists of five categories of red flags that are used as triggers to alert the organization to a potential identity theft; the categories are: (1) alerts, notifications, or warnings from a consumer reporting agency; (2) suspicious documents; (3) suspicious personally identifying information such as a suspicious address; (4) unusual use of, or suspicious activity relating to, a covered account; (5) Notices from customers, victims of identity theft, law enforcement authorities, or other businesses about possible identity theft in connection with an account

Referent power The ability of the team members to identify with leaders who have desirable resources or personal traits

Referred outpatient An outpatient who is provided special diagnostic or therapeutic services by a hospital on an ambulatory basis but whose medical care remains the responsibility of the referring physician

Registered health information administrator (RHIA) A type of certification granted after completion of an AHIMA-accredited four-year program in health information management and a credentialing examination

Registered health information technician (RHIT) A type of certification granted after completion of an AHIMA-accredited two-year program in health information management and a credentialing examination

Registration The act of enrolling

Registration-Admission, Discharge, Transfer (R-ADT) A type of administrative information system that stores demographic information and performs functionality related to registration, admission, discharge, and transfer of patients within the organization

Registry A collection of care information related to a specific disease, condition, or procedure that makes health record information available for analysis and comparison

Regression equation Type of inferential statistics that are used to determine if there is a relationship between variables and to identify what type of relationship is present

Reimbursement Compensation or repayment for healthcare services

Relational database A type of database that stores data in predefined tables made up of rows and columns

Reliability A measure of consistency of data items based on their reproducibility and an estimation of their error of measurement

Remittance advice An explanation of payments (for example, claim denials) made by third-party payers

Request for production Type of discovery that notifies an individual or organization the need to provide documents or other item

Requirements specification Determining and documenting the detailed features and functions desired in the system in order to meet the organization's specific goals

Requisition Request for the health record

Research An inquiry process aimed at discovering new information about a subject or revising old information

Research methodologies Research studies that can range from exploratory or descriptive studies that strive to generate new hypotheses based on data collected to experimental studies that provide interventions or treatments that can reduce the spread of an existing disease

Resident assessment instrument (RAI) In skilled nursing facilities, the care plan is based on a format required by federal regulations

Resource allocation A process and strategy of deciding where resources should be used to accomplish the mission, values, and goals of the organization

Resource-based relative value scale (RBRVS) A scale of national uniform relative values for all physicians' services. The relative value of each service must be the sum of relative value units representing the physicians' work, practice expenses net of malpractice insurance expenses, and the cost of professional liability insurance

Respect Appreciation of the value of differing perspectives, enjoyable experiences, courteous interaction, and celebration of achievements that advance our common cause

Results management An EHR application that enables diagnostic study results (primarily lab results) to be reviewed in a report format and the data within the reports to be processed

Retrospective documentation Healthcare providers add documentation after care has been given, possibly for the purpose of increasing reimbursement or avoiding a medical legal action

Retrospective review The part of the utilization review process that concentrates on a review of clinical information following patient discharge

Retrospective study A type of research conducted by reviewing records from the past (for example, birth and death certificates or health records) or by obtaining information about past events through surveys or interviews

Revenue The recognition of income earned and the use of appropriated capital from the rendering of services during the current period

Revenue cycle 1. The process of how patient financial and health information moves into, through, and out of the healthcare facility, culminating with the facility receiving reimbursement for services provided 2. The regularly repeating set of events that produce revenue

Revenue cycle management (RCM) Refers to the entire process of creating, submitting, analyzing, and obtaining payment for healthcare services

Reward power Power based on the leader's ability to give rewards to team members for commendable work, such as letters of recommendation, compliments, additional training or responsibilities, and additional compensation for working on the team

Right of access Allows an individual to inspect and obtain a copy of his or her own PHI contained within a designated record set, such as a health record

Right to request accounting of disclosures An individual has the right to receive an accounting of certain disclosures made by a covered entity

Right to request amendment One may request that a covered entity amend PHI or a record about the individual in a designated record set

Right to request confidential communications Healthcare providers and health plans must give individuals the opportunity to request that communications of PHI be routed to an alternative location or by an alternative method

Right to request restrictions of PHI An individual can request that a covered entity restrict the uses and disclosures of PHI to carry out treatment, payment, or healthcare operations

Right-to-work laws Federal legislation dealing with labor rights (examples include workers' compensation, child labor, and minimum wage laws)

Risk 1. The probability of incurring injury or loss 2. The probable amount of loss foreseen by an insurer in issuing a contract 3. A formal insurance term denoting liability to compensate individuals for injuries sustained in a healthcare facility

Risk analysis The process of identifying possible security threats to the organization's data and identifying which risks should be proactively addressed and which risks are lower in priority

Risk management A comprehensive program of activities intended to minimize the potential for injuries to occur in a facility and to anticipate and respond to ensuring liabilities for those injuries that do occur. The processes in place to identify, evaluate, and control risk, defined as the organization's risk of accidental financial liability

Risk management program A comprehensive program of activities intended to minimize the potential for injuries to occur in a facility and to anticipate and respond to ensuring liabilities for those injuries that do occur. The processes in place to identify, evaluate, and control risk, defined as the organization's risk of accidental financial liability

Role-based access control (RBAC) A control system in which access decisions are based on the roles of individual users as part of an organization

Root-cause analysis A technique used in performance improvement initiatives to discover the underlying causes of a problem. Analysis of a sentinel event from all aspects (human, procedural, machinery, material) to identify how each contributed to the occurrence of the event and to develop new systems that will prevent recurrence

Rootkit A computer program designed to gain unauthorized access to a computer and assume control of and modify the operating system

Rules and regulations Operating documents that describe the rules and regulations under which a healthcare organization operates

Rules-based algorithm Algorithm that assigns weights to specific data elements and uses those weights to compare one record to another

Rules engine Special server that supplies the rules that govern clinical decision support

Run chart A type of graph that shows data points collected over time and identifies emerging trends or patterns

RxNorm A clinical drug nomenclature developed by the Food and Drug Administration, the Department of Veterans Affairs, and HL7 to provide standard names for clinical drugs and administered dose forms

RxNorm concept unique identifier (RXCUI) The drug name and all of its synonyms, which represent a single concept

S

Safety net hospital (SNH) A hospital with the highest number of inpatient stays paid by Medicaid

Sale of information Addressed specifically by ARRA, which prohibits a covered entity or BA from selling (receiving direct or indirect compensation) in exchange for an individual's PHI without that individual's authorization; the authorization must also state whether the individual permits the recipient of the PHI to further exchange the PHI for compensation

Scales of measurement A reference standard for data collection and classification

Scatter charts A graph that visually displays the linear relationships among factors

Scorecards Reports of outcome measures to help leaders know what they have accomplished

Scribe An individual who enters clinical documentation into the EHR to reduce administrative burden on the physician

SCRIPT The NCPDP standard developed for electronically transmitting a prescription

Secondary data source Data derived from the primary patient record, such as an index or a database

Secondary purpose How the health record is used for healthcare purposes not directly related to patient care

Security 1. The means to control access and protect information from accidental or intentional disclosure to unauthorized persons and from unauthorized alteration, destruction, or loss 2. The physical protection of facilities and equipment from theft, damage, or unauthorized access; collectively, the policies, procedures, and safeguards designed to protect the confidentiality of information, maintain the integrity and availability of information systems, and control access to the content of these systems

Security breach Unauthorized data or system access

Security threat A situation that has the potential to damage a healthcare organization's information system

Selection The act or process of choosing

Selection test Assessment that identifies job skills, abilities, or job-related attitudes that may not surface in an interview

Self-awareness the ability to know one's self, to understand one's strengths and weakness and personal values and the effect that has on others

Self-regulation the ability to control or direct impulses and moods

Semantic interoperability Mutual understanding of the meaning of data exchanged between information systems

Semi-automated review Reviews that start with an automated review but also incorporate health record documents analyzed by humans

Sentinel event According to the Joint Commission, an unexpected occurrence involving death or serious physical or psychological injury, or the risk thereof. Serious injury specifically includes loss of limb or function. The phrase "or risk thereof" includes any process variation for which a recurrence would carry a significant chance of serious adverse outcome. Such events are called "sentinel" because they signal the need for immediate investigation and response

Serial numbering system System where a patient is issued a unique numeric identifier for every encounter at the healthcare facility; if a patient is admitted to the healthcare facility five times, he or she will have five different health record numbers

Serial-unit numbering system A combination of the serial and unit numbering systems; the patient is issued a new health record number with each encounter but all of the documentation is moved from the last number to the new number

Serial work division Tasks or steps in a process that are handled separately in sequence by individual workers, as with a factory assembly line, to complete a process

Sexual harassment A type of harassment that may include verbal comments, unwanted physical contact, sexual advances, or requests for sexual favors

Simulation A training technique for experimenting with real-world situations by means of a computerized model that represents the actual situation

Single-key encryption Two or more computers share the same secret key and that key is used to both encrypt and decrypt a message; however, the key must be kept secret and if it is compromised in any way, the security of the data is likely to be eliminated; *see also* private key infrastructure

Single sign-on A type of technology that allows a user access to all disparate applications through one authentication procedure, thus reducing the number and variety of passwords a user must remember and enforcing and centralizing access control

Situational leadership Involves the leader who changes the approach based on the needs of the team and situation

Six Sigma Disciplined and data-driven methodology for getting rid of defects in any process

Skilled nursing facility (SNF) A facility that primarily provides inpatient skilled nursing care and related services to patients who require medical, nursing, or rehabilitative services but does not provide the level of care or treatment available in a hospital

Skilled nursing facility prospective payment system A per-diem reimbursement system implemented in July 1998 for costs (routine, ancillary, and capital) associated with covered skilled nursing facility services furnished to Medicare Part A beneficiaries

Smart card A small plastic card with an embedded microchip that can store multiple identification factors for a specific user

SMART goals Statements that identify results that are: Specific, Measurable, Attainable, Relevant, and Time-based

Sniffers A software security product that runs in the background of a network, examining and logging packet traffic and serving as an early warning device against crackers

SNOMED CT identifier A unique integer assigned to each SNOMED CT component

Social determinants of health (SDOH) Conditions such as environment and age that impact a wide range of health, functioning, and quality-of-life outcomes and risks

Social engineering The manipulation of individuals (or targets) to freely disclose personal information or account credentials to hackers

Social media Websites or applications that provide an avenue for personal networking and the sharing of information

Social skill The ability to build relationships and rapport with people

Software as a Service (SaaS) Arrangement that is similar to an application service provider with generally less custom configuration ability and that offers a pay-as-you-go model, where there is payment for only the actual time using the system; may be delivered via dedicated communications technology or cloud computing

Source data The location from which the data originates such as a database or a data set

Source-oriented health record A system of health record organization in which information is arranged according to the patient care department that provided the care

Source systems 1. A system in which data were originally created 2. Independent information system application that contributes data to an EHR, including departmental clinical applications (for example, laboratory information system, clinical pharmacy information system) and specialty clinical applications (for example, intensive care, cardiology, labor and delivery)

Span of control The number of employees a person manages

Spear phishing A type of phishing where the hacker researches the individual being targeted

Special-cause variation An unusual source of variation that occurs outside a process but affects it

Speech dictation Method of collecting information in an information system through spoken word

Spoliation The act of destroying, changing, or hiding evidence intentionally

Spyware A computer program that tracks an individual's activity on a computer system

Staffing Decisions about the types of employees needed, how many employees are needed, how work will be organized, and how employees are scheduled

Stage of the neoplasm Pathological data characterizing the cancer, specifically the amount of metastasis, if any

Standard 1. A scientifically based statement of expected behavior against which structures, processes, and outcomes can be measured 2. A model or example established by authority, custom, or general consent or a rule established by an authority as a measure of quantity, weight, extent, value, or quality 3. Under HITECH, a technical, functional, or performance-based rule, condition, requirement, or specification that stipulates instructions, fields, codes, data, material, characteristics, or actions (45 CFR 170.102 2012) 4. As amended by HITECH at section 160.103, a rule, condition, or requirement: (1) describing the following information for products, systems, services, or practices: (i) classification of components; (ii) specification of materials, performance, or operations; or (iii) delineation of procedures; or (2) with respect to the privacy of protected health information (45 CFR 160.103 2013)

Standard deviation A measure of variability that describes the deviation from the mean of a frequency distribution in the original units of measurement; the square root of the variance

Standard of care An established set of clinical decisions and actions taken by clinicians and other representatives of healthcare organizations in accordance with state and federal laws, regulations, and guidelines; codes of ethics published by professional associations or societies; regulations for accreditation published by accreditation agencies; usual and common practice of equivalent clinicians or organizations in a geographical region

Standards development organization A private or government agency involved in the development of healthcare informatics standards at a national or international level

Standing orders Orders the medical staff or an individual physician has established as routine care for a specific diagnosis or procedure

Statistical packages Software that can be used to facilitate the data collection and analysis process; these packages simplify the statistical analysis of data and are often used in addition to spreadsheet software

Statistical process control chart A type of run chart that includes both upper and lower control limits and indicates whether a process is stable or unstable

Statistics A branch of mathematics concerned with collecting, organizing, summarizing, and analyzing data

Statistics-based modeling The use of analytical and graphical techniques to assist in the display and interpretation of raw data

Statute A piece of legislation written and approved by a state or federal legislature and then signed into law by the state's governor or the president

Statute of limitations A specific time frame allowed by a statute or law for bringing litigation

Statutory law Written law established by federal and state legislatures

Steering committee An overarching committee comprised of key stakeholders to health information systems in general, or, less commonly, a steering committee will be convened for each specific health information system project and include only stakeholders associated with that project

Stem and leaf plots A visual display that organizes data to show its shape and distribution, using two columns with the stem in the left-hand column and all leaves associated with that stem in the right-hand column; the "leaf" is the ones digit of the number, and the other digits form the "stem"

Stem codes A standalone code and can be a single entity or a combination of clinical detail (WHO 2018)

Stereotyping An assumption that everyone within a certain group is the same

Storage area network Type of network that supports the ability to retrieve data from any storage location for use in the EHR

Storage management The process of determining on what type of media to store data, how rapidly data must be accessible, arranging for replication of storage for backup and disaster recovery, and where storage systems should be maintained

Straight numeric filing system A health record filing system in which health records are arranged in ascending numerical order

Strategic information systems planning The process of identifying and prioritizing various upgrades and changes that might be made in an organization's information systems

Strategic plan The document in which the leadership of a healthcare organization identifies the organization's overall mission, vision, and goals to help set the long-term direction of the organization as a business entity

Strategic planning Involves how the organization will react to changes in the external environment in the foreseeable future

Strategy A course of action designed to produce a desired (business) outcome

Strike A temporary work stoppage called in an effort to express an employment contract negotiation demand

Structure indicators Indicators that measure the attributes of the setting, such as number and qualifications of the staff, adequacy of equipment and facilities, and adequacy of organizational policies and procedures

Structured brainstorming A group problem-solving technique wherein the team leader asks each participant to generate a list of ideas for the topic under discussion and then report them to the group in a nonjudgmental manner

Structured data Binary, machine-readable data in discrete fields; data able to be processed by the computer

Student membership AHIMA membership level that includes any student who does not have an AHIMA credential, has not previously been an active member of AHIMA, and who is formally enrolled in a Professional Certificate Approval Program or Approved Committee for Certificate Programs, or in a CAHIIM-accredited HIM program

Subacute care Offers patients access to constant nursing care while recovering at home

Subjective, objective, assessment, plan (SOAP) Documentation method that refers to how each progress note contains documentation relative to subjective observations, objective observations, assessments, and plans

Subpoena A command to appear at a certain time and place to give testimony on a certain matter

Subpoena ad testificandum A subpoena that seeks testimony

Subpoena duces tecum A written order commanding a person to appear, give testimony, and bring all documents, papers, books, and records described in the subpoena. The devices are used to obtain documents during pretrial discovery and to obtain testimony during trial

Summons An instrument used to begin a civil action or special proceeding and is a means of acquiring jurisdiction over a party

Sunsetting No longer selling or supporting a product

Supervisory management Management level that oversees the organization's efforts at the staff level and monitors the effectiveness of everyday operations and individual performance against preestablished standards

Supply management Management and control of the supplies used within an organization

Supreme courts The highest courts in a system, which hear final appeals from intermediate courts of appeal

Surgical operation One or more surgical procedures performed at one time for one patient via a common approach or for a common purpose

Surgical procedure Any single, separate, systematic process upon or within the body that can be complete in itself; is normally performed by a physician, dentist, or other licensed practitioner; can be performed either with or without instruments; and is performed to restore disunited or deficient parts, remove diseased or injured tissues, extract foreign matter, assist in obstetrical delivery, or aid in diagnosis

SWOT analysis Analysis tool used to outline the organization's strengths (S) and weaknesses (W), which are internal to the organization, and the opportunities (O) and threats (T) external to the organization

System Refers to all the components (technology, standards, people, policy, and process) that must work together to achieve a desired goal (interoperability)

System build The creation of data dictionaries, tables, decision support rules, templates for data entry, screen layouts, and reports used in a system; also known as *system configuration*

System characterization The process of creating an inventory of all systems that contain data, including documenting where the data are stored, what type of data are created or stored, how they are managed, with what hardware and software they interact, and providing basic security measures for the systems

System configuration The creation of data dictionaries, tables, decision support rules, templates for data entry, screen layouts, and reports used in a system; also known as *system build*

System integration A translation process that hardwires the applications together in order to be able to interoperate and exchange data seamlessly across the different applications

Systems development life cycle (SDLC) A model used to represent the ongoing process of developing (or purchasing) information systems

Systems thinking An objective way of looking at work-related ideas and processes with the goal of allowing people to uncover ineffective patterns of behavior and thinking and then finding ways to make lasting improvements

T

t-test Type of inferential statistic that measures the different between means

Table An organized arrangement of data, usually in columns and rows

Taft-Hartley Act Federal legislation passed in 1947 that imposed certain restrictions on unions while upholding their right to organize and bargain collectively

Tailgating A social engineering technique that allows a hacker, imposter, or other unauthorized individual to use an authorized individual's access privileges to gain access to a restricted physical area

Target data The location from which the data is mapped or to where it is sent

Team building The process of organizing and acquainting a team and building skills for dealing with later team processes

Team charter A document that explains the issues the team was initiated to address, describes the team's goal or vision, and lists the initial members of the team and their respective departments

Team leader A performance improvement team role responsible for championing the effectiveness of performance improvement activities in meeting customers' needs and for the content of a team's work

Team member A performance improvement team role responsible for participating in team decision-making and plan development; identifying opportunities for improvement; gathering, prioritizing, and analyzing data; and sharing knowledge, information, and data that pertain to the process under study

Team norms The rules, both explicit and implied, that determine acceptable and unacceptable behavior for a group

Technical component The portion of radiological and other procedures that is facility based or nonphysician based (for example, radiology films, equipment, overhead, endoscopic suites, and so on)

Technical interoperability The most basic form of interoperability. Technical interoperability refers to the exchange of any data element across information systems

Technical safeguards As amended by HITECH, the Security Rule means the technology and the policy and procedures for its use that protect electronic protected health information and control access to it

Telecommuting A work arrangement in which at least a portion of the employee's work hours is spent outside the office (usually in the home) and the work is transmitted back to the employer via electronic means

Telehealth A telecommunications system that links healthcare organizations and patients from diverse geographic locations and transmits text and images for (medical) consultation and treatment

Template A pattern used in computer-based patient records to capture data in a structured manner

Terminal-digit filing system A system of health record identification and filing in which the last digit or group of digits (terminal digits) in the health record number determines file placement

Termination The act of ending something (for example, a job)

Termination at will Recognizes that the employer or the employee can terminate employment for any reason unless prohibited by law (SHRM 2018d). However, employees do have protections against wrongful discharge based on statutes

Theory X and Y A management theory developed by McGregor that describes pessimistic and optimistic assumptions about people and their work potential

Third-party administrator 1. An entity required to make or responsible for making payment on behalf of a group health plan 2. A business associate that performs claims administration and related business functions for a self-insured entity

Third-party payer An insurance company (for example, Blue Cross/Blue Shield) or healthcare program (for example, Medicare) that pays or reimburses healthcare providers (second party) or patients (first party) for the delivery of medical services

3D printing Technology that will create a three-dimensional item using a printer

Time ladders Tools that support the collection of data that must be oriented by time; they specify intervals of time necessary to address the problem under consideration listed down the right side of one, two, or three columns; then, as the data collector observes, he or she records them next to the time of occurrence

Timekeeper A performance improvement team role responsible for notifying the team during meetings of time remaining on each agenda item in an effort to keep the team moving forward on its performance improvement project

Title VII of the Civil Rights Act of 1964 The federal legislation that prohibits discrimination in employment on the basis of race, religion, color, sex, or national origin (Public Law 88-352 1964)

Token A small electronic device programmed to generate and display new passwords at certain intervals

Tort An action brought when one party believes that another party caused harm through wrongful conduct and seeks compensation for that harm

Total length of stay (discharge days) The sum of length of stay for all patients discharged for a given period of time

Traditional fee-for-service reimbursement A reimbursement method involving third-party payers who compensate providers after the healthcare services have been delivered; payment is based on specific services provided to subscribers

Training A set of activities and materials that provide the opportunity to acquire job-related skills, knowledge, and abilities

Trait theory Proposes that leaders possess a collection of traits or qualities that distinguish them from nonleaders

Transaction As amended by HITECH, under HIPAA, the transmission of information between two parties to carry out financial or administrative activities related to health care. It includes the following types of information transmissions: (1) Health care claims or equivalent encounter information; (2) Health care payment and remittance advice; (3) Coordination of benefits; (4) Health care claim status; (5) Enrollment and disenrollment in a health plan; (6) Eligibility for a health plan; (7) Health plan premium payments; (8) Referral certification and authorization; (9) First report of injury; (10) Health claims attachments; (11) Health care electronic funds transfers (EFT) and remittance advice; (12) Other transactions that the secretary may prescribe by regulation (45 CFR 160.103 2013)

Transactional leadership Refers to the role of the manager who strives to create an efficient workplace by balancing task accomplishment with interpersonal satisfaction

Transfer record A review of the patient's acute stay that includes the patient's current status, discharge and transfer orders, and any additional instructions, and that accompanies the patient when he or she is transferred to another facility

Transformational leadership The leadership of a visionary who strives to change an organization

Transitional model Model created by William Bridges that defines three stages: (1) ending, losing, and letting go; (2) a neutral zone; and (3) new beginnings; each stage identifies the different emotions employees have as their daily work is either changed or replaced

Traumatic injury A wound or other injury caused by an external physical force such as an automobile accident, a shooting, a stabbing, or a fall

Treatment, payment, and operations (TPO) The Privacy Rule provides a number of exceptions for PHI that is being used or disclosed for TPO purposes; *treatment* means providing, coordinating, or managing healthcare or healthcare-related services by one or more healthcare providers; *payment* includes activities by a health plan to obtain premiums, billing by healthcare providers or health plans to obtain reimbursement, claims management, claims collection, review of the medical necessity of care, and utilization review; the Privacy Rule provides a broad list of activities that are healthcare *operations* that includes quality assessment and improvement, case management, review of healthcare professionals' qualifications, insurance contracting, legal and auditing functions, and general business management functions such as providing customer service and conducting due diligence

Trial court The lowest tier of state court, usually divided into two courts: the court of limited jurisdiction, which hears cases pertaining to a particular subject matter or involving crimes of lesser severity or civil matters of lower dollar amounts; and the court of general jurisdiction, which hears more serious criminal cases or civil cases that involve large amounts of money

TRICARE The federal healthcare program that provides coverage for the dependents of armed forces personnel and for retirees receiving care outside military treatment facilities in which the federal government pays a percentage of the cost; formerly known as Civilian Health and Medical Program of the Uniformed Services

Trigger events Review of access logs, audit trails, failed log-ins, and other reports generated to monitor compliance with the policies and procedures

Trojan horse A program that gains unauthorized access to a computer and masquerades as a useful function

Turnaround time In an ROI system, the time between receipt of request and when the information is sent to requester

Turnover The rate at which employees leave a firm and have to be replaced

Two-factor authentication A signature type that includes at least two of the following three elements: something known, such as a password; something held, such as a token or digital certificate; and something that is personal, such as a biometric in the form of a fingerprint, retinal scan, or other

U

Unbundling The practice of using multiple codes to bill for the various individual steps in a single procedure rather than using a single code that includes all of the steps of the comprehensive procedure

Unified Medical Language System (UMLS) A program initiated by the National Library of Medicine to build an intelligent, automated system that can understand biomedical concepts, words, and expressions and their interrelationships; includes concepts and terms from many different source vocabularies

Unintended consequence An unanticipated and undesired effect of implementing

Union An organization formed by employees for the purpose of acting as a unit when dealing with management regarding work issues

Unit numbering system A health record identification system in which the patient receives a unique medical record number at the time of the first encounter that is used for all subsequent encounters

Unity of command The management concept where each employee reports to one manager

Universal chart order A system in which the health record is maintained in the same format while the patient is in the facility and after discharge

Unsecured electronic protected health information (ePHI) ePHI that has not been made unusable, unreadable, or indecipherable to unauthorized persons

Unsecured PHI HIPAA concept where PHI has not been made unusable

Unstructured brainstorming method A group problem-solving technique wherein the team leader solicits spontaneous ideas for the topic under discussion from members of the team in a free-flowing and nonjudgmental manner

Unstructured data Nonbinary, human-readable data

Upcoding The practice of assigning diagnostic or procedural codes that represent higher payment rates than the codes that actually reflect the services provided to patients

Use As amended by HITECH, with respect to individually identifiable health information, the sharing, employment, application, utilization, examination, or analysis of such information within an entity that maintains such information (45 CFR 160.103 2013)

Use case A technique that develops scenarios based on how users will use information to assist in developing information systems that support the information requirements

User-based access control (UBAC) A security mechanism used to grant users of a system access based on identity

Usual, customary, and reasonable (UCR) charges Type of retrospective fee-for-service payment method in which the third-party payer pays for fees that are usual, customary, and reasonable, wherein "usual" is usual for the individual provider's practice; "customary" means customary for the community; and "reasonable" is reasonable for the situation

Utilization management (UM) 1. A collection of systems and processes to ensure that facilities and resources, both human and nonhuman, are used maximally and are consistent with patient care needs 2. A program that evaluates the healthcare facility's efficiency in providing necessary care to patients in the most effective manner

Utilization review The process of determining whether the medical care provided to a specific patient is necessary according to preestablished objective screening criteria at time frames specified in the organization's utilization management plan

Utilization Review Act Legislation in 1977 that made it a requirement for hospitals to conduct continued-stay reviews for Medicare and Medicaid patients

V

Validity 1. The extent to which data correspond to the actual state of affairs or that an instrument measures what it purports to measure 2. A term referring to a test's ability to accurately and consistently measure what it purports to measure

Value Refers to the combination of quality and cost

Value-based care (VBC) Reimbursement strategy designed to improve the quality of care and reduce healthcare costs

Value-based purchasing (VBP) CMS incentive plan that links payments more directly to the quality of care provided and rewards providers for delivering high-quality and efficient clinical care. It incorporates clinical process-of-care measures as well as measures from the Hospital Consumer Assessment of Healthcare Providers and Systems (HCAHPS) survey on how patients view their care experiences

Values The social and cultural belief system of a person or a healthcare organization

Variable costs Resources expended that vary with the activity of the organization, for example, medication expenses vary with patient volume

Variance A disagreement between two parts; the square of the standard deviation; a measure of variability that gives the average of the squared deviations from the mean; in financial management, the difference between the budgeted amount and the actual amount of a line item; in project management, the difference between the original project plan and current estimates

Vendor selection Formal process by a healthcare organization that is just starting to acquire health information systems or replacing an entire set of components with new components; steps in the process include needs identification, requirements specification, request for proposal (RFP), analysis of RFP responses, due diligence, and contract negotiation

Version control Identifies which version(s) of the documents is available to the user

Veterans Health Administration (VA) The nation's largest integrated healthcare system with more than 1,700 hospitals, clinics, community living centers, domiciliaries, readjustment counseling centers, and other facilities operated by the US Department of Veterans Affairs

Virtual private network (VPN) An encrypted tunnel through the internet that enables secure transmission of data

Vital statistics Data related to births, deaths, marriages, and fetal deaths

Vocabulary A list or collection of clinical words or phrases with their meanings

Voice recognition technology A method of encoding speech signals that do not require speaker pauses (but uses pauses when they are present) and of interpreting at least some of the signals' content as words or the intent of the speaker; also called continuous speech recognition; continuous speech technology

Voir dire Process of jury selection

W

Warrant A judge's order that authorizes law enforcement to seize evidence and conduct a search

Waste The overutilization or inappropriate utilization of services and misuse of resources, and typically is not a criminal or intentional act

Web services architecture (WSA) An architecture that utilizes web-based tools to permit communication among different software applications

Willful neglect As amended by HITECH, conscious, intentional failure or reckless indifference to the obligation to comply with the administrative simplification provision violated (45 CFR 160.401 2013)

Worker Adjustment and Retraining Notification (WARN) Act A 1988 Act that requires organizations of more than 100 employees to provide at least 60-days advance notice of a workforce layoff or downsizing

Workers' compensation Insurance that employers are required to have to cover employees who get sick or injured on the job

Workstations on wheels (WOWs) Notebook computers mounted on carts that can be moved through the facility by users

Work analysis The process of gathering information about what it takes to get a job done

Work distribution analysis This is a process of data collection to determine the type and appropriateness of a unit's work assignments, the time allowed for the tasks, and the employees doing the work. This analysis can be accomplished by having employees log time spent on key tasks or functions (as outlined in job descriptions) during a given period of time

Work measurement Assessment of internal data collected on actual work performed within the organization and the calculation of time it takes to do the work

Workflow Any work process that must be handled by more than one person

Workflow analysis A technique used to study the flow of operations for automation

Workforce As amended by HITECH, employees, volunteers, trainees, and other persons whose conduct, in the performance of work for a covered entity or business associate, is under the direct control of such covered entity or business associate, whether or not they are paid by the covered entity or business associate (45 CFR 160.103 2013)

Workforce planning Reviewing national demographic, social, and economic data and trends and relating these to an organization's local staffing needs

World Health Organization (WHO) The United Nations specialized agency created to ensure the attainment by all peoples of the highest possible levels of health; responsible for a number of international classifications, including ICD-10 and ICF

Wrongful discharge Unfair dismissal of employment due to failure of the employer to comply with law, organizational policy, or a contract

X

XML Language used to share information such as on the internet

Index

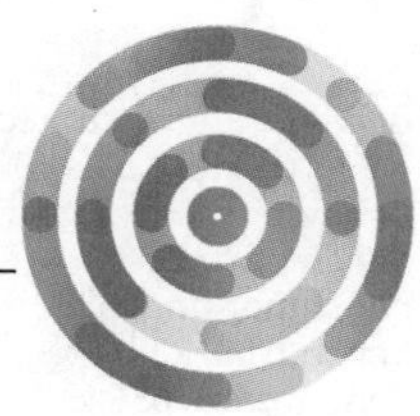

A

B

D

I

N

O

P

Q

R